D1859983

THE PRINCIPLES AND PRACTICE OF MEDICINE

Owing to the antiquity and rarity of this book, certain pages are regrettably absent, and readability is compromised due to the blurring of the original text. If you possess any insights regarding the availability of these missing sections, kindly inform us. Your assistance is crucial in ensuring the completion of this significant work for the benefit of future generations.

THE PRINCIPLES AND PRACTICE OF MEDICINE

DESIGNED FOR THE USE OF PRACTITIONERS AND STUDENTS OF MEDICINE

WILLIAM OSLER, THOMAS MCCRAE

GYAN

Published by

Gyan Publishing House
5, Ansari Road
Daryaganj, New Delhi-110002
Phone: 011-47034999, 9811692060
E-mail: books@gyanbooks.com

Distribution Network
gyanbooks.com
India, USA, Canada, UK, Australia

© Publisher

All rights reserved. No part of this work may be reproduced, stored, adapted, or transmitted in any form or by any means, electronic, mechanical, photocopying, micro-filming, recording or otherwise, or translated in any language, without the prior written permission of the copyright owner and the publisher.

ISBN: 978-93-6780-085-0 (PB)

First Published, 1892

2nd Impression 2025

Printed at: Gyan Press, Delhi.

The book is sold subject to the condition that it shall not, by way of trade or otherwise, be lent, resold, hired out, or otherwise circulated without the prior publisher's written consent.

THE PRINCIPLES AND PRACTICE OF MEDICINE
Author: WILLIAM OSLER, THOMAS MCCRAE

THE PRINCIPLES AND PRACTICE OF MEDICINE

THE PRINCIPLES AND PRACTICE OF MEDICINE

DESIGNED FOR THE USE OF PRACTITIONERS AND STUDENTS OF MEDICINE

BY

SIR WILLIAM OSLER, BT., M.D., F.R.S.

FELLOW OF THE ROYAL COLLEGE OF PHYSICIANS, LONDON; REGIUS PROFESSOR OF MEDICINE, OXFORD UNIVERSITY; HONORARY PROFESSOR OF MEDICINE, JOHNS HOPKINS UNIVERSITY, BALTIMORE; FORMERLY PROFESSOR OF THE INSTITUTES OF MEDICINE, McGILL UNIVERSITY, MONTREAL, AND PROFESSOR OF CLINICAL MEDICINE IN THE UNIVERSITY OF PENNSYLVANIA, PHILADELPHIA

EIGHTH EDITION—WITH THE ASSISTANCE OF

THOMAS McCRAE, M.D.

FELLOW OF THE ROYAL COLLEGE OF PHYSICIANS, LONDON; PROFESSOR OF MEDICINE, JEFFERSON MEDICAL COLLEGE, PHILADELPHIA; FORMERLY ASSOCIATE PROFESSOR OF MEDICINE, JOHNS HOPKINS UNIVERSITY

NEW YORK AND LONDON
D. APPLETON AND COMPANY
1918

TO THE

Memory of my Teachers:

WILLIAM ARTHUR JOHNSON,

PRIEST OF THE PARISH OF WESTON, ONTARIO.

JAMES BOVELL,

OF THE TORONTO SCHOOL OF MEDICINE, AND OF THE UNIVERSITY OF TRINITY COLLEGE, TORONTO.

ROBERT PALMER HOWARD,

DEAN OF THE MEDICAL FACULTY AND PROFESSOR OF MEDICINE, MCGILL UNIVERSITY, MONTREAL.

PREFACE TO THE EIGHTH EDITION.

In the twenty years that have passed since the publication of the first edition, triennial revisions have appeared regularly, with one exception—to secure protection against an edition pirated in Great Britain, a fifth edition had to be issued not long after the fourth. Comparing the first edition with the present, very little remains of the original work. The essential groundwork has been, as far as possible, my personal experience in hospital and private practice, correlated with the general experience of the profession, as expressed in its literature. To try to keep the book up to date has been a pleasure and an ambition. Adequately to express my appreciation of the generous support accorded by my colleagues is impossible. The printed page has brought me "mind to mind" with men in all parts of the world; and to feel that I may have been helpful in promoting sound knowledge is my greatest satisfaction.

This edition has been rearranged and largely rewritten. I have grouped the infectious diseases in a different order, and considered apart those of which the specific germs are doubtful or undiscovered. The extraordinary growth of our knowledge of this department has necessitated the incorporation of much new matter in every section, particularly in typhoid fever, typhus fever, pneumonia, tuberculosis and syphilis. Properly to present the recent advances many chapters have had to be recast. New sections deal with Leishmaniasis, the Sporotrichoses, the Colon infections, Poliomyelitis, Pellagra, Disorders of Metabolism, Caisson disease, Ochronosis, Hæmochromatosis, the disorders of the organs of internal secretion, and the diseases of the blood.

Dr. A. G. Gibson of Oxford has helped in the rewriting of the section on the heart and arteries. To Dr. H. M. Thomas and Dr. Harvey Cushing I am indebted for aid in the revision of the section on nervous diseases.

My former associate at the Johns Hopkins Hospital, Dr. Thomas McCrae, has revised the sections on treatment, and the section on diseases of the organs of locomotion. He has also seen the work through the press.

Messrs. Appleton have provided a new font of type and a new page.

William Osler.

Oxford.

PREFACE

The need for a reprinting has given the opportunity to make a considerable number of alterations. Many of these are in the section dealing with infectious diseases. The experiences of war have added much to our knowledge of these diseases and the present one is no exception, particularly in reference to paratyphoid fever and cerebrospinal fever. Additional proof has been given of the efficiency of inoculation against typhoid fever.

Additions have been made to the description of typhoid and paratyphoid fever, with especial reference to the latter, the serum changes and the subject of protective inoculation. Recent work on the pneumococcus infections, with its bearing on the problems of immunity, demands attention. Our knowledge of cerebrospinal fever has been increased by the studies of recent epidemics, particularly as regards the different strains of the organism. Additions have been made to the subject of poliomyelitis, especially in the study of the anomalous forms. There has been additional light thrown on the food deficiency diseases, for example—pellagra. The treatment of diabetes mellitus has been changed by the important advances of recent work. The convenient diet tables brought out by E. P. Joslin are included.

Throughout the book many minor changes have been made to incorporate the advances in our knowledge.

William Osler.

CONTENTS

SECTION I

Specific Infectious Diseases

SECTION II

Diseases Due to Physical Agents

SECTION III

The Intoxications

SECTION IV

Diseases of Metabolism

SECTION V

Diseases of the Digestive System

SECTION VI

Diseases of the Respiratory System

SECTION VII

Diseases of the Kidneys

SECTION VIII

Diseases of the Blood

SECTION IX

Diseases of the Circulatory System

SECTION X

Diseases of the Ductless Glands

SECTION XI

Diseases of the Nervous System

SECTION XII

Diseases of the Locomotor System

CHARTS AND ILLUSTRATIONS

THE PRINCIPLES AND PRACTICE OF MEDICINE

SECTION I

SPECIFIC INFECTIOUS DISEASES

A. BACTERIAL DISEASES

I. TYPHOID FEVER

Definition.—A general infection caused by the bacillus typhosus, characterized anatomically by hyperplasia and ulceration of the intestinal lymph-follicles, swelling of the mesenteric glands and spleen, and parenchymatous changes in the other organs. There are cases in which the local changes are slight or absent, and there are others with intense localization in the lungs, spleen, kidneys, or cerebro-spinal system. Clinically the disease is marked by fever, a rose-colored eruption, diarrhœa, abdominal tenderness, tympanites, and enlargement of the spleen; but these symptoms are extremely inconstant, and even the fever varies in its character.

Historical Note.—Huxham, in his remarkable Essay on Fevers, had "taken notice of the very great difference there is between the *putrid malignant* and the *slow nervous fever.*" In 1813 Pierre Bretonneau, of Tours, distinguished "dothiénentérite" as a separate disease; and Petit and Serres described entero-mesenteric fever. In 1829 Louis' great work appeared, in which the name "typhoid" was given to the fever. At this period typhoid fever alone prevailed in Paris and many European cities, and it was universally believed to be identical with the continued fever of Great Britain, where in reality typhoid and typhus coëxisted. The intestinal lesion was regarded as an accidental occurrence in the course of ordinary typhus. Louis' students returning to their homes in different countries, had opportunities for studying the prevalent fevers in the thorough and systematic manner of their master. Among these were certain young American physicians, to one of whom, Gerhard, of Philadelphia, is due the great honor of having first clearly laid down the differences between the two diseases. His papers in the American Journal of the Medical Sciences, 1837, are the first which give a full and satisfactory account of their clinical and anatomical distinctions. The studies of James Jackson, Sr. and Jr., of Enoch Hale and of George C. Shattuck, of

Boston, and of Alfred Stillé and Austin Flint made the subject very familiar in American medicine. In 1842 Elisha Bartlett's work appeared, in which, for the first time in a systematic treatise, typhoid and typhus fever were separately considered with admirable clearness. In Great Britain the recognition of the difference between the two diseases was very slow, and was due largely to A. P. Stewart, and, finally, to the careful studies of Jenner between 1849 and 1850.

Etiology.—General Prevalence.—Typhoid fever prevails especially in temperate climates, in which it constitutes the most common continued fever. Widely distributed throughout all parts of the world, it probably presents everywhere the same essential characteristics, and is everywhere an index of the sanitary intelligence of a community. *Imperfect sewerage* and *contaminated water-supply* are two special conditions favoring the distribution of the bacilli; *filth, overcrowding,* and *bad ventilation* are accessories in lowering the resistance of the individuals exposed. While from an infected person the disease may be spread by *fingers, food* and *flies.*

In *England and Wales* in 1910 the disease was fatal to 1,848 persons, a mortality of 46 per million of living persons. It destroys more lives in proportion to population in towns than in the country. The rate was lower in 1910 than in any year since 1869. Compared with the quinquennial average, there was a very marked reduction.

In *India* the disease is very prevalent; no race or creed is exempt, and 80 per cent. of the cases of continued fever lasting three weeks prove to be typhoid fever (L. Rogers).

In the *United States* typhoid fever continues to be disgracefully prevalent. From 1900 to 1909 the death rate in the registration areas was 29.5 per 100,000. It is estimated that from 35,000 to 40,000 persons die of it every year, so that at a moderate estimate nearly one half-million people are attacked annually. It is more prevalent in country districts than in cities, and, as Fulton has shown, the propagation is largely from the country to the town. What is needed both in Canada and the United States is a realization by the public that certain primary laws of health must be obeyed.

In *Germany* the larger cities have comparatively little typhoid fever. The story of Hamburg, as told by Reincke (Lancet, i, 1904), should be read by all interested in the disease. During the past twenty-five years the death rate in Prussia has been reduced from an average of over 6 to less than 2 per 10,000 of the population. It is still very prevalent in some of the country districts.

Typhoid fever has been one of the great scourges of the armies, and kills and maims more than powder and shot. The present war shows the results of preventive inoculation in a striking way.

In the Spanish-American War the report of the Commission (Reed, Vaughan, and Shakespeare) shows that one-fifth of the soldiers in the national encampments had typhoid fever—among 107,973 men there were 20,738 cases, with 1,580 deaths. In 90 per cent. of the volunteer regiments the disease broke out within eight weeks after going into camp. In the opinion of the Commission the most important factors were camp pollution, flies as carriers of contagion, and the contamination through the air in the form of dust.

In the South African War the British army, 557,653 officers and men, had

57,684 cases of enteric fever, with 8,225 deaths (Simpson), while only 7,582 men died of wounds received in battle. As in America, the disease was essentially one of the standing camps; troops constantly on the move were rarely much affected. While contaminated water was no doubt an important factor, as it always is in camp pollution, yet certain of the conditions in Africa were peculiar. Fæcal and urinary contamination must have been very common, as in the cooking, performed in the open air, sand "entered largely into every article of food." As there was a perfect plague of flies, they were without doubt a very important factor in the infection of both food and drink.

On the other hand, the Japanese and Russian War demonstrated the remarkable efficiency of modern hygiene, if carried out in an intelligent manner. In the great war at present raging typhoid fever has not prevailed to any extent in the Western armies. The efficacy of inoculation has been demonstrated. The large proportion of paratyphoid cases is remarkable.

Season.—Almost without exception the disease is everywhere more prevalent in the autumn, hence the old popular name autumnal fever. The exhaustive study of this question by Sedgwick and Winslow shows everywhere a striking parallelism between the monthly variations in temperature and the prevalence of the disease. In a few cities the curves are irregular, showing, in addition to the usual summer rise, two secondary maxima in the winter and spring, and these authors suggest that epidemics at these seasons are characteristic of cities whose water-supply is most subject to pollution. In their opinion "the most reasonable explanation of the seasonal variations of typhoid fever is a direct effect of the temperature upon the persistence in nature of the germs which proceed from previous victims of the disease."

Of 1,500 cases at the Johns Hopkins Hospital (upon the study of which this section is based), 840 were in August, September, and October.

Sex.—Males and females are equally liable to the disease, but males are much more frequently admitted into hospitals, 2.4 to 1 in our series.

Age.—Typhoid fever is a disease of youth and early adult life. The greatest susceptibility is between the ages of fifteen and twenty-five. Of 1,500 cases treated in my wards at the Johns Hopkins Hospital there were under fifteen years of age, 231; between fifteen and twenty, 253; between twenty and thirty, 680; between thirty and forty, 227; between forty and fifty, 88; between fifty and sixty, 8; above sixty, 11; age not given, 1. Cases are rare over sixty, although Manges believes that they are more common than the records show. As the course is often atypical the diagnosis may be uncertain and the disease not recognized until autopsy. It is not very infrequent in childhood, but infants are rarely attacked. Murchison saw a case at the sixth month. There is definite evidence that the disease may be conveyed to the fetus, the bacillus passing through the placenta.

Immunity.—Not all exposed to the infection take the disease. Some families seem more susceptible than others. One attack usually protects. Two attacks have been described within a year. "Of 2,000 cases of enteric fever at the Hamburg General Hospital, only 14 persons were affected twice and only 1 person three times" (Dreschfeld). In 500 of our cases in which special inquiry was made as to a previous attack, it was found to have occurred in 11 (2.2 per cent.). The interval varied from nine months to thirty years. It is well known that usually within a short time after recovery the immune substances disappear from the blood, yet in most cases the relative immunity lasts a long time, frequently for life. An experimental explanation for this fact has been given in the demonstration that animals which have once reacted to the typhoid infection, react in throwing out immune substances more quickly and in larger amounts when danger again threatens (Cole).

BACILLUS TYPHOSUS.—The researches of Eberth, Koch, Gaffky, and others have shown that there is a special micro-organism *constantly* associated with typhoid fever.

(*a*) *General Characters.*—It is a rather short, thick, flagellated, motile bacillus, with rounded ends, in one of which, sometimes in both (particularly in cultures), there can be seen a glistening round body, at one time believed to be a spore; but these polar structures are probably only areas of degenerated protoplasm. It grows readily on various nutritive media, and can now be differentiated from *Bacillus coli,* with which, and with certain other bacilli, it is apt to be confounded. This organism now fulfills all the requirements of Koch's law—it is constantly present, and it grows outside the body in a specific manner; the third requirement, the production of the disease experimentally, has been successfully met by the conveyance of the disease to chimpanzees. The bacilli or their toxins inoculated in large quantities into the blood of rabbits are pathogenic, and in some instances ulcerative and necrotic lesions in the intestine may be produced. But similar intestinal lesions may be caused by other bacteria, including *Bacillus coli.*

Cultures are killed within ten minutes by a temperature of 60° C. They may live for eighteen weeks at —5° C., although most die within two weeks, and all within twenty-two weeks (Park). The typhoid bacillus resists ordinary drying for months, unless in very thin layers, when it is killed in five to fifteen days. The direct rays of the sun completely destroy them in from four to ten hours' exposure. Bouillon cultures are destroyed by carbolic acid, 1 to 200, and by corrosive sublimate, 1 to 2,500.

(*b*) *Distribution in the Body.*—During recent years our ideas in regard to the distribution of the typhoid bacilli have been much modified, owing to the demonstration that in practically all cases the bacilli enter the circulating blood and are carried throughout the body. During life they may be demonstrated in the circulating blood in a large proportion of cases, in 75 per cent. of 604 collected cases (Coleman and Buxton). They occur in the urine in from 25 to 30 per cent. of the cases. They may be isolated from the stools in practically all cases at some stage. They are probably always present in the rose spots. They are reported to have been cultivated from the sweat, and they undoubtedly occur with considerable frequency in the sputum (Richardson, Rau, and others). At autopsy they are found widely distributed, most numerous and constant usually in the mesenteric glands, spleen, and gall-bladder, but are found in almost all organs, even the muscles, uterus, and lungs (von Drigalski). Cultures made from the intestines at autopsy (according to Jürgens, and also von Drigalski) show that they are very few or can not be cultivated from the rectum up to the cæcum, but above this they increase in number, being very numerous in the duodenum and jejunum, and practically constant in cultures made from the mucous membrane of the stomach. They are also present in the œsophagus and frequently on the tongue and tonsils. From endocardial vegetations, from meningeal and pleural exudates and from foci of suppuration in various parts of the body, the bacilli have also been isolated. A most important and remarkable fact is that at times they may be present in the stools of persons who show no symptoms of typhoid fever, but who have lived in very close association with typhoid-fever patients. This is especially true of children.

(*c*) *The Bacilli outside the Body.*—In sterile water the bacilli retain their vitality for weeks, but under ordinary conditions, in competition with saprophytes, disappear within a few days. The question of the longevity of the typhoid bacillus in water is of great importance, and has been much discussed in connection with the supposed pollution of the water of the Mississippi by the Chicago drainage canal. The experiments of E. O. Jordan would indicate that the vitality was retained as a rule not longer than three days after infection. Whether an increase can occur in water is not finally settled. Their detection in the water is difficult, and although they undoubtedly have been found, many such discoveries previously reported are not certain on account of the inaccurate differentiation of the typhoid bacillus and varieties of intestinal bacilli closely resembling it. Both Prudden and Ernst have found it in water filters.

There are cities deriving their ice supply from polluted streams with low death rates from typhoid fever. Sedgwick and Winslow conclude from their careful study that very few typhoid germs survive in ice. The Ogdensburg epidemic in 1902-'03 was apparently due to infection from ice. Typhoid bacilli were grown from frozen material in it (Hutchins and Wheeler).

In *milk* the bacilli undergo rapid development without changing its appearance. They may persist for three months in sour milk, and may live for several days in butter made from infected cream.

Robertson has shown that under entirely natural conditions typhoid bacilli may live in the upper layers of the soil for eleven months. Von Drigalski says if stools which contain typhoid bacilli are kept at room temperature the *B. typhosus* disappears in a few days.

The direct infection by dust of exposed food-stuffs, such as milk, is very probable. The bacilli retain their vitality for many weeks; in garden earth twenty-one days, in filter-sand eighty-two days, in dust of the street thirty days, on linen sixty to seventy days, on wood thirty-two days; on thread kept under suitable conditions for a year.

Modes of Conveyance.—(*a*) *Contagion.*—Direct aerial transmission does not seem probable. Each case should be regarded as a possible source of infection, and in houses, hospitals, schools, and barracks a widespread epidemic may arise from it. Fingers, food, and flies are the chief means of local propagation. It is impossible for a nurse to avoid finger contamination, and without scrupulous care the germs may be widely distributed in a ward or throughout a house. Cotton or rubber gloves are used in some institutions. Even with special precautions and an unusually large proportion of nurses to patients, it was not possible to avoid "house" infection at the Johns Hopkins Hospital. T. B. Futcher has analyzed the 31 cases contracted in the hospital among our first 1,500 cases; physicians, 5 * among a total of

---

* Only three of these were in attendance on typhoid cases. Two of the five died.—Oppenheimer and Ochsner.

288; nurses, 15 of a total of 407; patients, 8 out of a total of 47,956 admissions; 4 of these occurred in a small ward epidemic. Two orderlies were infected while caring for typhoid patients, and one woman in charge of a supply room, where she only handled clean linen. Newman concludes from his study of typhoid fever in London that direct personal infection, and infection through food are the two common channels for its propagation.

(*b*) *Infection of water* is the most common source of widespread epidemics, many of which have been shown to originate in the contamination of a well or a spring. A very striking one occurred at Plymouth, Pa., in 1885, which was investigated by Shakespeare. The town, with a population of 8,000, was in part supplied with drinking-water from a reservoir fed by a mountain stream. During January, February, and March, in a cottage by the side of and at a distance of from 60 to 80 feet from this stream, a man was ill with typhoid fever. The attendants were in the habit at night of throwing out the evacuations on the ground toward the stream. During these months the ground was frozen and covered with snow. In the latter part of March and early in April there was considerable rainfall and a thaw, in which a large part of the three months' accumulation of discharges was washed into a brook, not 60 feet distant. At the very time of this thaw the patient had numerous and copious discharges. About the 10th of April cases of typhoid fever broke out in the town, appearing for a time at the rate of fifty a day. In all about 1,200 people were attacked. An immense majority of all the cases were in the part of the town which received water from the infected reservoir.

The experience of Maidstone in 1897 illustrates the widespread and serious character of an epidemic when the water-supply becomes badly contaminated. The outbreak began about the middle of September, and within the first two weeks 509 cases were reported. By October 27th there were 1,748 cases, and by November 17th 1,848 cases. In all, in a population of 35,000, about 1,900 persons were attacked.

(*c*) *Typhoid Carriers.*—The bacilli may persist for years in the bile passages and intestines of persons in good health. They have been found by Young in the urinary bladder, and by Hunner in the gall-bladder, ten and twenty years after the fever, and there have been cases of typhoid bone lesion from which the bacilli were isolated many years after the primary attack. Within the past few years the work of Strassburg observers has called attention to a group of chronic typhoid carriers of the first importance in the spread of the disease. One woman, a baker, had typhoid fever ten years previously. The bacilli were found in large numbers in her stools. Every new employee in the bakery sooner or later became seriously ill with typhoid-like symptoms, and in two persons the disease proved fatal. Several localized epidemics have been traced to these carriers, particularly in asylums, as determined by the Strassburg observers. Soper reports an instance in which a cook, apparently in perfect health, but in whose stools bacilli had been present in large numbers, had been responsible for the occurrence of typhoid in seven households in five years. Apparently there is no limit to the length of time in which the bacilli may remain in the bile passages and pass into the stools. Dean reports a case of a carrier of twenty-nine years' standing, and instances of even longer duration are recorded. The paratyphoid bacillus may be carried in the same way. An epidemic of 19 cases in a French barrack was traced to a cook who was infected with a paratyphoid bacillus.

(*d*) *Infection of Food.*—Milk may be the source of infection. One of the most thoroughly studied epidemics due to this cause was that investigated by Ballard in Islington. The milk may be contaminated by infected water used in cleaning the cans. The milk epidemics have been collected by Ernest Hart and by Kober.

The germs may be conveyed in ice, salads of various sorts, etc. The danger of eating celery and other uncooked vegetables, which have grown in soil on which infected material has been used as a fertilizer, must not be forgotten.

Much attention has been paid of late years to the *oyster* as a source of infection. In several epidemics, such as that in Middletown, reported by Conn, that in Naples, by Lavis, and in the outbreak which occurred at Winchester, the chain of circumstantial evidence seems complete. Most suggestive sporadic cases have also been recorded by Broadbent and others. Foote showed that oysters taken from the feeding-grounds in rivers contain a larger number of micro-organisms of all sorts than those from the sea. Chantemesse found typhoid bacilli in oysters which had lain in infected sea-water, even after they had been transferred to and kept in fresh water for a time. C. W. Field, working in the laboratories of the Department of Health, New York (1904), confirms the observations of both Foote and Chantemesse, but he could not determine that the bacilli were able to multiply within the oysters. Mosny, in his report to the French Government (1900), admits the possibility of oyster infection, but he thinks that the oyster plays a very small *rôle* in relation to the total morbidity of the disease. Mussels have also been found contaminated with typhoid bacilli, and it is stated that dried fish have carried the infection.

(*e*) *Flies.*—The importance of flies in the transmission of the disease was brought out very strongly in the Spanish-American War in 1898. The Report of the Commission (Reed, Vaughan, and Shakespeare) states that "flies were undoubtedly the most active agents in the spread of typhoid fever. Flies alternately visited and fed on the infected fæcal matter and the food in the mess-tent. . . . Typhoid fever was much less frequent among members of the messes who had their mess-tents screened than it was among those who took no such precautions." In the South African War there was a perfect plague of flies, particularly in the typhoid fever tents, and among the army surgeons the opinion was universal that they had a great deal to do with the dissemination of the disease. Firth and Horrocks demonstrated the readiness with which flies, after feeding on typhoid stools or fresh cultures of typhoid bacilli, could infect sterile media. One of the most interesting studies on the question was made in the Chicago epidemic of 1902 by Alice Hamilton. Flies caught in two undrained privies, on the fences of two yards, on the walls of two houses, and in the room of a typhoid-fever patient, were used to inoculate eighteen tubes, and from five of these tubes typhoid bacilli were isolated.

(*f*) *Contamination of the Soil.*—Filth, bad sewers, or cesspools can not in themselves cause typhoid fever, but they furnish the conditions suitable for the preservation of the bacillus, and possibly for its propagation.

Dust may be an important factor, though it has been shown that the bacilli die very quickly when desiccated. In the dust storms during the South African War the food was often covered with dust. Possibly, too, as Barringer suggests, the dust on the railway tracks may become contaminated. Men working on the tracks are very liable to infection.

Types of Infection.—We may recognize the following groups: (*a*) *Ordinary typhoid fever with marked enteric lesions.* An immense majority of all the cases are of this character; and while the spleen and mesenteric glands are involved the lymphatic apparatus of the intestinal walls bears the brunt of the attack. (*b*) *Cases in which the intestinal lesions are very slight,* and may be found only after a very careful search. In reviewing the cases of "typhoid fever without intestinal lesions," Opie and Bassett call attention to the fact that in many negative cases slight lesions really did exist, while in others death occurred so late that the lesions might have healed. In some cases the disease is a general septicæmia with symptoms of severe intoxication and high fever and delirium. In others the main lesions may be in organs—liver, gall-bladder, pleura, meninges, or even the endocardium. (*c*) *Cases in which the typhoid bacillus enters the body without causing any lesion of the intestine.* In a number of the earlier cases reported as such the demonstration of the typhoid bacillus was inconclusive. In others the intestine showed tuberculous ulcers, through which the organisms may have entered. But after excluding all these, a few cases remain in which the demonstration of the typhoid bacillus was conclusive, cases in which death occurred early, and yet after a very careful search no intestinal lesions could be found. There were 4 cases in this series. Undoubtedly the intestinal lesions may be so slight as not to be recognizable at autopsy. (*d*) *Mixed infections.* It is well to distinguish, as Dreschfeld pointed out, between double infections, as with bacillus tuberculosis, the diphtheria bacillus, and the plasmodia of Laveran, in which two different diseases are present and can be readily distinguished, and the true mixed or secondary infections, in which the conditions induced by one organism favor the growth of other pathogenic forms; thus in ordinary typhoid fever secondary infection with the colon bacillus, the streptococcus, staphylococcus, or the pneumococcus, is quite common. (*e*) *Paratyphoid infections.* Described first by Achard in 1896 and then by Gwyn, from my clinic, in 1898, these infections have been shown to play an important part in the story of typhoid fever. They have increased in frequency in the United States during the past decade and in the present great war the cases in France have outnumbered those of ordinary typhoid fever. Until the return of the soldiers from France and the East these infections have been rare in England. The two forms Paratyphoid A and Paratyphoid B are distinguished from each other and from *B. typhosus* by well-marked cultural and serological differences. An attack of one does not protect against the others, nor does inoculation against *B. typhosus* protect against para-A or para-B. Of the two varieties para-B is the more prevalent in Europe and more important, as in a larger percentage of recoveries carriers are present. Clinically the paratyphoid infections represent a milder type of typhoid, with a much lower death rate. In the cases I have seen, enlargement of the spleen has been constant, rose spots have been frequent, and intestinal symptoms, even hæmorrhages, have occurred; perforation has been rare. Many cases have a very brief but acute course, resembling food poisoning. The sequelæ of ordinary typhoid fever may occur, and the paratyphoid organisms have been isolated from the lesions of osteomyelitis, an inflamed testis, and a chondrosternal abscess. Anatomically there are three groups, (1) a septicæmia with little or no change in the bowels; (2) cases not distinguishable from ordinary typhoid, and (3) a dysenteric form, in which the lesions are chiefly in the large bowel. In Dawson and Whittingden's recent study of 17 fatal cases, the large bowel was involved in 10. For practical purposes typhoid and paratyphoid may be considered the same. The differences are bacteriological, and the diagnosis rests upon the cultural peculiarities of the organism and upon the agglutination tests. (*f*) *Local infections.* The typhoid bacillus may cause a local abscess, cystitis, or cholecystitis without evidence of a general infection. (*g*) *Terminal typhoid infections.* In rare instances the bacillus causes a fatal infection towards the end of other diseases. The subjects may, of course, be typhoid carriers. In two cases of malignant disease at the Johns Hopkins Hospital the bacilli were isolated from the blood, and there were no intestinal lesions.

Products of the Growth of the Bacilli.—Brieger isolated from cultures a poison belonging to the group of ptomaines—typhotoxin. Later he and Fraenkel isolated a poison belonging to the group of toxalbumins. According to Pfeiffer, the chief poison belongs to the intracellular group of toxins. Sidney Martin has isolated a poison which is in the nature of a secretion, but does not differ from that contained within the bacterial cell. Injected into animals it causes lowering of temperature, diarrhœa, loss of weight, and degeneration of the myocardium. Its chemical nature is not known. Similar, but weaker, poisons may also be isolated from cultures of *Bacillus coli* and other members of this group. No toxins have yet been isolated which cause changes in animals at all comparable to typhoid fever in human beings. Macfadyen and Rowland, by mechanically breaking up the bacilli after they had been frozen by means of liquid air, obtained toxins, which injected into monkeys had both antitoxic and antibacterial properties.

Morbid Anatomy.—Intestines.—A catarrhal condition exists throughout the small and large bowel. Specific changes occur in the lymphoid elements, chiefly at the lower end of the ileum. The alterations which occur are most conveniently described in four stages:

(*a*) *Hyperplasia,* which involves the glands of Peyer in the jejunum and ileum, and to a variable extent those in the large intestine. The follicles are swollen, grayish-white, and the patches may project 3 to 5 mm., or may be still more prominent. The solitary glands, which range in size from a pin's head to a pea, are usually deeply imbedded in the submucosa, but project to a variable extent. Occasionally they are very prominent, and may be almost pedunculated. Microscopic examination shows at the outset a condition of hyperæmia of the follicles. Later there is a great increase and accumulation of cells of the lymph-tissue which may even infiltrate the adjacent mucosa and the muscularis; and the blood-vessels are more or less compressed, which gives the whitish, anæmic appearance to the follicles. The cells have all the characters of ordinary lymph-corpuscles. Some of them, however, are larger, epithelioid, and contain several nuclei. Occasionally cells containing red blood-corpuscles are seen. This so-called medullary infiltration, which is always more intense toward the lower end of the ileum, reaches its height from the eighth to the tenth day and then undergoes one of two changes, *resolution* or *necrosis*. Death very rarely takes place at this stage. Resolution is accomplished by a fatty and granular change in the cells, which are destroyed and absorbed. A curious condition of the patches is produced at this stage, in which they have a reticulated appearance, the *plaques à surface réticulée*. The swollen follicles in the patch undergo resolution and shrink more rapidly than the surrounding framework, or what is more probable the follicles alone, owing to the intense hyperplasia, become necrotic and disintegrate, leaving the little pits. In this process superficial hæmorrhages may result, and small ulcers may orginate by the fusion of these superficial losses of substance.

Except histologically there is nothing distinctive in the hyperplasia of the lymph-follicies; but apart from typhoid fever we rarely see in adults a marked affection of these glands with fever. In children, however, it is not uncommon when death has occurred from intestinal affections, and it is also met with in measles, diphtheria, and scarlet fever.

(*b*) *Necrosis and Sloughing.*—When the hyperplasia of the lymph-follicles reaches a certain grade, resolution is no longer possible. The blood-vessels become choked, there is a condition of anæmic necrosis, and sloughs form which must be separated and thrown off. The necrosis is probably due in great part to the direct action of the bacilli. According to Mallory, there occurs a proliferation of endothelial cells due to the action of a toxin. These cells are phagocytic in character, and the swelling of the intestinal lymphoid tissue is due almost entirely to their formation. The necrosis, he thinks, is due to the occlusion of the veins and capillaries by fibrinous thrombi, which owe their origin to degeneration of phagocytic cells beneath the lining endothelium of the vessels. The process may be superficial, affecting only the upper part of the mucous coat, or it may extend to and involve the submucosa. The "slough" may sometimes lie upon the Peyer's patch, scarcely involving more than the epithelium (Marchand). It is always more intense toward the ileo-cæcal valve, and in very severe cases the greater part of the mucosa of the last foot of the ileum may be converted into a brownish-black eschar. The necrotic area in the solitary glands forms a yellowish cap which often involves only the most prominent point of a follicle. The extent of the necrosis is very variable. It may pass deep into the muscular coat, reaching to or even perforating the peritoneum.

(*c*) *Ulceration.*—The separation of the necrotic tissue—the sloughing—is gradually effected from the edges inward, and results in the formation of an ulcer, the size and extent of which are directly proportionate to the amount of necrosis. If this be superficial, the entire thickness of the mucosa may not be involved and the loss of substance may be small and shallow. More commonly the slough in separating exposes the submucosa and muscularis, particularly the latter, which forms the floor of a majority of all typhoid ulcers. It is not common for an entire Peyer's patch to slough away, and a perfectly ovoid ulcer opposite to the mesentery is rarely seen. Irregularly oval and rounded forms are most common. A large patch may present three or four ulcers divided by septa of mucous membrane. The terminal 6 or 8 inches of the mucous membrane of the ileum may form a large ulcer, in which are here and there islands of mucosa. The edges of the ulcer are usually swollen, soft, sometimes congested, and often undermined. At a late period the ulcers near the valve may have very irregular sinuous borders. The base of a typhoid ulcer is smooth and clean, being usually formed of the submucosa or of the muscularis.

There may be large ulcers near the valve and swollen hyperæmic patches of Peyer in the upper part of the ileum.

(*d*) *Healing.*—This begins with the development of a thin granulation tissue which covers the base. Occasionally an appearance is seen as if an ulcer had healed in one place and was extending in another. The mucosa gradually extends from the edge, and a new growth of epithelium is formed. The glandular elements are reformed; the healed ulcer is somewhat depressed and is usually pigmented. In death during relapse healing ulcers may be seen in some patches with fresh ulcers in others.

We may say, indeed, that healing begins with the separation of the sloughs, as, when resolution is impossible, the removal of the necrosed part is the first step in the process of repair. In fatal cases, we seldom meet with evidences of cicatrization, as the majority of deaths occur before this stage is reached. It is remarkable that no matter how extensive the ulceration has been, healing is never associated with stricture, and typhoid fever does not appear as one of the causes of intestinal obstruction. Within a very short time all traces of the old ulcers disappear.

Large Intestine.—The cæcum and colon are affected in about one-third of the cases. Sometimes the solitary glands are greatly enlarged. The ulcers are usually larger in the cæcum than in the colon.

Perforation of the Bowel.—*Incidence at Autopsy.*—J. A. Scott's figures, embracing 9,713 cases from various English, Canadian, and American sources, give 351 deaths from perforation among 1,037 deaths from all causes, a percentage of 33.8 of the deaths and 3.6 of the cases. The German statistics give a much lower proportion of deaths from perforation; Munich in 2,000 autopsies, 5.7 per cent. from perforation; Basle in 2,000 autopsies, 1.3 per cent. from perforation; Hamburg in 3,686 autopsies, 1.2 per cent. from perforation (Hector Mackenzie, Lancet, 1903). At the Johns Hopkins Hospital among 1,500 cases of typhoid fever there were 43 with perforation. Twenty of these were operated upon, with 7 recoveries. One other case died of the toxæmia on the eighth day after operation. At the Pennsylvania Hospital there were 139 cases of perforation among 5,891 cases. Chomel remarks that "the accident is sometimes the result of ulceration, sometimes of a true eschar, and sometimes it is produced by the distention of the intestine, causing the rupture of tissues weakened by disease." As a rule, sloughs are adherent about the site of perforation. The site is usually in the ileum, 232 times in Hector Mackenzie's collection of 264 cases; the jejunum twice, the large intestine 22 times, and the appendix 9 times in his series. As a rule, the perforation occurs within twelve inches of the ileo-cæcal valve. There may be two or three separate perforations. J. A. Scott described two distinct varieties: first, the more common single, circular, pin-point in size, due to the extension of a necrotic process through the base of a small ulcer. The second variety, produced by a large area of tissue becoming necrotic, ranges in size from the finger-tip to 3 cm. in diameter.

Death from hæmorrhage occurred in 99 of the Munich cases, and in 12 of 137 deaths in my 1,500 cases. The bleeding seems to result directly from the separation of the sloughs. I was not able in any instance to find the bleeding vessel. In one case only a single patch had sloughed, and a firm clot was adherent to it. The bleeding may also come from the soft swollen edges of the patch.

The *mesenteric glands* show hyperæmia and subsequently become greatly swollen. Spots of necrosis are common. In several of my cases suppuration had occurred, and in one a large abscess of the mesentery was present. The rupture of a softened or suppurating mesenteric gland, of which there are only a few cases in the literature, may cause either fatal hæmorrhage or peritonitis. LeConte has successfully operated upon the latter condition. The bunch of glands in the mesentery, at the lower end of the ileum, is especially involved. The retroperitoneal glands are also swollen.

The *spleen* is invariably enlarged in the early stages of the disease. In 11 of my series it exceeded 20 ounces (600 grams) in weights, in one 900 grams. The tissue is soft, even diffluent. Infarction is not infrequent. Rupture may occur spontaneously or as a result of injury. In the Munich autopsies there were 5 instances of rupture of the spleen, one of which resulted from a gangrenous abscess.

The *bone-marrow* shows changes very similar to those in the lymphoid tissues, and there may be foci of necrosis (Longcope).

The *liver* shows signs of parenchymatous degeneration. Early in the disease it is hyperæmic, and in a majority of instances it is swollen, somewhat pale, on section turbid, and microscopically the cells are very granular and loaded with fat. Nodular areas (miscroscopic) occur in many cases, as described by Hanford. Reed, in Welch's laboratory, could not determine any relation between the groups of bacilli and these areas (Studies II). Some of the nodules are lymphoid, others are necrotic. In 12 of the Munich autopsies liver abscess was found, and in 3, acute yellow atrophy. In 3 of this series liver abscess occurred. Pylephlebitis may follow abscess of the mesentery or perforation of the appendix. Affections of the gall-bladder are not uncommon, and are fully described under the clinical features.

Kidneys.—Cloudy swelling, with granular degeneration of the cells of the convoluted tubules, less commonly an acute nephritis, may be present. Rayer, Wagner, and others described the occurrence of numerous small areas infiltrated with round cells, which may have the appearance of lymphomata, or may pass on to softening and suppuration, producing the so-called *miliary abscesses,* of which there were 7 cases in this series. The typhoid bacilli have been found in these areas. They may also be found in the urine. The kidneys in cases of typhoid bacilluria may show no changes other than cloudy swelling. Diphtheritic inflammation of the pelvis of the kidney may occur. It was present in 3 of my cases, in one of which the tips of the papillæ were also affected. Catarrh of the bladder is not uncommon. Diphtheritic inflammation of this viscus may also occur. Orchitis is occasionally met with.

Respiratory Organs.—Ulceration of the larynx occurs in a certain number of cases; in the Munich series it was noted 107 times. It may come on at the same time as the ulceration in the ileum. It occurs in the posterior wall, at the insertion of the cords, at the base of the epiglottis, and on the ary-epiglottidean folds. The cartilages are very apt to become involved. In the later periods ulcers may be present.

Œdema of the glottis was present in 20 of the Munich cases, in 8 of which tracheotomy was performed. Diphtheritis of the pharynx and larynx is not very uncommon. It occurred in a most extensive form in 2 of my cases. Lobar pneumonia may be found early in the disease (see Pneumo-typhus), or it may be a late event. Hypostatic congestion and the condition of the lung spoken of as splenization occur. Gangrene of the lung occurred in 40 cases in the Munich series; abscess of the lung in 14; hæmorrhagic infarction in 129. Pleurisy is not a very common event. Fibrinous pleurisy occurred in about 6 per cent. of the Munich cases, and empyema in nearly 2 per cent.

Changes in the Circulatory System.—*Heart Lesions.—Endocarditis,* while not a common complication, is probably more frequent than is generally supposed. It was present without being suspected in 3 out of 105 autopsies in this series, while in 3 other cases of my series the clinical symptoms suggested its presence. The typhoid bacilli have been found in the vegetations. *Pericarditis* was present in 14 cases of the Munich autopsies. *Myocarditis* is not very infrequent. In protracted cases the muscle-fibre is usually soft, flabby, and of a pale yellowish-brown color. The softening may be extreme, though rarely of the grade described by Stokes in typhus fever, in which, when held apex up by the vessels, the organ collapsed over the hand, forming a mushroom-like cap. Microscopically, the fibres may show little or no change, even when the impulse of the heart has been extremely feeble. A granular parenchymatous degeneration is common. Fatty degeneration may be present, particularly in long-standing cases with anæmia. The hyaline change is not common. The segmenting myocarditis, in which the cement substance is softened so that the muscles separate, has also been found, but probably as a post-mortem change.

Lesions of the Blood-vessels.—Changes in the arteries are not infrequent. In 21 of 52 cases in our series, in which there were notes on the state of the aorta, fresh endarteritis was present, and in 13 of 62 cases in which the condition of the coronary arteries was noted similar changes were found (Thayer). Arteritis of a peripheral vessel with thrombus formation is not uncommon. Bacilli have been found in the thrombi. The artery may be blocked by a thrombus of cardiac origin—an embolus—but in the great majority of instances they are autochthonous and due to arteritis, obliterating or partial. Thrombosis in the veins is very much more frequent than in the arteries, but is not such a serious event. It is most frequent in the femoral, and in the left more often than the right. The consequences are fully considered under the *symptoms.*

Nervous System.—There are very few obvious changes met with. Meningitis is extremely rare. It occurred in only 11 of the 2,000 Munich cases. The exudation may be either serous, sero-fibrinous, or purulent, and typhoid bacilli have been isolated. Five cases of serous and one of purulent meningitis occurred in our series (Cole). Optic neuritis, which occurs sometimes in typhoid fever, has not, so far as I know, been described in connection with the meningitis. The anatomical lesion of the aphasia—seen not infrequently in children—is not known, possibly it is an encephalitis. Parenchymatous changes have been met with in the peripheral nerves, and appear to be not very uncommon, even when there have been no symptoms of neuritis.

The *voluntary muscles* show, in certain instances, the changes described by Zenker, which occur, however, in all long-standing febrile affections, and are not peculiar to typhoid fever. The muscle substance within the sarcolemma undergoes either a granular degeneration or a hyaline transformation. The abdominal muscles, the adductors of the thighs, and the pectorals are most commonly involved. Rupture of a rectus abdominis has been found post mortem. Hæmorrhage may occur. Abscesses may develop in the muscles during convalescence.

Symptoms.—In a disease so complex as typhoid fever it will be well first to give a general description, and then to study more fully the symptoms, complications, and sequelæ according to the individual organs.

General Description.—The period of incubation lasts from "eight to fourteen days, sometimes twenty-three" (Clinical Society), during which there are feelings of lassitude and inaptitude for work. The onset is rarely abrupt. In the 1,500 cases chills occurred at onset in 334, headache in 1,117, anorexia in 825, diarrhœa (without purgation) in 516, epistaxis in 323, abdominal pain in 443, constipation in 249, pain in right iliac fossa in 10. The patient at last takes to his bed, from which event, in a majority of cases, the definite onset of the disease may be dated. During the *first week* there is, in some cases (but by no means in all, as has long been taught), a steady rise in the fever, the evening record rising a degree or a degree and a half higher each day, reaching 103° or 104°. The pulse is not rapid when compared with the temperature, full in volume, but of low tension and often dicrotic; the tongue is coated and white; the abdomen is slightly distended and tender. Unless the fever is high there is no delirium, but the patient complains of headache, and there may be mental confusion at night. The bowels may be constipated, or there may be two or three loose movements daily. Toward the end of the week the spleen becomes enlarged and the rash appears in the form of rose-colored spots, seen first on the skin of the abdomen. Cough and bronchitic symptoms are not uncommon at the outset.

In the *second week,* in cases of moderate severity, the symptoms become aggravated; the fever remains high and the morning remission is slight. The pulse is rapid and loses its dicrotic character. There is no longer headache, but there are mental torpor and dulness. The face looks heavy; the lips are dry; the tongue, in severe cases, becomes dry also. The abdominal symptoms, if present—diarrhœa, tympanites, and tenderness—become aggravated. Death may occur during this week, with pronounced nervous symptoms, or, toward the end of it, from hæmorrhage or perforation. In mild cases the temperature declines, and by the fourteenth day may be normal.

In the *third week,* in cases of moderate severity, the pulse ranges from 110 to 130; the temperature now shows marked morning remissions, and there is a gradual decline in the fever. The loss of flesh is now more noticeable, and the weakness is pronounced. Diarrhœa and meteorism may now occur for the first time. Unfavorable symptoms at this stage are the pulmonary complications, increasing feebleness of the heart, and pronounced delirium with muscular tremor. Special dangers are perforation and hæmorrhage.

With the *fourth week*, in a majority of instances, convalescence begins. The temperature gradually reaches the normal point, the diarrhœa stops, the tongue cleans, and the desire for food returns. In severe cases the fourth and even the fifth week may present an aggravated picture of the third; the patient grows weaker, the pulse is more rapid and feeble, the tongue dry, and the abdomen distended. He lies in a condition of profound stupor, with low muttering delirium and subsultus tendinum, and passes the fæces and urine involuntarily. Failure of the circulation and secondary complications are the chief dangers of this period.

In the *fifth and sixth weeks* protracted cases may still show irregular fever, and convalescence may not set in until after the fortieth day. In this period we meet with relapses in the milder forms or slight recrudescence of the fever. At this time, too, occur many of the complications and sequelæ.

Special Features and Symptoms.—*Mode of Onset.*—As a rule, the symptoms come on insidiously, and the patient is unable to fix definitely the time at which he began to feel ill. The following are the most important deviations from this common course:

(*a*) *Onset with Pronounced, Sometimes Sudden, Nervous Manifestations.*—Headache, of a severe and intractable nature, is by no means an infrequent initial symptom. Again, a severe facial neuralgia may for a few days put the practitioner off his guard. In cases in which the patients have kept about and, as they say, fought the disease, the very first manifestation may be pronounced delirium. Such patients may even leave home and wander about for days. In rare cases the disease sets in with the most intense cerebro-spinal symptoms, simulating meningitis—severe headache, photophobia, retraction of the head, twitching of the muscles, and even convulsions. Occasionally drowsiness, stupor, and signs of basilar meningitis may exist for ten days or more before the characteristic symptoms develop; the onset may be with mania and marked mental symptoms.

(*b*) *With Pronounced Pulmonary Symptoms.*—The initial bronchial catarrh may be of great severity and obscure the other features of the disease. More striking still are those cases in which the disease sets in with a single chill, with pain in the side and all the characteristic features of lobar pneumonia, or of acute pleurisy; or tuberculosis is suspected.

(*c*) *With Intense Gastro-intestinal Symptoms.*—The incessant vomiting and pain may lead to a suspicion of poisoning, or the patient may be sent to the surgical wards for appendicitis.

(*d*) *With symptoms of an acute nephritis,* smoky or bloody urine, with much albumin and tube-casts.

(*e*) *Ambulatory Form.*—Deserving of especial mention are those cases of typhoid fever in which the patient keeps about and attempts to do work, or perhaps takes a long journey to his home. He may come under observation for the first time with a temperature of 104° or 105°, and with the rash well out. Many of these cases run a severe course, and in general hospitals they contribute largely to the total mortality. Finally, there are rare instances in which typhoid is unsuspected until perforation or a profuse hæmorrhage from the bowels occurs.

Facial Aspect.—Early in the disease the cheeks are flushed and the eyes bright. Toward the end of the first week the expression becomes more

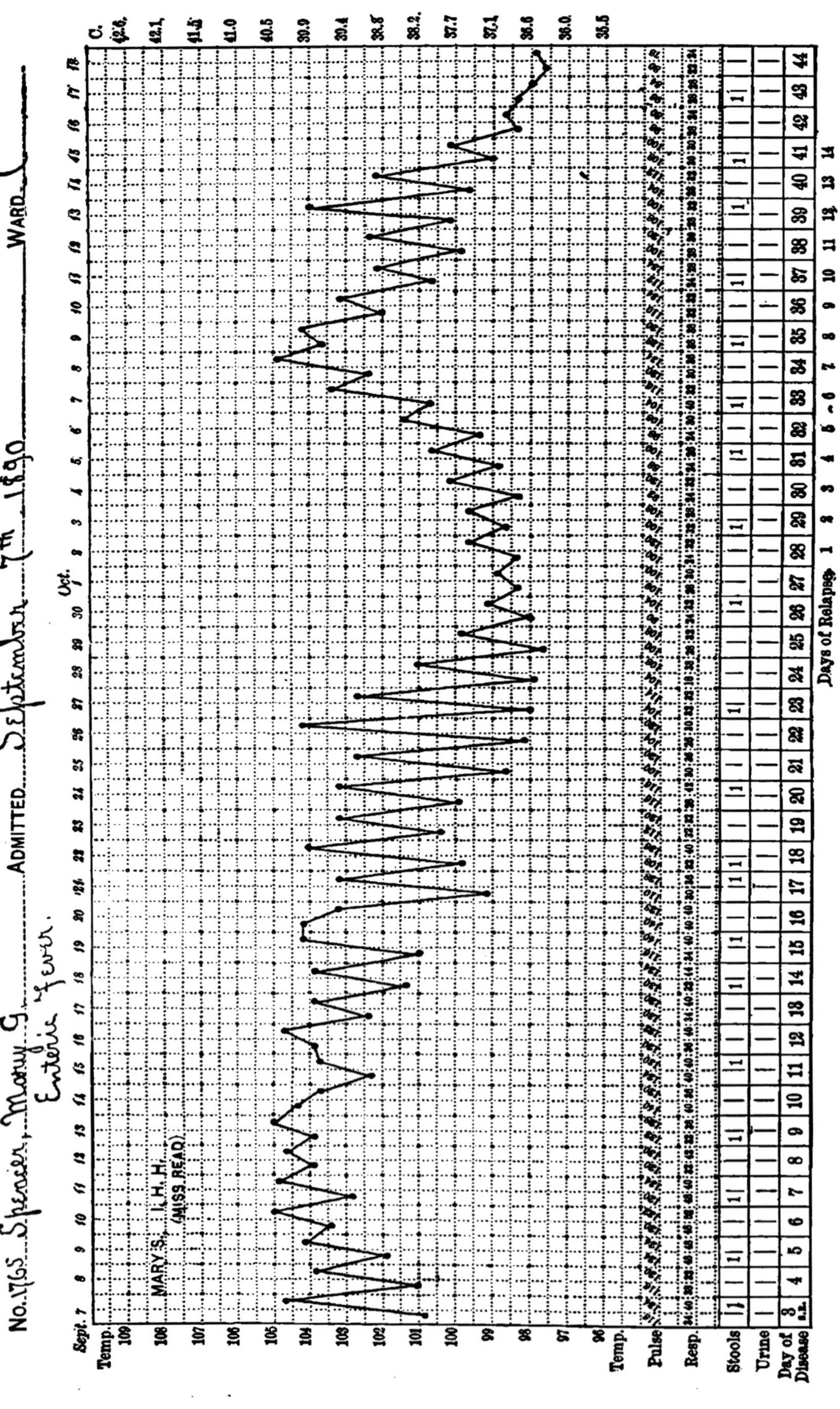

CHART I.—TYPHOID FEVER WITH RELAPSE.

listless, and when the disease is well established the patient has a dull and heavy look. There is never the rapid anæmia of malarial fever, and the color of the lips and cheeks may be retained even to the third week.

Fever.—(*a*) *Regular Course.* (Chart I.)—In the stage of invasion the fever rises steadily during the first five or six days. The evening temperature is about a degree or a degree and a half higher than the morning remission, so that a temperature of 104° or 105° is not uncommon by the end of the first week. Having reached the fastigium or height, the fever then persists with very slight daily remissions. The fever may be singularly persistent and but little influenced by bathing or other measures. At the end of the second and throughout the third week the temperature becomes more distinctly remittent. The difference between the morning or evening record may be 3° or 4°, and the morning temperature may even be normal. It falls by lysis, and the temperature is not considered normal until the evening record is at 98.4°.

(*b*) *Variations from the typical temperature curve* are common. We do not always see the gradual step-like ascent in the early stage; the patients do not often come under observation at this time. When the disease sets in with a chill, or in children with a convulsion, the temperature may rise at once to 103° or 104°. In many cases defervescence occurs at the end of the second week and the temperature may fall rapidly, reaching the normal within twelve or twenty hours. An inverse type of temperature, high in the morning and low in the evening, is occasionally seen, but has no especial significance.

Sudden falls in the temperature may occur; thus, as shown in Chart II, a drop of 6.4° may follow an intestinal hæmorrhage, and the fall may be very apparent even before the blood has appeared in the stools. Sometimes during the anæmia which follows a severe hæmorrhage from the bowels there are remarkable oscillations in the temperature. Hyperpyrexia is rare. In only 58 of 1,500 cases did the fever rise above 106°. Before death the fever may rise; the highest I have known was 109.5°.

(*c*) *Post-typhoid Variations.*—(1) *Recrudescences.*—After a normal temperature of perhaps five or six days, the fever may rise suddenly to 102° or 103°, without constitutional disturbance, furring of the tongue, or abdominal symptoms. After persisting for from two to four days the temperature falls. Of 1,500 cases, 92 presented these post-typhoid elevations, brief notes of which are given in the Studies on Typhoid Fever. Constipation, errors in diet, or excitement may cause them. These attacks are a frequent source of anxiety to the practitioner. They are very common, and it is not always possible to say upon what they depend. In some cases typhoid or colon bacilli are found in the blood. As a rule, if the rise in temperature is the result of a complication, such as pleurisy or thrombosis, there is an increase in the leucocytes. Naturally one suspects at the outset a relapse, but there is an absence of the step-like ascent, and, as a rule, the fever falls after lasting a few days.

(2) *The Sub-febrile Stage of Convalescence.*—In children, in very nervous patients, and in cases of anæmia, the evening temperature may keep up for weeks after the tongue has cleaned and the appetite has returned. This may usually be disregarded, and is often best treated by allowing the patient to get up, and by stopping the use of the thermometer. Of course, it is important not to overlook any latent complications.

(3) *Hypothermia.*—Low temperatures in typhoid fever are common, following the tubs, or spontaneously in the third and fourth week in the periods of marked remissions, and following hæmorrhage. An interesting form is the persistent hypothermia of convalescence. For ten days or more, particularly in the protracted cases with great emaciation, the temperature may be 96.5° or 97°. It is of no special significance.

(*d*) *The Fever of the Relapse.*—This is a repetition in many instances of the original fever, a gradual ascent and maintenance for a few days at a certain height and then a decline. It is usually shorter than the original pyrexia, and rarely continues more than two or three weeks. (Chart I.)

(*e*) *Afebrile Typhoid.*—There are cases described in which the chief features of the disease have been present without the existence of fever. They are extremely rare in this country. I have seen a case, afebrile at the thirteenth day, and in which the rose spots and other features persisted till the twenty-eighth day.

(*f*) Chills occur (1) sometimes with the fever of onset; (2) occasionally at intervals throughout the course of the disease, and followed by sweats (so-called sudoral form); (3) with the advent of complications, pleurisy, pneumonia, otitis media, phlebitis, etc.; (4) with active antipyretic treatment by the coal-tar remedies; (5) occasionally during the period of defervescence without relation to any complication, probably due to a septic infection; (6) after the injection of vaccines or serum; (*e*) according to Herringham, chills may result from constipation. There are cases in which throughout the latter half of the disease chills recur with great severity. (See Chills in Typhoid Fever, Studies II, Johns Hopkins Reports.)

Skin.—The characteristic rash consists of hyperæmic spots, which appear from the seventh to the tenth day, usually at first upon the abdomen. They are slightly raised, flattened papules, which can be felt distinctly, of a rose-red color, disappearing on pressure, and ranging in diameter from 2 to 4 mm. They were present in 93.2 per cent. of the white patients and 20.6 per cent. of the colored. They come out in successive crops, and after persisting for two or three days they disappear, occasionally leaving a brownish stain. The spots may be present upon the back, and not upon the abdomen. The eruption may be very abundant over the whole skin of the trunk, and on the extremities. There were 81 in which they occurred on the arms, 17 on the forearms, 43 on the thighs, legs 15, face 5, hands 3. The cases with very abundant eruption are not necessarily more severe. As already noted, the typhoid bacilli have been found in the spots. Of variations in the rash, frequently the spots are capped by small vesicles. A profuse miliary or sudaminal rash is not uncommon. In 38 cases in my series there were purpuric spots. Three of the cases were true hæmorrhagic typhoid fever. The rash may not appear until the relapse. In 21 cases in our series the rose spots came out after the patient was afebrile.

A branny desquamation is not rare in children, and common in adults after hydrotherapy. Occasionally the skin peels off in large flakes. A yellow color of the palms of the hands and soles of the feet is not uncommon.

Among other skin lesions the following may be mentioned:

Erythema.—It is not very uncommon in the first week of the disease to find a diffuse erythematous blush—E. typhosum. Sometimes the skin may have a peculiar mottled pink and white appearance. E. exudativum, E. nodosum, and urticaria may be present.

Herpes.—Herpes is certainly rare in typhoid fever in comparison with its great frequency in malarial fever and in pneumonia. It was noted in 20 of our 1,500 cases, usually on the lips.

The Tâches bleuâtres—Peliomata—Maculæ ceruleæ.—These are pale-blue or steel-gray spots, subcuticular, from 4 to 10 mm. in diameter, and of irregular outline. They are due to lice (see PEDICULOSIS).

Skin Gangrene.—Areas of superficial gangrene may follow the prolonged use of an ice-bag. In children noma may occur; as reported by McFarland in the Philadelphia epidemic of 1898, there were many cases with multiple areas of gangrene of the skin. The nose, ears, and genitals may be attacked.

Sweats.—At the height of the fever the skin is usually dry. Profuse sweating is rare, but it is not very uncommon to see the abdomen or chest moist with perspiration, particularly in the reaction which follows the bath. Sweats in some instances constitute a striking feature and may occasionally be associated with chilly sensations or actual chills. Jaccoud and others in France have especially described this *sudoral* form of typhoid fever. There may be recurring paroxysms of chill, fever, and sweats (even several in twenty-four hours), and the case may be mistaken for one of malarial fever. Profuse sweats may occur with hæmorrhage or perforation.

Œdema of the skin occurs: (1) As the result of vascular obstruction, most commonly of a vein, as in thrombosis of the femoral vein. (2) In connection with nephritis, very rarely. (3) In association with the anæmia and cachexia. *The hair* falls out after the attack, but complete baldness is rare. I have once seen permanent baldness. The nutrition of the nails suffers, and during and after convalescence tranverse ridges may occur. A peculiar *odor* is exhaled from the skin in some cases. Whether due to a cutaneous exhalation or not, there certainly is a very distinctive smell connected with many patients. Nathan Smith describes it as of a "semi-cadaverous, musty character."

Lineæ atrophicæ.—Lines of atrophy may appear on the skin of the abdomen, lateral aspects of the thighs and about the knees, similar to those seen after pregnancy. They have been attributed to neuritis, and Duckworth has reported a case in which the skin adjacent to them was hyperæsthetic.

Bed-sores are not uncommon in protracted cases, with great emaciation. As a rule, they result from pressure and are seen upon the sacrum, more rarely the ilia, the shoulders, and the heels. These are less common, I think, since the introduction of hydrotherapy. Scrupulous care and watchfulness do much for their prevention, but it is to be remembered that in cases with profound involvement of the nerve centres acute bed-sores of the back and heels may occur with very slight pressure, and with astonishing rapidity.

Boils and superficial abscesses constitute a common and troublesome sequel.

CIRCULATORY SYSTEM.—The *blood* presents important changes. The following statements are based on studies which W. S. Thayer has made in my wards (Studies I and III): During the first two weeks there may be little or no change in the blood. Profuse sweats or copious diarrhœa may, as Hayem has shown, cause the corpuscles—as in the collapse stage of cholera—to rise above normal. In the third week a fall usually takes place in corpuscles and hæmoglobin, and the number may sink rapidly even to 1,300,000 per c. mm., gradually rising to normal during convalescence. When the patient first gets up, there may be a slight fall in the number of corpuscles. The average maximum loss is about 1,000,000 to the c. mm.

The amount of hæmoglobin is always reduced, and usually in a greater relative proportion than the number of red corpuscles, and during recovery the normal color standard is reached at a later period. Leucopenia is present throughout the course. Cold baths increase temporarily the number of leucocytes in the peripheral circulation. The absence of leucocytosis may be at times of real diagnostic value in distinguishing typhoid fever from various septic fevers and acute inflammatory processes. The polymorphonuclear leucocytes are normal in number, while the large mononuclears are relatively increased. When an acute inflammatory process occurs in typhoid fever the leucocytes show an increase in the polynuclear forms, and this may be of great diagnostic moment.

The post-typhoid anæmia may reach an extreme grade. In one of my patients the blood-corpuscles sank to 1,300,000 per c. mm. and the hæmoglobin to about 20 per cent. These severe grades of anæmia are not common in my experience. In the Munich statistics there were 54 cases with general and extreme anæmia. Of changes in the blood plasma very little is known.

The *pulse* in typhoid fever presents no special characters. It is increased in rapidity, but not always in proportion to the height of the fever, and this may be a very special feature in the early stages. There is no acute disease with which, in the early stage, a dicrotic pulse is so frequently associated. Even with high fever the pulse may not be greatly accelerated. As the disease progresses the pulse becomes more rapid, feebler, and small. In 15 per cent. of our cases the pulse rate rose above 140. In the extreme prostration of severe cases it may reach 150 or more, and is a mere undulation—the so-called running pulse. The lowered arterial pressure is manifest in the dusky lividity of the skin and coldness of the hands and feet.

During convalescence the pulse gradually returns to normal, and occasionally becomes very slow. After no other acute fever do we so frequently meet with bradycardia. I have counted the pulse as low as 30, and instances are on record of still fewer beats to the minute. Tachycardia, while less common, may be a very troublesome and persistent feature of convalescence.

Blood Pressure.—This is usually from 115-125 mm. Hg. (Riva-Rocci instrument) in systole. The diastolic pressure has the normal relationship to the systolic, and averages 85-100 mm. Hg. There is a gradual fall during the course to about 100-110 mm. Hg. at the beginning of apyrexia. In two or three weeks later the pressure has usually returned to normal. Hæmorrhage usually produces a marked fall both in the systolic and diastolic pressure. In some cases of perforation there is a sharp rise in systolic pressure. Tubs and ice sponges usually cause a rise of 10-20 mm. Hg.

The *heart-sounds* may be normal throughout the course. In severe cases, the first sound becomes feeble and there is often to be heard, at the apex and along the left sternal margin, a soft systolic murmur, which was present in 22 per cent. of our cases. Absence of the first sound is rare. Gallop rhythm is not uncommon. In the extreme feebleness of the graver forms, the first and second sound become very similar, and the long pause is much shortened (embryocardia).

Of cardiac complications, *pericarditis* is rare and has been met with chiefly in children and in association with pneumonia. It was present in three of my series and occurred in only 14 of the 2,000 Munich post mortems. *Endocarditis* was found post mortem in three cases, and the physical signs suggested its presence in three other cases in the series. *Myocarditis* is more common, and is indicated by a progressive weakening of the heart-sounds and enfeeblement of the action of the organ.

Complications in the Arteries.—Arteritis with thrombus formation occurred in four cases in the series, one in the branches of the middle cerebral, two in the femoral, and one in the brachial. In one case gangrene of the leg followed. I saw a similar case with Roddick, in Montreal, in which obliteration of the left femoral artery occurred on the sixteenth day, and of the vessel on the right side on the twentieth day, with gangrene of both feet. Pain, tenderness, and swelling occur over the artery, with diminution or disappearance of the pulsations and coldness and blueness of the extremity. In two of the cases these symptoms gradually disappeared, and the pulsation returned not only in the peripheral, but in the affected vessels (Thayer). Keen refers to 46 cases of arterial gangrene, of which 8 were bilateral, 19 on the right side, and 19 on the left.

Thrombi in the Veins.—In our series there were 43 instances, distributed in the following veins: femoral 23, popliteal 5, iliac 5, veins of the calf 5, internal saphenous 3, pulmonary artery and common iliac 1, axillary vein 1 (Thayer). I saw one case in the right circumflex iliac vein. Femoral thrombosis is the most common, and almost invariably in the left vessel, due, as Liebermeister suggests, to the fact that the left iliac vein is crossed by the right iliac artery, and the blood flow is not so free. The symptoms of this complication are very definite—the fever may increase or recur. Chills occurred in 11 of all the cases. Pain and swelling at the site are constantly present, and the thrombotic mass can be felt, not always at first, nor is it well to feel for it. Swelling of the leg follows as a rule, but it is rarely so extreme, and never, I think, so painful as the puerperal phlegmasia alba dolens. In the iliac thrombosis the pain may be severe and lead to the suspicion of perforation, as in one of our cases. Leucocytosis is usually present, in 12 cases it rose above 10,000. Five of the 43 cases died, 2 only as a result of the thrombus; in the case of axillary thrombosis from pulmonary embolism, in one embolism of the inferior cava and right auricle from the dislocation of a piece of thrombus from the left iliac vein. Thayer examined 16 of the patients at varying periods after convalescence, and found in every case more or less disability from the varices and persistent swelling. In some cases, however, the recovery is complete.

Digestive System.—Loss of appetite is early, and, as a rule, the relish for food is not regained until convalescence. Thirst is constant, and should be fully and freely gratified. The *tongue* presents the changes inevitable in a prolonged fever. Early in the disease it is moist, swollen, and coated with a thin white fur, which, as the fever progresses, becomes denser. It may remain moist throughout. In severe cases, particularly those with delirium, the tongue becomes very dry, partly owing to the fact that such patients breathe with the mouth open. It may be covered with a brown or brownish-black fur, or with crusts between which are cracks and fissures. In these cases the teeth and lips may be covered with a dark brownish matter called *sordes*—a mixture of food, epithelial *débris*, and micro-organisms. By keeping the mouth and tongue clean from the outset, the fissures, which are extremely painful, may be prevented. Acute glossitis occurred in one case at the onset of the relapse. During convalescence the tongue gradually becomes clean, and the fur is thrown off, almost imperceptibly or occasionally in flakes.

The secretion of saliva is often diminished; salivation is rare.

Parotitis was present in 45 of the 2,000 Munich cases. It occurred in 14 cases in my series; of these, 5 died. It is most frequent in the third week in very severe cases. Extensive sloughing may follow in the tissues of the neck. Usually unilateral, and in a majority of cases going on to suppuration, it is regarded as a very fatal complication, but recovery has followed in nine of my cases. It undoubtedly may arise from extension of inflammation along Steno's duct. This is probably not so serious a form as when it arises from metastatic inflammation. In four cases the submaxillary glands were involved alone, in one a cellulitis of the neck extended from the gland and proved fatal. Parotitis may occur after the fever has subsided. A remarkable localized sweating in the parotid region is an occasional sequel of the abscess.

The *pharynx* may be the seat of catarrh or ulceration. Sometimes the fauces are deeply congested. Membranous pharyngitis, a serious and fatal complication, may come on in the third week. Difficulty in swallowing may result from ulcers of the œsophagus, and in one of our cases stricture followed.* Thyroiditis may occur with abscess formation.

The *gastric symptoms* are extremely variable. Nausea and vomiting are not common. There are instances, however, in which vomiting, resisting all measures, is a marked feature from the outset, and may directly cause death from exhaustion. Vomiting does not often occur in the second and third weeks, unless associated with some serious complication. Ulcers have been found in the stomach. Hæmatemesis occurred in 4 of our cases.

Intestinal Symptoms.—Diarrhœa is a very variable symptom, occurring in from 20 to 30 per cent. of the cases. Of 1,500 cases, 516 had diarrhœa before entering, 260 during their stay in hospital. It frequently follows the giving of purgatives and the small percentage in the hospital may be due to the fact that we use no purges or intestinal antiseptics. Its absence must not be taken as an indication that the intestinal lesions are of slight extent. I have seen, on several occasions, the most extensive infiltration and ulceration of the Peyer's glands of the small intestine, with the colon filled with solid fæces. The diarrhœa is caused less by the ulcers than by the associated catarrh, and, as in tuberculosis, it is probable that when this is in the large intestine the discharges are more frequent. It is most common toward the end of the first and throughout the second week, but it may not occur until the third or even the fourth week. The number of discharges ranges from 3 to 8 or 10 in the twenty-four hours. They are usually abundant, thin, grayish-yellow, granular, of the consistency and appearance of pea-soup, and resemble very much, as Addison remarked, the normal contents of the small bowel. The reaction is alkaline and the odor offensive. On standing, the discharges separate into a thin serous layer, containing albumin and salts,

---

* Mitchell, Œsophageal Complications in Typhoid Fever (Studies II).

and a lower stratum, consisting of epithelial *débris*, remnants of food, and numerous crystals of triple phosphates. Blood may be in small amount, and only recognized by the microscope. Sloughs of the Peyer's glands occur either as grayish-yellow fragments or occasionally as ovoid masses, an inch or more in length, in which portions of the bowel tissue may be found. The

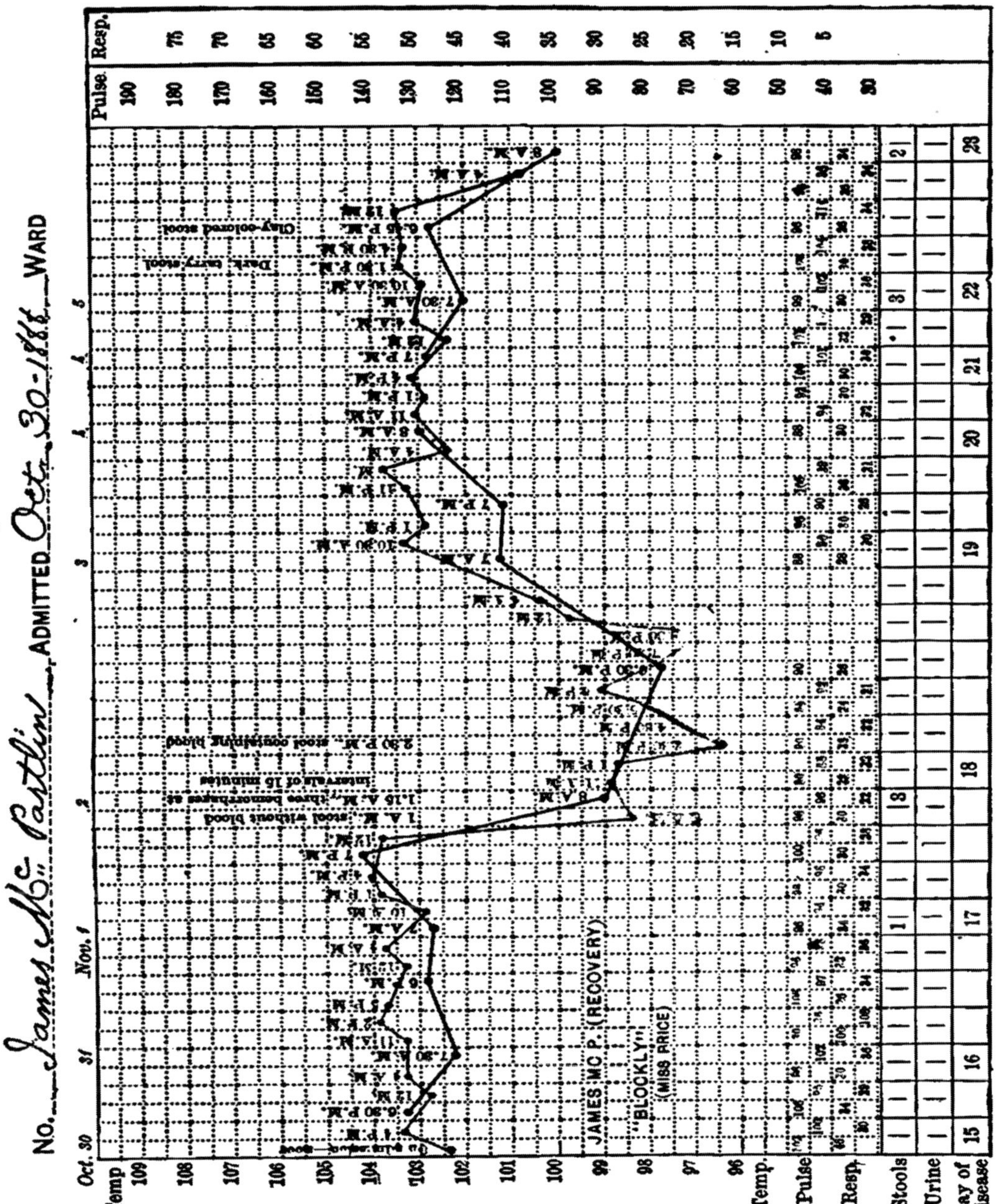

CHART II.—HÆMORRHAGE FROM THE BOWELS. RAPID FALL OF TEMPERATURE.

bacilli are not found in the stools until the end of the first or the middle of the second week. Constipation was present in 51 per cent. of this series.

Hæmorrhage from the bowels is a serious complication, occurring in about 7 per cent. of all cases. It had occurred in 99 of the 2,000 fatal Munich cases. In 1,500 cases treated in my wards hæmorrhage occurred in 118, and in 12 death followed the hæmorrhage. It occurred in 1,641 (7 per cent.) of

23,721 collected cases (McCrae). There may be only a slight trace of blood in the stools, but often it is a profuse, free hæmorrhage. It occurs most commonly between the end of the second and the beginning of the fourth week, the time of the separation of the sloughs. Occasionally, early in the course, it results simply from the intense hyperæmia. It usually comes on without warning. A sensation of sinking or collapse is experienced by the patient, the temperature falls, and may, as in the annexed chart, drop 6° or 7° in a few hours. Fatal collapse may supervene before the blood appears in the stool. Hæmorrhage usually occurs in cases of considerable severity, but Graves and Trousseau held that it was not a very dangerous symptom.

It must not be forgotten that melæna may also be part of a general hæmorrhagic tendency (to be referred to later), in which case it is associated with petechiæ and hæmaturia. There may be a special family predisposition to intestinal hæmorrhages in typhoid fever.

Meteorism, a frequent symptom, is not serious if of moderate grade, but when excessive is usually of ill omen. Owing to defective tone in the walls, in severe cases to their infiltration with serum, gas accumulates in the stomach, small and large bowel, particularly in the last. Pushing up the diaphragm, it interferes very much with the action of the heart and lungs, and may also favor perforation. Gurgling in the right iliac fossa exists in a large proportion of the cases, and indicates simply the presence of gas and fluid fæces in the colon and cæcum.

Abdominal pain and tenderness were present in three-fifths of a series of 500 cases studied with special reference to the point by T. McCrae. In some it was only present at the onset. Pain occurred during the course in about one-third of the cases. This is due in some instances to conditions apart from the bowel lesions, such as pleurisy, distention of the bladder, and phlebitis. It may be associated with diarrhœa, severe constipation, perisplenitis, or acute abdominal complications. Pain occurs with some cases of hæmorrhage, but is most constantly present with perforation. In a large group no cause could be found for the pain, and if other symptoms be associated the condition may lead to error in diagnosis. Operation for appendicitis has been performed in the early stage of typhoid fever, owing to the combination of pain in the right iliac fossa, fever and constipation.

Perforation.—From one-fourth to one-third of the deaths are due to perforation, and as there were 35,379 deaths from typhoid fever in the United States in the year 1900, this gives between 9,000 and 12,000 deaths from this cause. Among 34,916 collected cases perforation occurred in 3.1 per cent. (McCrae). While it may occur as early as the first week, in the great majority it is at the height of the disease in the third week, and much more frequently in the severe cases, particularly those associated with tympanites, diarrhœa, and hæmorrhage. It may occur, however, in very mild attacks and with great suddenness, when the patient is apparently progressing favorably.

Symptoms of Perforation.—By far the most important single indication is a sudden, sharp pain of increasing severity, often paroxysmal in character. It is rarely absent, except in the small group of cases with profound toxæmia. The situation is most frequent in the hypogastric region and to the right of the middle line. Tenderness on pressure is present in the great majority of cases, usually in the hypogastric and right iliac regions, sometimes diffuse;

it may only be brought out on deep pressure. As LeConte points out, when the perforation happens to be in contact with the parietal peritoneum the local features on palpation are much more marked than when the perforated ulcer is next to a coil or to the mesentery. There may be early irritability of the bladder, with frequent micturition, and pain extending toward the penis. A third important sign is muscle rigidity, increased tension, and spasm on any attempt to palpate. The temperature may rise for a few hours to fall later or may drop at once. The pulse and respiration rate are usually increased. Following these features in a few hours there is usually a reaction, and then the features of general peritonitis become manifest to a more or less marked degree. Among the general features, the facies of the patient shows changes; there is increased pallor, a pinched expression of the face, and as the symptoms progress and toward the end a marked Hippocratic facies, a dusky suffusion, and the forehead bathed in a clammy perspiration. The temperature rises with the increase of the peritonitis. The pulse quickens, is running and thready, the heart's action becomes progressively more feeble, and there is an increase in the frequency of the respiration. Vomiting is a variable feature; it is present in a majority of the cases. Hiccough is common and may occur early, but more frequently late.

The local abdominal features are often more important than the general, as it is surprising to notice how excellent the condition of a patient may be with perforative peritonitis. Limitation of the respiratory movements is usually present, perhaps confined to the hypogastric area. Increasing distention is the rule, but perforation and peritonitis may occur, it is to be remembered, with an abdomen flat or even scaphoid. Increasing pain on pressure, increasing muscle spasm and tension of the wall are important signs. Percussion may reveal a flat note in the flanks, due to exudate. A friction may be present within a few hours of the onset of the perforation. Obliteration of the liver flatness in the nipple line may be caused by excessive tympany, but rapid obliteration of liver flatness in a flat, or a not much distended abdomen, is a valuable sign. Examination of the rectum may show fullness or tenderness in the pelvis. Advance in the abdominal signs is an important point.

In a majority of all cases there is a rise in the leucocytes, and when present may be a valuable help, but it is not constant. Increase in the blood pressure is not constant.

General peritonitis, without perforation of the bowel, may occur by extension from an ulcer, or by rupture of a softened mesenteric gland, or, as in one recent case in my series, from inflammation of the Fallopian tubes. It was present in 2.2 per cent. of the Munich autopsies.

Perforation is almost invariably fatal. In a few cases healing takes place spontaneously, as is beautifully shown in one of the Pennsylvania Hospital specimens, or the orifice may be closed by a tag of omentum, as in a remarkable case reported by J. Milton Miller. There is a group of cases in which hæmorrhage complicates the perforation and adds to the difficulty in diagnosis. In 7 of our 43 cases hæmorrhage accompanied the perforation; in 3 others the hæmorrhage had occurred some days before.

The diagnosis of perforation, easy enough at times, is not without serious difficulties. The conditions for which it has been mistaken in my wards have been: appendicitis, occurring during the course of the typhoid fever, phlebitis of the iliac vein with great pain, hæmorrhage, and in one case a local peritonitis without perforation, for which no cause was found. Recovery followed the exploratory operation, which was made in all but one (hæmorrhage case) of the cases. Exploration is justifiable and better than delay in suspicious cases.

ASCITES occurs in rare instances (McPhedran).

The SPLEEN is usually enlarged, and the edge was felt below the costal margin in 71.6 per cent. of my cases. Percussion is uncertain, as, owing to distension of the stomach and colon, even the normal area of dulness may not be obtainable. Enlargement is often not marked in elderly patients.

LIVER.—Symptoms on the part of this organ are rare.

(*a*) *Jaundice* was present in only 8 cases of my series. Catarrh of the ducts, toxæmia, abscess, and occasionally gall-stones are the usual causes.

(*b*) *Abscess.*—Solitary abscess is exceedingly rare and occurred in but 3 cases in my series. It may occur early in the disease, but most frequently is a sequel. von Eberts has collected 30 cases, in 9 of which the typhoid bacillus was isolated from the pus. In about half the cases the right lobe was affected. Eighteen of the patients recovered. Abscess may follow the intestinal lesion or a complication as parotitis. Suppuratve pylephlebitis may follow perforation of the appendix. Suppurative cholangitis has been described.

(*c*) *Cholecystitis* occurred in 19 cases of the series. Pain in the region of the gall-bladder is the most constant symptom. Tenderness, muscle spasm with rigidity, and a gall-bladder tumor are present in a majority of the cases. Jaundice is inconstant. Leucocytosis usually occurs. With perforation there may be a marked drop in the fever and the onset of signs of peritonitis. In simple cholecystitis the urgency of the symptoms may abate, and recovery follow. Suppuration may occur with infection of the bile passages. Months or years after (eighteen years in Hunner's case) the bacilli may cause cholecystitis or gall-stones. Typhoid bacilli have been found as a cause of cholecystitis in patients who never had typhoid fever.

(*d*) *Gall-stones.*—Bernheim called attention to the frequency of cholelithiasis after typhoid fever. It is probably associated with the presence of typhoid bacilli in the gall-bladder (see under Gall-Stones).

PANCREAS.—Hæmorrhagic pancreatitis has occurred rarely.

RESPIRATORY SYSTEM.—*Epistaxis,* an early symptom, precedes typhoid fever more commonly than any other febrile affection. It is occasionally profuse and serious and may occur during the course.

Laryngitis is not very common. The ulcers and the perichondritis have already been described. Œdema, apart from ulceration, is rare. In the United States the laryngeal complications of typhoid fever seem much less frequent than on the Continent. I have twice seen severe perichondritis; both of the cases recovered, one after the expectoration of large portions of the thyroid cartilage. Keen and Lüning have collected 221 cases of serious surgical complications of the larynx. General emphysema may follow the perforation of an ulcer. Stenosis is a very serious sequence. It would appear that paralysis of the laryngeal muscles is more common than we have supposed. Przedborski (Volkmann's Sammlung, No. 182) systematically examined the larynx in 100 consecutive cases and found 25 with paralysis. The condition is nearly always due to neuritis, sometimes in connection with affections of other nerves.

Bronchitis is one of the most frequent initial symptoms. It is indicated by the presence of sibilant râles. The smaller tubes may be involved, producing urgent cough and even slight cyanosis. Collapse and lobular pneumonia may also occur.

Lobar pneumonia is met with under two conditions:

(*a*) At the outset, the *pneumo-typhus* of the Germans. This occurred in three of our cases. After an indisposition of a day or so, the patient is seized with a chill, has high fever, pain in the side, and within forty-eight hours there are signs of consolidation and the evidences of an ordinary lobar pneumonia. The intestinal symptoms may not occur until toward the end of the first week or later; the pulmonary symptoms persist, crisis does not occur; the aspect of the patient changes, and by the end of the second week the clinical picture is that of typhoid fever. Spots may then be present and doubts as to the nature of the case are solved. In other instances, in the absence of a characteristic eruption, the case remains doubtful, and it is impossible to say whether the disease has been pneumonia, in which the so-called typhoid symptoms have developed, or whether it was typhoid fever with early implication of the lungs. This condition may depend upon an early localization of the typhoid bacillus in the lung.

(*b*) Lobar pneumonia forms a serious and by no means infrequent complication of the second or third week—in 19 of our cases. It was present in over 8 per cent. of the Munich cases. The symptoms are usually not marked. There may be no rusty sputum, and, unless sought for, the condition is frequently overlooked. The etiological agent in these cases is still in dispute. Typhoid bacilli have been isolated from the sputum by Jehle, Rau, and others. They have also been isolated from the consolidated lungs at autopsy, but in such cases the pneumococci may have been originally present, and the typhoid bacilli secondary invaders. In all cases of pneumonia during typhoid fever occurring in the Johns Hopkins Hospital and coming to autopsy, the pneumococcus could be demonstrated in the consolidated lung. Infarction, abscess, and gangrene are occasionally pulmonary complications.

Hypostatic congestion of the lungs and œdema, due to enfeebled circulation, occur in the later periods of the disease. The physical signs are defective resonance at the bases, feeble breath-sounds, and, on deep inspiration, moist râles.

Hæmoptysis may occur. Creagh reports a case in which it caused death.

Pleurisy was present in about 8 per cent. of the Munich autopsies. It occurred in 2 per cent. of my series. It may occur at the outset—pleuro-typhoid—or slowly during convalescence, in which case it is almost always purulent and due to the typhoid bacillus.

Pneumothorax is rare. Hale White has reported two cases, in both of which pleurisy existed. After death, no lesions of the lungs or bronchi were discovered. The condition may be due to straining, or to the rupture of a small pyæmic abscess. It may occur also during convalescence.

NERVOUS SYSTEM.—*Cerebro-spinal Form.*—As already noted, the disease may set in with intense and persisting headache, or an aggravated form of neuralgia. There are cases in which the effect of the poison is manifested on the nervous system early and with the greatest intensity. There are headache, photophobia, retraction of the neck, marked twitchings of the muscles, rigidity, and even convulsions. In such cases the diagnosis of meningitis is invariably made. The cases showing marked *meningeal features* during the course of the disease may be divided into three groups. First, those with symptoms suggestive of meningitis, but without localizing features and without at post mortem the anatomical lesions of meningitis. In every series of cases numerous such examples occur. Secondly, the cases of so-called serous meningitis. There is a localization of typhoid bacilli in the cerebro-spinal fluid and a mild inflammatory reaction, but without suppurative meningitis. Cole has collected thirteen such cases, five of them occurring in our series. Probably more frequent lumbar punctures will show that this occurs not infrequently. Thirdly, true typhoid suppurative meningitis due to *B. typhosus.* Only one such case occurred in our series, and Cole has collected thirteen from the literature. Meningitis in typhoid fever is occasionally due to other organisms, as the tubercle bacillus, or the micrococcus intracellularis. Marked convulsive movements, local or general, with coma and delirium, are seen also in thrombosis of the cerebral veins and sinuses.

Delirium, usually present in very severe cases, is certainly less frequent under a rigid plan of hydrotherapy. It may exist from the outset, but usually does not occur until the second and sometimes not until the third week. It may be slight and only nocturnal. It is, as a rule, a quiet delirium, though there are cases in which the patient is very noisy and constantly tries to get out of bed, and, unless carefully watched, may escape. The patient does not often become maniacal. In heavy drinkers the delirium may have the character of delirium tremens. Even in patients who have no positive delirium, the mental processes are usually dulled and the aspect is listless and apathetic. In severe cases the patient passes into a condition of unconsciousness. The eyes may be open, but he is oblivious to all surrounding circumstances and neither knows nor can indicate his wants. The urine and fæces are passed involuntarily. In this pseudo-wakeful state, or coma vigil, as it is called, the eyes are open and the patient is constantly muttering. The lips and tongue are tremulous; there are twitchings of the fingers and wrists—subsultus tendinum and carphologia. He picks at the bedclothes or grasps at invisible objects. These are among the most serious symptoms of the disease and always indicate danger.

Convulsions in typhoid fever are rare. There were 7 instances in my series. They occur: first, at the onset of the disease, particularly in children; secondly, as a manifestation of the toxæmia; and thirdly, as a result of severe cerebral complications—thrombosis, meningitis, or acute encephalitis. Occasionally in convalescence convulsions may occur from unknown causes. Of the 7 cases 3 died.

Neuritis, which is not uncommon—11 cases in the series—may be local or a widespread affection.

Multiple neuritis comes on usually during convalescence. The legs may be affected, or the four extremities. The cases are often difficult to differentiate from those with subacute poliomyelitis. Recovery is the rule.

Local Neuritis.—This may occur during the height of the fever or after convalescence is established. It may set in with agonizing pain, and with sensitiveness of the affected nerve trunks. The local neuritis may affect the nerves of an arm or of a leg, and involve chiefly the extensors, so that there is wrist-drop or foot-drop. The arm or leg may be much swollen and the skin over it erythematous. A curious condition, probably a local neuritis, is that which was first described by Handford as *tender toes*, and which appears to be more common after the bath treatment. The tips and pads of the toes, rarely the pads at their bases, become exquisitely sensitive, so that the patient can not bear the weight of the bedclothes. There is no discoloration and no swelling, and it disappears usually within a week or ten days.

Painful muscles are not uncommon, particularly in the calves. I have reported a series of cases (Studies III). Painful cramps may also occur. In some of the cases of painful legs the condition is a myositis; in others the swelling and pain may be due to thrombosis in the deeper veins.

Poliomyelitis may occur with the symptoms of acute ascending paralysis and prove fatal in a few days. More frequently it is less acute, and causes either a paraplegia or a limited atrophic paralysis of one arm or leg.

Hemiplegia is a rare complication. Smithies (1907) collected 40 cases in 26 of which aphasia occurred and in 10 the hemiplegia was preceded by convulsions. In 21 cases the paralysis was on the right side. The lesion is usually thrombosis of the arteries, less often a meningo-encephalitis. The aphasia usually disappears.

Aphasia, apart from hemiplegia, occurs rarely and usually in children. The prognosis is good.

True *tetany* occurs sometimes, and has been reported in connection with certain epidemics. It may set in during the height of the disease.

Typhoid Psychoses.—There are three groups of cases: first, an initial delirium, which may be serious, and cause the patient to wander away from his home, or he may even become maniacal; secondly, the psychosis associated directly with the pyrexia and the toxæmia; in a few cases this outlasts the disappearance of the fever for months or even years; and, lastly, the asthenic psychosis of convalescence, more common after typhoid than after any other fever. The prognosis is usually good. Edsall has studied the condition in children, finding 69 cases, of which 43 recovered.

There is a distressing post-typhoid neurasthenia, in which for months or even for years the patient is unable to get into harmony with his surroundings.

Special Senses.—*Eye.*—Conjunctivitis, simple or phlyctenular, sometimes with keratitis and iritis, may develop. Panophthalmitis has been reported in one case in association with hæmorrhage (Finlay). Loss of accommodation may occur, usually in the asthenia of convalescence. Oculo-motor paralysis has been seen, due probably to neuritis. Retinal hæmorrhages may occur alone or in association with other hæmorrhagic features. Double optic neuritis has been described in the course of the fever. It may be independent of meningitis. Atrophy may follow, but these complications are excessively rare. Cataract may follow inflammation of the uveal tract. Other rare complications are thrombosis of the orbital veins and orbital hæmorrhage. (See de Schweinitz in Keen's monograph for full consideration of the subject.)

Ear.—Otitis media is not infrequent, 2.5 per cent. in Hengst's collected cases. We have never found the typhoid bacillus in the discharge. Serious results are rare; only one case of mastoid disease occurred in our series. The otitis may set in with a chill and an aggravation of the fever.

Renal System.—*Retention of urine* is an early symptom and may be the cause of abdominal pain. It may recur throughout the attack. *Suppression of urine* is rare. The urine is usually diminished at first, has the ordinary febrile characters, and the pigments are increased. Later in the disease it is more abundant and lighter in color.

Polyuria is not very uncommon. While most common during convalescence, the increase may be sudden in the second week at the height of the fever, as in a case reported by Fussell. The amount of urine depends very much on the fluid taken. Patients treated by what is known as the washing-out method, in which large quantities of water are taken, may pass enormous amounts, 18 or 19 litres. One of my patients passed as much as 23 litres in one day!

The Diazo-reaction of Ehrlich was found in 894 of 1,467 cases. It may be present previous to the occurrence of the rash, and as late as the twenty-second day. The value of the test is lessened by its occurrence in cases of miliary tuberculosis, in malarial fever, and occasionally in the acute diseases associated with high fever. In cases passing large quantities of urine, the diazo-reaction is very feeble or even absent. The urotoxic coefficient in typhoid fever is high and is said to be increased by the tubs.

Bacilluria caused by the typhoid bacilli occurs in about one-third of the cases. The urine may be turbid from their presence and in the test-tube give a peculiar shimmer. There may be millions of bacilli to the cubic millimetre without pyuria or any symptoms of renal or bladder trouble. The routine administration of hexamine diminishes the occurrence of typhoid bacilluria. The bacilli may be present in the urine for years after the attack (see Gwyn, Studies III). Of 51 cases during the session of 1900-1901 in my clinic, Cole found typhoid bacilli in the urine in 16.

The renal complications in typhoid fever may be thus grouped:

(*a*) Febrile albuminuria is common and of no special significance. It was present in 999 of 1,500 cases, 66 per cent. Tube casts were present in 568 cases, 37.8 per cent. *Hæmoglobinuria* occurred in one case.

(*b*) Acute nephritis at the onset or during the height of the disease—the *nephro-typhus* of the Germans, the *fièvre typhoïd à forme rénale* of the French—may set in, masking in many instances the true nature of the malady. After an indisposition of a few days there may be fever, pain in the back, and the passage of a small amount of bloody urine.

(*c*) Nephritis during convalescence is rare, and is usually associated with anæmia and œdema. Chronic nephritis is a most exceptional sequel.

(*d*) The lymphomatous nephritis, described by E. Wagner, and already referred to in the section on morbid anatomy, produces, as a rule, no symptoms.

(*e*) *Pyuria,* a not uncommon complication, may be associated with the typhoid or the colon bacillus, less often with staphylococci. It disappears during convalescence. It is usually due to a simple catarrh of the bladder, rarely to an intense cystitis.

(*f*) *Post-typhoid Pyelitis.*—One or both kidneys may be involved, either at the height of the disease or during convalescence. There may be blood and pus at first, later pus alone, varying in amount. A severe pyelonephritis may follow. The colon bacillus is often the organism present. *Perinephric abscess* is a rare sequel.

Generative System.—*Orchitis* is occasionally met with. Kinnicutt has collected 53 cases in the literature. It is usually associated with a catarrhal urethritis. Induration or atrophy may occur, and more rarely suppuration. It was present in 4 cases in my series. In 1 case double hydrocele developed suddenly on the nineteenth day (Dunlap). *Prostatitis* occurs rarely.

Acute mastitis, which may go on to suppuration, is a rare complication. It was present in 3 cases of my series during the fever and in one late in convalescence.

Osseous System.—Among the most troublesome of the sequelæ are the *bone lesions* which in a few cases occur at the height of the disease or even earlier. A boy was admitted in the second week of an attack of typhoid fever with acute periostitis of the frontal bone and of one rib. Of 237 cases collected by Keen there was periostitis in 110, necrosis in 85, and caries in 13. They are, I am sure, much more frequent than the figures indicate. Six cases came under my notice in the course of a year, and formed the basis of Parsons' paper (Studies II). The legs are chiefly involved. In Keen's series the tibia was affected in 91 cases, the ribs in 40. The typhoid bone lesion is apt to form what the old writers called a cold abscess. Only a few of the cases are acute. Chronicity, indolence, and a remarkable tendency to recurrence are perhaps the three most striking features. A bony node may be left by the typhoid periostitis.

Arthritis was present in 8 cases of my series. Keen has collected 84 cases from the literature. It may be monarticular or polyarticular. One of the most important points relating to it is the frequency with which spontaneous dislocations occur, particularly of the hip.

Typhoid Spine (Gibney).—During the disease but more often during convalescence, the patient complains of pain in the lumbar and sacral regions, perhaps after a slight jar or shock. Stiffness of the back, pain on movement, sometimes radiating, and tenderness on pressure are the chief features, but there are in addition marked nervous manifestations. There is rigidity and fixation of the spine, usually in the lower part. Kyphosis occurs in some cases. The X-ray plates may show definite bony change. There is usually spondylitis or perispondylitis. The duration is weeks or months, but the outlook is good.

The *muscles* may be the seat of the degeneration already referred to, but it rarely causes any symptoms. Hæmorrhage occasionally occurs into the muscles, and late in protracted cases abscesses may follow. Rupture of a muscle, usually the rectus abdominis, may occur, possibly associated with acute hæmorrhagic myositis.

Post-typhoid Septicæmia and Pyæmia.—In very protracted cases there may recur after defervescence a slight fever (100°-101° F.), with sweats, which is possibly septic. In other cases for two or three weeks there are recurring chills, often of great severity. They are usually of no moment in the absence of signs of complication. (See Studies II and III.)

Typhoid pyæmia is not very uncommon. (*a*) Extensive furunculosis may be associated with irregular fever and leucocytosis. (*b*) Following the fever there may be multiple subcutaneous "cold" abscesses, often with a dark, thin bloody pus. A score or more of these may appear in different parts. Pratt has isolated the bacillus in pure culture from the subcutaneous abscesses. (*c*) A crural thrombus may suppurate and cause a widespread pyæmia. (*d*) In rare instances suppuration of the mesenteric glands, of a splenic infarct, a sloughing parotid bubo, a perinephric or perirectal abscess, acute necrosis of the bones, or a multiple suppurative arthritis may cause pyæmia. In other cases following bed-sores or a furunculosis there occurs a general infection with pyogenic organisms with fatal result. In three such cases in our series staphylococci were cultivated from the blood. In one case with many chills late in the disease, and the general condition excellent, typhoid bacilli were cultivated from the blood. The colon bacillus may also be found in blood cultures.

Association of Other Diseases.—Erysipelas is a rare complication, most commonly met with during convalescence. Measles or scarlet fever may develop during the fever or in convalescence. Chicken-pox and noma have been reported in children. Pseudo-membranous inflammations may occur in the pharynx, larynx, or genitals.

Malarial and typhoid fevers may be associated, but a majority of the cases of so-called typho-malarial fever are either remittent malarial fever or true typhoid. It is interesting to note that among 1,500 cases of typhoid fever plasmodia were found in the blood in only 3 cases. (See Lyon, Studies III.) Many of the typhoid fever patients came from malarious regions.

The symptoms of influenza may precede the typhoid fever, or the two diseases may run concurrently. There are cases of chronic influenza which simulate typhoid fever very closely.

Typhoid Fever and Tuberculosis.—(*a*) The diseases may coexist. A person with chronic tuberculosis may contract the fever. Of 105 autopsies in typhoid fever, 7 presented marked tuberculous lesions. Miliary tuberculosis and typhoid fever may occur together. (*b*) Cases of typhoid fever with pulmonary and pleuritic symptoms may suggest tuberculosis at the onset. (*c*) There are five types of tuberculous infection which may simulate typhoid fever: the acute miliary form; tuberculous meningitis; tuberculous peritonitis; the acute toxæmia of certain local lesions; and forms of ordinary pulmonary tuberculosis. And, lastly, pulmonary tuberculosis may follow typhoid. In a large majority of such cases from the onset the disease has been tuberculosis, which has begun with a low fever and features suggestive of typhoid fever.

In epilepsy and in chronic chorea the fits and movements usually cease during an attack, and in typhoid fever in a diabetic subject the sugar may be absent during the height of the disease.

Varieties of Typhoid.—Typhoid fever presents an extremely complex symptomatology. Mary forms have been described, some of which present exaggeration of common symptoms, others modification in the course, others again greater intensity of action of the poison on certain organs. As we have seen, when the nervous system is specially involved, it has been called the cerebrospinal form; when the kidneys are early and severly affected, nephro-typhoid; when the disease begins with pulmonary symptoms, pneumo-typhoid; with pleurisy, pleuro-typhoid; when the disease is charactérized throughout by profuse sweats, the sudoral form of the disease. It is enough to remember that typhoid has no fixed and constant course, that it may set in occasionally with symptoms localized in certain organs, and that many of its symptoms are extremely variable—in one epidemic uniform and text-book-like, in another slight or not met with. This diversified symptomatology has led to many clinical errors, and in the absence of the salutary lessons of morbid anatomy it is not surprising that practitioners have so often been led astray. We may recognize the following varieties:

(*a*) The *mild* and *abortive* forms. Much attention has been paid of late to the milder varieties of typhoid fever—the typhus levissimus of Griesinger. Woodruff, of the United States Army, has called special attention to the great danger of neglecting these mild forms, which are often spoken of as mountain fever and malarial fever, "acclimation," "ground," and "miasmatic" fevers. During the prevalence of an epidemic there may be cases of fever so mild that the patient does not go to bed. The onset may be sudden, particularly in children. The general symptoms are slight, the pulse rate not high, the fever rarely above 102°. Rose spots ars usually present, with splenic enlargement. Diarrhœa is rare. The Widal reaction is present in a majority of the patients. There may be a marked tendency to relapse. While infrequent, characteristic complications and sequelæ may give the first positive clue to the nature of the trouble. J. B. Briggs has studied 44 of these mild cases from my clinic, in which the fever lasted 14 days or less. Rose spots were present in 24, and the Widal reaction in 26. There were three relapses. It can not be too forcibly impressed upon the profession that it is just by these mild cases, to which so little attention is paid, that the disease may be kept up in a community.

(*b*) The *grave* form is usually characterized by high fever and pronounced nervous symptoms. In this category come the very severe cases, setting in with pneumonia and nephritis, and with the very intense gastro-intestinal or cerebro-spinal symptoms.

(*c*) The *latent* or *ambulatory* form of typhoid fever, which is particularly common in hospital practice. The symptoms are usually slight, and the patient scarcely feels ill enough to go to bed. He has languor, perhaps slight diarrhœa, but keeps about and may even attend to his work throughout the entire attack. In other instances delirium sets in. The worst cases of this form are seen in sailors, who keep up and about, though feeling ill and feverish. When brought to the hospital they often have symptoms of a most severe type of the disease. Hæmorrhage or perforation may be the first marked symptom of this ambulatory type. Sir W. Jenner called attention to the dangers of this form, and particularly to the grave prognosis in the case of persons who have travelled far with the disease in progress.

(*d*) Hæmorrhagic Typhoid Fever.—This is excessively rare. Among Ouskow's 6,513 cases there were 4 fatal cases with general hæmorrhagic features. Only three instances were present in our series. Hæmorrhages may be marked from the outset, but more commonly they come on during the course of the disease. The condition is not ncessarily fatal. Several of those reported by Nicholls from the Royal Victoria Hospital, Montreal, recovered. (See Hamburger, Studies III.)

(*e*) An *afebrile* typhoid fever is recognized by authors. Liebermeister says that the cases were not uncommon at Basel. The patients presented lassitude, depression, headache, furred tongue, loss of appetite, slow pulse, and even the spots and enlarged spleen. I have seen the temperature normal on the sixteenth day, while the spots did not come out until later.

TYPHOID FEVER IN CHILDREN.—Griffith collected a series of 325 cases in children under two and a half years; 111 of these were in the first year. Out of a total of 278 cases in which the result was recorded, 142 died. The cases are not very uncommon. The high mortality in Griffith's paper was probably due to the fact that only the more serious cases are reported. The abdominal symptoms are usually mild; fatal hæmorrhage and perforation are rare. Among sequelæ, aphasia, noma, and bone lesions are stated to be more common in children than in adults. Two of our cases were under one year of age.

TYPHOID FEVER IN THE AGED.—After the sixtieth year the disease runs a less favorable course, and the mortality is very high. The fever is not so high, but complications are more common, particularly pneumonia and heart-failure.

TYPHOID FEVER IN PREGNANCY.—Pregnancy affords no immunity against typhoid. In 1,500 of our cases to September 10, 1904, 438 of which were females, there were 6 cases. Goltdammer noted 26 pregnancies in 600 cases of typhoid fever in the female. It is more commonly seen in the first half of pregnancy, The pregnancy is interrupted in about 65 per cent. of the cases, usually in the second week of the disease. In the obstetrical department of the Johns Hopkins Hospital (J. W. Williams) there have been (to January, 1905) three cases of puerperal infection with bacillus typhosus. One case showed a localized lesion of the chorion, from which cultures were obtained (Little).

TYPHOID FEVER IN THE FETUS.—From the recent studies of Fordyce, J. L. Morse, and F. W. Lynch, we may conclude that the typhoid bacillus may pass through the placenta to the child, causing a typhoid septicæmia, without intestinal lesions. Lynch has recently collected 16 such cases. Infection of the fetus does not necessarily follow, but when infected the child dies, either in utero or shortly after birth. The Widal reaction has been obtained with fetal blood. Its presence does not indicate that the child has survived infection in utero, as the agglutinating substances may filter through the placenta. They may also be transmitted to the nursling through the milk, and cause a transient reaction. The reaction could not be obtained with fetal blood from which typhoid bacilli were cultivated (Lynch).

RELAPSE.—Relapses vary in frequency in different epidemics, and, it would appear, in different places. The percentages of different authors range from 3 per cent. to 15 or 18 per cent. (Immermann). In 1,500 cases there were 172 relapses, 11.4 per cent. Among 28,057 collected cases 8.8 per cent. had a relapse (McCrae).

We may recognize the ordinary, the intercurrent, and the spurious relapse.

The *ordinary relapse* sets in after complete defervescence. The average duration of the interval in Irvine's cases was a little over five days.

In one of my cases there was complete apyrexia for twenty-three days, followed by a relapse of forty-one days' duration; then apyrexia for forty-two days, followed by a second relapse of two weeks' duration. As a rule, two of the three important symptoms—step-like temperature at onset, roseola, an enlarged spleen—should be present to justify the diagnosis of a relapse. The intestinal symptoms are variable. The onset may be abruptly with a chill, or the temperature may have a typical ascent, as shown in Chart I. The number of relapses ranges from 1 to 5. In a case at the Pennsylvania Hospital in 1904 the disease lasted eleven months and four days, during which there were six relapses. The relapse is usually less severe, of shorter duration and the mortality is low.

The *intercurrent relapse* is common, often most severe, and is responsible for a great many of the most protracted cases. The temperature drops and the patient improves; but after remaining between 100° and 102° for a few days, the fever again rises and the patient enters upon another attack, which may be more protracted, and of much greater intensity than the original one.

Spurious relapses are very common. They have already been mentioned as post-typhoid elevations of temperature. They are recrudescences of the fever due to a number of causes. It is not always easy to determine whether a relapse is present, particularly in cases in which the fever persists for only five or seven days without rose-spots and without enlargement of the spleen.

Undoubtedly a reinfection from within, yet of the conditions favoring the occurrence of relapse we as yet know little. Durham has advanced an interesting theory: Every typhoid infection is a complex phenomenon caused by groups of bacilli alike in species but not identical, as shown by their serum reactions. The antibodies formed in the blood during the primary attack neutralizes only one (or several) groups, the remaining groups still preserving their pathogenic power. Following an error in diet, or some indiscretion, these latter groups may multiply sufficiently to cause a reinfection. Multiple relapses may be similarly explained.

Diagnosis.—There are several points to note. In the first place, typhoid fever is the most common of all continued fevers. Secondly, it is extraordinarily variable in its manifestations. Thirdly, there is no such hybrid malady as typho-malarial fever. Fourthly, errors in diagnosis are inevitable, even under the most favorable conditions.

Data for Diagnosis.—(*a*) *General.*—No single symptom or feature is characteristic. The onset is often suggestive, particularly the occurrence of epistaxis, and (if seen from the start) the ascending fever. The steadiness of the fever for a week or longer after reaching the fastigium is an important point. The irregular remittent character in the third week, and the intermittent features with chills, are common sources of error. While there is nothing characteristic in the pulse, dicrotism is so much more common early in typhoid fever that its presence is always suggestive. The rash is the most valuable single sign, and with the fever usually clinches the diagnosis. The enlarged spleen is of less importance, since it occurs in all febrile conditions, but with the fever and the rash it completes a diagnostic triad. The absence of leucocytosis and the presence of Ehrlich's reaction are valuable accessory signs.

(*b*) *Specific.*—(1) *Isolation of Typhoid Bacilli from the Blood.*—New methods have given better results in this procedure, which is especially useful early in the disease, in doubtful cases and in the acute septic forms. The hypodermic puncture of a vein for the blood causes little or no pain.

(2) *Isolation of Typhoid Bacilli from the Stools.*—Cultures from the stools have proved of diagnostic value. A satisfactory method is that of von Drigalski and Conradi (Zeit. f. Hygiene, Bd. 39), largely used in the campaign against typhoid in Germany, with which those familiar with bacteriologic methods are able to isolate the bacilli in a majority of the cases.

(3) *Isolation of Typhoid Bacilli from the Urine.*—Neumann, Horton-Smith, Richardson, and Gwyn have shown the great frequency of typhoid bacilli in the urine. In some cases they may be obtained before the Widal test is positive. Routine cultures do not offer great difficulties, and may frequently be of diagnostic value.

(4) *Isolation of Typhoid Bacilli from the Rose-spots.*—Neufeld, Cursch-

mann, and Richardson have demonstrated the presence of the bacilli in rose-spots in 32 of 40 cases examined. As the procedure causes considerable discomfort it can not be used as a routine method.

(5) *The Agglutination Test.*—In 1894 Pfeiffer showed that cholera spirilla, when introduced into the peritoneum of an immunized animal, or when mixed with the serum of immunized animals, lose their motion and break up. This "Pfeiffer's phenomenon" was thoroughly studied by Durham and the specificity of the reaction demonstrated. A. S. Grünbaum and Widal made the method available in clinical work.

Macroscopic Method.—This may be done with living or dead organisms and has the advantage of use away from a laboratory. The diluted serum and organisms are mixed in a tube of small calibre (dilution 1 to 50 or 1 to 100). With a positive reaction there should be complete precipitation leaving a clear fluid above in twenty-four hours.

Microscopic Method.—The serum is mixed with a young bouillon culture of the typhoid bacillus, or with a suspension of a young agar culture, in such a manner as to dilute the serum to the required degree. A hanging-drop preparation of the mixture is made, and if the reaction is positive the bacilli will within a given time lose their motility and collect in clumps. With Dreyer's method of standard cultures of constant and known sensitiveness it is possible to follow the patient's serum changes in typhoid or paratyphoid infection.

Whatever be the infection the agglutination for that bacillus will show (*a*) a marked rise in an early stage and (*b*) a marked fall later in the infection. If the patient's serum already contains agglutinins for one or more of the bacilli (owing to inoculation), the following phenomena will be noted (*a*) there is no change in the inoculation agglutinins or (*b*) a slight rise occurs, followed by a slight fall—an alteration which may be caused by a number of non-specific stimuli.

A well marked rise or fall of the titre is the only positive evidence of active infection that can be obtained with the agglutination test and is probably the best evidence afforded by any test except a successful blood culture.

On the whole the serum reaction is of great value, in spite of certain difficulties and objections, and with the newer methods the reactions of equal importance in inoculated and uninoculated persons and in the paratyphoids.

(6) *Ophthalmo-Reaction.*—A solution of one-third to one-half of a milligram of "typho-protein" derived from many different strains of typhoid bacilli is instilled into the conjunctival sac. A typical reaction is marked by deep congestion of the conjunctiva of the lower lid and the caruncle. It reaches its maximum in six hours. A positive reaction is obtained most often during the febrile period, frequently before the agglutination reaction is given. The simplicity of the method and the absence of discomfort are valuable features. A cutaneous method has also been employed.

Common Sources of Error in Diagnosis.—An early and intense localization of the infection in certain organs may give rise to doubt at first.

Cases coming on with severe headache, photophobia, delirium, twitching of the muscles and retraction of the head are almost invariably regarded as *cerebro-spinal meningitis.* Under such circumstances it may for a few days be impossible to make a satisfactory diagnosis. I have thrice performed autopsies on cases of this kind in which no suspicion of typhoid fever had been present, the intense cerebro-spinal manifestations having dominated the scene. Until the appearance of abdominal symptoms, or the rash, it may be quite impossible to determine the nature of the case. Cerebro-spinal meningitis is, however, a rare disease; typhoid fever a very common one, and the onset with severe nervous symptoms is by no means infrequent. The lumbar puncture is now a great help.

I have already spoken of the misleading pulmonary symptoms, which occasionally occur at the very outset of the disease. The bronchitis rarely causes error, though it may be intense and attract the chief attention. More difficult are the cases setting in with chill and followed rapidly by *pneumonia.* I have brought such a case before the class one week as typical pneumonia, and a fortnight later shown the same case as undoubtedly one of typhoid fever. There is less danger of mistaking the pneumonia which occurs at the height of the disease, and yet this is possible, as in a case admitted a few years ago to my wards—a man aged seventy, insensible, with a dry tongue, tremor, ecchymoses upon the wrists and ankles, no rose-spots, enlargement of the spleen, and consolidation of his right lower lobe. It was very natural, particularly since there was no history, to regard such a case as senile pneumonia with profound constitutional disturbance, but the autopsy showed the characteristic lesions of typhoid fever. Early involvement of the pleura or the kidneys may for a time obscure the diagnosis.

Of diseases with which typhoid fever may be confounded, malaria, certain forms of pyæmia, acute tuberculosis, and tuberculous peritonitis are the most important.

From *malarial fever,* typhoid is, as a rule, readily recognized. There is no such disease as typho-malarial fever—that is, a separate and distinct malady. Typhoid fever and malarial fever may coexist in the same patient. In patients returning from Cuba and Porto Rico during the late war the two conditions were often found together, but in the United States it is excessively rare. The term typho-malarial fever should be abandoned. The autumnal type of malarial fever may present a striking similarity in its early days to typhoid fever. Differentiation may be made only by the blood examination. There may be no chills, the remissions may be extremely slight, there is a history perhaps of *malaise,* weakness, diarrhœa, and sometimes vomiting. The tongue is furred and white, the cheeks flushed, the spleen slightly enlarged, and the temperature continuous, or with very slight remissions. The æstivo-autumnal variety of the malarial parasite may not be present in the circulating blood for several days. Every year in Baltimore we had one or two cases in which the diagnosis was in doubt for a few days.

Pyæmia.—The long-continued fever of obscure, deep-seated suppuration, without chills or sweats, may simulate typhoid. The more chronic cases of ulcerative endocarditis are usually diagnosed typhoid fever. The presence or absence of leucocytosis is an important aid. The Widal reaction and the blood cultures now offer additional and valuable help.

Acute miliary tuberculosis is not infrequently mistaken for typhoid fever. The points in differential diagnosis will be discussed under that disease.

Tuberculous peritonitis in certain of its forms may closely simulate typhoid fever, and will be referred to in another section.

The early abdominal pain, etc., may lead to the diagnosis of appendicitis.

The "disease" described by Brill (a mild form of typhus fever) may be regarded as typhoid fever, but the character of the rash, the absence of the agglutination reaction, negative results of blood cultures and the course are against this. However, the majority of cases are probably diagnosed as typhoid fever.

Prognosis.—(*a*) DEATH-RATE.—The mortality is very variable, ranging in private practice from 5 to 12 and in hospital practice from 7 to 20 per cent. In some large epidemics the death-rate has been very low. In the Maidstone epidemic it was between 7 and 8 per cent. In recent years the mortality from typhoid fever has certainly diminished, and, under the influence of Brand, the reintroduction of hydrotherapy has reduced the death-rate in institutions in a remarkable manner, even as low as 5 or 6 per cent. Of the 1,500 cases treated in my wards, 9.1 per cent died. The mortality in the Spanish-American War was very low—7 per cent.—and may be attributed to the picked set of men and to the care and attention which the patients received.

(*b*) SPECIAL FEATURES IN PROGNOSIS.—Unfavorable symptoms are high fever, toxic symptoms with delirium, meteorism, and hæmorrhage. Perforation renders the outlook hopeless unless operation is done early. Fat subjects stand typhoid fever badly. The mortality in women is greater than in men. The complications and dangers are more serious in the ambulatory form in which the patient has kept about for a week or ten days. Early involvement of the nervous system is a bad indication; and the low, muttering delirium with tremor means a close fight for life. Prognostic signs from the fever alone are deceptive. A temperature above 104° may be well borne for many days if the nervous system is not involved.

(*c*) SUDDEN DEATH.—It is difficult in many cases to explain this most lamentable of accidents in the disease. There are cases in which neither cerebral, renal, nor cardiac changes have been found; there are instances too in which it does not seem likely that there could have been a special localization of the toxins in the pneumogastric centres. McPhedran, in reporting a case of the kind, in which the post-mortem showed no adequate cause of death, suggests that the experiments of McWilliam on sudden cardiac failure probably explain the occurrence of death in certain of the cases in which neither embolism nor uræmia is present. Under conditions of abnormal nutrition there is sometimes induced a state of *delirium cordis,* which may occur spontaneously, or, in the case of animals, on slight irritation of the heart, with the result of extreme irregularity and finally failure of action. Sudden death occurs more frequently in men than in women, according to Dewèvre's statistics, in a proportion of 114 to 26. It may occur at the height of the fever, and, as pointed out by Graves, may also happen during convalescence. There were four cases in my series.

Prophylaxis.—In cities the prevalence of typhoid fever is directly proportionate to the inefficiency of the drainage and the water-supply. With their improvement the mortality has been reduced one-half or even more. Fulton has shown that in the United States, at least, the disease exists to a proportionately greater extent in the country than it does in the city, and that the propagation of this disease is in general from the country to the town. In the water-supply of the latter the chances for dilution of the contaminating fluids are so much greater than in the country, where the privy vault is often in such close proximity to the well.

But it is not only through water that the disease is transmitted. Other methods play an important though not so frequent rôle. The bacilli may be carried by milk, oysters, uncooked vegetables, etc. Flies play an important part in the spread of the disease. Many cases undoubtedly arise by direct infection. But through whatever channel the infection occurs, for new cases to arise the virus must be obtained from another patient. It has been demonstrated by Jordan, Russell, Zeit and others that under ordinary circumstances the bacilli do not live and thrive long outside the body. To stamp out typhoid fever requires (1) *the recognition of all cases, including the typhoid carriers* and (2) *the destruction of all typhoid bacilli as they leave the patient.* It is as much a part of the physician's duty to look after these points as to take care of the patient. Mild cases of fever are to be regarded with suspicion.

From the standpoint of prophylaxis, the question practically narrows down to disinfection of the urine, stools, sputum (in the few cases where bacilli are present), and of objects which may accidentally be contaminated by these excretions. The nurse or attendant should be taught to regard every specimen of urine as a pure culture of typhoid bacilli, and to exercise the greatest care in preventing the scattering of drops of urine over the patient, bedding or floor, or over the hands of the attendant.

To disinfect the urine the best solutions are carbolic acid, 1-20, in an amount equal to that of the urine, or bichloride of mercury, 1-1,000, in an amount one-fifteenth that of the fluid to be sterilized. These mixtures with the urine should stand at least two hours. Hexamine causes disappearance of the bacilli from the urine when bacilluria is present, but under no circumstances should its administration permit the disinfection of the urine to be neglected.

For the stools, heat is the most efficient means and can be employed in hospitals by special hoppers in which steam is used. Of solutions, carbolic acid or freshly prepared milk of lime is most useful. The stool should be mixed with at least thrice its volume of these solutions and allowed to stand for several hours.

With hydrotherapy the disinfection of the bath water offers a somewhat difficult problem. E. Babucke found chloride of lime the best substance to use, and that even when the water contains coarse fæcal matter, 250 gm. (one-half pound) of chloride of lime will render the ordinary bath of 200 litres sterile in one-half hour.

If there be any expectoration, the sputum should receive the same care as in tuberculosis. It is best to collect it in small cloths, which may be burned.

All the linen leaving the patient's bed or person should be soaked for two hours in 1-20 carbolic acid solution or 1-2000 bichloride solution, and then sent to the laundry, where it should be boiled. All dishes should be boiled before leaving the patient's room.

The nurse should wear a rubber apron when giving tubs or working over a typhoid patient, and this should be washed frequently with a carbolic acid or bichloride of mercury solution. The nurse should wear rubber gloves when giving tubs, or else soak her hands throughly in 1-1,000 bichloride solution after she has finished.

It is impossible here to deal with all the possible modes of spread of the infection. Keeping in mind that everything leaving the patient should be sterilized whenever there is a chance of its having been contaminated by the discharges, a nurse of ordinary intelligence, even one of the family, can carry out very satisfactory prophylaxis.

Should the typhoid fever patient be isolated? To prevent direct infection of other members of the family a moderate degree of isolation should be carried out, though this need not be absolute as in the exanthemata. The windows should have fly screens in summer. After recovery the room should be disinfected.

An important question is as to the necessity for the isolation of typhoid patients in special wards in hospitals. At present this is not generally done in the United States. When, however, in a hospital with as good sanitary arrangements as the Johns Hopkins possesses, and in which all possible precautions are taken to prevent the infection spreading from patient to patient, 1.81 per cent. of all the cases have been of hospital origin, the advisability of isolation of typhoid fever patients is certainly worth considering. On the other hand, in the general hospital, with students in the wards, the cases are more thoroughly studied, and in the graver complications, as perforation, it is of the greatest advantage to have the early co-operation of the house surgeon.

During the past few years an active campaign has been started in Germany with the object of ultimately stamping out this disease by means of early diagnosis and the institution of rigid measures for preventing the distribution of the infecting agent from the patients so diagnosed. With a corps of assistants Koch fitted up a laboratory in Trier, a locality where the disease had a firm hold. By bacteriological methods he was able to demonstrate that 72 persons were suffering from typhoid infection. So soon as the nature of a case was established, isolation and vigorous disinfection were practiced. The result was that within three months no more typhoid bacilli were discoverable, the patients were cured, no fresh cases arose, and, so far as that group of villages was concerned, typhoid was exterminated.

When epidemics are prevalent the drinking-water and the milk used in families should be boiled. Travellers should drink light wines or mineral water rather than ordinary water or milk. Care should be taken to thoroughly cook oysters which have been fattened or freshened in streams contaminated with sewage.

While in camps it is easy to boil and filter the water, with troops on the march it is a very different matter, and it is impossible to restrain men from relieving their thirst the moment they reach water. Various chemical methods have been recommended of which chlorination (the use of calcium hypochlorite, 5 to 15 pounds for each million gallons of water) has proved the most satisfactory.

Anti-typhoid Inoculation.—Introduced by Wright the method has proved of inestimable value in the United States Army, in India and during the present war. The material used is a bouillon or agar culture of bacilli heated to a temperature of 53° to 55° C. in order to kill them. Lysol or tricresol may be added. Three inoculations are given at intervals of ten days.

A triple vaccine against typhoid and paratyphoid A and B is now prepared and should be used. Untoward results are rare. Of 31,000 inoculated at the Valcartier camp, Quebec, only one had a local abscess and there were no serious sequels. The inoculation fever begins in from four to six hours and may reach 101° or even 103° to 104°. Headache, chilliness, pains in the back and limbs, and vomiting may occur. In many there is only a transient indisposition. More severe symptoms may occur, such as arthritis, fugitive erythema, diarrhœa, abdominal pains, septicæmia, with pneumonia, pleurisy and pericarditis. In a few cases a fever resembling typhoid has followed. I was not able to find a fatality due directly to the inoculation. A light diet, avoidance of stimulants and rest lessen the possibility of serious sequels. The evidence so far points to a persistence of the protective effect for at least two years after inoculation.

Treatment.—(*a*) General Management.—The profession was long in learning that typhoid fever is not a disease to be treated mainly with drugs. Careful nursing and a regulated diet are the essentials in a majority of the cases. The patient should be in a well-ventilated room (or in summer out of doors during the day), strictly confined to bed from the outset, and there remain until convalescence is well established. The bed should be single, not too high, and the mattress should not be too hard. The woven wire bed, with soft hair mattress, upon which are two folds of blanket, combines the two great qualities of a sick-bed, smoothness and elasticity. A rubber cloth should be placed under the sheet. An intelligent nurse should be in charge. When this is impossible, the attending physician should write out specific instructions regarding diet and treatment of the discharges and bed-linen.

(*b*) Diet.—More liberality in diet is now generally practiced, as was advised years ago by Austin Flint and strongly supported by Shattuck, Kinnicutt and others. The patient should be nourished as well as possible and food given with a value of 2,500 to 3,000 calories and containing about 70 grams of protein if conditions permit. The bulk of the food should be liquid and milk or its modifications form the largest part. Milk in any form, cream, ice cream, cocoa, tea or coffee with cream, strained soups, eggs, either the white or the whole egg, raw or soft boiled, gruels and jellies may be given. The milk may be boiled or diluted, or some modification given—peptonised milk, fermented milk, malted milk, buttermilk or whey. Soft food is often permissible, such as milk toast, custard, junket, crackers and milk, bread and butter, and mashed potatoes. It is important to give carbohydrate freely to spare the body proteins, and this is aided by the addition of milk sugar to the diet; a teaspoonful can be given with each feeding of milk. Sugar can also be given freely in lemonade. The food should be chosen for each patient and a routine diet not allowed. In case of digestive disturbance—undigested food in the stools, diarrhœa, meteorism—the diet should be made very simple, buttermilk, whey, peptonised milk or albumin water usually being suitable. The beef extracts, meat juices, and artificially prepared foods are unnecessary, and in private practice among people in moderate circumstances add greatly to the expense of the illness. Water should be given freely at fixed intervals. A good plan is to have a jug of water beside the patient and tubing with a glass mouth-piece, so that he can drink as much as he wishes. It is desirable to have the patient take at least four litres of water daily and larger amounts are an advantage. The water causes polyuria, and is a sort of internal hydrotherapy by which the toxins may be washed out. Barley water, lemonade, soda water, or iced-tea may be used.

Special care must be given to the mouth, which should be cleaned after each feeding. A mouth wash should be used freely (such as carbolic acid ʒ i, 4 c. c., glycerine ℥ i, 30 c. c., and boric acid, saturated solution, to ℥ x, 300 c. c.).

Alcohol is unnecessary in a great majority of the cases. Of late years I have used it much less freely; but when the heart is feeble and the toxic symptoms are severe, eight to twelve ounces of whisky may be given in the twenty-four hours.

(*c*) Hydrotherapy.—The use of water, inside and outside, was no new treatment in fevers at the end of the eighteenth century, when James Currie (a friend of Burns and the editor of his poems) wrote his Medical Reports on the Effects of Water, Cold and Warm, as a Remedy in Fevers and other Diseases. In this country it was used with great effect and recommended strongly by Nathan Smith, of Yale. Since 1861 the value of bathing in fevers has been specially emphasized by the late Dr. Brand, of Stettin.

Hydrotherapy may be carried out in several different ways, of which, in typhoid fever, the most satisfactory are sponging, the wet pack, and the full bath.

(1) *Cold Sponging.*—The water may be tepid, cold, or ice-cold, according to the height of the fever. A thorough sponge-bath should take from fifteen to twenty minutes. The ice-cold sponging is not quite as formidable as the full bath, for which, when there is an insuperable objection in private practice, it is an excellent alternative. But frequently it is difficult to get the friends to appreciate the advantages of the sponging. When such is the case, and in children and delicate persons, it can be made a little less formidable by sponging limb by limb and then the back and abdomen.

(2) The *cold pack* is not so generally useful in typhoid fever, but in cases with very pronounced nervous symptoms, if the tub is not available, the patient may be wrapped in a sheet wrung out of water at 60° or 65°, and then cold water sprinkled over him with an ordinary watering-pot.

(3) *The Bath.*—The tub should be long enough so that the patient can be completely covered except his head. Our rule for some years has been to give a bath every third hour when the temperature was above 102.5°. The patient remains in the tub for fifteen or twenty minutes, is taken out, wrapped in a dry sheet, and covered with a blanket. While in the tub the limbs and trunk are rubbed thoroughly, either with the hand or with a suitable rubber. It is well to give the first one or two baths at a temperature of 80° to 85°. There is no routine temperature and that between 70° and 85° which suits best is chosen. It is important to see that the canvas supports are properly arranged, and that the rubber pillow is comfortable for the patient's head. The first bath should not be given at night, and it should be superintended by the physician. The amount of complaint made by the patient is largely dependent upon the skill and care with which the baths are given. Food is usually given, sometimes a stimulant, after the bath. The blueness and shiv-

ering, which often follow the bath, are not serious features. The rectal temperature is taken immediately after the bath, and again three-quarters of an hour later. Contra-indications are peritonitis, hæmorrhage, phlebitis, severe abdominal pain, and great prostration.

The good effects of the baths are: (i) The influence on the nervous system; delirium lessens, tremor diminishes and toxic features are less marked. (ii) Increased excretion of toxins by the kidney. (iii) The tonic effect on the circulation; the heart rate falls, the pulse becomes smaller and harder, and the blood pressure rises. Vaso-motor paresis is lessened. (iv) With hydrotherapy the initial bronchitis is benefitted, and there is less chance of passive congestion of the bases of the lungs. (v) The liability to bed-sores is diminished and the frequent cleansing of the skin is beneficial. The addition of half a pound of alum to the water is an advantage. Should boils occur, one bath-tub should be used for that patient alone. (vi) Reduction of the temperature may occur but is not an important effect. (vii) The mortality is reduced. In general hospitals from six to eight patients in every hundred are saved by this plan of treatment. At the Brisbane Hospital, where F. E. Hare used it so thoroughly, the mortality was reduced from 14.8 per cent. to 7.5. There is a remarkable uniformity in the death-rate of institutions using the method—usually from 6 to 8 per cent.

(*d*) Medicinal Treatment.—There is no specific drug treatment, but it is usually advisable to give hexamine after the second week, twenty to thirty grains (1.3 to 2 gm.) daily. In private practice it may be safer, for the young practitioner especially, to order an acid or a mild fever mixture. The question of medicinal antipyretics is important: they are used far too often and too rashly in typhoid fever. An occasional dose of antifebrin or antipyrin may do no harm, but the daily use of these drugs is most injurious. Quinine in moderate doses is still much employed, but its value is doubtful. In the various antiseptic drugs which have been advised I have no faith. Most of them do no harm, except that in private practice their use has too often diverted the practitioner from more rational and safer courses.

(*e*) Vaccine and Serum Therapy.—Treatment by vaccines during the height of the disease is still in an experimental stage. Various forms of vaccines are used and given subcutaneously or intravenously. Doses varying from 50 to 500 million bacilli are given, usually three or four days apart. As patients react very differently, the smaller doses are safer at first, especially if given intravenously. In long-continued attacks when progress is slow, for complications due to the presence of typhoid bacilli in organs or tissues, and for carriers vaccine therapy is helpful. No serum of proved value has been obtained.

(*f*) Treatment of Special Symptoms.—For severe *toxæmia* water should be given freely by mouth if possible, otherwise by the bowel or by infusion. Hydrotherapy should be used actively, best by tub baths. Whisky is generally indicated, four to ten ounces being given in the twenty-four hours. For headache and delirium an ice-bag or cold compresses should be kept to the head. If the patient is very delirious and restless a dose of morphia hypodermically is the best treatment. Lumbar puncture is also useful, the fluid being allowed to run as long as it flows under pressure. Every delirious patient should be constantly watched. It is important to secure sleep in the case of these patients, for which morphia is most reliable. Hydrotherapy, internal and external, is our greatest aid in the treatment of the nervous conditions. The abdominal *pain* and *tympanites* are best treated with fomentations or turpentine stupes. The latter, if well applied, give great relief. Sir William Jenner used to lay great stress on the advantages of a well-applied turpentine stupe. He directed it to be applied as follows: A flannel roller was placed beneath the patient, and then a double layer of thin flannel, wrung out of very hot water, with a drachm of turpentine mixed with the water, was applied to the abdomen and covered with the ends of the roller. When the stomach is greatly distended the passage of a stomach tube gives relief. When the gas is in the large bowel, a tube may be passed or a turpentine enema given. For tympanites, with a dry tongue, turpentine may be given, ♏ xv (1 c. c.) every three hours, or the oil of cinnamon, ♏ iii-v, every two hours (Caiger). If whey and albumen-water are substituted for milk, the distension lessens. Charcoal, bismuth, β-naphthol, and eserine, $\frac{1}{60}$ gr. hypodermically, may be tried. Opium should not be given.

For the *diarrhœa,* if severe—that is, if there are more than three or four stools daily—a starch and opium enema may be given; or, by the mouth, a combination of bismuth, in large doses, with Dover's powder; or the acid diarrhœa mixture, acetate of lead (gr. ii), dilute acetic acid (♏ xv-xx), and acetate of morphia (gr. $\frac{1}{6}$–$\frac{1}{8}$). The amount of food should be reduced, and whey and albumen-water in small amounts be substituted for the milk. An ice-bag or cold compresses relieve the soreness which sometimes accompanies the diarrhœa.

Constipation is present in many cases, and though I have never seen it do harm, yet it is well every second day to give an ordinary enema. The addition of turpentine (℥ ss, 15 c. c.) is advisable if there is meteorism.

Hæmorrhage.—As absolute rest is essential, the greatest care should be taken in the use of the bed-pan. It is perhaps better to allow the patient to pass the motions into a large pad. Ice may be given, and a light ice-bag placed on the abdomen. The amount of food should be restricted for eight or ten hours. If there is a tendency to collapse, stimulants should be given, and, if necessary, hypodermic injections of camphor. Injection of salt solution beneath the skin or directly into a vein may revive a failing heart, but should only be done in case of emergency. Turpentine is warmly recommended by certain authors. Should opium be given? One-fifth of the cases of perforation occur with hæmorrhage, and the opium may obscure the features upon which alone the diagnosis of perforation may be made. Opium increases any tendency to tympanites. We have abandoned the use of opium and have given calcium lactate in doses of gr. xv (1 gm.) every four hours. The injection of blood serum is sometimes of value.

Perforation and Peritonitis.—Early diagnosis and early operation mean the saving of one-third of the cases of this heretofore uniformly fatal complication. The aim should be to operate for the perforation, and not to wait until a general peritonitis diminishes by one-half the chances of recovery. An incessant, intelligent watchfulness on the part of the medical attendant and the early co-operation of the surgeon are essentials. Every case of more than ordinary severity should be watched with special reference to this complication. Thorough preparation by early observation, careful notes, and knowledge of the conditions will help to prevent needless exploration. No case is too desperate; we have had one recovery after three operations. Twenty cases of perforation in my series were operated upon with seven recoveries; in an eighth case the patient died of the toxæmia on the eighth day after the laparotomy. In doubtful cases it is best to operate, as experience shows that patients stand an exploration very well.

Cholecystitis.—A majority of the cases recover, but if the symptoms are very severe and progressive, operation should be advised. For chronic cholecystitis hexamine should be given in large doses and the vaccine treatment employed.

With signs of failure of the *circulation*, hydrotherapy should be carried on actively and strychnine given hypodermically (gr. $\frac{1}{60}$ to $\frac{1}{20}$, 0.001 to 0.003 gm.) every three hours. Saline infusions (500 c. c.) are useful especially if the patient is not taking much water by mouth. Alcohol is generally of value. Digitalis may be given as the tincture (mxv, 1 c. c.) or digitaline (gr. $\frac{1}{30}$, 0.002 gm.) intramuscularly. For collapse, camphor (gr. ii, 0.13 gm.) or ether hypodermically should be given. The bath treatment is the best preventive of circulatory failure. For *phlebitis* the limb should be kept absolutely at rest and wrapped in raw cotton. The application of a sedative lotion may relieve pain.

Bacilluria.—When bacilli are present, as demonstrated by cultures or shown by the microscope, hexamine may be given in ten-grain doses and kept up, if necessary, for several weeks. A patient should not be discharged with bacilli in his urine.

For *orchitis, mastitis, parotitis,* etc., an ice-bag should be applied. Incision and drainage are advisable on the first signs of suppuration.

In protracted cases very special care should be taken to guard against *bed-sores.* Absolute cleanliness and careful drying of the parts after an evacuation should be enjoined. Pressure should be avoided by the use of rubber rings. The patient should be turned from side to side and propped with pillows, and the back can then be sponged with alcohol.

Bone Lesions.—The use of a typhoid vaccine is well worthy of trial. Typhoid periostitis does not always go on to suppuration, though, as a rule, it requires operation. This should be done very thoroughly and the diseased parts completely removed, as otherwise recurrence is inevitable. For *typhoid spine* fixation by a plaster jacket or some form of apparatus is advisable. Trauma should be guarded against. In the milder cases active counter-irritation is useful. If pain is severe, large doses of sedatives are necessary.

(*g*) The Management of Convalescence.—Convalescents from typhoid fever frequently cause greater anxiety than patients in the attack. The question of food has to be met at once, as the patient acquires a ravenous appetite and clamors for a fuller diet. My custom has been not to allow solid food until the temperature has been normal for ten days. This is, I think, a safe rule, leaning perhaps to the side of extreme caution; but, after all, with the many soft foods, the patient can take a fairly varied diet. Many leading practitioners allow solid food to a patient so soon as he desires it. I had a lesson in this matter which I have never forgotten. A young lad in the Montreal General Hospital, in whose case I was much interested, passed through a tolerably sharp attack of typhoid fever. Two weeks after the evening temperature had been normal, and only a day or two before his intended discharge he ate several mutton chops, and within twenty-four hours was in a state of collapse from perforation. A small transverse rent was found at the bottom of an ulcer which was in process of healing. It is not easy to say why solid food, particularly meats, should disagree, but in so many instances an indiscretion in diet is followed by slight fever, the so-called *febris carnis*, that it is in the best interests of the patient to restrict the diet for some time after the fever has fallen. Whether an error in diet may cause relapse is doubtful. The patient may be allowed to sit up for a short time about the end of the first week of convalescence, and the period may be prolonged with a gradual return of strength. He should move about slowly, and when the weather is favorable should be in the open air as much as possible. He should be guarded at this period against all unnecessary excitement. Emotional disturbance not infrequently is the cause of recrudescence of the fever. Constipation is not uncommon in convalescence and is best treated by enemata. A protracted diarrhœa, which is usually due to ulceration in the colon, may retard recovery. In such cases the diet should be restricted to milk and the patient confined to bed; large doses of bismuth and astringent injections will prove useful. The recrudescence of the fever does not require special measures. The treatment of the relapse is essentially that of the original attack.

Post-typhoid insanity requires the judicious care of an expert. The cases usually recover. The swollen leg after phlebitis is a source of great worry. A bandage or a well-fitting elastic stocking should be worn during the day. The outlook depends on the completeness with which the collateral circulation is established. In a good many cases there is permanent disability.

The *post-typhoid neuritis*, a cause of much alarm and distress, usually gets well, though it may take months, or even a couple of years, before the paralysis disappears. After the subsidence of the acute symptoms systematic massage of the paralyzed and atrophic muscles is the most satisfactory treatment.

Typhoid Carriers.—Treatment of these is difficult. Hexamine should be given persistently and in large doses. Drainage of the gall bladder and X-ray exposures over it have been successful in some cases. The employment of an autogenous vaccine offers the best chance of success. Doses increasing from 25 to 1,000 or 1,500 million bacilli are given at intervals of 10 days.

Lastly, no patient should be discharged from observation until we are certain that he can not infect others.

II. COLON BACILLUS INFECTIONS

The colon bacillus, or more properly speaking the group of colon bacilli, in their biological and pathological peculiarities are closely related to the organisms of the typhoid group. Normal inhabitants of the intestines, where in all probability they serve a useful function, the *bacillus coli communis* may be taken as the typical member of the group. The ærogenic, the food-poisoning, the paratyphoid and the dysenteric groups must be excluded. There are great difficulties in determining the extent of the lesions caused by this organism, which varies extraordinarily in virulence. To it has been attributed a host of maladies from appendicitis to old age, but more conservative pathologists limit very much its pathogenic scope. It is not easy to separate the effects of the *B. coli* from those of other organisms with which it is so often associated. The needful bacteriological distinction must be considered in connection with agglutination and opsonic tests.

Recognized infections may be classed as follows:

A. General Hæmic Infections.—There are several groups of cases:

(*a*) *Terminal Infections.*—After death the colon bacillus swarms in the body, invading the blood and contaminating all parts. In protracted illnesses, in acute intestinal and peritoneal affections it may be present in the blood some time before death and may be responsible for the terminal fever.

(*b*) Cases running a course resembling typhoid fever. To this group much attention has been paid of late and there are now some 50 cases in the literature (Draper).

(*c*) Cases of general infection with secondary abscesses.

B. Sub-infections.—Adami has suggested that a large number of chronic diseases have their origin in a mild, continuous infection with *B. coli* and he has brought forward evidence to show that such affections as anæmia and cirrhosis of the liver may be due to it. Metchnikoff induced the lesions of early cirrhosis and of arterio-sclerosis by administering the products of the growth of the *B. coli.* The question is under discussion and is far from settled.

C. Local Infections.—Here we are on safer ground and we know of three definite lesions produced by the organism.

(*a*) *Peritonitis.*—In perforation of the bowel, in strangulated hernia, in obstruction in various types of ulcer, the associated peritonitis may be due to *B. coli.*

(*b*) *Cholecystitis* and *cholangitis,* either of the simple catarrhal type or suppurative, may be caused by it.

(*c*) *Infection of the Urinary Tract.*—The bladder and the pelves of the kidneys are chiefly affected. There are three possible channels of infection—by the ureter, the blood stream, and the lymphatics. The first route is probably the common one in women and children; but lymphatic infection from the bowel plays a very important role in a great many of the cases. Bowel troubles have been present, constipation or diarrhœa. It has been shown experimentally that with very slight abrasion of the mucosa of the colon the bacilli may enter the lymphatics. An interesting point is the relative frequency of involvement of the right kidney; Franke states that the cæcum and ascending colon are connected by a train of lymphatics with the right kidney, an anatomical communication not present with the left. Clinically there are three important groups of cases. (1) In children, in whom it seems by no means uncommon. In Jeffrey's study of 60 cases at the Hospital for Sick Children a large proportion occurred in females (53). Death followed in 9 cases. (2) In connection with pregnancy. The cases are common and important and may occur at any time during pregnancy or follow delivery. The pelvis of the right kidney is most often attacked. (3) The group of cases in adults, men and women, in whom, without any obvious cause, and in the majority of cases that I have seen, without any previous intestinal trouble, acute pyelitis or pyelocystitis comes on. The infection is obstinate and very difficult to treat, even with vaccines. An interesting and distressing sequel is a chronic arthritis. In one instance the condition was very similar to that of a gonorrhœal synovitis and periarthritis. The clinical picture presents nothing peculiar. (4) Intestines. To the *bacillus coli* almost all the diseases of the bowels from ulcers of the duodenum to appendicitis have been attributed. Ulcers of the stomach and of the duodenum have been produced by feeding cultures of *B. coli* to dogs, and from the peptic ulcers of very young infants Helmholz has isolated the organism in pure culture. The not infrequent association of appendicitis and peptic ulcer has been attributed to toxins from the appendix and large bowel. There is great difficulty in determining the precise etiological relationship of *B. coli* to the various lesions of the gastro-intestinal tract. (5) Other local infections with which the *colon bacillus* has been associated are acute meningitis, abscess of the brain, endocarditis, and suppuration in various parts. Only in a small proportion of these cases has the association been demonstrated by cultural and biological tests.

III. THE PYOGENIC INFECTIONS

(*Septicœmia, Sapræmia, Pyæmia*)

Definition.—A group of non-specific diseases, induced by a number of micro-organisms, of which the pyogenic cocci are the most important, characterized by fever, chills, leucocytosis, often a profound intoxication and sometimes by foci of suppuration.

A hard-and-fast line can not be drawn between an infection and an intoxication, but agents of infection alone are capable of reproduction, whereas those of intoxication are chemical poisons, some of which are produced by the agency of bacteria, or by vegetable and animal cells. Infectious diseases which are communicated directly from one person to another are termed contagious, and the infecting agent is sometimes spoken of as a contagium. "Whether or not an infectious disease is contagious in the ordinary sense depends upon the nature of the infectious agent, and especially upon the manner of its elimination from and reception by the body. Most but not all contagious diseases are infectious. Scabies is a contagious disease, but it is not infectious" (Welch).

There are three chief clinical types of pyogenic infection:

1. LOCAL INFECTIONS WITH THE DEVELOPMENT OF TOXINS

This is the common mode of invasion of many of the infectious diseases. Tetanus, diphtheria, erysipelas, and pneumonia are diseases which have sites of local infection in which the pathogenic organisms develop; but the constitutional effects are caused by the absorption of the poisonous products. The diphtheria toxin produces all the general symptoms, the tetanus toxin every feature of the disease without the presence of their respective bacilli. Certain of the symptoms following the absorption of the toxins are general to all; others are special and peculiar, according to the organism which produces them. A chill, fever, general malaise, prostration, rapid pulse, restlessness, and headache are the most frequent. With but few exceptions the febrile disturbance is the most common feature. The most serious effects are upon the nervous system and upon the circulation, and the gravity of the symptoms on the part of these organs is to some extent a measure of the intensity of the intoxication. The organisms of certain local infections produce poisons which have special actions; thus, the diphtheria toxin, besides having the effects already referred to, is especially prone to attack the nervous system and to cause peripheral neuritis. The tetanus toxin has a specific action on the motor neurones.

2. SEPTICÆMIA

Formerly, and in a surgical sense, the term "septicæmia" was used to designate the invasion of the blood and tissues of the body by the organisms of suppuration, but in the medical sense the term may be applied to any condition in which, with or without a local site of infection, there is microbic invasion of the blood and tissues, but without metastatic foci of suppuration. Owing to the great development of bacteria in the blood, and in order to separate it sharply from local infectious processes with toxic invasion of the body, it is proposed to call this condition bacteræmia; toxæmia denotes the latter state.

(a) Progressive Septicæmia from Local Infection.—The common streptococcus and staphylococcus infection is, as a rule, first local, and the toxins alone pass into the blood. In other instances the cocci appear in the blood and throughout the tissues, causing a septicæmia which intensifies greatly the severity of the case. Other infections in which the bacterial invasion, local at first, may become general are pneumonia, anthrax, gonorrhœa, and puerperal fever.

The clinical features of this form are well seen in the cases of puerperal septicæmia or in dissection wounds, in which the course of the infection may be traced along the lymphatics. The symptoms usually set in within twenty-four hours, and rarely later than the third or fourth day. There is a chill or chilliness, with moderate fever at first, which gradually rises and is marked by daily remissions and even intermissions. The pulse is small and compressible, and may reach 120 or higher. Gastro-intestinal disturbances are common, the tongue is red at the margin, and the dorsum is dry and dark. There may be early delirium or marked mental prostration and apathy. As the disease progresses there may be pallor of the face or a yellowish tint. Capillary hæmorrhages are not uncommon.

In streptococcus cases we are beginning to recognize the fact that these infections are not always so serious as we thought. Death may occur within twenty-four hours or be delayed for several days, even for weeks, and recovery may occur. One patient showed streptococci in the blood for six weeks, but ultimately recovered (Cole). On post-mortem examination there may be no gross focal lesions in the viscera, and the seat of infection may present only slight changes. The spleen is enlarged and soft, the blood may be extremely dark in color, and hæmorrhages are common, particularly on the serous surfaces. Neither thrombi nor emboli are found. Certain clinical features separate the streptococcus from the staphylococcus infection, chiefly in the absence of delirium, a rather abnormal mental acuteness, and in the presence of a greater degree of anæmia.

Many instances of septicæmia are combined infections; thus, in diphtheria streptococcus septicæmia is a common, and the most serious, event. The local disease and the symptoms produced by absorption of the toxins dominate the clinical picture; but the features are usually much aggravated by the systemic invasion. A similar infection may occur in typhoid fever and in tuberculosis, and may obscure the typical picture. These secondary septicæmias are caused most frequently by the streptococcus, but may result from the invasion of other bacteria.

(b) General Septicæmia without Recognizable Local Infection.—*Cryptogenetic Septicæmias.*—This is a group of very great interest to the physician, the full importance of which we are only now beginning to recognize.

The subjects when attacked may be in perfect health; more commonly they are already weakened by acute or chronic illness. The pathogenic organisms are varied. *Streptococcus pyogenes* is the most common; the forms of staphylococcus more rare. Other occasional causal agents are *Micrococcus lanceolatus* (pneumococcus), *Bacillus proteus, Bacillus pyocyaneus* and *Bacillus influenzæ.* Between May 1, 1892, and June 1, 1895, there were examined in the post-mortem room from my wards 21 cases of general infection, of which 13 were due to *Streptococcus pyogenes,* 2 to *Staphylococcus pyogenes,* and 6 to the pneumococcus. In 19 of these cases the patients were already the subjects of some other malady, which was aggravated, or in most instances terminated, by the general septicæmia. The symptoms vary somewhat with the character of the micro-organisms. In the streptococcus cases there may be chills with high, irregular fever, and a more characteristic *septic* state than in the pneumococcus infection.

These cases come correctly under the term "cryptogenetic septicæmia" as employed by Leube, inasmuch as the local focus of infection is not evident during life and may not be found after death. Although most of these cases are terminal infections, yet it is well to bear in mind that there are instances of this type of affection coming on in apparently healthy persons. The fever may be extremely irregular, characteristically septic, and persist for many weeks. Foci of suppuration may not develop, and may not be found even at autopsy. I have on several occasions met with cases of an intermittent pyrexia persisting for weeks, in which it seemed impossible to give any explanation of the phenomena, and some which ultimately recovered, and in which tuberculosis and malaria could be almost positively excluded. These cases require to be carefully studied bacteriologically. Dreschfeld has described them as idiopathic intermittent fever of pyæmic character. Local symptoms may be absent, though in three of his cases there was enlargement of the liver, and in two the condition was a diffuse suppurative hepatitis. The pyocyanic disease, or cyano-pyæmia, is an extremely interesting form of infection with *Bacillus pyocyaneus,* of which a large number of cases have been reported.

3. SEPTICO-PYÆMIA

The pathogenic micro-organisms which invade the blood and tissues may settle in certain foci and there cause suppuration. When multiple abscesses are thus produced in connection with a general infection, the condition is known as pyæmia or, perhaps better, septico-pyæmia. There are no specific organisms of suppuration, and the condition of pyæmia may be produced by organisms other than the streptococci and staphylococci, though these are the most common. Other forms which may invade the system and cause foci of suppuration are *Micrococcus lanceolatus,* the gonococcus, *Bacillus coli, Bacillus typhosus, Bacillus proteus, Bacillus pyocyaneus, Bacillus influenzæ.* In a large proportion of all cases of pyæmia there is a focus of infection, either a suppurating external wound, an osteomyelitis, a gonorrhœa, an otitis media, an empyema, or an area of suppuration in a lymph-gland or about the appendix. In a large majority of all these cases the common pus cocci are present.

In a suppurating wound, for example, the pus organisms induce hyaline necrosis in the smaller vessels with the production of thrombi and purulent phlebitis. The entrance of pus organisms in small numbers into the blood does not necessarily produce pyæmia. Commonly the transmission to various parts from the local focus takes place by the fragments of thrombi which pass as emboli to different parts, where, if the conditions are favorable, the pus organisms excite suppuration. A thrombus which is not septic or contaminated, when dislodged and impacted in a distant vessel, produces at most only a simple infarction; but, coming from an infected source and containing pus microbes, an independent centre of infection is established wherever the embolus may lodge. These independent suppurative centres in pyæmia, known as *embolic* or *metastatic abscesses,* have the following distribution:

(*a*) In external wounds, in osteo-myelitis, and in acute phlegmon of the skin, the embolic particles very frequently excite suppuration in the lungs, producing the well-known wedge-shaped pyæmic infarcts; from these, or rarely by paradoxical embolism, or direct passage of bacteria or minute emboli through the pulmonary capillaries, metastatic foci of inflammation may occur in other parts.

(*b*) Suppurative foci in the territory of the portal system, particularly in the intestines, produce metastatic abscesses in the liver with or without suppurative pylephlebitis.

Endocarditis is an event which is very liable to occur in all forms of septicæmia, and modifies materially the character of the clinical features. Streptococci and staphylococci are the most common organisms present in the vegetations, but pneumococci, gonoccocci, tubercle bacilli, typhoid bacilli, anthrax bacilli, and other forms have been isolated. The vegetations which grow at the site of the valve lesion become covered with thrombi, particles of which may be dislodged and carried as emboli to different parts of the body, causing multiple abscesses or infarcts.

Symptoms of Septico-pyæmia.—In a case of wound infection, prior to the onset of the characteristic symptoms, there may be signs of local trouble, and in the case of a discharging wound the pus may change in character. The onset of the disease is marked by a severe rigor, during which the temperature rises to 103° or 104° and is followed by a profuse sweat. These chills are repeated at intervals, either daily or every other day. In the intervals there may be slight pyrexia. The constitutional disturbance is marked and there are loss of appetite, nausea, and vomiting, and, as the disease progresses, rapid emaciation. Transient erythema is not uncommon. Local symptoms usually occur. If the lungs become involved there are dyspnœa and cough. The physical signs may be slight. Involvement of the pleura and pericardium is common. The anæmia, often profound, causes great pallor of the skin, which later may be bile-tinged. The spleen is enlarged, and there may be intense pain in the side, pointing to perisplenitis from embolism. Usually in the rapid cases a typhoid state supervenes, and the patient dies comatose.

In the chronic cases the disease may be prolonged for months; the chills recur at long intervals, the temperature is irregular, and the condition of the patient varies from month to month. The course is usually slow and progressively downward.

Diagnosis.—Pyæmia is a disease frequently overlooked and often mistaken for other affections.

Cases following a wound, an operation, or parturition are readily recognized. On the other hand, the following conditions may be overlooked:

Osteo-myelitis.—Here the lesion may be limited, the constitutional symptoms severe, and the course of the disease very rapid. The cause of the trouble may be discovered only post mortem.

So, too, acute septico-pyæmia may follow *gonorrhœa* or a *prostatic abscess.*

Cases are sometimes confounded with *typhoid fever,* particularly the more chronic instances, in which there are diarrhœa, great prostration, delirium, and irregular fever. The spleen, too, is often enlarged. The marked leucocytosis is an important differential point.

In some of the instances of *ulcerative endocarditis* the diagnosis is very difficult, particularly in what is known as the typhoid, in contradistinction to the septic, type of this disease. In *acute miliary tuberculosis* the symptoms occasionally resemble those of septicæmia, more commonly those of typhoid fever.

The *post-febrile arthritides,* such as occur after scarlet fever and gonorrhœa, are really instances of mild septic infection. The joints may sometimes suppurate and pyæmia develop. So, also, in *tuberculosis of the kidneys* and *calculous pyelitis* recurring rigors and sweats due to septic infection are common. In some latitudes septic and pyæmic processes are too often confounded with *malaria.* In early tuberculosis, or even when signs of excavation are present in the lungs, and in cases of suppuration in various parts, particularly empyema and abscess of the liver, the diagnosis of malaria is made. The practitioner may take it as a safe rule, to which he will find very few exceptions, that *an intermittent fever which resists quinine is not malaria.*

Other conditions associated with chills which may be mistaken for pyæmia are profound anæmia, certain cases of Hodgkin's disease, the hepatic intermittent fever associated with the lodgment of gall-stones at the orifice of the common duct, rare cases of essential fever in nervous women, and the intermittent fever sometimes seen in rapidly growing cancer.

Treatment.—(*a*) GENERAL.—Nourishment should be given as liberally as possible. Water should be forced and it is well to give it by the drop method into the bowel and by infusion if there is any difficulty in taking it by mouth. Hydrotherapy by tub baths is useful. Alcohol is generally indicated, and with severe toxæmia should be given in full doses.

(*b*) SURGICAL.—In pyæmia, when the pus is accessible, free evacuation and drainage is often the only treatment required. In a case of empyema with weeks of high and irregular fever the day after operation the temperature may be normal, and remain so. In some cases with a local infection Bier's method of hyperæmia has been used with success, but where the focus of manufacture of the poison is accessible the knife should be used. Unfortunately, in only too many cases the focus of infection is not accessible; it then is a septicæmia, and for such cases the bacteriologists have introduced the treatment with vaccines.

(*c*) Vaccine Treatment.—By blood cultures or by cultures from the focus of infection the organism is isolated, then a vaccine is prepared, and, if Wright's method is followed, the use and dose are regulated by the opsonic index of the patient. "Stock" vaccines may be used, but are not as useful as an autogenous vaccine. In many cases in which the germ cannot be isolated and the condition is one of septic fever the ordinary antistreptococcus serum or one of the polyvalent serums is used. Good results are not infrequently obtained.

(*d*) Drugs.—There are none which control septic fever. The coal-tar products are of doubtful service. Quinine may be used. The intravenous injection of antiseptic drugs has not been proved to be of value.

4. TERMINAL INFECTIONS

There is truth in the paradoxical statement that persons rarely die of the disease with which they suffer. Secondary, *terminal* infections carry off many incurable cases. Flexner analyzed 255 cases of chronic renal and cardiac disease in which complete bacteriological examinations were made at autopsy. Excluding tuberculous infection, 213 gave positive and 42 negative results. The infections may be local or general. The former are extremely common, and are found in a large proportion of all cases of Bright's disease, arterio-sclerosis, heart disease, cirrhosis of the liver, and other chronic disorders. Affections of the serous membranes (acute pleurisy, pericarditis, or peritonitis), meningitis, and endocarditis are the most frequent lesions. It is perhaps safe to say that the majority of cases of advanced arterio-sclerosis and of Bright's disease succumb to these intercurrent infections. The infective agents are very varied. The streptococcus is the most common, but the pneumococcus, staphylococcus and gonococcus, and the proteus, pyocyaneus, and gas bacillus are also found. It is surprising in how many instances of arterio-sclerosis, of chronic heart disease, of Bright's disease, and particularly of cirrhosis of the liver in Flexner's series the fatal event was determined by an acute tuberculosis of the peritoneum or pleura.

The general terminal infections are somewhat less common. Of 85 cases of chronic renal disease in which Flexner found micro-organisms at autopsy, 38 exhibited general infections; of 48 cases of chronic cardiac disease, in 14 the distribution of bacteria was general. The blood-serum of persons suffering from advanced chronic disease was found by him to be less destructive to the staphylococcus aureus than normal human serum. Other diseases in which general terminal infection may occur are Hodgkin's disease, leukæmia, and chronic tuberculosis.

And, lastly, probably of the same nature is the terminal entero-colitis so frequently met with in chronic disorders.

IV. ERYSIPELAS

Definition.—A special pyogenic infection caused by the *streptococcus erysipelatis,* characterized by inflammation of the skin with fever and toxæmia.

Etiology.—Erysipelas is a widespread affection, endemic in most communities, and at certain seasons epidemic. We are as yet ignorant of the atmospheric or telluric influences which favor the diffusion of the poison.

It is particularly prevalent in the spring of the year. Of 2,012 cases collected by Anders, 1,214 occurred during the first five months of the year. April had the largest number of cases. The affection prevails extensively in old, ill-ventilated hospitals and institutions in which the sanitary conditions are defective. With the improved sanitation of late years the number of cases has materially diminished. It has been observed, however, to break out in new institutions under the most favorable hygienic circumstances. Erysipelas is both contagious and inoculable; but, except under special conditions, the poison is not very virulent and does not seem to act at any great distance. It can be conveyed by a third person. The poison attaches itself to the furniture, bedding, and walls of rooms in which patients have been confined.

The disposition to the disease is widespread, but the susceptibility is specially marked in the case of individuals with wounds or abrasions of any sort. Recently delivered women and persons who have been the subjects of surgical operations are particularly prone to it. A wound, however, is not necessary, and in the so-called idiopathic form, although it may be difficult to say that there was not a slight abrasion about the nose or lips, in very many cases there certainly is no observable external lesion. In some cases the infection apparently spreads through the tissues from the nasal cavity to the skin.

Chronic alcoholism, debility, and Bright's disease are predisposing agents. Certain persons show a special susceptibility to erysipelas, and it may recur in them repeatedly. There are instances, too, of a family predisposition.

The specific agent of the disease is a streptococcus growing in long chains, which is included under the group name *Streptococcus pyogenes,* with which *Streptococcus erysipelatis* appears to be identical. The fever and constitutional symptoms are due in great part to the toxins; the more serious visceral complications are the result of secondary metastatic infection.

Morbid Anatomy.—Erysipelas is a simple inflammation. In its uncomplicated forms there is seen, post mortem, little else than inflammatory œdema. Investigations have shown that the cocci are found chiefly in the lymph-spaces and most abundantly in the zone of spreading inflammation. In the uninvolved tissue beyond the inflamed margin they are to be found in the lymph-vessels, and it is here, according to Metschnikoff and others, that an active warfare goes on between the leucocytes and the cocci (phagocytosis). In more extensive and virulent forms of the disease there is usually suppuration.

Infarcts occur in the lungs, spleen, and kidneys, and there may be the general evidences of pyæmic infection. Some of the worst cases of malignant endocarditis are secondary to erysipelas; thus, of 23 cases, 3 occurred in connection with this disease. Septic pericarditis and pleuritis also occur. The disease may in rare cases extend to and involve the meninges. Pneumonia is not a very common complication. Acute nephritis is also met with; it is often ingrafted upon an old chronic trouble.

Symptoms.—The following description applies specially to erysipelas of the face and head, the form of the disease which the physician is most commonly called upon to treat.

The *incubation* is variable, probably from three to seven days.

The stage of *invasion* is often marked by a rigor, and followed by a rapid rise in the temperature and other characteristics of an acute fever. When there is a local abrasion, the spot is slightly reddened; but if the disease is idiopathic, there is seen within a few hours slight redness over the bridge of the nose and on the cheeks. The swelling and tension of the skin increase and within twenty-four hours the external symptoms are well marked. The skin is smooth, tense, and œdematous. It looks red, feels hot, and the superficial layers of the epidermis may be lifted as small blebs. The patient complains of an unpleasant feeling of tension in the skin; the swelling rapidly increases; and during the second day the eyes are usually closed. The first-affected parts gradually become pale and less swollen as the disease extends at the periphery. When it reaches the forehead it progresses as an advancing ridge perfectly well defined and raised; and often, on palpation, hardened extensions can be felt beneath the skin which is not yet reddened. Even in a case of moderate severity, the face is enormously swollen, the eyes are closed, the lips greatly œdematous, the ears thickened, the scalp is swollen, and the patient's features are quite unrecognizable. The formation of blebs is common on the eyelids, ears, and forehead. The cervical lymph-glands are swollen, but are usually masked in the œdema of the neck. The temperature keeps high without marked remissions for four or five days and then defervescence takes place by crisis. Leucocytosis is present. Kirkbride has noted the presence in one case of leucin and tyrosin in the urine. The general condition of the patient varies much with his previous state of health. In old and debilitated persons, particularly in those addicted to alcohol, the constitutional depression from the outset may be very great. Delirium is present, the tongue becomes dry, the pulse feeble, and there is marked tendency to death from toxæmia. In the majority of cases, however, even with extensive lesions, the constitutional disturbance, considering the height of the fever range, is slight. The mucous membrane of the mouth and throat may be swollen and reddened. The erysipelatous inflammation may extend to the larynx, but the severe œdema of this part occasionally met with is commonly due to the extension of the inflammation from without inward.

There are cases in which the inflammation extends from the face to the neck, and over the chest, and may gradually migrate or wander over the greater part of the body (*E. migrans*).

The close relation between the erysipelas coccus and the pus organisms is shown by the frequency with which suppuration occurs in facial erysipelas. Small cutaneous abscesses are common about the cheeks and forehead and neck, and beneath the scalp large collections of pus may accumulate. Suppuration seems to occur more frequently in some epidemics than in others, and at the Philadelphia Hospital during one year nearly all the cases in the erysipelas wards presented local abscesses.

Complications.—Meningitis is rare. The cases in which death occurs with marked brain symptoms do not usually show, post mortem, meningeal affection.

Pneumonia is an occasional complication. Ulcerative endocarditis and septicæmia are more common. Albuminuria is almost constant, particularly in persons over fifty. True nephritis is occasionally seen. Da Costa has called attention to curious irregular returns of the fever which occur during convalescence without any aggravation of the local condition.

Diagnosis.—The diagnosis rarely presents any difficulty. The mode of onset, the rapid rise in fever, and the characters of the local disease are quite distinctive.

Prognosis.—Healthy adults rarely die. The general mortality in hospitals is about 7 per cent.; in private practice about 4 per cent. (Anders). In the new-born, when the disease attacks the navel, it is almost always fatal. In drunkards and in the aged erysipelas is a serious affection, and death may result either from the intensity of the fever or, more commonly, from toxæmia. The wandering or ambulatory erysipelas, which has a more protracted course, may cause death from exhaustion.

Treatment.—Isolation should be strictly carried out, particularly in hospitals. A practitioner in attendance upon a case of erysipelas should not attend cases of confinement.

The disease is self-limited and a large majority of the cases get well without any internal medication. The diet should be nutritious and light. Large amounts of water should be given. Stimulants are not required except in the old and feeble. For the restlessness, delirium, and insomnia, chloral or the bromides may be given; or, if these fail, opium. When the fever is high the patient may be bathed or sponged, or, in private practice, if there is an objection to this, antipyrin or antifebrin may be given.

Antistreptococcic serum may be tried or, better still, an autogenous vaccine, with the use of which good results have been obtained.

Of internal remedies believed to influence the disease, the tincture of the perchloride of iron has been highly recommended. At the Montreal General Hospital this was the routine treatment, and doses of half a drachm to a drachm were given every three or four hours. I am by no means convinced that it has any special action; nor, so far as I know, has any medicine, given internally, a definite control over the course of the disease.

Of local treatment, the injection of antiseptic solutions at the margin of the spreading areas has been much practised. Two-per-cent. solutions of carbolic acid, corrosive sublimate (1 to 4,000), and the biniodide of mercury have been much used. The injection should be made not into but just a little beyond the border of the inflamed patch. F. P. Henry has treated a large number of cases at the Philadelphia Hospital with the last-mentioned drug, and this mode of practice is certainly most rational.

Of local applications, ichthyol is at present much used (as a salve, 1 to 4 of lanolin). Bichloride of mercury solution (1 to 5,000), salicylic acid (1 to 500), collodion, or ichthyol in collodion (1 to 4), may be used. Painting the skin ahead of the advancing area with tincture of iodine is sometimes effectual. Perhaps as good an application as any is cold water, which was highly recommended by Hippocrates.

V. DIPHTHERIA

Definition.—A specific infectious disease, characterized by a local fibrinous exudate, usually upon the mucous membrane of the throat, and by constitutional symptoms due to toxins produced at the site of the lesion. The presence of the Klebs-Loeffler bacillus is the etiological criterion by which true diphtheria is distinguished from other forms of membranous inflammation.

Cases of angina, diagnosed as diphtheria, may be due to other organisms and to these the term diphtheroid is applied. Though usually milder, severe constitutional disturbance, and even paralysis, may follow these diphtheroid forms.

History.—Known in the East for centuries, and referred to in the Babylonian Talmud, it is not until the first century A. D. that an accurate clinical account appears in the writings of Aretæus. The paralysis of the palate was recognized by Ætius (sixth century A. D.) Throat pestilences are mentioned in the Middle Ages. Severe epidemics occurred in Europe in the sixteenth and seventeenth centuries, particularly in Spain. In England in the latter part of the eighteenth century it was described by Fothergill and Huxham, and in America by Bard. Washington died of the disease. Ballonius recognized the affection of the larynx and trachea in 1762, Home in Scotland described it as croup. The modern description dates from Bretonneau, of Tours (1826), who gave to it the name *diphthérite*. Throughout the nineteenth century it prevailed extensively in all known countries, and it is at present everywhere epidemic. After innumerable attempts, in which Klebs took a leading part, the peculiar organism of the disease was isolated by Loeffler. The toxin was determined by the work of Roux, Yersin, and others, and finally the antitoxin was discovered by Behring.

Etiology.—Everywhere endemic in large centres of population, the disease becomes at times epidemic. It is more prevalent on the continent of Europe than in Great Britain, and Ireland has less than other countries. In England and Wales in 1909, 5,476 persons died of the disease, the lowest mortality since 1859. The large cities of the United States have been much afflicted, and widespread epidemics have occurred in country districts. In the tropics it is not a very serious disease. Pandemics occur cyclically, at irregular intervals, under conditions as yet imperfectly known. Dry seasons seem to favor the disease, which, like typhoid fever, shows an autumnal prevalence.

Modes of Infection.—The disease is highly contagious. The bacilli may be transmitted (*a*) from one person to another; few diseases have proved more fatal to physicians and nurses. (*b*) Infected articles may convey the bacilli, which may remain alive for many months; scores of well-attested instances have been recorded of this mode of transmission. (*c*) Persons suffering from atypical forms of diphtheria may convey the disease; nasal catarrh, membranous rhinitis, mild tonsillitis, otorrhœa may be caused by the diphtheria bacilli, and from each of these sources cases have been traced. (*d*) From the throats of healthy contacts—diphtheria carriers, persons who present no signs of the disease—the bacilli have been obtained by culture. (*e*) Even healthy children without any naso-pharyngeal catarrh, who have not been in contact with the disease, may in large cities harbor the bacilli. In 1,000 children from the New York tenements Shelley found 18 with virulent and 38 with non-virulent bacilli, and the percentage in Chicago has been sometimes much higher. Long after recovery has taken place virulent bacilli have been isolated from the throat. It is important to bear in mind under *d* and *e* that it is only persons who harbor the virulent forms who are capable of transmitting the disease. In schools the interchange of articles, such as sweets, pencils, etc., and the habit which children have of putting everything into their mouths afford endless opportunities for the transmission of the disease. As Westbrook remarks, diphtheria is transmitted usually by almost direct exchange of the flora of the nose and mouth. (*f*) Numerous epidemics have been traced to milk, since Power in 1878 determined this method of spread. Virulent bacilli have been found in the milk, and Dean and Todd and Ashby have found virulent organisms in the acquired lesions on the teats of cows. (*g*) A few instances of accidental infection from cultures and through animals are on record.

Predisposing Causes.—Age is the most important. Sucklings are not often attacked, but Jacobi saw three cases in the new-born. Early in the second year the disposition increases rapidly, and continues at its height until the fifth year. At Baginsky's clinic, Berlin, among 2,711 cases, 1,235 occurred from the second to the fifth years inclusive. In New York between 1891-1900 among the deaths 80.8 per cent. occurred under five, 17 per cent. between five and ten—figures which show the extraordinary preponderance of the disease among children. Girls are attacked in slightly larger numbers than boys. November, December, and January are the months of greatest prevalence in the United States; in London the months of October and November.

Soil and *altitude* have little or no influence on the prevalence of the disease; nor does race play an important rôle. Individual susceptibility is a very special factor; not only do very many of those exposed escape, but even those, too, in whose throats virulent bacilli lodge and grow. The Schick reaction (intradermic injection of diphtheria toxin) is of great value in determining the presence of immunity.

The Klebs-Loeffler Bacillus occurs in a large number of all suspected cases—72 per cent., based upon an analysis of 27,000 cases in the literature by Graham Smith. It is found chiefly in the false membrane, and does not extend into the subjacent mucosa. The organisms are localized, and only a few penetrate into the interior. Post mortem the bacilli may be found in the blood and in the internal organs. Occasionally they are found in the blood during life. It may be the predominating or sole organism in the broncho-pneumonia so common in the disease. Outside the throat, the Klebs-Loeffler bacillus has been found in diphtheritic conjunctivitis, in otitis media, sometimes in wound diphtheria, upon the genitals, in fibrinous rhinitis, and in ulcerative endocarditis.

Morphological Characters.—The bacillus is non-motile, varies from 2.5 to 3 μ in length and from 0.5 to 0.8 μ in thickness. In appearance it is multiform, varying from short, rather sharply pointed rods to irregular bizarre forms, with one or both ends swollen, and staining more or less unevenly and intensely. Westbrook recognizes three main types—granular, barred, and solid staining. Branching forms are occasionally met with. The bacillus stains in sections or on the cover-glass by the Gram method.

The bacillus is very resistant, and cultures have been made from a bit of membrane preserved for five months in a dry cloth. Incorporated with dust and kept moist, the bacilli were still cultivable at the end of eight weeks; kept in a dried state they no longer grew at the end of this period (Ritter).

The Klebs-Loeffler bacillus has very varying grades of virulence down even to complete absence of pathogenic effects. The name pseudo-bacillus of diphtheria should not be given to this avirulent organism.

The Presence of the Klebs-Loeffler Bacillus in Non-membranous Angina and in Healthy Throats.—The bacillus has been isolated from cases which show nothing more than a simple catarrhal angina, of a mild type without any membrane, with diffuse redness, and perhaps huskiness and signs of catarrhal laryngitis. In other cases the anatomical picture may be that of a lacunar tonsillitis. The organisms may be met with in perfectly healthy throats (diphtheria carriers), particularly in persons in the same house, or the ward attendants and nurses in fever hospitals. Following an attack of diphtheria the bacilli may persist in the throat or nose after all the membrane has disappeared for weeks or months—even 15 months. In explanation of this persistence Councilman has called attention to the frequency with which the antrum is affected.

Toxins of the Klebs-Loeffler Bacillus.—Roux and Yersin showed that a fatal result following the inoculation with the bacillus was not caused by any extension of the micro-organisms within the body; and they were enabled in bouillon cultures to separate the bacilli from the poison. The toxin so separated killed with very much the same effects as those caused by the inoculation of the bacilli; the pseudo-membrane, however, is not formed.

Susceptible animals may be rendered immune from diphtheritic infection by injecting weakened cultures of the bacillus or, what is better, suitable doses of the diphtheria toxin. The result of the injections is a febrile reaction which soon passes away and leaves the animal less susceptible to the poison or the living bacilli. By repeating and gradually increasing the quantity of poison injected a high degree of immunity can be produced in large animals (goat, horse).

The Bacteria Associated with the Diphtheria Bacillus.—The most common is the streptococcus pyogenes. Others, in addition to the organisms constantly found in the mouth, are the micrococcus lanceolatus, the bacillus coli, and the staphylococcus aureus and albus. Of these, probably the streptococcus pyogenes is the most important, as cases of general infection with this organism have been found in diphtheria. The suppuration in the lymph-glands and the broncho-pneumonia are usually (though not always) caused by this organism.

Pseudo-Diphtheria Bacillus; Bacillus Xerosis.—As mentioned above, the Klebs-Loeffler bacillus varies very much in its virulence, and it exists in a form entirely devoid of pathogenic properties. This organism should not, however, be designated pseudo-diphtheria bacillus. The name should be confined to bacilli, which, though resembling the diphtheria bacillus, differ from it not only by abscence of virulence, but also by cultural peculiarities. A similar bacillus, showing, however, certain cultural differences from the pseudo-diphtheria bacillus, has been repeatedly found in the conjunctival sac in health and disease (*B. xerosis*). *Hoffmann's Bacillus,* which is also spoken of as pseudo-diphtheria bacillus, is a common organism in the throats of healthy persons and is found also in cases of diphtheria; but how far it is responsible for pathological conditions is not yet settled. *Vincent's Bacillus* is a fusiform organism associated with a diphtheroid angina (Vincent's angina), which occurs in two forms: a membranous and an ulcerative and destructive. The fusiform bacilli have been found in healthy throats and also in association with true diphtheria.

Diphtheroid Inflammations.—Under the term diphtheroid may be grouped those membranous inflammations which are not associated with the Klebs-Loeffler bacillus. It is perhaps a more suitable designation than pseudo-diphtheria or secondary diphtheria. As in a great majority of cases the streptococcus pyogenes is the active organism, the term "streptococcus diphtheritis" is often employed. The name "diphtheritis" is best used in an anatomical sense to designate an inflammation of a mucous membrane or integumentary surface characterized by necrosis and a fibrinous exudate, whereas the term "diphtheria" should be limited to the disease caused by the Klebs-Loeffler bacillus. The proportion of cases of diphtheroid inflammation varies greatly in the different statistics. Of the large number of observations made by Park and Beebe (5,611) in New York, 40 per cent. were diphtheroid. Figures from other sources do not show so high a percentage.

Conditions under Which the Diphtheroid Affection Occurs.—Of 450 cases (Park and Beebe), 300 occurred in the autumn months and 150 in the spring; 198 occurred in children from the first to the seventh year. In a large proportion of all the cases the disease develops in children, and can be differentiated from diphtheria proper only by the bacteriological examination. It may be simply an acute catarrhal angina with lacunar tonsillitis. Some of the cases are due to Hoffmann's bacillus, a few to Vincent's fusiform bacillus. The diphtheroid inflammations are particularly prone to develop in connection with the acute fevers.

(*a*) *Scarlet Fever.*—In a large proportion of the cases of angina in scarlet fever the Klebs-Loeffler bacillus is not present. Booker has reported 11 cases complicating scarlet fever, in all of which the streptococci were the predominant organisms. Of the 450 cases of Park and Beebe, 42 complicated scarlet fever. The angina of this disease is not always, however, due to the streptococcus. Where diphtheria is prevalent and opportunities are favorable for exposure, a large proportion of the cases of membranous throats in scarlet fever may be genuine diphtheria.

(*b*) *Measles.*—Membranous angina is much less common in this disease. It occurred in 6 of the 450 diphtheroid cases in New York. Of 4 cases with severe membranous angina at the Boston City Hospital, 1 only presented the Klebs-Loeffler bacillus.

(*c*) *Whooping-cough* may also be complicated with membranous angina. Escherich records 4 cases, in all of which the Klebs-Loeffler bacillus was found.

(*d*) *Typhoid Fever.*—Membranous inflammations in this disease are not very infrequent; they may occur in the throat, the pelvis of the kidney, the bladder, or the intestines. The complication may be caused by the Klebs-Loeffler bacillus, but it is frequently a streptococcus infection. Ernst Wagner has remarked upon the greater frequency of these membranous inflammations in typhoid fever when diphtheria is prevailing.

Clinical Features of the Diphtheroid Affection.—The cases, as a rule, are milder, and the mortality is low, only 2.5 per cent. in the 450 cases of Park and Beebe. The diphtheroid inflammations complicating the specific fevers are, however, often very fatal, and a general streptococcus infection is by no means infrequent. As in the Klebs-Loeffler angina, there may be only a simple catarrhal process. In other instances the tonsils are covered with a creamy, pultaceous exudate, without any actual membrane. An important group may begin as a simple lacunar tonsillitis, while in others the entire fauces and tonsils are covered by a continuous membrane, and there is a foul sloughing angina with intense constitutional disturbance.

Are the diphtheroid cases contagious? General clinical experience warrants the statement that the membranous angina associated with the fevers is rarely communicated to other patients. The health department of New York does not keep the diphtheroid cases under supervision. Their investigation of the 450 diphtheroid cases seems to justify this conclusion. Park and Beebe say that "it did not seem that the secondary cases were any less liable to occur when the primary case was isolated than when it was not."

Sequelæ of the Diphtheroid Angina.—The usual mildness of the disease is in part, no doubt, due to the less frequent systemic invasion. Some of the worst forms of general streptococcus infection are, however, seen in this disease. There are no peculiarities, local or general, which can be in any way regarded as distinctive; and even the most extensive paralysis may follow an angina caused by it.

Morbid Anatomy.—DISTRIBUTION OF MEMBRANE.—A definite membrane was found in 127 of the 220 fatal Boston cases, distributed as follows: tonsils, 65 cases; epiglottis, 60; larynx, 75; trachea, 66; pharynx, 51; mucous membrane of nares, 43; bronchi, 42; soft palate, including uvula, 13; œsophagus, 12; tongue, 9; stomach, 5; duodenum, 1; vagina, 2; vulva, 1; skin of ear, 1; conjunctiva, 1. An interesting point in the Boston investigation was the great frequency with which the accessory sinuses of the nose were found to be infected. In the fatal cases, the exudation is very extensive, involving the uvula, the soft palate, the posterior nares, and the lateral and posterior walls of the pharynx. These parts are covered with a dense pseudo-membrane, in places firmly adherent, in others beginning to separate. In extreme cases the necrosis is advanced and there is a gangrenous condition of the parts. The membrane is of a dirty greenish or gray color, and the tonsils and palate may be in a state of necrotic sloughing. The erosion may be deep enough in the tonsils to open the carotid artery, or a false aneurism may be produced in the deep tissues of the neck. The nose may be completely blocked by the false membrane, which may also extend into the conjunctivæ and through the Eustachian tubes into the middle ear. In cases of laryngeal diphtheria the exudate in the pharynx may be extensive. In many cases, however, it is slight upon the tonsils and fauces and abundant upon the epiglottis and the larynx, which may be completely occluded by false membrane. In severe cases the exudate extends into the trachea and to the bronchi of the third or fourth dimension.

In all these situations the membrane varies very much in consistence, depending greatly upon the stage at which death has taken place. If death has occurred early, it is firm and closely adherent; if late, it is soft, shreddy, and readily detached. When firmly adherent it is torn off with difficulty and leaves an abraded mucosa. In the most extreme cases, in which there is extensive necrosis, the parts look gangrenous. In fatal cases the lymphatic glands of the neck are enlarged, and there is a general infiltration of the tissues with serum; the salivary glands, too, may be swollen. In rare instances the membrane extends to the gullet and stomach.

On inspection of the larynx of a child dead of membranous croup the *rima* is seen filled with mucus or with a shreddy material which, when washed off carefully, leaves the mucosa covered by a thin grayish-yellow membrane, which may be uniform or in patches. It covers the ary-epiglottic folds and the true cords, and may be continued into the ventricles or even into the trachea. Above, it may involve the epiglottis. It varies much in consistency. I have seen fatal cases in which the exudation was not actually membranous, but rather friable and granular. It may form a thick, even stratified membrane, which fills the entire glottis. The exudation may extend down the trachea and into the bronchi, and may pass beyond the epiglottis to the fauces. Usually it is readily stripped off from the mucous membrane of the larynx and leaves exposed the swollen and injected mucosa. On examination it is seen that the fibrinous material has involved chiefly the epithelial lining and has not greatly infiltrated the subjacent tissues.

We owe largely to the labors of Wagner, Weigert, and more particularly to the splendid work of Oertel, our knowledge of the *histological changes* which take place in diphtheria. The beginning of the lesion is due to the toxic action of the bacilli growing in the throat. The primary lesion is a necrosis and degeneration of the epithelial tissues. The organisms grow, not in the living, but in the necrotic tissues. The first step is necrosis of the epithelium, often preceded by active proliferation of the nuclei of the cells, which become changed into refractive hyaline masses. From the structures below an inflammatory exudate rich in fibrin factors is poured out, and fibrin is formed when this comes in contact with the necrotic epithelium.

The following are the important changes in the other organs:

HEART.—Fatty degeneration is found in a majority of the cases. It may precede the more advanced degeneration, in which the sarcous elements become swollen and converted into hyaline masses. There is a primary, acute, interstitial myositis, and also a form secondary to degeneration of the heart muscle, to which it is possible that some of the cases of fibrous myocarditis are due. Pericarditis and endocarditis are rare; endocarditis was present in 7 of 220 cases at the Boston City Hospital. The diphtheria bacilli have been found in the vegetations.

The PULMONARY COMPLICATIONS are the most important, and death is due to them as often as to the throat lesion. Broncho-pneumonia, or, as Councilman terms it, acinous pneumonia, is the most common, and was present in 131 of the 220 Boston cases. Acute lobar pneumonia is rare. The pneumococcus is the principal agent in producing the lung infection. The streptococci and the diphtheria bacilli are frequently met with.

KIDNEYS.—The lesions, which are due to the action of the toxins, not to the presence of bacteria, vary from simple degeneration to an intense nephritis. There is no specific type of lesion. Interstitial and glomerular nephritis are most common in the older subjects. Degenerative changes are present in a large proportion of all the fatal cases.

The liver and the spleen show the degenerative lesions of the acute infections.

General infection is common, and is about equal with the streptococcus and the diphtheria bacillus. It occurs generally in the grave septic cases, in which type of cases the former organism is more frequently met with.

Symptoms.—The period of incubation is "from two to seven days, oftenest two."

The initial symptoms are those of an ordinary febrile attack—slight chilliness, fever, and aching pains in the back and limbs. In mild cases these symptoms are trifling, and the child may not feel ill enough to go to bed. Usually the temperature rises within the first twenty-four hours to 102.5° or 103° F.; in severe cases to 104° F. In young children there may be convulsions at the outset.

Pharyngeal Diphtheria.—In a typical case there is at first redness of the fauces, and the child complains of slight difficulty in swallowing. The membrane first appears upon the tonsils, and it may be a little difficult to distinguish a patchy diphtheritic pellicle from the exudate of the tonsillar crypts. The pharyngeal mucous membrane is reddened, and the tonsils themselves are swollen. By the third day the membrane has covered the tonsils, the pillars of the fauces, and perhaps the uvula, which is thickened and œdematous, and may fill completely the space between the swollen tonsils. The membrane may extend to the posterior wall of the pharynx. At first grayish-white in color, it changes to a dirty gray, often to a yellow-white. It is firmly adherent, and when removed leaves a bleeding, slightly eroded surface, which is soon covered by fresh exudate. The glands in the neck are swollen, and may be tender. The general condition of a patient in a case of moderate severity is usually good; the temperature not very high, in the absence of complications ranging from 102° to 103° F. The pulse range is from 100 to 120. The local condition of the throat is not of great severity, and the constitutional depression is slight. The symptoms gradually abate, the swelling of the neck diminishes, the membranes separate, and from the seventh to the tenth day the throat becomes clear and convalescence sets in.

Clinically atypical forms are extremely common, and I follow here Koplik's division:

(*a*) There may be no local manifestation of membrane, but a simple catarrhal angina associated sometimes with a croupy cough. The detection in these cases of the Klebs-Loeffler bacillus can alone determine the diagnosis. Such cases are of great moment, inasmuch as they may communicate the severer disease to other children.

(*b*) There are cases in which the tonsils are covered by a pultaceous exudate, not a consistent membrane.

(*c*) Cases presenting a punctate form of membrane, isolated, and usually on the surface of the tonsils.

(*d*) Cases which begin and often run their entire course with the local picture of a typical lacunar amygdalitis. They may be mild, and the local exudate may not extend, but in other cases there are rapid development of membrane, and extension of the disease to the pharynx and the nose, with severe septic and constitutional symptoms.

(*e*) Under the term "latent diphtheria" Heubner has described cases, usually secondary, occurring chiefly in hospital practice, in young persons the subject of wasting affections, such as rickets and tuberculosis. There are fever, naso-pharyngeal catarrh, and gastro-intestinal disturbances. Diphtheria may not be suspected until severe laryngeal complications develop, or the condition may not be determined until auptosy.

SYSTEMIC INFECTION.—The constitutional disturbance in mild diphtheria is very slight. There are instances, too, of extensive local disease without grave systemic symptoms. As a rule, the general features of a case bear a definite relation to the severity of the local disease. There are rare instances in which from the outset the constitutional prostration is extreme, the pulse frequent and small, the fever high, and the nervous phenomena are pronounced; the patient may sink in two or three days overwhelmed by the intensity of the toxæmia. There are cases of this sort in which the exudate in the throat may be slight, but usually the nasal symptoms are pronounced. The temperature may be very slightly raised or even subnormal. More commonly the severe systemic symptoms appear at a later date when the pharyngeal lesion is at its height. They are constantly present in extensive disease, and when there is a sloughing, fetid condition. The lymphatic glands become greatly enlarged; the pallor is extreme; the face has an ashen-gray hue; the pulse is rapid and feeble, and the temperature sinks below normal. In the most aggravated forms there are gangrenous processes in the throat, and in rare instances, when life is prolonged, extensive sloughing of the tissues of the neck.

Escherich accounts for the discrepancy sometimes observed between the severity of the constitutional disturbance and the intensity of the local process, by assuming varying degrees of susceptibility to the diphtheria bacillus on the one hand, and to its poison on the other hand. With high local susceptibility of a part to the action of the bacillus, with little general susceptibility to the toxin, there is extensive local exudate with mild constitutional symptoms, or *vice versa,* severe systematic disturbance with limited local inflammation.

A leucocytosis is present in diphtheria. Morse does not think it of any prognostic value, since it is present and may be pronounced in mild cases.

NASAL DIPHTHERIA.—In cases of pharyngeal diphtheria the Klebs-Loeffler bacillus is found on the mucous membrane of the nose and in the secretions, even when no membrane is present, but it may apparently produce two affections similar enough locally but widely differing in their general features.

In *membranous or fibrinous rhinitis,* a very remarkable affection seen usually in children, the nares are occupied by thick membranes, but there is an entire absence of any constitutional disturbance. The condition has been studied very carefully by Park, Abbott, Gerber and Podack, and others. Ravenel has collected 77 cases, in 41 of which a bacteriological examination was made, in 33 the Klebs-Loeffler bacillus being present. All the cases ran a benign course, and in all but a few the membrane was limited to the nose, and the constitutional symptoms were either absent or very slight. Remarkable and puzzling features are that the disease runs a benign course, and that infection of other children in the family is extremely rare.

On the other hand, nasal diphtheria is apt to present a most malignant type of the disease. The infection may be primary in the nose, and in a case in my wards there was otitis media, and the Klebs-Loeffler bacillus was separated from the discharge before the condition of nasal diphtheria was suspected. While some cases are of mild character, others are very malignant, and the constitutional symptoms most profound. The glandular inflammation is usually very intense, owing, as Jacobi points out, to the great richness of the nasal mucosa in lymphatics. From the nose the inflammation may extend through the tear-ducts to the conjunctivæ and into the antra.

LARYNGEAL DIPHTHERIA (*Membranous Croup*).—With a very large proportion of all the cases of membranous laryngitis the Klebs-Loeffler bacillus is associated; in a much smaller number other organisms, particularly the streptococcus, are found. Membranous croup, then, may be said to be either genuine diphtheria or diphtheroid in character. Of 286 cases in which the disease was confined to the larynx or bronchi, in 229 the Klebs-Loeffler bacilli were found. In 57 they were not present, but 17 of these cultures were unsatisfactory (Park and Beebe). The streptococcus cases are more likely to be secondary to other acute diseases.

Symptoms.—Naturally, the clinical symptoms are almost identical in the non-specific and specific forms of membranous laryngitis.

The affection begins like an acute laryngitis with slight hoarseness and rough cough, to which the term croupy has been applied. After these symptoms have lasted for a day or two with varying intensity, the child suddenly becomes worse, usually at night, and there are signs of impeded respiration. At first the difficulty in breathing is paroxysmal, due probably to more or less spasm of the muscles of the glottis. Soon the dyspnœa becomes continuous, inspiration and expiration become difficult, particularly the latter, and with the inspiratory movement the epigastrium and lower intercostal spaces are retracted. The voice is husky and may be reduced to a whisper. The color gradually changes and the imperfect aëration of the blood is shown in the lividity of the lips and finger-tips. Restlessness comes on and the child tosses from side to side, vainly trying to get breath. Occasionally, in a severer paroxysm, portions of membrane are coughed out. The fever in membranous laryngitis is rarely very high and the condition of the child is usually very good at the time of the onset. The pulse is always increased in frequency and if cyanosis be present is small. In favorable cases the dyspnœa is not very urgent, the color of the face remains good, and after one or two paroxysms the child goes to sleep and wakes in the morning, perhaps without fever and feeling comfortable. The attack may recur the following night with greater severity. In unfavorable cases the dyspnœa becomes more and more urgent, the cyanosis deepens, the child, after a period of intense restlessness, sinks into a semi-comatose state, and death finally occurs from poisoning of the nerve centres. In other cases the onset is less sudden and is preceded by a longer period of indisposition. As a rule, there are pharyngeal symptoms. The constitutional disturbance may be more severe, the fever higher, and there may be swelling of the glands of the neck. Inspection of the fauces may show the presence of false membranes on the pillars or on the tonsils. Bacteriological examination can alone determine whether these are due to the Klebs-Loffler bacillus or to the streptococcus. Fagge held that non-contagious membranous croup may spread upward from the larynx just as diphtheritic inflammation is in the habit of spreading downward from the fauces. Ware, of Boston, whose essay on croup is one of the most solid contributions to the subject, reported the presence of exudate in the fauces in 74 out of 75 cases of croup. These observations were made prior to 1840, during periods in which diphtheria was not epidemic to any extent in Boston. In protracted cases pulmonary symptoms may occur, which are sometimes due to the difficulty in expelling the muco-pus from the tubes; in others, the false membrane extends into the trachea and even into the bronchial tubes. During the paroxysm the vesicular murmur is scarcely audible, but the laryngeal stridor may be loudly communicated along the bronchial tubes.

DIPHTHERIA OF OTHER PARTS.—Primary diphtheria occurs occasionally in the *conjunctiva.* It follows in some instances the affection of the nasal mucous membrane. Some of the cases are severe and serious, but it has been shown by C. Fränkel and others that the diphtheria bacilli may be present in a conjunctivitis catarrhal in character, or associated with only slight croupous deposits.

Diphtheria of the *external auditory meatus* is seen in rare instances in which a diphtheritic otitis media has extended through the tympanic membrane.

Diphtheria of the *skin* is most frequently seen in the severer forms of pharyngeal diphtheria, in which the membrane extends to the mouth and lips, and invades the adjacent portions of the skin of the face. The skin about the anus and genitals may also be attacked. Pseudo-membranous inflammation is not uncommon on ulcerated surfaces and wounds. In very many of these cases it is a streptococcus infection, but in a majority, perhaps, in which the patient is suffering with diphtheria, the Klebs-Loeffler bacillus will be found in the fibrinous exudate. As proposed by Welch, the term "wound diphtheria" should be limited to infection of a wound by the Klebs-Loeffler bacillus. This "may manifest itself as a simple inflammation, or inflammation with superficial necrosis, or inflammation with more or less adherent pseudomembrane. The conditions as regards varying intensity and character of the infection, association with other bacteria, particularly streptococci, and the necessity of a bacteriological examination to establish the diagnosis, are in no way different in the diphtheria of wounds from those in diphtheria of mucous membranes. Wound diphtheria may occur without demonstrable connection with cases of diphtheria and without affection of the throat in the individual attacked, but such occurrences are rare" (Welch). Paralysis may follow wound diphtheria. Pseudo-membranous inflammations of wounds are caused more frequently by other micro-organisms, particularly the streptococcus pyogenes, than by the Klebs-Loeffler bacillus. The fibrinous membrane so common in the neighborhood of the tracheotomy wound in diphtheria is rarely associated with the Klebs-Loeffler bacillus. Diphtheria of the genitals is occasionally seen.

Complications and Sequelæ.—Of local complications, hæmorrhage from the nose or throat may occur in the severe ulcerative cases. Skin rashes are not infrequent, particularly the diffuse erythema. Occasionally there is urticaria and in the severe cases purpura. Fatal cases almost invariably show capillary bronchitis with broncho-penumonia and large patches of collapse, or the septic particles may reach the bronchi and excite gangrenous processes which may lead to severe and fatal hæmorrhage. Jaundice, usually a feature of the toxæmia, is rarely of serious import. Local gangrene may occur.

Albuminuria, present in all severe cases, is alarming only when the albumin is in considerable quantity and associated with epithelial or blood casts. *Nephritis* may appear quite early in the disease, setting in occasionally with complete suppression of the urine. In comparison with scarlet fever the renal changes lead less frequently to general dropsy. In rare instances there may be coma, and even convulsions, without albumin in the urine, and without dropsy.

Of the sequelæ, *paralysis* is by far the most important. It can be experimentally produced in animals by the inoculation of the toxins. The disease is a toxic neuritis, due to the absorption of the poison. The proportion of the cases in which it occurs ranges from 10 to 15 and even to 20 per cent. It is strictly a sequel, coming on usually in the second or third week of convalescence. It may follow very mild cases; indeed, the local lesion may be so trifling that the onset of the paralysis alone calls attention to the true nature of the trouble. It is proportionately less frequent in children than in adults. L. W. Rolleston's recent study of the subject indicates that the early use of antitoxin diminishes the liability to paralysis. In 494 cases collected by Woodhead, the palate was involved in 155, the ocular muscles in 197, in 10 other muscles. Ninety-one of the patients died.

Of the local paralyses the most common is that which affects the palate. This gives a nasal character to the voice, and, owing to a return of liquids through the nose, causes a difficulty in swallowing. The palate is seen to be relaxed and motionless, and the sensation in it is also much impaired. The affection may extend to the constrictors of the pharynx, and deglutition become embarrassed. Within two or three weeks or even a shorter time the paralysis disappears. In many cases the affection of the palate is only part of a general neuritis. Of other local forms perhaps the most common are paralyses of the eye-muscles, intrinsic and extrinsic. There may be strabismus, ptosis, and loss of power of accommodation. Facial paralysis is rare. The neuritis may be confined to the nerves of one limb, though more commonly the legs or the arms are affected together. Very often with the palatal paralysis is associated a weakness of the legs without definite palsy but with loss of the knee-jerk.

The multiple form of diphtheritic neuritis may begin with the palatal affection, or with loss of power of accommodation and loss of the tendon reflexes. This last is an important sign, which, as Bernard, Buzzard, and R. L. MacDonnell have shown, may occur early, but is not necessarily followed by other symptoms of neuritis. There is paraplegia, which may be complete or involve only the extensors of the feet. The paralysis may extend and involve the arms and face and render the patient entirely helpless. The muscles of respiration may be spared.

Heart.—Irregularity of the heart is common. It was present in 60 per cent. of the Boston cases of White and Smith. A murmur at the apex or base of the heart is present in 94 per cent. of all cases. This means, of course, that a majority of all young children with fever have a heart murmur. Only a few cases of diphtheria have serious heart symptoms, 36 out of the 946 cases specially studied. Rapid action of the heart with gallop rhythm and epigastric pain and tenderness are the most serious symptoms. The cases in which the pulse drops from 110 to 40 or 30 are usually very serious. Some are due to heart block. The heart symptoms are more common in the second or third week of the disease, and fatal dilatation of the heart may come on as late as the sixth or seventh week. It seems probable that the heart weakness is due to degeneration of the muscle. Possibly in some of the cases there is degeneration of the vagus, a view which is supported by the frequency of paralysis of the palate with vomiting and epigastric pain and tenderness.

Diagnosis.—The presence of the Klebs-Loeffler bacillus is regarded by bacteriologists as the sole criterion of true diphtheria, and as this organism may be associated with all grades of throat affections, from a simple catarrh to a sloughing, gangrenous process, it is evident that in many instances there will be a striking discrepancy between the clinical and the bacteriological diagnosis.

The bacteriological diagnosis is simple. The plan adopted by the New York Health Department is a model which may be followed with advantage in other cities. Outfits for making cultures, consisting of a box containing a tube of blood-serum and a sterilized swab in a test-tube, are distributed to stations at convenient points in the city. A list of these places is published, and a physician can obtain the outfit free of cost. The directions are as follows: "The patient should be placed in a good light, and, if a child, properly held. In cases where it is possible to get a good view of the throat, depress the tongue and rub the cotton swab gently but freely against any visible exudate. In other cases, including those in which the exudate is confined to the larynx, avoiding the tongue, pass the swab far back and rub it freely against the mucous membrane of the pharynx and tonsils. Without laying the swab down, withdraw the cotton plug from the culture-tube, insert the swab, and rub that portion of it which has touched the exudate gently but thoroughly all over the surface of the blood-serum. Do not push the swab into the blood-serum, nor break the surface in any way. Then replace the swab in its own tube, plug both tubes, put them in the box, and return the culture outfit at once to the station from which it was obtained." The culture-tubes which have been inoculated are kept in an incubator at 37° C. for twelve hours and are then ready for examination. Some prefer a method by which the material from the throat collected on a sterile swab, or, as recommended by von Esmarch, on small pieces of sterilized sponge, is sent to the laboratory where the cultures and microscopic examination are made by a bacteriologist.

An immediate diagnosis without the use of cultures is often possible by making a smear preparation of the exudate from the throat. The Klebs-Loeffler bacilli may be present in sufficient numbers, and may be quite characteristic to an expert. In this connection may be given the following statement by Park, who has had such an exceptional experience: "The examination by a competent bacteriologist of the bacterial growth in a blood-serum tube which has been properly inoculated and kept for fourteen hours at the body temperature can be thoroughly relied upon in cases where there is visible membrane in the throat, if the culture is made during the period in which the membrane is forming, and no antiseptic, especially no mercurial solution, has lately been applied. In cases in which the disease is confined to the larynx or bronchi, surprisingly accurate results can be obtained from cultures, but in a certain proportion of cases no diphtheria bacilli will be found in the first culture, and yet will be abundantly present in later cultures. We believe, therefore, that absolute reliance for a diagnosis can not be placed upon a single culture from the pharynx in purely laryngeal cases."

Where a bacteriological examination can not be made, the practitioner must regard as suspicious all forms of throat affections in children, and carry out measures of isolation and disinfection. In this way alone can serious errors be avoided. It is not, of course, in the severer forms of membranous angina that mistake is likely to occur, but in the various lighter forms, many of which are in reality due to the Klebs-Loeffler bacillus.

A large proportion of the cases of diphtheroid inflammation of the throat are due to the streptococcus pyogenes. They are usually milder, and the liability to general infection is less intense; still, in scarlet fever and other specific fevers some of the most virulent cases of throat disease which we see, with intense systemic infection, are caused by this micro-organism. These streptococcus cases are probably much less numerous than the figures given would indicate. The more careful examinations in the diphtheria pavilions of hospitals, particularly in Europe, have shown that in the large majority of cases admitted the Klebs-Loeffler bacillus is present. The question of the diagnosis between scarlet fever with severe angina and diphtheria is discussed in the section on scarlet fever.

Prognosis.—The outlook in any case depends on the promptness and thoroughness with which antitoxin treatment is carried out. In hospital practice the mortality was formerly from 30 to 50 per cent. In the Boston City Hospital the death-rate between 1888 and 1894 was only once below 40 per cent., and in 1892 and 1893 rose to nearly 50 per cent. Following the introduction of antitoxin from 1895 to 1912 the death-rate has not once been above 15 per cent., and in 6,080 recent cases has been 7.8 per cent. (McCollom). In country places the disease may display an appalling virulence. In cases of ordinary severity the outlook is usually good. Death results from involvement of the larynx, septic infection, sudden heart-failure, diphtheritic paralysis, occasionally from uræmia, and sometimes from broncho-pneumonia occurring during convalescence. In England and Wales in 1909 there were 5,476 deaths, compared with 9,130, the average number in the previous decennium (Tatham). Of late years the mortality has been steadily falling. In Boston during the twenty years ending 1894 the mortality per 10,000 of the living averaged 14.46. The mortality has greatly decreased, from 18.03 per 10,000 living in 1894 to 1.5 in 1912 (McCollom).

Prophylaxis.—Isolation of the sick, disinfection of the clothing and of everything that has come in contact with the patient, careful scrutiny of the milder cases of throat disorder, and more stringent surveillance in the period of convalescence are the essential measures to prevent the spread of the disease. Suspected cases in families or schools should be at once isolated or removed to a hospital for infectious disorders. When a death has occurred from diphtheria, the body should be wrapped in a sheet which has been soaked in a corrosive-sublimate solution (1 to 2,000), and placed in a closely sealed coffin. The funeral should always be private.

In cases of well-marked diphtheria these precautions are usually carried out, but the chief danger is from the milder cases, particularly the ambulatory form, in which the disease has perhaps not been suspected. But from such patients mingling with susceptible children the disease is often conveyed. The healthy children in a family in which diphtheria exists may carry the disease to their school-fellows. The question of the influence of isolation hospitals on the spread of the disease has, I think, been solved in Boston, a city which has suffered terribly from diphtheria. The ratio of mortality per 10,000 living in 1893 was 11+, and in 1894 it was 19+. In 1895 the infectious pavilion was opened. Prior to that year only about 10 per cent. of the reported cases were treated in hospital; in succeeding years 50 per cent. were treated in hospital. In 1898 the mortality per 10,000 had fallen to 3, and in 1899 it was 4.9.

A very important matter in the prophylaxis relates to the period of convalescence. It has been shown by numerous observations that, after all the membrane has cleared away, virulent bacilli may persist in the throat from periods ranging from six weeks to six months, or even longer. The disease may be communicated by these *carriers* and they should be isolated and the throat carefully treated, but there are cases very resistant to all forms of throat antiseptics. Antitoxin may be applied locally to the throat and spraying the throat and nose with a bouillon culture of *staphylococcus pyogenes aureus* is stated to be an efficient measure.

It cannot be too strongly emphasized that the important elements in the prophylaxis of diphtheria are the rigid scrutiny of the milder types of throat affection, and the thorough isolation and disinfection of the individual patients. During an epidemic there should be repeated examinations made of all those exposed to infection.

Careful attention should be given to the throats and mouths of childen, particularly to the teeth and tonsils, as Caillê has urged. Swollen and enlarged tonsils should be removed. Cats and dogs may carry infection and should be excluded from coming in contact with patients. In persons exposed, the antiseptic mouth washes, such as corrosive sublimate (1 to 10,000), hydrogen peroxide, or swabbing the throat with a diluted Loeffler's solution, should be employed. Physicians and nurses should wear gowns and caps, and cover the nose and mouth with gauze.

IMMUNIZATION.—The giving of antitoxin as a preventive measure has an important place. Its value is well shown in the children's hospitals in which it is given as a routine prophylactic measure. The usual dose for adults is 1,000 units, for older children 750 units, and for children under two years of age 500 units. The immunity lasts about three weeks. The same precautions should be taken as in giving antitoxin to those with the disease.

Treatment.—The important points are hygienic measures to prevent the spread of the malady, local treatment of the throat to destroy the bacilli, medication, general or specific, to counteract the effects of the toxins, and, lastly, to meet the complications and sequelæ.

(*a*) HYGIENIC MEASURES.—The patient should be in a room from which the carpets, curtains, and superfluous furniture have been removed. The temperature should be about 68°, and thorough ventilation should be secured. The air may be kept moist by a kettle or a steam-atomizer. If possible, only the nurse, the child's mother, and the doctor should come in contact with the patient. During the visit the physician should wear a gown and cap, and on leaving the room he should thoroughly wash his hands and face in a corrosive-sublimate solution. The strictest quarantine should be employed against other members in the house.

(*b*) LOCAL TREATMENT.—In mild cases the throat symptoms are alone prominent. Vigorous local treatment from the outset should be carried out, taking especial care in all instances to avoid mechanical injury to the tissues. A very large number of solutions have been recommended. They are best employed with a swab of cotton-wool or a soft sponge, or irrigation with hot antiseptic solutions may be used. The direct application with a swab of cotton-wool or sponge is, as a rule, effective. In many young children it is really a most trying procedure to carry out the treatment, and sometimes one is compelled to desist. In infants the disinfecting fluids are sometimes better applied through the nostrils, but the irrigating stream should be allowed to flow very gently. The following solutions may be employed:

Loeffler's solution: Menthol, 10 grams dissolved in toluol to 36 c. c.; Liq. Ferri sesquichlorati, 4 c. c.; alcohol absol., 60 c. c.

Corrosive sublimate, 1 to 1,000, either alone or with tartaric acid, 5 grams to the litre.

Carbolic acid, 3 per cent. in 30 per cent. alcohol solution, is much employed; some prefer to touch the small spots of exudate with pure carbolic acid.

Another solution is: The tincture of the perchloride of iron, a drachm and a half, in glycerine, one ounce, water, one ounce, with from 15 to 20 minims of carbolic acid. Chlorine water, boric acid, peroxide of hydrogen, iodoform, lactic acid, trypsin, and papain are also recommended.

In many cases the use of an alkaline solution or even of a saline solution is more satisfactory than antiseptics.

Nasal diphtheria requires prompt and thorough disinfection of the passages. Jacobi recommends chloride of sodium, saturated boric acid, or 1 part of bichloride of mercury, 35 of chloride of sodium, and 1,000 of water, or the 1-per-cent. solution of carbolic acid. Loeffler's solution may be diluted and applied with a syringe or spray. To be effectual the injection must be properly given. The nurse should be instructed to pass the nozzle of the syringe horizontally, not vertically; otherwise the fluid will return through the same nostril.

When the larynx becomes involved, a steam tent may be arranged upon the bed, so that the child may breathe an atmosphere saturated with moisture. When the signs of obstruction are marked there should be no delay in the performance of intubation or tracheotomy. The choice between these must depend on the circumstances in each case. Intubation may be regarded as the operation of choice in the majority of cases. Tracheotomy is preferable in adults and may be the operation of necessity. The patient requires more skillful care after intubation than after tracheotomy.

Hot applications to the neck are usually very grateful, particularly to young children, though in the case of older children and adults the ice poultices are to be preferred.

(*c*) GENERAL MEASURES.—Every effort should be made to nourish the patient. The food should be liquid—milk, beef juices, barley water, ice cream, albumen water, and soups. The patient should be encouraged to drink water freely. If there is difficulty in taking it by mouth, it should be given by the bowel or by infusion. The bowels should be freely opened, for which a calomel and saline purge is usually best. When the pharyngeal involvement is very great and swallowing painful, nutritive enemata should be used. In cases with severe constitutional symptoms stimulants should be given early.

Medicines given internally are of very little avail, but there is still a wide-spread belief in the profession that forms of mercury are beneficial. The tincture of the perchloride of iron is also very warmly recommended. We must rely on general measures of feeding and stimulation to support the strength.

(*d*) Antitoxin Treatment.—As the years go on additional experience has shown that, thoroughly carried out, this method of treatment is both safe and efficacious. There are no reasonable grounds for skepticism on the part of intelligent practitioners, and still less on the part of those in charge of the hospitals for infectious diseases.

The principle of action depends on the circumstance that the blood-serum of an animal rendered immune, when introduced into another animal, protects it from infection with the diphtheria bacilli, and has also an important curative influence upon diphtheria, whether artificially given to animals, or spontaneously acquired by man. In the preparation of the blood-serum a uniform standard strength is procured. The antitoxin unit is the amount of antitoxin which, injected into a guinea-pig of 250 grams in weight, neutralizes 100 times the minimum fatal dose of toxin of standard strength.

Dosage.—This is one of the most important questions relating to the use of the antitoxin. J. H. McCollom, of the Boston City Hospital, who probably had a richer experience with the disease than any man in the United States, insisted that the guiding practice in the use of the antitoxin is to give it until the characteristic effects are produced, whether 4,000 or 70,000 units be required for this result. He very rightly remarks that in the case of a patient ill with diphtheria there is no way of estimating the quantity of toxin generated by the membrane, and therefore one must administer the agent until the characteristic effect is produced—viz., the shriveling of the membrane, the diminution of the nasal discharge, the correction of the fetid odor, and a general improvement in the condition of the patient. No case, he says, in the acute stage should be considered hopeless. "When one sees a patient with membrane covering the tonsils and uvula, profuse sanious discharge from the nose, spots of ecchymosis on the body and extremities, cold, clammy hands and feet, a feeble pulse, and the nauseous odor of diphtheria, and finds that after the administration of 10,000 units of antitoxin in two doses the condition of the patient improves slightly; that after 10,000 units more have been given there is a marked abatement in the severity of the symptoms; that when an additional 10,000 units have been given the patient is apparently out of danger, and eventually recovers—one must believe in the curative power of antitoxin. When one sees a patient in whom the intubation tube has been repeatedly clogged, when the hopeless condition of the patient changes for the better after the administration of 50,000 units, one can not help but be convinced of the importance of giving large doses of antitoxin in the very severe and apparently hopeless cases. In the majority of instances these large doses are not required, particularly if the patients are seen early in the attack, 4,000 to 6,000 units being enough to produce the characteristic effect on the membrane." The initial dose in ordinary cases should be from 3,000 to 5,000 units and the result must determine the frequency of repetition. In severe cases and in laryngeal diphtheria the first dose should be from 5,000 to 10,000 units, repeated in six hours. The danger is in giving too small and not too large a dose.

Administration.—Antitoxin may be injected subcutaneously, intramuscularly or intravenously. The two last are advisable in severe cases. Intramuscular is usually better than subcutaneous injection. The skin and needle should be thoroughly clean.

Favorable effects are seen in the improvement in both the local and general condition. The swelling of the fauces subsides, the membrane begins to disappear, the temperature falls, and the pulse becomes slower.

Untoward Effects.—"Serum Disease."—This may appear in any normal individual and is due to the serum and not to the antitoxin. Following the injection after a varying interval, which varies from one to eighteen days, but is usually between seven and ten days, a local reaction appears which may be accompanied by general symptoms. The site of injection shows œdema, urticaria or erythema, which may become more or less general. Malaise, vomiting, fever, adenitis, albuminuria, and arthralgia may accompany this. The symptoms are usually not severe and disappear in three or four days. Calcium lactate (gr. xv, 1 gm. three times a day) may be given as a prophylactic or when the symptoms have appeared. There is another reaction which is much more serious. In individuals who have been given antitoxin previously, even at a long interval—who have been sensitized—in some who have had asthma and in some of those who are affected by the smell or proximity of horses, an acute dangerous condition may be caused by the injection of serum—anaphylaxis. This comes on very suddenly and with acute symptoms, among which are extreme distress, dyspnœa, cyanosis, œdema, collapse, respiratory failure and convulsions; death may follow rapidly. Fortunately this occurs rarely, but its possibility should be kept in mind, and before giving antitoxin the patient should be asked as to a history of asthma, an idiosyncrasy to horses and previous administration of antitoxin. If there is any reason to suspect the possibility of a reaction, the patient should be tested by the administration of two or three drops of antitoxin, which will not give a dangerous reaction. If he is susceptible a reaction usually occurs in an hour, but it is safer to wait three hours. The skin reaction may also be tried (Moss), but this demands twenty-four hours, too long to wait if the diphtheria is severe. If the patients are sensitive and the need of antitoxin is great, small doses should be given at short intervals. In the absence of reaction it is safe to give the usual dose, for a sensitized individual, after receiving a small dose, is refractory to larger doses some hours later. This must be kept in mind in the case of patients who have a relapse, as if seven days have elapsed since the first dose the patient may be sensitized. Children seem to be much less liable to sensitization than adults. If anaphylaxis should occur, morphia (gr. ¼) and atropine (gr. 1-100) hypodermically should be given at once. Artificial respiration should be done if there is respiratory failure.

Results.—Of 183,256 cases treated in 150 cities previous to the serum period, the mortality was 38.4 per cent. Since the introduction of serum among 132,548 cases, there was a mortality of 14.6 per cent. Leaving out those not treated with the serum, the mortality was 9.8 per cent. (Edwin Rosenthal). The figures of the Boston City Hospital are of special value, as the number of cases is large, the character severe, and the Director of the South Department, Dr. McCollom, had faith in the treatment and courage in carrying it out.

In Chicago, for fifteen years before antitoxin treatment, the death rate was 144, for the fifteen years after its introduction it was 38 (G. B. Young).

Convalescence.—This demands special care, particularly if there are signs of cardiac disturbance. In this event the patient should be kept absolutely at rest and this may be necessary for a long period. Nourishment should be given freely, strychnine administered in full doses, and iron with arsenic if there is anæmia. If swallowing becomes difficult it is wise to use the stomach tube for feeding. With the post-diphtheritic paralysis the patients should be kept in bed, fed liberally and given strychnine hypodermically. Antitoxin is valuable in doses of 1,000 to 3,000 units daily. In the chronic forms with muscular wasting, electricity and massage should be used. The patient should not be discharged from quarantine until two successive cultures from the throat and nose, two days apart, have been negative.

VI. THE PNEUMONIAS AND PNEUMOCOCCIC INFECTIONS

A variety of diseases are caused by the pneumococcus, among which lobar and lobular pneumonia are the most important. Various inflammatory affections of the lungs may be caused by other organisms, but the pneumococcus plays the important rôle in the common fibrinous pneumonia and in the ordinary broncho-pneumonia. It may set up also many local affections and is the cause of many terminal infections in chronic diseases.

A. LOBAR PNEUMONIA

(*Croupous or Fibrinous Pneumonia, Lung Fever*)

Definition.—An infection caused by the pneumococcus of Fraenkel, characterized by inflammation of the lungs, a toxæmia of varying intensity and a fever which usually terminates by crisis. Secondary infective processes are common.

History.—The disease was known to Hippocrates and the old Greek physicians, by whom it was confounded with pleurisy. Among the ancients, Aretæus gave a remarkable description. "Ruddy in countenance, but especially the cheeks; the white of the eyes very bright and fatty; the point of the nose flat; the veins in the temples and neck distended; loss of appetite; pulse, at first, large, empty, very frequent, as if forcibly accelerated; heat indeed, externally, feeble, and more humid than natural, but, internally, dry and very hot, by means of which the breath is hot; there is thirst, dryness of the tongue, desire of cold air, aberration of mind; cough mostly dry, but if anything be brought up it is a frothy phlegm, or slightly tinged with bile, or with a very florid tinge of blood. The blood-stained is of all others the worst." At the end of the seventeenth and the beginning of the eighteenth century Morgagni and Valsalva made many accurate clinical and anatomical observations on the disease. Our modern knowledge dates from Laënnec (1819), whose masterly description of the physical signs and morbid anatomy left very little for subsequent observers to add or modify.

Incidence.—One of the most widespread and fatal of all acute diseases, pneumonia has become the "Captain of the Men of Death," to use the phrase applied by John Bunyan to consumption. In England and Wales in 1913 there were 37,350 deaths from this cause; 8,055 were attributed to lobar pneumonia, 17,580 to broncho-pneumonia, while 11,715 were registered as from pneumonia without further qualification. In the United States in the registration area in 1913 there were 83,778 deaths. It is a disease of cities, in the overcrowded districts of which there has been an increase of late, particularly in America.

Careful studies of tropical pneumonia have been made at Panama. At the Ancon Hospital among 574 cases the mortality was 37 per cent.; among the mixed races, natives of the Isthmus, from 50 to 60 per cent. The same high death rate prevails at the Colon Hospital. Among the natives employed in the Transvaal mines the disease is very fatal, killing a larger number than any other disease, tuberculosis coming second. It is more particularly among the natives during the first month of work in the mines, 443 per thousand of all deaths during this period. There is a marked decline in succeeding periods of six months—from 16 per thousand in the first six months to 9.24 per thousand in the second six months, and 5.5 per thousand in the third six months. Of a total of 6,333 deaths in 1909-1910 in the labor area, 2,264, more than one-third, were due to pneumonia (G. D. Maynard). The case mortality is not extraordinarily high. In Johannesburg the deaths among the colored people fell from 1,196 in 1912-13 (a rate of 10.79 per 1,000 population) to 325 in 1913-14 (a rate of 3.09 per 1,000) coincident with improvement in the sanitary condition of the dwellings.

Etiology.—Age.—To the sixth year the predisposition to pneumonia is marked; it diminishes to the fifteenth year, but then for each subsequent decade it increases. For children Holt's statistics of 500 cases give: First year, 15 per cent.; from the second to the sixth year, 62 per cent.; from the seventh to the eleventh year, 21 per cent.; from the twelfth to the fourteenth year, 2 per cent. Lobar pneumonia has been met with in the new-born. The relation to age is well shown in the U. S. Census Report for 1900. The death-rate in persons from fifteen to forty-five years was 100.05 per 100,000 of population; from forty-five to sixty-five years it was 263.12; and in persons sixty-five years of age and over it was 733.77. Pneumonia may well be called the friend of the aged. Taken off by it in an acute, short, not often painful illness, the old escape those "cold gradations of decay" that make the last stage of all so distressing.

Sex.—Males are more frequently affected than females—533 to 125 in the Johns Hopkins Hospital series.

Race.—In the United States pneumonia is more fatal in negroes than among the whites. This was not so marked in our figures at the Johns Hopkins Hospital, but at the Charité Hospital, New Orleans, and at the Ancon and Colon hospitals of the Canal Zone the death rate among the negroes is much higher. It is rare among the Chinese.

Social Condition.—The disease is more common in the cities. Individuals who are much exposed to hardship and cold are particularly liable to the disease. Newcomers and immigrants are stated to be less susceptible than native inhabitants.

Personal Condition.—Debilitating causes of all sorts render individuals more susceptible. Alcoholism is perhaps the most potent predisposing factor. Robust, healthy men are, however, often attacked.

Previous Attack.—No other acute disease recurs in the same individual with such frequency. Instances are on record of individuals who have had ten or more attacks. The percentage of recurrences has been placed as high as 50. Netter gives it as 31, and he has collected the statistics of eleven observers who place the percentage at 26.8. Among the highest figures for recurrences are those of Benjamin Rush, 28, and Andral, 16.

Trauma—Contusion-pneumonia.—Pneumonia may follow directly upon injury, particularly of the chest, without necessarily any lesion of the lung. Litten gives 4.4 per cent., Stern 2.8 per cent. Stern describes three clinical varieties: first, the ordinary lobar pneumonia following a contusion of the chest wall; secondly, atypical cases, with slight fever and not very characteristic physical signs; thirdly, cases with the physical signs and features of broncho-pneumonia. The last two varieties have a favorable prognosis. According to Ballard, workers in certain phosphate factories, where they breathe a very dusty atmosphere, are particularly prone to pneumonia.

Cold has been for years regarded as an important etiological factor. The frequent occurrence of an initial chill has been one reason for this widespread belief. As to the close association of pneumonia with exposure there can be no question. We see the disease occur either promptly after a wetting or a chilling due to some unusual exposure, or come on after an ordinary catarrh of one or two days' duration. Cold is now regarded simply as a factor in lowering the resistance of the bronchial and pulmonary tissues.

Climate and Season.—Climate does not appear to have very much influence, as pneumonia prevails equally in hot and cold countries. It is stated to be more prevalent in the Southern than in the Northern States, but an examination of the Census Reports shows that there is very little difference in the various State groups.

The disease is less prevalent in England than in the United States, where the dry, overheated air of the houses favors catarrhal processes in the air passages, though I know of no figures which show a greater incidence of pneumococci in the mouths and throats of the inhabitants of the latter country.

Much more important is the influence of *season*. Statistics are almost unanimous in placing the highest incidence of the disease in the winter and spring months. In Montreal, January, the coldest month of the year, but with steady temperature, has usually a comparatively low death-rate from pneumonia. The large statistics of Seitz from Munich and of Seibert of New York give the highest percentage in February and March.

Bacteriology of Acute Lobar Pneumonia.—(*a*) Micrococcus lanceolatus, Pneumococcus or Diplococcus pneumoniæ of Fraenkel and Weichselbaum.—In September, 1880, Sternberg inoculated rabbits with his own saliva and isolated a micrococcus. The publication was not made until April, 1881. Pasteur discovered the same organism in the saliva of a child dead of hydrophobia in December, 1880, and the priority of the discovery belongs to him, as his publication is dated January, 1881. There was, however, no suspicion that this organism was concerned in the etiology of lobar pneumonia, and it was not really until April, 1884, that Fraenkel determined that the organism found by Sternberg and Pasteur in the saliva, and known as the coccus of sputum septicæmia, was the most frequent germ in pneumonia.

The organism is a somewhat elliptical, lance-shaped coccus, usually occurring in pairs; hence the term diplococcus. About the organism in the sputum a capsule can always be demonstrated. Its kinship to *Streptococcus pyogenes* is regarded by many as very close. R. Cole and his co-workers recognize four groups based upon well defined immunological differences. The numerous strains conform to one or other of these types but until they are worked out thoroughly we shall not have a rational basis for immunotherapy in the various pneumococcal infections. They differ in virulence, and Type IV which is responsible for only one-fifth of the cases is the commonest form found in the mouths of healthy individuals. A fifth well-marked strain has been determined in South Africa by Lister.

Distribution in the Body.—In the bronchial secretions and in the affected lung the pneumococcus is readily demonstrated in smears, and in the latter in sections. With the more recent methods it is possible to isolate the pneumococcus from the blood in a large proportion of all cases.

(*b*) Pneumococcus Under Normal Conditions.—(1) *In the Mouth.*—The pneumococcus is present in the mouths of a large proportion of healthy individuals, the various observers giving 80 to 90 per cent. of positive results. The virulence is not always uniform, and Longcope and Fox were able to show that the saliva of the same individual increased in virulence during the winter months. Some persons always harbor a virulent variety. Buerger at the Mt. Sinai Hospital studied the communicability of the organism from one person to another and it was found repeatedly that normal individuals—*i. e.*, persons in whose mouths the pneumococcus was proved by repeated examinations to be absent—acquired the organisms by association with cases of pneumonia, or with healthy persons in whose saliva pneumococci were present.

(2) *Outside the Body.*—The viability of the pneumococcus is not great. It has been found occasionally in the dust and sweepings of rooms, but Wood has shown (New York Commission Report) that the germs exposed to sunlight die in a very short time—an hour and a half being the limit. In moist sputum kept in a dark room the germs lived ten days, and in a badly ventilated room in which a person with pneumonia coughed, the germs suspended in the air retained their vitality for several hours.

(*c*) Bacillus pneumoniæ of Friedländer.—This is a larger organism than the pneumococcus, and appears in the form of plump, short rods. It also shows a capsule, but presents marked biological and cultural differences from Fraenkel's pneumococcus. It may cause broncho-pneumonia and other affections, and is not a cause of genuine lobar pneumonia. The exudate caused by this bacillus is usually more viscid and poorer in fibrin than that in diplococcus pneumonia.

(*d*) Other Organisms.—Various bacteria may be associated with the pneumococcus in lobar pneumonia, the most common of these being *Streptococcus pyogenes,* the pyogenic staphylococci, and Friedländer's pneumobacillus; but while these latter may cause broncho-pneumonia, they have not been satisfactorily demonstrated to be other than secondary invaders in lobar pneumonia. Likewise the pneumonias caused by *Bacillus typhosus*, *Bacillus diphtheriæ*, and the influenza bacillus are not to be identified with true lobar pneumonia.

Clinically, the *infectious nature* of pneumonia was recognized long before we knew anything of the pneumococcus. It may occur in endemic form, localized in certain houses, in barracks, jails, and schools. As many as ten occupants of one house have been attacked. I have seen three members of a family consecutively attacked with a most malignant type of pneumonia. Among the more remarkable endemic outbreaks is that reported by W. B. Rodman, of Frankfort, Ky. In a prison with a population of 735 there occurred in one year 118 cases of pneumonia with 25 deaths. The disease may assume epidemic proportions. In the Middlesborough epidemic, so carefully studied by Ballard, there were 682 persons attacked, with a mortality of 21 per cent. During some years pneumonia is so prevalent that it is practically pandemic. Direct contagion is suggested by the fact that a patient in the next bed to a pneumonia case may take the disease, or 2 or 3 cases may follow in rapid succession in a ward. It is very exceptional, however, for nurses or doctors to be attacked.

Infection, the Symptoms and Immunity.—A majority of persons harbor the germ in mouth, nose, or throat, but the virulence of the ordinary mouth form is low and varies with the season. A virulent germ may be constant and such persons are true carriers and play an important rôle in the spread of the disease. Some individuals are less resistant, and in no other acute disease may so many successive attacks occur in the same person. The negro race in the United States, in the Canal Zone, and in South Africa shows an extreme susceptibility; on the other hand the Chinese workmen, when in South Africa, showed an extraordinary resistance to the disease.

There are three phases in the infection—a period of incubation and onset, the clinical manifestations, and the immunization characterized by the crisis. The attack is usually attributed to lowered general resistance, but experimentally there is basis for the view that local conditions in the lung, such as the catarrhal processes, favor the development of pneumococci. Changes leading to lobar consolidation may be regarded as local defensive reactions. The explosive onset bears a certain resemblance to the anaphylactic reaction.

The clinical features are a toxæmia, plus disturbances of respiratory and circulatory functions. The intoxication bears no proportion to the local lesion. There are profound general infections with little or no pulmonary involvement. Some of the most toxic cases, particularly in the aged, have very slight lesions, while a lung may be solid and the patient show no signs of poisoning. The nature of the toxæmia is unknown, nor whether due to absorption of the products of digestion of the local exudate, which does not seem likely, as the symptoms abate after crisis when this absorption is most active. To regard the symptoms as due to absorption of a toxin is natural but no special substance has been discovered in the culture fluids of pneumococci; the problem is still under discussion. Metabolic studies on the oxygen and carbon dioxide contents of the blood by Peabody show no change in the reaction of the body tissues beyond the mild grade of acidosis present in all fevers. Probably, as

Pfeifer suggests, it is an endotoxin produced from the bodies of the pneumococci.

The explanation of the crisis is obscure. Immune bodies are not constantly increased after it, or they may not appear for several days. Upon what the neutralization of the toxins depends is doubtful.

The serum of a horse actively immunized will protect a mouse against a million lethal doses when injected together; but if injected only a few hours after the lethal dose it is not possible to save the animal (Cole). Insufficient dosage may account for the common failure and in each case the special strain must be determined. A univalent serum was efficient to protect animals against about 40 per cent. of cultures obtained from the blood of patients. Up to the present serums have been found useful in the treatment of infections with Types I and II. No effective serum has been obtained for Type III (*Pneumococcus Mucosus*).

Morbid Anatomy.—Since the time of Laënnec, pathologists have recognized three stages in the inflamed lung: engorgement, red hepatization, and gray hepatization.

In the stage of *engorgement* the lung tissue is deep red in color, firmer to the touch, and more solid, and on section the surface is bathed with blood and serum. It still crepitates, though not so distinctly as healthy lung, and excised portions float. The air-cells can be dilated by insufflation from the bronchus. The capillary vessels are greatly distended, the alveolar epithelium swollen, and the air-cells occupied by a variable number of blood corpuscles and detached alveolar cells. In the stage of *red hepatization* the lung tissue is solid, firm, and airless. If the entire lobe is involved it looks voluminous, and shows indentations of the ribs. On section, the surface is dry, reddish-brown in color, and has lost the deeply congested appearance of the first stage. One of the most remarkable features is the friability; in striking contrast to the healthy lung, which is torn with difficulty. The surface has a granular appearance due to the fibrinous plugs filling the air-cells. The distinctness of this appearance varies greatly with the size of the alveoli, which are about 0.10 mm. in diameter in the infant, 0.15 or 0.16 in the adult, and from 0.20 to 0.25 in old age. On scraping the surface with a knife a reddish viscid serum is removed, containing small granular masses. The smaller bronchi often contain fibrinous plugs. If the lung has been removed before the heart, it is not uncommon to find solid moulds of clot filling the blood-vessels. Microscopically, the air-cells are seen to be occupied by coagulated fibrin in the meshes of which are red blood-corpuscles, mononuclear and polynuclear leucocytes, and alveolar epithelium. The alveolar walls are infiltrated and leucocytes are seen in the interlobular tissues. Cover-glass preparations from the exudate, and thin sections show, as a rule, the diplococci already referred to, many of which are contained within cells. Staphylococci and streptococci may also be seen in some cases. In the stage of *gray hepatization* the tissue has changed from a reddish-brown to a grayish-white color. The surface is moister, the exudate obtained on scraping is more turbid, the granules in the acini are less distinct, and the lung tissue is still more friable. The air-cells are densely filled with leucocytes, the fibrin network and the red blood-corpuscles have largely disappeared. A more advanced condition of gray hepatization is that known as *purulent infiltration,* in which the lung tissue is softer and bathed with a purulent fluid. Small abscess cavities may form, and by their fusion larger ones, though this is a rare event in ordinary pneumonia.

Resolution.—The changes in the exudate which lead to its resolution are due to an autolytic digestion by proteolytic enzymes which are present much more abundantly in gray hepatization than in the preceding stage. The dissolved exudate is for the most part excreted by the kidneys. By following the nitrogen excess in the urine the progress of resolution may be followed and even an estimate formed of the amount of the exudate thus eliminated. In a study from my clinic H. W. Cook found in cases of delayed resolution that the nitrogen excess in the urine (which persisted until the lung was clear) was very large, and he suggests that delayed resolution may really be a matter of continued exudation.

General Details of the Morbid Anatomy.—In 100 autopsies, made by me at the General Hospital, Montreal, in 51 cases the right lung was affected, in 32 the left, in 17 both organs. In 27 cases the entire lung, with the exception, perhaps, of a narrow margin at the apex and anterior border, was consolidated. In 34 cases, the lower lobe alone was involved; in 13 cases, the upper lobe alone. When double, the lower lobes were usually affected together, but in three instances the lower lobe of one and the upper lobe of the other were attacked. In 3 cases, also, both upper lobes were affected. Occasionally the disease involves the greater part of both lungs; thus, in one instance the left organ with the exception of the anterior border was uniformly hepatized, while the right was in the stage of gray hepatization, except a still smaller portion in the corresponding region. In a third of the cases, red and gray hepatization existed together. In 22 instances there was gray hepatization. As a rule the unaffected portion of the lung is congested or œdematous. When the greater portion of a lobe is attacked, the uninvolved part may be in a state of almost gelatinous œdema. The unaffected lung is usually congested, particularly at the posterior part. This, it must be remembered, may be largely due to post mortem subsidence. The uninflamed portions are not always congested and œdematous. The upper lobe may be dry and bloodless when the lower lobe is uniformly consolidated. The average weight of a normal lung is about 600 grams, while that of an inflamed organ may be 1,500, 2,000, or even 2,500 grams.

The bronchi contain, as a rule, at the time of death a frothy serous fluid, rarely the tenacious mucus so characteristic of pneumonic sputum. The mucous membrane is usually reddened, rarely swollen. In the affected areas the smaller bronchi often contain fibrinous plugs, which may extend into the larger tubes, forming perfect casts. The bronchial glands are swollen and may even be soft and pulpy. The pleural surface of the inflamed lung is invariably involved when the process becomes superficial. Commonly, there is only a thin sheeting of exudate, producing slight turbidity of the membrane. The pleura was not involved in only two of the hundred instances. In some cases the fibrinous exudate may form a creamy layer an inch in thickness. A serous exudation of variable amount is not uncommon.

Lesions in Other Organs.—The heart, particularly its right chamber, is distended with firm, tenacious coagula, which can be withdrawn from the vessels as dendritic moulds. In no other acute disease do we meet with coagula of such solidity. The spleen is often enlarged, though in only 35 of the 100 cases was the weight above 200 grams. The kidneys show parenchymatous swelling, turbidity of the cortex, and, in a very considerable proportion of the cases—25 per cent.—chronic interstitial changes.

Pericarditis was present in 35 of 658 cases in my series (Chatard). *Endocarditis* occurred in 16 of my 100 post mortems. In 5 of these the endocarditis was of the simple character; in 11 the lesions were ulcerative. Of 209 cases of malignant endocarditis which I collected from the literature, 54 occurred in pneumonia. Kanthack found an antecedent pneumonia in 14.2 per cent. of cases of infective endocarditis. In the recent figures collected by E. F. Wells, of 517 fatal cases of acute endocarditis, 22.3 per cent. were in pneumonia. It is more common on the left than on the right side of the heart. Among 658 cases of pneumonia in the Johns Hopkins Hospital endocarditis occurred in 15 (Marshall). *Myocarditis* and fatty degeneration of the heart may be present in protracted cases.

Meningitis, which is not infrequent, may be associated with malignant endocarditis. It was present in 8 of the 100 autopsies. Of 20 cases of meningitis in ulcerative endocarditis 15 occurred in pneumonia. The meningitis is usually of the convex.

Croupous or diphtheritic inflammation may occur in other parts. A *croupous colitis,* as pointed out by Bristowe, is not very uncommon. It occurred in 5 of my 100 post mortems. It is usually a thin, flaky exudation, most marked on the tops of the folds of the mucous membrane. In one case there was a patch of *croupous gastritis,* covering an area 2 by 8 cm., situated to the left of the cardiac orifice.

The liver shows parenchymatous changes, and often extreme engorgement of the hepatic veins.

Symptoms.—Course of the Disease in Typical Cases.—We know but little of the incubation period in lobar pneumonia. It is probably very short. There are sometimes slight catarrhal symptoms for a day or two. As a rule, the disease sets in abruptly with a severe chill, which lasts from fifteen to thirty minutes or longer. In no acute disease is an initial chill so constant or so severe. The patient may be taken abruptly in the midst of his work, or may awaken out of a sound sleep in a rigor. The temperature taken during the chill shows that the fever has already begun. If seen shortly after the onset, the patient has usually features of an acute fever, and complains of headache and general pains. Within a few hours there is pain in the side, often of an agonizing character; a short, dry, painful cough begins, and the respirations are increased in frequency. When seen on the second or third day, the picture in typical pneumonia is more distinctive than that presented by any other acute disease. The patient lies flat in bed, often on the affected side; the face is flushed, particularly one or both cheeks; the breathing is hurried, accompanied often with a short expiratory grunt; the alæ nasi dilate with each inspiration; herpes is usually present on the lips or nose; the eyes are bright, the pupils are often unequal, the expression is anxious, and there is a frequent short cough which makes the patient wince and hold his side. The expectoration is blood-tinged and extremely tenacious. The temperature may be 104° or 105°. The pulse is full and bounding and the pulse-respiration ratio much disturbed. Examination of the lungs shows the physical signs of consolidation with blowing breathing and fine râles. After persisting for from seven to ten days the crisis occurs, and with a fall in the temperature

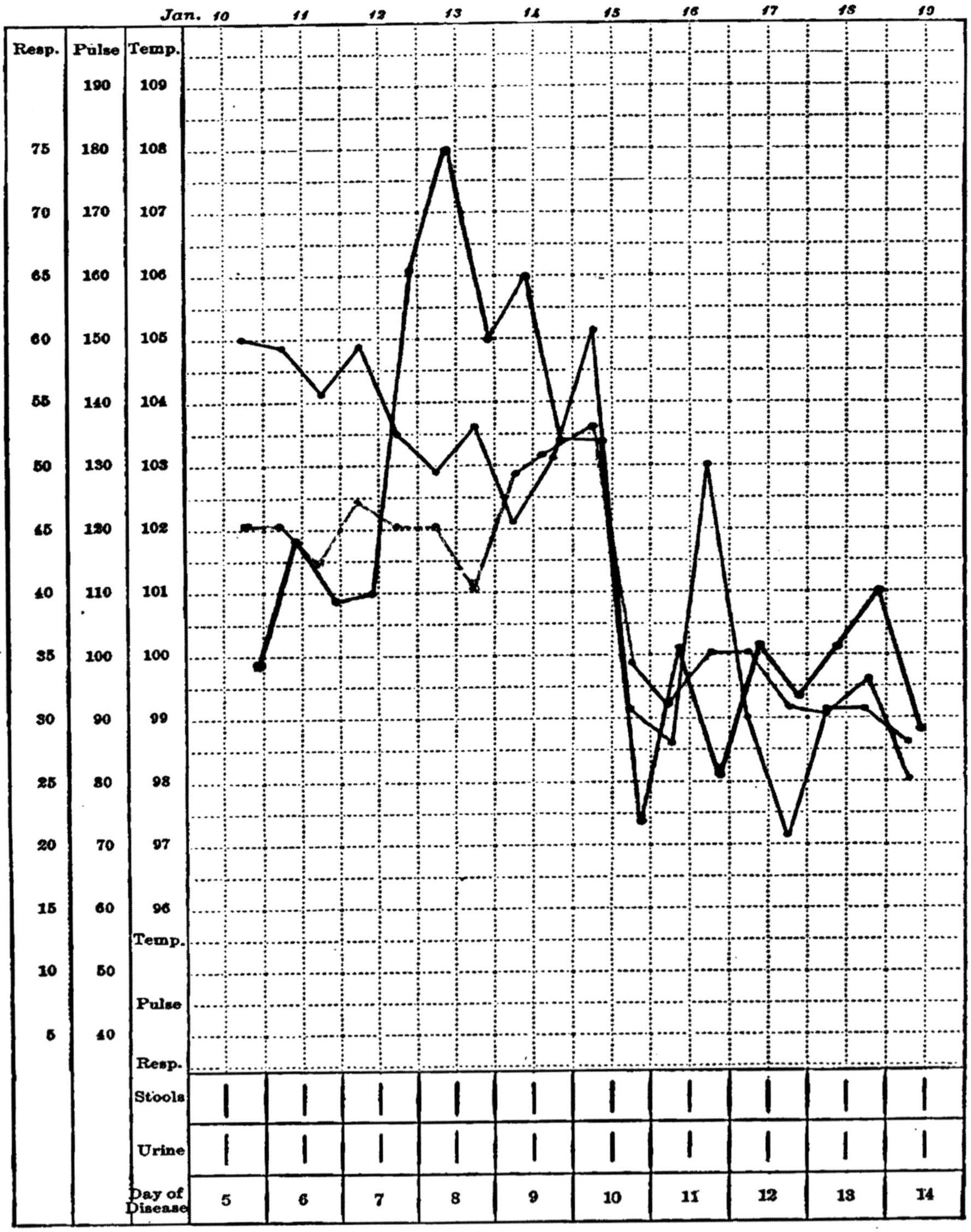

BLACK, TEMPERATURE; RED, PULSE; BLUE, RESPIRATION.

CHART III.—FEVER, PULSE AND RESPIRATION IN LOBAR PNEUMONIA

the patient passes from the condition of extreme distress and anxiety to one of comparative comfort.

SPECIAL FEATURES.—*The fever* rises rapidly, and the height may be 104°

F. or 105° F. within twelve hours. Having reached the fastigium, it is remarkably constant. Often the two-hour temperature chart will not show for two days more than a degree of variation. In children and in cases without chill the rise is more gradual. In old persons and in drunkards the temperature range is lower than in children and in healthy individuals; indeed, one occasionally meets with an afebrile pneumonia.

The Crisis.—After the fever has persisted for from five to nine or ten days there is an abrupt drop, known as the crisis, which is one of the most characteristic features of the disease. The day of the crisis is variable. It is very uncommon before the third day, and rare after the twelfth. I have seen it as early as the third day. From the time of Hippocrates it has been thought to be more frequent on the uneven days, particularly the fifth and seventh; the latter has the largest number of cases (Musser and Norris). A *precritical rise* of a degree or two may occur. In one case the temperature rose from 105° to nearly 107°, and then in a few hours fell to normal. Not even after the chill in malarial fever do we see such a prompt and rapid drop in the temperature. The usual time is from five to twelve hours, but often in an hour there may occur a fall of six or eight degrees (S. West). The temperature may be subnormal after the crisis, as low as 96° or 97°. Usually there is an abundant sweat, and the patient sinks into a comfortable sleep. The day after the crisis there may be a slight post-critical rise. A *pseudo-crisis* is not very uncommon, in which on the fifth or sixth day the temperature drops from 104° or 105° to 102°, and then rises again. When the fall takes place gradually within twenty-four hours it is called a protracted crisis. If the fever persists beyond the twelfth day, the fall is likely to be by lysis. In children this mode of termination is common, and occurred in one-third of a series of 183 cases reported by Morrill. Occasionally in debilitated individuals the temperature drops rapidly just before death; more frequently there is an ante-mortem elevation. In cases of delayed resolution the fever may persist for six or eight weeks. The crisis, the most remarkable phenomenon of pneumonia, appears to represent the stage of active immunity to the toxin of the pneumococcus. The fever, dyspnœa and the general symptoms disappear when the immunity reaches a certain stage. With the fall in the fever the respirations become reduced almost to normal, the pulse slows, and the patient passes from perhaps a state of extreme hazard and distress to one of safety and comfort, and yet, so far as the physical examination indicates, there is with the crisis no special change in the local condition in the lung. For a study of the problem see Emerson, The Johns Hopkins Hospital Reports, Vol. XV.

Pain.—There is early a sharp, agonizing pain, generally referred to the region of the nipple or lower axilla of the affected side, and much aggravated on deep inspiration and on coughing. It is associated, as Aretæus remarks, with involvement of the pleura. It is absent in central pneumonia, and much less frequent in apex pneumonia. The pain may be severe enough to require a hypodermic injection of morphia. As has been recognized for many years, the pain may be altogether abdominal, either central or in the right iliac fossa, suggesting appendicitis. Crozer Griffith, calling attention to the frequency of the simulation in children, reports 8 cases, and has collected 34 cases from the literature, many in adults. The operation for appendicitis has been performed.

Dyspnœa is an almost constant feature. Even early in the disease the respirations may be 30 in the minute, and on the second or third day between 40 and 50. The movements are shallow, evidently restrained, and if the patient is asked to draw a deep breath he cries out with the pain. Expiration is frequently interrupted by an audible grunt. At first with the increased respiration there may be no sensation of distress. Later this may be present in a marked degree. In children the respirations may be 80 or even 100. Many factors combine to produce the shortness of breath—the pain in the side, the toxæmia, the fever, and the loss of function in a considerable area of the lung tissue. Sometimes there appear to be nervous factors at work. That it does not depend upon the consolidation is shown by the fact that after the crisis, without any change in the local condition of the lung, the number of respirations may drop to normal. The ratio between the respirations and the pulse may be 1 to 2 or even 1 to 1.5, a disturbance rarely so marked in any other disease.

Cough.—This usually comes on with the pain in the side, and at first is dry, hard, and without any expectoration. Later it becomes very characteristic—frequent, short, restrained, and associated with great pain in the side. In old persons, in drunkards, in the terminal pneumonias, and sometimes in young children, there may be no cough. After the crisis the cough usually becomes much easier and the expectoration more easily expelled. The cough is sometimes persistent, continuous, and by far the most aggravated and distressing symptom of the disease. Paroxysms of coughing of great intensity after the crisis suggest a pleural exudate.

Sputum.—A brisk hæmoptysis may be the initial symptom. At first the sputum may be mucoid, but usually after twenty-four hours it becomes blood-tinged, viscid, and very tenacious. At first quite red from the unchanged blood, it gradually becomes rusty or of an orange yellow. The tenacious viscidity of the sputum is remarkable; it often has to be wiped from the lips of the patient. When jaundice is present it may be green or yellow. In low types of the disease the sputum may be fluid and of a dark brown color, resembling prune juice. The amount is very variable, ranging from 100 to 300 c. c. in the twenty-four hours. In 100 cases in my clinic studied by Emerson, in 16 there was little or no sputum; in 32 it was typically rusty; in 33 blood-streaked; in 3 cases the sputum was very bloody. In children and very old people there may be no sputum whatever. After the crisis the quantity is variable, abundant in some cases, absent in others.

Microscopically, the sputum consists of leucocytes, mucus corpuscles, red blood-corpuscles in all stages of degeneration, and bronchial and alveolar epithelium. Hæmatoidin crystals are occasionally met with. Of micro-organisms the pneumococcus is usually present, and sometimes Friedländer's bacillus, the influenza bacillus, streptococci, both pyogenes and mucosus, and the colon bacillus. Very interesting constituents are small cell moulds of the alveoli and the fibrinous casts of the bronchioles; the latter may be plainly visible to the naked eye, and sometimes may form good-sized dendritic casts. Chemically, the expectoration is particularly rich in calcium chloride.

PHYSICAL SIGNS.—*Inspection.*—The position of the patient is not constant. He usually rests more comfortably on the affected side, or he is propped up with the spine curved toward it. Orthopnœa is rare.

In a small lesion no differences may be noted between the sides; as a rule, movement is much less on the affected side, which may look larger. With involvement of a lower lobe, the apex on the same side may show greater movement. The compensatory increased movement on the sound side is sometimes very noticeable even before the patient's chest is bared. The intercostal spaces are not usually obliterated. When the cardiac lappet of the left upper lobe is involved there may be a marked increase in the area of visible cardiac pulsation. Pulsation of the affected lung may cause a marked movement of the chest wall (Graves). Other points to be noticed in the inspection are the frequency of the respiration, the action of the accessory muscles, such as the sterno-cleido-mastoids and scaleni, and the dilatation of the nostrils with each inspiration.

Mensuration may show a definite increase in the volume of the side affected, rarely more, however, than 1 or 1½ cm.

Palpation.—The lack of expansion on the affected side is sometimes more readily perceived by touch than by sight. The pleural friction may be felt. On asking the patient to count, the voice fremitus is greatly increased in comparison with the corresponding point on the healthy side. It is to be remembered that if the bronchi are filled with thick secretion, or if, in what is known as massive pneumonia, they are filled with fibrinous exudate, the tactile fremitus may be diminished. It is always well to ask the patient to cough before testing the fremitus.

Percussion.—In the stage of engorgement the note is higher pitched and may have a somewhat tympanitic quality, the so-called Skoda's resonance. This can often be obtained over the lung tissue just above a consolidated area. L. A. Conner calls attention to a point which all observers must have noticed, that, when the patient is lying on his side, the percussion at the dependent base is "deeper and more resonant than that of the upper side," which by contrast may seem abnormal, and there may even be a faint tubular element added to the vesicular breathing on the compressed side. When the lung is hepatized, the percussion note is dull, the quality varying a good deal from a note which has in it a certain tympanitic quality to one of absolute flatness. There is not the wooden flatness of effusion and the sense of resistance is not so great. During resolution the tympanitic quality of the percussion note usually returns. For weeks or months after convalescence there may be a higher-pitched note on the affected side. Wintrich's change in the percussion note when the mouth is open may be very well marked in pneumonia of the upper lobe. Occasionally there is an almost metallic quality over the consolidated area, and when this exists with a very pronounced amphoric quality in the breathing the presence of a cavity may be suggested. In deep-seated pneumonias there may be for several days no change in the percussion note.

Auscultation.—Quiet, suppressed breathing in the affected part is often a marked feature in the early stage, and is always suggestive. Only in a few cases is the breathing harsh or puerile. Very early there is heard at the end of inspiration the fine crepitant râle, a series of minute cracklings heard close to the ear, and perhaps not audible until a full breath is drawn. This is possibly a fine pleural crepitus, as J. B. Leaming maintained; it is usually believed to be produced in the air-cells and finer bronchi by the separation of the sticky exudate. In the stage of red hepatization and when dulness is well defined, the respiration is tubular. It is heard first with expiration (a point noted by James Jackson, Jr.), and is soft and of low pitch. Gradually it becomes more intense, and finally presents an intensity unknown in any other pulmonary affection—of high pitch, perfectly dry, and of equal length with inspiration and expiration. It is simply the propagation of the laryngeal and tracheal sounds through the bronchi and the consolidated lung tissue. The permeability of the bronchi is essential to its production. Tubular breathing is absent in the excessively rare cases of massive pneumonia in which the larger bronchi are completely filled with exudation. When resolution begins mucous râles of all sizes can be heard. At first they are small and have been called the *redux-crepitus.* The voice-sounds and the expiratory grunt are transmitted through the consolidated lung with great intensity. This bronchophony may have a curious nasal quality, to which the term ægophony has been given. There are cases in which the consolidation is deeply seated—so-called central pneumonia, in which the physical signs are slight or even absent, yet the cough, the rusty expectoration, and general features make the diagnosis certain.

Circulatory Symptoms.—During the chill the *pulse* is small, but in the succeeding fever it becomes full and bounding. In cases of moderate severity it ranges from 100 to 116. It is not often dicrotic. In strong, healthy individuals and in children there may be no sign of failing pulse throughout the attack. With extensive consolidation the left ventricle may receive a very much diminished amount of blood and the pulse in consequence may be small. In the old and feeble it may be small and rapid from the outset. The pulse may be full, soft, very deceptive, and of no value whatever in prognosis.

Blood Pressure.—During the first few days there is no change. The extent of involvement seems to have no effect upon the peripheral blood pressure. In the toxic cases the pressure may begin to fall early; a drop of 15-20 mm. Hg. is perfectly safe, but a progressive fall indicates the need of stimulation. A sudden drop is rarely seen except just before death. A slow, gradual fall of more than 20 mm. Hg. means cardio-vascular asthenia, and calls for an increase in the stimulation. The crisis has no effect on the blood pressure. The opinion commonly held, that when the blood pressure as expressed in millimeters of Hg. does not fall below the pulse rate expressed in beats per minute, the outlook is good, and *vice versa,* is by no means always correct. The *heart sounds* are usually loud and clear. During the intensity of the fever, particularly in children, *bruits* are not uncommon both in the mitral and in the pulmonic areas. The second sound over the pulmonary artery is accentuated. Attention to this sign gives a valuable indication as to the condition of the lesser circulation. With distention of the right chambers and failure of the right ventricle to empty itself completely, the pulmonary second sound becomes much less distinct. When the right heart is engorged there may be an increase in the dulness to the right of the sternum. With gradual heart weakness and signs of dilatation the long pause is greatly shortened, the sounds approach each other in tone and have a fetal character (embryocardia).

There may be a sudden early collapse of the heart with very feeble, rapid pulse and increasing cyanosis. I have known this to occur on the third day. Even when these symptoms are very serious recovery may take place. In other instances without any special warning death may occur even in robust, previously healthy men. The heart weakness may be due to paralysis of the vaso-motor centre and consequent lowering of the general arterial pressure. The soft, easily compressed pulse, with the gray, ashy facies, cold hands and feet, the clammy perspiration, and the progressive prostration tell of a toxic

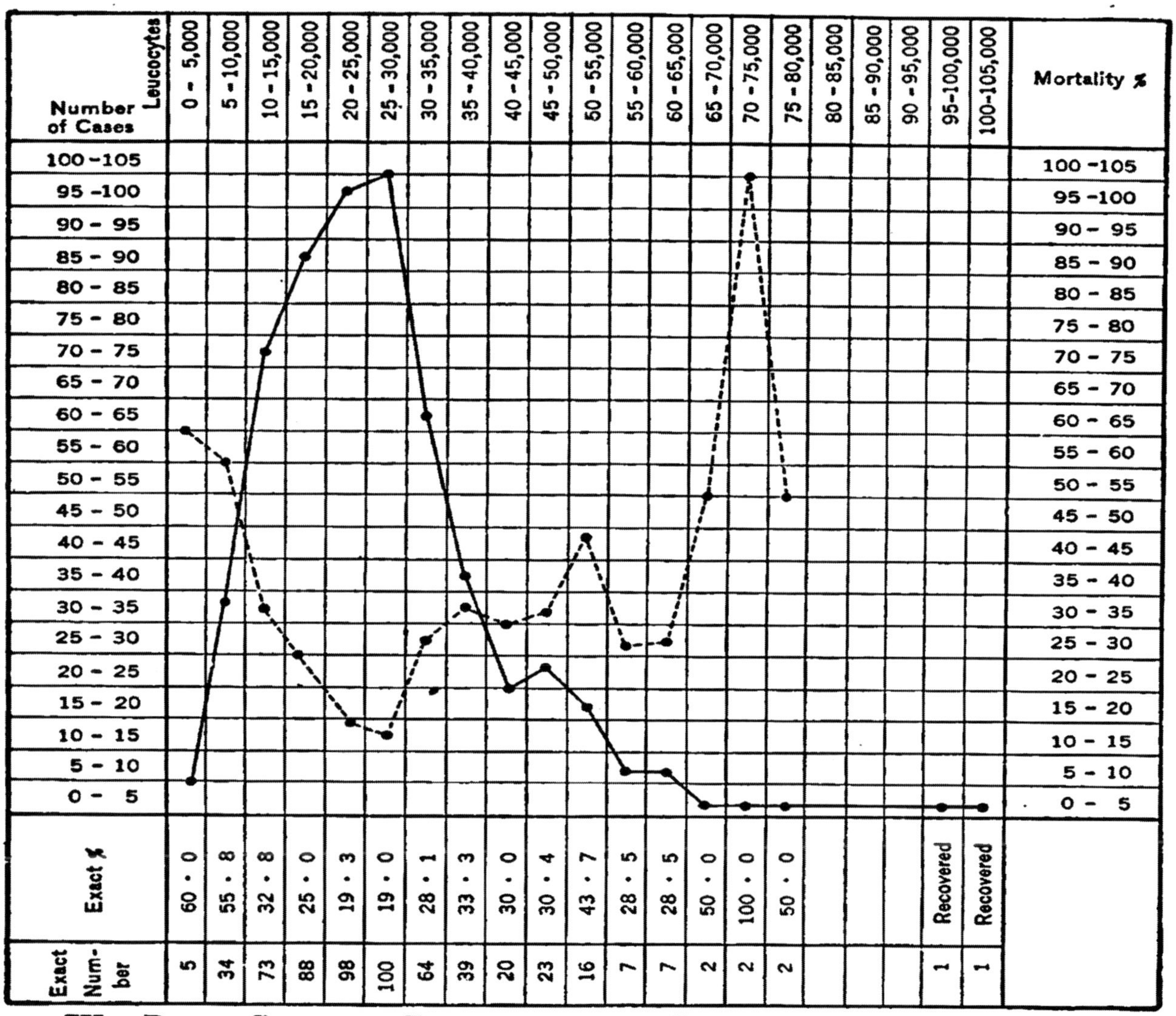

CHART IV.—BLOOD COUNT IN PNEUMONIA AND COMPARATIVE MORTALITY. CONTINUOUS LINE REPRESENTS NUMBER OF CASES OF PNEUMONIA. BROKEN LINE REPRESENTS MORTALITY PERCENTAGE OF SAME.

action on the vaso-motor centres. Endocarditis and pericarditis will be considered under complications.

Blood.—Pneumococci are present in the blood in a large proportion of all cases. Anæmia is rare. A decrease in the red cells may occur at the time of the crisis. There is in most cases a leucocytosis, which appears early, persists, and disappears with the crisis. The leucocytes may number from 12,000 to 40,000 or even 100,000 per cubic millimetre. The fall in the leucocytes is often slower than the drop in the fever, particularly when resolution is delayed or complications are present. The annexed chart gives a study of the leucocytes in 582 cases at the Johns Hopkins Hospital by Chatard. More than half of the patients, about 350, had a leucocytosis of between 15,000 and 35,000, and nearly one-third (198) between 20,000 and 30,000. The broken line represents the mortality which is high when the leucocytes are below 10,000, but steadily decreases and is lowest when they are between 20,000 and 30,0000. With the leucocytes between 30,000 and 60,000 the mortality is again higher. The two patients with the highest leucocytosis of the series, 95,000 and 105.000 respectively, recovered. A striking feature in the blood-slide is the richness and density of the fibrin network. This corresponds to the great increase in the fibrin elements, the proportion rising from 4 to 10 parts per thousand. The blood-plates are greatly increased.

Digestive Organs.—The tongue is white and furred, and in severe toxic cases rapidly becomes dry. Vomiting is not uncommon at the onset in children. The appetite is lost. Constipation is more common than diarrhœa. A distressing and sometimes dangerous symptom is meteorism. Fibrinous, pneumococcic exudates may occur in the conjunctivæ, nose, mouth, prepuce, and anus (Cary). The liver may be depressed by the large right lung, or enlarged from the engorged right heart or as a result of the infection. The spleen is usually enlarged, and the edge can be felt during a deep inspiration.

Skin.—Among *cutaneous* symptoms one of the most interesting is the association of herpes with pneumonia. Not excepting malaria, we see labial herpes more frequently in this than in any other disease, occurring, as it does, in from 12 to 40 per cent. of the cases. It is supposed to be of favorable prognosis, and figures have been quoted in proof of this assertion. It may also occur on the nose, genitals, and anus. Its significance and relation to the disease are unknown. At the height of the disease sweats are not common, but at the crisis they may be profuse. Redness of one cheek is a phenomenon long recognized in connection with pneumonia, and is usually on the same side as the disease. A diffuse erythema is occasionally seen, and in rare cases purpura. Jaundice is referred to among the complications.

Urine.—Early in the disease it presents the usual febrile characters of high color, high specific gravity, and increased acidity. A trace of albumin is very common. There may be tube-casts, and in a few instances the existence of albumin, tube-casts, and blood indicates the presence of an acute nephritis. The urea and uric acid are usually increased at first, but may be much diminished before the crisis, to increase greatly with its onset. Robert Hutchison's researches show that a true retention of chlorides within the body takes place, the average amount being about 2 grams daily. It is a more constant feature of pneumonia than of any other febrile disease, and this being the case, a diminution of the chlorides in the urine may be of value in the diagnosis from pleurisy with effusion or empyema. It is to be remembered that in dilatation of the stomach chlorides may be absent. Hæmaturia is a rare complication.

Cerebral Symptoms.—Headache is common. In children convulsions occur frequently at the outset. Apart from meningitis, which will be considered separately, one may group the cases with marked cerebral features into:

First, the so-called cerebral pneumonias of children, in which the disease sets in with a convulsion, and there are high fever, headache, delirium, great irritability, muscular tremor, and perhaps retraction of the head and neck.

The diagnosis of meningitis is usually made, and the local affection may be overlooked.

Secondly, the cases with maniacal symptoms. These may occur at the very outset, and there may be no suspicion whatever that the disease is other than acute mania.

Thirdly, alcoholic cases with the features of delirium tremens. It should be an invariable rule, even if fever be not present, to examine the lungs in a case of *mania a potu*.

Fourthly, cases with toxic features, rather resembling those of uræmia. Without a chill and without cough or pain in the side, a patient may have fever, a little shortness of breath, and then gradually grow dull mentally, and within three days be in profound toxæmia with low, muttering delirium.

It is stated that apex pneumonia is more often accompanied with severe delirium. Occasionally the cerebral symptoms occur immediately after the crisis. Mental disturbance may persist during and after convalescence, and in a few instances delusional insanity follows, the outlook in which is favorable.

Hemiplegia may be due to thrombosis, embolism, abscess or œdema. Withington has called attention to a form associated with encephalitis. It may be transient and recovery complete. Transient *aphasia*, with or without hemiplegia, may also occur and there are cases in which no gross lesions have been found, so that it has been suggested that it is due to œdema or to a relative ischæmia.

Complications.—Compared with typhoid fever, pneumonia has but few complications and still fewer sequelæ. The most important are the following:

Pleurisy is an inevitable event when the inflammation reaches the surface of the lung, and thus can scarcely be termed a complication. But there are cases in which the pleuritic features take the first place. The exudation may be sero-fibrinous with copious effusion, differing from that of an ordinary acute pleurisy in the greater richness of the fibrin, which may form thick, tenacious, curdy layers. Pneumonia on one side with extensive pleurisy on the other is sometimes a puzzling complication to diagnose, and an aspirating needle may be required to settle the question. *Empyema* is a most common complication occurring in 2.2 per cent. of clinical cases collected by Musser and Norris and in 3.6 per cent. of the Johns Hopkins Hospital series. During the eight years, 1883-'90, there were at Guy's Hospital 7 cases of empyema among 445 cases of pneumonia, while in the eight years, 1891-'98, there were 38 cases among 896 cases of pneumonia (Hale White). Influenza may be responsible for the increase. The pneumococcus is usually present; in a few the streptococcus, in which case the prognosis is not so good. Recurrence of the fever after the crisis or persistence of it after the tenth day, with sweats, leucocytosis, and an aggravation of the cough, are suspicious symptoms. The dulness persists at the base, or may extend. The breathing is feeble and there are no râles. Such a condition may be closely simulated, of course, by a thickened pleura. Exploratory aspiration may settle the question at once. There are obscure cases in which the pus has been found only after operation, as the collection may be very small. The X-rays often give aid.

Pericarditis, one of the most serious of complications was present in 35 of 658 patients in my wards at the Johns Hopkins Hospital (Chatard). It is often a terminal affair and overlooked. The mortality is very high; 31 of the

35 patients died. It was most frequently associated with pneumonia of the right lung. In only three instances was the amount of fluid above 500 c. c. Pleurisy is an almost constant accompaniment, being present in 28 of the 29 autopsies in my series.

Endocarditis.—The valves on the left side are more commonly attacked, and particularly if the seat of arterio-sclerosis. It is especially liable to attack persons with old valvular disease. There may be no symptoms indicative of this complication even in very severe cases. It may, however, be suspected in cases (1) in which the fever is protracted and irregular; (2) when signs of septic mischief arise, such as chills and sweats; (3) when embolic phenomena appear. The frequent complication of meningitis with the endocarditis of pneumonia, which has already been mentioned, gives prominence to the cerebral symptoms in these cases. The physical signs may be very deceptive. There are instances in which no cardiac murmurs have been heard. In others the occurrence under observation of a loud, rough murmur, particularly if diastolic, is extremely suggestive.

Ante-mortem clotting in the heart, upon which the old writers laid great stress, is very rare. *Thrombosis* in the peripheral veins is also uncommon. Three cases occurred at my clinic, which have been reported by Steiner, who was able to collect only 54 cases from the literature. In 35 out of 44 cases which were fully reported, the thrombosis occurred during convalescence. It is almost always in the femoral veins. A rare complication is *embolism* of one of the larger arteries. I saw in Montreal an instance of embolism of the femoral artery at the height of pneumonia, which necessitated amputation at the thigh. The patient recovered. *Aphasia* has been met with in a few instances, setting in abruptly with or without hemiplegia.

Meningitis is perhaps the most serious complication of pneumonia. It varies very much at different times and in different regions. My Montreal experience is rather exceptional, as 8 per cent. of the fatal cases had this complication. In twenty years at the Johns Hopkins Hospital there were 25 cases of pneumococcus meningitis, in 18 of which pneumonia was present. In 16 of the cases the organism was demonstrated in the cerebro-spinal fluid. Endocarditis was present in 7 of the 18 cases. The percentage of meningitis in the pneumonia cases was 2.4, which is lower than the figures of Musser and Norris of 3.5 per cent. in 4,883 autopsies. It usually comes on at the height of the fever, and in the majority of the cases is not recognized unless, as before mentioned, the base is involved, which is not common. Occurring later in the disease, it is more easily diagnosed. The prognosis is bad; all of our patients died. A few instances of recovery are on record.

Peripheral neuritis is a rare complication, of which several cases have been described.

Gastric complications are rare. Fussell has recently drawn attention to the occurrence of acute *dilatation of the stomach.* Persistent vomiting, sudden abdominal distention and collapse are the most common features. A croupous gastritis has already been mentioned. The *croupous colitis* may induce severe diarrhœa.

It is by no means uncommon to have early *pain,* either in the region of the umbilicus or in the right iliac fossa, and a suspicion of appendicitis is aroused; indeed, a catarrhal form of this disease may occur coincidently with the pneumonia. In other instances so localized may the pain be in the region of the pancreas, associated with meteorism and high fever, that the diagnosis of acute hæmorrhagic pancreatitis is made. Such a case occurred in February, 1905, in the wards of my colleague Dr. Halsted. The patient was admitted in a desperate condition, all the symptoms were abdominal, and the apex pneumonia was not discovered. *Peritonitis* is a rare complication, of which we have had only two or three instances. It is sometimes in the upper peritoneum, and a direct extension through the diaphragm. It is usually in the severer cases and not easy to recognize. In one case, indeed, in which there was a friction along the costal border, which we thought indicated a peritonitis; it was communicated from the diaphragmatic pleura. *Meteorism* is not infrequent, and is sometimes serious. In some cases it may be due to a defect in the mechanical action of the diaphragm, in others to an acute septic catarrh of the bowels, or to a toxic paresis of the walls, occasionally to peritonitis. *Jaundice* occurs with curious irregularity in different outbreaks of the disease. In Baltimore it was more common among the negro patients. It sets in early, is rarely very intense, and has not the characters of obstructive jaundice. There are cases in which it assumes a very serious form. The mode of production is not well ascertained. It does not appear to bear any definite relation to the degree of hepatic engorgement, and it is not always due to catarrh of the ducts. Possibly it may be, in great part, hæmatogenous.

Parotitis occasionally occurs, commonly in association with endocarditis. In children, middle-ear disease is not an infrequent complication.

Bright's disease does not often follow pneumonia.

Arthritis occurred in 5 of 658 cases at the Johns Hopkins Hospital (Howard). It may precede the onset, and the pneumonia, possibly with endocarditis and pleurisy, may occur as a complication. In other instances at the height of an ordinary pneumonia one or two joints may become red and sore. On the other hand, after the crisis has occurred pain and swelling may come on in the joints. It is a serious complication as recovery is often slow and a stiff joint may follow.

Relapse.—There are cases in which from the ninth to the eleventh day the fever subsides, and after the temperature has been normal for a day or two a rise occurs and fever may persist for another ten days or even two weeks. Though this might be termed a relapse, it is more correct to regard it as an instance of an anomalous course or delayed resolution. Wagner, who has studied the subject carefully, says that in his large experience of 1,100 cases he met with only 3 doubtful cases. When it does occur, the attack is usually abortive and mild. In the case of Z. R. (Medical No. J. H. H., 4223), with pneumonia of the right lower lobe, crisis occurred on the seventh day, and after a normal temperature for thirteen days he was discharged. That night he had a shaking chill, followed by fever, and he had recurring chills with reappearance of the pneumonia. In a second case (Medical No. J. H. H., 4538) crisis occurred on the third day, and there was recurrence of pneumonia on the thirteenth day.

Recurrence is more common in pneumonia than in any other acute disease. Rush gives an instance in which there were 28 attacks. Other authorities narrate cases of 8, 10, and even more attacks.

Convalescence in pneumonia is usually rapid, and sequelæ are rare. After the crisis, sudden death has occurred when the patient has got up too soon. With the onset of fever and persistence of the leucocytosis the affected side should be very carefully examined for pleurisy. With a persistence of the dulness the physical signs may be obscure, but the use of a small exploratory needle or the X-rays will help to clear the diagnosis.

Clinical Varieties.—Local variations are responsible for some of the most marked deviations from the usual type.

Apex pneumonia is said to be more often associated with adynamic features and with marked cerebral symptoms. The expectoration and cough may be slight.

Migratory or *creeping pneumonia*, a form which successively involves one lobe after the other.

Double pneumonia has no peculiarities other than the greater danger connected with it.

Massive pneumonia is a rare form, in which not alone the air-cells but the bronchi of an entire lobe or even of a lung are filled with the fibrinous exudate. The auscultatory signs are absent; there is neither fremitus nor tubular breathing, and on percussion the lung is absolutely flat. It closely resembles pleurisy with effusion. The moulds of the bronchi may be expectorated in violent fits of coughing.

Central Pneumonia.—The inflammation may be deep-seated at the root of the lung or centrally placed in a lobe, and for several days the diagnosis may be in doubt. It may not be until the third or fourth day that a pleural friction is detected, or that dulness or blowing breathing and râles are recognized. I saw in 1898 with Drs. H. Adler and Chew a young, thin-chested girl in whom at the end of the fourth day all the usual symptoms of pneumonia were present without any physical signs other than a few clicking râles at the left apex behind. The thinness of the patient greatly facilitated the examination. The general features of pneumonia continued, and the crisis occurred on the seventh day.

PNEUMONIA IN INFANTS.—It is sometimes seen in the new-born. In infants it very often sets in with a convulsion. The apex of the lung seems more frequently involved than in adults, and the cerebral symptoms are more marked. The torpor and coma, particularly if they follow convulsions, and the preliminary stage of excitement, may lead to the diagnosis of meningitis. Pneumonic sputum is rarely seen in children.

PNEUMONIA IN THE AGED.—The disease may be latent and set in without a chill; the cough and expectoration are slight, the physical signs ill-defined and changeable, and the constitutional symptoms out of all proportion to the extent of the local lesion.

PNEUMONIA IN ALCOHOLIC SUBJECTS.—The onset is insidious, the symptoms masked, the fever slight, and the clinical picture usually that of delirium tremens. The thermometer alone may indicate the presence of an acute disease. Often the local condition is overlooked, as the patient makes no complaint of pain, and there may be very little shortness of breath, no cough, and no sputum.

TERMINAL PNEUMONIA.—The wards and the post mortem room show a very striking contrast in their pneumonia statistics, owing to the occurrence of what may be called terminal pneumonia. During the winter months patients with chronic pulmonary tuberculosis, arterio-sclerosis, heart disease, Bright's disease, and diabetes are not infrequently carried off by a pneumonia which may give few or no signs of its presence. In the Johns Hopkins Hospital series of 658 cases, there were 35 cases of this variety, 20 of which were associated with cardio-vascular and 14 with renal disease. It is nearly always of the lobar form. There may be a slight elevation of temperature, with increase in the respirations, but the patient is near the end and perhaps not in a condition in which a thorough physical examination can be made. In our series the right lung was involved in 19 cases and 9 had a low leucocyte count. In diabetic patients the disease often runs a rapid and severe course, and may end in abscess or gangrene.

SECONDARY PNEUMONIA.—These are met with chiefly in the specific fevers, particularly diphtheria, typhoid fever, typhus, influenza, and the plague. Anatomically, they rarely present the typical form of red or gray hepatization. The surface is smoother, not so dry, and it is often a pseudo-lobar condition, a consolidation caused by closely set areas of lobular involvement. Histologically, they are characterized in many instances by a more cellular, less fibrinous exudate, which may also infiltrate the alveolar walls. Bacteriologically, the pneumococcus may be the dominant organism; but Friedländer's bacillus, streptococci, staphylococci, the influenza and colon bacillus have been found.

The symptoms of the secondary pneumonias often lack the striking definiteness of the primary croupous pneumonia. The pulmonary features may be latent or masked altogether. There may be no cough and only a slight increase in the number of respirations. The lower lobe of one lung is most commonly involved, and the physical signs are obscure and rarely amount to more than impaired resonance, feeble breathing, and a few crackling râles.

EPIDEMIC PNEUMONIA has already been referred to. It is, as a rule, more fatal, and often displays minor complications which differ in different outbreaks. In some the cerebral manifestations are very marked; in others, the cardiac; in others again, the gastro-intestinal.

LARVAL PNEUMONIA.—Mild, abortive types are seen, particularly in institutions when pneumonia is prevailing extensively. A patient may have the initial symptoms of the disease, a slight chill, moderate fever, a few indefinite local signs, and herpes. The whole process may only last for two or three days; some authors recognize even a one-day pneumonia.

ASTHENIC, TOXIC, OR TYPHOID PNEUMONIA.—The toxæmic features dominate the scene throughout. The local lesions may be slight in extent and the subjective phenomena of the disease absent. The nervous symptoms usually predominate. There are delirium, prostration, and early weakness. Very frequently there is jaundice. Gastro-intestinal symptoms may be present, particularly diarrhœa and meteorism. In such a case, seen about the end of the first week, it may be difficult to say whether the condition is one of asthenic pneumonia or one of typhoid fever which has set in with early localization in the lung. Here the Widal reaction and cultures from the blood are important aids. The pneumococcus may sometimes be isolated from the blood. Possibly, too, there is a mixed infection, and the streptococcus pyogenes may be in large part responsible for the toxic features of the disease.

ASSOCIATION OF PNEUMONIA WITH OTHER DISEASES.—(*a*) *With Malaria.* —A malarial pneumonia is described by many observers and thought to be particularly prevalent in some parts of the United States. One hears of it, indeed, even where true malaria is rarely seen. Pneumonia is a common disease in the tropics and often attacks the subjects of malaria. The prognosis is bad in the æstivo-autumnal infections. A special form of pneumonia due to the malarial parasite is unknown. Yet there are cases reported by Craig and others in which in an acute malarial infection the features suggest pneumonia at the onset, but the parasites are found in the blood, and under the use of quinine the fever drops rapidly and the pneumonia symptoms clear up. Such a case as the following we see occasionally: A patient was admitted, March 16, 1894, with tertian malarial fever. The lungs were clear. A pneumonia began thirty-six hours after admission. Quinine was given that evening, and the malarial organisms rapidly disappeared from the blood. There was successive involvement of the right lower, the middle, and the left lower lobe. The temperature fell by crisis on the 24th, and there were no features in the disease whatever suggestive of malaria. In other instances we have found a chill in the course of an ordinary pneumonia to be associated with a malarial infection, and quinine has rapidly and promptly caused the disappearance of the parasites from the blood.

(*b*) *Pneumonia and Acute Arthritis.*—We have already spoken under complications of this association, which is more frequently seen in children.

(*c*) *Pneumonia and Tuberculosis.*—Many subjects of chronic pulmonary tuberculosis die of an acute croupous pneumonia. A point to be specially borne in mind is the fact that acute tuberculous pneumonia may set in with all the features and physical signs of fibrinous pneumonia.

For the consideration of the association of pneumonia with typhoid fever and influenza, the reader is referred to the sections on those diseases.

Post-operation Pneumonia.—Before the days of anæsthesia, lobar pneumonia was a well-recognized cause of death after surgical injuries and operations. Norman Cheevers, in an early number of the Guy's Hospital Reports, calls attention to it as one of the most frequent causes of death after surgical procedures, and Erichsen states that of 41 deaths after surgical injuries 23 cases showed signs of pneumonia. In the statistics collected by Homans the mortality due to lung complications after laparotomies ranged from 0.56 to 12.5. Operations on the stomach seem to be peculiarly liable to be followed by pneumonia. The low figure, 0.56, in Krönlein's clinic may be attributed to the use of ether by the open method, to the absence of all preparation on the table and to shortening as much as possible the period of anæsthesia. The cases may be divided into three groups: (1) Inhalation or anæsthesia pneumonia, characterized by areas of broncho-pneumonia or a lobar pneumonia. (2) Hypostatic pneumonia due to enfeebled circulation. (3) Embolic cases with sudden onset. The route may be lymphatic or through the veins.

Anæsthesia Pneumonia.—The cases appear to be quite as frequent after chloroform as after ether. The vapor of the anæsthetic may itself have a damaging influence on the bronchial and alveolar epithelium, but a more important influence is the aspiration of mucus and saliva into the air passages during the anæsthesia. Neuwerck, and subsequently Whitney, have suggested thorough disinfection of the mouth and throat before operation. Pneumonia is the most frequent complication, next a diffuse bronchitis. W. Pasteur has called attention to a condition of massive collapse of the lungs due to deflation of the lower lobes, owing to imperfect action or paralysis of the diaphragm. He has published the statistics of lung complications at the Middlesex Hospital; following 3,559 abdominal operations there were 201 pulmonary complications, with 45 deaths. Among these pneumonia heads the list with 88 cases and 31 deaths. The complications are much more numerous in operations above the umbilicus. The pneumonia is usually patchy, involving both lungs; sometimes it is lobar, and as a rule the signs are well marked within the first two days after operation. The collapse, to which Pasteur calls attention, may involve both lower lobes or only one lung, and it may simulate pneumonia very closely, or may initiate it. When unilateral, the mediastinum and heart are drawn towards the affected side. It may come on with great suddenness, and when widespread it may prove fatal.

Delayed Resolution in Pneumonia.—The lung is restored to its normal state by the liquefaction and absorption of the exudate. There are cases in which resolution takes place rapidly without any increase in (or, indeed, without any) expectoration; on the other hand, during resolution it is not uncommon to find in the sputum the little plugs of fibrin and leucocytes which have been loosened from the air-cells and expelled by coughing. A variable time is taken in the restoration of the lung. Sometimes within a week or ten days the dulness is greatly diminished, the breath-sounds become clear, and, so far as physical signs are any guide, the lung seems perfectly restored. Delayed resolution occurs in from 3 to 4 per cent. of cases. Of 40 cases at the Johns Hopkins Hospital studied by McCrae, 33 were males and 7 females; 23 of the patients were negroes, a very high incidence. The lower lobe is most frequently involved, 37 cases in this series, usually the right one and as a rule only one lobe. The duration was to the fourth week 5 cases, fifth week 10 cases, sixth week 4 cases, ninth week 3 cases, tenth, eleventh and twelfth weeks each one case. I saw a patient in whom the left lung, except a small portion of the upper lobe, remained solid for eleven weeks and then cleared perfectly.

Clinically, there are several groups of cases: First, those in which the crisis occurs naturally, the temperature falls and remains normal; but the local features persist—well-marked flatness with tubular breathing and râles. Resolution may occur very slowly and gradually, taking from two to three weeks. In a second group of cases the temperature falls by lysis, and with the persistence of the local signs there is slight fever, sometimes sweats and rapid pulse. The condition may persist for three or four weeks and during all this time there may be little or no sputum. The practitioner is naturally much exercised, and he dreads lest tuberculosis should supervene. In a third group the crisis occurs or the fever falls by lysis; but the consolidation persists, and there may be intense bronchial breathing, with few or no râles, or the fever may recur and the patient may die exhausted.

Termination in Chronic Pneumonia.—The exudate may organize and the alveolar walls thicken with the production gradually of a chronic interstitial or fibroid pneumonia. In one of my pneumonia autopsies on a patient aged 58, dead on the thirty-second day from the initial chill, the right lung was solid and the cut surface grayish in color with a smooth, translucent appearance. This termination is most frequently seen as a sequence of delayed resolution in debilitated subjects. In a recent study Milne found 10 instances of organization of the exudate among 150 fatal cases. The shortest duration in the series was twenty-three days.

Ordinary fibrinous pneumonia never terminates in tuberculosis. The instances of caseous pneumonia and softening which have followed an acute pneumonic process have been from the outset tuberculous.

TERMINATION IN ABSCESS.—This occurred in 4 of my 100 autopsies. Usually the lung breaks down in limited areas and the abscesses are not large, but they may fuse and involve a considerable proportion of a lobe. The condition is recognized by the sputum, which is usually abundant and contains pus and elastic tissue, sometimes cholesterin crystals and hæmatoidin crystals. The cough is often paroxysmal and of great severity; usually the fever is remittent, or in protracted cases intermittent in character, and there may be pronounced hectic symptoms. When a case is seen for the first time it may be difficult to determine whether it is one of abscess of the lung or a local empyema which has perforated the lung.

GANGRENE.—This is most commonly seen in old debilitated persons. It was present in 3 of my 100 autopsies. It very often occurs with abscess. The gangrene is associated with the growth of the saprophytic bacteria on a soil made favorable by the presence of the pneumococcus or the streptococcus. Clinically, the gangrene is rendered very evident by the horribly fetid odor of the expectoration and its characteristic features. In some instances the gangrene may be found post mortem when clinically there has not been any evidence of its existence.

Prognosis.—Pneumonia is one of the most fatal of all acute diseases, killing more than diphtheria, and outranking even consumption as a cause of death. In America the mortality appears to be increasing.

The statistics of my clinic at the Johns Hopkins Hospital from 1889 to 1905 have been analyzed by Chatard. There were 658 cases with 200 deaths, a mortality of 30.4 per cent. Excluding 35 cases of terminal pneumonia the percentage is 26.4. The death rate among 245 negroes was very little above that of the whites. Greenwood and Candy in a study of the pneumonia statistics at the London Hospital from 1854-1903, a total of 5,097 cases, conclude that the fatality of the disease has not appreciably changed in this period. In comparing the collected figures of these authors with those from other institutions, there is an extraordinary uniformity in the mortality rate. Between the ages of 21-30 the mortality is everywhere about 20 per cent.; between the ages of 31-40, 30 per cent.; and then after each decade it rises, until above the age of 60 more than one-half of the persons attacked die.

The mortality in private practice varies greatly. R. P. Howard treated 170 cases with only 6 per cent. of deaths. Fussell has reported 134 cases with a mortality of 17.9 per cent. The mortality in children is sometimes very low. Morrill has reported 6 deaths in 123 cases of frank pneumonia. On the other hand, Goodhart had 25 deaths in 120 cases.

The following are among the circumstances which influence the prognosis:

Age.—As Sturges remarks, the old are likely to die, the young to recover. Under one year it is more fatal than between two and five. Of 50 cases under 10 years of age 4 died; of 119 cases under 20, 16 died (Chatard). Above sixty the death rate is very high, amounting to 60 or 80 per cent.; 33 of 44 cases in my series. From the reports of its fatality in some places, one may say that to die of pneumonia is almost the natural end of old people.

Previous habits of life and the condition of bodily health at the time of the attack form the most important factors in the prognosis of pneumonia. In analyzing a series of fatal cases one is very much impressed with the number of cases in which the organs show signs of degeneration. In 25 of my 100 autopsies at the Montreal General Hospital the kidneys showed extensive interstitial changes. Individuals debilitated from sickness or poor food, hard drinkers, and that large class of hospital patients, composed of robust-looking laborers between the ages of forty-five and sixty, whose organs show signs of wear and tear, and who have by excesses in alcohol weakened the reserve power, fall an easy prey to the disease. Very few fatal cases occur in robust, healthy adults. Some of the statistics given by army surgeons show better than any others the low mortality from pneumonia in healthy picked men. The death rate in the German army in over 40,000 cases was only 3.6 per cent.

Certain *complications* and terminations are particularly serious. The meningitis of pneumonia is almost always fatal. Endocarditis is extremely grave, much more so than pericarditis. Much stress has been laid of late upon the factor of *leucocytosis* as an element in the prognosis. A very slight or complete absence of a leucocytosis is rightly regarded as very unfavorable.

Toxæmia is the important prognostic feature in the disease, to which in a majority of the cases the degree of pyrexia and the extent of consolidation are entirely subsidiary. It is not at all proportionate to the degree of lung involved. A severe and fatal toxæmia may occur with the consolidation of only a small part of one lobe. On the other hand, a patient with complete solidification of one lung may have no signs of a general infection. The question of individual resistance seems to be the most important one, and one sees robust-looking individuals fatally stricken within a few days.

Death is rarely due to direct interference with the function of respiration, even in double pneumonia. Sometimes it seems to be caused by the extensive involvement with œdema of the other parts of the lungs, an engorgement with progressive weakness of the right heart. But death is most frequently due to the action of the poisons on the vaso-motor centres, with progressive lowering of the blood pressure. This is a much more serious factor than direct weakness of the heart muscle itself.

Diagnosis.—No disease is more readily recognized in a large majority of the cases. The external characters, the sputum, and the physical signs combine to make one of the clearest of clinical pictures. The ordinary lobar pneumonia of adults is rarely overlooked. Errors are particularly liable to occur in the intercurrent pneumonias, in those complicating chronic affections, and in the disease as met with in children, the aged, and drunkards. Tuberculo-pneumonic phthisis is frequently confounded with pneumonia. Pleurisy with effusion is not often mistaken except in children. The diagnostic points will be referred to under pleurisy.

In diabetes, Bright's disease, chronic heart-disease, pulmonary phthisis, and cancer, an acute pneumonia often ends the scene, and is frequently overlooked. In these cases the temperature is perhaps the best index, and should, more particularly if cough occurs, lead to a careful examination of the lungs.

The absence of expectoration and of pulmonary symptoms may make the diagnosis very difficult.

In children there are two special sources of error; the disease may be entirely masked by the cerebral symptoms and the case mistaken for one of meningitis. It is remarkable in these cases how few indications there are of pulmonary trouble. The other condition is pleurisy with effusion, which in children often has deceptive physical signs. The breathing may be intensely tubular and tactile fremitus may be present. The exploratory needle is sometimes required to decide the question. In the old and debilitated a knowledge that the onset of pneumonia is insidious, and that the symptoms are ill-defined and latent, should put the practitioner on his guard and make him very careful in the examination of the lungs in doubtful cases. In chronic alcoholism the cerebral symptoms may completely mask the local process. As mentioned, the disease may assume the form of violent mania, but more commonly the symptoms are those of delirium tremens. In any case, rapid pulse, rapid respiration, and fever are symptoms which should invariably excite suspicion of inflammation of the lungs. Under cerebro-spinal meningitis will be found the points of differential diagnosis between pneumonia and that disease.

Pneumonia is rarely confounded with pulmonary tuberculosis, but to differentiate acute tuberculo-pneumonic phthisis is often difficult. The attack may set in with a chill. It may be impossible to determine which condition is present until softening occurs and elastic tissue and tubercle bacilli appear in the sputum. A similar mistake is sometimes made in children. With typhoid fever, pneumonia is not infrequently confounded. There are instances of pneumonia with the local signs well marked in which the patient rapidly sinks into what is known as the typhoid state, with dry tongue, rapid pulse, and diarrhœa. Unless the case is seen from the outset it may be very difficult to determine the true nature of the malady. On the other hand, there are cases of typhoid fever which set in with symptoms of lobar pneumonia—the so-called pneumo-typhus. It may be impossible to make a differential diagnosis in such a case unless the characteristic eruption occurs, a blood culture is positive, or the Widal reaction is given.

Prophylaxis.—We do not know the percentage of individuals who harbor the pneumococcus normally in the secretions of the mouth and throat. In a great majority of cases it is an auto-infection, and the lowered resistance due to exposure or to alcohol, or a trauma or anæsthetization, simply furnishes conditions which favor the spread and growth of an organism already present. Individuals who have already had pneumonia should be careful to keep the teeth in good condition, and the mouth and throat in as healthy a state as possible. Antiseptic mouth washes may be used.

We know practically nothing of the conditions under which the pneumococcus lives outside the body, or how it gains entrance in healthy individuals. The sputum of each case should be very carefully disinfected. In institutions the patients should be isolated.

Treatment.—Pneumonia is a self-limited disease, which can neither be aborted nor cut short by any known means at our command. Even under the most unfavorable circumstances it may terminate abruptly and naturally. So also, under the favoring circumstances of good nursing and careful diet, the experience of many physicians in different lands has shown that pneumonia runs its course in a definite time, terminating sometimes spontaneously on the third or the fifth day, or continuing until the tenth or twelfth.

Morgenroth and Levy claim for optochin, a quinine derivative, a specific action on the pneumococcus. It has a well-marked protective action against experimental infection in mice; encouraging, but scarcely good enough results to use the term specific have been reported clinically.

(*a*) General Management of a Case.—The same careful hygiene of the bed and of the sick-room should be carried out as in typhoid fever. Everything should be done to make the patient comfortable and to save him exertion. Whenever possible the patient should be in the open air. In cold weather he should have sufficient covering to keep him warm, but should not be overburdened by a heavy weight of clothes. A blanket and rubber sheet, under the mattress, which can be folded up over the bed prevent chilling from below. A hot-water bag should be kept at the feet. The patient is brought indoors when necessary for hydrotherapy. For the heavy flannel undershirts should be substituted a thin, light flannel jacket, open in front, which enables the physician to make his examinations without unnecessarily disturbing the patient. If the patient is indoors the room should be bright and light, letting in the sunshine if possible, and thoroughly well ventilated. Only one or two persons should be allowed in the room at a time. Even when not called for on account of the high fever, the patient should be carefully sponged each day with tepid water. This should be done with as little disturbance as possible. Special care should be taken to keep the mouth and nose clean.

(*b*) Diet.—Plain water, a pleasant table water, or lemonade should be given freely. When the patient is delirious the water should be given at fixed intervals and by the bowel or by infusion if it is not taken by mouth. The food should be liquid, consisting chiefly of milk, either alone or, better, mixed with food prepared from some one of the cereals, and eggs, either soft boiled or raw. Carbohydrate, as milk sugar, can be added to each feeding of milk, and as cane sugar to lemonade.

(*c*) Bowels.—At the onset it is well to give a calomel and saline purge. The bowels can be kept open by salines or enemata. Drastic purgation is not advisable. It is important to prevent *meteorism*, if possible, by care in the diet, giving water freely and preventing constipation. If present, measures for relief should be begun at once. Turpentine stupes, turpentine (℥ ss, 15 c. c.) added to an enema, and the use of the rectal tube, are helpful. Strychnine and pituitary extract hypodermically are also useful. If the stomach is distended a stomach tube should be passed.

(*d*) Bleeding.—The reproach of Van Helmont, that "a bloody Moloch presides in the chairs of medicine," can not be brought against this generation of physicians. Before Louis' iconoclastic paper on bleeding in pneumonia it would have been regarded as almost criminal to treat a case without venesection. We employ it nowadays much more than we did a few years ago, but more often late in the disease than early. To bleed at the very onset in robust, healthy individuals in whom the disease sets in with great intensity and high fever is, I believe, a good practice. Late in the course marked dilatation of the right heart is the common indication. The quantity of blood removed must be decided by the effect; small amounts are often sufficient.

(*e*) Antipneumococcic Serum.—The value of this method of treatment is on trial. With prompt and accurate means to determine the variety of pneumococcus causing the attack much may be expected. Good results have been obtained by the early use of large doses, particularly in Type I.

(*f*) Hydrotherapy.—This—internal and external—is our principal means of combatting toxæmia and circulatory failure. Cold sponging is usually the best measure, done every three hours and with the least possible disturbance of the patient. With marked toxæmia or hyperpyrexia a bath at 80° with constant friction may be given for five minutes if it does not increase distress or dyspnœa. The application of linen compresses covered by flannel is an excellent measure. They should be cut to the size of the body, in the shape of a jacket, with the opening at one side instead of in the front, which can be applied from the side of the body with the patient turned, and fastened over the other shoulder and in the axilla. They should be wrung out of water at 50° to 60° and be changed every hour. The compress should cover the thorax and upper abdomen. A large flat ice bag may be kept to the side or back constantly, unless it causes distress. Probably the best effect of hydrotherapy is its effect on the vaso-motor system.

(*g*) Symptomatic Treatment.—(1) *To Relieve the Pain.*—The stitch in the side at onset, which is sometimes so agonizing, is best relieved by a hypodermic injection of a quarter of a grain of morphia. When the pain is less intense and diffuse over one side, the Paquelin cautery applied lightly is very helpful, but the ice bag is usually efficacious. When the disease is fairly established the pain is not, as a rule, distressing, except when the patient coughs, and for this codeia may be used in half-grain doses, or morphia given hypodermically (gr. 1/12 to 1/6), according to the patient's needs. Hot poultices, formerly so much in use, relieve the pain, though not more than the cold applications. For children they are often preferable.

(2) *To Combat the Toxæmia.*—Abundance of water should be given to promote the flow of urine, and the saline infusion seems to act helpfully in this way, but care must be taken not to give too large an amount if the circulation is failing; 500 c. c. is usually sufficient. External hydrotherapy should be kept up actively. Alcohol is generally advisable, best as whisky in amounts of four to twelve ounces in the twenty-four hours. The bowels should be kept freely open by saline laxatives.

(3) An all-important indication is *to support the circulation.* Hydrotherapy and keeping the patient out of doors are of great value for this. Mechanical disturbance, as from meteorism, should be prevented if possible. Drugs should not be given in any routine way and not until they are required. Strychnine is useful (also for its effects on the respiratory centre). It should be given hypodermically and in full doses (gr. 1/40 to 1/20 and even gr. 1/10 for short periods) every two or three hours. Digitalis can be given by mouth as the infusion (ʒ ii, 8 c. c.), the tincture (♏ xv, 1 c. c.), or digitalin intramuscularly (gr. 1/30) every four hours. For severe circulatory failure, camphor gr. ii, 0.13 gm. (dissolved in ♏ x of olive oil) hypodermically, digitalin (gr. 1/30) hypodermically, and caffeine (sodiobenzoate) gr. v (0.3 gm.) hypodermically may be tried. Pituitary extract (posterior lobe) has been warmly recommended. An injection of hot saline solution given high in the bowel or a saline infusion is helpful.

(4) *Respiratory Tract.*—The most comfortable position, avoidance of ex-

ertion, and abundance of fresh air are important aids in preventing dyspnœa. Pain should be relieyed as much as possible. The value of the administration of oxygen is doubtful. If used, it should be given very slowly and through a funnel held over the mouth and nose. The effect is the best guide as to its continuance. Expectorant drugs are not indicated and often upset the stomach. When the cough is severe it is well to give sedatives, of which codeia (gr. 1/4 to 1/2) or heroin (gr. 1/20 to 1/10) are the best. Morphia in small doses may be required, but these drugs should be given only when necessary. For *œdema* of the lungs strychnine (gr. 1/20) and atropine (gr. 1/100) should be given hypodermically. Venesection is advisable if the right heart be dilated.

(5) *Nervous System.*—The patient with delirium should be constantly watched. An ice bag to the head and frequent ice packs or cold sponges are useful. *Sleep* is important for every patient and the need for this is often forgotten. While such drugs as the bromides and chloral hydrate may be effectual, it is wiser, as a rule, to give morphia hypodermically in a sufficient dose (gr. 1/6 to 1/4) to secure rest and sleep.

(6) *Crisis.*—As this approaches constant watch should be kept for signs of collapse. If sweating is profuse and the patient feeble, atropine (gr. 1/100) should be given hypodermically.

(*h*) TREATMENT OF COMPLICATIONS.—If the fever persists it is important to look out for pleurisy, particularly for the meta-pneumonic empyema. The exploratory needle should be used if necessary. A sero-fibrinous effusion should be aspirated, a purulent opened and drained. In a complicating pericarditis with a large effusion aspiration may be necessary. Delayed resolution is a difficult condition to treat. Fibrolysin, 2.5 c. c. every other day, has been used successfully in a few cases (Crofton). The use of the X-rays is perhaps the most effective treatment.

(*i*) CONVALESCENCE.—The diet should be increased as rapidly as possible, the patient kept out of doors and after an ordinary attack allowed up in about a week. If the heart has suffered rest should be more prolonged.

B. BRONCHO-PNEUMONIA

(*Lobular Pneumonia, Capillary Bronchitis*)

Definition.—A bacterial infection of the finer bronchi and their related lobules.

The process begins with inflammation of the bronchioles and smaller bronchi, a capillary bronchitis, which extends to the alveoli and the whole lobule or a group of lobules becomes filled with exudate, cellular and hæmorrhagic but distinctly less fibrinous than in lobar pneumonia.

Etiology.—Broncho-pneumonia occurs either as a primary or as a secondary affection. The relative frequency in 443 cases is thus given by Holt: Primary, without previous bronchitis, 154; secondary to bronchitis of the larger tubes, 41; to measles, 89; to whooping-cough, 66; to diphtheria, 47; to scarlet fever, 7; to influenza, 6; to varicella, 2; to erysipelas, 2; and to acute ileo-colitis, 19. The proportion of primary to secondary forms as shown in this list is probably too low.

PRIMARY ACUTE BRONCHO-PNEUMONIA, like the lobar form, attacks children in good health, usually under two years but is not uncommon in adults. The etiological factors are very much those of ordinary pneumonia, and probably the pneumococcus is more often associated with it.

SECONDARY BRONCHO-PNEUMONIA occurs in two great groups: (*a*) As a sequence of the infectious fevers—measles, diphtheria, influenza, whooping-cough, scarlet fever, and, less frequently smallpox, erysipelas, and typhoid fever. In children it forms the most serious complication of these diseases, and in reality causes more deaths than are due directly to the fevers. In large cities it ranks next in fatality to infantile diarrhœa. Following, as it does, the contagious diseases which principally affect children, we find that a large majority of cases occur during early life. According to Morrill's Boston statistics, it is most fatal during the first two years of life. The number of cases in a community increases or decreases with the prevalence of measles, scarlet fever, and diphtheria. It is most prevalent in the winter and spring months. In the febrile affections of adults broncho-pneumonia is not very common. Thus in typhoid fever it is not so frequent as lobar pneumonia, though isolated areas of consolidation at the bases are by no means rare in protracted cases of this disease. In old people it may follow debilitating causes of any sort, and is met with in the course of chronic Bright's disease and various acute and chronic maladies.

(*b*) In the second division of this affection are embraced the cases of so-called aspiration or deglutition pneumonia. Whenever the sensitiveness of the larynx is benumbed, as in the coma of apoplexy or uræmia, minute particles of food or drink are allowed to pass the *rima,* and, reaching finally the smaller tubes, excite an intense inflammation similar to the vagus pneumonia which follows the section of the pneumogastrics in the dog. Cases are very common after operations about the mouth and nose, after tracheotomy, and in cancer of the larynx and œsophagus. The aspirated particles in some instances induce such an intense broncho-pneumonia that suppuration or even gangrene supervenes. The ether pneumonia, already described, is often lobular in type.

An aspiration broncho-pneumonia may follow hæmoptysis, the aspiration of material from a bronchiectatic cavity, and occasionally the material from an empyema which has ruptured into the lung. A common and fatal form of broncho-pneumonia is that excited by the tubercle bacillus.

Among general predisposing causes may be mentioned age. As just noted, it is prone to attack infants, and a majority of cases of pneumonia in children under five years of age are of this form. Of 370 cases in children under five years of age, 75 per cent. were broncho-pneumonia (Holt). At the opposite extreme of life it is also common, in association with influenza and with various debilitating circumstances and with the chronic diseases incident to the old. In children, rickets and diarrhœa are marked predisposing causes, and broncho-pneumonia is one of the most frequent post mortem lesions in infants' homes and foundling asylums. The disease prevails most extensively among the poorer classes.

Morbid Anatomy.—On the pleural surfaces, particularly toward the base, are seen depressed bluish or blue-brown areas of collapse, between which the lung tissue is of a lighter color. Here and there are projecting portions over which the pleura may be slightly turbid or granular. The lung is fuller and firmer than normal, and, though in great part crepitant, there can be felt in places throughout the substance solid, nodular bodies. The dark depressed areas may be isolated or a large section of one lobe may be in the condition of collapse. Gradual inflation by a blow-pipe inserted in the bronchus will distend a great majority of these collapsed areas. On section, the general surface has a dark reddish color and usually drips blood. Projecting above the level of the section are lighter red or reddish-gray areas representing the patches of broncho-pneumonia. These may be isolated and separated from each other by tracts of uninflamed tissue or they may be in groups; or the greater part of a lobe may be involved. Study of a favorable section of an isolated patch shows: (*a*) A dilated central bronchiole full of tenacious purulent mucus. A fortunate section parallel to the long axis may show a racemose arrangement—the alveolar passages full of muco-pus. (*b*) Surrounding the bronchus for from 3 to 5 mm. or even more, an area of grayish-red consolidation, usually elevated above the surface and firm to the touch. Unlike the consolidation of lobar pneumonia, it may present a perfectly smooth surface, though in some instances it is distinctly granular. In a late stage of the disease small grayish-white points may be seen, which on pressure may be squeezed out as purulent droplets. A section in the axis of the lobule may present a somewhat grape-like arrangement, the stalks and stems representing the bronchioles and alveolar passages filled with a yellowish or grayish-white pus, while surrounding them is a reddish-brown hepatized tissue. (*c*) In the immediate neighborhood of this peribronchial inflammation the tissue is dark in color, smooth, airless, at a somewhat lower level than the hepatized portion, and differs distinctly in color and appearance from the other portions of the lung. This is the condition to which the term *splenization* has been given. It really represents a tissue in the early stage of inflammation, and it perhaps would be as well to give up the use of this term and also that of *carnification*, which is only a more advanced stage.

There are three groups of cases: (1) Those in which the bronchitis and bronchiolitis are most marked, and in which there may be no definite consolidation, and yet on microscopic examination many of the alveolar passages and adjacent air-cells appear filled with inflammatory products. (2) The disseminated broncho-pneumonia, in which there are scattered areas of peribronchial hepatization with patches of collapse, while a considerable proportion of the lobe is still crepitant. This is by far the most common condition. (3) The pseudo-lobar form, in which the greater portion of the lobe is consolidated, but not uniformly, for intervening strands of dark congested lung tissue separate the groups of hepatized lobules.

Microscopically, the centre of the bronchus is seen filled with a plug of exudation, consisting of leucocytes and swollen epithelium. Section in the long axis may show irregular dilatations of the tube. The bronchial wall is swollen and infiltrated with cells. Under a low power it is readily seen that the air-cells next the bronchus are mostly densely filled, while toward the periphery the alveolar exudation becomes less. The contents of the air-cells are made up of leucocytes and swollen epithelial cells in varying proportions. Red corpuscles are not often present and a fibrin network is rarely seen, though it may be present in some alveoli. In the swollen walls are seen distended capillaries and numerous leucocytes. As Delafield has pointed out, the interstitial inflammation of the bronchi and alveolar walls is the special feature of broncho-pneumonia.

The histological changes in the aspiration or deglutition broncho-pneumonia differ from the ordinary post-febrile form in a more intense infiltration of the air-cells with leucocytes, producing suppuration and foci of softening; even gangrene may be present.

Bacteriology.—The organisms most commonly found in broncho-pneumonia are *Micrococcus lanceolatus, Streptococcus pyogenes* (either alone or with the pneumococcus), *Staphylococcus aureus et albus,* Friedländer's *Bacillus pneumoniæ,* and the influenza bacillus. The Klebs-Loeffler bacillus is not infrequently found in the secondary lesions of diphtheria. Except the pneumococcus these microbes are rarely found in pure cultures. In the lobular type the streptococcus is the most constant organism, in the pseudo-lobar the pneumococcus. Mixed infections are almost the rule in broncho-pneumonia.

Terminations of Broncho-pneumonia.—(*a*) In *resolution,* which when it once begins goes on more rapidly than in fibrinous pneumonia. Broncho-pneumonia of the apices, in a child, persisting for three or more weeks, particularly if it follow measles or diphtheria, is often tuberculous. In these instances, when resolution is supposed to be delayed, caseation has in reality taken place. (*b*) In *suppuration,* which is rarely seen apart from the aspiration and deglutition forms, in which it is extremely common. (*c*) In *gangrene,* which occurs under the same conditions. (*d*) In *fibroid changes—chronic broncho-pneumonia*—a rare termination in the simple, a common sequence of the tuberculous, disease. Formerly it was thought that one of the most common changes in broncho-pneumonia, particularly in children, was caseation; but this is really a tuberculous process, the natural termination of an originally specific broncho-pneumonia. It is of course quite possible that a broncho-pneumonia, simple in its origin, may subsequently be the seat of infection by *Bacillus tuberculosis.*

Symptoms.—The *primary* form sets in abruptly with a chill or a convulsion. The child has not had a previous illness, but there may have been slight exposure. The temperature rises rapidly and is more constant; the physical signs are more local and there is not the widespread diffuse catarrh of the smaller tubes. Many cases are mistaken for lobar pneumonia. In others the pulmonary features are in the background or are overlooked in the intensity of the general or cerebral symptoms. The termination is often by crisis, and the recovery is prompt. The mortality of this form is slight. S. West has called attention to the importance of recognizing these primary cases and to their resemblance in clinical features to acute lobar pneumonia. The *secondary* form begins usually as a bronchitis of the smaller tubes. Much confusion has arisen from the description of capillary bronchitis as a separate affection, whereas it is only a part, though a primary and important one, of broncho-pneumonia. At the outset it may be said that if in convalescence from measles or whooping-cough a child has an accession of fever with cough, rapid pulse, and rapid breathing, and if, on auscultation, fine râles are heard at the bases, or widely spread throughout the lungs, even though neither consolidation nor blowing breathing can be detected, the diagnosis of broncho-pneumonia may safely be made. I have never seen in a fatal case after diphtheria or measles a capillary bronchitis as the sole lesion. The onset is rarely sudden, or with a distinct chill; but after a day or so of indisposition the child becomes feverish and begins to cough and be short of breath. The fever is extremely variable; a range of from 102° to 104° F. is common. The skin is very dry and hot. The cough is hard, distressing, and may be painful. Dyspnœa gradually becomes a prominent feature. Expiration may be jerky and grunting. The respirations may rise as high as 60 or even 80 per minute. Within the first forty-eight hours the percussion resonance is not impaired; the note, indeed, may be very full at the anterior borders of the lungs. On auscultation, many râles are heard, chiefly the fine subcrepitant variety, with sibilant rhonchi. There may really be no signs indicating that the parenchyma of the lung is involved, and yet even at this early stage, within forty-eight hours of the onset of the pulmonary symptoms, I have repeatedly, after diphtheria, found scattered nodules of lobular hepatization. Northrup, in a case in which death occurred within the first twenty-four hours, in addition to the extensive involvement of the smaller bronchi, found the intralobular tissue also involved in places. The dyspnœa is constant and progressive and soon signs of deficient aëration of the blood are noted. The face becomes a little suffused and the finger-tips bluish. The child has an anxious expression and gradually enters upon the most distressing stage of asphyxia. At first the urgency of the symptoms is marked, but soon the influence of the toxins on the nerve-centres is seen and the child no longer makes strenuous efforts to breathe. The cough subsides, and, with a gradual increase in lividity and a drowsy restlessness, the right ventricle becomes more and more distended, the bronchial râles become more liquid as the tubes fill with mucus, and death follows. These are symptoms of a severe case of broncho-pneumonia, or what the older writers called *suffocative catarrh*.

The PHYSICAL SIGNS may at first be those of capillary bronchitis, as indicated by the absence of dulness and the presence of fine subcrepitant and whistling râles. In many cases death takes place before any definite pneumonic signs are detected. When these exist they are much more frequent at the bases, where there may be areas of impaired resonance or even of positive dulness. When numerous foci involve the greater part of a lobe the breathing may become tubular, but in the scattered patches of ordinary broncho-pneumonia, following the fevers, the breathing is more commonly harsh than blowing. In grave cases there is retraction of the base of the sternum and of the lower costal cartilages during inspiration, pointing to deficient lung expansion.

Diagnosis.—With lobar pneumonia it may readily be confounded if the areas of consolidation are large and merged together. It is to be remembered, as Holt's figures well show, that broncho-pneumonia occurs chiefly in children under one year, whereas lobar pneumonia is more common after the third year. No writer has so clearly brought out the difference between pneumonia at these periods as Gerhard,* of Philadelphia, whose papers on this subject have the freshness and accuracy which characterized all the writings of that eminent physician. Between lobar pneumonia and the secondary form of broncho-pneumonia the diagnosis is easy. The mode of onset is essentially different in the two infections, the one developing insidiously in the course or at the conclusion of another disease, the other setting in abruptly in a

* American Journal of Medical Sciences, vols. xiv and xv.

child in good health. In lobar pneumonia the disease is usually unilateral, in broncho-pneumonia bilateral. The chief trouble arises in cases of primary broncho-pneumonia, which by aggregation of the foci involves the greater part of one lobe. Here the difficulty is very great, and the physical signs may be practically identical, but in broncho-pneumonia it is much more likely that a lesion, however slight, will be found on the other side.

A still more difficult question to decide is whether an existing broncho-pneumonia is simple or tuberculous. In many instances the decision cannot be made, as the circumstances under which the disease occurs, the mode of onset, and the physical signs may be identical. It has often been my experience that a case has been sent down from the children's ward to the dead house with the diagnosis of post-febrile broncho-pneumonia in which there was no suspicion of the existence of tuberculosis; but on section there were found tuberculous bronchial glands and scattered areas of broncho-pneumonia, some of which were distinctly caseous, while others showed signs of softening. It is well to emphasize the fact that there are many cases of broncho-pneumonia in children which time alone enables us to distinguish from tuberculosis. The existence of extensive disease at the apices or central regions is a suggestive indication, and signs of softening may be detected. In the vomited matter, which is brought up after severe spells of coughing, sputum may be picked out and elastic tissue and tubercle bacilli detected.

It must not be forgotten that, as in lobar pneumonia, cerebral symptoms may mask the true nature of the disease, and may even lead to the diagnosis of meningitis. I recall more than one instance in which it could not be satisfactorily determined whether the infant had tuberculous meningitis or a cerebral complication of an acute pulmonary affection.

Prognosis.—In the primary form the outlook is good. In children enfeebled by constitutional disease and prolonged fevers broncho-pneumonia is terribly fatal, but in cases coming on in connection with whooping-cough or after measles recovery may take place in the most desperate cases. It is in this disease that the truth of the old maxim is shown—"Never despair of a sick child." The death rate in children under five has been variously estimated at from 30 to 50 per cent. After diphtheria and measles thin, wiry children seem to stand broncho-pneumonia much better than fat, flabby ones. In adults the aspiration or deglutition pneumonia is a very fatal disease.

Prophylaxis.—Much can be done to reduce the probability of attack after febrile affections. Thus, in the convalescence from measles and whooping-cough, it is very important that the child should not be exposed to cold, particularly at night, when the temperature of the room naturally falls. The use of light flannel "combinations" obviates this nocturnal chill, which is, I am sure, an important factor in the colds and pulmonary affections of young children. The catarrhal troubles of the nose and throat should be carefully attended to, and during fevers the mouth should be washed two or three times a day with an antiseptic solution.

Treatment.—The frequency and the seriousness of broncho-pneumonia render it a disease which taxes to the utmost the resources of the practitioner. There is no acute pulmonary affection over which he at times so greatly despairs. On the other hand, there is not one in which he will be more gratified in saving patients who have seemed past all succor. The general measures are much as in lobar pneumonia. The patient should be in the open air if possible; if indoors, the windows should be wide open with the patient protected from drafts.

(*a*) DIET.—As much food as possible should be given. Milk and its modifications, ice cream, eggs, broths, cocoa, and gruels are suitable. Water should be given freely by mouth and if this is not possible by the bowel or by infusion. Alcohol is usually indicated and best given as whisky to adults and brandy to young children. The *bowels* should be opened by castor oil or calomel and care taken to secure a daily movement.

(*b*) HYDROTHERAPY.—This may be given by various methods to be chosen for each patient, depending on the condition and results. Sponges may be given to any patient. Packs are useful, hot if there is much restlessness or cold if the temperature is high, or baths may be given to children for short periods, using water at 95° F. and gradually reducing to 75° or 80° F. Applying small amounts of cold water to the chest during the bath is sometimes useful, particularly if the respirations are shallow. Compresses, made out of linen covered by flannel or of flannel alone, wrung out of water at 60° to 70°, are particularly indicated and should be changed every one or two hours. They should not be covered by oiled silk. A mustard bath is of value for children, especially early in the attack. Alternate douches of hot and cold water are useful, particularly in children, when the condition is severe. Hydrotherapy is especially indicated for patients with high fever, delirium or stupor, severe toxæmia, or circulatory failure.

(*c*) LOCAL APPLICATIONS.—Poultices have gone out of fashion but are sometimes of value. They should be light and are best kept in place by being slipped in pockets in a flannel jacket which is constantly worn so that the poultice can be replaced without disturbing the patient. The use of dry cups is often advised; they should be applied frequently. The ice bag should be used if it gives comfort.

(*d*) MEDICINAL.—The indications must be carefully studied and drugs which may disturb the stomach given with care. If cough is distressing the use of the compound tincture of benzoin in an inhalation should be tried. The expectorant drugs may aid and of these ammonium chloride (gr. ii to v, 0.13 to 0.3 gm.) and the wine of ipecacuanha (♏ x to xx, 0.6 to 1.3 c. c.) are the most useful. To these a sedative, such as paregoric (ʒ i, 4 c. c.), codeia (gr. ¼, 0.016 gm.) or heroin (gr. 1-20, 0.0032 gm.) should be added if the cough is very distressing. Strychnine hypodermically (gr. 1-40 to 1-20, 0.0016 to 0.0032 gm.) is an aid to the respiratory centre and to the circulation. For circulatory failure the treatment is the same as described under lobar pneumonia. With increasing difficulty in getting up the secretions an emetic may be given, but only to robust patients. Ipecacuanha or apomorphine hypodermically should be employed. Inhalations of oxygen are advisable if they give relief to the dyspnœa and lessen cyanosis.

In old persons early stimulation is usually advisable and every effort should be made to persuade them to take nourishment. Cold applications or sponges must be used with caution and the use of heat is generally better. At all ages frequent change in position is advisable and in young children this may be done by taking them out of bed and holding them in the arms.

C. OTHER PNEUMOCOCCIC INFECTIONS

The organism is widely distributed and causes a number of important affections other than pulmonary, of which the following are the most important:

1. **Acute Septicæmia.**—A few instances have been reported in which without any recognized local lesion there has been a general infection with the pneumococcus. In Townsend's case, a girl, aged six, had pain in the abdomen, vomiting and a temperature of 104.2° F. without any throat affection. Death occurred in thirty hours, and a general infection with the organism was found in the blood, spleen, lungs and kidneys.

2. **Local Affections.**—The local affections caused by the pneumococcus are very numerous and will be described under their appropriate sections. In the *mouth,* erosions, gingivitis and glossitis; in the *pharynx,* inflammation and tonsillitis; in the *ear,* acute and chronic suppuration; in the accessory sinuses, of which it is a common habitat, inflammation and suppuration; in the *membrane of the brain* it is a common cause of primary and secondary meningitis; in the *bronchi* it has been found associated with acute and chronic bronchitis, and bronchiectasis; in the *lungs,* in addition to the two important diseases already considered, it may cause acute œdema and is associated with tuberculosis and many chronic affections. It has been found in acute pleurisy and it is one of the common causes of empyema; acute arthritis, primary and secondary forms; acute peritonitis, particularly in children; appendicitis; endocarditis; pyelitis and local abscesses in various parts may be caused by it.

VII. CEREBRO-SPINAL FEVER

Definition.—An infectious disease, occurring sporadically and in epidemics, caused by the *Diplococcus intracellularis,* characterized by inflammation of the cerebro-spinal meninges and a clinical course of great irregularity.

The affection is also known by the names of malignant purpuric fever, petechial fever, spotted fever and epidemic cerebro-spinal meningitis.

History.—Vieusseux first described a small outbreak in Geneva in 1805. In 1806 L. Danielson and E. Mann (Medical and Agricultural Register, Boston) gave an account of "a singular and very mortal disease which lately made its appearance in Medfield, Mass." The Massachusetts Medical Society, in 1809, appointed James Jackson, Thomas Welch, and J. C. Warren to investigate it. Elisha North's little book (1811) gives a full account of the early epidemics. Stillé's monograph (1867) and the elaborate section in vol. i of Joseph Jones' works contain details of the later American outbreaks. In his Geographical Pathology, Hirsch divides the outbreaks into four periods: From 1805 to 1830, in which the disease was most prevalent throughout the United States; a second period, from 1837 to 1850, when the disease prevailed extensively in France, and there were a few outbreaks in the United States; a third period, from 1854 to 1874, when there were outbreaks in Europe and several extensive epidemics in America. During the Civil War there were comparatively few cases. It prevailed extensively in the Ottawa Valley early in the seventies. In the fourth period, from 1875 to the present time, the disease has broken out in a great many regions. In the United

States, during 1898-1899, it prevailed in mild form in 27 states. Since 1899 there have been extensive outbreaks in Silesia, and in the cities of the United States on the Atlantic coast. In New York in 1904-5 there were 6,755 cases and 3,455 deaths. In Glasgow in 1907 there were nearly 1,000 cases with 595 deaths (Chalmers). In Belfast in the eighteen months ending June, 1908, there were 725 cases with 548 deaths (Robb). There were only 130 deaths in England and Wales in 1909, but there has been a rapid rise during the war. In the winter of 1914-15 the disease appeared among the Canadian troops and was carried by them to England. It broke out in many home camps and, spreading to the civil population, for the first time in its history the disease prevailed widely in England.

Etiology.—Cerebro-spinal fever occurs in epidemic and in sporadic forms. The *epidemics* are localized and are rarely very widespread. Only in the tropics have there been extensive killing pandemics. As a rule, country districts have been more afflicted than cities. Mining districts and seaports have suffered most severely. The outbreaks have occurred most frequently in the winter and spring. The concentration of individuals, as of troops in large barracks, is a special factor; recruits and young soldiers are specially liable. In civil life children and young adults are most susceptible. Over-exertion, long marches in the heat, depressing mental and bodily surroundings, and the misery and squalor of the large tenement houses in cities are predisposing causes. The disease is not highly contagious, and is probably not transmitted by clothing or the excretions. It is very rare to have more than one or two cases in a house, and in a city epidemic the distribution of the cases is very irregular. Meningitis carriers play an important rôle in transmitting the disease. They are found also when the disease is not epidemic.

Sporadic cerebro-spinal fever.—The disease lingers indefinitely after an outbreak, and in all large cities cases occur. There are two types, one the posterior basic meningitis of Gee and Barlow, which has very distinctive features, and the other the meningococcus meningitis of young adults met with in periods during which the disease is not specially prevalent; two, three, and even five cases may occur in succession in one family. The meningitis in children, known as the *simple* or *posterior basic,* is the sporadic form. It has two suggestive features of similarity in the seasonal incidence and in the fact that patients recover. Still determined the identity of the organism with the meningococcus, and the view has been confirmed by Koplik and many others.

Bacteriology.—In 1877 Weichselbaum described the meningococcus or *Diplococcus intracellularis meningitidis.* In the tissues the organism is almost constantly within the polynuclear leucocytes. Recent investigations have shown that there are two distinct types distinguishable from one another by immune reactions. In the recent outbreak both types were found widely distributed. The so-called parameningococcus is not, as was thought, a rare cause but it and the ordinary forms are equally responsible as causative agents and correspond exactly to the different types of pneumococci causing pneumonia (Ellis). The organism is found in the blood and in the various lesions of the disease. Three important facts have been brought out—the presence of the germ in fully half the cases in the naso-pharynx, the existence of it in healthy contacts, and the preparation of a curative serum.

Morbid Anatomy.—In malignant cases there may be no characteristic changes, the brain and spinal cord showing only extreme congestion, which was the lesion described by Vieusseux. In a majority of the acutely fatal cases death occurs within the first week. There is intense injection of the pia-arachnoid. The exudate is usually fibrino-purulent, most marked at the base of the brain, where the meninges may be greatly thickened and plastered over with it. On the cortex there may be much lymph along the larger fissures and in the sulci; sometimes the entire cortex is covered with a thick, purulent exudate. It deserves to be recorded that Danielson and Mann made five autopsies and were the first to describe "a fluid resembling pus between the dura and pia mater." The cord is always involved with the brain. The exudate is more abundant on the posterior surface, and involves, as a rule, the dorsal and lumbar regions more than the cervical portion.

In the more chronic cases there is general thickening of the meninges and scattered yellow patches mark where the exudate has been. The ventricles in the acute cases are dilated and contain a turbid fluid, or in the posterior cornua pure pus. In the chronic cases the dilatation may be very great. The brain substance is usually a little softer than normal and has a pinkish tinge; foci of hæmorrhage and of encephalitis may be found. The cranial nerves are usually involved, particularly the second, fifth, seventh, and eighth. The spinal nerve roots are also found imbedded in the exudate.

Microscopically, the exudate consists largely of polynuclear leucocytes closely packed in a fibrinous material. In some instances there are foci of purulent infiltration and hæmorrhage. The neuroglia cells are swollen, with large, clear, and vesicular nuclei. The ganglion cells show less marked changes. Diplococci are found in variable numbers in the exudate, being more numerous in the brain than in the cord.

The nasal secretion during life may show diplococci. The sphenoidal sinuses may be full of pus and the surrounding bone inflamed. The frequency of catarrhal and other changes in the naso-pharynx and sinuses suggests that the infection reaches the meninges through this route.

Pneumonia and pleurisy have been described in the disease. Councilman reports that in 13 cases there was congestion with œdema, in 7 broncho-pneumonia, in 2 characteristic croupous pneumonia with pneumococci; in 8 pneumonia due to the diplococcus intracellularis was present.

The *spleen* varies a good deal in size. In only three of the Boston fatal cases was it found much enlarged. The *liver* is rarely abnormal. Acute *nephritis* is sometimes present. The intestines show sometimes swelling of the follicles.

Symptoms.—Cases differ remarkably in their characters. Many different forms have been described. These are perhaps best grouped into three classes:

(*a*) MALIGNANT FORM.—This fulminant or apoplectic type is found with variable frequency in epidemics. It may occur sporadically. The onset is sudden, usually with violent chills, headache, somnolence, spasms in the muscles, great depression, moderate elevation of temperature, and feeble pulse, which may fall to fifty or sixty in the minute. Usually a purpuric rash develops. In a Philadelphia case, in 1888, a young girl, apparently quite well, died within twenty hours of this form. There are cases on record in which death has occurred within a shorter time. Stillé tells of a child of five years, in whom death occurred after an illness of ten hours; and refers to a case reported by Gordon, in which the entire duration of the illness was only five hours. Two of Vieusseux's cases died within twenty-four hours.

(*b*) Ordinary Form.—The stage of incubation is not known. The disease usually sets in suddenly. There may be premonitory symptoms: headache, pains in the back, and loss of appetite. More commonly, the onset is with headache, severe chill, and vomiting. The temperature rises to 101° or 102°. The pulse is full and strong. An early and important symptom is a painful stiffness of the muscles of the neck. The headache increases, and there are photophobia and great sensitiveness to noises. Children become very irritable and restless. In severe cases the contraction of the muscles of the neck sets in early, the head is drawn back, and when the muscles of the back are also involved, there is orthotonos, which is more common than opisthotonos. The pains in the back and in the limbs may be very severe. The motor symptoms are most characteristic. Tremor of the muscles may be present, with tonic or clonic spasms in the arms or legs. Rigidity of the muscles of the back or neck is very common, and the patient lies with the body stiff and the head drawn so far back that the occiput may be between the shoulder-blades. Except in early childhood convulsions are not common. Strabismus is a frequent and important symptom. Spasm of the muscles of the face may also occur. Cases have been described in which the general rigidity and stiffness was such that the body could be moved like a statue. Paralysis of the trunk muscles is rare, but paralysis of the muscles of the eye and the face is not uncommon.

Of sensory symptoms, headache is the most dominant and persists from the outset. It is chiefly in the back of the head, and the pain extends into the neck and back. There may be great sensitiveness along the spine, and in many cases there is general hyperæsthesia.

The psychical symptoms are pronounced. Delirium occurs at the onset, occasionally of a furious and maniacal kind. The patient may display marked erotic symptoms at the onset. The delirium gives place in a few days to stupor, which, as the effusion increases, deepens to coma.

The temperature is irregular and variable. Remissions occur frequently, and there is no uniform or typical curve during the disease. In some instances there has been little or no fever. In others the temperature may reach 105° or 106° F., or, before death, 108° F. The pulse may be very rapid in children; in adults it is at first usually full and strong. In some cases it is remarkably slow, and may not be more than fifty or sixty in the minute. Sighing respirations and Cheyne-Stokes breathing are met with in some instances. Unless there is pneumonia the respirations are not often increased in frequency.

The cutaneous symptoms of the disease are important. Herpes occurs with a frequency almost equal to that in pneumonia or intermittent fever. The petechial rash, which has given the name spotted fever to the disease, is very variable. Stillé states that of 98 cases in the Philadelphia Hospital, no eruption was observed in 37. In the Montreal cases petechiæ and purple spots were common. They appear to have been more frequent in the epidemics in America than in Europe. The petechiæ may be numerous and cover the entire skin. An erythema or dusky mottling may be present. In some instances there have been rose-colored hyperæmic spots like the typhoid rash.

Urticara or erythema nodosum, ecthyma, pemphigus, and in rare instances gangrene of the skin have been noted.

Leucocytosis is an early and constant feature, and ranges from 25,000 to 40,000 per cubic millimetre. It persists even in the most protracted cases. The diplococcus intracellularis has been isolated from the blood during life and demonstrated in the leucocytes.

As already stated, vomiting may be a special feature at the onset; but, as a rule, it gradually subsides. In some instances, however, it persists and becomes the most serious and distressing of the symptoms. Diarrhœa is not common, the bowels being usually constipated. The abdomen is not tender. In the acute form the spleen is usually enlarged.

The urine is sometimes albuminous and the quantity may be increased. Glycosuria has been noted in some instances, and in the malignant types hæmaturia.

The duration of the disease is extremely variable. Hirsch rightly states that it may range between a few hours and several months. More than half of the deaths occur within the first five days. In favorable cases, after the symptoms have persisted for five or six days, improvement is indicated by a lessening of the spasm, reduction of the fever, and a return of the intelligence. A sudden fall in the temperature is of bad omen. Convalescence is extremely tedious, and may be interrupted by complications and sequelæ to be noted.

(*c*) Anomalous Forms.—(1) *Abortive Type.*—The attack sets in with great severity, but in a day or two the symptoms subside and convalescence is rapid. Strümpell would distinguish between this abortive variety, which begins with such intensity, and the mild ambulant cases described by certain writers. He reports a case in which the meningeal symptoms set in with the greatest intensity and persisted for four days, the temperature rising to 105.6° F. On the fifth day the patient entered upon a rapid and satisfactory convalescence. In the mild cases, as distinguished from the abortive, the patients complain of headache, nausea, sensations of discomfort in the back and limbs, and stiffness in the neck. There is little or no fever, and only moderate vomiting. These cases could be recognized only during the prevalence of an epidemic.

(2) *An intermittent* type has been observed in many epidemics, and is recognized by von Ziemssen and Stillé. It is characterized by exacerbations of fever, which may recur daily or every second day, or follow a curve of an intermittent or remittent character. The pyrexia resembles that of pyæmia rather than malaria.

(3) *Chronic Form.*—Heubner states that this is a relatively frequent form, though it does not seem to be recognized by many writers on the subject. An attack may be protracted for from two to five or even six months, and may cause the most intense marasmus. It is characterized by a series of recurrences of the fever, and may present the most complex symptomatology. It is not improbable that in these protracted cases chronic hydrocephalus or abscess of the brain is present. This form differs distinctly from the intermittent type. Three cases in our series were of this chronic form; in one the disease persisted for ninety days.

Complications.—Pleurisy, pericarditis, and parotitis are not uncommon.

Pneumonia is described as frequent in certain outbreaks. Immermann found, during the Erlangen epidemic, many instances of the combination of pneumonia with meningitis, but it does not seem possible to determine whether, in such cases, pneumonia is the primary disease and the meningitis secondary, or *vice versa*. The frequency with which inflammation of the meninges of the brain complicates pneumonia is well known. Councilman suggests that the pneumonia of the disease is not the true croupous form, but due to the diplococcus meningitidis. This was found in eight of the Boston cases, and in one it was so extensive that it could have been mistaken for the ordinary croupous pneumonia. Cerebro-spinal fever sometimes prevails extensively with ordinary pneumonia, as in New York in the winter of 1903-'04. *Arthritis* has been the most frequent complication in certain epidemics. Many joints are affected simultaneously, and there are swelling, pain, and exudation, sometimes serous, sometimes purulent. This was first observed by James Jackson, Sr., in the epidemic which he described. Enteritis is rare.

Headache may persist for months or years after an attack. Chronic hydrocephalus occurs in certain instances in children. The symptoms of this are "paroxysms of severe headache, pains in the neck and extremities, vomiting, loss of consciousness, convulsions, and involuntary discharges of fæces and urine" (von Ziemssen). Mental feebleness and aphasia have occasionally been noted.

Paralysis of individual cranial nerves or of the lower extremities may persist for some time. In some of these cases there may be peripheral neuritis, as Mills suggested.

Special Senses.—*Eye.*—Optic neuritis may follow involvement of the nerve in the exudation at the base. Acute papillitis was found in 6 out of 40 cases examined by Randolph. The inflammation may extend directly into the eye along the pia-arachnoid of the optic nerve, causing purulent choroido-iritis or even keratitis. A neuritis of the fifth nerve may be followed by keratitis and purulent conjunctivitis.

Ear.—Deafness very often follows inflammation of the labyrinth. Otitis media, with mastoiditis, may occur from direct extension. In 64 cases of meningitis which recovered, Moos found that 55 per cent. were deaf. He suggests that the abortive form of the disease may be responsible for many cases of early acquired deafness. In children this not infrequently leads to deaf-mutism. Von Ziemssen states that in the deaf and dumb institutions of Bamberg and Nuremberg, in 1874, a majority of the pupils had become deaf from epidemic cerebro-spinal meningitis.

Nose.—Coryza is not infrequent early in the disease, and Strümpell says that in many of his cases nasal catarrh preceded the meningitis. He suggests that the latter may be caused by infection from the nose. Certainly the nasal secretion appears frequently to contain the diplococci—in 18 cases examined by Scherrer, and in 10 out of 15 of the Boston cases.

Diagnosis.—Much has been done of late to enable the practitioner to recognize definitely the existence of meningitis and of the various forms.

(*a*) General Features.—The fever, headache, delirium, retraction of the neck, tremor, and rigidity of the muscles are most important signs. As already mentioned, in the meningitis of cerebro-spinal fever the spinal symptoms are very much more marked than in the other forms. One has constantly to bear in mind that certain cases of typhoid fever and of pneumonia closely simulate cerebro-spinal meningitis.

(*b*) Among the SPECIAL DIAGNOSTIC FEATURES may be mentioned:

Kernig's Sign.—When the thigh is flexed at right angles to the abdomen, the leg can be extended upon the thigh nearly in a straight line. If meningitis be present, strong contractures of the flexors prevent the full extension of the leg on the thigh.

Brudzinski's Sign.—Flexing the head on the chest causes flexion of the legs at the hip and knee joints, and flexing one leg on the trunk produces the same movement in the other leg.

Lumbar Puncture.—The procedure is quite harmless, and in a majority of the cases can be done without general anæsthesia, with the aid of a local freezing mixture. As a rule, it is best in children to give a whiff or two of chloroform. The patient is turned on the side with the back bowed and the knees drawn up. As a rule, there is no difficulty in finding the spinal processes, and with the thumb or index finger of the left hand as a guide, a small aspirator needle is inserted slightly to one side of the median line and thrust deeply into the third lumbar interspace in an upward and inward direction. At a variable distance, according to the age and musculature, the needle enters the spinal canal—about two and a half centimetres in infants and from four to six centimetres in adults. The fluid runs, as a rule, drop by drop, and when meningitis is present it is usually turbid, sometimes purulent, occasionally bloody. Meningitis may be present with a clear fluid. The pressure under which the fluid flows may reach 250-300 mm., the normal being about 120 mm. The cytology of the fluid is important. The polymorphonuclear leucocytes are in great excess while in the tuberculous form the lymphocytes are the more abundant. In the late stages and throughout the course of the posterior basic form the formula may be reversed. There is rarely any difficulty in determining between the pneumococcus and the diplococcus intracellularis. Careful search will usually show tubercle bacilli in cases of tuberculous meningitis or a guinea-pig may be inoculated.

Prognosis.—Hirsch states that the mortality has ranged in various epidemics from 20 to 75 per cent. In children the death rate is much higher than in adults. The earlier the serum is given the better the outlook.

Prophylaxis.—The patient should be isolated, seen only by the doctor, nurses, and one or two special members of the family. Cultures from the nasopharynx of those in immediate contact should be taken and, if possible, carriers should be isolated. The throats of carriers should be thoroughly treated, irrigated with salt solution, and sprayed with a 1 per cent. solution of peroxide or with a solution of iodine and glycerine. Some carriers prove very resistant; in others the germs disappear after a few days. Hexamine, 30 to 50 grains daily, may be given. Protective vaccination has been tried extensively in the last English epidemic.

Treatment.—The patient should be kept as quiet as possible, handled gently, and all causes of irritation removed. Special attention should be given to the care of the skin owing to the danger of bedsores. The hair should be clipped close and an ice-bag applied to the head. The diet should be liquid, as concentrated as possible, and given at short intervals. If swallowing is difficult the patient can be fed through a tube. Water should be given freely.

The bowels are to be opened by a calomel and saline purge, and laxatives or enemata used later if necessary. For severe headache, general pains or vomiting, morphia hypodermically is usually best. The administration of hexamethylenamine, sixty grains (4 gm.) a day, is worthy of a trial.

SERUM THERAPY.—The serum should be given as early as possible and also in doubtful cases. Whenever the fluid obtained by lumbar puncture is purulent the serum should be given, but repeated only if the meningococcus is found. Before giving the serum as much cerebro-spinal fluid as possible should be withdrawn. If this has been large in amount (over 40 c. c.) and in severe cases, 45 c. c. of the serum should be introduced through the needle. In ordinary cases 30 c. c. of the serum should be given. In all cases with abnormal resistance to the injection of serum after an amount equal to the fluid removed has been injected, it is well to stop. If the symptoms are very severe or increasing, the injection should be repeated in twelve hours. Otherwise the usual dose (30 c. c.) should be given daily for four days. If diplococci are found after this, daily injections should be continued. Continuance or exacerbation of the symptoms demands further injections. If the condition remains stationary after four days' interval, the four daily injections should be given again and this repeated until the diplococci disappear and the symptoms abate. The failure of the serum in many hands during the recent epidemic may have been due to its preparation from different strains. In the chronic forms the serum should be given if diplococci are present and in the posterior basic form in the hope of benefit.

HYDROTHERAPY.—This may give relief to the symptoms. Hot baths or hot packs may be given for fifteen minutes every three hours.

LUMBAR PUNCTURE.—Done for injection of the serum it is often of value in itself. Severe headache and marked cerebral features are indications. As much fluid as possible should be removed and if it escapes under high pressure early repetition is advisable. It should be done early and frequently with signs of accumulation of fluid in the ventricles.

COMPLICATIONS.—Conditions due to extension to the cranial nerves are not influenced by treatment. *Otitis* requires early incision and *arthritis* rest, local applications and incision if suppuration occurs. With signs of dilatation of the ventricles, drainage with injection of serum may be tried. In the chronic cases every effort should be made to nourish the patient well and especial precautions taken against bed-sores. For the pain and stiffness sometimes occurring in convalescence, hot baths and massage are useful.

VIII. INFLUENZA

(*La Grippe*)

Definition.—A pandemic disease, appearing at irregular intervals, characterized by extraordinary rapidity of extension and the large number of people attacked. Following the pandemic there are, as a rule, for several years endemic, epidemic, or sporadic outbreaks in different regions. Clinically, the disease has protean aspects, but a special tendency to attack the respiratory mucous membranes. A special organism, *Bacillus influenzæ,* is found.

History.—Great pandemics have been recognized since the sixteenth century. There were four with their succeeding epidemics during the last century—1830-'33, 1836-'37, 1847-'48, and 1889-'90. The last pandemic seems to have begun, as many others had before, in the far East. It may have started in May, 1889, in Buchara, reaching Moscow in September, the Caucasus and St. Petersburg in October. By the middle of November Berlin was attacked. By the middle of December it was in London, and by the end of the month it had invaded New York, and was widely distributed over the entire continent. Within a year it had visited nearly all parts of the earth.

The duration of an epidemic in any one locality is from six to eight weeks. With the exception, perhaps, of dengue, there is no disease which attacks indiscriminately so large a portion of the inhabitants, about 40 per cent., as a rule. Fortunately, as in dengue, the rate of mortality is very low. Of 55,263 cases reported in the German army, 60 died, or about 0.1 per cent. As might be expected, in the civil population the mortality is somewhat higher, reaching 133, or about 0.5 per cent. of the 22,972 cases reported in Munich. Over one-half of these deaths were due to pneumonia. In 1909 the deaths in England and Wales numbered 8,992. The opportunity for studying the disease in the last epidemic has thrown much light upon many problems. Among the most notable productions were the work of Pfeiffer on the etiology of the disease, the elaborate Berlin report by von Leyden and Senator, and the Local Government Board's report by Parsons. Leichtenstern's article in Nothnagel's Handbuch is the most masterly and systematic consideration of the disease in the literature.

Etiology.—What relation has the epidemic influenza to the ordinary influenza cold or catarrhal fever (commonly also called the *grippe*), which is constantly present in the community? Leichtenstern answers this question by making the following divisions: (*a*) Epidemic *influenza vera,* caused by Pfeiffer's bacillus; (*b*) endemic-epidemic *influenza vera,* which often occurs for several years in succession after a pandemic, also caused by the same bacillus; (*c*) endemic *influenza nostras,* pseudo-influenza or catarrhal fever, commonly called the *grippe,* is caused by various organisms, alone or in combination, and bears the same relation to the true influenza as cholera nostras does to Asiatic cholera.

Since the last pandemic we have not been free from local outbreaks in some part of the world. In some places the disease seems to have been continually present.

Ruhemann reports 1,979 cases of typical grippe between 1895 and 1902. In 115 he demonstrated the influenza bacillus. Lord (in Boston) demonstrated influenza bacilli in about 30 per cent. of 100 unselected cases of acute and chronic bronchitis. Yet during this period there was no epidemic of influenza in the city. The reports are sufficiently numerous to show that the influenza bacillus is probably constantly with us. Many observations show that it is a frequent invader of the respiratory tract in the inter-epidemic periods and is probably responsible for many of the cases of Leichtenstern's influenza nostras. Indeed, it seems to bear a similar relation to the acute infections of the respiratory tract as other common organisms. It is still unexplained why it should stand in a different relation to the epidemics of influenza as the sole cause of the disease.

The disease is highly contagious; it spreads with remarkable rapidity, which, however, is not greater than modern methods of conveyance. In the great pandemic of 1889-'90 some of the large prisons escaped entirely. The outbreak of epidemics is independent of all seasonal and meteorological conditions, except perhaps sunshine. The worst have been in the colder seasons of the year. One attack does not necessarily protect from a subsequent one. A few persons appear not to be liable to the disease.

Bacteriology.—In 1892 Pfeiffer isolated a bacillus from the nasal and bronchial secretions, which is recognized as the cause of the disease. It is a small, non-motile organism, which stains well in Loeffler's methylene blue, or in a dilute, pale-red solution of carbol-fuchsin in water. The bacilli are present in enormous numbers in the nasal and bronchial secretions of patients, in the latter almost in pure cultures. They persist often after the severe symptoms have subsided.

The much-discussed question whether during the presence of an epidemic human influenza attacks animals must be answered in the negative. In great pandemics of influenza the general rule seems to hold that other diseases do not prevail to the same extent, but it may be that other diseases are wrongly included under influenza.

Symptoms.—The incubation period is "from one to four days; oftenest three to four days." The onset is usually abrupt, with fever and its associated phenomena.

Types of the Disease.—The manifestations are so extraordinarily complex that it is best to describe them under types of the disease.

(*a*) Respiratory.—The mucous membrane of the respiratory tract from the nose to the air-cells of the lungs may be regarded as the seat of election of the influenza bacilli. In the simple forms the disease sets in with coryza, and presents the features of an acute catarrhal fever, with perhaps rather more prostration and debility than is usual. In other cases after catarrhal symptoms bronchitis occurs, the fever increases, there is delirium and much prostration, and the picture may even be that of severe typhoid fever. The graver respiratory conditions are bronchitis, pleurisy, and pneumonia. The bronchitis has really no special peculiarities. The sputum is supposed by many to be distinctive. Sometimes it is in extraordinary amounts, very thin, and containing purulent masses. Pfeiffer regards sputum of a greenish-yellow color and in coin-like lumps as almost characteristic of influenza. In other cases there may be a dark red, bloody sputum. It occasionally happens that the bronchitis is of great intensity and reaches the finer tubes, so that the patient becomes cyanosed or even asphyxiated.

Influenza pneumonia is one of the most serious manifestations, and may depend upon Pfeiffer's bacillus itself, or is the result of a mixed infection. The true influenza pneumonia is most commonly lobular or catarrhal, probably never croupous. Much of the mortality of the disease depends upon the fatal character of this complication. The clinical course of the cases is often irregular and the symptoms are obscure or masked.

Influenza pleurisy is more rare, but cases of primary involvement of the pleura are reported. It is very apt to lead to empyema. Pulmonary tuberculosis is usually much aggravated by an attack of influenza.

(*b*) Nervous Form.—Without any catarrhal symptoms there are severe headache, pain in the back and joints, with profound prostration. Among the more serious complications may be mentioned meningitis and encephalitis, the latter leading to hemiplegia or monoplegia. Abscess of the brain has followed in acute cases. Myelitis, with symptoms like an acute Landry's paralysis, has occurred, and spastic paraplegia or a pseudo-tabes may follow an attack.

The influenza bacillus has been demonstrated by lumbar puncture during life and in the meninges after death. All forms of neuritis are not uncommon, and in some cases are characterized by marked disturbance of motion and sensation. Judging from the accounts in the literature, almost every form of disease of the nervous system may follow influenza.

Among the most important of the nervous sequelæ are depression of spirits, melancholia, and in some cases dementia.

(*c*) Gastro-intestinal Form.—With the onset of the fever there may be nausea and vomiting, or the attack may set in with abdominal pain, profuse diarrhœa, and collapse. In some epidemics jaundice has been a common symptom. In a considerable number of the cases there is enlargement of the spleen, depending chiefly upon the intensity of the fever. This was a very rare form in the United States.

(*d*) Febrile Form.—The fever in influenza is very variable, but it is important to recognize that it may be the only manifestation of the disease. It is sometimes markedly remittent, with chills; or in rare cases there is a protracted, continued fever of several weeks' duration, which simulates typhoid closely. Sometimes the fever resembles that of a tertian malaria.

Complications.—The *pericarditis* is apt to be latent. Of *endocarditis,* a number of cases have been reported in which micro-organisms morphologically like influenza bacilli have been isolated from the vegetations. The malignant form may occur. Myocarditis may follow, and has been a cause of sudden death. Functional disturbances are common, palpitation, bradycardia, tachycardia, and angina-like attacks. Phlebitis and thrombosis of various vessels have been described.

Septicæmia has been demonstrated in a number of cases by the cultivation of influenza bacilli from the circulating blood.

Peritonitis is rare. *Cholelithiasis* may follow an attack. The increased prevalence of *appendicitis* has been attributed to influenza.

Various renal affections have been noted. G. Baumgarten has called attention to the frequency of nephritis. Orchitis has been also seen. Herpes is common. A diffuse erythema sometimes occurs, occasionally purpura. Catarrhal conjunctivitis is a frequent event. Iritis, and in rare instances optic neuritis, have been met with. Acute otitis media is a common complication. I have seen severe and persistent vertigo follow influenza, probably from involvement of the labyrinth. Bronchiectasis may follow. I have seen several cases; in a fatal one of three years' duration the influenza bacilli were present in the sputum.

Since the late severe epidemics it has been the fashion to date various ailments or chronic ill health from influenza. In many cases this is correct. It is astonishing the number of people who have been crippled in health for years after an attack.

Diagnosis.—During a pandemic the cases offer but slight difficulty. The profoundness of the prostration, out of all proportion to the intensity of the disease, is one of the most characteristic features. In the respiratory form the diagnosis may be made by the bacteriological examination of the sputum, a procedure which should be resorted to early in a suspected epidemic. The differentiation of the various forms has been already sufficiently considered.

Treatment.—Isolation should be practised when possible, and old people should be guarded against all possible sources of infection. The secretions, nasal and bronchial, should be thoroughly disinfected. In every case the disease should be regarded as serious, and the patient should be confined to bed until the fever has completely disappeared. In this way alone can serious complications be avoided. From the outset the treatment should be supporting, and the patient should be carefully fed and well nursed. The bowels should be opened by a dose of calomel or a saline draught. At night 10 grains of Dover's powder may be given. At the onset a warm bath is sometimes grateful in relieving the pain in the back and limbs, but great care should be taken to have the bed well warmed, and the patient should be given after it a drink of hot lemonade. If the fever is high and there is delirium, small doses of antipyrin or aspirin (gr. x, 0.6 gm.) may be given and an ice-cap applied to the head. The medicinal antiypyretics should be used with caution, as profound prostration sometimes occurs after their employment. Too much stress should not be laid upon the mental features. Delirium may be marked even with slight fever. In the cases with great cardiac weakness stimulants should be given freely, and during convalescence strychnia in full doses.

The intense bronchitis, pneumonia, and other complications should receive their appropriate treatment. The convalescence requires careful management, and it may be weeks or months before the patient is restored to full health. A good nutritious diet, change of air, and pleasant surroundings are essential. The depression of spirits following this disease is one of its most unpleasant and obstinate features.

IX. WHOOPING COUGH

Definition.—A specific affection due in all probability to the Bordet bacillus, characterized by catarrh of the respiratory passages and a series of convulsive coughs which end in a long-drawn inspiration or "whoop."

History.—Ballonius, in his *Ephemerides,* describes the disease as it appeared in 1578. Glisson and Sydenham in the following century gave brief accounts. Willis (Pharmaceutice Rationalis, second part, 1674) gave a much better description and called it an "epidemical disorder."

Etiology.—The disease occurs in epidemic form, but sporadic cases appear in a community from time to time. It is directly contagious from person to person; but dwelling-rooms, houses, school-rooms, and other localities may be infected by a sick child. It is, however, in this way less contagious than other diseases, and is probably most often taken by direct contact. Epidemics prevail for two or three months, usually during the winter and spring, and have a curious relation to other diseases, often preceding or following epidemics of measles, less frequently of scarlet fever.

Children between the first and second dentitions are most liable to be attacked. Sucklings are, however, not exempt, and I have seen very severe attacks in infants under six weeks. Congenital cases are described. It is stated that girls are more subject to the disease than boys. Adults and old people are sometimes attacked, and in the aged it may be a very serious affection. It appears to be most contagious in the catarrhal period. A natural immunity has been mentioned, but it must be remembered that a child may have the disease in a very mild form. As a rule, one attack protects; second attacks are rare. The disease is more than twice as fatal in the negro race as in others. There were 7,182 deaths from it in 1909 in England.

An organism has been described by Bordet and Gengou, *Bacillus pertussis,* resembling in certain features the influenza bacillus. In convalescents the deviation of complement reaction is present and the serum is stated to agglutinate the organism. Apes have been inoculated with the production of a characteristic pertussis.

Morbid Anatomy.—Whooping cough itself has no special pathological changes. In fatal cases pulmonary complications, particularly broncho-pneumonia, are usually present. Collapse and compensatory emphysema, vesicular and interstitial, are found, and the tracheal and bronchial glands are enlarged. There is a constant lesion of the trachea with the presence of bacilli between the columnar cells.

Symptoms.—There is a variable period of incubation of from seven to ten days. Catarrhal and paroxysmal stages can be recognized. In the *catarrhal stage* the child has the symptoms of an ordinary cold, which may begin with slight fever, running at the nose, injection of the eyes, and a bronchial cough, usually dry, and sometimes giving indications of a spasmodic character. Trousseau calls attention to the *incessant* character of the early cough. The fever is usually not high, and slight attention is paid to the symptoms, which are thought to be those of a simple catarrh. After lasting for a week or ten days, instead of subsiding, the cough becomes worse and more convulsive in character.

The *paroxysmal stage,* marked by the characteristic cough, dates from the first appearance of the "whoop." The fit begins with a series of from fifteen to twenty forcible short coughs of increasing intensity, between which no inspiratory effort is made. The child gets blue in the face, and then with a deep inspiration the air is drawn into the lungs, making the "whoop," which may be heard at a distance, and from which the disease takes its name. A deep inspiration may precede the series of spasmodic expiratory efforts. Several coughing fits may succeed each other until a tenacious mucus is ejected, usually small in amount, but after a series of coughing spells a considerable quantity may be expectorated. Vomiting often takes place at the end of a paroxysm, and may recur so frequently in the day that the child does not get enough food and becomes emaciated. There may be only four or five attacks in the day, or in severe cases they may recur every half-hour. In severe and fatal cases the paroxysms may exceed one hundred daily. During the paroxysm the thorax is very strongly compressed by the powerful expiratory efforts, and, as very little air passes in through the glottis, there are signs of defective aëration of the blood; the face becomes swollen and congested, the veins are prominent, the eyeballs protrude, and the conjunctivæ become deeply engorged. Suffocation indeed seems imminent, when with a deep, crowing inspiration air enters the lungs and the color is quickly restored. The child knows for a few moments when the attack is coming on, and tries in every way to check it, but failing to do so, runs terrified to the nurse or mother to be supported, or clutches anything near by. Few diseases are more painful to witness. In severe paroxysms the sphincters may be opened. The urine is said to be of high specific gravity (1022-1032), pale yellow, and to contain much uric acid.

An ulcer may form under the tongue from rubbing on the teeth (Riga's disease).

During the attack, if the chest be examined, the resonance is defective in the expiratory stage, full and clear during the deep, crowing inspiration; but on auscultation during the latter there may be no vesicular murmur heard, owing to the slowness with which the air passes the narrowed glottis. Bronchial râles are occasionally heard.

Among circumstances which precipitate a paroxysm are emotion, such as crying, and any irritation about the throat. Even the act of swallowing sometimes seems sufficient. In a close dusty atmosphere the coughing fits are more frequent. After lasting for three or four weeks the attacks become lighter and finally cease. In cases of ordinary severity the course of the disease is rarely under six weeks.

Complications and Sequelæ.—The complications and sequelæ of whooping cough are important. During the extensive venous congestion, hæmorrhages are very apt to occur in the form of petechiæ, particularly about the forehead, ecchymosis of the conjunctivæ, and even bleeding tears of blood (Trousseau) from the rupture of the vessels, epistaxis, bleeding from the ears, and occasionally hæmoptysis. Hæmorrhage from the bowels is rare. Convulsions are not very uncommon, due perhaps to the extreme engorgement of the cerebral cortex. Death has occurred from spasm of the glottis. Sudden death has been caused by extensive subdural hæmorrhage. Paralysis is a rare event. It was associated with 3 of my series of 120 cases, but in none of them did the hemiplegia come on during the paroxysm, as in a case reported by S. West. Valentine (1901) has collected 79 cases, chiefly hemiplegias. A spastic paraplegia may follow. Acute polyneuritis is a rare sequel.

The persistent vomiting may induce marked anæmia and wasting. The pulmonary complications are extremely serious. During the severe coughing spells interstitial emphysema may be induced, more rarely pneumothorax. I saw one instance in which rupture occurred, evidently near the root of the lung, and the air passed along the trachea and reached the subcutaneous tissues of the neck, a condition which has been known to become general. Capillary bronchitis, lobular and pseudo-lobar pneumonia are the dangerous complications, responsible for nine out of ten deaths in the disease. In some cases the process is tuberculous. Pleurisy is sometimes met with and occasionally lobar pneumonia. Enlargement of the bronchial glands is very common in whooping cough, and has been thought to cause the disease. It may sometimes be sufficient to produce dulness over the manubrium. During the spasm the radial pulse is small, the right heart engorged, and during and after the attack the cardiac action is very much disturbed. Serious damage may result, and possibly some of the cases of severe valvular disease in children who have had neither rheumatic nor scarlet fever may be attributed to the terrible heart strain during a prolonged attack. Koplik regards the swelling about the face and eyes as an important sign of the heart strain. Serious renal complications are very uncommon, but albumin sometimes and sugar frequently are found in the urine. A distressing sequel in adults is asthma, which may recur at intervals for a year or more. An unusually marked leucocytosis appears early, chiefly of the lymphocytes (Meunier).

Diagnosis.—So distinctive is the "whoop" of the disease that the diagnosis is very easy; but occasionally there are doubtful cases, particularly during epidemics, in which a series of expiratory coughs occurs without any inspiratory crow. The spasmodic cough due to enlarged bronchial glands may cause difficulty.

Prognosis.—If we include its complications, whooping cough is a very fatal affection, ranking one of the first among the acute infections as a cause of death in children under five years of age.

Prophylaxis.—The disease should be placed on the list of reportable infections. When possible the sputum should be collected and disinfected. As the organism usually disappears within two weeks from the appearance of the characteristic cough it is probable that there is little danger of contagion in the later stages. A prophylactic vaccine has been used.

Treatment.—The gravity of the disease is scarcely appreciated by the public. Children with the disease should not be sent to school or exposed in public in any way. There is more reprehensible neglect in connection with this than with any other disease. The patient should be isolated, and if the paroxysms are at all severe, at rest in bed. Fresh air, night and day, is important, but in cities in the winter this is not easy to manage. The treatment is notoriously unsatisfactory. Stock vaccine has been used for treatment with some benefit. A few patients are promptly cured. Antiseptic measures have been extensively tried. Quinine holds its own with many practitioners; a sixth of a grain may be given three times a day for each month of age, and a grain and a half for each year in children under five. The use of benzoin inhalations is often helpful. For the catarrhal symptoms moderate doses of ipecac are probably the most satisfactory. Sedatives are by far the most trustworthy drugs in severe cases, and paregoric may be given freely, particularly to give rest at night. Codeia and heroin in doses proper for the age often give much relief. Jacobi advises belladonna in full doses, as much as one-sixth of a grain of the extract to a child of six or eight months three times a day. Children can often be taught to inhibit an attack.

Other remedies, such an antipyrin and chloral hydrate, may be tried. In older children and in adults it would be worth while, I think, to try the intratracheal injections of olive-oil and iodoform, which are sometimes so useful in allaying severe paroxysmal cough. The wearing of a tight abdominal binder is sometimes of value.

After the severity of the attack has passed and convalescence has begun, the child should be watched with the greatest care. It is just at this period that the fatal broncho-pneumonias are apt to develop. The cough sometimes persists for months and the child remains weak and delicate. Change of air should be tried. Such a patient should be fed with care and given tonics and cod-liver oil.

X. GONOCOCCUS INFECTION

Definition.—An acute infection with a primary lesion, usually blennorrhagia, and numerous secondary and systemic manifestations, of which prostatitis and epididymitis, salpingitis, arthritis, synovitis and endocarditis are the most important. The *Micrococcus gonorrhœæ* (gonococcus) was described by Neisser, in 1879.

Gonorrhœa, one of the most widespread and serious of infectious diseases, presents many features for consideration. It is not a killing disease; only 39 fatal cases are recorded in the Registrar General's Report, 1909, for England and Wales, but as a cause of ill-health and disability the gonococcus occupies a position of the very first rank among its fellows. While the local lesion is too often thought to be trifling, in its singular obstinacy, in the possibilities of permanent sexual damage to the individual himself and still more in the "grisly troop" which may follow in its train, gonorrhœa does not fall very far short of syphilis in importance.

Etiology.—The organism is a biscuit-shaped micrococcus, occurring in pairs, usually within the leucocytes, and is always found in the primary and systemic lesions. It is capable of cultivation, and the disease has been reproduced by inoculation of the pure culture.

The disease is seen in men and women as a result of impure sexual intercourse, and in the new-born from vaginal contamination, and in older children by accidental infection. Ophthalmia neonatorum is one of the great causes of blindness, but an active campaign of education is rapidly reducing the number of cases.

The gonococcus vaginitis and the ophthalmia are very serious diseases in children's hospitals and in infants' homes. The story of the gonococcus infection in the Babies' Hospital, New York, for eleven years, as told by Holt (N. Y. Med. Jour., March, 1905), illustrates the singular obstinacy of the infection. In spite of the greatest care and precaution, there were, in 1903, 65 cases of vaginitis, with 2 of ophthalmia and 12 of arthritis. In 1904 there were 52 cases of vaginitis, only 16 of which would have been recognized without the bacteriological examination. In all, in the eleven years, there were 273 cases of vaginitis, only 6 with ophthalmia and 26 with arthritis. Other institutions have had equally sad experiences. Isolation and prolonged quarantine are the only measures to combat successfully the disease.

The immediate and remote effects of the gonococcus may be considered under—

I. The primary infection.
II. The spread in the genito-urinary organs by direct continuity.
III. Systemic gonococcus infection.

The primary lesion we need not here consider, but we may call attention to the frequency of the complications, such as periurethral abscess, gonorrhœal prostatitis in the male, and vaginitis, endocervicitis, and inflammation of the glands of Bartholini in the female.

Perhaps the most serious of all the sequels are those which result from **the spread** by direct continuity of tissue. Gonococcus salpingitis has been shown to be not infrequent. Metritis and ovaritis are also occasionally met with, and peritonitis. The gonococcus has been found in pure culture in cases of acute general peritonitis. Equally important is the cystitis, which is probably much more frequently the result of a mixed infection than due to the gonococcus itself. There is some danger of extension upward through the ureters to the kidneys. The pyelitis, like the cystitis, is usually a mixed infection.

Systemic Gonococcus Infection.—(1) Gonococcus Septicæmia and Pyæmia.—Thayer and Blumer first cultivated the gonococci from the blood in a case in my wards, and the septicæmia has been thoroughly studied by them and by Cole, who has divided the cases into four groups: (1) Those with *endocarditis,* 11 of the 29 cases collected by him. The clinical features are those of malignant endocarditis; two of the cases recovered. (2) Cases with *local suppuration* and the general features of a *pyæmia*—of the six cases three died. The septicæmia associated with a small focus of suppuration may be very intense. I examined the body of a young man who ten days after the onset of urethritis had chills and high fever; he became profoundly toxæmic and died on the morning of the fourth day from the chill. There was a small prostatic abscess and a dark tarry fluid blood, unlike anything I have ever seen. (3) Cases *with no metastatic local affections* or perhaps only slight arthritis. In a remarkable case at the Johns Hopkins Hospital, three months after an acute gonorrhœa the patient had a fever resembling typhoid, which lasted seven weeks. Gonococci were cultivated from the blood. He recovered and, as Cole suggests, such cases are probably more common than we suspect. (4) Cases of *gonorrheal puerperal septicæmia,* of which several instances have been reported. Of the 29 cases in which the septicæmia was demonstrated by the cultivation of the organism from the blood, 12 died. The endocarditis will be considered later.

(2) Gonococcus Arthritis.—In many respects this is the most damaging, disabling, and serious of all the complications of gonorrhœa, occurring in from 2 to 5 per cent. of the cases. It occurs more frequently in males than in females; 43 to 7 in one series at the Johns Hopkins Hospital (Cole). In a series of 252 cases collected by Northrup, 230 were in males; 130 cases were between twenty and thirty years of age. It occurs, as a rule, during an acute attack of gonorrhœa. In 208 of Northrup's series there was a urethral discharge while in hospital. It may occur as the attack subsides, or even when it has become chronic. A gonorrhœal arthritis of great intensity may occur in a newly married woman infected by an old gleet in her husband. In women it is not always easy to find evidence of local infection. As a rule, many joints are affected. In an analysis by Cole and McCrae of the involvement of the joints in gonococcus arthritis and in rheumatic fever, the average number in the former was double that in the latter. In Northrup's series three or more joints were affected in 175 cases, one joint in 56 cases. It is peculiar in attacking certain joints which are rarely involved in rheumatic fever, as the sterno-clavicular, the inter-vertebral, the temporo-maxillary and sacro-iliac.

The *anatomical changes* are variable. The inflammation is often peri-articular, and extends along the sheaths of the tendons. When effusion occurs in the joints it rarely becomes purulent. It has more commonly the characters of a synovitis. About the wrist and hand suppuration sometimes occurs in the sheaths. The gonococcus itself is present in the inflamed joint or in the peri-arthritic exudate, and may often be obtained in pure culture. Sometimes the cultures are negative. Mixed infection with staphylococci or streptococci is very rare.

Clinical Course.—Variability and obstinacy are the two most distinguishing features. The following are the most important clinical forms:

(*a*) *Arthralgic,* in which there are wandering pains about the joints, without redness or swelling. These persist for a long time.

(*b*) *Polyarthritic,* in which several joints become affected. The fever is slight; the local inflammation may fix itself in one joint, but more commonly several become swollen and tender. In this form cerebral and cardiac complications may occur.

(*c*) *Acute gonococcus arthritis,* in which a joint, usually the knee, becomes suddenly involved. The pain is severe, the swelling extensive, and due chiefly to peri-articular œdema. The general fever is not at all proportionate to the intensity of the local signs. The exudate usually resolves, though suppuration occasionally supervenes.

(*d*) *Chronic Hydrarthrosis.*—This is usually mono-articular, and is particularly apt to involve the knee. It comes on often without pain, redness, or swelling. Formation of pus is rare. It occurred only twice in 96 cases tabulated by Nolen.

(*e*) *Bursal and Synovial Form.*—This attacks chiefly the tendons and their sheaths and the bursæ and the periosteum. The articulations may not be affected. The bursæ of the patella, the olecranon, and the tendo Achillis are most apt to be involved.

(*f*) *Septicæmic.*—In which with an acute arthritis the gonococci invade the blood, and the picture is that of an intense septico-pyæmia, usually with endocarditis.

(*g*) The *Painful Heel of Gonorrhœa.*—This is a remarkable form of pododynia due to local periosteal thickening and exostosis on the os calcis, causing pain and great disability. Baer has demonstrated the gonococcus in the periosteal lesion.

Complications.—Iritis is not infrequent and may recur with successive attacks. The visceral complications are serious. Endocarditis, pericarditis, and pleurisy may occur.

Treatment.—The primary infection—usually urethritis—should be actively treated. Of special measures, the use of antigonococcus serum and vaccine treatment are worthy of trial; either will help some cases, both fail in many. Good food, fresh air, and open bowels are important. Drugs are of little value, especially sodium salicylate and potassium iodide. Phenacetine or aspirin may be given for the pain.

The local treatment is very important. In acute cases, fixation of the joints is very beneficial, and in the chronic forms, massage and passive motion. Counter-irritation by the cautery or blisters, active hyperæmia by baking or passive by the Bier method are all useful. A distended joint may be tapped and then tightly bandaged. The surgical treatment is more satisfactory in severe cases and good results usually follow incision and irrigation.

XI. BACILLARY DYSENTERY

Definition.—A form of intestinal flux, usually of an acute type, occurring sporadically and in severe epidemics, attacking children as well as adults, characterized by pain, frequent passages of blood and mucus, and due to the action of a specific bacillus, of which there are various strains.

Etiology.—Owing to improved sanitation, dysentery has become less frequent. In temperate climates sporadic cases occur from time to time, and at intervals epidemics prevail, particularly in overcrowded institutions. The statistics of general hospitals for the past twenty years show a decided increase in the number of cases admitted. Records of widespread epidemics have been collected by Woodward. The most serious was that which prevailed from 1847 to 1856. In Great Britain and Ireland epidemics of the disease have become less frequent. In institutions, particularly in overcrowded asylums, dysentery is very common, and this form has been made the subject of a valuable report by Mott and Durham. In the tropics "dysentery is a destructive giant compared to which strong drink is a mere phantom" (Macgregor). Dysentery is one of the great camp diseases, and it has been more destructive to armies than powder and shot. In the Federal service during the civil war, according to Woodward,* there were 259,071 cases of acute and 28,451 cases of chronic dysentery. The disease prevails in Porto Rico, the Philippines, and to a less extent in Cuba. In the South African campaign dysentery prevailed widely. For many years a very fatal form of dysentery has prevailed in Japan, particularly in the summer and autumn months, having a mortality of from 26 to 27 per cent.; in 1899 there were 125,989 cases, with 26,709 deaths (Eldridge). It is now generally conceded that the severe epidemics of acute dysentery occurring in the tropics are of the bacillary type, and the same form prevails in temperate climates.

Bacillus Dysenteriæ.—In 1898, Shiga, a Japanese observer, found in the dysentery prevailing in his country a bacillus with special characters, which he considered to be the specific cause of the disease.

Flexner and Barker, of the Johns Hopkins Commission for the Study of Tropical Diseases, found in the dysentery in the Philippine Islands an identical organism, and it has been made the subject of very careful study by Flexner, and also by R. P. Strong, Musgrave, and Craig, of the United States army. It has also been found in cases of dysentery from Porto Rico. The organism appears to be constantly present in the acute dysentery of the tropics. In Manila, according to Strong and Musgrave, of 1,328 cases, 712 were of the acute specific variety, 55 suspected specific cases, and 561 of amœbic dysentery. Kruse, in an outbreak at Laar, in Germany, in which 300 persons were attacked, has isolated an identical bacillus. Vedder and Duval demonstrated that sporadic cases in adults in Philadelphia, as well as epidemics of dysentery in the Lancaster County Asylum, Pennsylvania, and in the almshouse at New Haven, were due to this organism. Duval and Bassett demonstrated that certain forms of summer diarrhœas of infants were

* Medical and Surgical History of the War of the Rebellion, Medical, vol. ii. The most exhaustive treatise extant on intestinal fluxes—an enduring monument to the industry and ability of the author.

due to infection with *B. dysenteriæ.* The Rockefeller Institute conducted a collective investigation into the cause of infantile diarrhœas in Boston, New York, Philadelphia, and Baltimore. Several observers, under Flexner's direction, studied 412 cases and found the dysentery bacillus present in 279 or 63.2 per cent.

The strain of the bacillus most frequently found in the United States is the "Flexner-Harris" type. It is now conceded that a number of strains of the bacillus occur. This fact has been determined by the relative agglutinative power of immune serum upon the bacilli isolated, as well as by the action of the latter upon various sugars. The lesions produced by the different strains are identical. The organism agglutinates with the blood serum of cases with acute dysentery as well as with the serum of immunized animals.

Infection takes place by the mouth. The organisms are widely distributed by the fæces of persons suffering with the disease and also by dysentery "carriers." In institutions food and drink readily become contaminated. Possibly, too, the germs are distributed by flies and dust.

Morbid Anatomy.—In the acute cases, when death has occurred on the fourth to the seventh day, the mucous membrane of the large intestine is swollen, of a deep-red color, and presents elevated, coarse corrugations and folds. In addition to the intense hyperæmia there are spots of hæmorrhage scattered through the swollen mucosa. Over the surface there is usually a superficial necrotic layer, which can be brushed off lightly with the finger. This may be in patches, or uniform over large areas. There is no ulceration, only the superficial, general necrosis of the mucosa. The solitary follicles are swollen and red, but the prominence is obscured in the involvement of the entire mucosa. In cases of great intensity the entire coats of the colon may be stiff and thick, and the mucous membrane enormously increased in thickness, grayish black in color, extensively necrotic, and, in places, gangrenous. The serous surface is often deeply injected. The ileum is, in many cases, involved, having a deeply hæmorrhagic mucosa, with a superficial necrosis. In the subacute cases there is not the same great thickening of the intestinal wall, the solitary follicles are more swollen, there is less necrosis, and, while there are no ulcers, there are superficial erosions.

Symptoms.—According to Strong and Musgrave, the period of incubation is not more than forty-eight hours. The onset, which is usually sudden, is characterized by slight fever, pain in the abdomen, and frequent stools. At first mucus is passed, but within twenty-four hours blood appears with it, or there is pure blood. There is a constant desire to go to stool, with great straining and tenesmus; every hour or half hour there may be a small amount of blood and mucus passed. The temperature rises and may reach 103° or 104°. The pulse increases in frequency, and in the severer cases becomes very small. The tongue is coated with a white fur, and there is excessive thirst. In the very acute cases the patient becomes seriously ill within forty-eight hours, the movements increase in frequency, the pain is of great intensity, the patient becomes delirious, and death may occur on the third or fourth day. In cases of moderate severity the urgency of the symptoms abates, the stools lessen, the temperature falls, and within two or three weeks the patient is convalescent. The mortality in the severe forms is very high. There is a subacute form which lasts for many weeks or months. The patients become greatly emaciated, having from three to five stools in the twenty-four hours. The *Bacillus dysenteriæ* is found in the stools, and it agglutinates readily with the blood serum.

Other Clinical Types.—The foregoing account describes the essential features of bacillary dysentery as seen in Japan, the Philippines, and the tropics. The clinical features of bacillary dysentery in adults in temperate climates differ in no essential manner from those already described. Although the evidence hardly warrants us at present in making the sweeping statement that all non-amœbic cases of dysentery are bacillary in origin, yet experience will probably demonstrate eventually that this is the case. What is known as the acute catarrhal dysentery is probably a sporadic form due to the *Bacillus dysenteriæ.* Diphtheritic dysentery is a type of the bacillary form with great necrosis and infiltration of the mucosa. There may be rapid gangrene and a fatal termination within twenty-four hours. A secondary diphtheritic dysentery is a common terminal event in many acute and chronic diseases, and a bacillus of the Shiga type has been isolated from these cases. Vedder and Duval have demonstrated that the bacillus is present in them.

Complications and Sequelæ.—*Peritonitis* is rare, due either to extension through the wall of the bowel or to perforation. When this occurs about the cæcal region, perityphlitis results; when low down in the rectum, periproctitis. In 108 autopsies collected by Woodward perforation occurred in 11. Abscess of the liver, so common in the amœbic form, is very rare. It is interesting to note, as illustrating the probable type of the disease, how comparatively rare abscess of the liver was during the American civil war. Very few cases occurred in the South-African War (Rolleston).

In the tropics malaria and acute dysentery very often coexist. With reference to typhoid fever, as a complication, Woodward mentions that the combination was exceedingly frequent during the civil war, and characteristic lesions of both diseases coexisted. In civil practice it is extremely rare.

Sydenham noted that dysentery was sometimes associated with rheumatic pains, and in certain epidemics joint swellings have been especially prevalent. They are not of the nature of rheumatic fever, but rather analogous to those of gonorrhœal arthritis. In severe cases there may be pleurisy, thrombosis, pericarditis, endocarditis, and occasionally pyæmic manifestations, among which may be mentioned pylephlebitis. Chronic nephritis is also an occasional sequel. In protracted cases there may be an anæmic œdema. An interesting sequel of dysentery is paralysis. Woodward reports 8 cases. Weir Mitchell mentions it as not uncommon, occurring chiefly in the form of paraplegia. As in other acute fevers, this is due probably to a neuritis. Remlinger, in two cases of non-amœbic dysentery in Tunis, observed an epididymitis during convalescence. Gonorrhœa was excluded. In a third case the dysentery was complicated by an abscess of the spleen, which ruptured, causing death. Intestinal stricture is a rare sequence—so rare that no case was reported at the Surgeon-General's office during the civil war. It appears to be not uncommon in the East. Among the sequelæ of chronic dysentery, in persons who have recovered a certain measure of health, may be mentioned persistent dyspepsia and irritability of the bowels.

Diagnosis.—In the acute specific form the blood serum agglutinates the dysentery bacillus. The "Flexner-Harris" type of the organism agglutinates in dilutions of from 1 to 1,000 up to 1 to 1,500. This is the form of the organism that prevails in the United States. The "Shiga" type agglutinates less readily. The blood serum of a dysenteric patient will agglutinate both types, but the former more readily than the latter. In all non-amœbic dysenteries efforts should be made to isolate the dysentery bacillus from the stools.

Treatment.—Flint has shown that sporadic dysentery is, in its slighter grades at least, a self-limited disease, which runs its course in eight or nine days. Reading the report of his cases, one is struck, however, with their comparative mildness.

PROPHYLACTIC.—The same prophylactic precautions should be followed as are adopted in typhoid fever. Flexner and Gay have shown that animals can be protected from infection by a previous treatment with immune horse serum. Protective and curative serums have been prepared and are now on the market.

I. ACUTE DYSENTERY.—The patient should be absolutely at rest in bed. He should be kept warm and have a flannel abdominal binder applied. The diet should be very simple—whey, egg albumen, barley or rice water, and strained gruels. Enough water should be given to relieve thirst. If vomiting occurs, nothing should be given by mouth for some hours, and if the patient requires fluid this can be given by infusion. Hot applications to the abdomen are useful. If the patient is seen early in the attack, free purgation is advisable, for which sodium sulphate and Rochelle salts are best. Either may be given in doses of two drachms (8 gm.) for two doses an hour apart and later half the amount every three hours until the bowels have moved freely. By this treatment the course is sometimes cut short. If the attack is well established, the use of purgatives must be determined by the conditions present. If solid fæcal matter is being passed, a purgative is indicated, castor oil being the best (ʒ vi, 25 c. c.). Until the bowels have been thoroughly cleared, purgation is indicated.

Medicinal.—Bismuth in large doses often has a beneficial effect. Thirty to sixty grains (2 to 4 gm.) should be given every hour. Minute doses of bichloride of mercury, one hundredth of a grain every two hours, were recommended by Ringer. For the relief of pain and to quiet the bowel, morphia is the most useful drug and is to be preferred to opium by mouth. It should be given hypodermically in large doses (gr. 1-4 to 1-3, 0.016 to 0.022 gm.), and repeated according to the needs of the patient. If tenesmus is not marked, opium can be given as the starch and laudanum enema, in which thirty minims (2 c. c.) of laudanum are given. The ipecacuanha treatment is not so suitable for the bacillary as for the amœbic form, with which it will be considered.

Local Treatment.—During the acute stages this may be out of the question, but should be employed whenever possible. Normal saline or sodium bicarbonate (1 per cent.) solution at the body temperature can be used. This should be given very gently and with the hips elevated. If there is rectal irritation, a cocaine or morphia suppository should be given beforehand. As the symptoms lessen, the quantity of fluid can be increased and other solutions used, such as boric acid (5 per cent.), salicylic acid (1 per cent.) or alum (1 to 200).

With convalescence the diet should be increased very gradually and only simple foods allowed. The patient should be kept quiet until all danger of a relapse is over. This is most important in the prevention of a chronic dysentery.

Serum Therapy.—Shiga produced a polyvalent serum by immunizing horses, by which he claims to have reduced the mortality in "endemic" dysentery in Japan from about 35 per cent. to 9 per cent. Good results have been reported from the use of the Pasteur Institute and Lister Institute serums, which should be given in doses of 20 c. c. two or three times a day.

II. CHRONIC DYSENTERY.—The patient should be at rest in bed and on simple diet, milk, boiled, peptonized or fermented, whey, beef juice, and eggs. In some cases milk may have to be given well diluted or in small amounts, but it usually agrees well. It is well to give an occasional purge (castor oil, ℥ ss, 15 c. c.) to empty the bowels. Drugs by mouth are not of great value. Bismuth, if used, should be in large doses (ʒ i, 4 gm.) every three hours while the patient is awake. Opium should not be given as a routine measure, as there is great danger of forming a habit. If employed, it is best given in the starch and laudanum enema.

Local Treatment.—This is most rational and should be carried out thoroughly. If the rectum is irritable, a cocaine or morphine suppository should be given half an hour previously. The irrigation, at the body temperature, should be given very gently, the patient encouraged to retain it as long as possible, and the amount gradually increased up to two litres if possible. One irrigation a day is usually enough. Silver nitrate solution is probably the best (1 to 5,000 at first and increased to 1 to 500). Boric acid (5 per cent.), salicylic acid (2 per cent.), alum, or tannic acid (3 per cent.) may also be used. With any of these an occasional irrigation of saline solution is useful. With improvement the frequency of the irrigations should be reduced. In the obstinate cases an appendicostomy may be done and the bowel irrigated through the opening.

XII. MALTA FEVER

(*Undulant Fever, Mediterranean Fever*)

Definition.—A specific fever, caused by the *Micrococcus melitensis*, characterized by undulatory pyrexial relapses, profuse sweats, rheumatic pains, arthritis, and an enlarged spleen. It is spread, as a rule, through the agency of goat's milk.

Distribution.—The disease prevails in the Mediterranean littoral, and endemic foci exist in India, Africa, China, and Manila. In the goat raising sections of Texas the disease is endemic (Gentry and Ferenbaugh). In the Malta garrison in the seven years 1898-1904, there were 2,229 cases, with an average case duration of one hundred and twenty days and with 77 deaths. About the same number of cases occurred in the fleet. Since the introduction of prophylactic measures the disease has practically disappeared from the Army and Navy, and has diminished greatly in the civil population.

Etiology.—The greater part of our knowledge of this remarkable disease we owe to the work of British army surgeons stationed at Gibraltar and Malta, particularly to Marston, Bruce, and Hughes. In 1886 Bruce isolated an organism which he called *Micrococcus melitensis* from the spleen and blood. Hughes, Wright, Semple, and others confirmed this. In 1904-1905 a Government Commission began a study on the island of the problems of the disease in all its aspects. It was shown to be a septicæmia, due to the above-named organism, which had an unusually prolonged saprophytic existence. Zamit showed that the goats, the most important animals in the domestic life of Malta, were largely infected, from 10 to 15 per cent. having the micrococcus in their milk. Monkeys were successfully infected with milk which contained the organisms. Steps were at once taken to stop the use as far as possible of goat's milk for the troops, with the result that the number of cases fell from 750 in 1905 to 145 in 1906, and to 7 for nine months of 1907. There were no cases in 1907 in the Mediterranean fleet, and since this date the disease has disappeared in the garrison and in the fleet.

The micrococcus enters the system through the gastro-intestinal tract. Ross and Eyre think it may also be transmitted by mosquitoes. It may spread by the infection of food by flies or by the fingers.

Symptoms.—There is no specific fever which presents the same remarkable group of phenomena. The period of incubation is from six to ten days. "Clinically the fever has a peculiar irregular temperature curve, consisting of intermittent waves or undulations of pyrexia, of a distinctly remittent character. These pyrexial waves or undulations last, as a rule, from one to three weeks, with an apyrexial interval lasting for two or more days. In rare cases the remissions may become so marked as to give an almost intermittent character to the febrile curve, clearly distinguishable, however, from the paroxysms of paludic infection. This pyrexial condition is usually much prolonged, having an uncertain duration, lasting for even six months or more. Unlike paludism, its course is not markedly affected by the administration of quinine. Its course is often irregular and even erratic in nature. This pyrexia is usually accompanied by obstinate constipation, progressive anæmia, and debility. It is often complicated with and followed by neuralgic symptoms referred to the peripheral or central nervous system, arthritic effusions, painful inflammatory conditions of certain fibrous structures, of a localized nature, or swelling of the testicles" (Hughes). There is a malignant type, in which the disease may prove fatal within a week or ten days; an undulatory type—the common variety—in which the fever is marked by intermittent waves or undulations of variable length, separated by periods of apyrexia and freedom from symptoms. In this really lie the peculiar features of the disease, and the unfortunate victim may suffer a series of relapses which may extend from three months, the average time, to two years. Lastly, there is an intermittent type, in which the patient may simply have daily pyrexia toward evening, without any special complications, and may do well and be able to go about his work, and yet at any time the other serious features of the disease may develop.

The blood serum of a patient with Malta fever agglutinates the *Micrococcus melitensis*. For diagnosis, cultures from the blood may be made or, if other procedures fail, from the spleen.

The mortality is slight, only about 2 per cent. There are no characteristic morbid lesions, but the spleen is enlarged, dark and soft. Malta fever can now be readily differentiated from typhoid fever and malaria. The *prophy-*

laxis is self-evident, and the brilliant work of the commission has already reduced the incidence of the disease to a minimum. The disease has disappeared from Gibraltar since the importation of goats from Malta has been stopped.

Treatment.—General measures suitable to typhoid fever are indicated. Fluid food should be given during the febrile period. Vaccines may be used and good results have been reported. Hydrotherapy, either the bath or the cold pack, should be used every third hour when the temperature is above 103° F. Otherwise the treatment is symptomatic. No drugs appear to have any special influence on the fever. A change of climate seems to promote convalescence.

XIII. CHOLERA ASIATICA

Definition.—A specific, infectious disease, caused by the comma bacillus of Koch, and characterized clinically by violent purging and rapid collapse.

Historical Summary.—Cholera has been endemic in India from a remote period, but only within the last century did it make inroads into Europe and America. An extensive epidemic occurred in 1832, in which year it was brought in immigrant ships from Great Britain to Quebec. It travelled along the lines of traffic up the Great Lakes, and finally reached as far west as the military posts of the upper Mississippi. In the same year it entered the United States by way of New York. There were recurrences of the disease in 1835-'36. In 1848 it entered the country through New Orleans, and spread widely up the Mississippi Valley and across the continent to California. In 1849 it again appeared. In 1854 it was introduced by immigrant ships into New York and prevailed widely throughout the country. In 1866 and in 1867 there were less serious epidemics. In 1873 it again appeared in the United States, but did not prevail widely. In 1884 there was an outbreak in Europe, and again in 1892 and 1893. Although occasional cases have been brought by ship to the quarantine stations of Great Britain and the United States, the disease has not gained a foothold in either country since 1873. It has prevailed continuously in the Philippines since 1901, but is now, 1912, well under control. For the past ten years it has prevailed widely in the near and far East. Russia has suffered severely since 1907, but last year, 1911, there were comparatively few cases. In 1911 cholera prevailed in Italy, North Africa and Madeira. There were outbreaks in Asia Minor, Arabia and Turkey, and the usual prevalence in India. To the United States, during 1911, cholera was frequently conveyed by ships from Italy, but there was no difficulty in controlling it. A number of cholera "carriers" were found.

Etiology.—In 1884 Koch announced the discovery of the specific organism of this disease. Subsequent observations have confirmed his statement that the comma bacillus, as it is termed, occurs constantly in the true cholera, and in no other disease. It has the form of a slightly bent rod, which is thicker, but not more than about half the length of the tubercle bacillus, and sometimes occurs in corkscrew-like or S forms. The organisms grow upon a great variety of media and display distinctive and characteristic appearances. Koch found them in the water tanks in India, and they were isolated from the Elbe water during the Hamburg epidemic of 1892. During epidemics virulent bacilli may be found in the fæces of healthy persons. The bacilli are found in the intestine, in the stools from the earliest period of the disease, and very abundantly in the characteristic rice-water evacuations, in which they may be seen as an almost pure culture. They very rarely occur in the vomit. Post mortem, they are found in enormous numbers in the intestine. In acutely fatal cases they do not seem to invade the intestinal wall, but in those with a more protracted course they are found in the depths of the glands and in the still deeper tissues. Experimental animals are not susceptible to cholera germs administered per os. But if introduced after neutralization of the gastric contents, and if kept in contact with the intestinal mucosa by controlling peristalsis with opium, guinea-pigs succumb after showing cholera-like symptoms. The intestines are filled with thin, watery contents, containing comma bacilli in almost pure culture.

Cholera Toxin.—Koch in his studies of cholera failed to find the spirilla in the internal organs. He concluded that the constitutional symptoms of the disease resulted from the absorption of toxic bodies from the intestine. R. Pfeiffer has shown that the cholera toxin is intimately associated with the proteid of the bacterial cells, and, being of a very labile nature, can not be separated. Dead cultures are toxic; and the symptoms produced by the introduction of even minimal amounts are often comparable with those of the algid stage of cholera asiatica. The symptoms occur very rapidly, and death often results in eight to twelve hours; in non-fatal cases recovery is often equally as rapid. The intracellular cholera toxin is poisonous to animals if introduced into the blood, peritoneal cavity, or subcutaneous tissues. No absorption takes place from the intestine unless the epithelial layer has been injured.

Immunity.—Animals may be immunized by repeated injections of non-fatal doses of the dead and later of the living organisms. The serum of an animal thus immunized has a protective power when injected into a guinea pig along with five or ten times the fatal dose. This serum has also agglutinative and other antibacterial properties. The blood serum of convalescent patients also possesses these properties, and for therapeutic purposes anti-serums have been introduced and used widely in India, the Philippines and in Russia.

Modes of Infection.—As in other diseases, individual peculiarities count for much, and during epidemics virulent cholera bacilli have been isolated from the normal stools of healthy men. Cholera cultures have also been swallowed with impunity.

The disease is not highly contagious; physicians, nurses, and others in close contact with patients are not often affected. On the other hand, washerwomen and those who are brought into very close contact with the linen of the cholera patients, or with their stools, are particularly prone to catch the disease. There have been several instances of so-called "laboratory cholera," in which students, having been accidentally infected while working with the cultures, have taken the disease, and at least one death has resulted.

Vegetables which have been washed in the infected water, particularly lettuces and cresses, may convey the disease. Milk may also be contaminated. The bacilli live on fresh bread, butter, and meat, for from six to eight days. In regions in which the disease prevails the possibility of the infection of food by flies should be borne in mind, since it has been shown that the bacilli may live for at least three days in their intestines.

Infection through the air is not to be much dreaded, since the germs when dried die rapidly.

The disease is propagated chiefly by contaminated water used for drinking, cooking, and washing. The virulence of an epidemic in any region is in direct proportion to the imperfection of its water-supply. In India the demonstration of the connection between drinking-water and cholera infection is complete. The Hamburg epidemic is a most remarkable illustration. The unfiltered water of the Elbe was the chief supply, although taken from the river in such a situation that it was of necessity directly contaminated by sewage. It is not known accurately from what source the contagion came, whether from Russia or from France, but in August, 1892, there was a sudden explosive epidemic, and within three months nearly 18,000 persons were attacked, with a mortality of 42.3 per cent. The neighboring city of Altona, which also took its water from the Elbe, but which had a thoroughly well-equipped modern filtration system, had in the same period only 516 cases.

Two main types of epidemics of cholera are recognized: the first, in which many individuals are attacked simultaneously, as in the Hamburg outbreak, and in which no direct connection can be traced between the individual cases. In this type there is widespread contamination of the drinking-water. In the other the cases occur in groups, so-called cholera nests; individuals are not attacked simultaneously, but successively. A direct connection between the cases may be very difficult to trace. Again, both these types may be combined, and in an epidemic which has started in a widespread infection through water, there may be other outbreaks, which are examples of the second or chain-like type.

Cholera "carriers" have no doubt an important influence. In Manila nearly 8 per cent. of 376 healthy persons harbored the bacilli. The perennial outbreaks of this disease in the Manila prison were due to carriers, 17 of whom were found among those who had to do with the preparation of the food and drink of 3,000 prisoners.

The disease always follows the lines of human travel. In India it has, in many notable cases, been widely spread by pilgrims. It is carried also by caravans and in ships. It is not conveyed through the atmosphere.

Places situated at the sea-level are more prone to the disease than inland towns. In high altitudes the disease does not prevail so extensively. A high temperature favors the development of cholera, but in Europe and America the epidemics have been chiefly in the late summer and in the autumn.

The disease affects persons of all ages. It is particularly prone to attack the intemperate and those debilitated by want of food and by bad surroundings. Depressing emotions, such as fear, undoubtedly have a marked influence. It is doubtful whether an attack furnishes immunity against a second one.

Morbid Anatomy.—A post mortem diagnosis of the nature of the disease could be made by any competent bacteriologist, as the organism is distinctive. The body has the appearances associated with profound collapse. There is often marked post mortem elevation of temperature. The *rigor mortis* sets in early and may produce displacement of the limbs. The lower jaw has been seen to move and the eyes to rotate. Various movements of the arms and legs have also been noted. The blood is thick and dark, and there is a remarkable diminution in the amount of its water and salts. The peritoneum is sticky, and the coils of intestines are congested and look thin and shrunken. The small intestine usually contains a turbid serum, similar in appearance to that which was passed in the stools. The mucosa is, as a rule, swollen, and in very acute cases slightly hyperæmic; later the congestion, which is not uniform, is more marked, especially about the Peyer's patches. Post mortem the epithelial lining is sometimes denuded, but this is probably not a change which takes place freely during life. In the stools, however, large numbers of columnar epithelial cells have been described by Horner and others. The bacilli are found in the contents of the intestine and in the mucous membrane. The spleen is usually small. The liver and kidneys show cloudy swellings, and the latter extensive coagulation-necrosis and destruction of the epithelial cells.

Symptoms.—A period of incubation of uncertain length, probably not more than from two to five days, precedes the onset of the symptoms.

Three stages may be recognized in the attack: the preliminary diarrhœa, the collapse stage, and the period of reaction.

(*a*) THE PRELIMINARY DIARRHŒA may set in abruptly without any previous indications. More commonly there are, for one or two days, colicky pains in the abdomen, with looseness of the bowels, perhaps vomiting, with headache and depression of spirits. There may be no fever.

(*b*) COLLAPSE STAGE.—The diarrhœa increases, or, without any of the preliminary symptoms, sets in with the greatest intensity, and profuse liquid evacuations succeed each other rapidly. There are in some instances griping pains and tenesmus. More commonly there is a sense of exhaustion and collapse. The thirst becomes extreme, the tongue is white; cramps of great severity occur in the legs and feet. Within a few hours vomiting sets in and becomes incessant. The patient rapidly sinks into a condition of collapse, the features are shrunken, the skin has an ashy-gray hue, the eyeballs sink in the sockets, the nose is pinched, the cheeks are hollow, the voice becomes husky, the extremities are cyanosed, and the skin is shriveled, wrinkled, and covered with a clammy perspiration. The temperature sinks. In the axilla or in the mouth it may be from five to ten degrees below normal, but in the rectum and in the internal parts it may be 103° or 104°. The blood pressure falls greatly and is often below 70 mm. Hg. The pulse becomes extremely feeble and flickering, and the patient gradually passes into a condition of coma, though consciousness is often retained until near the end.

The fæces are at first yellowish in color, from the bile pigment, but soon they become grayish-white and look like turbid whey or rice-water; whence the term "rice-water stools." There are found in them numerous small flakes of mucus and granular matter, and at times blood. The reaction is usually alkaline. The fluid contains albumin and the chief mineral ingredient is chloride of sodium. Microscopically, mucus and epithelial cells and innumerable bacteria are seen, the majority of the latter being the comma bacilli.

The condition of the patient is largely the result of the concentration of the blood consequent upon the loss of serum in the stools. The specific gravity of the blood rises to 1060 to 1072. There is almost complete arrest of secretion, particularly of the saliva and the urine. On the other hand, the sweat-glands increase in activity, and in nursing women it has been stated that the lacteal flow is unaffected. This stage sometimes lasts not more than two or three hours, but more commonly from twelve to twenty-four.

(*c*) Reaction Stage.—When the patient survives the collapse, the cyanosis gradually disappears, the warmth returns to the skin, which may have for a time a mottled color or present a definite erythematous rash. The heart's action becomes stronger, the urine increases in quantity, the irritability of the stomach disappears, the stools are at longer intervals, and there is no abdominal pain. In the reaction the temperature may not rise above normal. Not infrequently this favorable condition is interrupted by a recurrence of severe diarrhœa and the patient is carried off in a relapse. Other cases pass into the condition of what has been called *cholera-typhoid,* a state in which the patient is delirious, the pulse rapid and feeble, and the tongue dry. Death finally occurs with coma. These symptoms have been attributed to uræmia.

During epidemics attacks are found of all grades of severity. There are cases of diarrhœa with griping pains, liquid, copious stools, vomiting, and cramps, with slight collapse. To these the term *cholerine* has been applied. They resemble the milder cases of *cholera nostras.* At the opposite end of the series there are the instances of *cholera sicca,* in which death may occur in a few hours after the onset, without diarrhœa. There are also cases in which the patients are overwhelmed with the poison and die comatose, without the preliminary stage of collapse.

Complications and Sequelæ.—The typhoid condition has already been referred to. The consecutive nephritis rarely induces dropsy. Diphtheritic colitis has been described. There is a special tendency to diphtheritic inflammation of the mucous membranes, particularly of the throat and genitals. Pneumonia and pleurisy may follow, and destructive abscesses may occur in different parts. Suppurative parotitis is not very uncommon. In rare instances local gangrene may occur. A troublesome symptom of convalescence is cramps in the muscles of the arms and legs.

Diagnosis.—The only affection with which Asiatic cholera could be confounded is the *cholera nostras,* the severe choleraic diarrhœa which occurs during the summer months in temperate climates. The clinical picture of the two affections is identical. The extreme collapse, vomiting, and rice-water stools, the cramps, the cyanosed appearance, are all seen in the worst forms of cholera nostras. In enfeebled persons death may occur within twelve hours. It is of course extremely important to be able to diagnose between the two affections. This can only be done by one thoroughly versed in bacteriological methods, and conversant with the diversified flora of the intestines.

Attacks very similar to Asiatic cholera are produced in poisoning by arsenic, corrosive sublimate, and certain fungi; but a difficulty in diagnosis could scarcely arise.

The *prognosis* is always uncertain, as the mortality ranges in different epidemics from 30 to 80 per cent. Intemperance, debility, and old age are unfavorable conditions. The more rapidly the collapse sets in, the greater is the danger, and as Andral truly says of the malignant form, "It begins where other diseases end—in death." Patients with marked cyanosis and very low temperature rarely recover.

Prophylaxis.—Preventive measures are all-important, and isolation of the sick and thorough disinfection have effectually prevented the disease entering England or the United States since 1873. During epidemics the greatest care should be exercised in the disinfection of the stools and linen of the patients. When an epidemic prevails, persons should be warned not to drink water unless previously boiled. The milk should be boiled and all food and drinks carefully protected from flies. Errors in diet should be avoided. Uncooked vegetables and salads should not be eaten. As the disease is not more contagious than typhoid fever, the chance of a person passing safely through an epidemic depends very much upon how far he is able to carry out thoroughly prophylactic measures. Digestive disturbances are to be treated promptly, and particularly the diarrhœa, which so often is a preliminary symptom. For this, opium and acetate of lead and large doses of bismuth should be given. Protective inoculation has been carried out extensively in India by Haffkine and in the Philippines by Strong, in both places and recently in Russia with good results.

Treatment.—The patient should be at rest in bed, kept warm, and given simple diet, boiled milk, whey and egg albumen. The patient may be allowed to take water freely. If vomiting occurs food should be withheld and the stomach washed with an alkaline solution. Hot applications to the abdomen should be used and hot baths given if they prove helpful. Early in the course the bowels should be moved by castor oil or calomel. During the initial stage, when the diarrhœa is not excessive but the abdominal pain is marked, opium is the most efficient remedy, and it should be given hypodermically as morphia. It is advisable to give at once a full dose, which may be repeated on the return of the pain. It is best not to attempt to give remedies by the mouth, as they disturb the stomach. Ice should be given, and brandy or hot coffee. In the collapse stage, writers speak strongly against the use of opium. Undoubtedly it must be given with caution, but, judging from its effects in cholera nostras, I should say that collapse *per se* was not a contraindication.

Irrigation of the bowel with a solution of tannic acid (2 per cent.) in hot water (105°) should be used. With a long, soft-rubber tube, as much as two litres may be slowly injected. Not only is the colon cleansed, but the small bowel may also be reached, as shown by the fact that the tannic acid solutions have been vomited.

Owing to the profuse serous discharges the blood becomes concentrated, and absorption takes place rapidly from the lymph-spaces. To meet this, intravenous injections were introduced by Latta, of Leith, in the epidemic of 1832. My preceptor, Bovell, first practised the intravenous injections of milk in Toronto, in the epidemic of 1854.

Saline injections, intravenous and into the bowel, have been much used and with great success by the method introduced by Leonard Rogers. The hypertonic solution is composed of sodium chloride, grains 120; potassium chloride, grains 6; calcium chloride, grains 4; water, 1 pint. It is best given intravenously, particularly if the specific gravity of the blood is over 1063. As much as four pints may be injected slowly. It may be repeated and in one case as much as twenty pints were injected. In Calcutta the mortality has been reduced from 60 to about 33 per cent. in the cases treated by this method and Rogers has had equally good results at Palermo in the summer of 1911.

In the stage of reaction special pains should be taken to regulate the diet and to guard against recurrences of the severe diarrhœa.

XIV. THE PLAGUE

Definition.—A specific, infectious disease, caused by *Bacillus pestis,* and occurring in two chief forms: a bubonic, involving the lymphatic glands, and a pneumonic, causing an acute and rapidly fatal inflammation of the lungs.

History and Geographical Distribution.—The disease was probably not known to the classical Greek writers. The earliest positive account dates from the second century of our era. The plague of Athens and the pestilence of the reign of Marcus Aurelius were apparently not this disease (Payne). From the great plague in the days of Justinian (sixth century) to the middle of the seventeenth century epidemics of varying severity occurred in Europe. Among the most disastrous was the famous "black death" of the fourteenth century, which overran Europe and destroyed a fourth of the population. In the seventeenth century it raged virulently, and during the great plague of London, in 1665, about 70,000 people died. During the eighteenth and nineteenth centuries the ravages of the disease lessened.

The revival of the plague is the most important single fact in modern epidemiology. Throughout the nineteenth century it waned progressively, outbreaks of some extent occurring in Turkey and Asia Minor and Astrakan; but we had begun to place it with sweating sickness and typhus among the diseases of the past. We knew that it slumbered in parts of China, and in northwest India, but the outbreak in 1894 at Hong-Kong startled the world and showed that the "black death" was still virulent. Since then it has spread in an ominous manner, reaching India, China, French Indo-China, Japan, Formosa, Australia, the Philippine Islands, South America, the West Indies, the United States, Cape Colony, Madagascar, Egypt, Asia Minor, and Russia in Asia. In Europe, cases have been carried to Marseilles and other Mediterranean ports and to Hamburg and Glasgow. In the latter city there was a small outbreak in 1900, 36 cases. In the next year there were two cases and in 1907 two cases—this without fresh importation. In San Francisco there was in 1907-1908 a recrudescence of the disease, and to March 15, 1908, there were 121 cases with 77 deaths. The rats are now no longer affected. The disease spread to the ground squirrels of the neighboring countries from which source eleven cases originated. Cases have occurred in New Orleans—the last in October, 1911.

In England there have been four sets of human cases in East Suffolk; at Shotley in 1906-07, 8 cases and 6 deaths; at Trimley, in December, 1909, and January, 1910, 8 cases and 5 deaths; at Freston in the autumn of 1910, 4 fatal cases; and a fourth case occurred in the autumn of 1911. The majority of these were of the pneumonic type. The serious feature is that there has been an infection of the rats in East Anglia, beginning in the region between Ipswich and the coast. The rats are entirely of the species *Mus decumanus* except in part of Ipswich. The infection is not very widespread.

as of 568 rats examined only 17 were found infected. The disease extended to rabbits, but not to any great extent. Some fleas from the rats were found to contain bacilli indistinguishable from plague. A much more extensive investigation of the prevalence of the plague in the rats of Suffolk and Essex was made by Petrie and Macalister; of 6,071 examined not one presented the appearance of plague. The disease has been introduced into Suffolk by ship rats from plague infected countries. More serious is the fact that during the past three years rats infected with the plague have been occasionally discovered at Wapping, but there does not seem to have been any widespread epidemic among them.

The immunity of the human population seems to be due to the fact that 50 per cent. of the rat fleas are of the variety *Pulex cheopis*, which rarely bites man, and the other rat flea, the *Ceratophyllus fasciatus*, does not bite man very freely. Then the common brown rat is not a house resident to any extent, so that conditions in England are not very favorable for epidemic prevalence.

The distribution in India is remarkable, chiefly in the Punjab, Bombay, and the United Provinces, which have a combined population of about 100 millions. In these three provinces between 1896 and the middle of 1911, about five and a half million deaths from plague have occurred. In the remaining provinces of India, with a population of some 200 millions, only about two millions of plague deaths have occurred. In the Presidency of Madras the disease has not been very severe, while Eastern Bengal and Assam have remained free, though cases have been repeatedly imported. During 1911 the returns for India for the first six months show 604,634 deaths. There have been recent outbreaks in China, a sharp outbreak in Hong-Kong, and the disease has been reported in Egypt, Japan, Straits Settlements, Java and Sumatra, Persia, Turkey in Asia, Astrakan, the Mauritius, and several of the South American countries. The Manchurian outbreak of pneumonic plague in the winter of 1810-11 was one of the most virulent on record, carrying off more than 4,500 persons in a few months.

Etiology.—The specific organism of the disease is a bacillus discovered by Kitasato. It resembles somewhat the bacillus of chicken cholera, and grows in a perfectly characteristic manner. *Bacillus pestis* occurs in the blood, in the organs of the body and in the sputum, and has also been found in the dust and in the soil of houses in which the patients have lived.

The disease prevails most frequently in hot seasons, though an outbreak may occur during the coldest weather. Persons of all ages are attacked. It spreads chiefly among the poor, in the slums of the great cities.

The following conclusions of the Plague Commission (1908) relate to bubonic plague: (*a*) Contagion occurs in less than 3 per cent. of the cases, playing a very small part in the general spread of the disease. (*b*) Bubonic plague in man is entirely dependent on the disease in the rat. (*c*) The infection is conveyed from rat to rat and from rat to man solely by means of the rat-flea. (*d*) A case in man is not in itself infectious. (*e*) A large majority of cases occur singly in houses. When more than one case occurs in a house, the attacks are generally nearly simultaneous. (*f*) Plague is usually conveyed from place to place by imported rat-fleas, which are carried by people on their persons or in their baggage. The human agent may himself escape infection. (*g*) Insanitary conditions have no relation to the occurrence of plague, except in so far as they favor infestation by rats. (*h*) The non-epidemic season is bridged over by acute plague in the rat, accompanied by a few cases among human beings.

In the pneumonic form personal infection from one person to another is the common way, as the bacilli are sprayed into the air by coughing. The possibility of the human flea as a carrier must be considered.

Clinical Forms.—PESTIS MINOR.—In this variety, also known as the ambulant, the patient has a few days of fever. with swelling of the glands of the groin, and possibly suppuration. He may not be ill enough to seek medical relief. These cases, often found at the beginning and end of an epidemic, are a very serious danger, as the urine and fæces contain bacilli.

BUBONIC PLAGUE.—This constitutes the common variety, 77.65 per cent. of 11,600 cases of plague treated in the Arthur Road Hospital, Bombay (N. H. Choksy). The stage of invasion is characterized by headache, backache, stiffness of the limbs, a feeling of anxiety and restlessness, and great depression of spirits. There is a steady rise in the fever until the evening of the third or fourth day, when there is a drop of two or three degrees. There is then a secondary fever, as some writers describe it, in which the temperature reaches a still higher point. The tongue becomes brown, collapse symptoms are apt to supervene, and in very severe infections the patient may die at this stage. In at least two-thirds of all cases there are glandular swellings or buboes. An analysis of 9,500 cases of buboes gave more than 54 per cent. with the glands of the groin affected. The swelling appears usually from the third to the fifth day. Resolution may occur, or suppuration, or in rare cases gangrene. Suppuration is a favorable feature, as noted by De Foe in his graphic account of the London plague.

Petechiæ very commonly show themselves, and may be very extensive. These have been called the "plague spots," or the "tokens of the disease," and gave to it in the middle ages the name of the Black Death. Hæmorrhages from the mucous membranes may also occur; in some epidemics hæmoptysis has been especially frequent.

SEPTICÆMIC PLAGUE.—In this, the most rapid form, the patient succumbs in three or four days with a virulent infection before the buboes appear. This form constituted 14.25 per cent. of the 11,600 cases. Hæmorrhages are common. The bacilli can be obtained from the blood.

PNEUMONIC PLAGUE.—In the ordinary bubonic type, inflammation of the lungs is not an uncommon complication, but the true pneumonic plague begins abruptly with fever, shortness of breath, cough, and sometimes pain in the chest. The fever increases, the signs of the involvement of the lung occur early; there may be impaired resonance at both bases with harsh and tubular breathing; the sputum becomes bloody and stained and more fluid than in ordinary pneumonia. Cyanosis is an early feature; the pulse is small and rapid, the patient becomes profoundly prostrate; the spleen enlarges rapidly, as early as the second day, and a fatal result follows in from two to four days. Recovery is very rare.

In other varieties the chief manifestations may be in the skin and subcutaneous tissues, or in the intestines, causing diarrhœa and sometimes the features of typhoid fever.

Diagnosis.—At the early stage of an outbreak plague cases are easily overlooked, but if the suspicious cases are carefully studied by a competent bacteriologist, there is no disease which can be more positively identified. The San Francisco epidemic illustrates this. The nature of the cases was recognized by Kellog and by Kinyoun, but with an amazing stupidity (which was shared by not a few physicians, who should have known better) the Governor of the State refused to recognize the presence of plague, and the United States Government had to intervene and send a board of experts to settle the question. In the early Glasgow cases Colvin, while suspecting typhoid fever, saw that there was something unusual, and at once took precautionary measures. Probably, too, the association of four cases in one family made him suspicious. The limitation of the outbreak was due to the prompt and effective measures taken by A. K. Chalmers and his associates. The wide-spread prevalence of the disease makes it the imperative duty of the health authorities to have on hand, in connection with large ports, skilled men who can promptly make the bacteriological diagnosis. There are dangers from the cultures in laboratories, as shown by the experiences of Vienna and Ann Arbor, but with proper precautions they may be reduced to a minimum. Acute, rapidly fatal pneumonia should arouse suspicion as in the Suffolk cases.

Prophylaxis.—Wherever plague exists an organized staff, an intelligent policy, and a long purse are needed. In India, where fifteenth-century conditions prevail, and where the scale of the epidemic is so enormous, the problem of prophylaxis looks hopeless. Simpson's recommendation of a specially trained plague service, organized on proper lines and on a liberal basis, should be carried out. A careful watch should be kept on the mortality of rats. When found infected, energetic measures should be taken to stamp out the disease in them. Three things are necessary—the cleansing of premises, particularly stables and outhouses, so that the rats cannot find nesting places or food; systematic rat destruction; and making houses rat proof. Certain measures prevent the access of plague to healthy ports; fumigation of ships to destroy the rats, careful inspection of passengers and crew, and detention over a period which covers the incubation of the disease.

When a centre becomes infected, the sanitary organization should be arranged to carry out the segregation of the sick in hospitals, the disinfection of infected rooms with sulphur, destruction of infected bedding, and thorough cleansing of the entire district; old, badly infected buildings should be destroyed.

Treatment.—In a disease the mortality of which may reach as high as 80 or 90 per cent. the question of treatment resolves itself into making the patient as comfortable as possible, and following out certain general principles such as guide us in the care of fever patients. Cantlie recommends purgation and stimulation from the outset, and the use of morphia for the pain. The local treatment of the buboes is important. Ice may be applied to them, and good results apparently follow the injection of the bichloride of mercury. The pyrexia of the disease is best treated by systematic hydrotherapy.

A plague serum, chiefly the Lustig and the Yersin-Rouse, has been used. Choksy concludes that a reduction of 20-25 per cent. in the mortality may be obtained by its use.

Preventive Inoculation.—With Haffkine's serum in 12 districts, of 224,228 persons inoculated, 3,399 took the disease; of 639,600 uninoculated, 49,430 were attacked. C. J. Martin concludes that the chances of subsequent infection are reduced four-fifths, and the chances of recovery are two and a half times as great as in the case of the uninoculated. The recent reports from India are most favorable and in South America the value of this plan has been amply demonstrated. It is interesting to note that the laboratory staff at Bombay, 116 in number, have remained immune though in constant contact with plague infested rats.

XV. TETANUS

(*Lockjaw*)

Definition.—An infectious malady characterized by tonic spasms of the muscles with marked exacerbations. The virus is produced by a bacillus, *B. tetani* of Nicolaier, which occurs in earth, in putrefying fluids, and manure, and is a normal inhabitant of the intestines of many ruminants.

Etiology.—In the United States, according to Anders and Morgan, it is most frequent in the Hudson valley, in Long Island and in the Atlantic States. In 1909 there were 1,373 deaths from tetanus among 732,528 deaths in eighteen states; of which 30.7 per cent. were in children under one year. An extraordinary number of cases have followed the accidents of the July 4th celebrations, but the propaganda of the Journal of the American Medical Association has succeeded in reducing these fatalities in a remarkable way.

In England the disease is not very common, but has increased of late years. There were only 2,124 deaths in the twenty year period ending 1908. It is more prevalent in certain districts, e. g. the Thames valley. It is more frequent in the Radcliffe Infirmary, Oxford, than in any hospital with which I have been connected. It is more common in the summer months and males are more frequently attacked than females. In E. W. Hill's analysis of 3,038 cases in temperate climates 22.31 per cent. were in children under one year, 21 per cent. in the third and fourth decades.

In the tropics tetanus is a much more severe and common disease. In Jamaica and Cuba it is from five to six times more frequent as a cause of death than in the United States, and above 80 per cent. of the deaths are in infants. In the Canal Zone the disease has not been common, only 25 cases have been admitted to the Ancon and Colon Hospital (E. W. Hill) to 1910. It is not only in the tropics that tetanus is a very fatal disease in infants. On an island near Iceland all the children born died; and for years the island of St. Kilda, one of the Western Hebrides, had been scourged by the "eight days sickness" among the new born. Of 125 children, 84 died within fourteen days of birth. Since the discovery of the bacillus and the introduction of proper methods of treating the umbilical cord the disease has practically disappeared.

The tetanus bacillus has contaminated vaccines, and its presence in commercial gelatine is a grave danger. Owing to the careless preparation of the virus many cases of tetanus occurred in the neighborhood of Philadelphia in 1901 among vaccinated children. In 1902 nineteen persons who had been inoculated against the plague in the village of Mulkowal died of tetanus owing to accidental contamination of the cultures. Outbreaks have occurred in general hospitals following the use of catgut. The disease has occurred after prolonged use of the hypodermic needle to inject morphia or quinine, and it has followed the use of gelatine as a hæmostatic.

The disease usually follows an injury, often of a most trifling character, and particularly lacerated wounds of the hands which have been contaminated by dirt and splinters. It may occur without any recognizable wound, so-called idiopathic tetanus.

THE TETANUS BACILLUS.—The organism is widely diffused in nature, in garden mould, in and about stables and farmyards, and is a normal inhabitant of the intestines of many horses and of the herbivora. The disease has been produced by inoculating animals with garden earth. Living bacilli occur in the intestines of 5 per cent. of healthy men and up to 20 per cent. of ostlers and dairymen. It is a slender motile bacillus, one end of which is swollen and occupied by a spore. It is anaerobic and grows at ordinary temperatures. The spores are the most resistant known. From two steel nibs dipped in a tetanus culture in 1891 a growth of virulent bacilli was obtained from one in 1902 and from the other in 1909 (Semple). The toxin is perhaps the most virulent of known poisons. Whereas the fatal dose of strychnine for a man weighing 70 kilos is from 30 to 100 milligrammes, that of the tetanus toxin is estimated at 0.23 milligramme. Every feature of the disease can be produced by it experimentally without the presence of the bacilli. The symptoms do not arise immediately, as in the case of ordinary poisons, but slowly, and it has been found to be absorbed by the end plates in the muscles and to pass up the motor nerves to the spinal cord. What we speak of as the period of incubation is the time required for the toxins to travel along the nerves to the centres. A high degree of antitoxic immunity can be conferred on animals, which then yield a protective serum. It is, however, difficult to cure animals with this serum on account of the combination of the toxin with nerve-cells by the time symptoms appear.

Morbid Anatomy.—No characteristic lesions have been found in the cord or in the brain. Congestions occur in different parts, and perivascular exudations and granular changes in the nerve-cells have been found. The condition of the wound is variable. The nerves are often found injured, reddened, and swollen. In tetanus neonatorum the umbilicus may be inflamed.

Symptoms.—The incubation period is from one to twenty days. Of 1,092 cases analyzed by E. W. Hill, in 17.49 per cent. it was from one to five days and in 55.06 per cent. from five to ten days. In only 8 cases was the incubation as long as twenty days. The patient complains at first of slight stiffness in the neck, or a feeling of tightness in the jaws, or difficulty in mastication. Occasionally chilly feelings or actual rigors may precede these symptoms. Gradually a tonic spasm of the muscles of these parts produces the condition of trismus or lockjaw. The eyebrows may be raised and the angles of the mouth drawn out, causing the so-called sardonic grin—*risus sardonicus.* In children the spasm may be confined to these parts. Sometimes the attack is associated with paralysis of the facial muscles and difficulty in swallowing—the head-tetanus of Rose, which has most commonly followed injuries in the neighborhood of the fifth nerve. Gradually the process extends and involves the muscles of the body. Those of the back are most affected, so that during the spasm the unfortunate victim may rest upon the head and heels—a position known as *opisthotonos.* The rectus abdominis muscle has been torn across in the spasm. The entire trunk and limbs may be perfectly rigid—*orthotonos.* Flexion to one side is less common—*pleurothotonos;* while spasm of the muscles of the abdomen may cause the body to be bent forward—*emprosthotonos.* In very violent attacks the thorax is compressed, the respirations are rapid, and spasm of the glottis may occur, causing asphyxia. The paroxysms last for a variable period, but even in the intervals the relaxation is not complete. The slightest irritation is sufficient to cause a spasm. The paroxysms are associated with agonizing pain, and the patient may be held as in a vise, unable to utter a word. Usually he is bathed in a profuse sweat. The temperature may remain normal throughout, or show only a slight elevation toward the close. In other cases the pyrexia is marked from the outset; the temperature reaches 105° or 106° F., and before death 109° or 110° F. In rare instances it may go still higher. The course is sometimes very rapid, with fever and general spasms; death may take place on the third day. Death either occurs during the paroxysm from heart-failure or asphyxia, or is due to exhaustion.

The cephalic tetanus (*Kopftetanus* of Rose) originates usually from a wound of the head, and is characterized by stiffness of the muscles of the jaw and paralysis of the facial muscles on the same side as the wound, with difficulty in swallowing. There may be no other symptoms. This form has been called hydrophobic because of the spasm of the throat. The prognosis is good in the chronic cases; of those in Willard's table only 8 of 32 died; but in the acute form, of 45 cases, only 4 recovered.

Tetanus neonatorum.—This is a very common form, particularly in hot climates and in districts where the tetanus bacillus is very prevalent, as in the island of St. Kilda. The infection follows imperfect treatment of the navel. The symptoms may come on in a few days or be delayed for ten days. Trismus and difficulty in crying and taking food are the earliest symptoms, followed in a few days by more general spasms. It is a very fatal form. A form known as *visceral tetanus* is described by the French in which the disease originates in the intestines, and the possibility of this must be considered, as the spores have been found in human fæces. *Post-operative tetanus* occurs particularly after peritoneal operations. Paterson collected 150 cases in a large proportion of which catgut had been used. It is a very fatal form, with a short incubation and rapid course.

Diagnosis.—Well-marked cases following a trauma could not be mistaken for any other disease. The spasms are not unlike those of strychnia-poisoning, and in the celebrated Palmer murder trial this was the plea for the defence. The jaw-muscles, however, are never involved early, if at all, and between the paroxysms in strychnia-poisoning there is no rigidity. In tetany the distribution of the spasm at the extremities, the peculiar position, the greater involvement of the hands, and the condition under which it occurs are sufficient to make the diagnosis clear. In doubtful cases cultures should be made from the pus of the wound.

Escherich has described in children a form of generalized tonic contractures of the muscles of the jaw, neck, back, and limbs, usually a sequel of some acute infection, occasionally occurring as an independent malady. The contractures may be either intermittent or persistent. The condition may last from a week to a couple of months. The cases as a rule recover.

Prognosis.—Two of the Hippocratic aphorisms express tersely the general prognosis even at the present day: "The spasm supervening on a wound is fatal," and "such persons as are seized with tetanus die within four days, or if they pass these they recover." Of 1,264 cases analyzed by E. W. Hill only 414 recovered. If the disease lasts beyond the tenth day the patient has an even chance, and from this time the prognosis improves.

The mortality is greatest in children. Favorable indications are: late onset of the attack, localization of the spasms to the muscles of the neck and jaw, and an absence of fever.

Prophylaxis.—Suspicious wounds should be freely opened, thoroughly disinfected by hydrogen peroxide and cauterized with pure carbolic acid. In districts where the disease prevails, as in the Thames valley, special precautions should be taken with all injuries, and a prophylactic dose of antitetanic serum (500 to 1,000 units) administered. The experience in the United States with this treatment in the Fourth of July accidents has been most satisfactory. It should be carried out promptly in all street and infected injuries. As the serum is expensive, Boards of Health should arrange, if necessary, to provide it.

Treatment.—The patient should be kept in a darkened room, absolutely quiet, and attended by only one person. All possible sources of irritation should be avoided. Veterinarians appreciate the importance of this complete seclusion in treating horses.

When the lockjaw is extreme the patient may not be able to take food by the mouth, under which circumstances it is best to use rectal injections, or to feed by a catheter passed through the nose. The spasm should be controlled by chloroform, which may be repeatedly exhibited at intervals. It is more satisfactory to keep the patient thoroughly under the influence of morphia given hypodermically. Chloral hydrate, chloretone, bromide of potassium, Calabar bean, curare, Indian hemp, belladonna, and other drugs have been recommended, and recovery occasionally follows their use. Intraspinal injections of a solution of magnesium sulphate (25 per cent.) have been used (Meltzer); 1 c. c. is injected for every 25 pounds weight of the patient. Resection of the nerve and amputation of the limb have been advised. Although tetanus antitoxin of great strength can be obtained, its use in the treatment of human tetanus very often fails because it is given too late. Given at once and in sufficient doses, it should prove a specific. It may be given in various ways. The administration of 3,000 to 5,000 units intraspinally (repeated in 24 hours) and 10,000 units intravenously and 10,000 units subcutaneously three or four days later has given good results (Nicoll). The best results are obtained in subacute cases, but here the prognosis is relatively favorable.

XVI. GLANDERS

(*Farcy*)

Definition.—An infectious disease of the horse and ass, caused by *Bacillus mallei*, communicated occasionally to man. In the horse it is characterized by the formation of nodules, chiefly in the nares (glanders) and beneath the skin (farcy).

Etiology.—The disease belongs to the infective granulomata. The local manifestations in the nostrils and the skin of the horse are due to one and the same cause. The specific germ was discovered by Loeffler and Schutz. It is a short, non-motile bacillus, not unlike that of tubercle, but exhibits different staining reactions. It grows readily on the ordinary culture media. For the full recognition of glanders in man we are indebted to the labors of Rayer, whose monograph remains one of the best descriptions ever given of the disease. Man becomes infected by contact with diseased animals, and usually by inoculation on an abraded surface of the skin. The contagion may also be received on the mucous membrane. In a Montreal case a gentleman was probably infected by the material expelled from the nostril of his horse, which was not suspected of having the disease. It is a rare disease. Only 4 deaths were registered from this cause in England and Wales in 1909. Among laboratory workers the *Bacillus mallei* has caused more deaths than any other germ, and in working with it the greatest possible precautions should be taken.

Morbid Anatomy.—As in the horse, the disease may be localized in the nose (glanders) or beneath the skin (farcy). The essential lesion is the granulomatous tumor, characterized by the presence of numerous lymphoid and epithelioid cells, among and in which are seen the glanders bacilli. These nodular masses tend to break down rapidly, and on the mucous membrane result in ulcers, while beneath the skin they form abscesses. The glanders nodules may also occur in the internal organs.

Symptoms.—An acute and a chronic form of glanders may be recognized in man, and an acute and a chronic form of farcy.

Acute Glanders.—The period of incubation is rarely more than three or four days. There are signs of general febrile disturbance. At the site of infection there are swelling, redness, and lymphangitis. Within two or three days there is involvement of the mucous membrane of the nose, the nodules break down rapidly to ulcers, and there is a muco-purulent discharge. An eruption of papules, which rapidly become pustules, breaks out over the face and about the joints. It has been mistaken for variola. In a Montreal case this copious eruption led the attending physician to suspect smallpox, and the patient was isolated. There is a great swelling of the nose. The ulceration may go on to necrosis, in which case the discharge is very offensive. The lymph glands of the neck are usually much enlarged. Subacute pneumonia is very apt to occur. This form runs its course in about eight or ten days, and is invariably fatal. *Glanders pneumonia* may appear after subcutaneous infection (one case from infection with a hypodermic syringe stuck into the thumb). Grossly the lung appeared like a caseous pneumonia.

Chronic glanders is rare and difficult to diagnose, as it is usually mistaken for a chronic coryza. There are ulcers in the nose, and often laryngeal symptoms. It may last for months, or even longer, and recovery sometimes takes place. Tedeschi has described a case of chronic osteomyelitis, due to the *Bacillus mallei*, which was followed by a fatal glanders meningitis. The diagnosis may be extremely difficult. In such cases a suspension of the secretion, or of cultures upon agar-agar made from the secretion, should be injected into the peritoneal cavity of a male guinea-pig. At the end of two days, in positive cases, the testicles are found to be swollen and the skin of the scrotum reddened. The testicles continue to increase in size, and finally suppurate. Death takes place after the lapse of two or three weeks, and generalized glanders nodules are found in the viscera. The use of mallein for diagnostic purposes is highly recommended. The principles and methods of application are the same as for tuberculin. McFadyean and others have shown that, while the glanders bacilli are agglutinated in a dilution of 1 to 200 by normal horse serum, that of a glanders horse will agglutinate at 1 to 1,000. The test must be made before mallein is given.

Acute farcy in man results usually from the inoculation of the virus into the skin. There is an intense local reaction with a phlegmonous inflammation. The lymphatics are early affected, and along their course there are nodular subcutaneous enlargements, the so-called farcy buds, which may rapidly go on to suppuration. There are pains and swelling in the joints, and abscesses may form in the muscles. The symptoms are those of an acute infection, almost like an acute septicæmia. The nose is not involved and the superficial skin eruption is not common. The bacilli have been found in the urine in acute cases in man and animals.

The disease is fatal in a large proportion of the cases, usually in from twelve to fifteen days.

Chronic farcy is characterized by the presence of localized tumors which break down into abscesses, and sometimes form deep ulcers, without much inflammatory reaction and without special involvement of the lymphatics. The disease may last for months or even years. Death may result from pyæmia, or occasionally acute glanders develops. The celebrated French veterinarian Bouley had it and recovered.

The disease is transmissible also from man to man. Washerwomen have been infected from the clothes of a patient. In the diagnosis of this affection the occupation is very important. Nowadays, in cases of doubt the inoculation should be made in animals, as in this way the disease can be readily determined. Mallein, a product of the growth of the bacilli, is now used for the purpose of diagnosing glanders in animals. Several instances of cured glanders have been reported in animals treated with small and repeated doses of mallein (Pilavios, Babes).

Treatment.—If seen early, the wound should be either cut out or thoroughly destroyed by caustics and an antiseptic dressing applied. The farcy buds should be early opened. In the acute cases there is very little hope. In the chronic cases recovery is possible, though often tedious.

XVII. ANTHRAX

(*Splenic Fever; Charbon; Wool-sorter's Disease*)

Definition.—An acute infectious disease caused by *Bacillus anthracis*, occurring in three forms, cutaneous (malignant pustule), pulmonary, and intestinal. In animals, particularly in sheep and cattle, the disease has the character of an acute septicæmia with enlargement of the spleen—hence the name *splenic* fever. In man it occurs sporadically or as a result of accidental inoculations with the virus.

Etiology.—The infectious agent is a non-motile, rod-shaped organism, *Bacillus anthracis*, which has, by the researches of Pollender, Davaine, Koch, and Pasteur, become the best known perhaps of all pathogenic microbes. The bacillus has a length of from 2 to 25 μ; the rods are often united. The bacilli themselves are readily destroyed, but the spores are very resistant, and survive after prolonged immersion in a 5-per-cent. solution of carbolic acid, or withstand for some minutes a temperature of 212° F. They are capable also of resisting gastric digestion. Outside the body the spores are in all probability very durable.

In Animals.—Geographically and zoölogically the disease is the most widespread of all infections. It is much more prevalent in Europe and in Asia than in America. Its ravages among the herds of cattle in Russia and Siberia, and among sheep in certain parts of Europe, are not equalled by any other animal plague. In the United States anthrax is not very widespread. In France from 6 to 10 per cent. of the sheep and about 5 per cent. of the cattle formerly died of it.

The disease is conveyed sometimes by direct inoculation, as by the bites and stings of insects, by feeding on carcasses of animals which have died of the disease, but more commonly by grazing in pastures contaminated by the germs. Pasteur thought that the earthworm played an important part in bringing to the surface and distributing the bacilli which had been propagated in the buried carcass of an infected animal. Certain fields, or even farms, may thus be infected for an indefinite period of time. It seems probable, however, that, if the carcass is not opened or the blood spilt, spores are not formed in the buried animal and the bacilli quickly die.

In man the disease does not occur spontaneously. It results always from infection, either through the skin or intestines, or in rare instances through the lungs. Workers in wool and hair, and persons whose occupations bring them into contact with animals or animal products, as stablemen, shepherds, tanners, and butchers, are specially liable to the disease. In the United States the disease is usually found in the workers in hides, in butchers, and in veterinarians. It is rare in general hospital work. There was only one case in sixteen years at the Johns Hopkins Hospital. In England and Wales in 1909 there were 15 deaths from this cause in man. Ponder states that 40 per cent. of all the cases of anthrax in British leather workers are due to handling Chinese or East Indian goods; 80 per cent. of the cases are malignant pustule from skin infection while handling hides at the docks or in the tanneries.

Various forms of the disease have been described, and two chief groups may be recognized: the external anthrax and the internal anthrax, of which there are pulmonary and intestinal forms.

Symptoms.—(*a*) External Anthrax.—(1) *Malignant Pustule.*—At the site of inoculation, usually on an exposed surface—the hands, arms, or face—there are, within a few hours, itching and uneasiness, and the gradual formation of a small papule, which soon becomes vesicular. Inflammatory induration extends around this, and within thirty-six hours at the site of inoculation there is a dark brownish eschar, at a little distance from which there may be a series of small vesicles. The brawny induration may be extreme. The œdema produces very great swelling of the parts. The inflammation extends along the lymphatics, and the neighboring lymph-glands are swollen and sore. The fever at first rises rapidly, and the concomitant phenomena are marked. Subsequently the temperature falls, and in many cases becomes subnormal. Death may take place in from three to five days. In cases which recover the constitutional symptoms are slighter, the eschar gradually sloughs out, and the wound heals. The cases vary much in severity. In the mildest form there may be only slight swelling. At the site of inoculation a papule is formed, which rapidly becomes vesicular and dries into a scab, which separates in the course of a few days.

(2) *Malignant Anthrax Œdema.*—This form occurs in the eyelid, and also in the head, hand, and arm, and is characterized by the absence of the papule and vesicle forms, and by the most extensive œdema, which may follow rather than precede the constitutional symptoms. The œdema reaches such a grade of intensity that gangrene results, and may involve a considerable surface. The constitutional symptoms then become extremely grave, and the cases invariably prove fatal.

The greatest fatality is seen in cases of inoculation about the head and face, where the mortality, according to Nasarow, is 26 per cent.; the least in infection of the lower extremities, where it is 5 per cent.

In a case at the Johns Hopkins Hospital in 1895, in a hair-picker, there were most extensive enteritis, peritonitis, and endocarditis, which last lesion has been described by Eppinger.

A feature in both these forms of malignant pustule, to which many writers refer, is the absence of feeling of distress or anxiety on the part of the patient, whose mental condition may be perfectly clear. He may be without any apprehension, even though the condition be most critical.

The *diagnosis* in most instances is readily made from the character of the lesion and the occupation of the patient. When in doubt, the examination of the fluid from the pustule may show the presence of the anthrax bacilli. Cultures should be made, or a mouse or guinea-pig inoculated from the local lesion. It is to be remembered that the blood may not show the bacilli in numbers until shortly before death.

(*b*) Internal Anthrax.

(1) *Intestinal Form, Mycosis Intestinalis.*—In these cases the infection usually is through the stomach and intestines, and results from eating the flesh or drinking the milk of diseased animals; it may, however, follow an external infection if the germs are carried to the mouth. The symptoms are those of intense poisoning. The disease may set in with a chill, followed

by vomiting, diarrhœa, moderate fever, and pains in the legs and back. In acute cases there are dyspnœa, cyanosis, great anxiety and restlessness, and toward the end convulsions or spasms of the muscles. Hæmorrhage may occur from the mucous membranes. Occasionally there are on the skin small phlegmonous areas or petechiæ. The spleen is enlarged. The blood is dark and remains fluid for a long time after death. Late in the disease the bacilli may be found in the blood.

This is one of the forms of acute poisoning which may affect many individuals together. Thus, Butler and Karl Huber describe an epidemic in which twenty-five persons were attacked after eating the flesh of an animal which had had anthrax. Six died in from forty-eight hours to seven days.

(2) *Wool-sorter's Disease, Pulmonary Anthrax, Anthracœmia.*—This important form occurs in the large establishments in which wool or hair is sorted and cleansed. The hair and wool imported into Europe from Russia and South America appear to have induced the largest number of cases. Many of these show no external lesion. The infective material has been swallowed or inhaled with the dust. There are rarely premonitory symptoms. The patient is seized with a chill, becomes faint and prostrated, has pains in the back and legs, and the temperature rises to 102° or 103°. The breathing is rapid, and he complains of much pain in the chest. There may be a cough and signs of bronchitis. So prominent in some instances are these bronchial symptoms that a pulmonary form of the disease has been described. The pulse is feeble and very rapid. There may be vomiting, and death may occur within twenty-four hours with symptoms of profound collapse and prostration. Other cases are more protracted, and there may be diarrhœa, delirium, and unconsciousness. The cerebral symptoms may be most intense; in at least four cases the brain seems to have been chiefly affected, and its capillaries stuffed with bacilli (Merkel). The recognition of wool-sorter's disease as a form of anthrax is due to J. H. Bell, of Bradford.

In certain instances these profound constitutional symptoms of internal anthrax are associated with the external lesions of malignant pustule.

The *rag-picker's disease* has been made the subject of an exhaustive study by Eppinger (Die Hadernkrankheit, Jena, 1894), who has shown that it is a local anthrax of the lungs and pleura, with general infection.

Prophylaxis.—This is important, and should be carried out by a most rigid disinfection of the hides, hair, and rags before they are placed in the hands of the workmen. It is suggested to soak the hides for 24 hours in a solution of 1 per cent. formic acid and 0.02 per cent. of mercuric perchloride. Animals may be immunized against the disease and Pasteur's method of vaccination has been extensively employed in France with good results. The immunity is lost within a year in nearly 50 per cent. of the animals.

Treatment.—In malignant pustule the site of inoculation should be excised and, after the cautery or pure carbolic acid is applied, powdered bichloride of mercury sprinkled over the exposed surface. The local development of the bacilli about the site of inoculation may be prevented by the subcutaneous injections of solutions of carbolic acid (3 per cent.) or bichloride of mercury (1 to 1,000). The injections should be made at various points around the pustule, and may be repeated two or three times a day. The internal treatment should be confined to the administration of stimulants and plenty of nutritious food.

In malignant forms, particularly the intestinal cases, little can be done. Active purgatives may be given at the outset, so as to remove the infecting material. Quinine in large doses has been recommended.

An anti-anthrax serum has been prepared by Sclavo, for which good results are claimed.

XVIII. LEPROSY

Definition.—A chronic infectious disease caused by *Bacillus lepræ,* characterized by the presence of tubercular nodules in the skin and mucous membranes (tubercular leprosy) or by changes in the nerves (anæsthetic leprosy). At first these forms may be separate, but ultimately both are combined, and in the characteristic tubercular form there are disturbances of sensation.

History.—The disease appears to have prevailed in Egypt even so far back as three or four thousand years before Christ. The Hebrew writers make many references to it, but, as is evident from the description in Leviticus, many different forms of skin disease were embraced under the term leprosy. Both in India and in China the affection was also known many centuries before the Christian era. The old Greek and Roman physicians were perfectly familiar with its manifestations. Evidence of a pre-Columbian existence of leprosy in America has been sought in the old pieces of Peruvian pottery representing deformities suggestive of this disease, but Ashmead denies their significance. Throughout the middle ages leprosy prevailed extensively in Europe, and the number of leper asylums has been estimated as at least 20,000. During the sixteenth century it gradually declined.

Geographical Distribution.—In Europe leprosy prevails in Iceland, Norway and Sweden, parts of Russia, particularly about Dorpat, Riga, and the Caucasus, and in certain provinces of Spain and Portugal. In Great Britain the cases are now all imported.

In the United States there were 139 cases in 1909, of which 50 were in Louisiana, 20 in Florida, 16 in Minnesota, and 12 in Texas. In the Dominion of Canada there are foci of leprosy in two or three counties of New Brunswick, settled by French Canadians, and in Cape Breton, Nova Scotia. The disease appears to have been imported from Normandy about the end of the 18th century. The number has gradually lessened, and now only a few cases remain in the lazaretto at Tracadie.

Leprosy is endemic in the West India Islands. It also occurs in Mexico and throughout the Southern States. In the Sandwich Islands it spread rapidly after 1860, and strenuous attempts have been made to stamp it out by segregating all lepers on the island of Molokai. In the Philippine Islands, in a population of over six millions, there are 2,330 lepers.

In British India, according to the Leprosy Commission, there are 100,000 lepers. This is probably a low estimate. In China leprosy prevails extensively. In South Africa it has increased rapidly. In Australia, New Zealand, and the Australasian islands it also prevails, chiefly among the Chinese. The essays of Ashburton Thompson and James Cantlie deal fully with leprosy in China, Australia, and the Pacific islands. In Egypt the census of 1907 gave 6,000 lepers.

Etiology.—*Bacillus lepræ,* discovered by Hansen, of Bergen, in 1871, is universally recognized as the cause of the disease. It has many points of resemblance to the tubercle bacillus, but can be readily differentiated. It has been cultivated, but with difficulty, and is stated to have a pleomorphism of which the bacillus as seen in the tissues is only one phase.

Modes of Infection.—(*a*) *Inoculation.*—While it is highly probable that leprosy may be contracted by accidental inoculation, the experimental evidence is as yet inconclusive. With one possible exception, negative results have followed the attempts to reproduce the disease in man. The Hawaiian convict, under sentence of death, who was inoculated on September 30, 1884, by Arning, four weeks later had rheumatoid pains and gradual painful swelling of the ulnar and median nerves. The neuritis gradually subsided, but there developed a small lepra tubercle at the site of the inoculation. In 1887 the disease was quite manifest, and the man died of it six years after inoculation. The case is not regarded as conclusive, as he had leprous relatives and lived in a leprous country.

(*b*) *Heredity.*—For years it was thought that the disease was transmitted from parent to child, but the general opinion, as expressed in the recent Leprosy Congress in Berlin, was decidedly against this view. Of course, the possibility of its transmission cannot be denied, and in this respect leprosy and tuberculosis occupy very much the same position, though men with very wide experience have never seen a new-born leper. The youngest cases are rarely under three or four years of age.

(*c*) *By Contagion.*—The bacilli are given off from the open sores; they are found in the saliva and expectoration of the cases with leprous lesions in the mouth and throat, and occur in very large numbers in the nasal secretion. Sticker found in 153 lepers, subjects of both forms of the disease, bacilli in the nasal secretion in 128, and herein, he thinks, lies the chief source of danger. Schaffer was able to collect lepra bacilli on clean slides placed on tables and floors near to lepers whom he had caused to read aloud. The bacilli have also been isolated from the urine and the milk of patients. It seems probable that they may enter the body in many ways through the mucous membranes and through the skin. Sticker believes that the initial lesion is in an ulcer above the cartilaginous part of the nasal septum. One of the most striking examples of the contagiousness of leprosy is the following: "In 1860, a girl who had hitherto lived at Holstfershof, where no leprosy existed, married and went to live at Tarwast with her mother-in-law, who was a leper. She remained healthy, but her three children (1, 2, 3) became leprous, as also her younger sister (4), who came on a visit to Tarwast and slept with the children. The younger sister developed leprosy after returning to Holstfershof. At the latter place a man (5), fifty-two years old, who married one of the 'younger sister's' children, acquired leprosy; also a relative (6), thirty-six years old, a tailor by occupation, who frequented the house, and his wife (7), who came from a place where no leprosy existed. The two men last mentioned are at present (1897) inmates of the leper asylum at Dorpat." There is certain evidence to show that the disease may be spread through infected clothing, and the high percentage of washerwomen among lepers is also suggestive.

Conditions Influencing Infection.—The disease attacks persons of all ages. We do not yet understand all the conditions necessary. Evidently the closest and most intimate contact is essential. The doctors, nurses, and Sisters of Charity who care for the patients are very rarely attacked. In the lazaretto at Tracadie not one of the Sisters who for more than fifty years have so faithfully nursed the lepers has contracted the disease. Father Damian, in the Sandwich Islands, and Father Boblioli, in New Orleans, both fell victims in the discharge of their priestly duties. There has long been an idea that possibly the disease may be associated with some special kind of food, and Jonathan Hutchinson believes that a fish diet is the *tertium quid,* which either renders the patient susceptible or with which the poison may be taken.

Morbid Anatomy.—The leprosy tubercles consist of granulomatous tissue made up of cells of various sizes in a connective-tissue matrix. The bacilli in extraordinary numbers lie partly between and partly in the cells. The process gradually involves the skin, giving rise to tuberous outgrowths with intervening areas of ulceration or cicatrization, which in the face may gradually produce the so-called *facies leontina.* The mucous membranes, particularly the conjunctiva, the cornea, and the larynx, may gradually be involved. In many cases deep ulcers form which result in extensive loss of substance or loss of fingers or toes, the so-called *lepra mutilans.* In anæsthetic leprosy there is a peripheral neuritis due to the development of the bacilli in the nerve-fibres. Indeed, this involvement of the nerves plays a primary part in the etiology of many of the important features, particularly the trophic changes in the skin and the disturbances of sensation.

Clinical Forms.—(*a*) TUBERCULAR LEPROSY.—Prior to the appearance of the nodules there are areas of cutaneous erythema which may be sharply defined and often hyperæsthetic. This is sometimes known as *macular* leprosy. The affected spots in time become pigmented. In some instances this superficial change continues without the development of nodules, the areas become anæsthetic, the pigment gradually disappears, and the skin gets perfectly white—the *lepra alba.* Among the patients at Tracadie it was particularly interesting to see three or four in this early stage presenting on the face and forearms a patchy erythema with slight swelling of the skin. The diagnosis of the condition is perfectly clear, though it may be a long time before any other than sensory changes develop. The eyelashes and eyebrows and the hairs on the face fall out. The mucous membranes finally become involved, particularly of the mouth, throat, and larynx; the voice becomes harsh and finally aphonic. Death results not infrequently from the laryngeal complications and aspiration pneumonia. The conjunctivæ are frequently attacked, and the sight is lost by a leprous keratitis.

(*b*) ANÆSTHETIC LEPROSY.—This remarkable form has, in characteristic cases, no external resemblance whatever to the other variety. It usually begins with pains in the limbs and areas of hyperæsthesia or of numbness. Very early there may be trophic changes, seen in the formation of small bullæ (Hillis). Maculæ appear upon the trunk and extremities, and after persisting for a variable time gradually disappear, leaving areas of anæsthesia, but the loss of sensation may come on independently of the outbreak of maculæ. The nerve-trunks, where superficial, may be felt to be large and nodular. The trophic disturbances are usually marked. Pemphigus-like bullæ develop in the affected areas, which break and leave ulcers which may be very destructive. The fingers and toes are liable to contractures and to necrosis, so that in chronic cases the phalanges are lost. The course of anæsthetic leprosy is extraordinarily chronic and may persist for years without leading to much deformity. I knew a prominent clergyman who had anæsthetic leprosy for more than thirty years, which did not seriously interfere with his usefulness, and not in the slightest with his career.

Diagnosis.—Even in the early stage the dusky erythematous maculæ with hyperæsthesia or areas of anæsthesia are very characteristic. In an advanced grade neither the tubercular nor anæsthetic forms could possibly be mistaken for any other affection. In a doubtful case the microscopic examination of an excised nodule is decisive.

Treatment.—Vaccines have been prepared and good results are claimed by various observers. The Finsen light, X-rays, and radium do good to the local lesions. Nastin, a fatty principle extracted from cultures of a lepra-streptothrix combined with benzoyl chloride, has come into vogue and the Calcutta report is favorable. The gurjun and chaulmoogra oils have been recommended, the former in doses of from 5 to 10 minims, the latter in 2-drachm doses, but their use must be continued for at least two years. Calmette's antivenene, 20 to 30 c. c., subcutaneously, has been followed by remarkable results in a few cases. Segregation should be compulsory in all cases except where the friends can show that they have ample provision in their own home for the complete isolation and proper care of the patient.

XIX. TUBERCULOSIS

I. GENERAL ETIOLOGY AND MORBID ANATOMY

Definition.—An infection caused by *Bacillus tuberculosis,* the lesions of which are characterized by nodular bodies, tubercles, and diffuse infiltrations, which either undergo caseation, necrosis, and ulceration, or heal with sclerosis and calcification.

The very varied clinical features depend upon the organ involved, the intensity of the infection, and the degree of resistance offered by the body.

History.—The Greek physicians made many observations upon the clinical features of pulmonary tuberculosis, and our description of the symptoms and of the consumptive "type" dates from Hippocrates. Galen recognized its contagious nature. In the 17th century F. Sylvius indicated the connection between the tuberculous nodule and phthisis, and Richard Morton, a friend and contemporary of Sydenham, wrote (1689) the first modern treatise on the subject, in which the clinical side of the disease was well considered. He regarded it as contagious. Pierre Desault, William Stark, and Matthew Baillie laid the foundation of our knowledge of the coarse characters of tubercle as the anatomical basis of consumption. Our real knowledge of the disease is a 19th century contribution, beginning with the work of Bayle on the structure of the tubercle and on its identity in the widely distributed lesions. With the Traité d'Auscultation Médiate (1819) Laennec laid the foundation not only of our modern knowledge of tuberculosis, but of modern clinical medicine. This work (easily to be had also in an English translation) should be read from cover to cover by every young doctor, and, when possible, by every senior student. The unity of the forms of the tubercle—the miliary granule, the infiltration, and the caseous mass—was recognized, and for the first time physical signs and anatomical features were correlated, and the course of the disease carefully studied. Virchow led a battle against the unity of tuberculous lesions, and held that the products of any simple inflammation might become caseous, and that the ordinary so-called catarrhal pneumonia might terminate in phthisis.

The contagiousness of the disease, a belief in which had all along been held by individuals, and was widely spread in certain countries—as in Italy—was emphasized and confirmed by the brilliant work of Villemin, who first placed the infective nature of the disease on a solid experimental basis. There is nothing more masterly in the literature of experimental medicine than his work. Then came the demonstration by Robert Koch (in 1882) of the *Bacillus tuberculosis*. The preliminary article in the Berliner klin. Wochenschrift (1882) and the more complete work (Mitteilungen a. d. k. Gesundheitsamte, Bd. 2) should be studied by all who wish to appreciate the value of scientific methods. The thoroughness of Koch's work is manifested by the fact that, in the years that have elapsed, the innumerable workers have amplified and extended, but in no way essentially modified his original position.

During the past thirty years we have been gradually getting accommodated to the new views, the most important single effect of which has been a worldwide crusade against tuberculosis as a preventable disease.

Distribution.—The disease is widely spread zoologically.

(*a*) In Animals.—Of animals the cold-blooded are rarely affected. In birds the disease is not uncommon, particularly in fowls, but there are minor differences between the avian and mammalian forms. In the domestic animals tuberculosis is a common disease, particularly in cattle. In sheep, goats, and horses it is rare. In pigs it is not uncommon in certain parts of Europe. Cats and dogs are not prone to the disease. In monkeys in confinement it is very common. The most important single fact in the distribution of the disease in animals is its widespread prevalence in bovines, from which nearly all the milk and a large proportion of our meat are derived.

(*b*) In Man.—Tuberculosis is his most universal scourge, well deserving the epithet bestowed upon it by Bunyan of the "Captain of the Men of Death." It is estimated that at least one-seventh of all deaths are due to it. In England and Wales there were 54,435 deaths from tuberculosis in 1909. In the United States it is estimated that it is responsible for about one-ninth of the deaths annually. There has been a remarkable reduction in England in the death-rate within the past forty years, as shown by the following figures:

1871-1880	rate	per	100,000	of	population,	219
1881-1890	"	"	"	"	"	178
1891-1900	"	"	"	"	"	139
1901-1910	"	"	"	"	"	117

It has dropped nearly 50 per cent. in 40 years.

In London the death-rate from consumption has declined 33 per cent. between 1901 and 1910, and other forms of tuberculosis show a similar fall.

In 1909, 54,435 deaths from tuberculosis occurred, 38,699 of which were from pulmonary consumption. Had the death-rate been as high in 1909 as during an average year of the 1871-1880 period the number of deaths from phthisis would have been 78,308, instead of 38,639 (Newsholme). The mortality has been cut in half! To a less striking degree, but practically everywhere in the civilized world, there has been a reduction in the death-rate—the most encouraging feature of modern sanitation. To what is this to be attributed? *First.* To the improved social condition of the people, better housing, better food, better habits. The falling death-rate began before the present campaign against the disease. *Secondly.* The education of the people, which has made great strides, and a larger proportion are striving to lead hygienic lives. There are less drunkenness, less overcrowding, better air, and better food. The habit of spitting in public has been checked, and we may say confidently that the seeds of the disease are not spread so broadcast. *Thirdly.* As Newsholme points out, segregation has done much to protect the healthy from the sick. In the year 1910, 20.5 per cent. of the deaths in England and Wales and 43.4 per cent. of the deaths in London occurred in public institutions for the sick. In America, in Germany, and in France this factor also holds good. *Fourthly.* The cases are seen earlier and the condition is recognized before it is hopeless. Unquestionably in a larger number of persons with pulmonary disease the diagnosis is made at a stage when complete healing is possible. The two important elements then are, fewer seeds, more stony soil. The economic loss from tuberculosis has been estimated by various writers. Baldwin puts it for the United States at from 150 to 200 millions of dollars annually.

Etiology: the Bacillus tuberculosis.—(*a*) THE SEED.—The *Bacillus tuberculosis* is a minute rod-shaped organism slightly bent or curved, with an average length of from 3 to 4 μ. When stained it may present a beaded appearance; whether due to spores or vacuoles is doubtful. Aberrant forms are not uncommon, i. e., long filaments or branched forms. It stains in a characteristic way with aniline dyes, and in cultures the mode of growth is very distinctive.

Specific varieties are recognized. As already stated, the avian form has well-marked peculiarities, but the great point of discussion has been the relation of the bacillus causing human to that which causes bovine tuberculosis. Differences in the character of the tubercles of these two classes had long been recognized, and Theobald Smith pointed out special differences between the human and the bovine bacilli. But the matter was brought to a focus in 1901 by Koch's statement that the bacilli of bovine tuberculosis did not cause human tuberculosis, and *vice versa.* The question has now been submitted to the test by a number of commissions, and it is generally recognized that there are differences between the two forms. The recent report of the English commission confirms the view that the bovine organism is capable of producing the disease in man, in whom it may often be recognized as a special form.

The virulence of the individual strains varies, a factor of great importance in all specific infections.

In the Body.—The bacilli are found in all tuberculous lesions, particularly in those actively growing, but in the chronic disease of the lymph glands and of the joints they are scanty. In all caseous foci they are few in number.

In the sputum in pulmonary tuberculosis they may be present in countless myriads. They are found in the blood, particularly in cases of miliary tuberculosis.

Outside the Body.—The tubercle bacilli are widely scattered and are found in varying numbers wherever human beings are crowded together. There are two chief sources—the expectoration of persons with advanced disease of the lungs and the milk of tuberculous cows.

From a patient in my wards at the Johns Hopkins Hospital, with moderately advanced disease, Nuttall estimated that from 1½ to 4 1-3 billions of bacilli were thrown off each twenty-four hours. Allowed to dry, the sputum becomes dust and is distributed far and wide. Scores of experiments have shown the presence of the bacilli in dust samples from hospital wards, from public buildings, streets, railway carriages, and various localities. So widely spread are the bacilli that in cities at least few individuals pass a week without affording opportunity for their lodgment, usually in the throat or air passages, inhaled with dust. They may readily contaminate food. The hands of tuberculous subjects are almost always contaminated. From the street, tuberculous sputum may be brought into the house on shoes, on the long skirts of women, on the hair of dogs, etc. It is interesting to note that in some of the places most frequented by tuberculous subjects, e. g., the sanatoria, the dust (as shown by experiments at Saranac) may be free from bacilli.

Bovine bacilli are distributed by means of the milk, rarely by the flesh, and still more rarely by contact with the animals. A proportion of all cases of infection in childhood are with this variety. A careful study by Park and Krumwiede showed that bovine tuberculosis is practically negligible in adults but in young children it causes from 6 to 10 per cent. of the deaths from tuberculosis.

So widely spread everywhere is the seed, that the soil, the conditions suitable for its growth, is practically of equal moment.

(*b*) The Soil.—Many years ago I drew the parallel between infection in tuberculosis and the parable of the sower, which though now somewhat hackneyed illustrates in an effective way the importance of the nature of the ground upon which the seed falls. *"Some seeds fell by the wayside and the fowls of the air came and devoured them up."* These are the bacilli scattered broadcast outside the body, an immense majority of which die. *"Some fell upon stony places."* These are the bacilli that find lodgment in many of us, perhaps, with the production of a small focus, but nothing comes of it; they wither away "because they have no root." *"Some fell among thorns, and the thorns sprang up and choked them."* This represents the cases of tuberculosis, latent or active, in which the seed finds the soil suitable and grows, but the conditions are not favorable, as the thorns, representing the protecting force of the body, get the better in the struggle. *"But others fell on good ground and sprang up and bare fruit an hundredfold."* Of this fourth group were the 54,435 who died of the disease in 1909 in England—the soil suitable, the protecting forces feeble.

What makes a good soil? Fortunately the human body is not a very good culture medium for the tubercle bacillus. The adult human individual in normal health seems to be practically immune to natural infection (Baldwin). And yet one-seventh of the human race dies of tuberculosis, but a large proportion of all individuals become infected before reaching adult life and never have the disease. The studies of Naegli, Burkhardt, and others show that in fully 90 per cent. of the bodies of city-dwellers who have died of disease other than tuberculosis small tuberculous lesions are present. This is probably too high an estimate for England or the United States. Franz has shown that over 60 per cent. of healthy young adults react to the subcutaneous tuberculin test. Using more delicate tuberculin tests it is found that nearly all adults react, and according to Hamburger, who has employed the subcutaneous-local reaction, over 90 per cent. of children are infected before reaching the twelfth year of life. This means, of course, that in a very small proportion of those upon whom the seed falls is the soil suitable for active growth—only a natural immunity keeps the race alive.

What this suitable soil is has been the subject of much discussion. From the time of Hippocrates the profession has recognized a tuberculous habitus, which has been variously described as disposition, diathesis, dyscrasia, temperament, constitution, or by the German word "Anlage." These terms are not always regarded as interchangeable, but here for practical purposes Ribbert's definition suffices, that a disposition is "that peculiarity in the organism which allows of the effective working of the exciting causes of a disease." Manifestly, such a disposition or constitution of the body may be inherited or acquired. The studies of Pearson indicate the very great importance of heredity in the phthisical soil. He concludes that "the diathesis of pulmonary tuberculosis is certainly inherited, and the intensity of the inheritance is sensibly the same as that of any normal physical character yet investigated in man. Infection probably plays a necessary part, but in the artisan classes of the urban populations of this country (England) it is doubtful if their members can escape the risks of infection, except by the absence of diathesis—i. e., the inheritance of what amounts to a counter-disposition."

Hippocrates defines the *habitus phthisicus* in the following words: "The form of body peculiar to subjects of phthisical complaints was the smooth, the whitish, that resembled the lentil; the reddish, the blue-eyed, the leucophlegmatic, and that with the scapulæ having the appearance of wings." The so-called scrofulous type has broad coarse features, opaque skin, large thick bones, and heavy figure.

Acquired disposition may arise through a lowering of the resistance of the body forces. Dwellers in cities in the dark, close alleys, and tenement houses, workers in cellars and ill-ventilated rooms, persons addicted to drink, are much more prone to the disease. The influence of environment was never better demonstrated than in the well-known experiment of Trudeau, who found that rabbits inoculated with tuberculosis if confined in a dark, damp place, without sunlight and fresh air, rapidly succumbed, while others treated in the same way, but allowed to run wild, either recovered or showed very slight lesions. The occupants of prisons, asylums, and poorhouses, too often, indeed, in barracks and large workshops, are in the position of Trudeau's rabbits in the cellar, and under the conditions most favorable to foster the development of the bacilli which may have lodged in their tissues.

No age is exempt. The disease is met with in the suckling and in the octogenarian, but fatal tuberculosis is, as Hippocrates pointed out, more common between the eighteenth and thirty-fifth year. The influence of sex is very slight. On the other hand the influence of race is important. It is a very fatal disease in the negroes, particularly in the southern United States, and in the North American Indians. The Irish, both at home and in the United States, are more prone to the disease than other European races. The Jews everywhere have a low mortality from tuberculosis.

Occupation has an influence, in so far as insanitary surroundings, exposure to dust, close confinement, long, irregular hours, and low rates of wages, favor the prevalence of the disease. Certain local conditions influence the soil very greatly. Catarrh of the respiratory passages appears to lower the resistance and favor the conditions which enable the bacilli to enter the system, or to grow in the tissues. The specific fevers, particularly measles and whooping-cough, predispose to tuberculosis; and any lowering disease may do so, but in such cases it is very often not a fresh infection, but the blazing of a smouldering fire. As is well known, the soil of diabetes is very favorable to the growth of the tubercle bacilli. Many chronic affections lower the resistance and make the soil more favorable. It is notorious in hospital practice how often the fatal event in arterio-sclerosis, cirrhosis of the liver, etc., is a terminal acute tuberculosis.

Trauma, as for example a blow on the chest, injury to the knee, a blow upon the head, may be followed by local tuberculosis. The injured part for a time is a *locus minoris resistentiæ,* and the bacilli already present grow in the favorable conditions caused by the injury.

(*c*) Specific Reactions of the Bacilli.—In its growth the bacillus so far as we know does not form soluble toxins, at least not in the cultures. It causes (1) a local tissue reaction which results in the formation of a new growth, the tubercle; (2) changes in the metabolism of the body fluids. The local tissue reactions will be considered later; here we may speak of the phenomena grouped under the term immunity.

(1) *Tuberculin Reaction.*—An animal inoculated subcutaneously with tubercle bacilli, or with dead cultures, has a local reaction associated with the formation of a tubercle; the neighboring lymph glands become involved, and in susceptible animals the disease generalizes and causes death. Koch found that if to a guinea-pig with a subcutaneous focus of tuberculosis so caused a second injection of the bacillus was given, healing occurred in the primary nodule, and the animal did not die. Upon these facts his famous tuberculin treatment was based. Tuberculin consists of the dead and macerated bacilli together with any substances formed in the cultures. If into a healthy person .25 c. c. of tuberculin is injected, there is a very slight fever with a little feeling of uneasiness which passes off in from twelve to twenty-four hours. If into an individual with a focus of tuberculosis doses of .015 c. c. of tuberculin are injected subcutaneously, there is an active local reaction about the tuberculous focus, with intense inflammation leading often to necrosis and, in the case of a skin tubercle, as lupus, in which the process can be followed, healing is seen to take place. This process, now known as the "tuberculin reaction," is used extensively for purposes of diagnosis. The chief methods in use are the ophthalmo-reaction, of Calmette and the cutaneous of von Pirquet. For the Calmette reaction Koch's old tuberculin is used, prepared in a special way. A drop of the solution, placed on the conjunctiva of a person with a focus of tuberculosis anywhere in the system, is followed in a

few hours by a deep injection of the blood-vessels, increased lachrymation, and a slight swelling of the membrane. This, known as a positive reaction, lasts for from twenty-four to thirty-six hours.

For the skin reaction of von Pirquet a couple of drops of tuberculin are placed on a disinfected region of the skin, and the epidermis is scarified through the drops without drawing blood. If positive, at the end of twenty-four hours there is an inflammatory reaction which reaches its maximum in from thirty-six to forty-eight hours. For clinical purposes the tuberculin reaction is to be relied on, but that it may be given by a small focus of latent disease in a healthy person and that it has been found to be positive in as large a proportion as 60 per cent. of apparently normal individuals are facts which diminish its practical value.

(2) *Immunity Changes.*—In an infected person certain changes occur in the blood serum, depending upon the development of so-called antibodies, the presence of which may be demonstrated by the method of complement fixation; and the serum also contains agglutinins which possess an agglutinating action on the tubercle bacilli. Either directly themselves or through the toxic products there are brought into play certain cellular and humoral reactions which are capable of destroying the infecting agents or of neutralizing their effects or of limiting their activities. There exist in the blood-serum antibodies, called by Wright opsonins, which have the power of stimulating phagocytosis. When these opsonins are abnormally low, the bacilli that gain entrance to the body can multiply at the point of infection. This increase is associated with a still further local reduction in the opsonins. Wright believes that the amount of opsonin in the serum is an indication of the defensive capacity of the individual, and he has established what he calls an "opsonic index," which is the ratio between the number of bacteria found within twenty to forty polymorpho-leucocytes in an emulsion made with the patient's serum and the number of bacteria found in the same number of similar leucocytes in an emulsion made with a normal serum, the latter being taken as 1.0. This index in tuberculous patients is usually low, varying from .1 to .8. When tuberculin is injected, the production of opsonins is stimulated, and the opsonic index rises. With the body fluids richer in opsonins than before, the phagocytes are more active and more bacilli are destroyed. Experimentally in animals, according to the virulence of the organism and the dose, all gradations of symptoms may be produced, from the slightest local reaction to the profoundest septicæmia with high fever and death. In a local tuberculous infection, such as happens to the great majority of us in some part of our bodies at some time in our lives, happily the protective mechanism suffices to localize and limit the invaders. It may amount only to a skirmish, such as is constantly going on at the frontiers of a great empire, but if the local infection is more virulent, or becomes wider spread, the products of the growth of the bacilli or the bacilli themselves enter the circulation, occasioning what is called an auto-inoculation, in which case the general metabolism is disturbed, fever is produced, and antibodies are formed to counteract the infective products. The rationale of the use of tuberculin is to stimulate the fighting forces of the body—to mobilize them, so to speak—in the fight that is going on in an infected area. The whole question of active immunization in tuberculosis is being thoroughly studied, and, while many have thrown doubt on

the trustworthiness and the usefulness of the opsonic index as a gauge of the progress of a case, there can be no question that Wright's researches have put us in the right path for a scientific treatment of the disease.

Recent studies on anaphylaxis or hypersensitiveness to foreign proteins have an important bearing on the question of immunity in tuberculosis. Baldwin of Saranac Lake, in a series of experiments, has demonstrated that sensitization to and subsequent intoxication by tubercle bacillus protein follow the general laws of anaphylaxis established for the parenteral introduction of horse serum. From his experiments we may now reasonably interpret the tuberculin reaction as an anaphylactic phenomenon. Undoubtedly hypersensitiveness to the tubercle bacillus protein is directly responsible for the so-called toxic symptoms of tuberculous disease. Koch in his original experiments that led up to the introduction of tuberculin observed a marked difference in the reaction of healthy and tuberculous animals to cutaneous inoculation with tubercle bacilli. In healthy animals the wound closes and for a few days seems to heal, but in from ten to fourteen days a hard nodule appears, which soon breaks down. General infection occurs and the ulcer remains open to the time of the death of the animal. In tuberculous animals extensive ulceration occurs on the second or third day after vaccination, but the ulcer heals quickly and permanently, without even the neighboring lymph glands becoming infected. Roemer has extended Koch's observations and has demonstrated that tuberculous animals may react in one of three ways to injections of tubercle bacilli: (1) If a small dose be given, a dose, however, surely fatal for healthy animals, infection does not occur. The animals are therefore highly resistant to re-infection. (2) If a large dose be given, the animals die promptly, with the symptoms of an intense intoxication. The condition is analogous to the anaphylactic shock. (3) If a moderate dose be given, the animals display the symptoms of a profound intoxication, but gradually recover, and, although infection follows, a mild and chronic form of the disease is produced. Upon the same principle depends the protective inoculation of calves, so successfully practiced by v. Behring and Koch. The animals receive injections of human tubercle bacilli and, although anatomically disease does not follow their introduction, the calves become highly sensitive to tuberculin and at the same time immune to doses of bovine tubercle bacilli fatal to unprotected calves. At the end of a year the tuberculin hypersensitiveness disappears, and the calves again become susceptible to infection. While we are not in a position to state that protection depends upon the same mechanism that produces hypersensitiveness to the tubercle bacillus protein, the two phenomena are undoubtedly closely related.

Antituberculous serums have been obtained from animals immunized by the tubercle bacillus or its products. The two most important are those of Marmorek and of Maragliano.

(*d*) Modes of Infection.—(1) *Hereditary Transmission.*—In order that the disease could be transmitted by the sperm it would be necessary that the tubercle bacilli should lodge in the individual spermatozoön which fecundates an ovum. The chances that such a thing could occur are extremely small, looking at the subject from a numerical point of view, although we know that bacilli do occasionally exist in the semen; they become still smaller when we consider that the spermatozoön is made up of nuclear material, which the tubercle bacillus is never known to attack. The possibility of transmission by the ovum must be accepted. Baumgarten has in one instance been able to detect the tubercle bacillus in the ovum of a female rabbit which he had artificially fecundated with tuberculous semen.

The almost constant method of transmission in congenital tuberculosis is through the blood current, the tubercle bacilli penetrating by way of the placenta. In these cases the placenta itself is usually the seat of tuberculosis; but there are undoubted instances in which, with an apparently sound placenta, both the placental blood and the fetal organs contained tubercle bacilli, notwithstanding the fact that the organs also appeared normal. The number of cases of congenital tuberculosis in man is very small; it is more common in cattle.

Possible Latency of the Tubercle Germs.—Baumgarten and his followers assume that the tubercle bacilli lie latent in the tissues and subsequently develop when, for some reason or other, the individual resistance is lowered. He likens such cases of latent tuberculosis to the late hereditary forms of syphilis, and explains the lack of development of the germs by the greater resisting power of the tissues of children. Baumgarten bases his belief in germ transmission upon two main factors—the great frequency of the disease in early life and the localization of tuberculous lesions in children.

Against this theory are the facts that the percentage of cases of congenital tuberculosis is extremely small, and that in the great majority of instances the organs of fetuses born of tuberculous mothers give negative results when inoculated into guinea-pigs.

(2) *Inoculation.—Cutaneous.*—The infective nature of tuberculosis was first demonstrated by Villemin, who showed in 1865 that it could be transmitted to animals by inoculation. The experiments of Cohnheim and Salomonsen, who produced tuberculosis in the eyes of guinea-pigs and rabbits by inoculating fresh tubercle into the anterior chamber, confirmed and extended Villemin's original observations and paved the way for the reception of Koch's announcement. This mode of infection is seen in persons whose occupation brings them in contact with the dead bodies or animal products. Demonstrators of morbid anatomy, butchers, and handlers of hides are subject to a local tubercle of the skin, which forms a reddened mass of granulation tissue, usually capping the dorsal surface of the hand or a finger. This is the so-called post mortem wart, the *verruca necrogenica* of Wilks. The demonstration of its nature is shown by the presence of tubercle bacilli, and by inoculation experiments in animals.

In the performance of the rite of circumcision children have been accidentally inoculated. Infection in these cases is probably always associated with disease in the operator, and occurs in connection with the habit of cleansing the wound by suction.

Other means of inoculation have been described: as the wearing of earrings, washing the clothes of phthisical patients, the bite of a tuberculous subject, or inoculation from a cut by a broken spit-glass of a consumptive; and Czerny has reported two cases of infection by transplantation of skin.

It has been urged by the opponents of vaccination that tuberculosis, as well as syphilis, may be thus conveyed, but of this there is no evidence. Lymph of revaccinated consumptives is non-infective. Lupus has originated at the site of vaccination in a few cases (C. Fox, Graham Little). It may be said, on the whole, that inoculation in man plays a trifling rôle in the transmission of tuberculosis.

Mucous membrane inoculation is probably important in childhood through abrasions of the lips, tongue or gums, though a primary focus is not often seen. The open door in the mouth and throat is more often by loss of the protective epithelium due to catarrhal and ulcerative processes.

(3) *Infection by Inhalation.*—A belief in the contagiousness of pulmonary tuberculosis originated with the early Greek physicians, and has persisted among the Latin races. The investigations of Cornet afford conclusive proof that the dust of a room or other locality frequented by patients with pulmonary tuberculosis is infective. The bacilli attached to fine particles of dust are inhaled and gain entrance to the system through the lungs.

Flügge denies that the bacillus-containing dust is the dangerous element in infection. Experimentally he has only succeeded in producing the disease when there is some lesion in the respiratory tract. He thinks that the danger of infection by the dry sputum is very improbable. On the other hand, he thinks that the infection is chiefly conveyed by the free, finely divided particles of sputum produced in the act of coughing, and that these tiny fragments are suspended in the atmosphere. Those who cough very much and with the mouth open are most liable to infect the surrounding air.

It is well remarked by Cornet, "The consumptive in himself is almost harmless, and only becomes harmful through bad habits." It has been fully shown that the expired air of consumptives is not infective. The virus is only contained in the sputum, which when dry is widely disseminated in the form of dust, and constitutes the great medium for the transmission of the disease.

Among the points urged in favor of the inhalation view are:

(*i*) Primary tuberculous lesions are in a majority of all cases connected with the respiratory system. The frequency with which foci are met with in the lungs and in the bronchial glands is extraordinary, and the statistics of the Paris morgue show that a considerable proportion of all persons dying of accident or by suicide present evidences of the disease in these parts. The post mortem statistics of hospitals show the same widespread prevalence of infection through the air passages. Biggs reports that more than 60 per cent. of his post mortems showed lesions of pulmonary tuberculosis. In 125 autopsies at the Foundling Hospital, New York, the bronchial glands were tuberculous in every case. In adults the bronchial glands may be infected and the individual remain in good health.

(*ii*) The greater prevalence of tuberculosis in institutions in which the residents are confined and restricted in the matter of fresh air and a free open life—conditions which would favor, on the one hand, the presence of the bacilli in the atmosphere, and, on the other, lower the vital resistance of the individual. The investigations of Cornet upon the death-rate from consumption among certain religious orders devoted to nursing give some striking facts in illustration of this. In a review of 38 cloisters, embracing the average number of 4,028 residents, among 2,099 deaths in the course of twenty-five years, 1,320 (62.88 per cent.) were from tuberculosis. In some cloisters more than three-fourths of the deaths are from this disease, and the mortality in all the residents, up to the fortieth year, is greatly above the average, the increase being due entirely to the prevalence of tuberculosis. It has been stated that nurses are not more prone to the disease than other individuals, but Cornet says that, of 100 nurses deceased, 63 died of tuberculosis. The more perfect the prophylaxis and hygienic arrangements of an asylum or institution, the lower the death-rate from tuberculosis. The mortality in prisons has been shown by Baer to be four times as great as outside. The death-rate from phthisis is estimated at 15 per cent. of the total mortality, while in prisons it constitutes from 40 to 50 per cent., and in some countries, as Austria, over 60 per cent. Flick has studied the distribution of the deaths from tuberculosis in a single city ward in Philadelphia for twenty-five years. His researches go far to show that it is a house disease. About 33 per cent. of infected houses have had more than one case. There are, however, opposing facts. The statistics of the Brompton Consumption Hospital show that doctors, nurses, and attendants are rarely attacked. Dettweiler claims that no case of tuberculosis has been contracted among his nurses or attendants at Falkenstein. Among 174 previously healthy sanitarium physicians whose average term of service was three years only two became tuberculous (Sangmann). On the other hand, in the Paris hospitals tuberculosis decimates the attendants.

(*iii*) Special danger is believed to exist when the contact is very intimate, as between man and wife. Until recently nearly all writers have held that under these circumstances the husband or wife is much more likely subsequently to die of tuberculosis. Upon the figures of the late Ernest Pope, of Saranac, Karl Pearson bases the following conclusions: (*a*) There is some sensible but slight infection between married couples; (*b*) this is largely obscured or forestalled by the fact of infection from outside sources; (*c*) the liability to the infection depends on the presence of the necessary diathesis; (*d*) assortative mating probably accounts for at least two-thirds, and infective action not more than one-third of the whole correlation observed in these cases. There are cases in which this source of infection seems to play an important rôle.

(4) *Infection by Ingestion.*—The work of the past few years has shown that there are two other channels, the tonsils and the intestines, both of great importance.

(*i*) *Tonsillar Infection.*—The frequency of involvement of these glands has been shown by Schlenker, Arthur Latham, and Walsham. The bacilli pass to the glands of the neck and of the mediastinum, and reach the circulation through the lymph-channels. Or an infected bronchial gland becomes adherent to a branch of the pulmonary artery; if a large number of bacilli escape, miliary tuberculosis follows; if only a small number, they reach the lungs, at the apices of which they find conditions suitable for their growth. Through this tonsillar-cervical route bacilli may gain entrance without causing local disease at the portal of entry. It is a common method of infection in children, causing the "scrofulous" glands of the neck.

(*ii*) *Intestinal Infection.*—Behring announced in 1903 that pulmonary tuberculosis could be induced through intestinal infection, and he further maintained that milk fed to infants was the chief cause of consumption in adults, the infection remaining latent. Behring's first contention was supported by Ravenel and others, who produced pulmonary tuberculosis in animals by feeding experiments, and it was demonstrated that the intestinal surface itself might remain intact. This does away with the objection raised by Koch that, if infection through the milk of tuberculous cattle were common, primary intestinal tuberculosis should be more frequent, whereas in ten years among 3,104 cases of tuberculosis in children there were only 16 of primary bowel infection. Recent experiments have shown in a striking manner how the lungs act as filters for particles absorbed from the intestines. Vansteenberghe and Grysez have produced anthracosis of the lungs by introducing china-ink emulsion directly into the stomach (see Anthracosis). They found a remarkable difference in young and adult guinea-pigs; in the former the carbon particles were filtered out by the mesenteric glands, while the lungs remained free; in the latter the glands were unaffected, but the lungs were carbonized. Calmette and Guérin, repeating the experiments of Ravenel with improved technique, have shown how easily the lungs may be infected through the intestinal route without leaving the slightest trace of disease of the bowel itself. Behring's view of the importance of infection through the intestinal route has thus received the strongest support, and many go so far as to maintain that a majority of all cases of phthisis originate in this manner. The truth is that this ubiquitous bacillus is not particular, and gains entrance through either portal, preferring the throat and intestines in childhood, the bronchi and lungs in adults. The important matter for the individual is the nature of the soil on which it falls.

Milk alone is a common source of intestinal infection, particularly in the large cities. In New York, Hess found tubercle bacilli in 16 per cent. of 107 specimens! The ordinary commercial pasteurization does not kill them. The flesh of tuberculous animals is rarely dangerous.

General Morbid Anatomy and Histology of Tuberculous Lesions.—(*a*) Distribution of the Tubercles in the Body.—The organs of the body are variously affected by tuberculosis. In adults, the lungs may be regarded as the seat of election; in children, the lymph-glands, bones, and joints. In 1,000 autopsies there were 275 cases with tuberculous lesions. With but two or three exceptions the lungs were affected. The distribution in the other organs was as follows: Pericardium, 7; peritoneum, 36; brain, 31; spleen, 23; liver, 12; kidneys, 32; intestines, 65; heart, 4; and generative organs, 8.

Among 8,873 surgical patients at the Würzburg clinic, 1,287 were tuberculous, with the following distribution of lesions: Bones and joints, 1,037; lymph-glands, 196; skin and connective tissues, 77; mucous membranes, 10; genito-urinary organs, 20.

(*b*) The Changes Produced by the Tubercle Bacilli.—*The Nodular Tubercle.*—A "tubercle" *presents in its early formation nothing distinctive or peculiar, either in its components or in their arrangement.* Identical structures are produced by other parasites, such as the actinomyces, and by the strongylus in the lungs of sheep.

The following changes occur in the evolution of a tubercle:

(1) The tubercle bacilli multiply and disseminate in the surrounding tissues, partly by growth, partly in the lymph currents.

(2) The fixed cells, especially those of connective tissue and the endothelium of the capillaries, multiply and form rounded, cuboidal, or polygonal

bodies with vesicular nuclei—the *epithelioid cells*—inside some of which the bacilli are soon seen.

(3) Leucocytes, chiefly polynuclear, migrate in numbers and accumulate about the focus of infection. They do not survive. Many undergo rapid destruction. Later, as the little tubercle grows, the leucocytes are chiefly of the mononuclear variety (lymphocytes), which do not undergo the rapid degeneration of the polynuclear forms.

(4) A retriculum of fibres is formed by the fibrillation and rarefaction of the connective-tissue matrix. This is most apparent, as a rule, at the margin of the growth.

(5) In some, but not all, tubercles *giant cells* are formed by an increase in the protoplasm and in the nuclei of an individual cell, or possibly by the fusion of several cells. The giant cells seem to be in inverse ratio to the number and virulence of the bacilli.

(*c*) THE DEGENERATION OF TUBERCLE.—(1) *Caseation.*—At the central part of the growth, owing to the direct action of the bacilli or their products, a process of coagulation necrosis goes on in the cells, which lose their outline, become irregular, no longer take stains, and are finally converted into a homogeneous, structureless substance. Proceeding from the centre outward, the tubercle may be gradually converted into a yellowish-gray body, in which, however, the bacilli are still abundant. No blood vessels are found in them. Aggregated together these form the cheesy masses so common in tuberculosis, which may undergo softening, fibroid limitation (encapsulation), or calcification.

(2) *Sclerosis.*—With the necrosis of the cell elements at the centre of the tubercle, hyaline transformation proceeds, together with great increase in the fibroid elements; so that the tubercle is converted into a firm, hard structure. Often the change is rather of a fibro-caseous nature; but the sclerosis predominates. In some situations, as in the peritoneum, this seems to be the natural transformation of tubercle, and it is by no means rare in the lungs.

In all tubercles two processes go on: the one—caseation—destructive and dangerous; and the other—sclerosis—conservative and healing. The ultimate result in a given case depends upon the capabilities of the body to fight the invaders. There are tissue-soils in which the bacilli are, in all probability, killed at once. There are others in which a lodgment is gained and more or less damage done, but finally the day is with the conservative, protecting forces. Thirdly, there are tissue-soils in which the bacilli grow luxuriantly, caseation and softening, not limitation and sclerosis, prevail, and the day is with the invaders.

The action of the bacilli injected directly into the blood-vessels illustrates many points in the histology and pathology of tuberculosis. If into the vein of a rabbit a pure culture of the bacilli is injected, the microbes accumulate chiefly in the liver and spleen. The animal dies usually within two weeks, and the organs apparently show no trace of tubercles. Microscopically, in both spleen and liver the young tubercles in process of formation are very numerous, and karyokinesis is going on in the liver-cells. After an injection of a more dilute culture, or one whose virulence has been mitigated by age, instead of dying within a fortnight the animal survives for five or six weeks, by which time the tubercles are apparent in the spleen and liver, and often in the other organs.

(*d*) THE DIFFUSED INFLAMMATORY TUBERCLE.—This is most frequently seen in the lungs and results from the fusion of many small foci of infection —so small indeed that they may not be visible to the naked eye, but which histologically are seen to be composed of scattered centres, surrounded by areas in which the air-cells are filled with the products of exudation and of the proliferation of the alveolar epithelium. Under the influence of the bacilli, caseation takes place, usually in small groups of lobules, occasionally in an entire lobe, or even the greater part of a lung. In the early stage of the process, the tissue has a gray gelatinous appearance, the *gray infiltration* of Laennec. The alveoli contain a sero-fibrinous fluid with cells, and the septa are also infiltrated. These cells accumulate and undergo coagulation necrosis, forming areas of caseation, the *infiltration tuberculeuse jaune* of Laennec, the scrofulous or cheesy pneumonia of later writers. There may also be a diffuse infiltration and caseation without any special foci, a widespread tuberculous pneumonia induced by the bacilli.

After all, the two processes are identical. As Baumgarten states: "There is no well-marked difference between miliary tubercle and chronic caseous pneumonia. Speaking histologically, miliary tuberculosis is nothing else than a chronic caseous miliary pneumonia, and chronic caseous pneumonia is nothing but a tuberculosis of the lungs."

(*e*) SECONDARY INFLAMMATORY PROCESSES.—(1) The irritation caused by the bacilli produces an inflammation which may, as has been described, be limited to exudation of leucocytes and serum, but may also be much more extensive, and vary with changing conditions. We find, for example, about the smaller tubercles in the lungs, pneumonia—either catarrhal or fibrinous—proliferation of the connective-tissue elements in the septa (which also become infiltrated with round cells), and changes in the blood and lymph-vessels.

(2) In processes of minor intensity the inflammation is of the slow reactive nature, which results in the production of a cicatricial connective tissue which limits and restricts the development of the tubercles and is the essential conservative element in the disease. It is to be remembered that in chronic pulmonary tuberculosis much of the fibroid tissue which is present is not in any way associated with the action of the bacilli.

(3) Suppuration. Do the bacilli themselves induce suppuration? In so-called cold tuberculous abscess the material is not histologically pus, but a *débris* consisting of broken-down cells and cheesy material. It is moreover sterile—that is, does not contain the usual pus organisms. The products of the tubercle bacilli are probably able to induce suppuration, as in joint and bone tuberculosis pus is frequently produced, although this may be due to a mixed infection. Tuberculin is one of the best agents for the production of experimental suppuration. In tuberculosis of the lungs the suppuration is largely the result of an infection with pus organisms.

II. ACUTE MILIARY TUBERCULOSIS

The modern knowledge of this remarkable form dates from the statement of Buhl (1856), that miliary tuberculosis is a specific infection dependent on the presence in the body of an unencapsulated yellow tubercle, or a tuberculous cavity in the lung; and that it bears the same relation to the primary lesion as pyæmia does to a focus of suppuration.

Carl Weigert established the truth of this brilliant conception by demonstrating the association of miliary tuberculosis with tuberculosis of the blood-vessels. There are two groups of vessel tubercle—the tuberculous periangitis in which there is invasion of the adventitia, and the endangitis in which the tubercles start in the intima. The parts most frequently affected are the pulmonary veins and the thoracic duct, less often the jugular vein, the supra-renal and the vena cava superior, and the sinuses of the dura mater, the aorta, and the endocardium. To the branches of the pulmonary veins it is not uncommon to find caseous glands adherent, penetrating the walls and showing a growth of miliary tubercles in the intima. A special interest belongs to tuberculosis of the thoracic duct, first accurately described by Sir Astley Cooper. Benda in a series of 19 cases of vessel tuberculosis found in many instances an enormous number of bacilli, particularly in the caseous tubercles of the thoracic duct.

The bacilli do not increase in the blood, but settle in the different organs, producing a generalized tuberculosis, of which Weigert recognizes three types or grades: I. The acute general miliary tuberculosis, in which the various organs of the body are stuffed with miliary and submiliary nodules. II. A second form characterized by a small number of tubercles in one or many organs. III. The occurrence of numerous tuberculous foci widely spread throughout the body, but in a more chronic form; the tubercles are larger and many are caseous. It is the chronic generalized tuberculosis of children. Transitional forms between these groups occur. In the first variety, which we are here considering, there is an eruption into the circulation of an enormous number of bacilli. Benda suggests in explanation of the profound toxæmia seen in certain cases (the typhoid form) that in addition the blood is surcharged with toxins from a large caseous focus which has eroded the vessel.

Clinical Forms

The cases may be grouped into those with the symptoms of an *acute general infection*—the typhoid form; cases in which pulmonary symptoms predominate; and cases in which the *cerebral* or *cerebro-spinal* symptoms are marked—tuberculous meningitis.

Other forms have been recognized, but this division covers a large majority of the cases.

Taking any series of cases it will be found that the meningeal form of acute tuberculosis exceeds in numbers the cases with general or marked pulmonary symptoms.

General or Typhoid Form.—Symptoms.—The patient presents the symptoms of a profound infection which simulates and is frequently mistaken for typhoid fever. After a period of failing health, with loss of appetite, he becomes feverish and weak. Occasionally the disease sets in more abruptly, but in many instances the anamnesis closely resembles that of typhoid fever. Nose-bleeding, however, is rare. The temperature increases, the pulse becomes rapid and feeble, the tongue dry; delirium becomes marked and the cheeks are flushed. The pulmonary symptoms may be very slight; usually bronchitis exists, but is not more severe than is common with typhoid fever. The pulse is seldom dicrotic, but is rapid in proportion to the pyrexia. Perhaps the most striking feature of the temperature is the irregularity; and if seen from the outset there is not the steady ascent noted in typhoid fever. There is usually an evening rise to 103° F., sometimes 104° F., and a morning remission of from two to three degrees. Sometimes the pyrexia is intermittent, and the thermometer may register below normal during the early morning hours. The inverse type of temperature, in which the rise takes place in the morning, is held by some writers to be more frequent in general tuberculosis than in other diseases. In rare instances there may be little or no fever. On two occasions I have had a patient admitted to my wards in a condition of profound debility, with a history of illness of from three to four weeks' duration, with rapid pulse, flushed cheeks, dry tongue, and very slight elevation in temperature, in whom (post mortem) the condition proved to be general tuberculosis. In one instance there was tolerably extensive disease at the right apex. Reinhold, from Bäumler's clinic, has called attention to these afebrile forms of acute tuberculosis. In 9 of 52 cases there was no fever, or only a transient rise.

In a considerable number of the cases the respirations are increased in frequency, particularly in the early stage, and there may be signs of diffuse bronchitis and slight cyanosis. Cheyne-Stokes breathing occurs toward the close.

Active delirium is rare. More commonly there are torpor and dullness, gradually deepening into coma, in which the patient dies. In some cases the pulmonary symptoms become more marked; in others meningeal or cerebral features occur.

Diagnosis.—The differential diagnosis between general miliary tuberculosis without local manifestations and typhoid fever is extremely difficult. A point of importance, to which reference has already been made, is the irregularity of the temperature curve. The greater frequency of the respirations and the tendency to slight cyanosis are much more common in tuberculosis. There are cases, however, of typhoid fever in which the initial bronchitis is severe and may lead to dyspnœa and disturbed oxygenation. The cough may be slight or absent. Diarrhœa is rare in tuberculosis; the bowels are usually constipated; but diarrhœa may occur and persist for days. In certain cases the diagnosis has been complicated still further by the occurrence of blood in the stools. Enlargement of the spleen occurs in general tuberculosis, but is neither so early nor so marked as in typhoid fever. In children, however, the enlargement may be considerable. The urine may show traces of albumin, and unfortunately Ehrlich's diazo-reaction, which is so constant in typhoid fever, is also met with in general tuberculosis. The absence of the characteristic roseola is an important feature. Occasionally in acute tuberculosis reddish spots may occur and for a time cause difficulty, but they do not come out in crops, and rarely have the characters of the true typhoid eruption. Herpes is perhaps more common in tuberculosis. Toward the close, petechiæ may appear on the skin, particularly about the wrists. A rare event is jaundice, due possibly to the eruption of tubercles in the liver. It is to be remembered that the lesions of acute tuberculosis and of typhoid fever have been demonstrated in the same body.

A negative Widal test or ophthalmo-reaction, and the absence of typhoid bacilli in blood-cultures may be of decisive importance in these doubtful cases. In very rare instances tubercle bacilli have been found in the blood. Leucocytosis is more common in miliary tuberculosis than in typhoid fever, in which leucopenia is the rule. Careful examination of the eyes may show choroidal tubercles, though I have never known a diagnosis made on their presence alone. In the fluid obtained by lumbar puncture the tubercle bacilli may be abundant, even when there is no active meningitis. In a few cases the bacilli have been found in the urine.

Pulmonary Form.—SYMPTOMS.—From the outset the pulmonary symptoms are marked. The patient may have had a cough for months or for years without much impairment of health, or he may be known to be the subject of chronic pulmonary tuberculosis. In other instances, particularly in children, the affection follows measles or whooping cough, and is of a distinctly broncho-pneumonic type. The disease begins with the symptoms of diffuse bronchitis. The cough is marked, the expectoration muco-purulent, occasionally rusty. Hæmoptysis has been noted in a few instances. From the outset dyspnœa is a striking feature and may be out of proportion to the intensity of the physical signs. There is more or less cyanosis of the lips and finger-tips, and the cheeks are suffused. Apart from emphysema and the later stages of severe pneumonia, I know of no other pulmonary condition in which the cyanosis is so marked. The physical signs are those of bronchitis. In children there may be defective resonance at the bases, from scattered areas of broncho-pneumonia; or, what is equally suggestive, areas of hyper-resonance. Indeed, the percussion note, particularly in the front of the chest, in some cases of miliary tuberculosis, is full and clear, and it will be noted (post mortem) that the lungs are unusually voluminous. This is probably the result of more or less widespread acute emphysema. On auscultation, the râles are either sibilant and sonorous or small, fine, and crepitant. There may be fine crepitation from the occurrence of tubercles on the pleura (Jürgensen). In children there may be high-pitched tubular breathing at the bases or toward the root of the lung. Toward the close the râles may be larger and more mucous. The temperature rises to 102° or 103° F., and may present the inverse type. The pulse is rapid and feeble. In the very acute cases the spleen is always enlarged. The disease may prove fatal in ten or twelve days, or may be protracted for weeks or even months.

DIAGNOSIS.—The diagnosis of this form offers less difficulty and is more frequently made. There is often a history of previous cough, or the patient is known to be the subject of local disease of the lung, or of the lymph glands, or of the bones. In children these symptoms following measles or whooping cough indicate in the majority of cases acute miliary tuberculosis, with or without broncho-pneumonia. Occasionally the sputum contains tubercle bacilli.

The choroidal tubercle occurs in a limited number of cases and may help the diagnosis. More important in an adult is the combination of dyspnœa with cyanosis and the signs of a diffuse bronchitis. In some instances the occurrence of cerebral symptoms at once gives a clew to the nature of the trouble.

Meningeal Form (*Tuberculous Meningitis, Basilar Meningitis*).—This affection, which is also known as acute hydrocephalus or "water on the brain," is essentially an acute tuberculosis in which the membranes of the brain, sometimes of the cord, bear the brunt of the attack. Our first accurate knowledge of this affection dates from the publication of Robert Whytt's Observations on the Dropsy of the Brain, Edinburgh, 1768. He studied 20 cases and divided the disease into three stages, according to the condition of the pulse.

Though Guersant had as early as 1827 used the name *granular meningitis* for this form of inflammation of the meninges, it was not until 1830 that Papavoine demonstrated the nature of the granules and noted their occurrence with tubercles in other parts.

In 1832 and 1833, W. W. Gerhard, of Philadelphia, made a very careful study of the disease in the Children's Hospital at Paris, and his publications, more than those of any other author, served to place the disease on a firm anatomical and clinical basis.

There are several special *etiological* factors in connection with this form. It is much more common in children than in adults. It occurs during the first year of life, but is more frequent between the second and the fifth years. In a majority of the cases a focus of old tuberculous disease will be found, commonly in the bronchial or mesenteric glands. In a few instances the affection seems to be primary in the meninges. It is very difficult, however, in an ordinary post mortem to make an exhaustive search, and the lesion may be in the bones, sometimes in the middle ear, or in the genito-urinary organs. In those instances in which no primary focus has been discovered it has been suggested that the bacilli reach the meninges through the cribriform plate of the ethmoid from the upper part of the nostrils, but this is not probable.

Morbid Anatomy.—The meninges at the base are most involved, hence the term basilar meningitis. The parts about the optic chiasm, the Sylvian fissures, and the interpeduncular space are affected. There may be only slight turbidity and matting of the membranes, and a certain stickiness with serous infiltration; but more commonly there is a turbid exudate, fibrino-purulent in character, which covers the structures at the base, surrounds the nerves, extends into the Sylvian fissures, and appears on the lateral, rarely on the upper, surfaces of the hemispheres. The tubercles may be very apparent, particularly in the Sylvian fissures, appearing as small, whitish nodules on the membranes. They vary much in number and size, and may be difficult to find. The amount of exudate bears no definite relation to the abundance of tubercles. The arteries of the anterior and posterior perforated spaces should be carefully withdrawn and searched, as upon them nodular tubercles may be found when not present elsewhere. In doubtful cases the middle cerebral arteries should be very carefully removed, spread on a glass plate with a black background, and examined with a lens. The tubercles are then seen as nodular enlargements on the smaller arteries. The lateral ventricles are dilated (acute hydrocephalus) and contain a turbid fluid; the ependyma may be softened, and the septum lucidum and fornix are usually broken down. The convolutions are often flattened and the sulci obliterated owing to the increased intra-ventricular pressure. The meninges are not alone involved, but the contiguous cerebral substance is more or less œdematous and infiltrated with leucocytes, so that anatomically the condition is in reality a *meningo-encephalitis.*

There are instances in which the acute process is associated with chronic meningeal tuberculosis; cases which may for months present the clinical picture of brain tumor. Although in a majority of instances the process is cerebral, the spinal meninges may also be involved, particularly those of the cervical cord. There are cases, indeed, in which the symptoms are chiefly spinal.

Symptoms.—Tuberculous meningitis presents an extremely complex clinical picture. It will be best to describe the form found in children.

Prodromal symptoms are common. The child may have been in failing health for some weeks, or may be convalescent from measles or whooping cough. In many instances there is a history of a fall. The child gets thin, is restless, peevish, irritable, loses its appetite, and the disposition may completely change. Symptoms pointing to the disease may then set in, either quite suddenly with a convulsion, or more commonly with headache, vomiting, and fever, three essential symptoms of the onset which are rarely absent. The pain may be intense and agonizing. The child puts its hand to its head and occasionally, when the pain becomes worse, gives a short, sudden cry, the so-called hydrocephalic cry. Sometimes the child screams continuously until utterly exhausted. The vomiting is without apparent cause, and is independent of taking of food. Constipation is usually present. The fever is slight, but gradually rises to 102° to 103° F. The pulse is at first rapid, subsequently irregular and slow. The respirations are rarely altered. During sleep the child is restless and disturbed. There may be twitchings of the muscles, or sudden startings; or the child may wake up from sleep in great terror. In this early stage the pupils are usually contracted. These are the chief symptoms of the initial stage, or, as it is termed, the *stage of irritation.*

In the second period of the disease these irritative symptoms subside; vomiting is no longer marked, the abdomen becomes retracted, boat-shaped, or *carinated.* The bowels are obstinately constipated, the child no longer complains of headache, but is dull and apathetic, and when roused is more or less delirious. The head is often retracted and the child utters an occasional cry. The pupils are dilated or irregular, and a squint may develop. Sighing respiration is common. Convulsions may occur, or rigidity of the muscles of one side or of one limb. The temperature is variable, ranging from 100° to 102.5° F. A blotchy erythema is not uncommon on the skin. If the finger-nail is drawn across the skin of any region a red line comes out quickly, the so-called *tache cérébrale,* which, however, has no diagnostic significance.

In the final period, or stage of *paralysis,* the coma increases and the child can not be roused. Convulsions are not infrequent, and there are spasmodic contractions of the muscles of the back and neck. Spasms may occur in the limbs of one side. Optic neuritis and paralysis of the ocular muscles may be present. The pupils become dilated, the eyelids are only partially closed, and the eyeballs are rolled up so that the corneæ are only uncovered in part by the upper eyelids. Diarrhœa may occur, the pulse becomes rapid, and the child may sink into a typhoid state with dry tongue, low delirium, and involuntary passages of urine and fæces. The temperature often becomes subnormal, sinking in rare instances to 93° or 94° F. In some cases there is an ante-mortem elevation of temperature, the fever rising to 106° F. The entire duration of the disease is from a fortnight to three or four weeks. A leucocytosis is not infrequently present throughout the disease.

There are cases of tuberculous meningitis which pursue a more rapid course. They set in with great violence, often in persons apparently in good health, and may prove fatal within a few days. In these instances, more commonly seen in adults, the convex surface of the brain is usually involved. There are again instances which are essentially chronic and display symptoms of a limited meningitis, sometimes with pronounced psychical symptoms, and sometimes with those of cerebral tumor.

There are certain features which call for special comment.

The irregularity and slowness of the pulse in the early and middle stages of the disease are points upon which all authors agree. Toward the close, as the heart's action becomes weaker, the pulsations are more frequent. The temperature is usually elevated, but there are instances in which it does not rise in the whole course of the disease much above 100° F. It may be extremely irregular, and the oscillations are often as much as three or four degrees in the day. Toward the close the temperature may sink to 95° F., occasionally to 94° F., or there may be hyperpyrexia. In a case of Bäumler's the temperature rose before death to 43.7° C. (110.7° F.).

The ocular symptoms of the disease are of special importance. In the early stages narrowing of the pupils is the rule. Toward the close, with increase in the intra-cranial pressure, the pupils dilate and are irregular. There may be conjugate deviation of the eyes. Of ocular nerves the third is most frequently involved, sometimes with paralysis of the face, limbs, and hypoglossal nerve on the opposite side (syndrome of Weber), due to a lesion limited to the inferior and internal part of the crus. The changes in the retinæ are very important. Neuritis is the most common. According to Gowers, the disk at first becomes full colored and has hazy outlines, and the veins are dilated. Swelling and striation become pronounced, but the neuritis is rarely intense. Of 26 cases studied by Garlick, in 6 the condition was of diagnostic value. The tubercles in the choroid are rare and much less frequently seen during life than post mortem figures would indicate. Thus, Litten found them (post mortem) in 39 out of 52 cases. They were present in only 1 of the 26 cases of tuberculous meningitis examined by Garlick. Heinzel examined with negative results 41 cases.

Among the motor symptoms convulsions are most common, but there are other changes which deserve special mention. A tetanic contraction of one limb may persist for several days, or a cataleptic condition. Tremor and athetoid movements are sometimes seen. The paralyses are either hemiplegias or monoplegias. Hemiplegia may result from disturbance in the cortical branches of the middle cerebral artery, occasionally from softening in the internal capsule, due to involvement of the central branches. Of monoplegias, that of the face is perhaps most common, and if on the right side it may occur with aphasia. In two of my cases in adults aphasia occurred. Brachial monoplegia may be associated with it. In the more chronic cases the symptoms persist for months, and there may be a characteristic Jacksonian epilepsy. Kernig's sign may be present, but is not constant. The Babinski reflex is sometimes found.

The DIAGNOSIS of tuberculous meningitis is rarely difficult, and points upon which special stress is to be laid are the existence of a tuberculous focus in the body, the mode of onset and the symptoms, and the evidence obtained on lumbar puncture. The fluid withdrawn is turbid, under increased pressure, and the protein content is increased. By centrifugalization, careful staining, and long search, tubercle bacilli can be found in a large proportion of cases—in 135 of 137 in one series (Hemenway). The cells are usually much increased in number and a large percentage (over 90 per cent.) are small mononuclear lymphocytes, though occasionally an excess of polymorphonuclear leucocytes is found.

The PROGNOSIS in this form of meningitis is always most serious. I have neither seen a case which I regarded as tuberculous recover, nor have I seen post mortem evidence of past disease of this nature. Cases of recovery have been reported by reliable authorities, but they are extremely rare, and there is always a reasonable doubt as to the correctness of the diagnosis. The differential features and treatment are considered in connection with acute meningitis.

III. TUBERCULOSIS OF THE LYMPHATIC SYSTEM

1. *Tuberculosis of the Lymph-glands* (*Scrofula*)

Scrofula is tubercle, as it has been shown that the bacillus of Koch is the essential element. Formerly special attention was given to different types of scrofula, of which two important forms were recognized—the sanguine, in which the child was slightly built, tall, with small limbs, a fine clear skin, soft silky hair, and was mentally very bright and intelligent; and the phlegmatic type, in which the child was short and thick-set, with coarse features, muddy complexion, and a dull, heavy aspect. It is not yet definitely settled whether the virus which produces the chronic tuberculous adenitis or scrofula differs from that which produces tuberculosis in other parts, or whether it is the local conditions in the glands which account for the slow development and milder course. The observations of Lingard are important as showing a variation in the virulence of the tubercle bacillus. Guinea-pigs inoculated with ordinary tubercle showed lymphatic infection within the first week, and the animals died within three months; infected with material from scrofulous glands, the lymphatic enlargement did not appear until the second or third week, and the animals survived for six or seven months. He showed, moreover, that the virulence of the infection obtained from the scrofulous glands increased in intensity by passing through a series of guinea-pigs. In a certain number of cases the infection is with the bovine germ, but exactly in what proportion, and with what special clinical features has not yet been determined.

Tuberculous adenitis, met with at all ages, is more common in children than in adults, and may occur in old age.

Tubercle bacilli are ubiquitous; all are exposed to infection, and upon the local conditions, whether favorable or unfavorable, depends the fate of those organisms which find lodgment in our bodies. A special predisposing factor in lymphatic tuberculosis is catarrh of the mucous membranes, which in itself excites slight adenitis of the neighboring glands. In a child with constantly recurring naso-pharyngeal catarrh, the bacilli which lodge on the mucous membranes find in all probability the gateways less strictly guarded and are taken up by the lymphatics and passed to the nearest glands. The importance of the tonsils as an infection-atrium has of late been urged. In conditions of health the local resistance, or, as some would put it, the phagocytes, would be active enough to deal with the invaders, but the irritation of a chronic catarrh weakens the resistance of the lymph-tissue, and the bacilli are enabled to grow and gradually to change a simple into a tuberculous adenitis. The frequent association of tuberculous adenitis of the bronchial glands with whooping cough and with measles, and the association of tubercle in the mesenteric glands in children with intestinal catarrh, find in this way a rational explanation.

The following are some of the features of interest in tuberculous adenitis:

(*a*) The local character of the disease. Thus, the glands of the neck, or at the bifurcation of the bronchi, or those of the mesentery, may be alone involved.

(*b*) The tendency to spontaneous healing. In a large proportion of the cases the battle which ensues between the bacilli and the protective forces is long; but the latter are finally successful, and we find in the calcified remnants in the bronchial and mesenteric lymph-glands evidences of victory. Too often in the bronchial glands a truce only is declared and hostilities may break out afresh in the form of an acute tuberculosis.

(*c*) The tendency of tuberculous adenitis to pass on to suppuration. The frequency with which, particularly in the glands of the neck, we find the tuberculous processes associated with suppuration is a special feature of this form of adenitis. In nearly all instances the pus is sterile. Whether the suppuration is excited by the bacilli or by their products, or whether it is the result of a mixed infection with pus organisms, which are subsequently destroyed, has not been settled.

(*d*) The existence of an unhealed tuberculous adenitis is a constant menace to the organism. It is safe to say that in three-fourths of the instances of acute tuberculosis the infection is derived from this source. On the other hand, it has been urged that "scrofula" in childhood gives immunity in adult life. We certainly do meet with many persons of exceptional bodily vigor who in childhood had enlarged glands, but the evidence which Marfan brings forward in support of this view is not conclusive.

Generalized Tuberculous Lymphadenitis.—In exceptional instances we find diffuse tuberculosis of nearly all the lymph-glands of the body with little or no involvement of other parts. The most extreme cases of it, which I have seen, have been in negro patients. Two well-marked cases occurred at the Philadelphia Hospital. In a woman, the chart from April, 1888, until March, 1889, showed persistent fever, ranging from 101° to 103° F., occasionally rising to 104° F. On December 16th the glands on the right side of the neck were removed. After an attack of erysipelas, on February 17th, she gradually sank and died March 5th. The lungs presented only one or two puckered spots at the apices. The bronchial, retro-peritoneal, and mesenteric glands were greatly enlarged and caseous. There was no intestinal, uterine, or bone disease. The continuous high fever in this case depended apparently upon the tuberculous adenitis, which was much more extensive than was supposed during life. In these instances the enlargement is most marked in the retro-peritoneal, bronchial, and mesenteric glands, but may be also present in the groups of external glands. Occurring acutely, it presents a picture resembling Hodgkin's disease. In a case which died in the Montreal General Hospital this diagnosis was made. The cervical and axillary glands were enormously enlarged, and death was caused by infiltration of the larynx. In infants and children there is a form of general tuberculous adenitis in which the various groups of glands are successively, more rarely simultaneously, involved, and in which death is caused either by cachexia or by an acute infection of the meninges.

Local Tuberculous Adenitis.—(*a*) CERVICAL.—This is the most common form met with in children. It is seen particularly among the poor and those who live continuously in the impure atmosphere of badly ventilated lodgings. Children in foundling hospitals and asylums are specially prone to the disease. In the United States it is most common in the negro race. As already stated, it is often met with in catarrh of the nose and throat, or chronic enlargement of the tonsils; or the child may have had eczema of the scalp or a purulent otitis.

The submaxillary glands are first involved, and are popularly spoken of as enlarged *kernels.* They are usually larger on one side than on the other. As they increase in size, the individual tumors can be felt; the surface is smooth and the consistence firm. They may remain isolated, but more commonly they form large, knotted masses, over which the skin is, as a rule, freely movable. In many cases the skin ultimately becomes adherent, and inflammation and suppuration occur. An abscess points and, unless opened, bursts, leaving a sinus which heals slowly. The disease is frequently associated with coryza, with eczema of the scalp, ear, or lips, and with conjunctivitis or keratitis. When the glands are large and growing actively there is fever. The subjects are usually anæmic, particularly if suppuration has occurred. The progress of this form of adenitis is slow and tedious. Death, however, rarely follows, and many aggravated cases in children get well. Not only the submaxillary group, but the glands above the clavicle and in the posterior cervical triangle, may be involved. In other instances the cervical and axillary glands are involved together, forming a continuous chain which extends beneath the clavicle and the pectoral muscle. With them the bronchial glands may also be enlarged and caseous. Not infrequently the enlargement of the supra-clavicular and axillary group of glands on one side precedes a tuberculous pleurisy or pulmonary tuberculosis.

(*b*) TRACHEO-BRONCHIAL.—The mediastinal lymph-glands constitute filters in which lodge the various foreign particles which escape the normal phagocytes of bronchi and lungs. Among these foreign particles, and probably attached to them, tubercle bacilli are not uncommon, and we find tubercles and caseous matter with great frequency in this group. Northrup found them involved in every one of 127 cases of tuberculosis at the New York Foundling Hospital. This tuberculous adenitis may, in the bronchial glands, attain the dimensions of a tumor of large size. In children the bronchial adenitis is apt to be associated with suppuration. The glands at the bifurcation of the trachea are first involved and chiefly on the right side—in 74 per cent. of Wollstein's cases. Irregular fever, failure of nutrition, loss of appetite, and lassitude may be caused by the absorption of toxins; pain is rare, though it is complained of sometimes in the mammary region. The cough is paroxysmal, often brassy, so that it has been mistaken for whooping cough. Stridor, when present, is more often expiratory. The physical signs are not very definite. Dilated veins over the anterior aspect of the thorax, absence of descent of the larynx during inspiration, and pain on pressure over the upper dorsal vertebræ are mentioned. Extension of the normal dulness over the upper four thoracic vertebræ to the fifth and sixth is of importance, and there may be para-vertebral dulness on delicate percussion. Some writers lay stress upon the bronchophony over the upper thoracic vertebræ, and a venous hum may be heard sometimes over the manubrium. The X-ray pictures are regarded by experts as distinctive, showing the shadow extending from either side of the spine.

Some of the more uncommon effects are the following: Compression of the superior cava, of the pulmonary artery, and of the azygos vein. The trachea and bronchi, though often flattened, are rarely seriously compressed. The pneumogastric nerve may be involved, particularly the recurrent laryngeal branch. More important really are the perforations of the enlarged and softened glands into the bronchi or trachea, or a sort of secondary cyst may be formed between the lung and the trachea. Asphyxia has been caused by blocking of the larynx by a caseous gland which has ulcerated through the bronchus (Voelcker), and Cyril Ogle has reported a case in which the ulcerated gland practically occluded both bronchi. Perforations of the vessels are much less common, but the pulmonary artery and the aorta have been opened. Perforation of the œsophagus has been described in several cases. One of the most serious effects is infection of the lung or pleura by the caseous glands situated deep along the bronchi. This may, as is often clearly seen, be by direct contact, and it may be difficult to determine in some sections where the caseous bronchial gland terminates and the pulmonary tissue begins. In other instances it takes place along the root of the lung and is subpleural. Among other sequences may be mentioned diverticulum of the œsophagus following adhesion of an enlarged gland and its subsequent retraction; and, in the case of the anterior mediastinal and aortic groups, the frequent production of pericarditis, either by contact or by rupture of a softened gland into the sac.

A serious danger is systemic infection, which takes place through the vessels.

(*c*) Mesenteric; Tabes mesenterica.—In this affection, the abdominal scrofula of old writers, the glands of the mesentery and retro-peritoneum become enlarged and caseate; more rarely they suppurate or calcify. A slight tuberculous adenitis is extremely common in children, and is often accidentally found (post mortem) when they have died of other diseases. It may be a primary lesion associated with intestinal catarrh, or it may be secondary to tuberculous disease of the intestines.

The statistics of abdominal tuberculosis show a great variation in different localities. The small percentage in New York, less than one per cent. of all cases (Bovaird and Mt. Sinai Hospital figures), contrasts with the high figures given for Scotland by John Thomson, 3.57 for Edinburgh and 4.51 for Glasgow. The general involvement of the glands interferes seriously with nutrition, and the patients are puny, wasted, and anæmic. The abdomen is enlarged and tympanitic; diarrhœa is a constant feature; the stools are thin and offensive. There is moderate fever, but the general wasting and debility are the most characteristic features. The enlarged glands can not often be felt, owing to the distended condition of the bowels. These cases are often spoken of as consumption of the bowels, but in a majority of them the intestines do not present tuberculous lesions. In a considerable number of the cases of tabes mesenterica the peritoneum is also involved, and in such the abdomen is large and hard, and nodules may be felt.

In adults tuberculous disease of the mesenteric glands may occur as a primary affection, or in association with pulmonary disease. Large tumors may exist without tuberculous disease in the intestines or in any other part.

2. *Tuberculosis of the Serous Membranes*

General Serous Membrane Tuberculosis (*Polyorrhomenitis*).—The serous membranes may be chiefly involved, simultaneously or consecutively, presenting a distinctive and readily recognizable clinical type of tuberculosis. There are three groups of cases. First, those in which an acute tuberculosis of the peritoneum and pleuræ occurs rapidly, caused by local disease of the tubes in women, or of the mediastinal or bronchial lymph-glands. Secondly, cases in which the disease is more chronic, with exudation into both peritoneum and pleuræ, the formation of cheesy masses, and the occurrence of ulcerative and suppurative processes. Thirdly, there are cases in which the pleuro-peritoneal affection is still more chronic, the tubercles hard and fibroid, the membranes much thickened, and with little or no exudate. In any one of these three forms the pericardium may be involved with the pleuræ and peritoneum. It is important to bear in mind that there may be no visceral tuberculosis in these cases.

Tuberculosis of the Pleura.—(*a*) Acute Tuberculous Pleurisy.—It is difficult in the present state of our knowledge to estimate the proportion of instances of acute pleurisy due to tuberculosis (see Acute Pleurisy). The cases are rarely fatal. Here, too, there are three groups of cases: (1) Acute tuberculous pleurisy with subsequent chronic course. (2) Secondary and terminal forms of acute pleurisy (these are not uncommon in hospital practice). And (3) a form of acute tuberculous suppurative pleurisy. A considerable number of the purulent pleurisies, designated as latent and chronic, are caused by tubercle bacilli, but the fact is not so widely recognized that there is an acute, ulcerative, and suppurative disease which may run a very rapid course. The pleurisy sets in abruptly, with pain in the side, fever, cough, and sometimes with a chill. There may be nothing to suggest a tuberculous process, and the subject may have a fine physique and come of healthy stock.

(*b*) The subacute and chronic tuberculous pleurisies are more common. The largest group of cases comprises those with sero-fibrinous effusion. The onset is insidious, the true character of the disease is frequently overlooked, and in almost every instance there are tuberculous foci in the lungs and in the bronchial glands. These are cases in which the termination is often in pulmonary tuberculosis or general miliary tuberculosis. In a few cases the exudate becomes purulent.

And, lastly, there is a *chronic adhesive pleurisy*, a primary proliferative form which is of long standing, may lead to very great thickening of the membrane, and sometimes to invasion of the lung.

Secondary tuberculous pleurisy is very common. The visceral layer is always involved in pulmonary tuberculosis. Adhesions usually form and a chronic pleurisy results, which may be simple, but usually tubercles are scattered through the adhesions. An acute tuberculous pleurisy may result from direct extension. The fluid may be sero-fibrinous or hæmorrhagic, or may become purulent. And, lastly, a very common event in pulmonary tuberculosis is the perforation of a superficial spot of softening, and the production of *pyo-pneumothorax.*

The general symptomatology of these forms will be considered under disease of the pleura.

Tuberculosis of the Pericardium.—Miliary tubercles may occur as a part of a general infection, but the term is properly limited to those cases in which, either as a primary or secondary process, there is extensive disease of the membrane. Tuberculosis is not so common in the pericardium as in the pleura and peritoneum, but it is certainly more common than the literature would lead us to suppose. George Norris found 82 instances among 1,780 post mortems in tuberculous subjects.

We may recognize four groups of cases: First, those in which the condition is entirely latent, and the disease is discovered accidentally in individuals who have died of other affections or of chronic pulmonary tuberculosis.

A second group, in which the symptoms are those of cardiac insufficiency following the dilatation and hypertrophy consequent upon a chronic adhesive pericarditis. The symptoms are those of cardiac dropsy, and suggest either idiopathic hypertrophy and dilatation, or, if there is a loud blowing systolic murmur at the apex, mitral valve disease, either insufficiency or stenosis. The condition of adherent pericardium is usually overlooked.

In a third group the clinical picture is that of an acute tuberculosis, either general or with cerebro-spinal manifestations, which has had its origin from the tuberculous pericardium or tuberculous mediastinal lymph-glands.

A fourth group, with symptoms of acute pericarditis, includes cases in which the affection is acute and accompanied with more or less exudation of a sero-fibrinous, hæmorrhagic, or purulent character. There may be no suspicion whatever of the tuberculous nature of the trouble.

Tuberculosis of the Peritoneum.—In connection with miliary and chronic pulmonary tuberculosis it is not uncommon to find the peritoneum studded with small gray granulations. They are constantly present on the serous surface of tuberculous ulcers of the intestines. Apart from these conditions the membrane is often the seat of extensive tuberculous disease, which occurs in the following forms:

(*a*) *Acute miliary tuberculosis* with sero-fibrinous or bloody exudation.

(*b*) *Chronic tuberculosis,* characterized by larger growths, which tend to caseate and ulcerate. The exudate is purulent or sero-purulent, and is often sacculated.

(*c*) *Chronic fibroid tuberculosis,* which may be subacute from the onset, or which may represent the final stage of an acute miliary eruption. The tubercles are hard and pigmented. There is little or no exudation, and the serous surfaces are matted together by adhesions.

The process may be primary and local, which was the case in 5 of 17 post mortems. In children the infection appears to pass from the intestines, and in adults this is the source in the cases associated with chronic phthisis. In women the disease extends commonly from the Fallopian tubes. In at least 30 or 40 per cent. of the instances of laparotomy in this affection reported by gynæcologists the infection was from them. The prostate or the seminal vesicles may be the starting-point. In many cases the peritoneum is involved with the pleura and pericardium, particularly with the former membrane.

It is interesting to note that certain morbid conditions of the abdominal organs predispose to the development of the disease; thus patients with cirrhosis of the liver very often die of an acute tuberculous peritonitis. The frequency with which the condition is met with in operations upon ovarian tumors has been commented upon by gynæcologists. Many cases have followed trauma of the abdomen. A very interesting feature is the occurrence of tuberculosis in hernial sacs. The condition is not very uncommon. In a majority of the instances it has been discovered accidentally during the operation for radical cure or for strangulation. In 7 instances the sac alone was involved.

It is generally stated that males are attacked oftener than females, but in the collected statistics I find the cases to be twice as numerous in females as in males; in the ratio, indeed, of 131 to 60.

Tuberculous peritonitis occurs at all ages. It is common in children associated with intestinal and mesenteric disease. The incidence is most frequent between the ages of twenty and forty. It may occur in advanced life. In one of my cases the patient was eighty-two years of age. Of 357 cases collected by me from the literature, there were under ten years, 27; between ten and twenty, 75; from twenty to thirty, 87; between thirty and forty, 71; from forty to fifty, 61; from fifty to sixty, 19; from sixty to seventy, 4; above seventy, 2. In America it is more common in the negro than in the white race. More blacks than whites, 77 to 70, were admitted to the Johns Hopkins Hospital (Hamman).

SYMPTOMS.—In certain special features the tuberculous varies considerably from other forms of peritonitis. It presents a symptom-complex of extraordinary diversity.

In the first place, the process may be *latent* and met with accidentally in the operation for hernia or for ovarian tumor. The *acute onset* is not uncommon. Four cases in our records were diagnosed appendicitis, two acute cholecystitis, and six had symptoms of intestinal obstruction, in two of these coming on with great abruptness (Hamman). The cases have been mistaken for strangulated hernia. Other cases set in acutely with fever, abdominal tenderness, and the symptoms of ordinary acute peritonitis. Cases with a slow onset, abdominal tenderness, tympanites, and low continuous fever are often mistaken for *typhoid fever*.

Ascites is frequent, but the effusion is rarely large. It is sometimes hæmorrhagic. In this form the diagnosis may rest between an acute miliary cancer, cirrhosis of the liver, and a chronic simple peritonitis—conditions which usually offer no special difficulties in differentiation. A most important point is the simultaneous presence of a pleurisy. The tuberculin test may be used. *Tympanites* may be present in the very acute cases, when it is due to loss of tone in the intestines owing to inflammatory infiltration; or it may occur in the old, long-standing cases when universal adhesion has taken place between the parietal and visceral layers. *Fever* is a marked symptom in the acute cases, and the temperature may reach 103° or 104°. In many instances the fever is slight. In the more chronic cases subnormal temperatures are common, and for days the temperature may not rise above 97°, and the morning record may be as low as 95.5°. An occasional symptom is pigmentation of the skin, which in some cases has led to the diagnosis of Addison's disease. A striking peculiarity of tuberculous peritonitis is the frequency with which the condition either simulates or is associated with *tumor*. This may be:

(*a*) *Omental,* due to puckering and rolling of this membrane until it forms an elongated firm mass, attached to the transverse colon and lying athwart the upper part of the abdomen. This cord-like structure is found also with cancerous peritonitis, but is much more common in tuberculosis. Gairdner has called special attention to this form of tumor, and in children has seen it undergo gradual resolution. A resonant percussion note may sometimes be elicited above the mass. Though usually situated near the umbilicus, the omental mass may form a prominent tumor in the right iliac region.

(*b*) *Sacculated exudation,* in which the effusion is limited and confined by adhesions between the coils, the parietal peritoneum, the mesentery, and the abdominal or pelvic organs. This encysted exudate is most common in the middle zone, and has frequently been mistaken for ovarian tumor. It may occupy the entire anterior portion of the peritoneum, or there may be a more limited saccular exudate on one side or the other. Within the pelvis it is associated with disease of the Fallopian tubes. Eighteen cases in the gynæcological wards (J. H. H.) were operated upon for pyosalpinx (Hamman).

(*c*) In rare cases the tumor formations may be due to great retraction or thickening of the *intestinal coils.* The small intestine is found shortened, the walls enormously thickened, and the entire coil may form a firm knot close against the spine, giving on examination the idea of a solid mass. Not the small intestine only, but the entire bowel from the duodenum to the rectum, has been found forming such a hard nodular tumor.

(*d*) *Mesenteric glands,* which occasionally form very large, tumor-like masses, more commonly found in children than in adults. This condition may be confined to the abdominal glands. Ascites may coexist. The condition must be distinguished from that in children, in which, with ascites or tympanites—sometimes both—there can be felt irregular nodular masses, due to large caseous formations between the intestinal coils. No doubt in a considerable number of cases of the so-called tabes mesenterica, particularly in those with enlargement and hardness of the abdomen—the condition which the French call *carreau*—there is involvement also of the peritoneum.

The *diagnosis* of these peritoneal tumors is sometimes very difficult. The omental mass is a less frequent source of error than any other; but, as already mentioned, a similar condition may occur in cancer. The most important problem is the diagnosis of the saccular exudation from ovarian tumor. In fully one-third of the recorded cases of laparotomy in tuberculous peritonitis the diagnosis of cystic ovarian disease had been made. The most suggestive points for consideration are the history of the patient and the evidence of old tuberculous lesions. The physical condition is not of much help, as in many instances the patients have been robust and well nourished. Irregular febrile attacks, gastro-intestinal disturbance, and pains are more common in tuberculous disease. Unless inflamed there is usually not much fever with ovarian cysts. The local signs are very deceptive, and in certain cases have conformed in every particular to those of cystic disease. The outlines in saccular exudation are rarely so well defined. The position and form may be variable, owing to alterations in the size of the coils of which in parts the walls are composed. Nodular cheesy masses may sometimes be felt at the periphery. Depression of the vaginal wall is mentioned as occurring in encysted peritonitis; but it is also found in ovarian tumor. Lastly, the condition of the Fallopian tubes, of the lungs and the pleuræ, should be thoroughly examined. The association of salpingitis with an ill-defined anomalous mass in the abdomen should arouse suspicion, as should also involvement of the pleura, the apex of one lung, or a testis in the male.

IV. PULMONARY TUBERCULOSIS

(*Phthisis, Consumption*)

Three clinical groups may be conveniently recognized: (1) *tuberculo-pneumonic phthisis*—acute phthisis; (2) *chronic ulcerative phthisis;* and (3) *fibroid phthisis.*

According to the mode of infection there are two distinct types of lesions:

(*a*) When the bacilli reach the lungs through the blood-vessels or lymphatics the primary lesion is usually in the tissues of the alveolar walls, in the capillary vessels, the epithelium of the air-cells, and in the connective-tissue framework of the septa. The irritation of the bacilli produces, within a few days, the small, gray miliary nodules, involving several alveoli and consisting largely of round, cuboidal, uninuclear epithelioid cells. Depending upon the number of bacilli which reach the lung in this way, either a localized or a general tuberculosis is excited. The tubercles may be uniformly scattered through both lungs and form a part of a general miliary tuberculosis, or they may be confined to the lungs, or even in great part to one lung. The changes which the tubercles undergo have already been referred to. The further stages may be: (1) Arrest of the process of cell division, gradual sclerosis of the tubercle, and ultimately complete fibroid transformation. (2) Caseation of the centre of the tubercle, extension at the periphery by proliferation of the epithelioid and lymphoid cells, so that the individual tubercles or small groups become confluent and form diffuse areas which undergo caseation and softening. (3) Occasionally as a result of intense infection of a localized region through the blood-vessels the tubercles are thickly set. The intervening tissue becomes acutely inflamed, the air-cells are filled with the products of a desquamative pneumonia, and many lobules are involved.

(*b*) When the bacilli reach the lung through the bronchi—inhalation or aspiration tuberculosis—the picture differs. The smaller bronchi and bronchioles are more extensively affected; the process is not confined to single groups of alveoli, but has a more lobular arrangement, and the tuberculous masses from the outset are larger, more diffuse, and may in some cases involve an entire lobe or the greater part of a lung. It is in this mode of infection that we see the characteristic peri-bronchial granulations and the areas of the so-called nodular broncho-pneumonia. These broncho-pneumonic areas, with on the one hand caseation, ulceration, and cavity formation, and on the other sclerosis and limitation, make up the essential elements in the anatomical picture of tuberculous phthisis.

1. *Acute Pneumonic Tuberculosis of the Lungs*

This form, known also by the name of *galloping consumption,* is met with both in children and adults. In the former many of the cases are mistaken for simple broncho-pneumonia.

Two types may be recognized, the *pneumonic* and *broncho-pneumonic.*

The Pneumonic Form.—In the *pneumonic form* one lobe may be involved, or in some instances an entire lung. The organ is heavy, the affected portion airless; the pleura is usually covered with a thin exudate, and on section the picture resembles closely that of ordinary hepatization. The following is an extract from the post mortem report of a case in which death occurred twenty-nine days after the onset of the illness, having all the characters of an acute pneumonia: "Left lung weighs 1,500 grams (double the weight of the other organ) and is heavy and airless, crepitant only at the anterior margins. Section shows a small cavity the size of a walnut at the apex, about which are scattered tubercles in a consolidated tissue. The greater part of the lung presents a grayish-white appearance due to the aggregation of tubercles which in some places have a continuous, uniform appearance, in others are surrounded by an injected and consolidated lung-tissue. Toward the margins of the lower lobe strands of this firm reddish tissue separate anæmic, dry areas. There are in the right lung three or four small groups of tubercles but no caseous masses. The bronchial glands are not tuberculous." Here the intense local infection was due to the small focus at the apex of the lung, probably an aspiration process.

Only the most careful inspection may reveal the presence of miliary tubercles, or the attention may be arrested by the detection of tubercles in the other lung or in the bronchial glands. The process may involve only one lobe. There may be older areas which are of a peculiarly yellowish-white color and distinctly caseous. The most remarkable picture is presented by cases of this kind in which the disease lasts for some months. A lobe or an entire lung may be enlarged, firm, airless throughout, and converted into a dry, yellowish-white, cheesy substance. Cases are met with in which the entire lung from apex to base is in this condition, with perhaps only a small, narrow area of air-containing tissue on the margin. More commonly, if the disease has lasted for two or three months, rapid softening has taken place at the apex with extensive cavity formation.

Males are much more frequently attacked than females. Of my series of 15 cases, 11 were males. The onset was acute in 13, with a chill in 9. Bacilli were found in the sputum in one case as early as the fourth day. Fraenkel and Troje believe that the cases are of bronchogenous origin, due to infection from a small focus somewhere in the lung. They found tubercle bacilli alone in 11 of their 12 cases. Tendeloo, who reports a fatal case on the sixth day, regards the infection as sometimes hæmatogenous.

SYMPTOMS.—The attack sets in abruptly with a chill, usually in an individual who has enjoyed good health, although in many cases the onset has been preceded by exposure to cold, or there have been debilitating circumstances. The temperature rises rapidly after the chill, there are pain in the side and cough, with at first mucoid, subsequently rusty-colored expectoration which may contain tubercle bacilli. The dyspnœa may become extreme and the patient may have suffocative attacks. The physical examination shows involvement of one lobe or of one lung, with signs of consolidation, dulness, increased fremitus, at first feeble or suppressed vesicular murmur, and subsequently well-marked bronchial breathing. The upper or lower lobe may be involved, or in some cases the entire lung.

At this time, as a rule, no suspicion enters the mind of the practitioner that the case is anything but one of frank lobar pneumonia. Occasionally there may be suspicious circumstances in the history of the patient or in his family; but, as a rule, no stress is laid upon them in view of the intense and characteristic mode of onset. Between the eighth and tenth day, instead of the expected crisis, the condition becomes aggravated, the temperature is irregular, and the pulse more rapid. There may be sweating, and the expectoration bcomes muco-purulent and greenish in color—a point of special importance, to which Traube called attention. Even in the second or third week, with the persistence of these symptoms, the physician tries to console himself with the idea that the case is one of unresolved pneumonia, and that all will yet be well. Gradually, however, the severity of the symptoms, the presence of physical signs indicating softening, the existence of elastic tissue and tubercle bacilli in the sputum present the mournful proofs that the case is one of acute pneumonic phthisis. Death may occur on the sixth day, as in a case of Tendeloo's. The earliest death in my series was on the thirteenth day. A majority of the cases drag on, and death does not occur until the third month. In a few cases, even after a stormy onset and active course, the symptoms subside and the patient passes into the chronic stage.

DIAGNOSIS.—Waters, of Liverpool, who gave an admirable description of these cases, called attention to the difficulty in distinguishing them from ordinary pneumonia. Certainly the mode of onset affords no criterion whatever. A healthy, robust-looking young Irishman, a cab-driver, who had been kept waiting on a cold, blustering night until three in the morning, was seized the next afternoon with a violent chill, and the following day was admitted to my wards at the University Hospital, Philadelphia. He was made the subject of a clinical lecture on the fifth day, when there was absent no single feature in history, symptoms, or physical signs of acute lobar pneumonia of the right upper lobe. It was not until ten days later, when bacilli were found in his expectoration, that we were made aware of the true nature of the case. I know of no criterion by which cases of this kind can be distinguished in the early stage. A point to which Traube called attention, and which is also referred to as important by Hérard and Cornil, is the absence of breath-sounds in the consolidated region; but this, I am sure, does not hold good in all cases. The tubular breathing may be intense and marked as early as the fourth day; and again, how common it is to have, as one of the earliest and most suggestive symptoms of lobar pneumonia, suppression or enfeeblement of the vesicular murmur! In many cases, however, there are suspicious circumstances in the onset: the patient has been in bad health, or may have had previous pulmonary trouble, or there are recurring chills. Careful examination of the sputum and a study of the physical signs from day to day can alone determine the true nature of the case. In one of my cases the bacilli were found on the fourth day. A point of some moment is the character of the fever, which in true pneumonia is more continuous, particularly in severe cases, whereas in this form of tuberculosis remissions of 1.5° or 2° are not infrequent.

Acute Tuberculous Broncho-pneumonia.—Acute tuberculous broncho-pneumonia is more common, particularly in children, and forms a majority of the cases of *phthisis florida*, or "galloping consumption." It is an acute caseous broncho-pneumonia, starting in the smaller tubes, which become blocked with a cheesy substance, while the air-cells of the lobule are filled with the products of a catarrhal pneumonia. In the early stages the areas have a grayish red, later an opaque white, caseous appearance. By the fusion of contiguous masses an entire lobe may be rendered nearly solid, but areas of crepitant air tissue can usually be seen between the groups. This is not an uncommon picture in the acute phthisis of adults, but it is still more frequent in children. The following is an extract from the post mortem report of a case on a child aged four months, who died in the sixth week of illness: "On section, the right upper lobe is occupied with caseous masses from 5 to 12 mm. in diameter, separated from each other by an intervening tissue of a deep red color. The bronchi are filled with cheesy substance. The middle and lower lobes are studded with tubercles, many of which are becoming caseous. Toward the diaphragmatic surface of the lower lobe there is a small cavity the size of a marble. The left lung is more crepitant and uniformly studded with tubercles of all sizes, some as large as peas. The bronchial glands are very large, and one contains a tuberculous abscess."

There is a form of tuberculous aspiration pneumonia, to which Bäumler has called attention, occurring as a sequence of hæmoptysis, and due to the aspiration of blood and the contents of pulmonary cavities into the finer tubes. There are fever, dyspnœa, and signs of a diffuse broncho-pneumonia. Some of these cases run a very rapid course, and are examples of galloping consumption following hæmoptysis. This accident may occur not only early in the disease, but may follow hæmorrhage in a well-marked pulmonary tuberculosis.

In children the enlarged bronchial glands usually surround the root of the lung, and even pass deeply into the substance, and the lobules are often involved by direct contact.

In other cases the caseous broncho-pneumonia involves groups of alveoli or lobules in different portions of the lungs, more commonly at both apices, forming areas from 1 to 3 cm. in diameter. The size of the mass depends largely upon that of the bronchus involved. There are cases which probably should come in this category, in which, with a history of an acute illness of from four to eight weeks, the lungs are extensively studded with large gray tubercles, ranging in size from 5 to 10 mm. In some instances there are cheesy masses the size of a cherry. All of these are grayish-white in color, distinctly cheesy, and between the adjacent ones, particularly in the lower lobe, there may be recent pneumonia, or the condition of lung which has been termed splenization. In a case of this kind at the Philadelphia Hospital death took place about the eighth week from the abrupt onset of the illness with hæmorrhage. There were no extensive areas of consolidation, but the cheesy nodules were uniformly scattered throughout both lungs. No softening had taken place.

Secondary infections are not uncommon; but Prudden was able to show that the tubercle bacillus could produce not only distinct tubercle nodules, but also the various kinds of exudative pneumonia, the exudates varying in appearance in different cases, which phenomena occurred absolutely without the intervention of other organisms. The fact that these latter had not subsequently crept in was shown by cultures at the autopsy on the affected animal.

SYMPTOMS.—The symptoms of acute broncho-pneumonic phthisis are very variable. In adults the disease may attack persons in good health, but overworked or "run down" from any cause. Hæmorrhage initiates the attack in a few cases. There may be repeated chills; the temperature is high, the pulse rapid, and the respirations are increased. The loss of flesh and strength is very striking.

The physical signs may at first be uncertain and indefinite, but finally there are areas of impaired resonance, usually at the apices; the breath sounds are harsh and tubular, with numerous râles. The sputum may early show elastic tissue and tubercle bacilli. In the acute cases, within three weeks, the patient may be in a marked typhoid state, with delirium, dry tongue, and high fever. Death may occur within three weeks. In other cases the onset is severe, with high fever, rapid loss of flesh and strength, and signs of extensive unilateral or bilateral disease. Softening takes place; there are sweats, chills, and progressive emaciation, and all the features of *phthisis florida*. Six or eight weeks later the patient may begin to improve, the fever lessens, the general symptoms abate, and a case which looked as if it would certainly terminate fatally within a few weeks drags on and becomes chronic.

In *children* the disease most commonly follows the infectious diseases, particularly measles and whooping cough. At least *three groups* of these tuberculous broncho-pneumonias may be recognized. In the *first* the child is taken ill suddenly while teething or during convalescence from fever; the temperature rises rapidly, the cough is severe, and there may be signs of consolidation at one or both apices with râles. Death may occur within a few days, and the lung shows areas of broncho-pneumonia, with perhaps here and there scattered opaque grayish-yellow nodules. Macroscopically the affection does not look tuberculous, but histologically miliary granulations and bacilli may be found. Tubercles are usually present in the bronchial glands, but the appearance of the broncho-pneumonia may be exceedingly deceptive, and it may require careful microscopic examination to determine its tuberculous character. The *second group* is represented by the case of the child previously quoted, who died at the sixth week with the ordinary symptoms of severe broncho-pneumonia. And the *third group* is that in which, during the convalescence from an infectious disease, the child is taken ill with fever, cough, and shortness of breath. The severity of the symptoms abates within the first fortnight; but there is loss of flesh, the general condition is bad, and the physical examination shows the presence of scattered râles throughout the lungs, and here and there areas of defective resonance. The child has sweats, the fever becomes hectic in character, and in many cases the clinical picture gradually passes into that of chronic phthisis.

2. *Chronic Ulcerative Tuberculosis of the Lungs.*

Under this heading may be grouped the great majority of cases of pulmonary tuberculosis, in which the lesions proceed to ulceration and softening, and ultimately produce the well-known picture of chronic phthisis.

Morbid Anatomy.—Inspection of the lungs shows a remarkable variety of lesions, comprising nodular tubercles, diffuse tuberculous infiltration, caseous masses, pneumonic areas, cavities of various sizes, with changes in the pleura, bronchi, and bronchial glands.

THE DISTRIBUTION OF THE LESIONS.—For years it has been recognized that the most advanced lesions are at the apices, and that the disease progresses downward, usually more rapidly in one of the lungs. This general statement, which has passed current in the text-books ever since the masterly description of Laennec, has been carefully elaborated by Kingston Fowler, who finds that the disease in its onward progress through the lungs follows, in a majority of the cases, distinct routes. In the upper lobe the primary lesion is not, as a rule, at the extreme apex, but from an inch to an inch and a half below the summit of the lung, and nearer to the posterior and external borders. The lesion here tends to spread downward, probably from inhalation of the virus, and this accounts for the frequent circumstance that examination behind, in the supra-spinous fossa, will give indications of disease before any evidences exist at the apex in front. Anteriorly this initial focus corresponds to a spot just below the centre of the clavicle, and the direction of extension in front is along the anterior aspect of the upper lobe, along a line running about an inch and a half from the inner ends of the first, second, and third interspaces. A second less common site of the primary lesion in the apex "corresponds on the chest wall with the first and second interspaces below the outer third of the clavicle." The extension is downward, so that the outer part of the upper lobe is chiefly involved.

In the middle lobe of the right lung the affection usually follows disease of the upper lobe on the same side. In the involvement of the lower lobe the first secondary infiltration is about an inch to an inch and a half below the posterior extremity of its apex, and corresponds on the chest wall to a spot opposite the fifth dorsal spine. This involvement is of the greatest importance clinically, as "in the great majority of cases, when the physical signs of the disease at the apex are sufficiently definite to allow of the diagnosis of phthisis being made, the lower lobe is already affected." Examination, therefore, should be made carefully of this posterior apex in all suspicious cases. In this situation the lesion spreads downward and laterally along the line of the interlobular septa, a line which is marked by the vertebral border of the scapula, when the hand is placed on the opposite scapula and the elbow raised above the level of the shoulder. Once present in an apex, the disease usually extends in time to the opposite upper lobe; but not, as a rule, until the apex of the lower lobe of the lung first affected has been attacked.

Of 427 cases above mentioned, the right apex was involved in 172, the left in 130, both in 111.

Lesions of the base may be primary, though this is rare. Percy Kidd makes the proportion of basic to apical phthisis 1 to 500, a smaller number than existed in my series. In very chronic cases there may be arrested lesions at the apex and more recent lesions at the base.

SUMMARY OF THE LESIONS IN CHRONIC ULCERATIVE PHTHISIS.—(*a*) *Miliary Tubercles.*—They have one of two distributions: (1) A dissemination due to aspiration of tuberculous material, the tubercles being situated in the air-cells or the walls of the smaller bronchi; (2) the distribution due to dissemination of tubercle bacilli by the lymph current, the tubercles being scattered about the old foci in a radial manner—the secondary crop of Laennec. Much more rarely there is a scattered dissemination from infection here and there of the smaller vessels, the tubercles then being situated in the vessel walls. Sometimes, in cases with cavity formation at the apex, the greater part of the lower lobes presents many groups of firm, sclerotic, miliary tubercles, which may indeed form the distinguishing anatomical feature—a chronic miliary tuberculosis.

(*b*) *Tuberculous Broncho-pneumonia.*—In a large proportion of the cases of chronic phthisis the terminal bronchiole is the point of origin of the process, consequently we find the smaller bronchi and their alveolar territories blocked with the accumulated products of inflammation in all stages of *caseation.* At an early period a cross-section of an area of tuberculous broncho-pneumonia gives the most characteristic appearance. The central bronchiole is seen as a small orifice, or it is plugged with cheesy contents, while surrounding it is a caseous nodule, the so-called peribronchial tubercle. The longitudinal section has a somewhat dendritic or foliaceous appearance. The condition of the picture depends much upon the slowness or rapidity with which the process has advanced. The following changes may occur:

Ulceration.—When the caseation takes place rapidly or ulceration occurs in the bronchial wall, the mass may break down and form a small cavity.

Sclerosis.—In other instances the process is more chronic, and fibroid changes gradually produce a sclerosis of the affected area. The sclerosis may be confined to the margin of the mass, forming a limiting capsule, within which is a uniform, firm, cheesy substance, in which lime salts are often deposited. This represents the healing of one of these areas of caseous broncho-pneumonia. It is only, however, when complete fibroid transformation or calcification has occurred that we can really speak of healing. In many instances the colonies of miliary tubercles about these masses show that the virus is still active in them. Subsequently, in ulcerative processes, these calcareous bodies—lung-stones, as they are sometimes called—may be expectorated.

(*c*) *Pneumonia.*—An important though secondary place is occupied by inflammation of the alveoli surrounding the tubercles, which become filled with epithelioid cells. The consolidation may extend for some distance about the tuberculous foci and unite them into areas of uniform consolidation. Although in some instances this inflammatory process may be simple, in others it is undoubtedly specific. It is excited by the tubercle bacilli and is a manifestation of their action. It may present a very varied appearance; in some instances resembling closely ordinary red hepatization, in others being more homogeneous and infiltrated, the so-called *infiltration tuberculeuse* of Laennec. In other cases the contents of the alveoli undergo fatty degeneration, and appear on the cut surface as opaque white or yellowish-white bodies. In early phthisis much of the consolidation is due to this pneumonic infiltration, which may surround for some distance the smaller tuberculous foci.

(*d*) *Cavities.*—A vomica is a cavity in the lung tissue, produced by necrosis and ulceration. The process usually begins in the wall of the bronchus in a tuberculous area. Dilatation is produced by retained secretion, and necrosis and ulceration of the wall occur with gradual destruction of the contiguous tissues. By extension of the necrosis and ulceration the cavity increases, contiguous ones unite, and in an affected region there may be a series of small excavations communicating with a bronchus. In nearly all instances the process extends from the bronchi, though it is possible for necrosis and softening to take place in the centre of a caseous area without primary involvement of the bronchial wall. Three forms of cavities may be recognized.

The *fresh ulcerative,* seen in acute phthisis, in which there is no limiting membrane, but the walls are made up of softened, necrotic, and caseous masses. A small vomica of this sort, situated just beneath the pleura, may rupture and cause pneumothorax. In cases of acute tuberculo-pneumonic phthisis they may be large, occupying the greater portion of the upper lobe. In the chronic ulcerative phthisis cavities of this sort are invariably present in those portions of the lung in which the disease is advancing. At the apex there may be a large old cavity with well-defined walls, while at the anterior margin of the upper lobes, or in the apices of the lower lobes, there are recent ulcerating cavities communicating with the bronchi.

Cavities with well-defined Walls.—A majority of the cavities in the chronic form of phthisis have a well-defined limiting membrane, the inner surface of which constantly produces pus. The walls are crossed by trabeculæ which represent remnants of bronchi and blood-vessels. Even the cavities with the well-defined walls extend gradually by a slow necrosis and destruction of the contiguous lung tissue. The contents are usually purulent, similar in character to the grayish nummular sputa coughed up. Not infrequently the membrane is vascular or it may be hæmorrhagic. Occasionally, when gangrene has occurred in the wall, the contents are horribly fetid. These cavities may occupy the greater portion of the apex, forming an irregular series which communicate with each other and with the bronchi, or the entire upper lobe except the anterior margin may be excavated, forming a thin-walled cavity. In rare instances the process has proceeded to total excavation of the lung, not a remnant of which remains, except perhaps a narrow strip at the anterior margin. In a case of this kind, in a young girl, the cavity held 40 fluid ounces, in another 42 ounces.

Quiescent Cavities.—When quite small and surrounded by dense cicatricial tissue communicating with the bronchi they form the *cicatrices fistuleuses* of Laennec. Occasionally one apex may be represented by a series of these small cavities, surrounded by dense fibrous tissue. The lining membrane of these old cavities may be quite smooth, almost like a mucous membrane. Cavities of any size do not heal completely.

Cases are often seen in which it has been supposed that a cavity has healed; but the signs of excavation are notoriously uncertain, and there may be pectoriloquy and cavernous sounds with gurgling resonant râles in an area of consolidation close to a large bronchus.

In the formation of cavities the blood vessels gradually become closed by an obliterating inflammation. They are the last structures to yield and may be completely exposed in a cavity, even when the circulation is still going on in them. Unfortunately, the erosion of a large vessel which has not yet been obliterated is by no means infrequent, and causes profuse and often fatal hæmorrhage. Another common event is the formation of aneurisms on the arteries running in the walls of cavities. These may be small, bunch-like dilatations, or they may form sacs the size of a walnut or even larger. Rasmussen, Douglas Powell, and others have called attention to their importance in hæmoptysis, under which section they are dealt with more fully.

And, finally, about cavities of all sorts, the connective tissue grows, tending to limit their extent. The thickening is particularly marked beneath the pleura, and in chronic cases an entire apex may be converted into a mass of fibrous tissue, inclosing a few small cavities.

(*e*) *Pleura.*—Practically, in all cases of chronic phthisis the pleura is involved. Adhesions take place which may be thin and readily torn, or dense and firm, uniting layers of from 2 to 5 mm. in thickness. This pleurisy may be simple, but in many cases it is tuberculous, and miliary tubercles or caseous masses are seen in the thickened membrane. Effusion is not at all infrequent, either serous, purulent, or hæmorrhagic. Pneumothorax is a common accident.

(*f*) Changes in the *smaller bronchi* control the situation in the early stages of tuberculous phthisis, and play an important rôle throughout the disease. The process very often begins in the walls of the smaller tubes and leads to caseation, distention with products of inflammation, and broncho-pneumonia of the lobules. In many cases the visible implication of the bronchus is an extension upward of a process which has begun in the smallest bronchiole. This involvement weakens the wall, leading to bronchiectasis, not an uncommon event. The mucous membrane of the larger bronchi, which is usually involved in a chronic catarrh, is more or less swollen, and in some instances ulcerated. Besides these specific lesions, they may be the seat, especially in children, of inflammation due to secondary invasion, most frequently by the *Micrococcus lanceolatus,* with the production of a broncho-pneumonia.

(*g*) The *bronchial glands,* in the more acute cases, are swollen and œdematous. Miliary tubercles and caseous foci are usually present. In cases of chronic tuberculosis the caseous areas are common, calcification may occur, and not infrequently purulent softening.

(*h*) *Changes in the Other Organs.*—Of these, tuberculosis is the most common. In my series of autopsies the brain presented tuberculous lesions in 31, the spleen in 33, the liver in 12, the kidneys in 32, the intestines in 65, and the pericardium in 7. Other groups of lymphatic glands besides the bronchial may be affected.

Amyloid change may occur in the liver, spleen, kidneys, and mucous membrane of the intestines. The *liver* is often the seat of extensive fatty infiltration, which may cause marked enlargement. The *intestinal tuberculosis* occurs in advanced cases and is responsible in great part for the troublesome diarrhœa.

Endocarditis is not very common, and was present in 12 of my post mortems and in 27 of Percy Kidd's 500 cases. Tubercle bacilli have been found in the vegetations. Tubercles may be present on the endocardium, particularly of the right ventricle.

The *larynx* is frequently involved, and ulceration of the vocal cords and destruction of the epiglottis are not at all uncommon.

Modes of Onset.—We have already seen that tuberculosis of the lungs may occur as the chief part of a general infection, or may set in with symptoms which closely simulate acute pneumonia. In the ordinary type of pulmonary tuberculosis the invasion is gradual and less striking, but presents an extraordinarily diverse picture, so that the practitioner is often led into error. Among the most characteristic modes of onset are the following:

(*a*) Latent Types.—It is probable that many slight, ill-defined ailments are due to a local unrecognized tuberculosis of the lung. In the history of patients with tuberculosis such attacks are not infrequently mentioned.

The disease makes considerable progress before there are serious symptoms to arouse the attention of the patient. In workingmen the disease may even advance to excavation of an apex before they seek advice. It is not a little remarkable how slight the lung symptoms may have been.

The symptoms may be masked by the existence of serious disease in other organs, as in the peritoneum, intestines, or bones.

(*b*) With Symptoms of Dyspepsia and Anæmia.—The gastric mode of onset is very common, and the early manifestations may be great irritability of the stomach with vomiting or a type of acid dyspepsia with eructations. In young girls (and in children) with this dyspepsia there is very frequently a pronounced chloro-anæmia, and the patient complains of palpitation of the heart, increasing weakness, slight afternoon fever, and amenorrhœa.

(*c*) Malarial Symptoms.—In a considerable number of cases the onset of pulmonary tuberculosis is with symptoms which suggest malarial fever. The patient has repeated paroxysms of chills, fevers, and sweats, which may recur with great regularity. In districts in which malaria prevails there is no more common mistake than to confound the initial rigors of pulmonary tuberculosis with it.

(*d*) Onset with Pleurisy.—The first symptoms may be a dry pleurisy over an apex, with persistent friction murmur. In other instances the pulmonary symptoms have followed an attack of pleurisy with effusion. The exudate gradually disappears, but the cough persists and the patient becomes feverish, and gradually signs of disease at one apex become manifest. About one-third of all cases of pleurisy with effusion subsequently have pulmonary tuberculosis.

(*e*) With Laryngeal Symptoms.—The primary localization may be in the larynx, though in a majority of the instances in which huskiness and laryngeal symptoms are the first noticeable features of the disease there are doubtless foci already existing in the lung. The group of cases in which for many months throat and larynx symptoms precede the manifestations of pulmonary tuberculosis is a very important one.

(*f*) Onset with Hæmoptysis.—Frequently the very first symptom is a brisk hæmorrhage from the lungs, following which the pulmonary symptoms may come on with great rapidity. In other cases the hæmoptysis recurs, and it may be months before the symptoms become well established. In a majority of these cases the local tuberculous lesion exists at the date of the hæmoptysis.

(*g*) WITH TUBERCULOSIS OF THE CERVICO-AXILLARY GLANDS.—Preceding the onset of pulmonary disease for months, or even for years, the lymph-glands of the neck or of the neck and axilla of one side may be enlarged. These cases are by no means infrequent, and they are of importance because of the latency of the pulmonary lesions. Nowadays, when operative interference is so common, it is well to bear in mind that in such patients the corresponding apex of the lung may be extensively involved.

(*h*) BRONCHIAL SYMPTOMS.—And, lastly, in by far the largest number of all cases the onset is with a *bronchitis,* or, as the patient expresses it, a neglected cold. There has been, perhaps, a liability to catch cold easily or the patient has been subject to naso-pharyngeal catarrh; then, following some unusual exposure, a cough begins, which may be frequent and very irritating. The examination of the lungs may reveal localized moist sounds at one apex and perhaps wheezing bronchitic râles in other parts. In a few cases the early symptoms are often suggestive of asthma with marked wheezing and diffuse piping râles.

Symptoms.—In discussing the symptoms it is usual to divide the disease into three periods: the first embracing the time of the growth and development of the tubercles; the second, when they soften; and the third, when there is a formation of cavities. Unfortunately, these anatomical stages can not be satisfactorily correlated with corresponding clinical periods, and we often find that a patient in the third stage with a well-marked cavity is in a far better condition and has greater prospects of recovery than a patient in the first stage with diffuse consolidation. It is therefore better perhaps to disregard them altogether.

LOCAL SYMPTOMS.—*Pain* in the chest may be early and troublesome or absent throughout. It is usually associated with pleurisy, and may be sharp and stabbing in character, and either constant or felt only during coughing. Perhaps the commonest situation is in the lower thoracic zone, though in some instances it is beneath the scapula or referred to the apex. The attacks may recur at long intervals. Intercostal neuralgia occasionally occurs in the course of ordinary pulmonary tuberculosis.

Cough is one of the earliest symptoms, and is present in the majority of cases from beginning to end. There is nothing peculiar or distinctive about it. At first dry and hacking, and perhaps scarcely exciting the attention of the patient, it subsequently becomes looser, more constant, and associated with a glairy, muco-purulent expectoration. In the early stages of the disease the cough is bronchial in its origin. When cavities have formed it becomes more paroxysmal, and is most marked in the morning or after a sleep. Cough is not a constant symptom, however, and a patient may present himself with well-marked excavation at one apex who will declare that he has had little or no cough. So, too, there may be well-marked physical signs, dulness and moist sounds, without either expectoration or cough. In well-established cases the nocturnal paroxysms are most distressing and prevent sleep. The cough may be of such persistence and severity as to cause vomiting, and the patient becomes rapidly emaciated from loss of food—Morton's cough (Phthisiologia, 1689, p. 101). The laryngeal complications give a peculiarly husky quality to the cough, and when erosion and ulceration have proceeded far in the vocal cords the coughing becomes much less effective.

Sputum.—This varies greatly in amount and character with the different stages. There are patients with well-marked local signs at one apex, with slight cough and moderately high fever, without from day to day a trace of expectoration. So, also, there are instances with the most extensive consolidation (caseous pneumonia) and high fever, but without enough expectoration to enable an examination for bacilli to be made. In the early stage of pulmonary tuberculosis the sputum is chiefly catarrhal and has a glairy, sago-like appearance, due to the presence of alveolar cells which have undergone the myeline degeneration. There is nothing distinctive or peculiar in this form of expectoration, which may persist for months without indicating serious trouble. The earliest trace of characteristic sputum may show the presence of small grayish or greenish-gray purulent masses. These, when coughed up, are always suggestive and should be the portions picked out for microscopic examination. As softening comes on, the expectoration becomes more profuse and purulent, but may still contain a considerable quantity of alveolar epithelium. Finally, when cavities exist, the sputum assumes the so-called nummular form; each mass is isolated, flattened, greenish-gray in color, quite airless, and, when spat into water, sinks to the bottom.

By the microscopic examination of the sputum we determine whether the process is tuberculous, and whether softening has occurred. The bacilli in stained preparations are seen as elongated, slightly curved, red rods, sometimes presenting a beaded appearance. They are frequently in groups of three or four, but the number varies considerably. Only one or two may be found in a preparation, or, in some instances, they are so abundant that the entire field is occupied. Repeated examinations may be necessary.

The continued presence of tubercle bacilli in the sputum is an infallible indication of the existence of tuberculosis.

One or two may possibly be due to accidental inhalation. A number may come from a spot of softening 3 by 3 cm. In the nummular sputa of later stages the bacilli are very abundant.

Elastic tissue may be derived from the bronchi, the alveoli, or from the arterial coats; and naturally the appearance of the tissue will vary with the locality from which it comes. In the examination for this it is not necessary to boil the sputum with caustic potash. For years I have used a simple plan which was shown to me at the London Hospital by Sir Andrew Clark. This method depends upon the fact that in almost all instances if the sputum is spread in a sufficiently thin layer the fragments of elastic tissue can be seen with the naked eye. The thick, purulent portions are placed upon a glass plate 15 × 15 cm. and flattened into a thin layer by a second glass plate 10 × 10 cm. In this compressed grayish layer between the glass slips any fragments of elastic tissue show on a black background as grayish-yellow spots and can either be examined at once under a low power or the uppermost piece of glass is slid along until the fragment is exposed, when it is picked out and placed upon the ordinary microscopic slide. Fragments of bread and collections of milk-globules may also present an opaque white appearance, but with a little practice they can readily be recognized. Fragments of epithelium from the tongue, infiltrated with micrococci, are still more deceptive, but the miscroscope at once shows the difference.

The bronchial elastic tissue forms an elongated network, or two or three long, narrow fibres are found close together. From the blood-vessels a somewhat similar form may be seen and occasionally a distinct sheeting is found as if it had come from the intima of a good-sized artery. The elastic tissue of the alveolar wall is quite distinctive; the fibres are branched and often show the outline of the arrangement of the air-cells. The elastic tissue from bronchi or alveoli indicates extensive erosion of a tube and softening of the lung-tissue.

Another occasional constituent of the sputum is blood, which may be present as the chief characteristic of the expectoration in hæmoptysis or may simply tinge the sputum. In chronic cases with large cavities, in addition to bacteria, various forms of fungi may be found, of which the aspergillus is the most important. Sarcinæ may also occur.

Calcareous Fragments.—Formerly a good deal of stress was laid upon their presence in the sputum, and Morton described a phthisis *a calculis in pulmonibus generatis.* Bayle also described a separate form of *phthisis calculeuse.* The size of the fragments varies from a small pea to a large cherry. As a rule, a single one is ejected; sometimes large numbers are coughed up in the course of the disease. They are formed in the lung by the calcification of caseous masses, and it is said also occasionally in obstructed bronchi. They may come from the bronchial glands by ulceration into the bronchi, and there is a case on record of suffocation in a child from this cause.

The daily amount of expectoration varies. In rapidly advancing cases, with much cough, it may reach as high as 500 c. c. in the day. In cases with large cavities the chief amount is brought up in the morning. The expectoration of tuberculous patients usually has a heavy, sweetish odor, and occasionally it is fetid, owing to decomposition in the cavities.

Hæmoptysis.—One of the most famous of the Hippocratic axioms says, "From a spitting of blood there is a spitting of pus." The older writers thought that the phthisis was directly due to the inflammatory or putrefactive changes caused by the hæmorrhage into the lung. Morton, however, in his interesting section, *Phthisis ab Hæmoptöe,* rather doubted this sequence. Laennec and Louis, and later in the century Traube, regarded the hæmoptysis as an evidence of existing disease of the lung. From the accurate views of Laennec and Louis the profession was led away by Graves, and particularly by Niemeyer, who held that the blood in the air-cells set up an inflammatory process, a common termination of which was caseation. Since Koch's discovery we have learned that many cases in which the physical examination is negative show, either during the period of hæmorrhage or immediately after it, tubercle bacilli in the sputum, so that opinion has veered to the older view, and we now regard the appearance of hæmoptysis as an indication of existing disease. In young, apparently healthy, persons cases of hæmoptysis may be divided into three groups. In the first the bleeding has come on without premonition, without overexertion or injury, and there is no family history of tuberculosis. The physical examination is negative, and the examination of the expectoration at the time of the hæmorrhage and subsequently shows no tubercle bacilli. Such instances are not uncommon, and, though one may suspect strongly the presence of some focus of tuberculosis, yet the individuals may retain good health for many years, and have no further trouble. Of the 386 cases of hæmoptysis noted by Ware in private practice 62 recovered, and pulmonary disease did not subsequently occur.

In a second group individuals in apparently perfect health are suddenly attacked, perhaps after a slight exertion or during some athletic exercises. The physical examination is also negative, but tubercle bacilli are found sometimes in the bloody sputum, more frequently a few days later.

In a third set of cases the individuals have been in failing health for a month or two, but the symptoms have not been urgent and perhaps not noticed by the patients. The physical examination shows the presence of well-marked tuberculous disease, and there are both tubercle bacilli and elastic tissue in the sputum.

A very interesting systematic study of the subject of hæmoptysis, particularly in its relation to the question of tuberculosis, has been completed in the Prussian army by Franz Stricker. During the five years 1890-'95 there were 900 cases admitted to the hospitals, which is a percentage of 0.045 of the strength (1,728,505). Of the cases, in 480 the hæmorrhage came on without recognizable cause. Of these, 417 cases, 86 per cent., were certainly or probably tuberculous. In only 221, however, was the evidence conclusive.

In a second group of 213 cases the hæmorrhage came on during the military exercise, and of these 75 patients were shown to be tuberculous.

In 118 cases the hæmorrhage followed certain special exercises, as in the gymnasium or in riding or in consequence of swimming. In 24 cases it occurred during the exercise of the voice in singing or in giving command or in the use of wind instruments. A very interesting group of 24 cases is reported in which the hæmorrhage followed trauma, either a fall or a blow upon the thorax. In 7 of these tuberculosis was positively present, and in 6 other cases there was a strong probability of its existence.

Among the conclusions which Stricker draws the following are the most important: namely, that soldiers attacked with hæmoptysis without special cause are in at least 86.8 per cent. tuberculous. In the cases in which the hæmoptysis follows the special exercises, etc., of military service at least 74.4 per cent. are tuberculous. In the cases which come on during swimming or as a consequence of direct injury to the thorax about one-half are not associated with tuberculosis.

Hæmoptysis occurs in from 60 to 80 per cent. of all cases of pulmonary tuberculosis. It is more frequent in males than in females.

In a majority of all cases the bleeding recurs. Sometimes it is a special feature throughout the disease, so that a hæmorrhagic form has been recognized. The amount of blood brought up varies from a couple of drachms to a pint or more. In 69 per cent. of 4,125 cases of hæmoptysis at the Brompton Hospital the amount brought up was under half an ounce.

A distinction may be drawn between the hæmoptysis early in the disease and that which occurs in the later periods. In the former the bleeding is usually slight, is apt to recur, and fatal hæmorrhage is very rare. In these cases the bleeding is usually from small areas of softening or from early erosions in the bronchial mucosa. In the later periods, after cavities have formed, the bleeding, is, as a rule, more profuse and is more apt to be fatal. Single large hæmorrhages, proving quickly fatal, are very rare, except in the advanced stages of the disease. In these cases the bleeding comes either from an erosion of a good-sized vessel in the wall of a cavity or from the rupture of an aneurism of the pulmonary artery.

The bleeding, as a rule, sets in suddenly. Without any warning the patient may notice a warm salt taste and the mouth fills with blood. It may come up with a slight cough. The total amount may not be more than a few drachms, and for a day or two the patient may spit up small quantities. When a large vessel is eroded or an aneurism bursts, the amount of blood brought up is large, and in the course of a short time a pint or two may be expectorated. Fatal hæmorrhage may occur into a very large cavity without any blood being coughed up. The character of the blood is, as a rule, distinctive. It is frothy, mixed with mucus, generally bright red in color, except when large amounts are expectorated, and then it may be dark. The sputum may remain blood-tinged for some days, or there are brownish-black streaks in it, or friable nodules consisting entirely of blood-corpuscles may be coughed up. Blood moulds of the smaller bronchi are sometimes expectorated.

The microscopic examination of the sputum in hæmorrhage cases is most important. If carefully spread out, there may be noted, even in an apparently pure hæmorrhagic mass, little portions of mucus from which bacilli or elastic tissue may be obtained. Flick and others have called attention to the frequency with which hæmoptysis is associated with the appearance or an increase of pneumococci and influenza bacilli in the sputum.

Dyspnœa is not a common accompaniment of ordinary tuberculosis. The greater part of one lung may be diseased and local trouble exist at the other apex without any shortness of breath. Even in the paroxysms of very high fever the respirations may not be much increased. Dyspnœa occurs (*a*) with the rapid extension in both lungs of a broncho-pneumonia; (*b*) with the occurrence of miliary tuberculosis; (*c*) sometimes with pneumothorax; (*d*) in old cases with much emphysema, and it may be associated with cyanosis; (*c*) and, lastly, in long-standing cases, with contracted apices or great thickening of the pleura, the right heart is enlarged, and the dyspnœa may be cardiac.

General Symptoms.—*Fever.*—It is well to bear in mind that the temperature varies slightly in normal individuals, and the afternoon range may be 99°, 99.5° or even 100° F. The difference between the mouth and rectal temperature may be a full degree, and in young full-blooded persons, in the nervous, and after exercise the normal rectal temperature may be 100.5° or even 101° F. To get a correct idea of the temperature range in pulmonary tuberculosis it is necessary to make observations every two hours at first. The usual 8 A. M. and 8 P. M. record is, in a majority of the cases, very deceptive, giving neither the minimum nor maximum. The former usually occurs between 2 and 6 A. M., and the latter between 2 and 6 P. M.

Fever, one of the earliest and most important symptoms, is due to the effect on the heat centres of the toxins or materials absorbed from the tuberculous focus. Later in the disease the hectic fever is caused in part by the absorption of the bacterial products of other organisms. From a small spot of disease not a sufficient amount of toxin may be produced to disturb the body metabolism, but in the lymph glands, lungs, and bones, from progressing areas of infection sufficient absorption takes place to cause fever. It is an auto-inoculation comparable with the fever produced by an injection of tuberculin. Anything that stimulates the local lymph and blood flow favors the discharge of the toxins and causes fever. A patient at rest may be afebrile; after exercise the temperature may be 102.5°, due to an auto-inoculation. In acute cases the fever is more or less continuous, resembling that of typhoid fever or pneumonia, with slight morning remissions. It may set in with a chill and be followed by sweats, and there are cases with a marked intermittent pyrexia from the onset. As a rule, the degree of activity of the local process may be gauged by the persistency and the range of the fever; and favorable cases are those in which the temperature yields rapidly to rest. In a few cases progress of the local disease continues and may even be rapid without fever. The temperature of consumptives is easily influenced by trivial causes which would not affect a normal person, such as mental excitement, exercise, constipation, etc. The patient is usually aware when fever is present and feels more comfortable with a temperature of 101°. Except the sweating, there are rarely any unpleasant feelings connected with it.

With breaking down of the lung-tissue and formation of cavities, associated as these processes always are with suppuration and mixed infection, the fever assumes a characteristically intermittent or hectic type. For a large part of the day the patient is not only afebrile, but the temperature is subnormal. In the annexed two-hourly chart, from a case of chronic tuberculosis of the lungs, it will be seen that, from 10 P. M. to 8 A. M. or noon, the temperature continuously fell and went as low as 95°. A slow rise then took place through the late morning and early afternoon hours and reached its maximum between 6 and 10 P. M. As shown in the chart, there were in the three days about forty-three hours of pyrexia and twenty-nine hours of apyrexia. The rapid fall of the temperature in the early morning hours is usually associated with sweating. This hectic, as it is called, which is a typical fever of septic infection, is met with when the process of cavity formation and softening is advanced and extending.

Sweating—Drenching perspirations are common in phthisis and constitute one of the most distressing features of the disease. They occur usually with the drop in the fever in the early morning hours, or at any time in the day when the patient sleeps. They may come on early in the disease, but are more persistent and frequent after cavities have formed. Some patients escape altogether.

The *pulse* is increased in frequency and usually in proportion to the height of the fever. Even when at rest and afebrile the pulse may be rapid, but the excitement of counting it may increase the rate 20 to 30 beats. The pulse is often remarkably full, soft and compressible; even after recovery it may remain rapid. Pulsation may sometimes be seen in the capillaries and in the veins on the back of the hand.

Emaciation is a pronounced feature, from which the two common names of the disease have been derived. The loss of weight is gradual and, if the disease is extending, progressive. The scales give one of the best indications of the progress of the patient. It is most rapid early in the disease, when the patient may lose at the rate of five or six pounds a week; and usually is in direct relation to the intensity and duration of the fever. With the arrest of the progress and the fall in temperature the patient usually begins to regain weight. The average gain in weight of 901 patients at the Adirondack Sanatorium was fourteen pounds (L. Brown). A gain of two pounds a week is satisfactory. Loss of strength may be out of proportion to and quite independent of loss of weight. Early debility may be a marked feature.

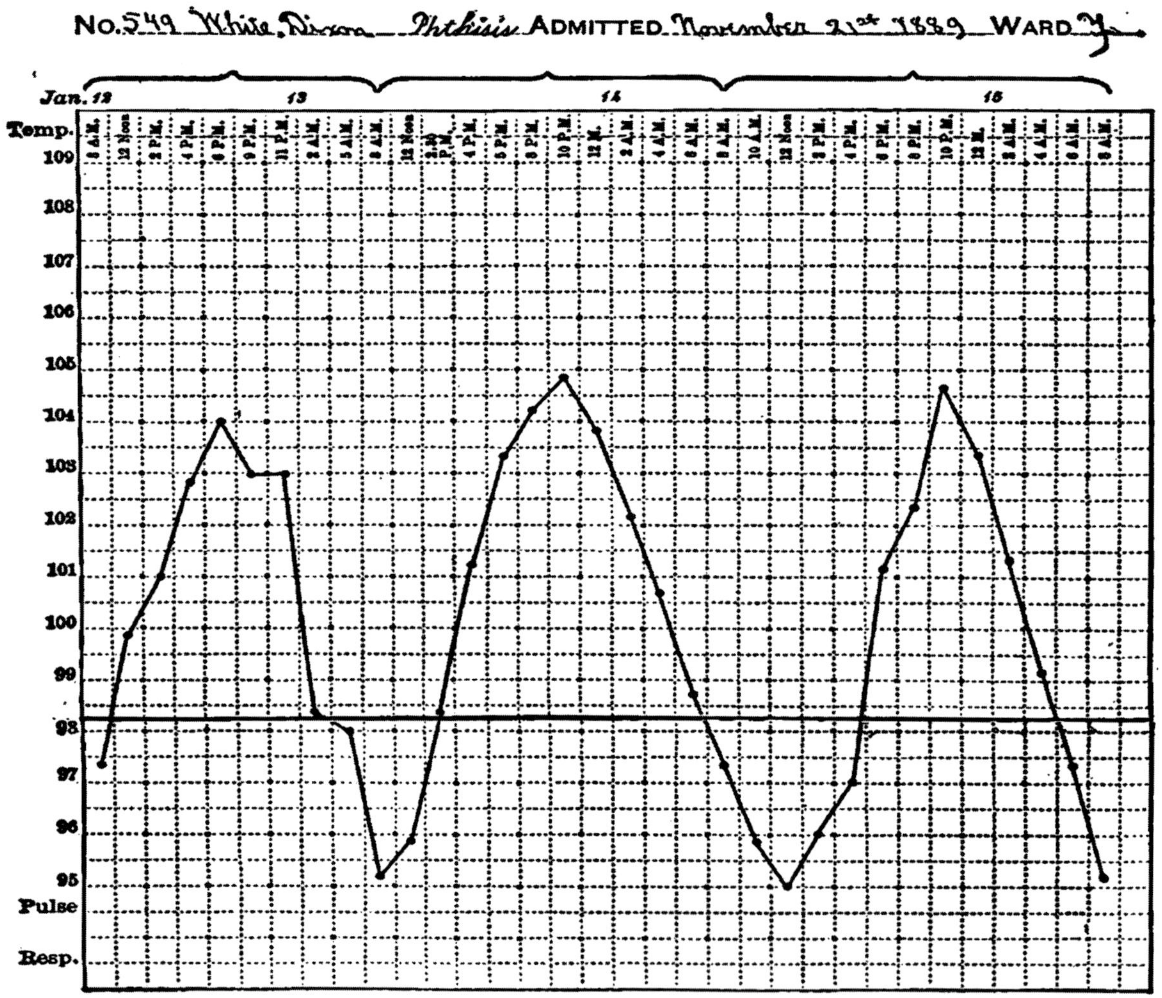

CHART V.—THREE DAYS. CHRONIC TUBERCULOSIS.

PHYSICAL SIGNS.—(*a*) *Inspection.*—The shape of the chest is often suggestive, though it is to be remembered that the disease may be met with in chests of any build. Practically, however, in a considerable proportion of cases the thorax is long and narrow, with very wide intercostal spaces, the ribs more vertical in direction, and the costal angle very narrow. The scapulæ are "winged," a point noted by Hippocrates. Another type of chest which is very common is that which is flattened in the antero-posterior diameter. The costal cartilages may be prominent and the sternum depressed. Occasionally the lower sternum forms a deep concavity, the so-called funnel breast (*Trichter-Brust*). Special examination should be made of the clavicular regions to see if one clavicle stands out more distinctly than the other, or if the spaces above or below it are more marked. Defective expansion at one apex is an early and important sign. The condition of expansion of the lower zone of the thorax may be well estimated by inspection. The condition of the præcordia should also be noted, as a wide area of impulse, particularly in the second, third, and fourth interspaces, often results from disease of the left apex. From a point behind the patient, looking over the shoulders, one can often better estimate the relative expansion of the apices. Atrophy of the muscles of the shoulder-girdle on the affected side is not uncommon, and a slight scoliosis may be present. Movement may be restricted on the affected side, particularly at the apex. Pleurisy with adhesions or with effusion, fibrosis, and pneumonic consolidation may limit the movement of one side. The Litten phenomenon (seen best on the right side) may be restricted in extent or absent. The chest expansion may be much reduced. It should be recorded carefully at the first examination.

(*b*) *Palpation.*—Deficiency in expansion at the apices or bases is perhaps best gauged by placing the hands in the subclavicular spaces and then in the lateral regions of the chest and asking the patient to draw slowly a full breath. Standing behind the patient and placing the thumbs in the supraclavicular and the fingers in the infraclavicular spaces one can judge accurately as to the relative mobility of the two sides. Disease at an apex, though early and before dulness is at all marked, may be indicated by deficient expansion. On asking the patient to count, the tactile fremitus is increased wherever there is local growth of tubercle or extensive caseation. In comparing the apices it is important to bear in mind that normally the fremitus is stronger over the right than the left. So, too, at the base, when there is consolidation of the lung, the fremitus is increased; whereas, if there is pleural effusion, it is diminished or absent. In the later stages, when cavities form, the tactile fremitus is usually much exaggerated over them. When the pleura is greatly thickened the fremitus may be diminished.

(*c*) *Percussion.*—Tubercles, inflammatory products, fibroid changes, and cavities produce important changes in the pulmonary resonance. There may be localized disease, even of some extent, without inducing much alteration, as when the tubercles are scattered there is air-containing tissue between them. In incipient cases percussion may be negative, 28 out of 201 in L. Brown's series. It requires a fair-sized area of infiltration to cause a change in the percussion note, 4 x 6 cm., according to Cornet. The personal equation is very important in estimating the early physical signs in pulmonary tuberculosis, and I remember a notable diagnosis of a cavity at the back of the left apex the size of a hickory nut, *with the shell on!* One of the earliest and most valuable signs is defective resonance upon and above a clavicle. In a considerable proportion of all cases of phthisis the dulness is first noted in these regions. The comparison between the two sides should be made also when the breath is held after a full inspiration, as the defective resonance may then be more clearly marked. In the early stages the percussion note is usually higher in pitch, and it may require an experienced ear to detect the difference. In recent consolidation from caseous pneumonia the percussion note often has a tympanitic quality. A wooden dulness is rarely heard except in old cases with extensive fibroid change at the apex or base. Over large, thin-walled cavities at the apex the so-called cracked-pot sound may be obtained. In thin subjects the percussion should be carefully practiced in the supraspinous fossæ and the interscapular space, as they correspond to very important areas early involved in the disease. By light percussion along the border of the trapezius and in the supraclavicular and supraspinous fossæ, areas of apical resonance may be mapped out (Kronig's apical resonance zones). Under normal conditions the areas are equal on the two sides. Consolidation or retraction of an apex causes definite narrowing of the zone on the affected side. The procedure requires considerable skill. It gives valuable information in the early stage of infiltration. Goldscheider uses a special pleximeter and percusses out the borders of the apex of the lung projecting above the clavicle. The method is less satisfactory than that of Kronig. In cases with numerous isolated cavities at the apex, without much fibroid tissue or thickening of the pleura, the percussion note may show little change, and the contrast between the signs obtained an auscultation and percussion is most marked. In the direct percussion of the chest, particularly in thin patients over the pectorals, one frequently sees the phenomenon known as *myoidema*, a local contraction of the muscle causing bulging, which persists for a variable period and gradually subsides. It has no special significance.

(*d*) *Auscultation.*—Feeble breath-sounds are among the most characteristic early signs, since not as much air enters the tubes and vesicles of the affected area. It is well at first always to compare carefully the corresponding points on the two sides of the chest without asking the patient either to draw a deep breath or to cough. With early apical disease the inspiration on quiet breathing may be scarcely audible. Expiration is usually prolonged. On the other hand, there are cases in which the earliest sign is a harsh, rude, respiratory murmur. On deep breathing it is frequently to be noted that inspiration is jerking or wavy, the so-called "cog-wheel" rhythm; which, however, is by no means confined to tuberculosis. With extension of the disease the inspiratory murmur is harsh, and, when consolidation occurs, whiffing and bronchial. With these changes in the character of the murmur there are râles. The patient should first breathe quietly, then take a full breath, and then cough. When heard with quiet breathing, if they persist and are present in one area only, they are of great importance. The fine rustling crepitus at one or both apices which is heard when the patient first takes a deep breath is of no moment. It may also be present at the bases. Râles at the end of deep inspiration which disappear on repeated breathing may also be disregarded. Râles which are brought out by coughing, which persist, and are repeatedly heard at the same spot are of the greatest importance. It is of equal import when moist, clicking râles are present with change in the percussion note. Attention to these brief rules will save many of the unnecessary diagnoses of pulmonary tuberculosis at present made on auscultatory signs alone.

When softening occurs the râles are louder and have a bubbling, sometimes a characteristic clicking quality. These "moist sounds," as they are called, when associated with change in the percussion resonance are extremely suggestive. When cavities form the râles are louder, more gurgling, and resonant in quality. When there is consolidation of any extent the breath sounds are tubular, and in the large excavations loud and cavernous, or have an amphoric quality. In the unaffected portions of the lobe and in the opposite lung the breath sounds may be harsh and even puerile. The vocal resonance is usually increased in all stages of the process, and bronchophony and pectoriloquy are met with in the regions of consolidation and over cavities. Pleuritic friction may be present at any stage and, as mentioned before, occurs very early. There are cases in which it is a marked feature throughout. When the lappet of lung over the heart is involved there may be a pleuro-pericardial friction, and when this area is consolidated there may be curious clicking râles synchronous with the heart-beat, due to the compression by the heart of this portion with expulsion of air from it. An interesting auscultatory sign met with in thin-chested persons, in nervous patients, and often in early pulmonary tuberculosis is the so-called cardio-respiratory murmur, a whiffing systolic bruit due to the propulsion of air out of the tubes by the impulse of the heart. It is best heard during inspiration and in the antero-lateral regions of the chest.

A systolic murmur is frequently heard in the subclavian artery on either side, the pulsation of which may be very visible. The murmur is in all probability due to pressure on the vessels by the thickened pleura.

The signs of cavity may be here briefly enumerated.

(1) When there is not much thickening of the pleura or condensation of the surrounding lung-tissue, the percussion sound may be full and clear, resembling the normal note. More commonly there is defective resonance or a tympanitic quality which may at times be purely amphoric. The pitch of the percussion note changes over a cavity when the mouth is opened or closed (Wintrich's sign), or it may be brought out more clearly on change of position. The cracked-pot sound is obtainable only over tolerably large cavities with thin walls. It is best elicited by a firm, quick stroke, the patient at the time having the mouth open. In those rare instances of almost total excavation of one lung the percussion note may be amphoric in quality. (2) On auscultation the so-called cavernous sounds are heard: (i) Various grades of modified breathing—blowing or tubular, cavernous or amphoric. There may be a curiously sharp hissing sound, as if the air was passing from a narrow opening into a wide space. In very large cavities both inspiration and expiration may be typically amphoric. (ii) There are coarse bubbling râles which have a resonant quality, and on coughing may have a metallic or ringing character. On coughing they are often loud and gurgling. In very large thin-walled cavities, and more rarely in medium-sized cavities, surrounded by recent consolidation, the râles may have a distinctly amphoric echo, simulating those of pneumothorax. There are dry cavities in which no râles are heard. (iii) The vocal resonance is greatly intensified, and whispered broncophony is clearly heard. In large apical cavities the heart-sounds are well heard, and occasionally there may be an intense systolic murmur, probably always transmitted to, and not produced, as has been supposed, in the cavity itself. In large excavations of the left apex the heart impulse may cause gurgling sounds or clicks synchronous with the systole. They may even be loud enough to be heard at a little distance from the chest wall. A large cavity with smooth walls and thin fluid contents may give the succussion sound when the trunk is abruptly shaken (Walshe), and even the coin sound may be obtained.

Pseudo-cavernous signs may be caused by an area of consolidation near a large bronchus. The condition may be most deceptive—the high-pitched or tympanitic percussion note, the tubular or cavernous breathing, and the resonant râles simulate closely the signs of cavity.

3. *Fibroid Phthisis*

In their monograph on Fibroid Diseases of the Lung, Clark, Hadley, and Chaplin make the following classification: 1. Pure fibroid—a condition in which there is no tubercle. 2. Tuberculo-fibroid disease—a condition primarily tuberculous, but which has run a fibroid course. 3. Fibro-tuberculous disease—a condition primarily fibroid, but which has become tuberculous. The tuberculo-fibroid form may come on gradually as a sequence of a chronic tuberculous broncho-pneumonia or follow a chronic tuberculous pleurisy. In other instances the process supervenes upon an ordinary ulcerative phthisis. The disease becomes limited to one apex, the cavity is surrounded by layers of dense fibrous tissue, the pleura is thickened, and the lower lobe is gradually invaded by the sclerotic change. Ultimately a picture is produced little if at all different from the condition known as cirrhosis of the lungs. It may even be difficult to say that the process is tuberculous, but in advanced cases the bacilli are usually present in the walls of the cavity at the apex, or old, encapsulated caseous areas are present, or there may be tubercles at the apex of the other lung and in the bronchial glands. Dilatation of the bronchi is present; the right ventricle, sometimes the entire heart, is hypertrophied.

The disease is chronic, lasting from ten to twenty or more years, during which time the patient may have fair health. The chief symptoms are cough, often paroxysmal in character and most marked in the morning, and dyspnœa on exertion. The expectoration is purulent, and in some instances, when the bronchiectasis is extensive, fetid. There is rarely any fever.

The physical signs are very characteristic. The chest is sunken and the shoulder lower on the affected side; the heart is often drawn over and displaced. If the left lung is involved there may be an unusually large area of cardiac pulsation in the third, fourth, and fifth interspaces. Heart murmurs are common. There are dulness and deficient tactile fremitus over the affected side, except over cavities where the fremitus is increased. At the apex there may be well-marked cavernous sounds; at the base, distant bronchial breathing. In some cases the other lung becomes involved, or the patient has repeated attacks of hæmoptysis, in one of which he dies. As a result of the chronic suppuration, amyloid degeneration of the liver, spleen, and intestines may take place; dropsy frequently supervenes from failure of the right heart.

A more detailed account is found under Cirrhosis of the Lung, with which this form is clinically identical.

Complications of Pulmonary Tuberculosis

In the Respiratory System.—The larynx is rarely spared in chronic pulmonary tuberculosis. The first symptom may be huskiness of the voice. There are pain, particularly in swallowing, and a cough which is often wheezing, and in the later stages very ineffectual. Aphonia and dysphagia are the two most distressing symptoms of the laryngeal involvement. When the epiglottis is seriously diseased and the ulceration extends to the lateral wall of the pharynx, the pain in swallowing may be very intense, or, owing to the imperfect closure of the glottis, there may be coughing spells and regurgitation of food through the nostrils. Bronchitis and tracheitis are almost invariable accompaniments.

Pneumonia is a not infrequent complication of pulmonary tuberculosis. It may run a perfectly normal course, while in other instances resolution may be delayed, and one is in doubt, in spite of the abruptness of the onset, as to the presence of a simple or a tuberculous pneumonia. In some cases a pneumonia is a terminal complication.

Emphysema of the uninvolved portions of the lung is a common feature, rarely producing any special symptoms. There are, however, cases of chronic tuberculosis in which emphysema dominates the picture, and in which the condition comes on slowly during a period of many years. (General subcutaneous emphysema, which has been met with in a few rare cases, is due either to perforation of the trachea or to the rupture of a cavity adherent to the chest wall.)

Gangrene of the lung is an occasional event in chronic pulmonary tuberculosis, due in almost all instances to sphacelus in the walls of the cavity, rarely in the lung-tissue itself.

Complications in the Pleura.—A dry pleurisy is a very common accompaniment of the early stages of tuberculosis. It is always a conservative, useful process. In some cases it is very extensive, and friction murmurs may be heard over the sides and back. The cases with dry pleurisy and adhesions are, of course, much less liable to the dangers of pneumothorax. Pleurisy with effusion more commonly precedes than occurs in the course of pulmonary tuberculosis. Still, it is common enough to meet with cases in which a sero-fibrinous effusion arises in the course of the chronic disease. There are cases in which it is a special feature, and it often, I think, favors chronicity. A patient may during a period of four or five years have signs of local disease at one apex with recurring effusion in the same side. Owing to adhesions in different parts of the pleura, the effusion may be encapsulated. Hæmorrhagic effusions, which are not uncommon in connection with tuberculous pleurisy, are comparatively rare in chronic phthisis. Chyliform or milky exudates are sometimes found. Purulent effusions are not frequent apart from pneumothorax. An empyema, however, may occur in the course of the disease or as a sequence of a sero-fibrinous exudate. *Pneumothorax* is an extremely common complication. Of 49 cases at the Johns Hopkins Hospital, 23 were tuberculous (Emerson). It may prove fatal in twenty-four hours. In other instances a pyo-pneumothorax follows and the patient lingers for weeks or months. In a third group of cases it seems to have a beneficial effect on the course of the disease, and is sometimes produced for the therapeutic effect.

Symptoms Referable to the Other Organs.—(*a*) *Cardio-vascular.*—The retraction of the left upper lobe exposes a large area of the heart. In thin-chested subjects there may be pulsation in the second, third, and fourth interspaces close to the sternum. Sometimes with much retraction of the left upper lobe the heart is drawn up. A systolic murmur over the pulmonary area and in the subclavian arteries is common in all stages of phthisis. Apical murmurs are also not infrequent and may be extremely rough and harsh without necessarily indicating that endocarditis is present. The association of heart disease with phthisis is not, however, very uncommon. As already mentioned, there were 12 instances of endocarditis in 216 autopsies. The arterial tension is usually low and the capillary resistance lessened so that the pulse is often full and soft even in the later stages of the disease. The capillary pulse is not infrequently found, and pulsation of the veins in the back of the hand is occasionally seen.

(*b*) *Blood Glandular System.*—The early anæmia has already been noted. It is often more apparent than real, a chloro-anæmia, and the blood-count rarely sinks below two millions per cubic millimetre.

The blood-plates are, as a rule, enormously increased and are seen in the withdrawn blood as the so-called Schultze's granule masses. Without any significance, they are of interest chiefly from the fact that every few years some tyro announces their discovery as a new diagnostic sign of tuberculosis. The leucocytes are greatly increased, particularly in the later stages.

(*c*) *Gastro-intestinal System.*—The tongue is usually furred, but may be clean and red. Small aphthous ulcers are sometimes distressing. A red line on the gums, a symptom to which at one time much attention was paid as a special feature of phthisis, occurs in other cachectic states. Extensive tuberculous disease of the pharynx, associated with a similar affection of the larynx, may interfere seriously with deglutition and prove a very distressing and intractable symptom. The saliva has very full digestive powers.

Tuberculosis of the stomach is rare. Ulceration may occur as an accidental complication and multiple catarrhal ulcers are not uncommon. Interstitial and parenchymatous changes in the mucosa are common (possibly associated with the venous stasis) and lead to atrophy, but these cannot always be connected with the symptoms, and they may be found when not expected. On the other hand, when the gastric symptoms have been most persistent the mucosa may show very little change. It is impossible always to refer the anorexia, nausea, and vomiting of consumption to local conditions. The hectic fever and the neurotic influences, upon which Immermann lays much stress, must be taken into account, as they play an important rôle. The organ is often dilated, and to muscular insufficiency alone may be due some of the cases of dyspepsia. The condition of the gastric secretion is not constant, and the reports are discordant. In the early stages there may be superacidity; later, a deficiency of acid.

Anorexia is often a marked symptom at the onset; there may be positive loathing for food, and even small quantities cause nausea. Sometimes, without any nausea or distress after eating, the feeding of the patient is a daily battle. When practicable, Debove's forced alimentation is of great benefit in such cases. Nausea and vomiting, though occasionally troublesome at an early period, are more marked in the later stages. The latter may be caused by the severe attacks of coughing. S. H. Habershon refers to four different causes of the vomiting in phthisis: (1) central, as from tuberculous meningitis; (2) pressure on the vagi by caseous glands; (3) stimulation from the peripheral branches of the vagus, either pulmonary, pharyngeal, or gastric; and (4) mechanical causes.

Of the *intestinal* symptoms diarrhœa is the most serious. It may come on early, but is more usually a symptom of the later stages, and is associated with ulceration, particularly of the large bowel. Extensive ulceration of the ileum may exist without any diarrhœa. The associated catarrhal condition may account in part for it, and in some instances the amyloid degeneration of the mucous membrane. Perforation occurred in 13 of 475 autopsies in chronic pulmonary tuberculosis.

(*d*) *Nervous System.*—(1) Focal lesions due to the development of coarse tubercles and areas of tuberculous meningo-encephalitis. Aphasia, for instance, may result from the growth of meningeal tubercles in the fissure of Sylvius, or even hemiplegia may occur. The solitary tubercles are more common in the chronic phthisis of children. (2) Basilar meningitis is an occasional complication. It may be confined to the brain, though more commonly it is a (3) cerebro-spinal meningitis, which may come on in persons without well-marked local signs in the chest. Twice have I known strong, robust men brought into hospital with signs of cerebro-spinal meningitis, in whom the existence of pulmonary disease was not discovered until the post mortem. (4) *Peripheral neuritis,* which is not common, may cause an extensor paralysis of the arm or leg, more commonly the latter, with foot-drop. It is usually a late manifestation. (5) Mental symptoms. It was noted, even by the older writers, that consumptives had a peculiarly hopeful temperament, and the *spes phthisica* forms a curious characteristic of the disease. Patients with extensive cavities, high fever, and too weak to move will often make plans for the future and confidently expect to recover.

Apart from tuberculosis of the brain, there is sometimes in chronic phthisis a form of insanity not unlike that which occurs in the canvalescence from acute affections.

(*e*) A remarkable *hypertrophy of the mammary gland* may occur in pulmonary tuberculosis, most commonly in males. It may be only on the affected side. It is a chronic interstitial, non-tuberculous mammitis (Allot). Mastitis adolescentium, not very uncommon, is not necessarily suggestive of pulmonary tuberculosis.

(*f*) *Genito-urinary System.*—The urine presents no special peculiarities in amount or constituents. Fever, however, has a marked influence upon it. Albumin is met with frequently and may be associated with the fever, or is the result of definite changes in the kidneys. In the latter case it is more abundant and more curd like. Amyloid disease of the kidneys is not uncommon. Its presence is shown by albumin and tube casts, and sometimes by a great increase in the amount of urine. In other instances there is dropsy, and the patients have all the characteristic features of chronic Bright's disease.

Pus in the urine may be due to disease of the bladder or of the pelves of the kidneys. In some instances the entire urinary tract is involved. In pulmonary phthisis, however, extensive tuberculous disease is rarely found in the urinary organs. Bacilli may occasionally be detected in the pus. Hæmaturia is not a very common symptom. It may occur occasionally as a result of congestion of the kidneys, and pass off, leaving the urine albuminous. In other instances it results from disease of the pelvis or of the bladder, and is associated either with early tuberculosis of the mucous membranes or more commonly with ulceration. In a medical clinic the routine inspection of the testes for tubercle will save two or three mistakes a year.

(*g*) *Cutaneous System.*—The skin is often dry and harsh. Local tubercles occasionally occur on the hands. There may be pigmentary staining, the *chloasma phthisicorum,* which is more common when the peritoneum is involved. Upon the chest and back the brown stains of *pityriasis versicolor* are very frequent. The hair of the head and beard may become dry and lanky. The terminal phalanges, in chronic cases, become clubbed and the nails incurvated—the Hippocratic fingers. Landouzy has called attention to a curious bending, usually of the ring and little fingers, which permits of flexion, but not of extension—a condition which he calls camptodactaly. A remarkable and unusual complication is general emphysema, which may result from ulceration of an adherent lung or perforation of the larynx.

Diagnosis of Pulmonary Tuberculosis.

With fever, well-marked physical signs and bacilli in the sputum, no disease is more easily diagnosed than pulmonary tuberculosis. Successful treatment depends largely upon early diagnosis, and special attention must be paid to the obscure, variable, and uncertain symptoms and signs of the initial stage. The active crusade against the disease has made both the public and the profession more alert, and we have, as so often happens, gone to an extreme, and are apt to see early tuberculosis in trivial complaints. I say this from an experience of cases seen in consultation, and it is borne out by the records of institutions. Hamman, in charge of the Phipps Tuberculosis Dispensary of the Johns Hopkins Hospital, makes the interesting confession that in the early days, when they depended on slight physical signs and the tuberculin reaction, there were innumerable early cases, but with a wider experience and greater confidence in clinical symptoms the outlook on these borderland cases has changed completely, and now, instead of condemning them peremptorily to a sanatorium, they are found to keep well under the ordinary conditions of life, in spite of the persistence of slight abnormal signs. How important this feature of tuberculosis work has become is also indicated by the figures for the first year at the Tuberculosis Dispensary of the Radcliffe Infirmary. Of the 580 cases, all sent by physicians, 243 were found not to be tuberculous! One lesson from the work of the past few years is that we should pay more attention to symptoms than to physical signs. The following are the points of special importance in the diagnosis of early cases:

History.—Tuberculosis in the family, "Phthisical habitus," unusual exposure, special debilitating circumstances, as worry, grief, dissipation, or a chronic illness.

Symptoms.—Loss of weight, loss of strength, and anæmia, if progressive and not to be accounted for by mental worries or prolonged indigestion, are of first importance. Fever is at once a most trustworthy and the most fallacious symptom. The thermometer has needlessly condemned many patients to the sanatorium. Regard should be had to the points already mentioned in speaking of the fever. In nervous persons, particularly in stout, flabby young girls, a temperature from 99.5° to 100.5° may mean nothing, and the rectal temperature is often very deceptive: if taken after exercise or excitement it may be a degree and a half above normal. In the case of a flabby, fat girl of ten, with an anxious mother, a foolish nurse, and an alarmist doctor, for months the rectal temperature was taken hourly during the day; the child had been in bed; there was no cough, and the only physical sign a few rustling râles at one apex. The *cure* followed rapidly on the breaking of the thermometer and getting rid of the nurse. In a suspicious case a two-hour temperature record should be taken during the day for ten days and the influence of exercise upon it carefully estimated.

A cough is always suspicious in the young, more in the winter than in the summer, and more in the morning than at other times in the day. Throat conditions should be carefully excluded, particularly the irritation from cigarette smoking. The spitting of blood has already been considered sufficiently, and its importance in the diagnosis of tuberculosis is universally recognised. A brisk, early hæmoptysis is often helpful, not only for the positive information it gives us, but for its useful moral effect on the patient. The greater the care with which the bloody sputum is examined the more likely will it be that bacilli are found.

Sputum.—The patient should be instructed to collect what is expectorated, particularly early in the morning, and everything brought up should be sent. The difficulty in private practice is that it requires a long series of examinations to exclude positively the presence of tubercle bacilli. Time and again with suspicious cases, or in pleurisy with effusion, I have asked a clinical clerk day by day "Any bacilli yet?", and in one instance there were none found until the twentieth examination! Of course, in private practice this is impossible, but it is well to bear in mind that one or two negative examinations are not sufficient. Various methods of digesting the sputum and examining the centrifugalized sediment are important when few bacilli are present. The antiformin method introduced by Uhlenhuth is simple and often reveals tubercle bacilli missed by an ordinary examination.

Physical Signs.—These raise the difficulty. At present, so far as the lungs are concerned, the position resembles that of twenty-five years ago in respect to the heart, when any murmur was regarded as serious. Now, if we see the apex beat within the nipple line and there is no shortness of breath, and the pulse is regular, we discount physical signs and tell the patient to live a rational life. This is what we should do with many cases of suspected early tuberculosis. If the symptoms above dealt with are not present, "discount" the physical signs. These have already been considered: change in the character of the respiratory murmur and the presence of râles are the two most important, as dulness is rarely present in early cases. Altogether too much stress has been laid upon roughened or impure inspiration associated with a few dry râles. Only upon repeated examination should a decision be reached. Practically, in these early cases, we have two groups—the one with symptoms and no physical signs, and the other with physical signs and no symptoms. Of the two, the former is of the greater importance.

Specific Reaction.—*Tuberculin Test.*—The experience of hundreds of observers in different parts of the world testifies to the value of the Calmette and the von Pirquet tests. But we must remember the reaction simply means that the organism has developed a responsive activity to tuberculous infection, and it by no means indicates that an individual has tuberculous disease, in the ordinary sense of the term "disease." From the careful studies made at the Phipps Dispensary, the conjunctival test was found of the greater value in indicating the presence of an active lesion. The following conclusions reached by Hamman and his colleagues appear to be sane: "When a patient fails to react to either test, and there are no striking symptoms or physical signs of pulmonary disease, we feel that the negative diagnosis has received a valuable confirmation. If the eye reaction is positive, this is a strong indication that the patient has an active tuberculous focus; if symptoms and signs are present it is an important aid in excluding other pulmonary conditions; if they are absent it marks the patient as a suspect. * * * None of these tests can replace in the slightest degree a carefully taken history and a well-made examination. They can never stand censor over these; rather their value must ultimately be judged by them. They are aids and nothing more."

While the cutaneous and conjunctival are the more important as a routine procedure, still in special instances in which it is desired to elicit a focal reaction the subcutaneous tuberculin test is invaluable.

X-ray Diagnosis.—In skilful hands the study of cases with the Röntgen rays is of great value. In a normal case the radiogram shows a shadow beneath and extending beyond the sternum due to the contents of the mediastinum. Extending from the mediastinum and radiating out into the various lobes is a series of shadows which may be likened to the branches of a tree, the thickest shadow being at the hilus and thinning toward the periphery of the lungs. In diseased conditions changes are seen in the hilus, shadows due to enlarged or calcified glands and to the increase in the fibrous and lymphatic tissues in the mediastinum. The pulmonary vessels with their contained blood play an important part in the production of the shadow. A study made at the Phipps' Dispensary by Dunham, Boardman, and Wolman showed that in a very large percentage of all the early cases, clinically found to be tuberculosis, these shadows showed certain changes which corresponded to the clinical findings. It is not proved, however, that other pulmonary conditions, such as those produced by the influenza bacillus, may not cause the same changes. The X-rays undoubtedly show very early changes in the lungs, but they can not determine the etiological factor. In the majority of cases the X-rays tell no more than a careful clinical examination, and they do not differentiate an active from a healed lesion. More than any others, radiographers need the salutory lessons of the dead house to correct their visionary interpretations of shadows, particularly of those radiating from the roots of the lungs.

Concurrent Infections and Diseases Associated with Pulmonary Tuberculosis

Concurrent Infections in Pulmonary Tuberculosis.—It has long been known that in pulmonary tuberculosis organisms other than the specific bacilli are present, particularly *Micrococcus lanceolatus, Streptococcus pyogenes,* the influenza bacillus, *Micrococcus catarrhalis,* and *Staphylococcus aureus;* less frequently *Bacillus pyocyaneus.*

Many cases of pulmonary tuberculosis are combined infections; streptococci and pneumococci may be found in the sputum, and the former have been isolated from the blood. Prudden, who has very carefully studied this question, arrives at the following conclusions: The pulmonary lesions of tuberculosis are subject to variations depending largely on the different modes of distribution of the bacilli, whether by the blood vessels or through the bronchi, and also whether a concurrent infection with other organisms has taken place. The pneumonia complicating tuberculosis may be the direct result of the tubercle bacillus or its toxins, or it may follow secondary infection with other germs, particularly the *Streptococcus pyogenes,* the *Micrococcus lanceolatus,* and the *Staphylococcus pyogenes.* An infection with the influenza bacillus or *Micrococcus catarrhalis* may be followed by increased fever and an aggravation of the general symptoms. The frequency of these secondary infections and the relative significance of their germs are not yet fully decided. It is very probable that in man the effect of contamination with the pus organisms is a very important one in hastening necrosis and softening, and also in the chronic cases they doubtless produce in large amounts the toxins which are responsible for many of the symptoms of the disease. The work of Hastings indicates that secondary infections are not so important as we had thought, and a study by Radcliffe at the King Edward Sanatorium points in this direction.

Diseases Associated with Pulmonary Tuberculosis.—*Lobar pneumonia* is a not uncommon cause of death. It is met with, most frequently, indeed, as a terminal event in the chronic cases. It may, however, occur early, and be difficult to distinguish from an acute caseous pneumonia. The sputum in the latter is rarely rusty, while the fever in the former is more continuous and higher, but in many cases it is impossible to differentiate between the two conditions.

The association of tuberculosis and *typhoid fever* has already been discussed (page 32).

Erysipelas not infrequently attacks old *poitrinaires* in hospital wards and almshouses. There are instances in which the attack seems to be beneficial, as the cough lessens and the symptoms ameliorate. It may, however, prove fatal.

The *eruptive fevers,* particularly measles, frequently precede but rarely occur in the course of pulmonary tuberculosis. In the revaccination of a tuberculous subject the vesicles run a normal course.

Fistula in ano, so often associated with pulmonary tuberculosis, in a majority of such cases is a tuberculous process. The general affection may progress rapidly after an operation. The question is considered in tuberculosis of the alimentary canal.

Heart Disease.—Cardiac hypoplasia seems uncommon in tuberculosis, though it was much referred to by the older writers. It was present in only 3 cases in 1,764 autopsies on tuberculous patients (Norris). Rokitansky taught that there was an antagonism between valvular lesions and aneurisms and tuberculosis. All forms of congenital heart disease predispose to it, particularly stenosis of the pulmonary artery. Mitral stenosis, on the other hand, has a distinctly inhibitory influence. The two conditions are rarely found associated. Endocarditis has already been referred to. A terminal acute tuberculosis, particularly of the serous membranes, is not at all uncommon in cardio-vascular diseases.

In chronic and arrested phthisis *arterio-sclerosis* and *phlebo-sclerosis* are not uncommon. Ormerod noted 30 cases of chronic renal disease in 100 post mortems.

The association of tuberculosis with *chronic arthritis,* upon which certain writers lay stress, finds its explanation in the lowered resistance of these patients and the greater liability to infection in the institutions in which so many of them live.

Peculiarities of Pulmonary Tuberculosis at the Extremes of Life

Old Age.—It is remarkable how common tuberculosis is in the aged, particularly in institutions. McLachlan noted 145 cases in which tuberculosis was the cause of death in old persons in Chelsea Hospital. All were over sixty years of age. The experience at the Salpêtrière is the same. Laennec met with a case in a person over ninety-nine years of age.

At the Philadelphia Hospital, in the bodies of aged persons sent over from the almshouse, it was extremely common to find either old or recent tuberculosis. A patient died under my care at the age of eighty-two with extensive peritoneal tuberculosis. Pulmonary tuberculosis in the aged is usually latent and runs a slow course. The physical signs are often masked by emphysema and by the coëxisting chronic bronchitis. The diagnosis may depend entirely upon the discovery of the bacilli and elastic tissue. Contrary to the opinion which was held some years ago, tuberculosis is by no means uncommon with senile emphysema. Some of the cases of tuberculosis in the aged are instances of quiescent disease which may have dated from an early period.

Infancy.—The occurrence of acute tuberculosis in children has already been mentioned, and also the fact that the disease is occasionally congenital. The incidence is very variable, from 13 to 42 per cent. in collected statistics. In Wollstein's study from the New York Babies' Hospital, among 1,131 autopsies in children under four years of age, in 192 tuberculosis was present; the percentage was: first year 1.8 per cent., second year 11 per cent., third year 16 per cent., and fourth year 23 per cent. Chronic ulcerative tuberculosis of the lungs is much more rare than in adults. In Parrot's series of 219 cases in children under three years of age, in only 57 were cavities found in the lungs.

Modes of Death in Pulmonary Tuberculosis

(a) By asthenia, a gradual failure of the strength. The end is usually peaceable and quiet, occasionally disturbed by paroxysms of cough. Consciousness is often retained until near the close.

(b) By asphyxia, as in some cases of acute miliary tuberculosis and in acute pneumonic phthisis. In chronic phthisis it is rarely seen, even when pneumothorax develops.

(c) By syncope. This is not common. I have known it to happen once or twice in patients who insisted upon going about when in the advanced stages of the disease. There may be, but not necessarily, fatty degeneration of the heart. Rapid syncope may follow hæmorrhage or may be due to thrombosis or embolism of the pulmonary artery, or to pneumothorax.

(d) From hæmorrhage. The fatal bleeding in chronic phthisis is due to erosion of a large vessel or rupture of an aneurism in a pulmonary cavity, most commonly the latter. Of 26 cases analyzed by S. West, in 11 the fatal hæmoptysis was due to aneurism, and, of 35 cases collected by Percy Kidd, aneurism was present in 30. In a case of Curtin's, at the Philadelphia Hospital, the bleeding proved fatal before hæmoptysis occurred, as the eroded vessel opened into a capacious cavity.

(e) With cerebral symptoms. Coma may be due to meningitis, less often to uræmia. Death in convulsions is rare. The hæmorrhagic pachy-meningitis which occurs in some cases of phthisis occasionally causes loss of consciousness, but is rarely a direct cause of death. In one of my cases death resulted from thrombosis of the cerebral sinuses with symptoms of meningitis.

V. TUBERCULOSIS OF THE ALIMENTARY CANAL

(a) Lips.—Tuberculosis of the lip is very rare. It occurs occasionally in the form of an ulcer, either alone or more commonly in association with laryngeal or pulmonary disease. The ulcer is usually very sensitive and may be mistaken for a chancre or an epithelioma. The diagnosis may be made in cases of doubt by inoculation or the examination of a portion for tubercle bacilli.

(b) Tongue.—The disease begins by an aggregation of small granular bodies on the edge or dorsum. Ulceration proceeds, leaving an irregular sore with a distinct but uneven margin, and a rough, often caseous base. The disease extends slowly and may form an ulcer of considerable size. I have known it to be mistaken for epithelioma and the tongue to be excised. It is rarely met with except when other organs are involved. The glands of the angle of the jaw are not enlarged and the sore does not yield to iodide of potassium, which are points of distinction between the tuberculous and the syphilitic ulcer. In doubtful cases the inoculation test should be made, or a portion excised for microscopic examination.

(c) Salivary Glands.—The salivary glands belong to that small group of organs of the body which seem to possess an immunity; a very few cases have been reported.

(d) Palate.—Tubercles of the hard or soft palate nearly always follow extension of the disease from neighboring parts.

(e) Tuberculosis of the Tonsils.—In 7 of 45 consecutive cases in children from three months to fifteen years, A. Latham demonstrated, by inoculation, the presence of tuberculosis of the tonsils either in organs removed by operation or post mortem. The observation is of interest in connection with the views of Schlenker, who claims that the majority of the cases of tuberculous cervical glands result from infection with tubercle bacilli which gain admission by way of the tonsil. A large number of his cases of tuberculous cervical adenitis were definitely of a descending variety and associated with tuberculosis of these glands. The majority also had pulmonary tuberculosis, and he regards surface infection of the tonsil by tuberculous food and sputum far more common than infection by way of the circulation. The disease may occur as a superficial ulceration. More commonly there is an infiltration of the tonsil with miliary tubercles, which produces a greater or less hypertrophy which it is practically impossible to distinguish from an ordinary enlargement of the tonsil without a microscopic examination.

(f) Pharynx.—In extensive laryngeal tuberculosis an eruption of miliary granules on the posterior wall of the pharynx is not very uncommon. In chronic phthisis an ulcerative pharyngitis, due to extension of the disease from the epiglottis and larynx, is one of the most distressing of complications, rendering deglutition acutely painful. Adenoids of the naso-pharynx may be tuberculous, as shown by Lermoyez. Macroscopically, they do not differ from the ordinary vegetations found in this situation.

(g) Œsophagus.—A few instances occur in the literature of tuberculosis of the œsophagus. The condition is a pathological curiosity, except in the slight extension from the larynx, which is not infrequent; but in a case in my wards, described by Flexner, the ulcer perforated and caused purulent pleurisy. The condition has been fully considered by Claribel Cone, who has described a second case from the Johns Hopkins Hospital (Bulletin, November, 1897).

(h) Stomach.—Many cases are reported which are doubtful. Primary disease is unknown. Perforation of the stomach occurred six times in the 12 cases collected by Marfan, thrice by a tuberculous gland. In Oppolzer's case an ulcer of the colon perforated the organ. In Musser's case there was a large tuberculous ulcer 3 by 1½ inches in extent. Three cases have been described from my wards by Alice Hamilton (J. H. H. Bulletin, April, 1897).

(i) Intestines.—The tubercles may be (1) primary in the mucous membrane, or more commonly (2) secondary to disease of the lungs, or in rare cases the affection may (3) pass from the peritoneum.

(1) Primary intestinal tuberculosis occurs most frequently in children, in whom it may be associated with enlargement and caseation of the mesenteric glands, or with peritonitis. As stated, there is great discrepancy in the statistics on this point, and the question needs careful study. Biedert gives 16 cases in 3,104 instances of tuberculosis in children. In adults primary intestinal tuberculosis is rare, occurring in but 1 instance in 1,000 autopsies upon tuberculous adults at the Munich Pathological Institute; but now and then cases occur in which the disease sets in with irregular diarrhœa, moderate fever, and colicky pains. In a few cases hæmorrhage has been the initial symptom. Regarded at first as a chronic catarrh, it is not until the emaciation becomes marked or the signs of disease appear in the lungs that the true nature is apparent. Still more deceptive are the cases in which the tuberculosis begins in the cæcum and there are symptoms of appendicitis—tenderness in the right iliac fossa, constipation, or an irregular diarrhœa and fever. These signs may gradually disappear, to recur again in a few weeks and still further complicate the diagnosis. Fatal hæmorrhage has occurred in several of my cases. Perforation may occur with the formation of a pericæcal abscess, or perforation into the peritoneum may take place, or in very rare instances there is partial healing with great thickening of the walls and narrowing of the lumen.

(2) Secondary involvement of the bowels is very common in chronic pulmonary tuberculosis, *e. g.*, in 566 of the 1,000 Munich autopsies in tuberculosis just referred to. In only three of these cases were the lungs not involved. The lesions are chiefly in the ileum, cæcum, and colon. The affection begins in the solitary and agminated glands, or on the surface of or within the mucosa. The caseation and necrosis lead to ulceration, which may be very extensive and involve the greater portion of the mucosa of the large and small bowels. In the ileum the Peyer's patches are chiefly involved and the ulcers may be ovoid, but in the jejunum and colon they are usually round or transverse to the long axis. The tuberculous ulcer has the following characters: (*a*) It is irregular, rarely ovoid or in the long axis, more

frequently girdling the bowel; (*b*) the edges and base are infiltrated, often caseous; (*c*) the submucosa and muscularis are usually involved; and (*d*) on the serosa may be seen colonies of young tubercles or a well-marked tuberculous lymphangitis. Perforation and peritonitis are not uncommon events in the secondary ulceration. Stenosis of the bowel from cicatrization may occur; the strictures may be multiple.

Localized chronic tuberculosis of the *ileo-cæcal region* is of great importance. The cæcum may present a chronic hyperplastic tuberculosis, which not uncommonly extends into the appendix. As a consequence of the changes produced a definite tumor-like mass is formed in the right iliac fossa. This varies in size, is usually elongated in a vertical direction, hard, slightly movable, or bound down by adhesions and very sensitive to pressure. The tumor simulates more or less closely a true neoplasm of this region, particularly carcinoma. The condition is characterized by gradual constriction of the lumen of the bowel, periodic attacks of severe pain, and alternating diarrhœa and constipation. The extremely localized character of the disease warrants an exploratory operation, as the results of enterectomy are remarkably favorable. Of 11 cases reported by F. M. Caird, 7 recovered. In a second form of this disease, occurring less frequently than the former, there is no definite tumor mass to be felt, but a general induration and thickening in the right iliac fossa similar to the local changes produced by a recurring appendicitis. In this variety a fistula discharging fæcal matter occasionally results. Both forms may be distinguished from the diseases they simulate by the finding of tubercle bacilli in the stools or in the discharge from the fistula when such exists.

Tuberculosis of the *rectum* has a special interest in connection with *fistula in ano,* which occurs in about 3.5 per cent. of cases of pulmonary disease. In many instances the lesion has been shown to be tuberculous. It is very rarely primary, but if the tissue on removal contains bacilli and is infective the lungs are almost invariably found to be involved. It is a common opinion that the pulmonary symptoms progress rapidly after the fistula is cut. This may have some basis if the operation consists in laying the tract open, and not in a free excision.

(3) Extension from the peritoneum may excite tuberculous disease in the bowels. The affection may be primary in the peritoneum or extend from the tubes in women or the mesenteric glands in children. The coils of intestines become matted together, caseous and suppurating foci develop between the folds, and perforation may take place between the coils.

VI. TUBERCULOSIS OF THE LIVER

This organ is very constantly involved in (*a*) *Miliary tuberculosis.* This is seen in acute generalized tuberculosis, though the granules may be small and have to be looked for very carefully. In chronic tuberculosis miliary tubercles are not at all uncommon in the liver. (*b*) *Solitary tubercle.* Occasionally large tuberculous masses are found in the organ, sometimes associated with perihepatitis, sometimes with tuberculous peritonitis, and in children with tuberculous adenitis. In a few cases the masses are very large, though it is only in exceptional cases that the tumor can be felt through the abdominal wall. The organ may be enlarged by numerous caseous masses and present the clinical picture of an enlarged rough tender liver with jaundice, as in a case reported by Thayer. The solitary tubercles become infected with pus organisms, soften, and form an abscess. (*c*) *Tuberculosis of the bile ducts.* This is by far the most characteristic tuberculous change in the organ, and is not uncommon. It was well described by Bristowe in 1858. The liver is enlarged, and section shows numerous small cavities, which look at first like multiple abscesses in suppurative pylephlebitis, but the pus is bile-stained and the whole process is a local tuberculous cholangitis. (*d*) *Tuberculous cirrhosis.* With the eruption of miliary tubercles there may be slight increase in the connective tissue, which is overshadowed by the fatty change. In all the chronic forms of tubercle in this organ there may be fibrous overgrowth. Hanot, who has described several varieties, states that the condition may be primary. Practically it is very rare, except in connection with chronic tuberculous peritonitis and perihepatitis, when the organ may be much deformed by a sclerosis involving the portal canals and the capsule, which may be greatly involved in a polyserositis.

VII. TUBERCULOSIS OF THE BRAIN AND CORD

Tuberculosis of the *brain* occurs as (*a*) an acute miliary infection causing meningitis and acute hydrocephalus; (*b*) as a chronic meningo-encephalitis, usually localized, and containing small nodular tubercles; and (*c*) as the so-called solitary tubercle. Between the last two forms there are all gradations, and it is rare to see the meninges uninvolved. The acute variety has already been considered. I shall here consider the chronic form, which comes on slowly and has the clinical characters of a tumor.

It is most common in the young. Of 148 cases collected by Pribram 118 were under fifteen years of age. Other organs are usually involved, particularly the lungs, the bronchial glands, or the bones. In rare instances no tubercles are found elsewhere. They occur most frequently in the cerebellum; next in the cerebrum, and then in the pons. The growths are often multiple, in 100 out of 183 cases (Gowers). They range in size from a pea to a walnut; large tumors occasionally occur, and sometimes an entire lobe of the cerebellum is affected. On section the tubercle presents a grayish-yellow, caseous appearance, usually firm and hard, and encircled by a translucent, softer tissue. The centre of the growth may be semi-diffluent. As in other localities the tubercle may calcify. The tumors are as a rule attached to the meninges, often to the pia at the bottom of a sulcus so that they look imbedded in the brain-substance. About the longitudinal fissure there may be an aggregation of the growths, with compression of the sinus, and the formation of a thrombus. The tuberculous tumor not infrequently excites acute meningitis. In localized meningo-encephalitis the pia is thickened, tubercles are adherent to the under surface and grow about the arteries. It is often combined with cerebral softening from interference with the circulation. Several of the most characteristic instances which I have seen were on the meninges covering the insula. This form may occur in pulmonary tuberculosis, causing hemiplegia or aphasia which may persist for months.

The symptoms of tuberculous growths in the brain are those of tumor, and will be considered in the section on the brain.

In the *spinal cord* the same forms are found. The acute tuberculous meningitis has been considered and is almost always cerebro-spinal. The solitary tubercle of the cord is rare. Herter reported 3 cases and collected 24 from the literature. It was secondary in all save one case. The symptoms are those of spinal tumor or meningitis.

VIII. TUBERCULOSIS OF THE GENITO-URINARY SYSTEM

The studies of the past few years, and particularly the work of surgeons and gynæcologists, have taught us the great importance of tuberculosis of this tract. Any part of the genito-urinary system may be invaded. The successive involvement of the organs may be so rapid that unless the case has been seen early it may be impossible to state with any degree of certainty which has been the primary seat of infection. There may be simultaneous involvement of various portions of the tract. In tuberculosis of the genito-urinary system one always has to bear in mind the possibility of latent disease elsewhere in the body. As Bollinger says, tubercle bacilli may gain admission at some part of the respiratory tract without producing any lesion at the point of entrance, and finally reach a bronchial gland, where they set up a tuberculous process of extremely slow development without producing any symptoms. From this point bacilli may enter the blood stream and lodge in the epididymis or testicle proper, and produce nodules which are readily discovered owing to the ease with which these parts are examined. Such a case might be quite easily mistaken for one of primary genital tuberculosis, whereas the true primary tuberculous focus is far distant.

Infection of the genito-urinary tract occurs in various ways:

(*a*) By Hereditary Transmission.—It has been met with in the fetus. The comparative frequency of tuberculosis of the testicle in very young children suggests very strongly that the uro-genital organs may be involved as a result of direct transmission of the disease.

(*b*) By Infection from Areas of Tuberculosis Already Existing in the Patient.—(1) *Infection through the Blood.*—In many cases uro-genital tuberculosis is found at autopsy associated with disease of some distant organ, particularly the lungs, and it would appear most probable that in them infection has been through the blood-vessels. Jani's observations, which were published by Weigert after the author's death, strongly support this theory. In studying sections of the genital organs of patients who died of pulmonary tuberculosis, he found tubercle bacilli in 5 out of 8 cases in the testicle, and in 4 out of 6 cases in the prostate, without in any instance finding microscopic evidences of tubercles in these organs. The bacilli lay, in the testis, partly within and partly close beside the cellular and granular contents of the seminal tubules, while in the prostate they were always situated in the neighborhood of the glandular epithelium.

(2) *Infection from the Peritoneum.*—This source of infection, in both men and women, is much more frequent than is commonly supposed. The intimate relationship between the peritoneum and bladder in both sexes, and with the vesiculæ seminales and vasa deferentia in the male, allows a ready way of invasion of these organs by direct extension of the disease. The peritoneum is a frequent source of genital tuberculosis in the female. No

doubt many cases of tuberculosis of the Fallopian tubes originate from this source. The fact that the fimbriated extremity of the tube is often most seriously involved points rather strongly in this direction, although the fact might be taken as a point in favor of blood infection, favored by its greater vascularity. Various observations go to show that the action of the cilia lining the lumina of the Fallopian tubes tends to attract particles introduced into the peritoneal cavity. Jani's observation is very interesting in this connection, as showing the possibility of tubercle bacilli entering the tubes from the peritoneal cavity without there being any tuberculous peritonitis. He found typical tubercle bacilli in the lumen, in sections of a normal Fallopian tube, in a woman who died of pulmonary and intestinal tuberculosis. The explanation advanced was that the bacilli made their way through the thin peritoneal coat from one of the intestinal ulcers, thus reaching the peritoneal cavity, and thence were attracted into the Fallopian tube by the current produced by the action of the cilia lining the lumen. The intimate relationship between tuberculous peritonitis and tuberculosis of the Fallopian tubes is shown in the fact that the latter are affected in from 30 to 40 per cent. of the cases.

(3) *Infection from Other Organs by Direct Extension.*—The occurrence of direct extension from the peritoneum has already been mentioned. In tuberculous ulceration of the intestine or rectum adhesions to the bladder in the male or to the uterus and vagina in the female may occur, with resulting fistulæ and a direct extension of the disease. Perirectal tuberculous abscesses may lead to secondary involvement of some portion of the genito-urinary tract. It must not be forgotten that tuberculosis of the vertebræ may be followed by tuberculosis of the kidney as a result of direct extension of the disease.

(*c*) By Infection from Without.—Whether uro-genital tuberculosis may occur as a result of the entrance of tubercle bacilli into the urethra or vagina is still a disputed question. That bacilli gain admission to these passages during coitus with a person the subject of uro-genital tuberculosis, or by the use of foul instruments or syringes, seems quite probable. The possibility of genital tuberculosis occurring in the female as a result of coitus with a male the subject of tuberculosis in some portion of the genito-urinary system was first suggested by Cohnheim, who stated, however, that it rarely, if ever, occurred.

In a patient with intestinal tuberculosis the tubercle bacilli might accidentally reach the urethra or vagina from the rectum.

Uro-genital tuberculosis is commonest between the ages of twenty and forty years—that is, during the period of greatest sexual activity. Males are affected much more frequently than females, the proportion being 3 to 1. This great difference is no doubt partly due to the more intimate relationship between the urinary and genital systems in the former than in the latter. In the male the urethra forms the common outlet for the two systems, while in the female there is a separate outlet for each.

Once the uro-genital tract has been invaded the disease is likely to spread rapidly, and the method of extension is an important one. Frequently there is direct extension, as when the bladder is involved secondarily to the kidney by passage of the disease along the ureter, or where the tuberculous process extends along the vas deferens to the vesiculæ seminales. No doubt surface inoculation occurs in some instances, and to this cause may be attributed a certain percentage of cases of vesical and prostatic disease following tuberculosis of the kidney. Although this probability is acknowledged, there is an element of doubt as to the possibility of the kidney becoming affected secondarily to the bladder or prostate by the direct passage of the bacilli up the lumen of one ureter; for in such a case we have to suppose that a nonmotile bacillus, contrary to the laws of gravity, ascends against an almost constant current of urine flowing in the opposite direction. The lymphatics may afford a means for the spreading of the disease, but in a greater number of cases than is generally supposed it takes place by way of the blood-vessels. Cystoscopic examinations of the bladder not infrequently show the presence of tubercles beneath the mucous membrane before there is any evidence of superficial ulceration—a fact suggesting strongly a blood infection.

The discovery of tubercle bacilli in the urine and the obtaining of tuberculous lesions in animals as a result of inoculation with the urinary sediment afford us the only positive evidence of genito-urinary tuberculosis. So far there are no authentic accounts of tubercle bacilli having been found in the semen of men with tuberculosis of the testicle or vesiculæ seminales. Owing to the fact that the smegma bacillus has the same staining reaction as the tubercle bacillus, and, morphologically is practically indistinguishable from it, the greatest care must be used in obtaining the specimen of urine for examination, to eliminate, if possible, all chances of contamination. Thus the urine examined must be a catheterized specimen, and even then one runs the risk of carrying back into the bladder on the end of the catheter a few bacilli which may be washed out in the stream of urine and be mistaken for tubercle bacilli in the sediment. One or more guinea-pigs should be inoculated with some of the suspected urine. If tubercle bacilli be present the animals will manifest tuberculous lesions in from three to five weeks.

Tuberculosis of the Kidneys (*Phthisis Renum*).—In general tuberculosis the kidneys frequently present scattered miliary tubercles. In pulmonary tuberculosis it is common to find a few nodules in the substance of the organ, or there may be pyelitis. In the first 17,000 admissions to the medical wards of the Johns Hopkins Hospital there were 1,085 cases of tuberculous infection. In 17 of these a clinical diagnosis of renal tuberculosis was made. Walker analyzed the first 1,369 autopsies in the same hospital and found that 784 had tuberculosis in some part of the body. In all there were 61 cases of renal tuberculosis. Of 482 cases of pulmonary tuberculosis showing symptoms during life, one or both kidneys were involved in 23. There were 36 cases of acute general miliary tuberculosis, and in every instance the kidney was affected. The 2 other cases of renal tuberculosis occurred in patients with latent disease. Primary tuberculosis of the kidneys is not very rare, but in no instance in the above series did Walker demonstrate a primary infection in the kidney. The tuberculous process was primary in some other part of the genito-urinary tract in 6 cases. In a majority of the cases the process involves the pelvis and the ureter as well, sometimes the bladder and prostate. It may be difficult to say in advanced cases whether the disease has started in the bladder, prostate, or vesicles, and crept up the ureters, or whether it started in the kidneys and proceeded downward. In a majority of cases, I believe, the latter is true, and the infection is through the blood. Walker thinks that a hæmatogenous infection takes place in 90 per cent. of the cases, and that this is the channel of infection in the majority of instances where renal follows vesical tuberculosis rather than along the ureter. One kidney alone may be involved, and the disease creeps down the ureter and may only extend a few millimetres on the vesical mucosa. A man with aortic insufficiency, who had no lesions in the lungs, presented a localized patch in the pelvis of the kidney, involving a pyramid, while the ureter, 5 cm. from the bladder and at its orifice, was thickened and tuberculous. The prostate showed an area of caseation. The process is most common between twenty and thirty years of age, but it may occur at the extremes of age. In a series of 386 cases collected by Walker in which the sex was stated 182 of the patients were males and 204 females. In the earliest stage, which may be met with accidentally, the disease is seen to begin in the pyramids and calyces. Necrosis and caseation proceed rapidly, and the colonies of tubercles start throughout the pyramids and extend upon the mucous membrane of the pelvis. As a rule, from the outset it is a tuberculous pyo-nephrosis. The renal infection may result from direct extension of the disease from a tuberculous vertebra. It may be confined to one kidney, or progress more extensively in one than in the other. At autopsy both organs are usually found enlarged. In only 3 of the 61 autopsies previously referred to was the disease unilateral. One kidney may be completely destroyed and converted into a series of cysts containing cheesy substance—a form of kidney which the older writers called scrofulous. In the putty-like contents of these cysts lime salts may be deposited. In other instances the walls of the pelvis are thickened and cheesy, the pyramids eroded, and caseous nodules are scattered through the organ, even to the capsule, which may be thickened and adherent. The other organ is usually less affected, and shows only pyelitis or a superficial necrosis of one or two pyramids. The ureters are usually thickened and the mucous membrane ulcerated and caseous. Involvement of the bladder, vesiculæ seminales, and testes is not uncommon in males.

The SYMPTOMS are those of pyelitis. The urine may be purulent for years, and there may be little or no distress. Even before the bladder becomes involved micturition is frequent, and many instances are mistaken for cystitis. The frequent micturition is in part due to an initial polyuria, in part to reflex irritation, but chiefly to a non-tuberculous inflammation over the trigone of the bladder. It is usually the earliest and most constant symptom. Hæmaturia, of a mild grade, occurs at some time during the course of the disease in the majority of the cases. Dull, aching pain in the lumbar region on one side is frequently complained of and may be the first symptom. The condition is for many years compatible with fair health. The curability is shown by the accidental discovery of the so-called scrofulous kidney, converted into cysts containing a putty-like substance. In cases in which the disease becomes advanced and both organs are affected constitutional symptoms are more marked. There is irregular fever, with chills and loss of weight and strength. General tuberculosis is common. In only one of my cases were the lungs uninvolved. In a case at the Montreal General Hospital a cyst perforated and caused fatal peritonitis.

Physical examination may detect special tenderness on one side, or the kidney may be palpable in front on deep pressure; but tuberculous pyelonephritis seldom causes a large tumor. Occasionally the pelvis becomes enormously distended; but this is rare in comparison with its frequency in calculous pyelitis. The urine presents changes similar to those of ordinary calculous pyelitis—pus-cells, epithelium, and occasionally definite caseous masses. It is nearly always acid in reaction. Albumin is, of course, present. Tubercle bacilli may be demonstrated by the ordinary methods. Tube-casts are not often seen.

Diagnosis.—To distinguish the condition from calculous pyelitis is often difficult. Hæmorrhage may be present in both, though not nearly so frequently in the tuberculous disease. Functional hæmaturia, to which Senator has given the name *essential renal hæmaturia*, and Klemperer that of *angioneurotic renal hæmaturia*, has been a source of error in diagnosis and has led to surgical interference. In this condition it is highly probable that bleeding from the kidney can occur in the absence of any definite lesion of the organ, although Israel denies the existence of such an anomaly. The subcutaneous injection of phenolsulphonephthalein, introduced by Rowntree and Geraghty, is of value in determining the kidney affected and its functional capacity. The diagnosis rests on three points: (1) The detection of some focus of tuberculosis, as in the testis; (2) the presence of tubercle bacilli in the sediment; and (3) the use of tuberculin. The kidney involved is now easily determined by catheterizing the ureters.

Tuberculosis of the suprarenal capsules will be considered under Addison's Disease.

Tuberculosis of the Ureter and Bladder.—This rarely occurs as a primary affection, but is nearly always secondary to involvement of other parts, particularly the pelvis of the kidney. In the case of uro-genital tuberculosis, above mentioned, in a patient who died of heart-disease, the ureter, just where it entered the bladder, showed a fresh patch of tuberculosis.

Protracted cystitis which has come on without apparent cause is always suggestive of tuberculosis. The renal regions, the testes, and the prostate should be examined with care. It may follow a pyelo-nephritis, or be associated with primary disease of the prostate or vesiculæ seminales. Primary tuberculosis of the posterior wall of the bladder may simulate stone.

Tuberculosis of the Prostate and Vesiculæ Seminales.—The prostate is frequently involved in tuberculosis of the uro-genital tract. In Krzyincki's cases, of 15 males the prostate was involved in 14 and the vesiculæ seminales in 11. In Orth's cases the prostate was involved in 18 of the 37 cases in males. These parts are much more frequently involved than ordinary post-mortem statistics indicate. *Per rectum* the prostatic lobes are felt to be occupied by hard nodules varying in size from a pea to a bean. There is great irritability of the bladder, and agonizing pain in catheterization. An extremely rare lesion is primary urethral tuberculosis, which may simulate stricture.

Tuberculosis of the Testes.—This somewhat common affection may be primary; or, more frequently, is secondary to tuberculous disease elsewhere. Many cases occur before the second year, and it is stated to have been met with in the fetus. In infants it is serious and usually associated with tuberculous disease in other parts. In 9 cases reported by Hutinel and Deschamps, in every one there was a general affection. In 20 cases reported by Jullien, 6 were under one year, and 6 between one and two years old. In 5 of the cases both testicles were affected. Koplik holds that most of the instances of this kind are congenital, in Baumgarten's sense. In the adult the tubercles begin within the substance of the gland, but in children the tunica albuginea is first affected. The tubercle does not always undergo caseation, but it may present a number of embryonic cells, not unlike a sarcoma.

Tubercle of the testes is most likely to be confounded with syphilis. In the latter the body of the organ is most often affected, there is less pain, and the outlines of the growth are more nodular and irregular. In obscure peritoneal disease the detection of tubercle in a testis has not infrequently led to a correct diagnosis. The association of the two conditions is not uncommon. The lesion in the testis may heal completely, or the disease may become generalized. General infection has followed operation. Too much stress can not be laid on the importance of a routine examination of the testes.

Tuberculosis of the Fallopian Tubes, Ovaries, and Uterus.—The *Fallopian tubes* are by far the most frequent seat of genital tuberculosis. The disease may be primary and produce a most characteristic form of salpingitis, in which the tubes are enlarged, the walls thickened and infiltrated, and the contents cheesy. Adhesion takes place between the fimbriæ and the ovaries, or the uterus may be invaded. The condition is usually bilateral. It may occur in young children. Although, as a rule, very evident to the naked eye, there are specimens resembling ordinary salpingitis, which show on microscopic examination numerous miliary tubercles (Welch and Williams). Tuberculous salpingitis may cause serious local disease with abscess formation, and it may be the starting-point of peritonitis.

Tuberculosis of the *ovary* is always secondary. There may be an eruption of tubercles over the surface in an extensive involvement of the stroma with abscess formation.

Tuberculosis of the *uterus* is very rare. Only three examples have come under my observation, all in connection with pulmonary phthisis. It may be primary. The mucosa of the fundus is thickened and caseous, and tubercles may be seen in the muscular tissue. Occasionally the process extends to the vagina.

Tuberculosis of the *placenta* is more common than has been supposed. Of 20 placentas from tuberculous women, 9 were affected; 5 of these were from cases of advanced disease of the lung. The lesions are easily overlooked.

IX. TUBERCULOSIS OF THE MAMMARY GLAND

Mandry (Bruns's Beiträge, viii) has collected 40 cases, 1 of which was in a male. The disease is most common between the fortieth and sixtieth years. The breast is frequently fistulous, unevenly indurated, and the nipple is retracted. The fistulæ and ulcers present a characteristic tuberculous aspect. There is also a cold tuberculous abscess of the breast. The axillary glands are affected in about two-thirds of the cases. The disease runs a chronic course of months or years. The diagnosis can be made by the general appearance of the fistulæ and ulcers, and by the existence of tubercle bacilli. The prognosis is not serious, if total eradication of the disease be possible.

In 1836 Bedor described an hypertrophy of the breast in the subjects of pulmonary tuberculosis. As a rule, if one gland is involved, usually on the side of the affected lung, as already mentioned, the condition is one of chronic interstitial mammitis, and is not tuberculous.

X. TUBERCULOSIS OF THE CIRCULATORY SYSTEM

Myocardium.—Scattered miliary tubercles are sometimes met with in the acute disease. Larger caseous tubercles are excessively rare. A. Moser found 46 cases on record. There is also a sclerotic tuberculous myocarditis. The infection often passes from a mediastinal gland.

Endocardium.—In 216 autopsies in cases of chronic phthisis I found endocarditis in 12. It was present in only 151 among more than 11,000 autopsies on tuberculous cases (G. W. Norris). As a rule, it is a secondary form, the result of a mixed infection, so common in pulmonary tuberculosis. A true tuberculous endocarditis does, however, occur, directly dependent upon infection with the bacillus of Koch. As a rule, it is a vegetative endocarditis, not to be distinguished from that caused by a streptococcus or staphylococcus. In rare cases, however, caseous tubercles develop.

Arteries.—Primary tuberculosis of the larger blood-vessels is very rare, and is usually the result of invasion from without. The disease may, however, occur in a large artery and not result from external invasion. In a case of chronic tuberculosis Flexner found a fresh tuberculous growth in the aorta, which had no connection with cheesy masses outside the vessel. Simmitsky has collected 18 cases of tuberculosis of the aorta.

In the lungs and other organs attacked by tuberculosis the *arteries* are involved in an acute infiltration which usually leads to thrombosis, or tubercles may develop in the walls and proceed to caseation and softening, frequently with a resulting hæmorrhage. By extension into vessels, particularly veins, the bacilli are widely distributed with the production of miliary tuberculosis.

XI. THE PROGNOSIS IN TUBERCULOSIS

The parable of the sower already referred to expresses better than in any other way the question of individual predisposition. There are five groups of cases of tuberculous infection. 1. Those who become infected and recover spontaneously without knowing they have been infected. 2. Mild infections which produce slight symptoms, recovery following after a few months of change of air or special treatment. 3. Cases with well-marked signs of lung disease in which thorough treatment is followed by complete recovery. 4. Cases with extensive local disease and cavity formation in which arrest takes place and the patients live for many years. 5. The cases in which the infection is of such a type that death follows no matter what is done. The late Austin Flint, *facile princeps* among American students of the disease, called attention to the self-limitation and intrinsic tendency to recovery in pulmonary tuberculosis. This natural tendency to cure is still more strikingly shown in lymphatic and bone tuberculosis.

The following may be considered favorable circumstances in the prognosis of pulmonary tuberculosis: An early diagnosis, a good family history, previous good health, a strong digestion, a suitable environment, and an insidious onset, without high fever, and without extensive pneumonic consolidation. Cases beginning with pleurisy seem to run a more protracted and more favorable course. Repeated attacks of hæmoptysis are unfavorable. When well established the course of tuberculosis in any organ is marked by intervals of weeks or months in which the fever lessens, the symptoms subside, and there is improvement in the general health.

In pulmonary cases the duration is extremely variable. Laennec placed the average duration at two years, and for the majority of cases this is perhaps a correct estimate. Pollock's large statistics of over 3,500 cases show a mean duration of the disease of over two years and a half. Williams's analysis of 1,000 cases in private practice shows a much more protracted course, as the average duration was over seven years.

Tuberculosis and Marriage.—Under the subject of prognosis comes the question of the marriage of persons who have had tuberculosis, or in whose family the disease prevails. The following brief statements may be made with reference to it:

(*a*) Subjects with healed lymphatic or bone tuberculosis marry with personal impunity and may beget healthy children. It is undeniable, however, that in such families scrofula, caries of the bone, arthritis, cerebral and pulmonary tuberculosis are more common. The risks, however, are such as may properly be taken.

(*b*) The question of marriage of a person who has arrested or cured lung tuberculosis is more difficult to decide. In a male the personal risk is not so great; and when the health and strength are good, the external environment favorable, and the family history not extremely bad, the experiment—for it is such—is often successful, and many healthy and happy families are begotten under these circumstances. In women the question is complicated with that of child-bearing, which increases the risks enormously. With a localized lesion, absence of hereditary taint, good physique, and favorable environment marriage might be permitted. When tuberculosis has existed, however, in a girl whose family history is bad, whose chest expansion is slight, and whose physique is below the standard, the physician should, if possible, place his veto upon marriage.

(*c*) With existing disease, fever, bacilli, etc., marriage should be prohibited. Pregnancy usually hastens the process, though it may be held in abeyance. After parturition the disease advances rapidly. There is much truth, indeed, in the remark of Dubois: "If a woman threatened with phthisis marries, she may bear the first accouchement well; a second, with difficulty; a third, never." Conception may occur in an advanced stage of the disease.

XII. PROPHYLAXIS IN TUBERCULOSIS

General.—Among the more important measures may be mentioned the following: *First,* education of the public. Much has been done in this direction by the antituberculosis crusade, which has resulted in the formation of many active societies, and has stimulated widespread interest in the disease. *Secondly,* the placing of pulmonary tuberculosis on the list of reportable diseases. This gives the board of health control of the situation, and, as the New York experience has demonstrated, is perhaps the most helpful measure in the prophylaxis. *Thirdly,* the improved sanitary condition of the poor, particularly with reference to the housing. *Fourthly,* direct preventive measures, such as the enactment of laws against spitting in public, the proper disinfection and cleaning of the rooms and houses which have been occupied by tuberculous patients, and the careful inspection of dairies and abattoirs. *Fifthly,* in the large cities, *organization* of sanatoria and hospitals for early curable and late incurable cases, and the establishment of separate dispensaries with a system of visiting the patients at their homes by specially assigned nurses. *Lastly,* the care of the sputum of the consumptive. Thorough boiling or putting it into the fire is sufficient. In hospitals it is well to have printed directions as to the care of the sputum, and also printed cards for out-patients, giving the most important rules. It should be explained to the patient that the only risk, practically, is from this source.

Individual.—Individual prophylaxis in the case of delicate children is most important. An infant born of tuberculous parents, or of a family in which consumption prevails, should be brought up with the greatest care and guarded most particularly against catarrhal affections of all kinds. Special attention should be given to the throat and nose, and on the first indication of mouth-breathing, or any obstruction of the naso-pharynx, a careful examination should be made for adenoid vegetations. The child should be clad in flannel and live in the open air as much as possible, avoiding close rooms. It is a good practice to sponge the throat and chest night and morning with cold water. Special attention should be paid to diet and to the mode of feeding. The meals should be at regular hours and the food plain and substantial. From the outset the child should be encouraged to drink freely of milk. Unfortunately, in these cases there seems to be an uncontrollable aversion to fats of all kinds. As the child grows older, systematically regulated exercise or a course of pulmonary gymnastics may be taken. In the choice of an occupation preference should be given to an out-of-door life. Families with a marked predisposition to tuberculosis should, if possible, reside in an equable climate. The possibility of a protective inoculation has been shown by the experiments of Webb and Williams, as monkeys so protected can be exposed successfully in situations favorable to infection. It is stated that the method has been used with success in children.

The trifling ailments of children should be carefully watched. In the convalescence from the fevers which so frequently prove dangerous the greatest caution should be exercised to prevent catching cold. Cod-liver oil, the syrup of the iodide of iron, and arsenic may be given. As mentioned, care of the throat in these children is very important. Enlarged tonsils should be removed.

XIII. TREATMENT OF TUBERCULOSIS

The Natural or Spontaneous Cure.—The spontaneous healing of local tuberculosis is an every-day affair. A majority of those infected never have the disease, *i. e.,* they recover without symptoms, without the slight lesion having disturbed the health. Many cases of adenitis and disease of the bone or of the joints terminate favorably. The healing of pulmonary tuberculosis is shown clinically by the recovery of patients in whose sputum elastic tissue and bacilli have been found; anatomically, by the presence of lesions in all stages of repair. In the granulation products and associated pneumonia a scar-tissue is formed, while the smaller caseous areas become impregnated with lime salts. To such conditions alone should the term healing be applied. When the fibroid change encapsulates but does not involve the entire tuberculous tissue, the tubercle may be termed involuted or quiescent, but is not destroyed. When cavities of any size have formed, healing, in the proper sense of the term, does not occur. I have yet to see a specimen which would indicate that a vomica had cicatrized. Cavities may be greatly reduced in size—indeed, an entire series of them may be so contracted by sclerosis of the tissue about them that an upper lobe, in which this process most frequently occurs, may be reduced to a third of its ordinary dimensions. Laennec understood thoroughly this natural process of cure in tuberculosis, and recognized the frequency with which old tuberculous lesions occurred in the lungs. He described *cicatrices complètes* and *cicatrices fistuleuses,* the latter being the shrunken cavities communicating with the bronchi; and remarked that, as tubercles growing in the glands, which are called scrofula, often heal, why should not the same take place in the lungs?

There is an old German axiom, *"Jedermann hat am Ende ein bischen Tuberculose,"* a statement partly borne out by the statistics showing the proportions of cases in persons dying of all disease in whom quiescent or tuberculous lesions are found in the lungs. We find at the apices the following conditions, which have been held to signify healed tuberculous processes: (*a*) Thickening of the pleura, usually at the posterior surface of the apex, with subadjacent induration for a distance of a few millimetres. This has, perhaps, no greater significance than the milky patch on the pericardium. (*b*) Puckered cicatrices at the apex, depressing the pleura, and on section showing a large pigmented, fibrous scar. The bronchioles in the neighborhood may be dilated, but there are neither tubercles nor cheesy masses. This may sometimes, but not always, indicate a healed tuberculous lesion. (*c*) Puckered cicatrices with cheesy or cretaceous nodules, and with scattered tubercles in the vicinity. (*d*) The *cicatrices fistuleuses* of Laennec, in which the fibroid puckering has reduced the size of one or more cavities which communicate directly with the bronchi.

General Measures.—The cure of tuberculosis is a question of nutrition; digestion and assimilation control the situation; as a rule, make a patient grow fat and strong, and the local disease may be left to take care of itself. There are three indications: First, to place the patient in surroundings most favorable for the maintenance of a maximum degree of nutrition; second, to take such measures as, in a local or general way, influence the tuberculous processes; third, to alleviate symptoms.

Open-air Treatment.—The value of fresh air and out-of-door life is well illustrated by an experiment of Trudeau. Inoculated rabbits confined in a dark, damp place rapidly succumbed, while others, allowed to run wild, either recovered or show slight lesions. It is the same in human tuberculosis. A patient confined to the house—particularly in the close, overheated, stuffy dwellings of the poor, or treated in a hospital ward—is in a position analogous to that of the rabbit confined to a hutch in the cellar; whereas a patient living in the fresh air and sunshine for the greater part of the day has chances comparable to those of the rabbit running wild.

The open-air treatment of tuberculosis may be carried out at home, by change of residence to a suitable climate, or in a sanatorium.

(*a*) *At Home.*—In a majority of all cases the patient has to be cared for in his own home, and, if in the city, under very disadvantageous circumstances. Much, however, may be done even in cities to promote arrest by insisting upon systematic treatment. How much may be done by care and instruction is shown by the success of J. H. Pratt's *tuberculosis classes.* As not five per cent. of the patients can be dealt with in sanatoria, it is surprising and gratifying to see how successful the home treatment may be. Even in cities the patients may be trained to sleep out of doors, and the results obtained by Pratt, Millett, and others are as good as any that have been published. *While there is fever the patient should be at rest in bed,* and night and day the windows should be open, so that he may be exposed freely to the fresh air. Low temperature is not a contra-indication. If there is a balcony or a suitable yard or garden, on the brighter days the patient may be wrapped up and put in a reclining chair or on a sofa. The important thing is for the physician to emphasize the fact that neither the cough, fever, night sweats, and not even hæmoptysis contra-indicate a full exposure to the fresh air. In country places this can be carried out much more effectively. In the summer the patient should be out of doors for at least eleven or twelve hours, and in winter six or eight hours. At night the room should be cool and thoroughly well ventilated. It may require several months of this rest treatment in the open air before the temperature falls to normal.

(*b*) *Treatment in Sanatoria.*—Perhaps the most important advance in the treatment of tuberculosis has been in the establishment in favorable localities of institutions in which patients are made to live according to strict rules. To Brehmer, of Göbersdorf, we owe the successful execution of this plan, which has been followed in Germany with most gratifying results. In the United States the zeal, energy, and scientific devotion of Edward L. Trudeau have demonstrated its feasibility, and the Saranac institution has become a model of its kind. The results at hundreds of institutions demonstrate the great importance of system and rigid discipline in carrying out a successful treatment of tuberculosis. Much has been done in the United States, Great Britain and the Continent to promote the sanatorium treatment of tuberculosis. The past ten years have been rich in experience. The good results have quite justified the heavy expenditure of money. In many places it has been demonstrated that with an inexpensive plant excellent results may be obtained. A reaction has naturally followed the "stuffing" plan of feeding, and more reasonable methods are now employed. The "absolute rest" plan has been modified to meet individual cases. The all-important matter is the establishment near to the large cities of public sanatoria for the treatment of cases in the early stages. There should be opened in the large general hospitals special out-patient departments for tuberculous patients, from which suitable cases could be sent to the sanatoria. Much discussion has taken place as to the result of sanatorium treatment. Personally I am stongly convinced of its extraordinary benefits in suitable cases. To pay a visit with Dr. Bardwell to the King Edward Sanatorium at Midhurst and see nearly every one of 100 early cases looking in good condition with fresh air, judicious rest, proper exercise and diet, without drugs and without tuberculin, impresses one immensely with the value of the method. Statistics are notoriously uncertain, but there is perhaps no institution of the English-speaking world in which greater care has been taken to trace the after-history of the patients than at the Adirondack Sanatorium, founded by Dr. Trudeau. The total number of patients from the years 1885 to 1909 inclusive was 2,878. It has been impossible to trace 206 of these. Of the remaining 2,672, 1,512 were living (1911) and 1,160 dead.

(*c*) *Climatic Treatment.*—This, after all, is only a modification of the open-air method. The first question to be decided is whether the patient is fit to be sent from home. In many instances it is a positive hardship. A patient with well-marked cavities, hectic fever, night sweats, and emaciation is much better at home, and the physician should not be too much influenced by the importunities of the sick man or his friends. The requirements of a suitable climate are a *pure atmosphere,* an *equable temperature* not subject to rapid variations, and a *maximum amount of sunshine.* Given these three factors, it makes little difference *where* a patient goes, so long as he lives *an outdoor life.* Major Woodruff believes that sunshine may be hurtful, and he has collected statistics to show that tuberculosis is more prevalent and more fatal among the dark races, who live where the sun shines the brightest. The point is one of interest, but I do not think the case against the sun is made out. The different climates may be grouped into the high altitudes, the dry, warm climates, and the moist, warm climates. Among high altitudes in the United States, the Colorado resorts are the most important. Of others, those in Arizona and New Mexico have been growing rapidly. The rarefaction of the air in high altitudes is of benefit in increasing the respiratory movements in pulmonary disease, but brings about in time a condition of dilatation of the air-vesicles and a permanent increase in the size of the chest which is a marked disadvantage when such persons attempt subsequently to reside at the sea-level. The great advantage of these western resorts is that they are in progressive, prosperous countries, in which a man may find means of livelihood and live in comfort. In Europe the chief resorts at high altitudes are Davos, Les Avants, and St. Moritz. Of resorts at a moderate altitude, Asheville and the Adirondacks are the best known in America. The Adirondack cure has become of late years quite famous. One very decided advantage is that after arrest of the disease the patient can return to the sea-level without any special risk. The cases most suitable for high altitudes are those in which the disease is limited, without much cavity formation, and without much emaciation. The thin, irritable patients with chronic tuberculosis and a good deal of emphysema are better at the sea-level. The cold winter climate seems to be of decided advantage in tuberculosis, and in the Adirondacks, where the temperature falls sometimes to 20° or even more below zero, the patients are able to lead an out-of-door life throughout the entire winter.

Of the moist, warm climates, in America Florida and the Bermudas, in Europe the Madeira Islands, and in Great Britain Eastbourne Bournemouth, Torquay, and Falmouth are the best known. Of the dry, warm climates, Southern California in the United States is the most satisfactory. Many of the health resorts in the Southern States, such as Aiken, Thomasville, and Summerville, are delightful winter climates for tuberculous cases. Egypt,

Algiers, and the Riviera are the most satisfactory resorts for patients from Europe.

Other considerations which should influence the choice of a locality are good accommodations and good food. It is also important to be under the care of a competent physician. Very much is said concerning the choice of locality in the different stages of pulmonary tuberculosis, but when the disease is limited to an apex, in a man of fairly good personal and family history, the chances are that he may fight a winning battle if he lives out of doors in any climate, whether high, dry, and cold, or low, moist, and warm. With bilateral disease and cavity formation there is but little hope of permanent cure, and the mild or warm climates are preferable.

Measures which, by their Local or General Action, Influence the Tuberculous Process.—Under this heading we may consider the specific, the dietetic, and the general medicinal treatment of tuberculosis.

(*a*) Specific Treatment.—Introduced by Koch in 1890, the tuberculin treatment soon fell into disfavor, but, in spite of the bad results that naturally followed its injudicious use, certain men (among them, particularly, Trudeau) continued to use it. Of late years there has been a reaction in its favor, and now tuberculin is again lauded by some fanatics as the one and only means of cure in the disease. Unquestionably in suitable cases it has a very beneficial influence; the difficulty is to decide which they are. At present so indiscriminate is its use that an estimation of the results is very difficult. The preliminary question arises as to what justifies the diagnosis of tuberculosis, and it is impossible to compare the results obtained by different observers. Anybody, by any method, can secure 100 per cent. of cures in the so-called "closed" pulmonary tuberculosis. As Hamman states very sensibly: "If in the case of every patient who presents himself for examination and shows some trifling deviation from the normal physical signs a diagnosis of tuberculosis is made, or if tuberculin is made the ultimate test of a correct diagnosis, similar results may be obtained with any or with no method." A variety of preparations come under the name Tuberculin: O. T. and T. R., which are Koch's old and new preparations; Deny's tuberculin, *bouillon filtré*, known as B. F., and a bacillary emulsion of Koch, B. E. If given in accordance with Wright's instructions, the smallest dose which will bring out a response should be used, 1/2000 or 1/1000 mgm. and re-inoculations are made at intervals of from one to two weeks. If the tuberculo-opsonic index rises, it is taken as an indication that the injections are helpful, and the amount is gradually increased when it is found that the dose previously given ceases to bring out a sufficient response. It is administered to afebrile patients. It is no longer thought desirable—quite the contrary, in fact—to get a severe general reaction, particularly as this may be associated with marked focal reactions. The aim striven for is to get as high a grade of tuberculin tolerance as possible. Trudeau, who had probably the longest individual experience of anyone using tuberculin, began with doses so small that no reaction is produced; then the dose is cautiously raised, avoiding the slightest reaction. On the other hand, Wilkinson begins with a very high dose, and uses the tuberculin in a much wider range of cases.

(*b*) Dietetic Treatment.—The outlook in tuberculosis depends much upon the digestion. It is rare to see recovery in a patient in whom there is persistent gastric trouble, and the physician should ever bear in mind the fact that in this disease the *primæ viæ* control the position. The early nausea and loss of appetite in many cases are serious obstacles. Many patients loathe food of all kinds. A change of air or a sea voyage may promptly restore the appetite. When either of these is impossible, and if, as is almost always the case, fever is present, the patient should be placed at rest, kept in the open air nearly all day, and fed at stated intervals with small quantities either of milk, buttermilk, or koumyss, alternating if necessary with meat juice and egg albumin. Some patients who are disturbed by eggs and milk do well on koumyss. It may be necessary to resort to Débove's method of over-alimentation or forced feeding. The stomach is first washed out with cold water, and then, through the tube, a mixture is given containing a litre of milk, an egg, and 100 grams of very finely powdered meat. This is given three times a day. Sometimes the patients will take this mixture without the unpleasant necessity of the stomach-tube, in which case a smaller amount may be given. Raw eggs are very suitable for the purpose of over-feeding, and may be taken in the intervals between the meals. Beginning with one three times a day the number may be increased to two, three, or even four at a time. In the German sanatoria a very special feature is this over-feeding, even when fever is present. R. W. Philip advises a raw meat diet—zomotherapy—half a pound three times a day, either minced or as a soup.

In many cases the digestion is not at all disturbed and the patient can take an ordinary diet. It is remarkable how rapidly the appetite and digestion improve with the fresh-air treatment, even in patients who have to remain in the city. Care should be taken that the medicines do not disturb the stomach. Not infrequently the sweet syrups used in the cough mixtures, cod-liver oil, creosote, and the hypophosphites produce irritation, and by interfering with digestion do more harm than good. On the other hand, the bitter tonics, with acids, and the various malt preparations are often most satisfactory. The indications for alcohol in tuberculosis are enfeebled digestion with fever, a weak heart, and rapid pulse. A routine administration is not advisable, and there is no evidence that its persistent use promotes fibroid processes in the tuberculous areas. In the advanced stages, particularly when the temperature is low between eight and ten in the morning, whisky and milk, or whisky, egg, and milk may be given with great advantage. The red wines are also beneficial in moderate quantities.

(*c*) Exercise.—It is found as a rule that the patient with fever does best at absolute rest, and that exercise should only be taken after an afebrile period, and then very gradually. It has long been known that following exercise the temperature is raised, and Paterson, of Frimly, has adopted a method of graded exercises which have yielded excellent results. The plan is based upon the view that physical exercise induces auto-inoculation, the extent of which may be controlled by the amount of muscular effort. By a study of the fever-chart, the body weight, the amount of sputum, and the appetite the rate of progress may be estimated. The febrile patient is regarded as one in whom the auto-inoculation is excessive. To overcome this the patient is immobilized in bed so far as possible, and not allowed to make any movements whatever. The effect of this is often remarkable in reducing the fever. Once afebrile, the principal element in the treatment is the induction of an auto-inoculation by exercises, which Paterson believes have very much the same effect as a dose of tuberculin. A scheme of graded labor has been devised, which has many advantages in sanatorium life, and the results obtained at Frimly are certainly very gratifying.

(*d*) IMMOBILIZING THE LUNG BY INDUCTION OF PNEUMOTHORAX.—Years ago Cayley induced pneumothorax in a case of hæmoptysis. The method never came into general use; but, on the principle of keeping an inflamed organ at rest, this method has been advocated in pulmonary tuberculosis by Forlanini and by J. B. Murphy. Sterile nitrogen is introduced into the pleural cavity through a thin, hollow needle. It is best to use a special apparatus with a water-manometer, so that measured quantities may be injected. At first from 200 to 300 c. c.; later as much as 500 c. c. are introduced, at intervals of a day or every other day, until the lung is completely collapsed, and until there is a positive interpleural pressure of from 5 to 10 cm. of water. The method has been widely practiced in America and on the Continent, with excellent results, it is claimed, in certain cases; but there are dangers, as hæmoptysis, serous effusion, and empyema, and a serious objection is the duration of the treatment, as the pleural cavity requires to be refilled every month or two.

(*e*) GENERAL MEDICAL TREATMENT.—No medicinal agents have any special or peculiar action upon tuberculous processes. The influence which they exert is upon the general nutrition, increasing the physiological resistance, and rendering the tissues less susceptible to invasion. The following are the most important remedies which seem to act in this manner:

Creosote, which may be administered in capsules, in increasing doses, beginning with 1 minim three times a day and, if well borne, increasing the dose to 8 or 10 minims. It may also be given in solution with tincture of cardamon and alcohol. It is an old remedy, strongly recommended by Addison, and the reports of Jaccoud, Fraentzel, and many others show that it has a positive value in the disease. It may be used as an inhalation. Guaiacol may be given as a substitute, either internally or hypodermically.

Cod-liver Oil.—In glandular and bone tuberculosis this remedy is undoubtedly beneficial in improving the nutrition. In pulmonary tuberculosis its action is less certain, and it is scarcely worthy of the unbounded confidence which it enjoyed for so many years. It should be given in small doses, not more than a teaspoonful three times a day after meals. It seems to act better in children than in adults. Fever and gastric irritation are contra-indications to its use. When it is not well borne, a dessertspoonful of rich cream three times a day is an excellent substitute. The clotted or Devonshire cream is preferable.

The Hypophosphites.—These in various forms are useful tonics, but it is doubtful if they have any other action. They certainly exercise no specific influence upon tubercle.

Arsenic.—There is no general tonic more satisfactory in cases of tuberculosis of all kinds than Fowler's solution. It may be given in 5-minim doses three times a day and gradually increased; stopping its use whenever unpleasant symptoms arise, and in any case intermitting it every third or fourth week. Recently intramuscular injections of the salts of cacodylic acid have been used to combat the anæmia so commonly present in tuberculous infections with, it is claimed, unusual success.

Treatment by compressed air is in many cases beneficial, and under its use the appetite improves, there is gain in weight and reduction of the fever. The air may be saturated with creosote.

Treatment of Special Symptoms in Pulmonary Tuberculosis.—(*a*) THE FEVER.—There is no more difficult problem in practical therapeutics than the treatment of the pyrexia of tuberculosis. The patient should be at absolute rest, and *in the open air night and day for some weeks.* Fever does not contra-indicate an out-of-door life, but it is well for patients with a temperature above 100.5° F. to be at rest. For the continuous pyrexia or the remittent type of the early stages, quinine, small doses of digitalis, and the salicylates may be tried; but they are uncertain and rarely reliable. In large doses quinine has a moderate antipyretic action, but it is just in these efficient doses that it is so apt to disturb the stomach.

Antipyrin and antifebrin may be used cautiously; but it is better, when the fever rises above 103° F. to rely upon cold sponging or the tepid bath, gradually cooled. When softening has taken place and the fever assumes the characteristic septic type, the problem becomes still more difficult. As shown by Chart V (which is not by any means an exceptional one), the pyrexia, at this stage, lasts only for twelve or fifteen hours. As a rule there are not more than from eight to ten hours in which the fever is high enough to demand antipyretic treatment. Sometimes antifebrin, given in 2-grain doses every hour for three or four hours before the rise in temperature takes place, either prevents entirely or limits the paroxysm. If the temperature begins to rise between two and three in the afternoon, the antifebrin may be given at eleven, twelve, one, and, if necessary, at two. It answers better in this way than given in the single doses. Careful sponging of the extremities for from half an hour to an hour during the height of the fever is useful. Quinine is of little benefit in this type of fever; the salicylates are of still less use.

(*b*) SWEATING.—Atropine, in doses of gr. $\frac{1}{120}$–$\frac{1}{60}$, and the aromatic sulphuric acid in large doses are the best remedies. When there are cough and nocturnal restlessness, an eighth of a grain of morphia may be given with the atropine. Muscarin (♏ v of a 1-per-cent solution), tincture of nux vomica (♏ xxx, 2 c. c.), picrotoxin (gr. $\frac{1}{60}$) may be tried. The patient should use light flannel night-dresses, as the cotton night-shirts, when soaked with perspiration, have a very unpleasant cold, clammy feeling.

(*c*) COUGH.—The *cough* is a troublesome, though necessary, feature in pulmonary tuberculosis. Unless very worrying and disturbing sleep at night, or so severe as to produce vomiting, it is not well to attempt to restrict it. When irritative and bronchial in character, inhalations are useful, particularly the tincture of benzoin or preparations of tar, creosote, or turpentine. The throat should be carefully examined, as some of the most irritable and distressing forms of cough in phthisis result from laryngeal erosions. The distressing nocturnal cough, which begin just as the patient gets into bed and is preparing to fall asleep, requires, as a rule, preparations of opium. Codeia, in quarter- or half-grain doses may be given. An excellent combination for the nocturnal cough of phthisis is morphia (gr. $\frac{1}{8}$–$\frac{1}{6}$), dilute hydrocyanic acid (♏ ij-iij), and syrup of wild cherry (ʒ j). The spirits of chloroform, B. P., or a mixture of chloroform and sedatives or Hoffman's anodyne, given in whisky before going to sleep, are efficacious. Mild counter-irritation, or the application of a hot poultice, will sometimes promptly relieve the cough. The morning cough is often much relieved by taking immediately after getting up a glass of hot milk or a cup of hot water, to which 15 grains of bicarbonate of soda have been added. In the later stages of the disease, when cavities have formed, the accumulated secretion must be expectorated and the paroxysms of coughing are now most exhausting. The sedatives, such as morphia and hydrocyanic acid, should be given cautiously. The aromatic spirit of ammonia in full doses helps to allay the paroxysm. When the expectoration is profuse, creosote internally, or inhalations of turpentine and iodine, or oil of eucalyptus, are useful. For the troublesome dysphagia a strong solution of cocaine (gr. x, 0.6 gm.) with boric acid (gr. v, 0.3 gm.) in glycerine and water (℥ j, 30 c. c.) may be used locally.

(*d*) Diarrhœa.—For the diarrhœa large doses of bismuth, combined with Dover's powder, and small starch enemata, with or without opium, may be given. The acetate of lead and opium pill often acts promptly, and the acid diarrhœa mixture, dilute acetic acid (♏ x-xv, 1 c. c.), morphia (gr. 1/8, 0.008 gm.), and acetate of lead (gr. j-ij, 0.1 gm.), may be tried.

(*e*) The treatment of the hæmoptysis will be considered in the section on hæmorrhage from the lungs. Dyspnœa is rarely a prominent symptom except in the advanced stages, when it may be very troublesome and distressing. Ammonia and morphia, cautiously administered, may be used.

If the pleuritic pains are severe, the side may be strapped, or painted with tincture of iodine. The dyspeptic symptoms require careful treatment, as the outlook in individual cases depends much upon the condition of the stomach. Small doses of calomel and soda often allay the distressing nausea of the early stage.

A last word on the subject of tuberculosis to the general practitioner. *The leadership of the battle against this scourge is in your hands. Much has been done, much remains to do. By early diagnosis and prompt, systematic treatment of individual cases, by striving in every possible way to improve the social condition of the poor, by joining actively in the work of the local and national antituberculosis societies you can help in the most important and the most hopeful campaign ever undertaken by the profession.*

B. NON-BACTERIAL FUNGUS INFECTIONS—THE MYCOSES

Much attention has been paid lately to the local and general infections caused by the group of fungoid organisms variously classed as Streptothrix, Actinomyces, Cladothrix and Leptothrix. The French workers, who have done so much lately, group the various diseases caused by these organisms under the term Mycoses, which is a convenient and useful designation. Four or five of these diseases are of sufficient importance to be considered in a work of this scope.

I. ACTINOMYCOSIS

Definition.—A chronic infective disorder produced by the actinomyces or ray-fungus, *Streptothrix actinomyces.*

Etiology.—The disease is widespread among cattle, and occurs also in the pig. It was first described by Bollinger in the ox, in which it forms the affection known in America as "big-jaw." The first accurate description of the disease in man was given by James Israel, and subsequently Ponfick insisted upon the identity of the disease in man and cattle.

In the United States and England the disease is less common than in Germany. It is nearly three times as common in men as in women.

The *parasite* belongs probably to the *Streptothrix* group. In both man and cattle it can be seen in the pus from the affected region as yellowish or opaque granules from one-half to two millimetres in diameter, which are made up of cocci and radiating threads, presenting bulbous, club-like terminations. The youngest granules are gray in color and semi-translucent; in these the bulbous extremities are wanting.

The parasite has been successfully cultivated, and in a few instances the disease has been inoculated both with the natural and artificially grown organism.

The Mode of Infection.—There is no evidence of direct infection with the flesh or milk of diseased animals. The streptothrix has not been detected outside the body. It seems highly probable that it is taken in with the food. The site of infection in a majority of cases in man and animals is in the mouth or neighboring passages. In the cow, possibly also in man, barley, oats, and rye have been carriers of the germ.

Morbid Anatomy.—As in tubercle, the first effect is the destruction of adjacent cells and the attraction of leucocytes—later the surrounding cells begin to proliferate. After the tumor reaches a certain size there is great proliferation of the surrounding connective tissue, and the growth may, particularly in the jaw, look like, and was long mistaken for, osteo-sarcoma. Finally suppuration occurs, which in man, according to Israel, may be produced directly by the streptothrix itself.

Clinical Forms.—(*a*) DIGESTIVE TRACT.—Israel is said to have found the fungus in the cavities of carious teeth. The jaw has been affected in a number of cases in man. The patient comes under observation with swelling of one side of the face, or with a chronic enlargement of the jaw which may simulate sarcoma.

The tongue has been involved in several cases, showing small growths, either primary or following disease of the jaw. In the intestines the disease may occur either as a primary or secondary affection. The most common seat is the region of the cæcum and appendix. An actinomycotic appendicitis has been described; primary actinomycosis of the large intestine with metastases has also been found. Ransom has found the actinomyces in the stools. Actinomycotic *peritonitis* due to infection through a gastrostomy wound has been described. Actinomycosis of the *liver* is rare. Auvray in 1903 could only collect 31 cases (Rolleston). It forms a most characteristic lesion, an alveolar honey-combed abscess—like a sponge soaked in pus. It is usually secondary to an intestinal lesion, but in a few cases no other focus has been found.

(b) Pulmonary Actinomycosis.—In September, 1878, James Israel described a remarkable mycotic disease of the lungs, which subsequent observation showed to be the affection described the year before by Bollinger in cattle. Since that date many instances have been reported in which the lungs were affected. It is a chronic infectious pulmonary disorder, characterized by cough, fever, wasting, and a muco-purulent, sometimes fetid, expectoration. The lesions are unilateral in a majority of the cases. Hodenpyl classifies them in three groups: (1) Lesions of chronic bronchitis; the diagnosis has been made by the presence of the actinomyces in the sputum. (2) Miliary actinomycosis, closely resembling miliary tubercle, but the nodules are seen to be made up of groups of fungi, surrounded by granulation tissue. This form of pulmonary actinomycosis is not infrequent in oxen with advanced disease of the jaw or adjacent structures. (3) The cases in which there is more extensive destructive disease of the lungs, broncho-pneumonia, interstitial changes, and abscesses, the latter forming cavities large enough to be diagnosed during life. Actinomycotic lesions of other organs are often present in connection with the pulmonary disease; erosion of the vertebræ, necrosis of the ribs and sternum, with node-like formations, subcutaneous abscesses, and occasionally metastases in all parts of the body.

Symptoms.—The fever is of an irregular type and depends largely on the existence of suppuration. The cough is an important symptom, and the diagnosis in 18 of the cases was made during life by the discovery of the actinomyces. Death results usually with septic symptoms. Occasionally there is a condition simulating typhoid fever. The average duration of the disease was ten months. Recovery is not very rare. Clinically the disease closely resembles certain forms of pulmonary tuberculosis and of fetid bronchitis. It is not to be forgotten in the examination of the sputum that, as Bizzozero mentions, certain degenerated epithelial cells may be mistaken for the organism. The radiating leptothrix threads about the epithelium of the mouth sometimes present a striking resemblance.

(*c*) Cutaneous Actinomycosis.—In more than half of the recorded cases the disease has involved the skin of the head and neck; the buccal, lingual and pharyngeal structures may be involved also. It is a very chronic affection resembling tuberculosis of the skin, associated with the growth of tumors which suppurate and leave open sores, which may remain for years.

(*d*) Cerebral Actinomycosis.—Bollinger has reported an instance of primary disease of the brain. The symptoms were those of tumor. A second remarkable case has been reported by Gamgee and Delepine. The patient was admitted to St. George's Hospital with left-sided pleural effusion. At the post mortem three pints of purulent fluid were found in the left pleura; there was an actinomycotic abscess of the liver, and in the brain there were abscesses in the frontal, parietal, and temporo-sphenoidal lobes which contained the mycelium, but no clubs. A third case, reported by O. B. Keller, had *empyema necessitatis,* which was opened and actinomycetes were found in the pus. Subsequently she had Jacksonian epilepsy, for which she was trephined twice and abscesses opened, which contained actinomyces grains. Death occurred after the second operation.

Diagnosis.—The disease is in reality a chronic pyæmia. The only test is the presence of the actinomyces in the pus. Metastases may occur as in pyæmia and in tumors. The tendency, however, is rather to the production of a local purulent affection which erodes the bones and is very destructive.

Treatment.—This is largely surgical and is practically that of pyæmia. Incision of the abscess, removal of the dead tissue, and thorough irrigation are appropriate measures. Thomassen has recommended iodide of potassium, which, in doses of from 40 to 60 grains (2.5 to 4 gm.) daily, has proved curative in a number of recent cases. The X-rays have been very beneficial in the cutaneous forms.

II. THE SPOROTRICHOSES

Definition.—A chronic infection characterized by cutaneous and internal lesions due to the growth of various forms of parasitic fungi of the sporotrichosis group.

History.—In November, 1896, a patient presented himself at Finney's outpatient clinic at the Johns Hopkins Hospital with an infection of the right arm, which had lasted for several weeks. There were ulcerations on the hand and indurations on the forearm. The condition was recognized as unusual and Schenck, who undertook its study, found on culture a branched mycelium with numerous spores or conidia. Its identification was made by the well-known expert, Erwin F. Smith, and it has been named *Sporotrichum schenckii.* Since this publication, the disease has become widely recognized, owing chiefly to the studies of Beurmann and Gougerot, and it is now recognized that the disease is widely distributed and one of the most clearly defined of the mycoses.

The Parasite.—In the tissues and in the pus the parasite is a large short rod from 3 to 5 μ long and from 2 to 3 μ in breadth. In cultures it grows in filaments of about 2 μ in diameter and forms characteristic ovoid spores. The points of differentiation between the forms are due largely to variation in the modes of sporulation. The parasite is introduced chiefly by accidental inoculation, and possibly through grains and fruit. The fungi have an identical action with the pathogenic bacteria, producing toxins towards which there are active humoral reactions. Widal and Abrami determined the agglutinating and fixation properties of the serum in individuals affected, and specific reactions have been determined. There are minor differences between the form described by Schenck and that described by Beurmann.

Clinical Forms.—Beurmann and Gougerot recognize three groups: First, the disseminated gummatous form in which in the subcutaneous tissues in various parts of the body there are small, firm, solid nodules, which break down and form small abscesses, ulcerating the skin. In the second, ulcerative, type the lesions are not unlike those of cutaneous tuberculosis, occurring commonly on the hands and arms, though they may appear on the legs or on the body. They may be single or in groups of two or three, and in several of the cases I had an opportunity of seeing in Paris they resembled very much eroded syphilitic gummata. In the third form there is a localized lesion, a hard chancroid body, eroded on the surface. Dissemination occurs through the lymphatics, the regional glands become involved and there may be a group of open sores along the arm or on the side of the head. Fourthly, there are certain extra-cutaneous forms—ulcerous lesions of the mucous membranes, gummata of the muscles and an ulcerative osteo-myelitis. The disease rarely generalizes in the internal organs but the parasite has been found in connection with a pyelonephrosis.

The disease is essentially chronic, lasting often for a year or two; sometimes disturbing the health very slightly, and other times leading to anæmia. There may be no fever, but instances of acute attacks have been reported.

Diagnosis.—This has to be made from tuberculosis, syphilis, and actinomycosis, which may be done by cultures (as the parasites grow in a very specific way) and by the methods of sporo-agglutination and the fixation reaction, the full details of which are given in Beurmann's and Gougerot's manual.

Treatment.—As a rule this is surgical, but the iodide of potassium has a most beneficial effect.

III. NOCARDIOSIS

J. H. Wright of Boston has separated this group from the actinomycoses and the streptothrix infections. On the one hand the parasites resemble bacteria, on the other hand the hypomycetes or moulds, in forming branching, thread-like filaments and in the production of fine conidia. They represent a transition between the bacteria and the lower fungi.

Wright states that there are not more than a dozen well reported human cases, the majority of which have had the signs and symptoms of pulmonary tuberculosis or of multiple abscesses. In the lungs nodules, caseous masses and lesions not unlike tubercle have been found. In three cases there was abscess of the brain.

The parasite may be recognized by the typically branched filaments and by the growth in cultures.

IV. OÏDIOMYCOSIS

Under this term is now described a form of infective dermatitis, of which some 50 or 60 cases have been reported, all, with few exceptions, in the United States. It has been called blastomycosis and saccharomycosis, and, as the parasites were at first thought to be protozoon, coccidioidal or protozoic dermatitis. The parasite grows as a spherical or oval budding cell which is capable of producing a mycelium with aerial hyphæ.

The essential lesion is a granuloma, resembling tuberculosis and involving the skin of the face as a rule, but sometimes the lesions are multiple and there is extensive ulceration from the breaking down of the nodules. In a few cases the lungs and other parts have been affected. A secondary meningitis has been described, and grayish nodular infiltrations have been found in the liver, spleen, lymph glands and other organs. The disease is chronic, lasting for many years.

The *diagnosis* is easily made by the microscopic examination of material from the small abscesses, or a fragment of the tissue.

When localized, recovery may take place, but when the lungs or internal organs are involved, or if the skin lesions are very extensive, death follows. For *treatment,* the actual cautery, excision, the X-rays and the internal administration of iodide of potassium may be tried.

V. MYCETOMA

(*Madura Disease*)

Vandyke Carter of Bombay, a pioneer in the study of tropical diseases, gave an admirable description of this affection, which prevails largely in certain districts of India, and sporadically in other parts of the world.

The disease, usually involving the foot, is characterized by great swelling, nodular growths and the formation of multiple abscesses. There are remarkable granules 1 mm. in diameter, usually of a black color, which occur in the discharges; in other cases the granules are yellow or brownish in color. In the pale variety a streptothrix has been found, which morphologically closely resembles actinomyces. It is held by most observers that this streptothrix maduræ and actinomyces are distinct species. From the black variety of granules a hypomycete has been grown, an organism closely allied to aspergillus.

The disease begins as a granuloma, with swelling of the foot, generally on the sole. The tumors gradually soften, others form, the foot increases enormously in bulk, becomes much deformed, numerous sinuses pass between the bones, the discharges are muco-purulent and contain the characteristic granules. The only satisfactory *treatment* is early excision or, in later stages, amputation of the foot.

VI. ASPERGILLOSIS

Bennett in 1842 described the parasite from the lungs, the *Aspergillus fumigatus,* a fungus widely distributed as a harmless parasite, having been found in the auditory canal, nose and throat. In birds, in cattle, more rarely in dogs, the aspergillus may cause lesions of the lungs resembling tuberculosis, and there have of late years been a good many cases reported in man, particularly in pigeon keepers and hair sorters. In the majority of cases the infection is secondary to some long-standing affection of the lungs, but it has been met with as a primary disease with lesions resembling broncho-pneumonia, which undergo necrosis and softening and the clinical picture is that of ordinary tuberculosis.

The symptoms are those of chronic pulmonary disease, cough, fever, and expectoration, in which the aspergillus is found. It is readily recognized by the character of its spores. In the case which I reported, at intervals of two or three months for twelve years the patient coughed up, usually with a good deal of difficulty, a grayish-brown mass the size of a small bean, which was made up entirely of the mycelium and spores of the aspergillus. The interesting point was that the patient had no symptoms, other than the cough, and was in excellent health.

In the majority of cases the outlook is bad, and the treatment is that of chronic tuberculosis.

C. PROTOZOAN INFECTIONS

I. PSOROSPERMIASIS

Though widely spread in invertebrates, pathogenic psorosperms are not common in mammals, and in man serious disease is very rarely caused by them.

One of the commonest and most readily studied forms of psorosperm is the so-called Rainey's tube, an ovoid body found in the muscle of the pig, within the sarcolemma, filled with small sickle-shaped unicellular organisms, *Sarcocystis miescheri*. In a few instances similar structures have been found in the muscles of man. The only human parasite of this group which has caused serious disease belongs to the *coccidia*.

Coccidiosis.—In a majority of the cases of this group the psorosperms have been found in the liver, producing a disease similar to that which occurs in rabbits. In Guebler's case there were tumors which could be felt during life, and they were determined by Leuckart to be due to coccidia. A patient of W. B. Haddon's was admitted to St. Thomas's Hospital with slight fever and drowsiness, and gradually became unconscious—death occurring on the fourteenth day of observation. Whitish neoplasms were found upon the peritoneum, omentum, and on the layers of the pericardium; and a few were found in the liver, spleen, and kidneys. A somewhat similar case, though more remarkable, as it ran a very acute course, is reported by Silcott. A woman, aged fifty-three, admitted to St. Mary's Hospital, was thought to be suffering from typhoid fever. She had had a chill six weeks before admission. There were fever of an intermittent type, slight diarrhœa, nausea, tenderness over the liver and spleen, and a dry tongue; death occurred from heart-failure. The liver was enlarged, weighed 83 ounces, and in its substance there were caseous foci, around each of which was a ring of congestion. The spleen weighed 16 ounces and contained similar bodies. The ileum presented six papule-like elevations. The masses resembled tubercles, but on examination coccidia were found.

The parasites are also found in the kidneys and ureters. Cases of this kind have been recorded by Bland Sutton and Paul Eve. In Eve's case the symptoms were hæmaturia and frequent micturition, and death took place on the seventeenth day. The nodules throughout the pelvis and ureters have been regarded as mucous cysts.

II. AMŒBIASIS

(Amœbic Dysentery, Amœbic Hepatitis)

Definition.—A colitis, acute or chronic, caused by the *Amœba dysenteriæ* with a special liability to the formation of abscesses of the liver.

Distribution.—The disease is widely prevalent in Egypt, in India and in tropical countries. In Europe sporadic cases occur, rarely small epidemics. It is an uncommon disease in Great Britain. It is a common variety throughout the United States, particularly in the Southern States, where it is endemic, increasing sometimes to such an extent as to form an epidemic. Sporadic cases occur in all temperate regions. The relative frequency of this form of dysentery in the tropics is illustrated by the Manila statistics as given by Strong; of 1,328 cases in the United States Army, 561 were of the amœbic variety. The cases of acute and chronic dysentery in the Johns Hopkins Hospital have been almost exclusively amœbic. To 1908 of 182 cases, 123 came from the State of Maryland.

AGE.—It is not uncommon in children but the greatest number of cases occur between the ages of 20 and 35.

SEX.—Males are much more frequently affected. Of 182 cases at the Johns Hopkins Hospital 171 were males (Futcher).

RACE.—The white race is more susceptible, 163 whites to 19 blacks in the Johns Hopkins Hospital series. In the Philippines the whites are more often attacked. In India the disease is common in the native races.

The Amœba.—The organism *Amœba dysenteriæ* was first described by Lanbl in 1859 and subsequently by Lösch in 1875. Kartulis in 1886 found them in the stools of the endemic dysentery in Egypt and in the liver abscesses. In 1890 I found them in a case of dysentery with abscess of the liver originating in Panama. Subsequently from my wards a series of cases was described by Councilman and Lafleur. The studies of Quincke and Roos, of Dock, Harris and others in the United States, of Strong and Musgrave in the Philippines, of Kruse and Pasquale in Egypt and of Leonard Rogers in India have put our knowledge of the disease on a firm basis. To find the amœbæ the little flakes of mucus or pus in the stools should be selected for examination or the mucus obtained by passing a soft rubber catheter. Musgrave holds that the best way is to give the patient a saline cathartic and then examine the fluid portion of the stool.

Amœba or *Entamœba dysenteriæ* is from 15 to 20 μ in diameter, has a clear outer zone (ectosarc) and a granular inner zone (endosarc), and contains a nucleus and one or two vacuoles. The movements are similar to those of the ordinary pond amœba, consisting of slight protrusions of the protoplasm. They vary a good deal, and usually may be intensified by having the slide heated. Not infrequently the amœbæ contain red blood corpuscles. In the tissues they are very readily recognized by suitable stains. They may be in enormous numbers, and sometimes the field of the microscope is completely occupied. In the pus of a liver abscess they may be very abundant, though in large, long standing abscesses they may not be found until after a few days, when the pus begins to discharge from the wall. In the sputum in the cases of pulmono-hepatic abscess they are readily recognized.

Amœbæ are frequently found in the stools of healthy persons, as Cunningham and Lewis pointed out. Schaudinn found them in from 20 to 60 per cent. in Germany, but they vary greatly in different localities. Among 300 persons in Manila, Musgrave found 101 infected with amœbæ, 61 of these had dysentery, the remaining 40 had no diarrhœa. In the next two months 8 of the 40 cases died and showed amœbic infection of the bowel. Within the next three months the remaining 32 had dysentery. Musgrave believes that at any time the amœba may become pathogenic. Schaudinn described two distinct forms—a non-pathogenic *Entamœba coli,* and a pathogenic larger form, the *Entamœba histolytica,* the same as the *Amœba dysenteriæ,* with a strongly refractile hyaline ectoplasm. The amœbæ can be cultivated, but with difficulty, and it is doubtful if they grow apart from certain bacteria. Resistant forms, somewhat analogous to the gamete forms of the malarial parasite, have been described. These "encysted amœbæ" are believed to be necessary, under certain conditions, for the transmission of the disease from one person to another, and are regarded by Musgrave and Clegg as the most dangerous forms of the organism. Cultures of amœbæ have been shown to withstand drying for from eleven to fifteen months.

Morbid Anatomy.—INTESTINES.—The lesions consist of ulceration, produced by preceding infiltration, general or local, of the submucosa, due to an œdematous condition and to multiplication of the fixed cells of the tissue. In the earliest stage these local infiltrations appear as hemispherical elevations above the general level of the mucosa. The mucous membrane over these becomes necrotic and is cast off, exposing the infiltrated submucous tissue as a grayish yellow gelatinous mass, which at first forms the floor of the ulcer, but is subsequently cast off as a slough. The individual ulcers are round, oval, or irregular, with infiltrated, undermined edges. The visible aperture is often small compared to the loss of tissue beneath it, the ulcers undermining the mucosa, coalescing, and forming sinuous tracts bridged over by apparently normal mucous membrane. According to the stage at which the lesions are observed, the floor of the ulcer may be formed by the submucous, the muscular, or the serous coat of the intestine. The ulceration may affect the whole or some portion only of the large intestine, particularly the cæcum, the hepatic and sigmoid flexures, and the rectum. In severe cases the whole of the intestine is much thickened and riddled with ulcers, with only here and there islands of intact mucous membrane. In 100 autopsies on this disease in Manila the appendix was involved in 7; perforation of the colon took place in 19.

The disease advances by progressive infiltration of the connective tissue layers of the intestine, which produces necrosis of the overlying structures. Thus, in severe cases there may be in different parts of the bowel sloughing *en masse* of the mucosa or of the muscularis, and the same process is observed, but not so conspicuously, in the less severe forms. In some cases a secondary diphtheritic inflammation complicates the original lesions. Healing takes place by the gradual formation of fibrous tissue in the floor and at the edges of the ulcers, which may ultimately result in partial and irregular strictures of the bowel.

Microscopic examination shows a notable absence of the products of purulent inflammation. In the infiltrated tissues polynuclear leucocytes are seldom found, and never constitute purulent collections. On the other hand, there is proliferation of the fixed connective tissue cells. Amœbæ are found more or less abundantly in the tissues at the base of and around the ulcers, in the lymphatic spaces, and occasionally in the blood vessels. The portal capillaries occasionally contain them, and this fact seems to afford the best explanation for the mode of infection of the liver.

LIVER.—The lesions are of two kinds: first, local necroses of the parenchyma, scattered throughout the organ, and possibly due to the action of chemical products of the amœbæ; and, secondly, abscesses. These may be single or multiple. There were 37 cases of hepatic abscess among the 182 cases of amœbic dysentery in my wards. Of these, 18 came to autopsy. In 10 the abscess was single and in 8 multiple. When single they are generally in the right lobe, either toward the convex surface near its diaphragmatic attachment or on the concave surface in proximity to the bowel. Multiple abscesses are small and generally superficial. There may be innumerable miliary abscesses containing amœbæ scattered throughout the organ. Although the hepatic abscess usually occurs within the first two months from the onset of the dysentery, in one of my cases the latter had lasted one and in another six years. In 5 cases the intestinal symptoms had been so slight that dysentery had never been complained of. In 2 fatal cases there were only scars of old ulcers and in 2 others the mucosa appeared normal. In an early stage the abscesses are grayish yellow, with sharply defined contours, and contain a spongy necrotic material, with more or less fluid in its interstices. The larger abscesses have ragged necrotic walls, and contain a more or less viscid, greenish yellow or reddish yellow purulent material mixed with blood and shreds of liver tissue. The older abscesses have fibrous walls of a dense, almost cartilaginous toughness. A section of the abscess wall shows an inner necrotic zone, a middle zone in which there are great proliferation of the connective-tissue cells and compression and atrophy of the liver-cells, and an outer zone of intense hyperæmia. There is the same absence of purulent inflammation as in the intestine, except in those cases in which a secondary infection with pyogenic organisms has taken place.

Lesions in the lungs are seen when an abscess of the liver—as so frequently happens—points toward the diaphragm and extends by continuity through it into the lower lobe of the right lung. This is the commonest situation for rupture to occur. Nine of my cases ruptured into the lung. In 3 cases rupture into the right pleura occurred, causing an empyema. In one of these the lung abscess ruptured into the pleura, producing a pyo-pneumothorax. Perforation may occur into *adjacent structures.* In 3 of the cases perforation took place into the inferior vena cava and in another the upper pole of the right kidney had been invaded. The abscess may rupture into the pericardium, peritoneum, stomach, intestine, portal and hepatic veins, or externally.

Symptoms.—Differing remarkably in their symptoms, three groups of cases may be recognized:

Mild Form.—Infection may be present for a month or two before the individual is aware of it. There may be vague symptoms—headache, lassitude, weakness, slight abdominal pains and occasional diarrhœa, features common enough in the tropics. Strong gives the case of a laboratory chemist who had slight diarrhœa for one day and asked to have the stools examined; an unusually rich infection with amœba was found. The next day he felt well. From August to December amœbæ were present in the stools, though he had no symptoms. Liver abscess may occur in these cases.

Acute Amœbic Dysentery.—Many cases have an acute onset. Pain and tenesmus are common. The stools are bloody, or mucus and blood occur together. In very severe cases there may be constant tenesmus, with pain of the greatest intensity, and the passage every few minutes of a little blood and mucus. In some cases large sloughs are passed. The temperature as a rule is not high. The patient may become rapidly emaciated; the heart's action becomes feeble, and death may occur within a week of the onset. Among other symptoms are hæmorrhage from the bowels, which occurred in three cases, and perforation of an ulcer with general peritonitis, which occurred in three cases. A majority of the patients recover; in others the disease drags on and becomes chronic. In a few cases, after the separation of the sloughs, there is extensive ulceration remaining, with thickening and induration of the colon, and the patient has constant diarrhœa, loses weight, and ultimately dies exhausted, usually within three months of the onset. With the exception of cancer of the œsophagus and anorexia nervosa, no such extreme grade of emaciation is seen. Extensive ulceration of the cornea may occur.

Chronic Amœbic Dysentery.—The disease may be subacute from the onset, and gradually passes into a chronic stage, the special characteristic of which is alternating periods of constipation and of diarrhœa. These may occur over a period of from six months to a year or more. Some of our patients have been admitted to the hospital five or six times within a period of two years. During the exacerbations there are pain, frequent passages of mucus and blood, and a slight rise of temperature. Many patients do not feel very ill, and retain their nutrition in a remarkable way; indeed, in the United States it is rare to see the extreme emaciation so common in the chronic cases from the tropics. Alternating periods of improvement with attacks of diarrhœa are the rule. The appetite is capricious, the digestion disordered, and slight errors in diet are apt to be followed at once by an increase in the number of stools. The tongue is often red, glazed, and beefy.

Complications and Sequelæ.—Liver Abscess.—A pre-suppurative stage lasting for several weeks or months is recognized by Rogers, characterized by fever of an intermittent type, moderate leucocytosis, and an enlarged and tender liver. Suppuration in the liver is the most serious and frequent complication. Abscess of the brain has occurred.

Perforation of the intestine and peritonitis occurred in three of my cases. Intestinal hæmorrhage occurred three times. The infrequency of this complication is probably due to the thrombosis of the vessels about the areas of infiltration. Occasionally an arthritis, probably toxic in origin, may occur. There was one case in my series. Five cases were complicated by malaria; 1 by typhoid fever; 1 by pulmonary tuberculosis; and 1 by a strongyloides intestinalis infection.

Diagnosis.—From the other forms of dysentery the disease is recognized by the finding of amœbæ in the stools. Unless one sees undoubted amœboid movement a suspected body should not be considered an amœba. A non-motile body containing one or more red cells is most probably an amœba, but should only lead to further search for motile organisms. Swollen epithelial cells are confusing, but the hyaline periphery is not amœboid in its action as is the ectosarc of the amœba. The trichomonads and cercomonads so frequently associated with amœbæ are not likely to give trouble. The extent of liver dulness should be watched throughout the course of a case, and any increase upward or downward should lead to the suspicion of a liver abscess. Hepatic abscess is usually accompanied by fever, sweats, or chills and local pain, but it may be entirely latent. Exploratory puncture is safe as a rule and, personally, I have never seen any ill effects, but severe hæmorrhage into the peritoneum, six cases of which were recorded by Hatch in India, may occur. A varying leucocytosis occurs in the abscess cases. The highest count in my series was 53,000, the average being 18,350. The average leucocyte count in the uncomplicated dysentery cases was 10,600. Hepato-pulmonary abscess is attended by local lung signs and the expectoration of "anchovy sauce" sputum in which amœbæ are almost invariably found.

Prognosis.—In many cases the disease yields to rest and intestinal medication. Tendency to a relapse of the dysenteric symptoms is one of the striking characteristics of the disease. One of my patients was admitted to the hospital five times in nine months.

Treatment.—Rest in bed is very important, even in mild attacks, and materially hastens recovery. The diet should be governed by the severity of the intestinal manifestations. In the very acute cases the patient should be given a liquid diet, consisting of milk, whey, and broths.

A return to the use of ipecacuanha is the most important event of late years in the treatment of this form of dysentery. It should always be tried, even in chronic cases. It must be given in salol-coated pills or keratin capsules so that it is not dissolved in the stomach. The patient should be on milk diet and without anything by mouth for three hours before the drug is given, the best time being at bedtime. One dose is given each night; the first may be 60 to 90 grains (4 to 6 gm.), which is reduced by five grains each night until it is down to ten grains (0.6 gm.). This course should be repeated in a week if amœbæ remain in the stools. Emetine hydrochloride hypodermically is generally preferable to ipecac by mouth. An average dose is ½ grain (0.03 gm.) three times a day for three to six days, and this repeated if necessary. Rogers advises ipecac to prevent liver abscess when there is a suspicion of hepatitis. Doses of 20 to 30 grains (1.3 to 2 gm.) are given daily and continued for two weeks after the temperature is normal.

Bismuth probably does more harm than good, owing to the fact that it coats the surface of the ulcers so that the solutions used in the injections can not reach the amœbæ in the ulcer walls. It is well in the chronic forms to give an occasional dose of saline or castor oil. Large injections of quinine solution in the strength of 1 to 5,000, gradually increasing to 1 to 500, have given the most satisfactory results of all the local remedies. The amœbæ are rapidly destroyed by the drug. The success of the treatment depends largely on the care with which the injections are given. The failures are undoubtedly, in many instances, due to the fact that sufficient care is not used to insure the solution reaching the cæcum and ascending colon, where the ulceration is often most severe. From a litre to two litres should be allowed to flow into the colon. The patient's hips should be elevated and he should change his position so as to allow the fluid to flow into all parts of the colon. The solution should be retained, if possible, for fifteen minutes. One or two injections may be given daily. Injections of silver nitrate solution (1 to 2,000, increased to 1 to 500) are useful in chronic cases, given in the same way. Tuttle has recently reported good results in the treatment of amœbic dysentery by the use of simple ice-water enemas, given frequently. When there is much tenesmus a small injection of thin starch and half a drachm to a drachm of laudanum gives great relief. Local application to the abdomen, in the form of light poultices, or turpentine stupes, are very grateful.

When medical treatment fails, colostomy may be tried or irrigations given through the appendix.

Hepatic abscess should be drained at once and the cavity irrigated by quinine solution (1 to 1,000). Ipecacuanha should be given persistently, as advised for the dysentery.

III. MALARIAL FEVER

Definition.—An infectious disease with: (*a*) paroxysms of intermittent fever of quotidian, tertian, or quartan type; (*b*) a continued fever with marked remissions; (*c*) certain pernicious, rapidly fatal forms; and (*d*) a chronic cachexia, with anæmia and enlarged spleen.

The hæmocytozoa described by Laveran, which are transmitted to man by the bite of the mosquito, are invariably associated with the disease. Malaria occurs as an endemic and epidemic disease, the latter prevailing in the tropics under favoring conditions. No infection except, perhaps, tuberculosis compares with it in the extent of its distribution or its importance as a killing and disabling disease.

Geographical Distribution.—In Europe, southern Russia and certain parts of Italy are now the chief seats of the disease. It is rare in Germany, France, and England, and the foci of epidemics are becoming yearly more restricted. In the United States malaria has progressively diminished in extent and severity during the past fifty years. From New England, where it once prevailed extensively, it has gradually disappeared, but there has of late years been a slight return in some places. In the city of New York even the milder forms of the disease are very rare. In Philadelphia and along the valleys of the Delaware and Schuylkill Rivers, formerly hot-beds of malaria, the disease has become much restricted. In Baltimore a few cases occur in the autumn, but a majority of the patients seeking relief are from the outlying districts and one or two of the inlets of Chesapeake Bay. Throughout the Southern States there are many regions in which malaria prevails; but here, too, the disease has diminished in prevalence and intensity. In temperate regions, like the central Atlantic States, there are only a few cases in the spring, usually in the month of May, and a large number of cases in September and October, and sometimes in November. In the Northwestern States malaria is almost unknown. It is rare on the Pacific coast. In the region of the Great Lakes malaria prevails only in the Lake Erie and Lake St. Clair regions. The St. Lawrence basin remains free from the disease.

In India the disease is very prevalent, particularly in the great river basins. Terrible epidemics occur. In the Punjab in 1908 there were more than three million deaths from fever, a large proportion of which were from malaria. In the months of October and November there were 307,317 deaths from the disease. In Burma and Assam severe types are met with. In Africa the malarial fevers form the great obstacle to European settlements on the coast and along the river basins. The *black-water* or West African fever of the Gold Coast is a very fatal type of malarial hæmoglobinuria. The Atlantic coast line of Central America is severely infected, and the Isthmus of Panama for centuries was known as the "white man's grave."

In the tropics there are minimal and maximal periods, the former corresponding to the summer and winter, the latter to the spring and autumn months.

Etiology: The Parasite.—HISTORY.—Parasites of the red blood corpuscles —hæmocytozoa—are very widespread throughout the animal series. They are met with in the blood of frogs, fish, birds, and among mammals in monkeys, bats, cattle, and man. In birds and in frogs the parasites appear to do no harm except when present in very large numbers.

In 1880 Laveran, a French army surgeon stationed at Algiers, noted in the blood of patients with malarial fever pigmented bodies, which he regarded as parasites, and as the cause of the disease. Richard, another French army surgeon, confirmed these observations. In 1885 Marchiafava and Celli described the parasites with great accuracy, and in the same year Golgi made the all-important observation that the paroxysm of fever invariably coincided with the sporulation or segmentation of a group of the parasites. In the following year (1886) Laveran's observations were brought before the profession of the United States by Sternberg. Councilman and Abbott had already, in the previous year, described the remarkable pigmented bodies in the red blood corpuscles in the blood vessels of the brain in a fatal case, and in 1886 Councilman confirmed the observations of Laveran in clinical cases. Stimulated by his work, I began studying the malarial cases in the Philadelphia Hospital, and soon became convinced of the truth of Laveran's discovery, and was able to confirm Golgi's statement as to the coincidence of the sporulation with the paroxysm. The work was taken up actively in the United States by Walter James, Dock, Koplik, Thayer, Hewetson, and others, and in a number of subsequent communications I tried to emphasize the extraordinary clinical importance of Laveran's discovery.*

Among British observers, Vandyke Carter alone, in India, seems to have appreciated at an early date the profound significance of Laveran's work.

The next important observation was the discovery by Golgi that the parasite of quartan malarial fever differed from the tertian. From this time on the Italian observers took up the work with great energy, and in 1889 Marchiafava and Celli determined that the organism of the severer forms of malarial fever differed from the parasite of the tertian and quartan varieties.

The idea that fever was transmitted by the bite of the mosquito prevailed widely in the West Indies and in the Southern States. King, of Washington, warmly advocated this view. The important rôle played by insects as an intermediate host had been shown in the case of the Texas cattle fever, in which Theobald Smith demonstrated that the hæmatozoa developed in, and the disease was transmitted by, ticks; but it remained for Manson to for-

* The following references to work on malaria which has been done in connection with my clinic, chiefly under the supervision of my colleague, Professor Thayer, may be of interest: Philadelphia Medical Times, 1886; British Medical Journal, March, 1887; Medical News, 1889, vol. i; Johns Hopkins Hospital Bulletin, 1889; the first edition of my Text-Book of Medicine, 1892; Thayer and Hewetson, Johns Hopkins Hospital Reports, 1895; Thayer, Lectures on Malarial Fever, 1897; W. G. MacCallum, Hæmatozoa of Birds, Jour. of Exp. Med., 1898; Opie, on the Hæmatozoa of Birds, 1898; Barker, on Fatal Cases of Malaria, Johns Hopkins Hospital Reports, 1899; MacCallum, on the Significance of the Flagella, Lancet, 1897; Thayer, Transactions American Medical Congress, vol. iv, 1900: Lazear, Structure of the Malarial Parasites, Johns Hopkins Hospital Reports, 1902.

mulate in a clear and scientific way the theory of infection in malaria by the mosquito. Impressed with the truth of this, Ross studied the problem in India, and showed that the parasites developed in the bodies of the mosquitoes, demonstrating conclusively that the infection in birds was transmitted by the mosquito. W. G. MacCallum suggested that the flagella were sexual elements, and observed the process of fertilization by them. Studies by Grassi, Bastianelli and Bignami, and many others, confirmed the observations of Ross and demonstrated the fact that the malarial parasites of human beings develop only in mosquitoes of the genus anopheles.

Then came the practical demonstration by Italian observers, and by the interesting experiments on Manson, Jr., of the direct transmission of the disease to man by the bite of infected mosquitoes. And lastly, as a practical conclusion of the whole matter, the anti-malarial campaigns so energetically advocated and carried out by Ross have shown that by protecting the individual from the bites of mosquitoes, by exterminating the insects, or by carefully treating all patients so that no opportunity may be offered for the parasite to enter the mosquito, malaria may be eradicated from any locality.

General Morphology of the Parasite.—Belonging to the sporozoa, it has received a large number of names. The term *Plasmodium,* inapt though it may be, must, according to the rules of zoological nomenclature, be applied to the human parasite. There are three well-marked varieties which exist in two separate phases or stages: (*a*) the parasite in man, who acts as the intermediate host, and in whom, in the cycle of its development, it causes symptoms of malaria; and (*b*) an extracorporeal cycle, in which it lives and develops in the body of the mosquito, which is its definitive host.

(*a*) *The Parasite in Man.*—(1) The Parasite of Tertian Fever (*Plasmodium vivax*).—The earliest form seen in the red blood corpuscle is round or irregular in shape, about 2 μ in diameter and unpigmented. It corresponds very much in appearance with the segments of the rosettes formed during the chill. A few hours later the body has increased in size, is still ring-shaped, and there is pigment in the form of fine grains. It has a relatively large nuclear body, consisting of a well-defined, clear area, in part almost transparent, in part consisting of a milk-white substance, in which there lies a small, deeply staining chromatin mass. At this period it usually shows active amœboid movements, with tongue-like protrusions. The pigment increases in amount and the corpuscle becomes larger and paler, owing to a progressive diminution of its hæmoglobin. There is a gradual growth of the parasite, which, toward the end of forty-eight hours, occupies almost all of the swollen red corpuscle. It is now much pigmented, and is in the stage of what is often called the full-grown parasite. Between the fortieth and forty-eighth hours many of the parasites are seen to have undergone the change known as segmentation, in which the pigment becomes collected into a single mass or block, and the protoplasm divides into a series of from fifteen to twenty spores, often showing a radial arrangement. Certain full-grown tertian parasites, however, do not undergo segmentation. These forms, which are larger than the sporulating bodies, and contain very actively dancing pigment granules, represent the sexually differentiated form of the parasite—gametocytes.

(2) The Parasite of Quartan Fever (*Plasmodium malariæ*).—The earliest form is very like the tertian in appearance, but as it increases in size the

earlier granules are coarser and darker and the movement is not nearly so marked. By the second day the parasite is still larger, rounded in shape, scarcely at all amœboid, and the pigment is more often arranged at the periphery of the parasite. The rim of protoplasm about it is often of a deep yellowish-green color or of a dark brassy tint. On the third day the segmenting bodies become abundant, the pigment flowing in toward the centre of the parasite in radial lines so as to give a star-shaped appearance. The parasites finally break up into from six to twelve segments. Here also, as in the case of the tertian parasite, some full-grown bodies persist without sporulating, representing the gametocytes.

(3) The Parasite of the Æstivo-Autumnal Fever (*Plasmodium falciparum*).—This parasite is considerably smaller than the other varieties; at full development it is often less than one-half the size of a red blood corpuscle. The pigment is much scantier, often consisting of a few minute granules. At first only the earlier stages of development, small, hyaline bodies, sometimes with one or two pigment granules, are to be found in the peripheral circulation; the later stages are ordinarily to be seen only in the blood of certain internal organs, the spleen and bone marrow particularly. The corpuscles containing the parasites become not infrequently shrunken, crenated, and brassy-colored. After the process has existed for about a week, larger, refractive, crescentic, ovoid, and round bodies, with central clumps of coarse pigment granules, begin to appear. These bodies are characteristic of æstivo-autumnal fever. The crescentic and ovoid forms are incapable of sporulation; they are analogous to the large, full-grown, non-sporulating bodies of the tertian and quartan parasites which have been mentioned above, and represent sexually differentiated forms—gametocytes. Within the human host they are incapable of further development, but upon the slide, or within the stomach of the normal intermediate host, the mosquito, the male elements (micro-gametocytes) give rise to a number of long, actively motile flagella (micro-gametes) which break loose, penetrating and fecundating the female forms—macro-gametes (W. G. MacCallum). The fecundated female form enters into the stomach wall of the intermediate host, the mosquito, where it undergoes a definite cycle of existence.

(*b*) *The Parasite within the Body of the Mosquito.*—The brilliant researches of Ross, followed by the work of Grassi, Bastianelli, Bignami, Stephens, Christophers, and Daniels, have proved that a certain genus of mosquito—anopheles—is not only the intermediate host of the malarial parasite, but also the sole source of infection. In the present state of our knowledge it would appear that all species of the genus anopheles may act as hosts of the parasite. The more common genera of mosquito in temperate climates are culex and anopheles. The different species of culex form the great majority of our ordinary house mosquitoes, and are apparently incapable of acting as hosts of the malarial parasite. All malarial regions, however, which have been investigated contain anopheles. Although this is apparently a positive rule, anopheles may, however, be present without the existence of malaria under two circumstances: first, when the climate is too cold for the development of the malarial parasite; and secondly, in a region which has not yet been infected. So far as is known, the parasite exists only in the mosquito and in man. It is apparently fair to state that regions in which mosquitoes of the genus anopheles are present may become malarious during the warm season.

A large number of species of anopheles have been described. In North America, however, only four have been positively recognized: *A. punctipennis* (Say), *A. maculipennis* (Wied.), *A. crucians* (Wied.), *A. argyritarsis* (Desv.). The commonest variety, and that which in all probability is most concerned in the spread of the disease, is *A. maculipennis,* which is, also, the most important agent in the spread of the disease in Europe. In parts of India, *e. g.* Bombay, the common anopheles, *Neocellia rossi,* plays no part, but the carrier is *N. stephensi.*

The culex lays its eggs in sinks, tanks, cisterns, and any collection of water about or in houses, while the anopheles lays its eggs in small, shallow puddles or slowly running streams, especially those in which certain forms of algæ exist. The culex is essentially a city mosquito, the anopheles a country insect.

Evolution in the Body of the Mosquito.—When a mosquito of the genus anopheles bites an individual whose blood contains sex-ripe forms (gametocytes) of the malarial parasite, flagellation and fecundation of the female element occur within the stomach of the insect. The fecundated element then penetrates the wall of the mosquito's stomach and begins a definite cycle of development in the muscular coat. Two days after biting there begin to appear small, round, refractive, granular bodies in the stomach wall of the mosquito, which contain pigment granules clearly identical with those previously contained in the malarial parasite. These develop until at the end of seven days they have reached a diameter of from 60 to 70 μ. At this period they may be observed to show a delicate radial striation due to the presence of great numbers of small sporoblasts. The mother oöcyst (zygote) then bursts, setting free into the body cavity of the mosquito an enormous number of delicate spindle-shaped sporozoids. These accumulate in the cells of the veneno-salivary glands of the mosquito, and, escaping into the ducts, are inoculated with subsequent bites of the insect. These little spindle-shaped sporozoids develop, after inoculation into the warm-blooded host, into fresh young parasites. The sporozoid which has developed in the oöcyst in the stomach wall of the mosquito is then the equivalent of the spore resulting from the asexual segmentation of the full-grown parasite in the circulation. Either one, on entering a red blood corpuscle, may give rise to the asexual or sexual cycle. As a rule the first several generations of parasites in the human body pursue the asexual cycle, the sexual forms developing later. These sexual forms, sterile while in the human host, serve as the means of preserving the life of the parasite and spreading infection when the individual is subjected to bites of anopheles.

Morbid Anatomy.—The changes result from the disintegration of the red blood corpuscles, accumulation of the pigment thereby formed, and possibly the influence of toxic materials produced by the parasite. Cases of simple malarial infection, ague, are rarely fatal, and our knowledge of the morbid anatomy of the disease is drawn from the pernicious malaria or the chronic cachexia. Rupture of the enlarged spleen may occur spontaneously, but more commonly from trauma. I have known fatal hæmorrhage to follow the exploratory puncture of an enlarged malarial spleen.

PERNICIOUS MALARIA.—The blood is hydræmic and the serum may even be tinged with hæmoglobin. The red blood corpuscles present the endoglobular forms of the parasite and are in all stages of destruction. The *spleen* is enlarged, often only moderately; thus, of two fatal cases in my wards the spleens measured 13×8 cm. and 14×8 cm. respectively. In a fresh infection the spleen is usually very soft, and the pulp lake-colored and turbid. The *liver* is swollen and turbid.

In some acute pernicious cases with choleraic symptoms the capillaries of the gastro-intestinal mucosa may be packed with parasites.

MALARIAL CACHEXIA.—In fatal cases of chronic paludism death occurs usually from anæmia or the hæmorrhage associated with it. The anæmia is profound, particularly if the patient has died of fever.

The spleen may weigh from five to ten pounds. The liver may be greatly enlarged, and presents to the naked eye a grayish-brown or slate color, due to the large amount of pigment. In the portal canals and beneath the capsule the connective tissue is impregnated with melanin. The pigment is seen in the Kupffer's cells and the perivascular tissue. The kidneys may be enlarged and present a grayish-red color, or areas of pigmentation may be seen. The peritoneum is usually of a deep slate color. The mucous membrane of the stomach and intestines may have the same hue, due to the pigment in and about the blood-vessels. In some cases this is confined to the lymph nodules of Peyer's patches, causing the shaven-beard appearance.

THE ACCIDENTAL AND LATE LESIONS OF MALARIAL FEVER.—(*a*) *The Liver.*—Paludal hepatitis plays a very important rôle in the history of malaria, as described by French writers. Only those cases in which the history of chronic malaria is definite, and in which the melanosis of both liver and spleen coexist, should be regarded as of paludal origin.

(*b*) *Pneumonia* is believed by many authors to be common in malaria, and even to depend directly upon the malarial poison, occurring either in the acute or in the chronic forms of the disease. I have no personal knowledge of such a special pneumonia.

(*c*) *Nephritis.*—Moderate albuminuria is a frequent occurrence, having occurred in 46.4 per cent. of the cases in my wards. Acute nephritis is relatively frequent in æstivo-autumnal infections, having occurred in over 4.5 per cent. of my cases. Chronic nephritis occasionally follows long-continued or frequently repeated infections.

Clinical Forms of Malarial Fever.—The relative frequency of the different forms varies in different regions. The tertian is the most common in temperate regions, the æstivo-autumnal in the tropics, the quartan is everywhere rare except in certain parts of India. In the Canal Zone the relative frequency of the different forms from 1904 to January 1st, 1910, was as follows: æstivo-autumnal, 22,089; tertian, 8,013; mixed infections, 677, and quartan, 20 cases. The quartan is relatively much more frequent in Baltimore; of 1,618 cases of malaria at my clinic, there were 15 instances (Thayer).

I. THE REGULARLY INTERMITTENT FEVERS.—(*a*) Tertian fever; (*b*) quartan fever. These forms are characterized by recurring paroxysms of what is known as ague, in which, as a rule, chill, fever, and sweat follow each other in orderly sequence. The stage of *incubation* is not definitely known; it probably varies much according to the amount of the infectious material absorbed. Experimentally the period of incubation varies from thirty-six hours to fifteen days, being a trifle longer in quartan than in tertian infections. Attacks have been reported within a very short time after the apparent exposure. On the other hand, the ague may be, as is said, "in the system," and the patient may have a paroxysm months after he has removed from a malarial region, though of course this can not be the case unless he has had the disease when living there.

Description of the Paroxysm.—The patient generally knows he is going to have a chill a few hours before its advent by unpleasant feelings and uneasy sensations, sometimes by headache. The paroxysm is divided into three stages—cold, hot, and sweating.

Cold Stage.—The onset is indicated by a feeling of lassitude and a desire to yawn and stretch, by headache, uneasy sensations in the epigastrium, sometimes by nausea and vomiting. Even before the chill begins the thermometer indicates a rise in temperature. Gradually the patient begins to shiver, the face looks cold, and in the fully developed rigor the whole body shakes, the teeth chatter, and the movements may often be violent enough to shake the bed. Not only does the patient look cold and blue, but a surface thermometer will indicate a reduction of the skin temperature. On the other hand, the axillary or rectal temperature may, during the chill, be greatly increased, and, as shown in the chart, the fever may rise meanwhile even to 105° or 106°. Of symptoms associated with the chill, nausea and vomiting are common. There may be intense headache. The pulse is quick, small, and hard. The urine is increased in quantity. The chill lasts for a variable time, from ten or twelve minutes to an hour, or even longer.

The *hot stage* is ushered in by transient flushes of heat; gradually the coldness of the surface disappears and the skin becomes intensely hot. The contrast in the patient's appearance is striking: the face is flushed, the hands are congested, the skin is reddened, the pulse is full and bounding, the heart's action is forcible, and the patient may complain of a throbbing headache. There may be active delirium. One of my patients in this stage jumped through a ward window and sustained fatal injuries. The rectal temperature may not increase much during this stage; in fact, by the termination of the chill the fever may have reached its maximum. The duration of the hot stage varies from half an hour to three or four hours. The patient is intensely thirsty and drinks eagerly of cold water.

Sweating Stage.—Beads of perspiration appear upon the face and gradually the entire body is bathed in a copious sweat. The uncomfortable feeling associated with the fever disappears, the headache is relieved, and within an hour or two the paroxysm is over and the patient usually sinks into a refreshing sleep. The sweating varies much. It may be drenching in character or it may be slight.

Chart VI*a* is from a case of double tertian infection with resulting quotidian paroxysms. Charts VI*b* and VI*c* give temperature curves in æstivo-autumnal forms. Chart VI*d* shows a quartan ague.

The total duration of the paroxysm averages from ten to twelve hours, but may be shorter. Variations in the paroxysm are common. Thus the patient may, instead of a chill, experience only a slight feeling of coldness. The most common variation is the occurrence of a hot stage alone, or with very slight sweating. During the paroxysm the spleen is enlarged and the edge can usually be felt below the costal margin. In the interval or intermission of the paroxysm the patient feels very well, and, unless the disease is unusually

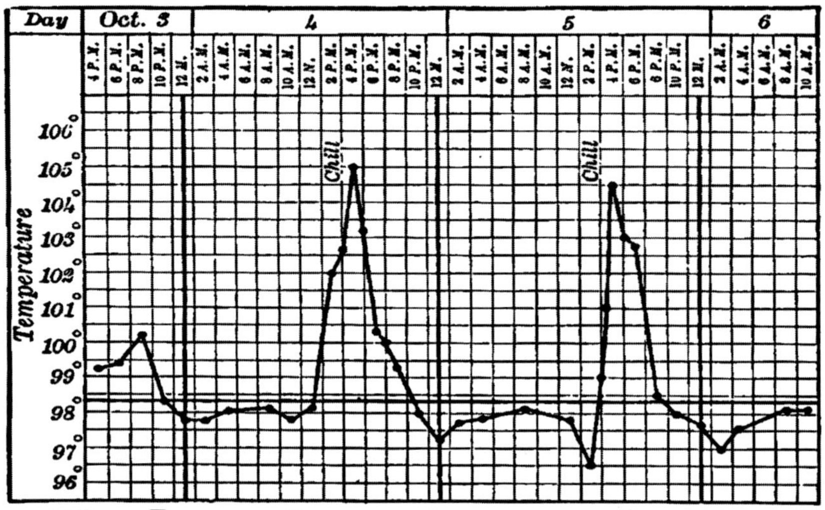

CHART VI*a*.—DOUBLE TERTIAN INFECTION.—QUOTIDIAN FEVER.

severe, he is able to be up. Bronchitis is a common symptom. Herpes, usually labial, is almost as frequent in malaria as in pneumonia.

Types of the Regularly Intermittent Fevers.—As has been stated in the description of the parasites, two distinct types of the regularly intermittent fevers have been separated. These are (*a*) tertian fever and (*b*) quartan fever.

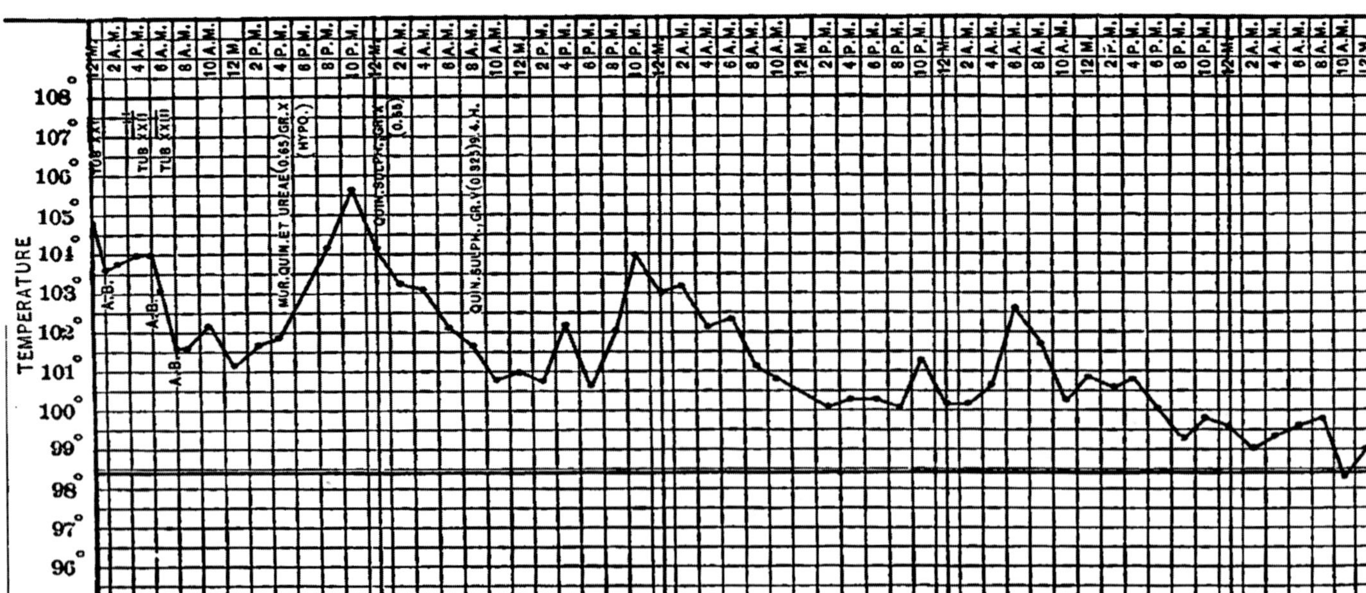

CHART VI*b*.—ÆSTIVO-AUTUMNAL INFECTION.—REMITTENT FEVER.
The case was treated for a week as one of typhoid fever.

(*a*) Tertian Fever.—This type of fever depends upon the presence in the blood of the tertian parasite, an organism which, as stated above, is usually present in sharply defined groups, whose cycle of development lasts approximately forty-eight hours, segmentation occurring every third day. In infections with one group of the tertian parasite the paroxysms occur synchronously with segmentation at remarkably regular intervals of about forty-

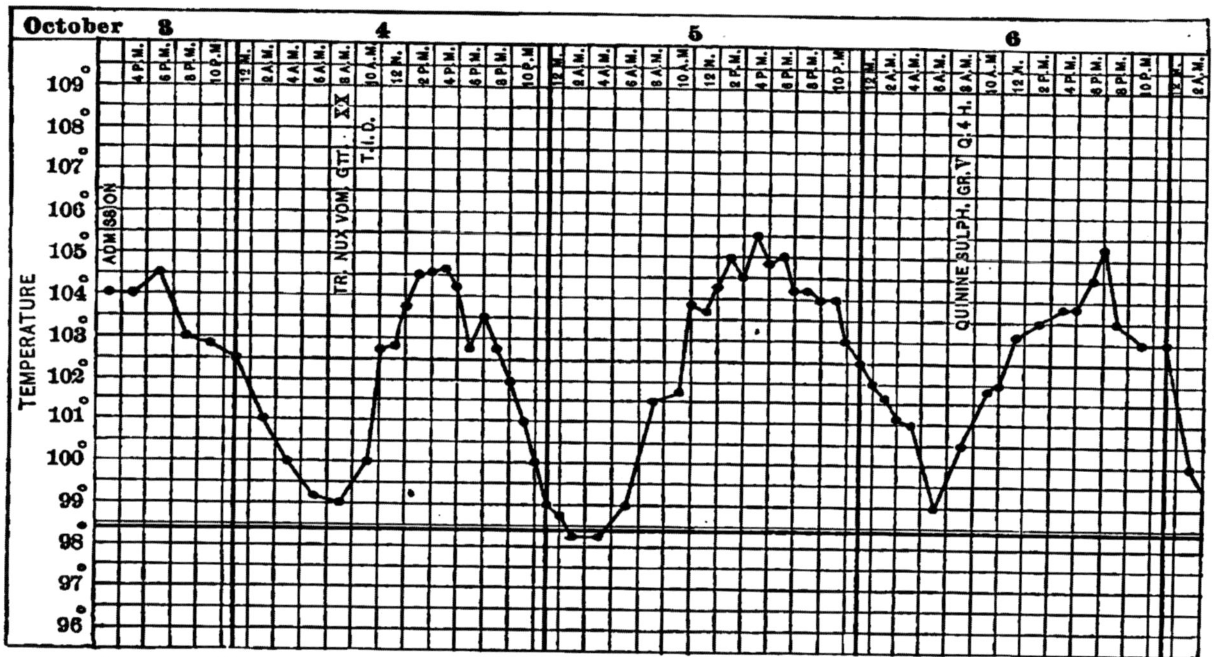

CHART VI*c*.—ÆSTIVO-AUTUMNAL FEVER.—QUOTIDIAN PAROXYSMS.

eight hours, every third day—hence the name *tertian*. Very commonly, however, there may be two groups of parasites which reach maturity on alternate days, resulting thus in daily (*quotidian*) paroxysms—*double tertian infection*.

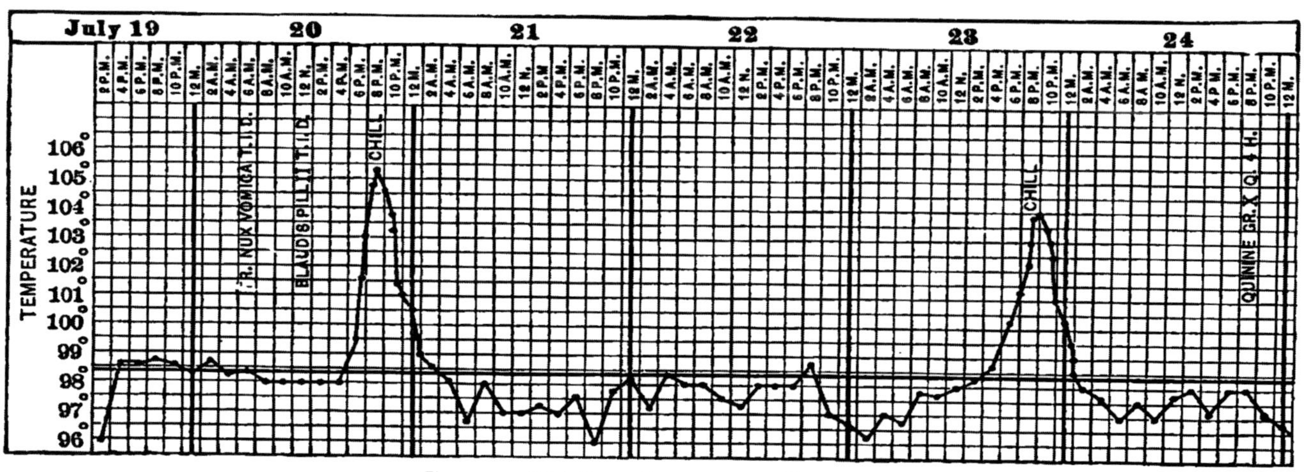

CHART VI*d*.—QUARTAN FEVER.

(*b*) Quartan Fever.—The symptoms resemble those of the tertian infection, but as a rule are milder. Paroxysms appear on the fourth day and correspond with the evolution of a parasitic cycle of seventy-two hours. In recent infections the recurrence of the paroxysm may be almost precisely the same hour every fourth day. The infection may be double, in which case there are two paroxysms followed by a day of intermission, or triple, in which there is a daily paroxysm. As pointed out by the old Greek physicians, the quartan infection is very difficult to cure. Disappearing for a time spontaneously, or yielding promptly to quinine, it has a singular proneness to relapse, even after the most energetic treatment.

Thus a quotidian intermittent fever may be due to infection with either the tertian or quartan parasites.

Course of the Disease.—After a few paroxysms, or after the disease has persisted for ten days or two weeks, the patient may get well without any special medication. I have repeatedly known the chills to stop spontaneously. Relapses are common. The infection may persist for years, and an attack may follow an accident, an acute fever, or a surgical operation. A resting stage of the parasite has been suggested in explanation of these long intervals. Persistence of the fever leads to anæmia and hæmatogenous jaundice, owing to the destruction of blood cells. Ultimately the condition may become chronic—malarial cachexia.

II. THE MORE IRREGULAR, REMITTENT, OR CONTINUED FEVERS.—(*a*) *Æstivo-autumnal Fever.*—This type of fever occurs in temperate climates, chiefly in the later summer and autumn; hence the term given to it by Marchiafava and Celli, *æstivo-autumnal fever.* The severer forms of it prevail in the Southern States and in tropical countries.

This type of fever is associated with the presence in the blood of the æstivo-autumnal parasite, an organism the length of whose cycle of development, ordinarily about forty-eight hours, is probably subject to considerable variations, while the existence of multiple groups of the parasite, or the absence of arrangement into definite groups, is not infrequent.

The *symptoms* are therefore, as might be expected, often irregular. In some instances there may be regular intermittent fever occurring at uncertain intervals of from twenty-four to forty-eight hours, or even more. In the cases with longer remissions the paroxysms are longer. Some of the quotidian intermittent cases may closely resemble the quotidian fever depending upon double tertian or triple quartan infection. Commonly, however, the paroxysms show material differences; their length averages over twenty hours, instead of from ten to twelve; the onset occurs often without chills and even without chilly sensations. The rise in temperature is frequently gradual and slow, instead of sudden, while the fall may occur by lysis instead of by crisis. There may be a marked tendency toward anticipation in the paroxysms, while frequently, from the anticipation of one paroxysm or the retardation of another, more or less continuous fever may result. Sometimes there is continuous fever without sharp paroxysms. In these cases of continuous and remittent fever the patient, seen fairly early in the disease, has a flushed face and looks ill. The tongue is furred, the pulse is full and bounding, but rarely dicrotic. The temperature may range from 102° to 103°, or is in some instances higher. The general appearance of the patient is strongly suggestive of typhoid fever—a suggestion still further borne out by the existence of acute splenic enlargement of moderate grade. As in intermittent fever, an initial bronchitis may be present. The course of these cases is variable. The fever may be continuous, with remissions more or less marked; definite paroxysms with or without chills may occur, in which the temperature rises to 105° or 106°F. Intestinal symptoms are usually absent. A slight hæmatogenous jaundice may arise early. Delirium of a mild type may occur. The cases vary very greatly in severity. In some the fever subsides at the end of the week, and the practitioner is in doubt whether he has had to do with a mild typhoid or a simple febricula. In other instances the fever persists for from ten days to two weeks; there are marked remissions, perhaps chills, with a furred tongue and low delirium. Jaundice is not infrequent. These are the cases to which the terms *bilious remittent* and *typho-malarial* fevers are applied. In other instances the symptoms become grave and assume the character of the pernicious type. It is in this form of malarial fever that so much confusion still exists. The similarity of the cases to typhoid fever is most striking, more particularly the appearance of the faces; the patient *looks* very ill. The cases occur, too, in the autumn, at the very time when typhoid fever occurs. The fever yields, as a rule, promptly to quinine, though here and there cases are met with—rarely indeed in my experience—which are refractory. Several of the charts in Thayer and Hewetson's monograph show how closely, in some instances, the disease may simulate typhoid fever.

The *diagnosis* may be definitely made by the examination of the blood. Repeated examinations at short intervals may be required before the parasites are found. The small, actively motile, hyaline forms of the æstivo-autumnal parasite are to be found, while, if the course has been over a week, the larger crescentic and ovoid bodies are often seen. In many cases in the tropics one is unable to distinguish between typhoid and continued malarial fever without a blood examination.

(*b*) *Pernicious Malarial Fever.*—This is fortunately rare in temperate climates, and the number of cases which now occur, for example, in Philadelphia and Baltimore, is very much less than it was thirty or forty years ago. Pernicious fever is always associated with the æstivo-autumnal parasite. The following are the most important types:

(1) Comatose Form.—The comatose form, in which a patient is struck down with symptoms of the most intense cerebral disturbance, either acute delirium or, more frequently, a rapidly developing coma. A chill may or may not precede the attack. The fever is usually high, and the skin hot and dry. The unconsciousness may persist for from twelve to twenty-four hours, or the patient may sink and die. After regaining consciousness a second attack may come on and prove fatal. In these instances, as has been stated, the special localization of the infection is in the brain, where actual thrombi of parasites with marked secondary changes in the surrounding tissues have been found.

(2) Algid Form.—In this the attack sets in usually with gastric symptoms; there are vomiting, intense prostration, and feebleness out of all proportion to the local disturbance. The patient complains of feeling cold, although there may be no actual chill. The temperature may be normal, or even subnormal; consciousness may be retained. The pulse is feeble and small, and the respirations are increased. There may be most severe diarrhœa, the attack assuming a choleriform nature. The urine is often diminished, or even suppressed. This condition may persist with slight exacerba-

tions of fever for several days and the patient may die in a condition of profound asthenia. This is essentially the same as described as the *asthenic* or *adynamic* form of the disease. In the cases with vomiting and diarrhœa the gastro-intestinal mucosa is often the seat of a special invasion by the parasites, actual thrombosis of the small vessels with superficial ulceration and necrosis occurring.

(3) Hæmorrhagic Forms—Black-water Fever—Hæmoglobinuric Fever—Malarial Hæmoglobinuria.—There are two types of hæmoglobinuria in malaria, the one associated with any severe pernicious malaria, in which an enormous number of red blood corpuscles are directly destroyed by parasites. Not very uncommon, we had a number of cases of this type at the Johns Hopkins Hospital. But in the true black-water fever there is a solution of red blood corpuscles by an unknown hæmolysin, not directly by the malarial parasites themselves.

The figures at Panama, based on five years' work at the Ancon Hospital, given by Deeks and James, show 230 cases in more than 40,000 cases of malaria. Their studies strongly favor the association of black-water fever with malaria, holding that there are three causes superadded to the previous malarial infection: (i) A renewed malarial attack with production of toxins sufficient to destroy many red blood corpuscles; (ii) a lowering of the bodily resistance; (iii) quinine, which appears to be the *tertium quid* necessary to produce the hæmolysin. The general experience at Panama is in favor of withholding quinine in the true erytholytic hæmoglobinuria. It is possible that we may find some measure to counteract the hæmolysis.

(*c*) *Malarial Cachexia.*—The general symptoms are those of secondary anæmia—breathlessness on exertion, œdema of the ankles, and hæmorrhages, particularly into the retina. Occasionally the bleeding is severe, and I have twice known fatal hæmatemesis to occur in association with the enlarged spleen. The fever is variable. The temperature may be low for days, not going above 99.5°. In other instances there may be irregular fever, and the temperature rises gradually to 102.5° or 103° F.

With careful treatment the outlook is good, and a majority of cases recover. The spleen is gradually reduced in size, but it may take several months, or, indeed, in some instances several years, before the "ague-cake" entirely disappears.

Rarer Complications.—Paraplegia may be due to a peripheral neuritis or to changes in the cord, and hemiplegia may occur in the pernicious comatose form, or occasionally at the very height of a paroxysm. Acute ataxia has been described, and there are remarkable cases with the symptoms of disseminated sclerosis (Spiller). Multiple gangrene may occur, as in an instance reported by me, in which a patient with æstivo-autumnal infection presented many areas on the skin. *Orchitis* has been described by Charvot in Algiers and Fedeli in Rome.

Relapse.—It is not easy to explain the relapse. Some think there is a resting stage of the parasite which remains in the spleen or the bone marrow. Schaudinn believed that there is a special parthenogenetic form which may remain latent for an indefinite period. This seems most likely, as there can be no question that months or even years may elapse between the primary infection and a relapse occurring under conditions that preclude the possibility of re-infection.

Diagnosis.—The endemic index of a country may be determined by the "parasite rate" or by the "spleen rate." It is best sought for in children, in whom, as is well known, the infection may occur without much disturbance of the health. To determine the index by examining the blood for the parasites is a laborious and almost impossible task; on the other hand, as the work of Ross in Greece and Mauritius has shown, the index may be readily gauged by an examination of the spleen. Thus, in the last-named island, of 31,022 children, 34.1 per cent. had enlarged spleen. In Bombay, among 50,000 children examined, the spleen index varied from 5.3 per cent. in the Hindoos to 23.2 per cent. in the Parsees (Bentley).

The individual forms of malarial infection are readily recognized, but it requires a long and careful training to become an expert in blood examination. Great progress has been made in the past twenty years, and a diagnosis of malaria is no longer a refuge for our ignorance. One lesson it is hard for the practitioner to learn—namely, that an intermittent fever which resists quinine is not malarial.

The malarial poison is supposed to influence many affections in a remarkable way, giving to them a paroxysmal character. A whole series of minor ailments and some more severe ones, such as neuralgia, are attributed to certain occult effects of paludism. The more closely such cases are investigated the less definite appears the connection with malaria.

Prophylaxis.—In the discovery of Laveran there lay the promise of benefits more potent than any gift science had ever offered to mankind—viz., the possibility of the extermination of malaria. By the persistent missionary efforts of Ross this promise has reached the stage of practical fulfilment, and one of the greatest scourges of the race is now under our command. The story of the Canal Zone, Panama, under Colonel Gorgas is a triumph of the application of scientific methods. Between 1881 and 1904 among the employees of the French Canal Company (a maximum in 1887 of 17,995, of whom 15,726 were negroes) the monthly mortality ranged from 60 to 70, and on seven occasions was above 100, once reaching the enormous figure of 176.97 per 1,000. With the measures given below, the mortality has fallen below that of temperate regions. For the year 1910 the death rate among 50,802 employees was, total deaths 558, from disease 381, from violence 177; the death rate from disease was 7.5 per 1,000. In August, 1911, among 49,710 employees the death rate from disease was 6.27!

This most successful campaign has been carried out on the following lines: (1) The eradication of mosquito propagation areas by drainage, and the filling of places where the larvæ exist. This has been done successfully in large districts.

(2) The control of propagation areas that are allowed to exist, or that cannot be economically and permanently treated. On small areas the larvæ are prevented from arriving at the adult stage by the use of crude oil or kerosene, and in large bodies of water by treating the edges where alone the mosquito larvæ exist. A concentrated larvacide of carbolic acid, resin, and caustic soda, so made as to form an emulsion with the water into which it is placed, has been found effective, when applied to the edges of large pools, ditches, wet

areas and streams. A barrel of oil with an automatic drip at the head of a stream has been found to work satisfactorily.

(3) Protection by screening of houses. On the Zone all the houses occupied by Americans are protected by copper-bronze screens of 18 mesh to the inch. Cotton bar treated with wax is also recommended as inexpensive. Screened vestibules decrease the chance of access of mosquitoes. Mosquito nets over the beds are found, as a rule, to be a failure, chiefly because few persons sleep through a whole night without an arm or leg coming in contact with the netting on which the anopheles settle.

(4) The destruction of adult anopheles. In two sets of barracks not far apart, with many anopheles, in one all the adult mosquitoes were killed daily, in the other they were not; in the latter during a period of several months there was forty-two times as much malaria. The mosquitoes are easily caught; they are usually in the corners, and very often within a foot of the floor.

Of the enormous importance of these anti-malarial measures there can now be no question. It requires system, organization, energy and perseverance. But the story of Havana, where malaria no longer exists, and the story of Ismalia, and, above all, the story of the Panama Canal Zone show what can be done. The following chart, taken from an article of Le Prince, the chief sanitary inspector of the Zone, gives a good idea of the results. The objection offered on the score of cost in the tropics has been shown by Gorgas to be fallacious.

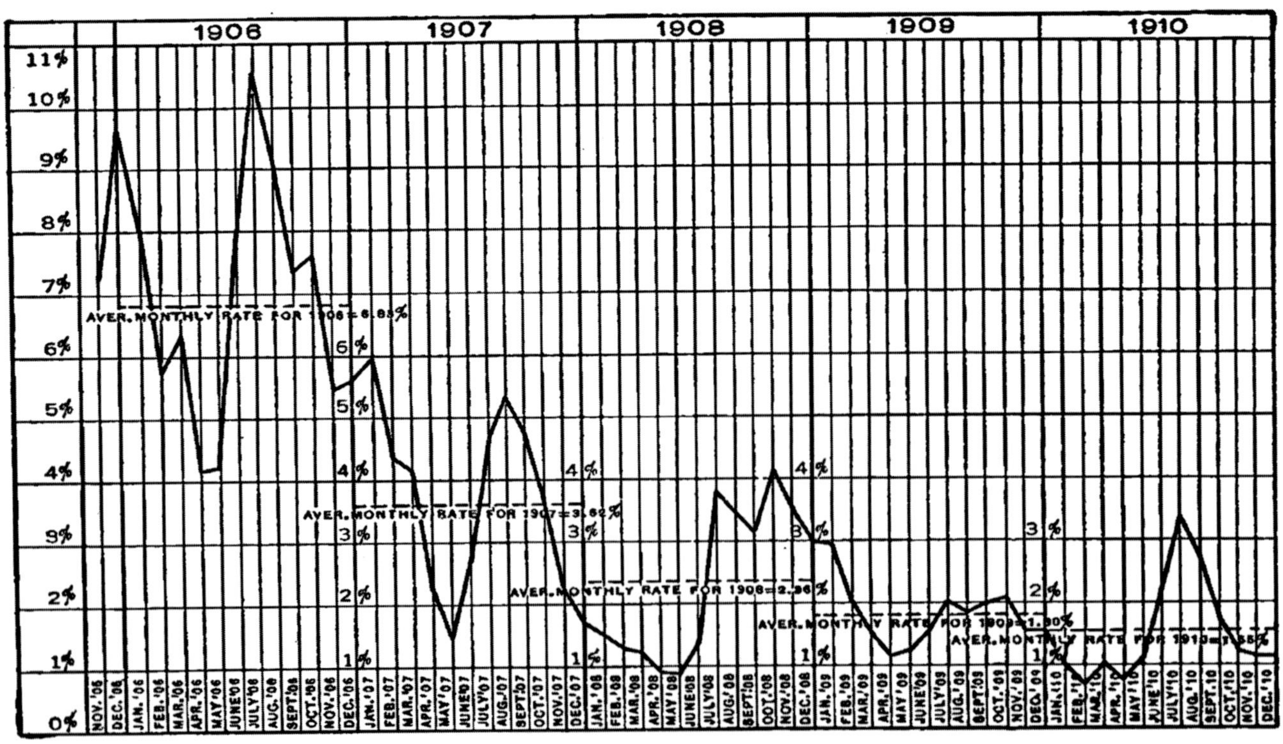

Chart VII.—Malaria Cases Among the Employees of the Isthmian Canal Commission, 1906-1910.

Every patient with malaria should be regarded as a centre of infection, and in a systematic warfare reported to the health authorities. In the tropics segregation of Europeans may do much to lessen the chances of infection.

Every patient should receive thorough and prolonged treatment with quinine. There is far too much carelessness on this point in the profession. Malarial infection is a difficult one to eradicate. Quinine is the only known drug which is an effective parasiticide. Patients should be told to resume the treatment in the spring and autumn for several years after the primary infection. In very malarial districts, as many persons harbor the parasites who do not show any (or at the most very few) signs, a systematic treatment with quinine should be instituted, particularly of the young children.

Patients with the disease should be protected from mosquitoes as far as possible. As a rule, anopheles are more likely to bite after sundown, so that in regions in which the disease prevails extensively mosquito netting should be used. Persons going to a malarial region should take about 10 grains (0.6 gm.) of quinine daily, though Sézary found that 2 grains (0.13 gm.) three times a day was a sufficient protection against the disease.

Treatment.—The patient should be in bed and given liquid or soft diet. The bowels should be moved freely, for which a calomel and saline purge is best. In quinine we possess a specific remedy against malarial infection. Experiment has shown that the parasites are most easily destroyed by quinine at the stage when they are free in the circulation—that is, during and just after segmentation. While in most instances the parasites of the regularly intermittent fevers may be destroyed, even in the intra-corpuscular stage, in æstivo-autumnal fever this is much more difficult. It should, then, be our object, if we wish to most effectively eradicate the infection, to have as much quinine in circulation at the time of the paroxysm and shortly before as is possible, for this is the period at which segmentation occurs. In the regularly intermittent fevers from 10 to 30 grains (0.6 to 2 gm.) in divided doses throughout the day will in many instances prevent any fresh paroxysms. If the patient comes under observation shortly before an expected paroxysm, the administration of a good dose of quinine just before its onset may be advisable to obtain a maximum effect upon the group of parasites. The quinine will not prevent the paroxysm, but will destroy the greater part of the group of organisms and prevent its recurrence. It is safer to give at least 20 to 30 grains (1.3 to 2 gm.) daily for the first three days, and then to continue the remedy in smaller doses for the next two or three weeks. In æstivo-autumnal fever larger doses may be necessary, though in relatively few instances is it necessary to give more than 30 grains (2 gm.) in the twenty-four hours. During the paroxysm the patient should, in the cold stage, be wrapped in blankets and given hot drinks. The reactionary fever is rarely dangerous even if it reaches a high grade. The body may, however, be sponged.

The quinine should be ordered in solution or in capsules. The pills and compressed tablets are more uncertain, as they may not be dissolved. Euquinin, in the same dosage, may be given to patients with whom quinine disagrees.

A question of interest is the efficient dose of quinine necessary to cure the disease. I have a number of charts showing that grain doses three times a day will in many cases prevent the paroxysm, but not always with the certainty of larger doses. In cases of æstivo-autumnal fever with pernicious symptoms it is necessary to get the system under the influence of quinine as rapidly as possible. In these instances the drug should be administered by injection into the muscles, as the dihydrochlorate in ten-grain (0.6 gm.) doses, in a freshly prepared solution (1 to 2) in sterile water and repeated in two hours. Further administration must be decided by the condition. The muriate of quinine and urea is also a good form in which to administer the drug hypodermically; 10-grain (0.6 gm.) doses may be given. In the most severe instances some observers advise the intravenous administration of quinine, for which the very soluble bimuriate is well adapted. Fifteen grains with 40 grains of sodium chloride may be injected in ten ounces of freshly distilled water. The intravenous administration is not without danger. For extreme restlessness in these cases opium is indicated, and cardiac stimulants, such as alcohol and strychnine, may be necessary. If in the comatose form the internal temperature is raised, the patient should be sponged or given a tub bath. For malarial anæmia iron and arsenic are indicated.

An interesting question is much discussed, whether quinine does not cause, or at any rate aggravate, hæmoglobinuria. We have not yet seen a case in which this condition has occurred as a result of the use of the drug, and Bastianelli states that it is not seen in the Roman malarial fevers. In any case of hæmoglobinuria if the blood shows parasites quinine should be administered cautiously. In the post-malarial forms quinine aggravates the attack. In an active malarial infection the patient runs less risk with the quinine.

In malarial cachexia the patient should have a change of climate, be given a liberal diet, and take quinine in small doses and iron and arsenic for some time.

IV. TRYPANOSOMIASIS

Definition.—A chronic disorder characterized by fever, lassitude, weakness, wasting, and often a protracted lethargy—sleeping sickness. *Trypanosoma gambiense* is the active agent in the disease.

Trypanosomes are flagellate infusoria, parasitic in a great many invertebrate and vertebrates. The life history is in two stages, a flagellate monadine phase, in which they live in the blood stream of vertebrates and in some of which they cause serious disease; the other is a gregarine non-flagellate phase which may also be parasitic and which is met with in forms of Kala-Azar.

History.—In 1843 Gruby found a blood parasite in the frog which he called *Trypanosoma sanguinis.* Subsequently it was found to be a very common blood parasite in fishes and birds. In 1878 Lewis found it in the rat—*T. lewisi*—in which it apparently does no harm. The pathological significance of the protozoa was first suggested in 1880 by Griffith Evans, who discovered *trypanosomes*—*T. evansi*—in the disease of horses and cattle in India known as *surra.* In 1895 Bruce made the important announcement that the tsetze fly disease or *nagana* of South Africa, which made whole districts impassable for cattle and horses, was really due to a trypanosome—*T. brucei.* Normally present in the blood of the big-game animals of the districts, and doing them no harm, it was conveyed by the tsetze fly to the non-immune horses and cattle imported into what were called the fly-belts. Other trypanosomes are the Philippine surra, studied by Musgrave, the *mal de caderas*—*T. equinum*—of South America and a harmless infection in cattle in the Transvaal caused by *Trypanosoma theileri.*

Human Trypanosomiasis.—In 1901 Dutton found a trypanosome in the blood of a West Indian. In 1903 Castellani found trypanosomes in the cerebro-spinal fluid and in the blood of five cases of the African sleeping sickness. The Royal Society Commission (Bruce and Nabarro) demonstrated the great frequency of the parasites in the cerebro-spinal fluid and in the blood in sleeping sickness, and suggested that it was a sort of human tsetze fly infection.

DISTRIBUTION.—For many years it had been known that the West African natives were subject to a remarkable malady known as the lethargy or sleeping sickness. It was also met with among the slaves imported into America. The demonstration of the association of the trypanosomes with the terrible sleeping sickness has been the most important recent "find" in tropical medicine. The disease prevails in Gambia, Sierra Leone, and Liberia, and is spreading rapidly in the Congo basin, Uganda, and Rhodesia. The recent opening up of equatorial Africa has led to intercommunication between the different districts which were formerly isolated, and the seriousness of the disease may be appreciated from the fact that within three years after its introduction 100,000 negroes died of it in Uganda. In the infected regions a large number of natives, not apparently suffering from the disease, harbor the parasites in the blood and suffer only with occasional attacks of fever, during which the trypanosomes are also found in the cerebro-spinal fluid.

The disease is not confined to negroes, and Europeans may be attacked. Persons particularly prone are those who live on the wooded shores of the lakes and rivers, such as fishermen and canoe men.

The parasite is introduced by the bite of a fly, the *Glossina palpalis,* and where this insect exists the disease is liable to prevail. The fly lives on the bushes on the lake shores or river banks, and feeds on the blood of crocodiles, antelopes, etc. The trypanosomes undergo changes in the body of the fly and the infectivity does not appear until the thirty-second day, but continues for at least 75 days (Bruce).

Symptoms.—There is stated to be a long latent period. The Uganda Commissioners divide the course of the disease into three stages: first, of fever with rapid pulse, dulling of the mind, and loss of weight; secondly, the stage of tremors in which the gait becomes shuffling, the speech slow, and there are tremors of the tongue and of the hands and feet; lastly, a stage in which the patient becomes lethargic with low temperature and presents the typical picture of the dreaded sleeping sickness. The parasites are found in the cerebrospinal fluid, less constantly in the blood. In the early stages the glands of the neck are involved, and Todd and Dutton recommend puncture of these glands for the purpose of diagnosis. Death is usually caused by some intercurrent infection, as purulent meningitis or suppuration of the lymph glands. The duration is seldom longer than eighteen months. To stay the ravages and prevent the spread of the disease will tax the energies of the nations interested in the settlement of tropical Africa. The hope appears to be in the extermination of the animals upon which the *Glossina palpalis* feeds (among which Koch holds the crocodile to be the most important), just as the killing off of the big game in other parts of Africa has saved the cattle from the ravages of the tsetze fly. Though a colossal task, the examination of natives of infected districts should be undertaken, isolation villages established, and the cases kept under observation and treatment.

Prognosis.—Nine cases in Europeans have been cured, and six of these have been without symptoms from three and one-half to seven years. The criteria of cure are the absence of symptoms, failure to find the trypanosomes, the absence of auto-agglutination, and negative inoculation of the blood into susceptible animals.

Treatment.—Atoxyl introduced by Wolferstan Thomas and Breinl appears to have given the most satisfactory results. The parasites seem to vary in their resistance to arsenic. In some places the arsenophenylglycin seems to have acted almost as a specific. Antimony has been used a good deal of late, and Kerandel, a member of the French Commission, has cured himself with it, injecting intravenously on successive days a solution of tartar emetic in seventeen 10-centigram doses. Salvarsan has been used with benefit, but we have not yet a full knowledge of its effects.

V. LEISHMANIASIS

(*Kala-Azar*)

Definition.—Leishmaniasis is an affection caused by parasites of the Leishmania group, of which there are three chief forms: the *Indian kala-azar*, the *infantile kala-azar*, and *tropical sore.*

Indian Kala-Azar.—An affection characterized by enlarged spleen, anæmia and irregularly remittent fever. Leishman in 1900 discovered the parasite, which was subsequently studied by Donovan. It is a protozoon of very constant form, living in the cells of the spleen and bone-marrow. It has been successfully cultivated by Rogers and others, and develops into a flagellate form.

Distribution.—The disease is widely spread in Asia, particularly in Assam, many parts of India, Burma, Indo-China, Ceylon and Syria. Europeans contract it rarely.

Etiology.—Rogers believes the bedbug of India is the chief agent in transmitting it, a view which Patton shares, as he found the ingested parasite in the bedbug underwent development into flagellate forms. Donovan suggests that the disease is transmitted by the plant-feeding bug, the conorrhinus, which is an occasional blood-sucker.

Symptoms.—Enlargement of the spleen is almost constant; there is irregular fever, which lasts for months and is sometimes characterized by a double rise in the twenty-four hours. The other features are those of a progressive anæmia of a secondary type. Recovery is possible, but the mortality is above 80 per cent.

Infantile Kala-Azar.—This form, separated by Nicole and his associates at Tunis, is the infantile splenic anæmia long recognized in the countries of the Mediterranean basin. It differs from the Indian form in attacking children almost exclusively, and in the presence of a parasite which differs from the *L. donovani,* and which is known as the *L. infantum.* Another special feature is that the disease may be reproduced in dogs and monkeys and a spontaneous infection of dogs exists in the endemic areas of infantile Kala-

Azar. Observations strongly suggest that the disease is transmitted to children through the dog flea, or through the human flea having bitten an infected dog.

Tropical Sore.—Under the various names Aleppo boil, Delhi boil, Bagdad sore, Nile sore and many others, has been described a form of disease characterized by ulcerating and non-ulcerating lesions, almost always on the exposed parts of the body. The parasite discovered by Homer Wright and known as *Leishmania tropica* has very much the same characters as the other forms, but there are slight differences, morphological and cultural. The mode of transmission has not been definitely determined.

Treatment.—For Indian kala-azar not much can be done. Quinine given in the ordinary way seems useless, but from hypodermic injections into the muscles good results are reported. Atoxyl has been freely used. In some regions the natives insert a dirty seton in the region of the spleen. Both for this and the infantile form salvarsan has been used, but with doubtful benefit. For the tropical sore dusting with potassium permanganate, and a few days later applying a 10 per cent. solution of Prussian blue, has been found useful.

VI. RELAPSING FEVER

(*Febris recurrens*)

Definition.—A group of specific infections caused by spirochætes, characterized by febrile paroxysms which usually last five or six days with remissions of about the same length of time. The paroxysms may be repeated three or even four times, whence the name relapsing, or recurring, fever.

European, Indian, American and African forms are described presenting clinically much the same features, but the parasites differ in certain peculiarities.

Etiology.—The European form, which has also the name "famine fever" and "seven-day fever," has been known since the early part of the eighteenth century, and has from time to time extensively prevailed, especially in Ireland. It is a very rare disease in England. In the United States the disease appeared in 1844, when cases were admitted to the Philadelphia Hospital, which are described by Meredith Clymer in his work on Fevers. Flint saw cases in 1850-'51. In 1869 it prevailed extensively in epidemic form in New York and Philadelphia; since when it has not reappeared. While clinically the same as the European form, the organism is different and has been called *S. novyi.*

In India, where the disease is very prevalent, the parasite called after Vandyke Carter, differs from the spirochæte of Obermeier. Possibly it may be transmitted by mosquitoes as well as bugs.

The *African relapsing fever,* known as *tick fever,* is a very serious and widespread affection, the parasite of which, *S. duttoni,* is distinct from the other forms. It is transmitted by the tick *Ornithodoros monbata,* but as Leishman has shown, not by direct inoculation with the salivary secretion, but from other secretions voided in the act of gorging. The symptoms are very similar to those of European relapsing fever, and as many as from five to seven relapses may take place. The mortality is not very high.

The *Spirillum* or spirochæte, described by Obermeier in 1873, was one of the first micro-organisms shown to be definitely associated with a specific fever. It is from 15 to 40 μ. in length, spirally arranged like a corkscrew, sometimes curved and twisted. The ends are tapering; whether furnished with flagella or not is doubtful. It is actively motile, and it is present in the blood during the febrile paroxysm, disappearing at intervals.

The mode of transmission of the disease is probably through lice and bed bugs. The disease has been reproduced by injecting into a healthy monkey blood sucked by a bug from an infected animal. The special conditions under which it occurs are similar to those of typhus fever. Neither age, sex, nor season seems to have any special influence. One attack does not confer immunity from subsequent attacks.

Morbid Anatomy.—There are no characteristic anatomical appearances in relapsing fever. If death takes place during the paroxysm the spleen is large and soft, and the liver, kidneys and heart show cloudy swelling. There may be infarcts in the kidneys and spleen. The bone-marrow has been found in a condition of hyperplasia. Ecchymoses are not uncommon.

Symptoms.—The *incubation* appears to be short; in some instances the attack occurs within twelve hours after exposure; more frequently, however, from five to seven days elapse.

The *invasion* is abrupt, with chill, fever, and intense pain in the back and limbs. In young persons there may be nausea, vomiting, and convulsions. The temperature rises rapidly and may reach 104° on the evening of the first day. Sweats are common. The pulse is rapid, ranging from 110 to 130. There may be delirium if the fever is high. Swelling of the spleen can be detected early. Jaundice is common in some epidemics. The gastric symptoms may be severe, but there are seldom intestinal symptoms. Cough may

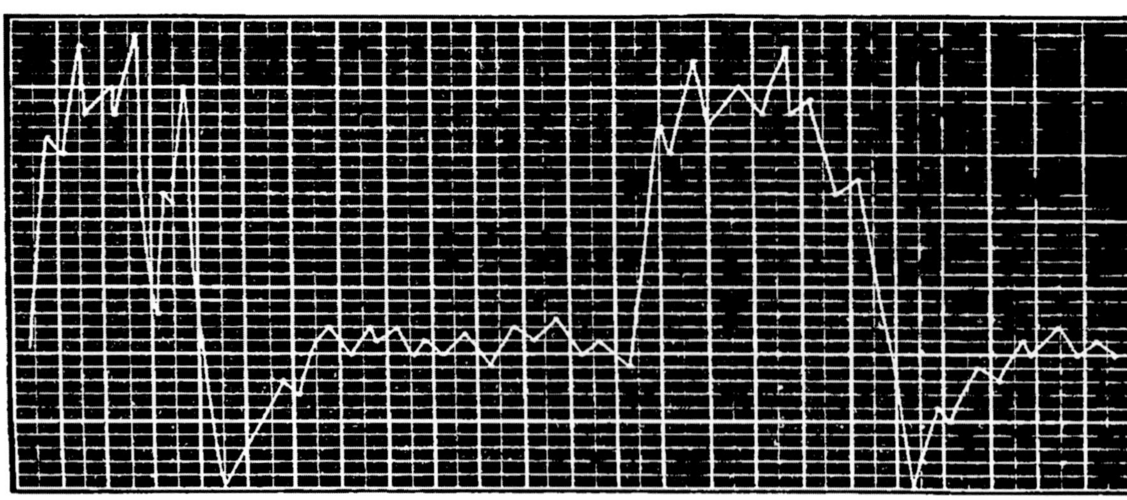

CHART VIII.—RELAPSING FEVER (Murchison).

be present. Occasionally herpes is noted, and there may be miliary vesicles and petechiæ. During the paroxysm the blood invariably shows the spirochæte, and there is usually a leucocytosis. After the fever has persisted with severity or even with an increasing intensity for five or six days the crisis occurs. In the course of a few hours, accompanied by profuse sweating, sometimes by diarrhœa, the temperature falls to normal or even subnormal, and the period of apyrexia begins.

The crisis may occur as early as the third day, or it may be delayed to the tenth; it usually comes, however, about the end of the first week. In delicate and elderly persons there may be collapse. The convalescence is rapid, and in a few days the patient is up and about. Then in a week, usually on the fourteenth day, he again has a rigor, or a series of chills; the fever returns and the attack is repeated. A second crisis occurs from the twentieth to the twenty-third day, and again the patient recovers rapidly. As a rule, the relapse is shorter than the original attack. A second and a third may occur, and there are instances on record of even a fourth and a fifth. In epidemics there are cases which terminate by crisis on the seventh or eighth day without the occurrence of relapse. In protracted cases the convalescence is very tedious, as the patient is much exhausted.

Relapsing fever is not a very fatal disease. Murchison states that the mortality is about 4 per cent., but it has been as high as 30 per cent. in India. In the enfeebled and old, death may occur at the height of the first paroxysm.

Complications are not frequent. In some epidemics hæmatemesis and hæmaturia have occurred. Pneumonia is not infrequent. The acute enlargement of the spleen may end in rupture. Post-febrile paralyses may occur. Ophthalmia has followed in certain epidemics, and may prove a very tedious and serious complication. In pregnant women abortion usually takes place. Convulsions occasionally follow. Dutton, the well-known worker on tropical diseases, died in *status epilepticus* some weeks after the attack.

Diagnosis.—The onset and general symptoms may not at first be distinctive. At the beginning of an epidemic the cases are usually regarded as anomalous typhoid; but once the typical course is followed in a case the diagnosis is clear. The blood examination is distinctive.

Prophylaxis.—As overcrowding is an important element in the transmission, the patient should be isolated. The bedding, clothing, and dwellings of infected persons should be thoroughly disinfected and care taken that all cracks and crevices in woodwork which may harbor bedbugs are treated with disinfectants.

Treatment.—The paroxysm can neither be cut short nor can its recurrence be prevented. The disease must be treated like any other continued fever, by careful nursing, a regular diet, and ordinary hygienic measures. Of special symptoms, pain in the back and in the limbs and joints demands opium. In enfeebled persons the collapse at the crisis may be serious, and stimulants with ammonia and digitalis should be given freely. The arsenical preparations may be tried, but they have not been very successful.

VII. SYPHILIS

I. HISTORY, ETIOLOGY AND MORBID ANATOMY

Definition.—A specific disease of slow evolution caused by *Treponema pallidum,* propagated by inoculation (acquired syphilis) or transmission through the mother (congenital syphilis).

History.—Whether the disease was known in Europe before 1493 is still discussed. Block, in the System of Syphilis, Vol. I, 1908, insists that there is no evidence of pre-Columbian syphilis in the Eastern hemisphere before the return of the Spanish sailors from Hayti, from whom it spread among the inhabitants of Barcelona. In 1493 it reached Italy with the army of Charles VIII. His soldiers syphilized Naples; the disease spread throughout Italy, and in a few years Europe was aflame. On the other hand, writers who contend for the antiquity of the disease in Asia and Europe rely on certain old Chinese records, on references in the Bible and in old medical writers to diseases resembling syphilis and on suggestive bone lesions in very old skeletons. The balance of evidence, according to the best syphilographers, is in favor of the American origin. At first it was called the Neapolitan disease, the French pox, or Morbus Gallicus; and in 1530 Fracastorius, in a poem entitled "Syphilis sive Morbus Gallicus," gave it the name by which it is now commonly known. The etymology of the name is uncertain.

At first the disease was thought to be transmitted like any other epidemic, but gradually the venereal nature was recognized, and Fernel, a famous Paris physician of the 16th century, insisted on the necessity of a primary inoculation. Paracelsus observed its hereditary character. Throughout the 16th century the symptoms were well described. The disease appears to have been of much greater severity then than at present. Mercury and guaiacum were introduced as the important remedies. In the 18th century Lancisi recognized the relations existing between syphilis and aneurism, and Morgagni described many of the visceral lesions. Hunter, misled by inoculations made on his own person, decided in favor of the unity of the venereal poisons, gonorrhœa, soft chancre and syphilis. Ricord clearly differentiated the soft and hard chancre, and throughout the 19th century the clinical and pathological lesions were so thoroughly studied that scarcely a feature of the disease remained unknown. But all efforts at discovering the cause had failed, until in 1905 Schaudinn demonstrated the presence of a spirochæte in the lesions. Since then his work has been amply verified, and in 1910 Ehrlich announced the discovery of a compound which would destroy the parasite and not damage the individual.

Etiology: The Parasite.—The treponema is a spiral, curved organism from 5 to 15 μ in length, showing active movements in fresh specimens. It is present in the primary sore, in the regional lymph glands, in the secondary lesions, in many gummata, and in special abundance in the congenital lesions, particularly in the liver. Its presence in the body has been demonstrated as long as 15 to 20 years after the primary infection. It is inoculable into monkeys, with the production of a disease resembling in most particulars that of man. The parasite has been successfully cultivated by Noguchi.

One of the most important results of the discovery of the parasite has been the application of the newer methods of serum diagnosis. What is called the Wassermann reaction is a special way of determining the presence of immune bodies in the blood of a patient suffering from any syphilitic infection. An enormous amount of work has been done upon it within the past few years with the general result of confirming its value in diagnosis. A positive result has been obtained in from 90 to 95 per cent. of all cases. It appears from the end of the second to the end of the fourth week, becomes more marked and may continue for an indefinite period. During active treatment it may be absent, to reappear again. Its intensity bears some relation to the activity of the lesions. A positive result has been found in a large proportion of cases of locomotor ataxia, and in paralysis of the insane.

Modes of Infection.—(*a*) In a large majority of all cases the disease is transmitted by *sexual congress,* but the designation *venereal* disease (*lues venerea*) is not always correct, as there are many other modes of inoculation. In the St. Louis Hospital collection there are illustrations of 26 varieties of extragenital chancres.

(*b*) *Accidental Infection.*—In surgical and in midwifery practice physicians are not infrequently inoculated. General infection may occur without a characteristic local sore. Midwifery chancres are usually on the fingers, but they may be on the back of the hand. The lip chancre is the most common of these erratic or extra-genital forms, and may be acquired in many ways apart from direct infection. Mouth and tonsillar sores result as a rule from improper practices. Wet-nurses are sometimes infected on the nipple, and it occasionally happens that relatives of a syphilitic child are accidentally contaminated.

(*c*) *Congenital Transmission.*—The disease is not directly inherited, but the fetus is infected through the placenta. It is a question entirely of intra-uterine infection. The mother herself may be, and often is, apparently quite healthy, but, as recent observations have shown, the Wassermann reaction is present and it is through her and not directly through the father that the disease is transmitted. We can now understand what is known as Beaumès' or Colles' law, which was thus stated by the distinguished Dublin surgeon: "That a child born of a mother who is without obvious venereal symptoms, and which, without being exposed to any infection subsequent to its birth, shows this disease when a few weeks old, this child will infect the most healthy nurse, whether she suckle it, or merely handle and dress it; and yet this child is never known to infect its own mother, even though she suckle it while it has venereal ulcers of the lips and tongue." So, too, a child showing no taint, but born of a woman suffering with syphilis, may with impunity be suckled by its mother (Profeta's law).

Morbid Anatomy.—The *primary lesion,* or chancre, shows: (*a*) A diffuse infiltration of the connective tissue with small, round cells. (*b*) Larger epithelioid cells. (*c*) Giant cells. (*d*) Changes in the small arteries and veins, chiefly thickening of the intima, and alterations in the nerve fibres going to the part. The sclerosis is due in part to this acute obliterative endarteritis. Associated with the initial lesions are changes in the adjacent lymph glands, which undergo hyperplasia, and finally become indurated.

The *secondary lesions* of syphilis are too varied for description here. They consist of condylomata, skin eruptions, affections of the eye, etc.

The *tertiary lesions* consist of circumscribed tumors known as gummata, various skin lesions, and a special type of arteritis.

Gummata.—Syphilomata occur in the bones or periosteum—here they are called nodes—in the muscles, skin, brain, lungs, liver, kidneys, heart, testes, and adrenals. They vary in size from small, almost microscopic bodies to large solid tumors from 3 to 5 cm. in diameter. They are usually firm and hard, but in the skin and on the mucous membranes they tend to break down rapidly and ulcerate. On cross-section a medium-sized gumma has a grayish-white, homogeneous appearance, presenting in the centre a firm, caseous substance, and at the periphery a translucent, fibrous tissue. Often there are groups of three or more surrounded by dense sclerotic tissue.

The arteritis will be considered in a separate section.

II. ACQUIRED SYPHILIS

Primary Stage.—This extends from the appearance of the initial sore until the onset of the constitutional symptoms, and has a variable duration of from six to twelve weeks. The initial sore appears within a month after inoculation, and it first shows itself as a small red papule, which gradually enlarges and breaks in the centre, leaving a small ulcer. The tissue about this becomes indurated so that it ultimately has a gristly, cartilaginous consistence—hence the name, hard or indurated chancre. The size attained is variable, and when small the sore may be overlooked, particularly if it is just within the urethra. The initial lesion has no invariable characteristic and may not be indurated. Syphilitic infection may occur with a chancroid. The glands in the lymph-district of the chancre enlarge and become hard. Suppuration both in the initial lesion and in the glands may occur as a secondary change. The general condition of the patient in this stage is good. There may be no fever and no impairment of health.

Secondary Stage.—The first constitutional symptoms are usually manifested within three months of the appearance of the primary sore. They rarely occur earlier than the sixth or later than the twelfth week:

(*a*) *Fever,* slight or intense, and very variable in character, may occur early before the skin rash; more frequently it is the "fever of invasion" with the secondary symptoms, or the fever may occur at any period. It may be a mild continuous pyrexia, or in other instances with marked remissions, but the most remarkable form is the intermittent, often mistaken for malaria. Such cases have been reported by Yeo and by Sidney Phillips. The fever may reach 105° and the paroxysms persist for months. I have had several cases in which typhoid fever was suspected, and in others tuberculosis.

(*b*) *Anæmia.*—In many cases the syphilitic poison causes a pronounced anæmia which gives to the face a muddy pallor, and there may even be a light-yellow tinging of the conjunctivæ or of the skin, a hæmatogenous icterus. This syphilitic cachexia may in some instances be extreme. The red blood corpuscles do not show any special alterations. The blood count may fall to three millions per cubic millimetre, or even lower. The anæmia may come on suddenly. In a case of syphilitic arthritis in a young girl, following three or four inunctions of mercury, the blood-count fell below two millions per cubic millimetre in a few days.

(*c*) *Cutaneous Lesions.*—The earliest and most common is a *macular syphilide* or *syphilitic roseola,* which occurs on the trunk, and on the front of the arms. The face is often exempt. The spots, which are reddish-brown and symmetrically arranged, persist for a week or two. There may be multiple relapses of roseola, sometimes at long intervals, even eleven years (Fournier). The *papular syphilide,* which forms acne-like indurations about the face and trunk, is often arranged in groups. Other forms are the *pustular rash,* which may closely simulate variola. A *squamous syphilide* occurs, not unlike ordinary psoriasis, except that the scales are less abundant. The rash is more copper-colored and not specially confined to the extensor surfaces.

In the moist regions of the skin, such as the perineum and groins, the axillæ, between the toes, and at the angles of the mouth, the so-called *mucous patches* occur, which are flat, warty outgrowths, with well-defined margins and surfaces covered with a grayish secretion. They are among the most distinctive lesions of syphilis.

Frequently the hair falls out (alopecia), either in patches or by a general thinning. Occasionally the nails become affected (syphilitic onychia).

(*d*) *Mucous Lesions.*—With the fever and the roseolous rash the throat and mouth become sore. The pharyngeal mucosa is hyperæmic, the tonsils are swollen and often present small, kidney-shaped ulcers with grayish-white borders. Mucous patches are seen on the inner surfaces of the cheeks and on the tongue and lips. Hypertrophy of the papillæ in various portions of the mucous membrane produces the syphilitic warts or condylomata which are most frequent about the vulva and anus.

(*e*) *Adenitis.*—The glands are hard, painless and not much enlarged. Involvement of the epitrochlear and posterior cervical glands is specially significant.

(*f*) *Arthritis* and pains in the limbs are common secondary symptoms. Occasionally the joint affection is severe and rheumatic fever is suspected.

(*g*) *Other Lesions.*—*Iritis* is common, and usually affects one eye before the other. It comes on from three to six months after the chancre. There may be only slight ciliary congestion in mild cases, but in severer forms there is great pain, and the condition is serious and demands careful management. *Choroiditis* and *retinitis* are rare secondary symptoms. Ear affections are not common in the secondary stage, but instances are found in which sudden deafness occurs, which may be due to labyrinthine disease; more commonly the impaired hearing is due to the extension of inflammation from the throat to the middle ear. Epididymitis and parotitis are rare. Jaundice may occur, the *icterus syphiliticus præcox.* The acute nephritis will be referred to later.

Tertiary Stage.—No hard and fast line can be drawn between the lesions of the secondary and those of the tertiary period; and, indeed, in exceptional cases, manifestations which usually appear late may set in even before the primary sore has properly healed. The special affections of this stage are certain skin eruptions, visceral gummata, and amyloid degenerations.

(*a*) The late *syphilides* show a greater tendency to ulceration and destruction of the deeper layers of the skin, so that in healing scars are left. They are also more scattered and seldom symmetrical. One of the most characteristic of the syphilides is *rupia,* the dry stratified crusts of which cover an ulcer which involves the deeper layers of the skin and in healing leaves a scar.

(b) *Gummata.*—These may occur in the skin, subcutaneous tissue, muscles, or internal organs. The general character has been already described. In the skin they tend to break down and ulcerate, leaving ugly sores which heal with difficulty. In the solid organs they undergo fibroid transformation and produce puckering and deformity. On the mucous membranes these tertiary lesions lead to ulceration, in the healing of which cicatrices are formed; thus, in the larynx great narrowing may result, and in the rectum ulceration with fibroid thickening and retraction may lead to stricture. Gummatous ulcers may be infective.

(*c*) *Amyloid Degeneration.*—Syphilis plays a most important rôle in the production of this affection. Of 244 instances analyzed by Fagge, 76 had syphilis, and of these 42 had no bone lesions. It follows the acquired form and is very common in association with rectal syphilis in women. In congenital lues amyloid degeneration is rare.

Quaternary Stage.—Long years it may be from the primary sore and from any active manifestations, certain diseases may follow, termed meta- or parasyphilitic affections, the chief of which are locomotor ataxia and dementia paralytica. Since the introduction of the Wassermann reaction these are regarded as definitely syphilitic, dependent upon the parasite itself or in some unknown way upon its poison.

III. CONGENITAL SYPHILIS

With the exception of the primary sore, every feature of the acquired disease may be seen in the congenital form.

The intra-uterine conditions leading to the death of the fetus do not here concern us. The child may be born healthy-looking, or with well-marked evidences of the disease. In the majority of instances the former is the case and within the first month or two the signs of the disease appear.

Symptoms.—(*a*) *At Birth.*—When the disease exists at birth the child is feebly developed and wasted, and a skin eruption is usually present, commonly in the form of bullæ about the hands and feet (pemphigus neonatorum syphiliticus). The child snuffles, the lips are ulcerated, the angles of the mouth fissured, and there is enlargement of the liver and spleen. The bone symptoms may be marked, and the epiphyses may even be separated. In such cases the children rarely survive long.

(*b*) *Early Manifestations.*—When born healthy the child thrives, is fat and plump, and shows no abnormity whatever; then from the fourth to the eighth week, rarely later, a nasal catarrh occurs, *syphilitic rhinitis,* which impedes respiration, and produces the characteristic symptom which has given the name *snuffles* to the disease. The discharge may be sero-purulent or bloody. The child nurses with great difficulty. In severe cases ulceration takes place with necrosis of the bone, leading to a depression at the root of the nose and a deformity characteristic of congenital syphilis. This coryza may be mistaken at first for an ordinary catarrh, but the coexistence of other manifestations usually makes the diagnosis clear. The disease may extend into the Eustachian tube and middle ears and lead to deafness.

The *cutaneous* lesions arise with or shortly after the onset of the snuffles. The skin often has a sallow, earthy hue. The eruptions are first noticed about the nates. There may be an erythema or an eczematous condition, but more commonly there are irregular reddish-brown patches with well-defined edges. A papular syphilide in this region is by no means uncommon. Fissures occur about the lips, either at the angles of the mouth or in the median line. These *rhagades,* as they are called, are very characteristic. There may be marked ulceration of the muco-cutaneous surfaces. The secretions from these mouth lesions are very virulent, and it is from this source that the wet-nurse is usually infected. Not only the nurse, but members of the family, may be contaminated. There are instances in which other children have been accidentally inoculated from a syphilitic infant. The hair of the head or of the eyebrows may fall out. The syphilitic *onychia* is not uncommon. Enlargement of the glands is not so frequent in the congenital as in the acquired disease. When the cutaneous lesions are marked the contiguous glands can usually be felt. As pointed out by Gee, the spleen is enlarged in many cases. The condition may persist for a long time. Enlargement of the liver, though often present, is less significant, since in infants it may be due to various causes. These are among the most constant symptoms of congenital syphilis, and usually arise between the third and twelfth weeks. Frequently they are preceded by a period of restlessness and wakefulness, particularly at night. Some authors have described a peculiar syphilitic cry, high-pitched and harsh. Among rarer manifestations are hæmorrhages—the *syphilis hæmorrhagica neonatorum*. The bleeding may be subcutaneous, from the mucous surfaces, or, when early, from the umbilicus. All of such cases, however, are not syphilitic, and the disease must not be confounded with the acute hæmoglobinuria of new-born infants. E. Fournier has described a remarkable enlargement of the subcutaneous veins.

(*c*) *Late Manifestations.*—Children with congenital syphilis rarely thrive. Usually they present a wizened, wasted appearance, and a prematurely aged face. In the patients who recover the general nutrition may remain good and the child may show no further manifestations of the disease; commonly, however, at the period of second dentition or at puberty the disease reappears. Although the child may have recovered from the early lesions, it does not develop like other children. Growth is slow, development tardy, and there are facial and cranial characteristics which often render the disease recognizable at a glance. A young man of nineteen or twenty may neither look older nor be more developed than a boy of ten or twelve. Fournier describes this condition as *infantilism*. The forehead is prominent, the frontal eminences are marked, and the skull may be very asymmetrical. The bridge of the nose is depressed, the tip *retroussé*. The lips are often prominent, and there are striated lines running from the corners of the mouth. The *teeth* are deformed and may present appearances which Jonathan Hutchinson claims are specific and peculiar. The upper central incisors of the permanent set are peg-shaped, stunted in length and breadth, and narrower at the cutting edge than at the root. On the anterior surface the enamel is well formed, and not eroded or honeycombed. At the cutting edge there is a single notch, usually shallow, sometimes deep, in which the dentine is exposed.

Among late manifestations, particularly apt to appear about puberty, is the interstitial *keratitis*, which usually begins as a slight steaminess of the corneæ, which present a ground-glass appearance. It affects both eyes, though one is attacked before the other. It may persist for months, and usually clears completely, though it may leave opacities, which prevent clear vision. *Iritis* may also occur. Of *ear affections*, apart from those which follow the pharyngeal disease, a form occurs, about the time of puberty or earlier, in which deafness comes on rapidly and persists in spite of all treatment. It is unassociated with obvious lesions, and is probably labyrinthine in character. *Bone lesions*, occurring oftenest after the sixth year, are not rare among the late manifestations of hereditary syphilis. The tibiæ are most frequently attacked. It is really a chronic gummatous periostitis, which gradually leads to great thickening of the bone. The nodes of congenital syphilis, which are often mistaken for rickets, are more commonly diffuse and affect the bones of the upper and lower extremities. They are generally symmetrical and rarely painful. They may occur late, even after the twenty-first year.

Joint lesions are rare. Clutton has described a symmetrical synovitis of the knee in hereditary syphilis. Enlargement of the spleen, sometimes with the lymph-glands, may be one of the late manifestations, and may occur either alone or in connection with disease of the liver.

Gummata of the liver, brain, and kidneys have been found in late hereditary syphilis. General paresis may follow.

Is syphilis transmitted to the third generation? Opinion on this subject is divided. Occasionally cases of pronounced congenital syphilis are met with in the children of parents who are perfectly healthy, and who have not, so far as is known, had syphilis; and yet, as remarked by Coutts in reporting such a group of cases, they do not always bear careful scrutiny. E. Fournier, in his *L'Hérédo-Syphilis Tardive* (1907), cites interesting examples which appear to prove the transmission to the third generation, and this appears to be the view of the French syphilographers. Sir Jonathan Hutchinson was opposed to this view.

IV. VISCERAL SYPHILIS

1. *Syphilis of the Brain and Cord*

Pathology.—There are three anatomical changes in the central nervous system—new growths, arteritis, and chronic degenerative (sclerotic) processes.

(*a*) The new formations or *gummata* form definite tumors, ranging in size from a pea to a walnut, usually multiple and attached to the pia mater, sometimes to the dura. Very rarely they are found unassociated with the meninges. When small they present a uniform, translucent appearance, but when large the centre undergoes a fibro-caseous change, while at the periphery there is a firm, translucent, grayish tissue. They may resemble large tuberculous tumors. The growths are most common in the cerebrum. They may be multiple and may even attain a considerable size without becoming caseous. Occasionally gummata undergo cystic degeneration. In the cord large growths are not so common.

In the neighborhood of the growths gummous meningitis occurs, in which all the membranes are involved. This is more common at the base, about the chiasma and the interpeduncular space, and along the Sylvian fissures.

(*b*) *Arteritis* occurs in the form of nodular tumors on the vessels, which may break down or lead to rupture, or there is a progressive obliterative endarteritis.

(*c*) *Degenerative fibroid changes,* not distinctive anatomically, but clinically directly connected with the disease, are known as post- or meta-syphilitic.

Secondary Changes.—In the brain gummatous arteritis is one of the common causes of softening, which may be extensive, as when the middle cerebral artery is involved, or when there is a large patch of meningitis. In such instances the process is really a meningo-encephalitis, and the symptoms are due to the secondary changes, not directly to the gumma. In the neighborhood of the gumma intense encephalitis or myelitis may occur, and within a few days change the clinical picture.

Syphilitic disease of the nerve-centres occurs usually in the acquired form. In the congenital cases the tumors usually occur early, but may be as late as the twenty-first year. Of late years it has been recognized that the nervous lesions may occur very early in the disease, even before the induration of the primary sore has gone. In a majority of the cases brain symptoms come on within three or four years after infection.

Symptoms.—The chief features of cerebral syphilis are those of tumor cerebri, which will be considered later. They may be classified here as follows:

(*a*) Psychical features. A sudden and violent onset of delirium may be the first symptom. In other instances prior to the occurrence of delirium there have been headache, alteration of character, and loss of memory. The condition may be accompanied by convulsions. There may be no neuritis, no palsy, and no localizing symptoms.

(*b*) More commonly following headache, giddiness, or an excited state which may amount to delirium, the patient has an epileptic seizure or a hemiplegic attack, or there is involvement of the nerves of the base. Some of these cases display a prolonged torpor, a special feature of brain syphilis to which both Buzzard and Huebner have referred, which may persist for a month.

(*c*) In some cases the clinical picture is that of dementia paralytica.

(*d*) Many cases of cerebral syphilis display the symptoms of brain tumor —headache, optic neuritis, vomiting, and convulsions. Of these symptoms convulsions are the most important, and both Fournier and Wood have laid great stress on the value of this symptom in persons over thirty. The first symptoms may, however, rather resemble those of embolism or thrombosis; thus there may be sudden hemiplegia, with or without loss of consciousness.

The symptoms of *spinal syphilis* are extremely varied and may be caused by large gummatous growths attached to the meninges, in which case the features are those of tumor, by gummatous arteritis with secondary softening, by meningitis with secondary cord changes, or by late scleroses. Syphilitic myelitis will be considered under affections of the spinal cord.

Diagnosis.—The history is of the first importance, but it may be extremely difficult to get a trustworthy account. Careful examination should be made for traces of the primary sore, for the cicatrices of bubo, for scars of the skin eruption or throat ulcers, and for bone lesions. The character of the symptoms is often of great assistance. They are multiform, variable, and often such as could not be explained by a single lesion; thus there may be anomalous spinal symptoms or involvement of the nerves of the brain on both sides. The Wassermann reaction in the blood and spinal fluid is of the greatest aid; the spinal fluid shows lymphocytosis (in 85-90 per cent.), a positive globulin reaction (in 90-95 per cent.) and the colloidal gold reaction (in 75-80 per cent.); and lastly the result of treatment has a definite bearing on the diagnosis, as the symptoms may clear up and disappear with the use of anti-syphilitic remedies.

2. *Syphilis of the Respiratory Organs*

Syphilis of the Trachea and Bronchi.—L. A. Conner has analyzed 128 recorded cases of syphilis of the trachea and bronchi. In 52 per cent. of the cases the trachea was alone involved. In only 10 per cent. were characteristic lesions of syphilis found in the lungs. Bronchial dilatation below the lesion was found in 15 per cent. of the cases. In ten of the cases the lesion occurred in congenital syphilis.

Syphilis of the Lung.—This is a very rare disease. In 2,800 post mortems at the Johns Hopkins Hospital there were 12 cases with syphilitic disease in the lungs; in 8 of these the lesions were in congenital syphilis. In 11 cases there were definite gummata. Clinically the presence of syphilis of the lung was suspected in three cases. Some years ago Fowler visited the museums of the London hospitals and the Royal College of Surgeons, and could find only twelve specimens illustrating syphilitic lesions of the lungs, two of which are doubtful. For the most full and satisfactory consideration of pulmonary syphilis, the reader is referred to chapter xxxvii of Fowler and Godlee's work on Diseases of the Lungs.

It occurs under the following forms:

(*a*) *The white pneumonia of the fetus.* This may affect large areas or an entire lung, which then is firm, heavy, and airless, even though the child may have been alive. On section it has a grayish-white appearance—the so-called white hepatization of Virchow. The chief change is in the alveolar walls, which are greatly thickened and infiltrated, and the section is like one of the pancreas—"pancreatization" of the lung. In the early stages, for example, in a seven or eight months' fetus, there may be scattered miliary foci of this induration chiefly about the arteries. The air-cells are filled with desquamated and swollen epithelium.

(*b*) In the form of definite *gummata,* which vary in size from a pea to a goose-egg. They occur irregularly scattered through the lung, but, as a rule, are more numerous toward the root. They present a grayish-yellow caseous appearance, are dry and usually imbedded in a translucent, more or less firm, connective tissue. In a case from my wards described by Councilman there was extensive involvement of the root of the lungs. Bands of connective tissue passed inward from the thickened pleura, and between these strands and surrounding the gummata there was in places a mottled red pneumonic consolidation. In the caseous nodules there is typical hyaline degeneration. In a few rare instances there are most extensive caseous gummata with softening and formation of bronchiectatic cavities, and clinically a picture of pulmonary tuberculosis without the presence of tubercle bacilli. In one case, a man aged twenty-seven, admitted in April, 1902, had had for a year cough and bloody expectoration and died of severe hæmoptysis. Bacilli were never found in the sputum. There were extensive caseous gummata throughout both lungs, with much fibrous thickening, and in the lower lobe of the right lung a cavity 3 by 5 cm. in diameter, on the wall of which a branch of the pulmonary artery was eroded. This is the only instance among my cases in which there was an extensive destruction of the lung tissue with the clinical picture simulating pulmonary phthisis.

(*c*) A majority of authors follow Virchow in recognizing the fibrous interstitial pneumonia at the root of the lung and passing along the bronchi and vessels as probably syphilitic. This much may be said, that in certain cases gummata are associated with these fibroid changes. Again, this condition alone is found in persons with well-marked syphilitic history or with other visceral lesions. It seems in many instances to be a purely sclerotic process, advancing sometimes from the pleura, more commonly from the root of the lung, and invading the interlobular tissue, gradually producing a more or less extensive fibroid change. It rarely involves more than a portion of a lobe or portions of the lobes at the root of the lung. The bronchi are often dilated.

Diagnosis.—It is to be borne in mind, in the first place, that hospital physicians and pathologists the world over bear witness to the extreme rarity of lung syphilis. In the second place, the therapeutic test upon which so much reliance is placed is by no means conclusive. With pulmonary tuberculosis there should be no confusion, owing to the readiness with which the presence of bacilli is determined. Bronchiectasis in the lower lobe of a lung, dependent upon an interstitial pneumonia of syphilitic origin, could not be distinguished from any other form of the disease. In persons with well-marked syphilitic lesions elsewhere, when obscure pneumonia with dilated bronchi and no tubercle bacilli are present, the condition may possibly be due to syphilis. So far as my experience goes, tuberculous phthisis occurring in a syphilitic subject has no special peculiarities. The lesions of syphilis and tuberculosis could of course coexist in a lung. The Wassermann reaction is helpful in a doubtful case.

3. *Syphilis of the Liver*

Varieties.—Inherited.—(*a*) *Congenital.*—Gubler in 1852 first described the diffuse hepatitis which occurs in a large percentage of all deaths in congenital lues. While there may be little or no macroscopic change, the liver preserves its form and is usually enlarged, hard and resistant, and has a yellowish color, compared by Trousseau to sole-leather, or by Gubler to that of flint. Small grayish nodules may be seen on the section. In other cases there are definite gummata with extensive sclerosis. The spirochætes are present in extraordinary numbers.

The child may be still-born or die shortly after birth, or it may be healthy when born and the liver enlarges within a few weeks. The organ is firm; the edge may be readily felt, usually far below the navel. The spleen is also enlarged. The general features are those of a hypertrophic cirrhosis, but jaundice and ascites are not common. Hochsinger states that of 45 cases recovery took place in 30.

(*b*) *Delayed Congenital Syphilis.*—The condition is by no means rare. Of 132 cases of syphilis hereditaria tarda collected by Forbes, in 34 the liver was involved. The children are nearly always ill-developed, sometimes with marked clubbing of the fingers and showing signs of infantilism. Jaundice is rare. The liver is usually enlarged, or it may show nodular masses.

Acquired Syphilis.—(*a*) In the *secondary stages* of the disease the liver is not often involved. Jaundice may occur coincident with the rash and with the enlargement of the superficial glands. Rolleston thinks it is probably due to a catarrhal condition of the smaller ducts, part of a general syphilitic hepatitis. There are cases in which it has passed on to a state of acute yellow atrophy. The liver is slightly enlarged. The prognosis is generally good.

(*b*) *Tertiary Lesions.*—The frequency with which the liver is involved in syphilis in adults is very variously estimated. J. L. Allen, quoted by Rolleston, found 37 cases of hepatic gummata among 11,629 autopsies at St. George's Hospital; in 27 cases cicatrices alone were present. Flexner at the Philadelphia Hospital found 88 cases of hepatic syphilis among 5,088 autopsies. Among 2,300 autopsies at the Johns Hopkins Hospital (Professor Welch) there have been 47 cases of syphilis of the liver, gummata in 19, scars in 16, cirrhosis in 21 cases; 6 of the cases were congenital. My experience coincides with that of Einhorn and of Stockton, who hold that in the United States the disease is by no means uncommon. In 21 cases the diagnosis of syphilis of the liver was made clinically.

Anatomically the lesions may be either gummata or scars or a syphilitic sclerosis. The gummata range in size from a pea to an orange. When small they are pale and gray; the larger ones present yellowish centres; but later there is a "pale, yellowish, cheese-like nodule of irregular outline, surrounded by a fibrous zone, the outer edge of which loses itself in the lobular tissue, the lobules dwindling gradually in its grasp. This fibrous zone is never very broad; the cheesy centre varies in consistence from a gristle-like toughness to a pulpy softness; it is sometimes mortar-like, from cretaceous change" (Wilks). They may form enormous tumors, as in the remarkable one figured on page 351 in Rolleston's work on Diseases of the Liver. They may be felt as large as an orange beneath the skin in the epigastrium and they may disappear with the same extraordinary rapidity as the subcutaneous or periosteal gumma. Macroscopically they may, indeed, at first look like massive cancer. Extensive caseation, softening and calcification may occur. The syphilitic scars are usually linear or star-shaped. They may be very numerous and divide the liver into small sections—the so-called botyroid organ, of which a remarkable example is figured in my *Lectures on Abdominal Tumors.* The syphilitic cirrhosis is usually combined with gummata, or with marked scarring in the portal canal, leading to lobulation of the organ, but the ordinary multilobular cirrhosis is not common.

Symptoms.—In the first place, the clinical picture may be that of cirrhosis —slight jaundice, fever, portal obstruction, ascites. There may not be the slightest suspicion of the syphilitic nature of the case. One of my patients had been tapped thirteen times before admission to the hospital. The diagnosis was made by finding gummata on the shins. She recovered promptly.

In a second group of cases the patient is anæmic, passes large quantities of pale urine containing albumin and tube-casts; the liver is enlarged, perhaps irregular, and the spleen also is enlarged. Dropsical symptoms may supervene, or the patient may be carried off by some intercurrent disease. Extensive amyloid degeneration of the spleen, the intestinal mucosa, and of the liver, with gummata, is found.

Thirdly, in a very important group the symptoms are those of tumor of the liver, causing pain and distress, and on examination an irregular mass is discovered. The tumor may be large, causing a prominent bulging in the epigastrium. Naturally carcinoma is thought of, as there may be nothing to suggest syphilis. In other cases the history or the presence of gummata elsewhere should aid in the diagnosis. In other instances the rapid disappearance under treatment even of a large visible tumor makes the syphilitic nature quite positive. Lastly, in a few cases the irregular fever with enlargement and irregularity of the liver may suggest suppuration, or the uniform great enlargement of the organ hypertrophic biliary cirrhosis, while there are some cases in which the spleen is so greatly enlarged, the anæmia so pronounced, and the liver so small and contracted that the diagnosis of splenic anæmia is made.

4. *Syphilis of the Digestive Tract*

The *œsophagus* is very rarely affected. Stenosis is the usual result. Syphilis of the *stomach* is excessively rare. Flexner reported a remarkable case in association with gummata of the liver, and collected 14 cases in the literature. Syphilitic ulceration has been found in the small intestine and in the cæcum.

The most common seat in this tract is the *rectum*. The affection is found most commonly in women, and results from the growth of gummata in the submucosa above the internal sphincter. The process is slow and tedious, and may last for years before it finally induces stricture. The symptoms are usually those of narrowing of the lower bowel. The condition is readily recognized by rectal examination. The history of gradual on-coming stricture, the state of the patient, and the fact that there is a hard, fibrous narrowing, not an elevated crater-like ulcer, usually render easy the diagnosis from malignant disease. In medical practice these cases come under observation for other symptoms, particularly amyloid degeneration; and the rectal disease may be entirely overlooked, and only discovered post mortem.

5. *Circulatory System*

Syphilis of the Heart.—A fresh, warty endocarditis due to syphilis is not recognized, though occasionally in persons dead of the disease this form is present, as is not uncommon in conditions of debility. Myocarditis is common; there may be fatty degeneration and fibroid changes. Pain, precordial tenderness, disturbance of rhythm and tachycardia are special features. There may be a soft apex systolic murmur, not transmitted and increased by exercise. Changes in the blood-vessels of the walls of the heart are common both in congenital and acquired syphilis, even in cases without clinical symptoms or gross lesions (Adler).

Rupture may take place, as in the cases reported by Dandridge and Nalty, or sudden death, as in the cases of Cayley and Pearce Gould; indeed, sudden death is frequent, occurring in 21 of 63 cases (Mracek).

Syphilis of the Arteries.—Syphilis plays an important rôle in arteriosclerosis and aneurism. Its connection with these processes will be considered later; here we shall refer only to the syphilitic affection of the smaller vessels, which occurs in two forms:

(*a*) An *obliterating endarteritis*, characterized by a proliferation of the subendothelial tissue. The new growth lies within the elastic lamina, and may gradually fill the entire lumen; hence the term obliterating. The media and adventitia are also infiltrated with small cells. This form of endarteritis described by Huebner is not, however, characteristic of syphilis, and its presence alone in an artery could not be considered pathognomonic. If, however, there are gummata in other parts, or if the condition about to be described exists in adjacent arteries, the process may be regarded as syphilitic.

(*b*) *Gummatous Periarteritis.*—With or without involvement of the intima, nodular gummata may develop in the adventitia of the artery, producing globular or ovoid swellings, which may attain considerable size. They are not infrequently seen in the cerebral arteries, which seem to be specially prone to this affection. This form is specific and distinctive of syphilis. Many observers have found *Treponema pallidum* in the syphilitic aortitis, and also in gummatous arteritis of the cerebral vessels.

6. *Renal Syphilis*

Gummata.—Gummata occasionally are found in the kidneys, particularly in cases in which there is extensive gummatous hepatitis. They are rarely numerous, and occasionally lead to scattered cicatrices. Clinically the affection is not recognizable.

Acute Syphilitic Nephritis.—This condition has been carefully studied by the French writers and by Lafleur of Montreal. It is estimated to occur in the secondary stage in about 3.8 per cent., and may occur in from three to six months, sometimes later, from the initial lesion. The outlook is good, though often the albuminuria may persist for months; more rarely chronic nephritis follows. In a few instances syphilitic nephritis has proved rapidly fatal in a fortnight or three weeks. The lesions are not specific, but are similar to those in other acute infections.

7. *Syphilitic Orchitis*

This affection is of special significance to the physician, as its detection frequently clinches the diagnosis in obscure internal disorders. Syphilis occurs in the testes in two forms:

(*a*) The gummatous growth, forming an indurated mass or group of masses in the substance of the organ, and sometimes difficult to distinguish from tuberculous disease. The area of induration is harder and it affects the body of the testes, while tubercle more commonly involves the epididymis. It rarely tends to invade the skin, or to break down, soften, and suppurate, and is usually painless.

(*b*) There is an *interstitial orchitis* regarded as syphilitic, which leads to fibroid induration of the gland and gradually to atrophy. It is a slow, progressive change, coming on without pain, usually involving one organ more than another.

V. DIAGNOSIS, TREATMENT, ETC.

Diagnosis.—General Diagnosis of Syphilis.—There is seldom any doubt concerning the recognition of syphilitic lesions; but the number of persons, without any evident sign of the disease, in whom a positive Wassermann reaction is found proves that a negative diagnosis cannot be based on the absence of history and clinical manifestations. Syphilis is common in the community, and is no respecter of age, sex, or station in life. It is possible that the primary sore may have been of trifling extent, or urethral and masked by a gonorrhœa, and the patient may not have had severe secondary symptoms, but such instances are extremely rare. Inquiries should be made into the history to ascertain if the patient has had skin rashes, sore throat, or if the hair has fallen out. Careful inspection should be made of the throat and skin for signs of old lesions. Scars in the groins, the result of buboes, are uncertain evidences of syphilitic infection. The cicatrices on the legs are often copper-colored, though this cannot be regarded as peculiar to syphilis. The bones should be examined for nodes. In doubtful cases the scar of the primary sore may be found, or there may be signs of atrophy or of hardening of the testes. In women special stress has been laid upon the occurrence of frequent miscarriages, which, in connection with other circumstances, are always suggestive.

In the congenital disease, the occurrence within the first three months of snuffles and skin rash is conclusive. Later, the characters of the syphilitic facies, already referred to, often give a clew to the nature of some obscure visceral lesion. Other distinctive features are the symmetrical development of nodes on the bones and the interstitial keratitis.

The *Treponema pallidum* may be studied from the fresh lesion. After cleaning carefully, serum is sucked out with a small Bier apparatus, and the living spirochætes may be seen in the special "dark field" apparatus used for the purpose.

SERUM DIAGNOSIS.—The Wassermann reaction in good hands may be accepted as a most valuable aid in diagnosis. It is obtained in from 80 to 90 per cent. of all cases of syphilis with manifestations. The results in tabes and dementia paralytica are very constant.

CUTANEOUS REACTION.—An emulsion or extract of pure cultures of *Treponema pallidum*—termed *luetin*—has been employed by Noguchi to obtain a skin reaction. The skin is sterilized and 0.05 c. c. injected intradermically. The local reaction is usually papular, and surrounded by a zone of redness, but may become pustular. There is very slight constitutional effect. The reaction is most constant and marked in tertiary and hereditary cases; it is infrequent, and, if present, mild in the primary and secondary stages, in which the Wassermann reaction is more constant. Treatment affects the Wassermann more than the cutaneous reaction.

THERAPEUTIC TEST.—In a doubtful case, as, for example, an obstinate skin rash or an obscure tumor in the abdomen, antisyphilitic treatment may prove successful, but this cannot always be relied upon.

Prophylaxis.—Irregular intercourse has existed from the beginning of recorded history, and unless man's nature wholly changes—and of this we can have no hope—will continue. Resisting all attempts at solution, the social evil remains the great blot upon our civilization, and inextricably blended with it is the question of the prevention of syphilis. Two measures are available—the one personal, the other administrative.

Personal purity is the prophylaxis which we, as physicians, are especially bound to advocate. Continence may be a hard condition (to some harder than to others), but it can be borne, and it is our duty to urge this lesson upon young and old who seek our advice in matters sexual. Certainly it is better, as St. Paul says, to marry than to burn, but if the former is not feasible there are other altars than those of Venus upon which a young man may light fires. He may practice at least two of the five means by which, as the physician Rondibilis counseled Panurge, carnal concupiscence may be cooled and quelled—hard work of body and hard work of mind. Idleness is the mother of lechery; and a young man will find that absorption in any pursuit will do much to cool passions which, though natural and proper, cannot in the exigencies of our civilization always obtain natural and proper gratification.

To carry out successfully any administrative measures seems hopeless, at any rate in our Anglo-Saxon civilization. The state accepts the responsibility of guarding citizens against small-pox or cholera, but in dealing with syphilis the problem has been too complex and has hitherto baffled solution. Inspection, segregation, and regulation are difficult, if not impossible, to carry out, and public sentiment is bitterly opposed to this plan. The compulsory registration of every case of gonorrhœa and syphilis, with greatly increased facilities for thorough treatment, offers a more acceptable alternative.

The patient should be warned of the various ways in which he may spread the disease and given directions regarding this. Measures for the prevention of infection after exposure can be carried out in the military and naval services more readily than in civil life. The most successful is the application of mercurial ointment mixed with lanolin soon after exposure.

Treatment.—That the later stages which come under the charge of the physician are so common results, in great part, from the carelessness of the patient, who, wearied with treatment, cannot understand why he should continue to take medicine after all the symptoms have disappeared; but, in part, the profession also is to blame for not insisting more urgently that acquired syphilis is not cured in a few months, but takes at least three years, during which time the patient should be under careful supervision.

The patient should lead a regular life, avoiding excess of all kinds. If there is fever rest in bed is advisable. The usual diet can be taken and the patient should drink large quantities of water. The use of alcohol and tobacco should be forbidden during active treatment. When mercury is being taken special care must be given to the mouth. A mouth wash and a potassium chlorate tooth paste should be used frequently. Treatment consists essentially in the use of three remedies, mercury, arsenic and iodide of potassium.

MERCURY.—It is usually well to push the administration of mercury so that the patient is brought under its influence as rapidly as possible, but salivation is to be avoided. Mercury may be given by the *mouth* in the form of gray powder, the hydrargyrum cum cretâ, which Hutchinson recommends to be given in pills, one-grain doses with a grain of Dover's powder. One pill from four to six times a day will usually suffice. I warmly endorse the excellent results which are obtained by this method, under which the patient often gains rapidly in weight, and the general health improves remarkably. It may be continued for months without any ill effects. Other forms given by the mouth are biniodide (gr. 1/16), the protoiodide (gr. 1/4), or the bichloride (gr. 1/16 to 1/8), three times a day.

Inunction is a still more effective means. A drachm of the ordinary mercurial ointment or the oleate of mercury is thoroughly rubbed into the skin, on areas free from hair, every evening for six days; on the seventh a warm bath is taken, and on the eighth the mercurial course is resumed. At least half an hour should be given to each inunction. It is well to apply it to different places on successive days. The sides of the chest and abdomen and the inner surfaces of the arms and thighs are the best positions. A course of thirty to forty inunctions should be given.

The mercury may be given by intramuscular *injection*. If proper precautions are taken in sterilizing the syringe, and if the injections are made into the muscles, not into the subcutaneous tissue, abscesses rarely result. Mercury salicylate as a 10 per cent. solution in albolene, of which ten minims are given every five to seven days, bichloride of mercury (gr. 1/20 to 1/10) in olive oil, the "gray oil," or calomel (gr. i) in equal parts of glycerine and water (1 of calomel to 10 of the mixture) are the usual preparations. A course of twenty to thirty injections should be given.

Intravenous injections are sometimes given in malignant cases. Fifteen minims of a .1 to .2 per cent. solution of the bichloride in sterile salt solution are administered.

Still another method in vogue in certain parts of the Continent and in institutions is *fumigation*. The patient sits on a chair wrapped in blankets, with the head exposed. Calomel (gr. xx, 1.3 gm.) is volatilized and deposited with the vapor on the patient's skin. The process lasts about twenty minutes, and the patient goes to bed wrapped in blankets without washing or drying the skin.

ARSENIC.—While atoxyl and cacodylate of sodium have been employed, the most useful preparations are salvarsan (dioxydiamido-arsenobenzol) and neo-salvarsan. We are not yet able to speak with finality regarding all the points with reference to them, but they are certainly a valuable addition to our treatment of syphilis. They should be given *intravenously* and only by those who are properly instructed in the method. The salt solution employed should be prepared from water *freshly* distilled not more than a few hours before from glass and not from metal. The solution is prepared as follows: To 30 c. c. of sterile freshly distilled water in a graduated sterile glass vessel the amount of salvarsan to be given is added and dissolved by vigorous shaking which may be aided by glass beads. When complete solution has occurred a 15 per cent. solution of sodium hydroxide solution is added drop by drop. This causes a precipitate to form and sufficient sodium hydroxide is then added drop by drop until this dissolves. Sterile salt solution (0.5 per cent.) is then added to bring the quantity up to 200 c. c. Salvarsan should be given well diluted (40 c. c. of solution to 0.1 gm. of salvarsan), and always in a freshly prepared solution. The solution is best injected into one of the veins at the elbow and may be given by a syringe with a three-way cock or by gravity through a funnel or from a glass cylinder. Some salt solution should be run in first to be sure that the needle is in the vein and the salvarsan solution then given. Salt solution should be given at the end. It is wise for the patient to remain in bed for a day after the injection.

The most suitable dosage is not yet determined. Some give two doses (0.5 gm., 7½ grains) at intervals of ten days, others one dose (0.5 gm.) followed by several smaller ones (0.2 gm., 3 grains), others repeated small doses (0.2 gm.) at intervals; half a gram may be regarded as an average maximum dose, but larger amounts are sometimes given. For young children doses of 0.1 to 0.2 gm. are used and for infants 0.02 to 0.1 gm. In determining the amount, the weight of the patient is a good indication. Changes in the eye grounds and severe circulatory and renal lesions may be contra-indications in some cases. Caution is advisable in the syphilitic lesions of the aorta and aortic valves; if salvarsan is used, small doses (0.2 gm.) should be given. Neo-salvarsan is given in about double the dose of salvarsan.

The conditions in which salvarsan is especially useful are: (1) at the onset when the diagnosis is made early; one dose (0.5 gm.) may be sufficient. (2) In patients with severe skin or mucous membrane lesions. (3) In intractable cases, in those resistant to or unable to take mercury. (4) In malignant cases. (5) In congenital syphilis. (6) In latent cases, in which without any signs of syphilis a Wasserman reaction is present. In visceral syphilis the drug is less useful. Its value in lesions of the nervous system is not settled; some patients are undoubtedly benefited and the same may be said of the para-syphilitic affections. In general the earlier in the course the drug is given the better the effect.

Mercury should always be given after salvarsan, which, except perhaps in a few cases given at the onset, can not be regarded as a complete remedy in itself. If the patient is seen early salvarsan should be given and followed by mercury, the first course of which should be by inunction or injection if possible, and after this by mouth. The mixed treatment should only be given after a thorough course of mercury. For one year mercury should be given as continuously as possible; during the second year intermissions are advisable, but not for more than one-quarter of the time.

In CONGENITAL SYPHILIS the treatment of cases born with bullæ and other signs of the disease is not satisfactory, and the infants usually die within a few days or weeks. The child should be nursed by the mother alone, or, if this is not feasible, should be hand-fed, but under no circumstances should a wet-nurse be employed. The child is most rapidly and thoroughly brought under the influence of the drug by inunction. The mercurial ointment may be smeared on the flannel roller. This is not a very cleanly method, and sometimes rouses the suspicion of the mother. It is preferable to give the drug by the mouth, in the form of gray powder, half a grain three times a day. In the late manifestations associated with bone lesions the combination of mercury and iodide of potassium is most suitable and is well given in the form of Gilbert's syrup, which consists of the biniodide of mercury (gr. j), of potassium iodide (℥ss.), and water (℥ij). Of this the dose for a child under three is from five to ten drops three times a day, gradually increased. Under these measures the cases of congenital syphilis usually improve with great rapidity. The medication should be continued at intervals for many months, and it is well to watch these patients carefully during the period of second dentition and at puberty, and if necessary to place them on specific treatment.

In the treatment of the VISCERAL LESIONS of syphilis, which come more distinctly within the province of the physician, iodide of potassium is of equal or even greater value than mercury. Under its use ulcers rapidly heal, gummatous tumors melt away, and we have an illustration of a specific action only equaled by that of mercury in the secondary stages, by iron in certain forms of anæmia, and by quinine in malaria. It is as a rule well borne in an initial dose of 10 grains (0.6 gm.); given in milk the patient does not notice the taste. It should be gradually increased to 30 or more grains three times a day. In syphilis of the nervous system it may be used in still larger doses.

When syphilitic hepatitis is suspected the combination of mercury and iodide of potassium is most satisfactory. If there is ascites, Addison's or Guy's pill (as it is often called) of calomel, digitalis, and squill will be found very useful. Occasionally the iodide of sodium is more satisfactory than the iodide of potassium. It is less depressing and agrees better with the stomach.

Syphilis and Marriage.—Upon this question the family physician is often called to decide. He should insist upon the necessity of two full years elapsing between the date of infection and the contracting of marriage. This, it should be borne in mind, is the earliest possible limit, and marriage should be allowed only if the treatment has been thorough and if at least a year has passed without any manifestation of the disease.

Syphilis and Life Insurance.—An individual with syphilis can not be regarded as a first-class risk unless he can furnish evidence of prolonged and thorough treatment and of immunity for two or three years from all manifestations. Even then, when we consider the extraordinary frequency of the cerebral and other complications in persons who have had this disease and who may even have undergone thorough treatment, the risk to the company is certainly increased (see Bramwell, Clinical Studies, vol. i).

VIII. DISEASES DUE TO PARASITIC INFUSORIA

Several flagellates are parasitic in man. The *Trichomonas vaginalis*, which measures 15 μ to 25 μ in length and has four flagella, which are as long as or longer than the body, is by no means uncommon in the acid vaginal mucus.

The *Trichomonas* or *Cercomonas hominis* lives in the intestines, and is met with in the stools under all sorts of conditions. Freund from Dock's clinic has reported a series of cases which show that the parasite may cause acute and chronic diarrhœa with severe abdominal pain, and anatomically an acute enteritis. In one of Dock's cases the parasites were associated with a hæmorrhagic cystitis without bacteria.

The *Lamblia intestinalis* is another intestinal monad, larger than the common trichomonas. Flagellates have also been found in the expectoration in cases of gangrene of the lung and of bronchiectasis, and in the exudate of pleurisy.

The *Balantidium coli*, oval in form, 70 μ to 100 μ long and 50 μ to 70 μ broad, may be pathogenic. It is common in pigs, and has been known to produce an epidemic dysentery in apes (Harlow Brooks). The pathological significance of this parasite has been demonstrated by Strong and Musgrave in the Philippines, where it is a cause of dysentery. It has not only been found in the stools and on the mucous membrane of the intestine, but the parasites have occurred in the mucosa itself and in the submucosa. Apparently they do not extend beyond the wall of the bowel.

D. DISEASES DUE TO METAZOAN PARASITES

I. DISEASES DUE TO FLUKES—DISTOMIASIS

The Trematoda or flukes are parasitic platyhelminths, usually with flattened or leaf-shaped bodies. The term *Distomiasis* is based upon Distoma, the term being used to designate the trematodes.

The following are the important clinical forms:

1. Pulmonary Distomiasis; Parasitic Hæmoptysis.—*Paragonimus* (Distoma) *westermanii*, the Asiatic lung or bronchial fluke, is from 8 to 16 mm. in length by 4 to 8 mm. broad, and of a pinkish or reddish-brown color.

It is found extensively in China and Japan, Formosa, and the Philippines, and cases are occasionally imported into Europe and America, and has been met with in the oriental population of the Pacific coast. It has been found in the United States in the cat, in the dog, and in the hog. One instance of pulmonary distomiasis has been reported caused by the giant liver fluke.

Clinically the disease, as described by Manson and Ringer, is characterized by a chronic cough, with rusty-brown sputum, and occasional attacks of hæmoptysis, usually trifling, but sometimes very severe. The disease is very apt to be mistaken for tuberculosis, but the diagnosis is easily made by microscopic examination of the sputum. The ova, which are abundant in the sputum, are oval, smooth, and measure from 80 μ to 100 μ in length by 40 μ to 60 μ in breadth. The parasites may affect other organs—the liver, the brain, and eyelid.

2. Hepatic Distomiasis.—Six species of liver flukes are known to occur in man. More specifically these are: (1) The common liver fluke—*Fasciola hepatica*—which is a very common parasite in the ruminants. It is a rare and accidental parasite in man, but in Syria a strange disease called *Halzoun* is caused by eating raw goat-liver infected with the parasite. (2) The lancet fluke—*Dicrocœlium* (*Distoma*) *lanceatum.* (3) *Opisthorchis* (*Distoma*) *felineus,* which is found in Prussia and Siberia, and by Ward in cats in Nebraska. (4) *Opisthorchis noverca—Distomum conjunctum*—the Indian liver fluke described in man by McConnell. (5) *Opisthorchis* (*Distoma*) *sinensis,* which is by far the most important of the liver flukes and occurs extensively in Japan, China, and India. It is 10 to 20 mm. long by 2 to 5 mm. broad. The eggs are oval, 27 μ to 30 μ by 15 μ to 17 μ, dark brown, with sharply defined operculum. A number of imported cases have been found in Canada and the United States. White found 18 cases in San Francisco.

The *symptoms* of hepatic distomiasis are best described in connection with the last form. The following account is abstracted from Wallace Taylor. Young children are the chief sufferers. Many members of a family are usually affected. In some villages a large proportion of the inhabitants are attacked. Among important symptoms is an irregular, intermittent diarrhœa; at first there may or may not be blood. The liver enlarges and a condition of cirrhosis gradually comes on. There may be pain and an intermittent jaundice. There is not much fever. After lasting for two or three years dropsy comes on, with anasarca and ascites. Even then transient recovery may take place, but as a rule there is a recurrence, and the patient dies after many years of illness. The ova of the parasite are readily found in the stools.

3. Intestinal Distomiasis.—In India the *Fasciolopsis* (*Distoma*) *buskii* has been found in a number of cases in the small intestines. The *Mesogonimus heterophyes* has been found in Egypt and Japan.

The *Asiatic Amphistome—Gastrodiscus* (*Amphistoma*) *hominis*—a not uncommon parasite in India—is easily recognized by its large posterior sucker.

4. Hæmic Distomiasis; Bilharziasis.—One of the most important of parasitic diseases, caused by the blood fluke, *Schistosomum hæmatobium* or *Bilharzia hæmatobia.* Endemic hæmaturia has been known for many years, particularly in Egypt, where in 1851 Bilharz discovered the parasite of the disease. It prevails in South and North Africa, particularly the latter, in Arabia, Persia, and the west coast of India. Imported cases are not very uncommon in Europe, and an occasional instance is met with in the United States. In Egypt, among 11,698 patients admitted to the Cairo Hospital, 1,270 were infected, practically 10 per cent. (Madden). Of 500 autopsies at the same hospital, in 8 per cent. death was due to the effects of Bilharzial disease. The seriousness of the condition in Egypt is well illustrated by the fact that in 7.5 per cent. of army recruits the ova are found in the urine. An Asiatic blood fluke, *Schistosomum japonicum,* has recently been discovered which differs in small details from the African variety.

The *parasite* is singular among flukes as having the sexes separate, and the male usually carries the female in a gynæcophorous canal. The mode of entrance into the body is unknown, whether by the mouth, the urethra, or through the skin. The eggs are very characteristic, oval in shape, 0.16 mm. by 0.06 mm., and one end has a terminal spine. The eggs hatch in water, but the further development of the free-swimming embryos has not been followed. Taken into the body, possibly with water or on cresses, it reaches the portal veins, in which the worms are most commonly found, usually young specimens and uncoupled. The males bearing the females creep to various parts, particularly the bladder and rectum. The vesciculæ seminales may be first attacked. The eggs are laid in the tissues, but wander, like other sharp foreign bodies, and escape with the urine and fæces. A majority of them remain in the tissues and cause irritation, fibroid changes, and papillomata in the bladder and rectum. Collecting in the bladder as foreign bodies they form the nuclei of calculi.

Symptoms.—As is so often the case with animal parasites, they may cause no inconvenience. Irritability of the bladder, dull pain in the perineum, and hæmaturia are the most frequent symptoms. A chronic cystitis follows when the walls of the bladder are much thickened by the irritation caused by the ova. The anæmia caused by the hæmorrhage is slight in comparison with that of ankylostomiasis. When the rectum is involved there are straining and tenesmus, with the passage of mucus and blood; in severe cases large papillomata form and a chronic ulcerative proctitis. There may be a chronic vaginitis.

Of the complications, calculi in kidney and bladder are the most important. Milton, Madden, and others of the Cairo School of Medicine have studied carefully the surgical aspects of the disease. Periurethral abscess and perineal fistulæ are very common in the chronic cases.

Few symptoms are caused by the presence of the parasites in the portal veins, but there may be an advanced cirrhosis of a Glissonian type due to an enormous thickening of the periportal tissues (Symmers). This author has also reported an instance of the Bilharzia in the pulmonary blood in a case of Bilharzial colitis, and the worms were found living in the pulmonary circulation.

The diagnosis is readily made by finding the characteristic ova in the bloody urine or in the blood and mucus from the rectum. The Bilharzia may be present in the body for years without producing serious damage, and in slight infections the symptoms may disappear (Sandwith), particularly in children.

5. Schistosoma japonicum vel cattoi.—In China and Japan and in the Philippines there is a disease characterized by cirrhosis of the liver, splenomegaly, ascites, dysentery, progressive anæmia, and sometimes by focalized epilepsy. It occurs extensively in one district of Japan, and is known as the "Katayama" disease. Woolley has met with it in the Philippines, and Catto in China. It seems that the so-called urticarial fever, which is not very uncommon in China and Japan, is associated with the presence of this parasite, and an eosinophilia with fever and urticaria should lead to a careful examination of the stools for its eggs. The parasite lives in the vessels of the alimentary canal; the ova are smaller than those of *S. hœmatobium,* and have not the characteristic spinous ends.

Treatment.—We know of nothing which can kill the parasites in the blood. Extract of male fern is recommended for the hæmaturia. The chronic cystitis and proctitis demand the usual measures for these disorders.

II. DISEASES CAUSED BY CESTODES—TÆNIASIS

Man harbors the adult parasites in the small intestine, the larval forms in the muscles and solid organs.

1. INTESTINAL CESTODES; TAPEWORMS

Tænia solium (Pork Tapeworm).—This is not a common form in the United States. It is not uncommon in Panama. It is more frequent in parts of Europe and Asia. When mature it is from 6 to 12 feet in length. The head is small, round, not so large as the head of a pin, and provided with four sucking disks and a double row of hooklets; hence it is called, in contradistinction to the other form in man, the armed tapeworm. To the head succeeds a narrow, thread-like neck, then the segments, or proglottides, as they are called. The segments possess both male and female generative organs, and at about the four-hundred-and-fiftieth they become mature and contain ripe ova. The worm attains its full growth in from three to three and a half months, after which time the segments are continuously shed and appear in the stools. The segments are about 1 cm. in length and from 7 to 8 mm. in breadth. Pressed between glass plates the uterus is seen as a median stem with about eight to fourteen lateral branches. There are many thousands of ova in each ripe segment, and each ovum consists of a firm shell, inside of which is a little embryo, provided with six hooklets. The segments are continuously passed, and if the ova are to attain further development they must be taken into the stomach, either of a pig, or of man himself. The egg-shells are digested, the six-hooked embryos become free, and passing from the stomach reach various parts of the body (the liver, muscles, brain, or eye), where they develop into the larvæ or cysticerci. A hog under these circumstances is said to be *measled,* and the cysticerci are spoken of as measles or bladder worms.

Tænia solium received its name because it was thought to exist as a solitary parasite in the bowel, but two or three or even more worms may occur.

Tænia saginata or Mediocanellata (Unarmed, Fat, or Beef Tapeworm.)—This is a longer and larger parasite than *Tænia solium.* It is certainly the common tapeworm of North America. Of scores of specimens which I have examined almost all were of this variety. According to Bérenger-Féraud it has spread rapidly in western Europe, owing probably to the importation of beef and live-stock from the Mediterranean basin. It may attain a length of 15 or 20 feet, or more. The head is large in comparison with that of *Tænia solium,* and measures over 2 mm. in breadth. It is square-shaped and provided with four large sucking disks, but there are no hooklets. The ripe segments are from 17 to 18 mm. in length and from 8 to 10 mm. in breadth. The uterus consists of a median stem with from fifteen to thirty-five lateral branches, which are given off more dichotomously than in *Tænia solium.* The ova are somewhat larger, and the shell is thicker, but the two forms can scarcely be distinguished by their ova. The ripe segments are passed as in *Tænia solium,* and are ingested by cattle, in the flesh or organs of which the eggs develop into the bladder worms or cysticerci.

Of other forms of tapeworm may be mentioned:

Dipylidium caninum (Tænia elliptica, Tænia cucumerina).—A small parasite very common in the dog and occasionally found in man; the larvæ develop in the lice and fleas of the dog.

Hymenolepis diminuta (Tænia flavo-punctata).—This small cestode was found in the intestine of a child in Boston, and has since been met with in twelve cases (Ransom). It is common in rats. The larvæ develop in *Lepidoptera* and in beetles.

Hymenolepis nana (Tænia nana) occurs not infrequently in Italy. It is not very uncommon in the United States (Stiles). The *Davainea madagascariensis* (*Tænia madagascariensis*) is a rare form.

Tænia confusa, a new species described by Ward.

Dibothriocephalus latus.—A cestode worm found only in certain districts bordering on the Baltic Sea, in parts of Switzerland, and in Japan. Nickerson has shown that it is common among the Finns in the Northwestern States, and it seems not improbable that the fish in the Great Lakes have become infected, as cases have increased of late years. The parasite is large and long, measuring from 25 to 30 feet or more. Its head is different from that of the tænia, as it possesses two lateral grooves or pits and has no hooklets. The larvæ develop in the peritoneum and muscles of the pike and other fish, and it has been shown experimentally that they grow into the adult worm when eaten by man.

Symptoms of Tapeworm Infection.—These parasites are found at all ages. They are not uncommon in children and are occasionally found in sucklings. W. T. Plant refers to a number of cases in children under two years, and there is one in the literature in which it is stated that the tapeworm was found in an infant five days old!

The parasites may cause no disturbance and are rarely dangerous. A knowledge of the existence of the worm is generally a source of worry and anxiety; the patient may have considerable distress and complain of abdominal pains, nausea, diarrhœa, and sometimes anæmia. Occasionally the appetite is ravenous. In women and in nervous patients the constitutional disturbance may be considerable, and we not infrequently see great mental depression and even hypochondria. Various nervous phenomena, such as chorea, convulsions, or epilepsy, are believed to be caused by the parasites. Such effects, however, are very rare. The *Dibothriocephalus* may cause a severe and even fatal form of anæmia, which has been described fully in the monograph of Schaumann, of Helsingfors. It has been suggested that the metabolic products of the worm may have in some cases a hæmolytic action. Eosinophilia may occur.

Diagnosis.—The diagnosis is never doubtful. The presence of the segments is distinctive. The ova, too, may be recognized in the stools. It makes but little difference as to the form of tapeworm, but the ripe segments of *Tænia saginata* are larger and broader, and show differences in the generative system as already mentioned.

Prophylaxis.—The prophylaxis is most important. Careful attention should be given to three points. First, all tapeworm segments should be burned; they should never be thrown into the water-closet or outside; secondly, careful inspection of meat at the abattoirs; and, thirdly, cooking the meat sufficiently to kill the parasites.

In the case of the beef measles, the distribution of the parasites, as given by Ostertag, shows that the muscles of the jaw are much more frequently affected than other parts—360 times—while other organs were infected but 55 times. Sometimes there are instances of general infection. In Berlin the proportion of cattle infected in 1892-'93 was about 1 to 672. Cold storage kills the cysticercus usually within three weeks. The measles are more readily overlooked in beef than in pork, as they do not present such an opaque white color.

In the examination of hogs for cysticerci "particular stress should be laid upon the tongue, the muscles of mastication, and the muscles of the shoulder, neck, and diaphragm" (Stiles). They may be seen very easily on the under surface of the tongue. American hogs are comparatively free. In Prussia one hog is infected in about every 637. Specimens have been found alive twenty-nine days after slaughtering. In the examination of 1,000 hogs in Montreal, Clement and I found 76 instances of cysticerci. For full details with reference to the inspection of meat for animal parasites, the practitioner is referred to the work of Dr. Stiles, in Bulletin No. 19, United States Department of Agriculture, 1898.

Treatment.—Three days should be given to preparation for treatment, whatever drug is employed. For two days the patient should take soft food and the third day liquids only. The bowels should be well moved by castor oil taken each evening and a saline in the morning if necessary. Unless the bowels have moved freely an enema should be given. On the third night a laxative, such as cascara, should be taken. There are many drugs, but male fern is usually the most reliable, given in the form of the ethereal extract. This is taken early in the morning of the fourth day before any food is taken. The usual dose is ʒi (4 c. c.), which is repeated in an hour. It may be given in capsules or in glycerine (℥ ss, 15 c. c.). If there is fear of nausea a cup of coffee may be taken before the drug. After taking the male fern the patient should remain quiet and resist any desire to vomit. One hour after the second dose of male fern a full dose of saline is taken (magnesium or sodium sulphate, or magnesium citrate), and an hour later a second dose if the bowels have not moved. Great care should be taken during the expulsion of the worm, which should be passed into a chamber containing water at about the body temperature, a practice recommended by Celsus.

The pomegranate root is a very efficient remedy, and may be given as an infusion of the bark, 3 ounces of which may be macerated in 10 ounces of water and then reduced to one-half by evaporation. The entire quantity is then taken in divided doses. It occasionally produces colic, but is a very effective remedy. The active principle, pelleticrine, is now much employed as the tannate, given in doses of 6 to 8 or even 10 grains (0.4 to 0.6 gm.), and followed in an hour by a purge.

Pumpkin seeds are sometimes very efficient. Three or four ounces should be carefully bruised and then macerated for twelve or fourteen hours, and the entire quantity taken and followed in an hour by a purge. Of other remedies, cusso, naphthalein (gr. v, 0.3 gm.), turpentine in ounce doses in honey, and kamala may be mentioned. Sometimes a combination of remedies is effectual when one fails. In children the use of pumpkin seeds or pelletierine is generally best. One cause of failure is the use of drugs which are old and inert.

Unless the head is brought away, the parasite continues to grow, and within a few months the segments again appear. Some instances are extraordinarily obstinate. Doubtless almost everything depends upon the exposure of the worm. The head and neck may be thoroughly protected beneath the valvulæ conniventes, in which case the remedies may not act. Owing to its armature *Tænia solium* is more difficult to expel. It is probable that no degree of peristalsis could dislodge the head, and unless the worm is killed it does not let go its extraordinarily firm hold on the mucous membrane. Owing to the danger of cysticercosis, treatment should not be delayed in case of infection with *Tænia solium.*

2. SOMATIC TÆNIASIS

Whereas adult tænia may give rise to little or no disturbance, and rarely, if ever, prove directly fatal, the affections caused by the larvæ or immature forms in the solid organs are serious and important. There are two chief cestode larvæ known to frequent man: (*a*) the *Cysticercus cellulosæ,* the larva of *Tænia solium,* and (*b*) the *Echinococcus,* the larva of *Tænia echinococcus.* The *Cysticercus tæniæ saginatæ* has been found only two or three times in man.

Cysticercus cellulosæ.—When man accidentally takes into his stomach the ripe ova of *Tænia solium* he is liable to become the intermediate host, a part usually played for this tapeworm by the pig. This accident may occur in an individual the subject of *Tænia solium*, in which case the mature proglottides either themselves wander into the stomach or, what is more likely, are forced into the organ in attacks of prolonged vomiting. Of course the accidental ingestion from the outside of a few ova is quite possible, and the liability of infection should always be borne in mind in handling the segments of the worm.

The symptoms depend entirely upon the number of ova ingested and the localities reached. In the hog the cysticerci produce very little disturbance. The muscles, the connective tissue, and the brain may be swarming with the measles, as they are called, and yet the nutrition is maintained and the animal does not appear to be seriously incommoded. In the invasion period, if large numbers of the parasites are taken, there is, in all probability, constitutional disturbance; certainly this is seen in the calf, when fed with the ripe segments of *Tænia saginata*.

In man a few cysticerci lodged beneath the skin or in the muscles give no trouble, and in time the larvæ die and become calcified. They are occasionally found in dissection subjects or in post mortems as ovoid white bodies in the muscles or subcutaneous tissue. In America they are very rare. I saw but one instance in my post mortem experience. Depending on the number and the locality specially affected, the symptoms may be grouped into general, cerebro-spinal, and ocular. In 155 cases compiled by Stiles, the parasite in 117 was found in the brain, in 32 in the muscles, in 9 in the heart, in 3 in the lungs, subcutaneously in 5, in the liver in 2.

1. General.—As a rule the invasion of the larvæ in man, unless in very large numbers, does not cause very definite symptoms. It occasionally happens, however, that a striking picture is produced. A patient was admitted to my wards very stiff and helpless, so much so that he had to be assisted upstairs and into bed. He complained of numbness and tingling in the extremities and general weakness, so that at first he was thought to have a peripheral neuritis. At the examination, however, a number of painful subcutaneous nodules were discovered, which proved on excision to be the cysticerci. Altogether 75 could be felt subcutaneously, and from the soreness and stiffness they probably existed in large numbers in the muscles. There were none in his eyes, and he had no brain symptoms.

2. Cerebro-spinal.—Remarkable symptoms may result from the presence of the cysticerci in the brain and cord. In the silent region they may be abundant without producing any symptoms. I have in my possession the brain of a pig containing scores of "measles," yet the animal in the few moments in which I saw it just prior to death did not present any symptoms to attract attention. In the ventricles of the brain the cysticerci may attain a considerable size, owing to the fact that in regions in which they are unrestrained in their growth, as in the peritoneum, the bladder-like body grows freely. When in the fourth ventricle remarkable irritative symptoms may be produced. In 1884 I saw with Friedländer in Berlin a case from Riess's wards in which during life there had been symptoms of diabetes and anomalous nervous symptoms. Post mortem, the cysticercus was found beneath the valve of Vieussens, pressing upon the floor of the fourth ventricle.

3. OCULAR.—Since von Graefe demonstrated the presence of the cysticercus in the vitreous humor many cases have been placed on record, as it is a condition easily recognized.

Except in the eye, the diagnosis can rarely be made; when the cysticerci are subcutaneous one may be excised. It is possible that when numerous throughout the muscles they may be seen under the tongue, in which situation they may exist in the pig in numbers.

Echinococcus Disease.—The hydatid worms or echinococci are the larvæ of *Tænia echinococcus* of the dog. This is a tiny cestode not more than 4 or 5 mm. in length, consisting of only three or four segments, of which the terminal one alone is mature, and has a length of about 2 mm. and a breadth of 0.6 mm. The head is small and provided with four sucking disks and a rostellum with a double row of hooklets. This is an exceedingly rare parasite in the dog. Cobbold states that he has never met with a natural specimen in England. Leidy had not one in his large collection. I did not meet with an instance in America; Curtice, of Washington, found it once in an American dog. The worms are so small that they may be readily overlooked, since they form small, white, thread-like bodies closely adherent among the villi of the small intestines. The ripe segment contains about 5,000 eggs, which attain their development in the solid organs of various animals, particularly the hog and ox, more rarely the horse and the sheep. In some countries man is a common intermediate host, owing to the accidental ingestion of the ova.

DEVELOPMENT.—The little six-hooked embryo, freed from the egg-shell by digestion, burrows through the intestinal wall and reaches the peritoneal cavity or the muscles; it may enter the portal vessels and be carried to the liver. It may enter the systemic vessels, and, passing the pulmonary capillaries, as it is protoplasmic and elastic, may reach the brain or other parts. Once having reached its destination, it undergoes the following changes: The hooklets disappear and the little embryo is gradually converted into a small cyst which presents two distinct layers—an external, laminated, cuticular membrane or capsule, and an internal, granular, parenchymatous layer, the endocyst. The little cyst or vesicle contains a clear fluid. There is more or less reaction in the neighboring tissues, and the cyst in time has a fibrous investment. When this primary cyst or vesicle has attained a certain size, buds develop from the parenchymatous layer, which are gradually converted into cysts, presenting a structure identical with that of the original cyst, namely, an elastic chitinous membrane lined with a granular parenchymatous layer. These secondary or daughter cysts are at first connected with the lining membrane of the primary cyst, but are soon set free. In this way the parent cyst as it grows may contain a dozen or more daughter cysts. Inside these daughter cysts a similar process may occur, and from buds in the walls granddaughter cysts are developed. From the granular layer of the parent and daughter cysts buds arise which develop into brood capsules. From the lining membrane the little outgrowths arise and gradually develop into bodies known as scolices, which represent in reality the head of the *Tænia echinococcus* and present four sucking disks and a circle of hooklets. Each scolex is capable when transferred to the intestines of a dog of developing into an adult tapeworm. The difference between the ovum of an ordinary tapeworm, such as *Tænia solium,* and *Tænia echinococcus* is in this way very striking. In the former case the ovum develops into a single larva—*Cysticercus cellulosæ* —whereas the egg of *Tænia echinococcus* develops into a cyst which is capable of multiplying enormously and from the lining membrane of which millions of larval tapeworms develop. Ordinarily in man the development of the echinococcus takes place as above mentioned and by an endogenous form in which the secondary and tertiary cysts are contained within the primary; but in animals the formation may be different, as the buds from the primary cyst penetrate between the layers and develop externally, forming the exogenous variety. A third form is the multilocular echinococcus, in which form the primary cyst buds develop which are cut off completely and are surrounded by thick capsules of a connective tissue, which join together and ultimately form a hard mass represented by strands of connective tissue inclosing alveolar spaces about the size of peas or a little larger. In these spaces are found the remnants of the echinococcus cyst, occasionally the scolices or hooklets, but they are often sterile.

The fluid is limpid, non-albuminous; specific gravity 1.005 to 1.009, occasionally higher. It may contain sugar and succinic acid, and, after repeated tapping of the cyst, albumin. When not degenerated the hydatid heads or the characteristic hooklets are found in the contents of the cyst.

Changes in the Cyst.—It is not known definitely how long the echinococcus remains alive, probably many years, possibly as long as twenty years. The most common change is death and the gradual inspissation of the contents and conversion of the cyst into a mass containing putty-like or granular material which may be partially calcified. Remnants of the chitinous cyst wall or hooklets may be found. These obsolete hydatid cysts are not infrequently found in the liver. A more serious termination is rupture, which may take place into a serous sac, or perforation may take place externally when the cysts are discharged, as into the bronchi or alimentary canal or urinary passages. More unfavorable are the instances in which rupture occurs into the bile-passages or into the inferior cava. Recovery may follow the rupture and discharge of the hydatids externally. Sudden death has been known to follow the rupture. A third and very serious mode of termination is suppuration, which may occur spontaneously or follow rupture and is found most frequently in the liver.

Geographical Distribution of the Echinococcus.—The disease prevails most extensively in those countries in which man is brought into close contact with the dog, particularly when, as in Australia, the dogs are used for herding sheep, the animal in which the larval form of *Tænia echinococcus* is most often found. In Iceland the cases are very numerous. In Europe the disease is not uncommon. In Great Britain and in North America it is rare, and a majority of the cases are in foreigners. Statistics of the prevalence of the disease in America have been published by Osler (1882), Sommer (1895-'96), and by Lyon (1902), who has collected 241 cases. Of these, 136 cases were in foreigners; in 92 the nationality was not stated; 10 were negroes; 2 Canadians, and only 1 a native American. Fifty-six cases occurred in Manitoba, in which province there is a large settlement of Icelanders, who have brought the disease with them. Only one instance is known in a Canadian-born offspring of an Icelandic emigrant.

Distribution in the Body.—Of 1,634 cases comprised in the statistics of Davaine, Böcker, Finsen, and Neisser, the parasite existed in the liver in 820; in the lung or pleura in 137; in the abdominal organs, including the kidneys, bladder, and genitalia, in 334; in the nervous system in 122; in the circulatory system in 42; in other organs 179. Of the 241 cases in Lyon's series in America the liver was the seat in 177, and the omentum, peritoneal cavity, and mesentery in 26. In 11 cases cysts were passed per rectum, in 7 cases cysts or hooklets were expectorated, and in 2 cases passed per urethram.

Symptoms.—1. *Hydatids of the Liver.*—Small cysts may cause no disturbance; large and growing cysts produce signs of tumor of the liver with great increase in the size of the organ. Naturally the physical signs depend much upon the situation of the growth. Near the anterior surface in the epigastric region the tumor may form a distinct prominence and have a tense, firm feeling, sometimes with fluctuation. A not infrequent situation is to the left of the suspensory ligament, the resulting tumor pushing up the heart and causing an extensive area of dulness in the lower sternal and left hypochondriac regions. In the right lobe, if the tumor is on the posterior surface, the enlargement of the organ is chiefly upward into the pleura and the vertical area of dulness in the posterior axillary line is increased. Superficial cysts may give what is known as the hydatid fremitus. If the tumor is palpated lightly with the fingers of the left hand and percussed at the same time with those of the right, there is felt a vibration or trembling movement which persists for a certain time. It is not always present, and it is doubtful whether it is peculiar to the hydatid tumors or is due, as Briançon held, to the collision of the daughter cysts. Very large cysts are accompanied by feelings of pressure or dragging in the hepatic region, sometimes actual pain. The general condition of the patient is at first good and the nutrition little, if at all, interfered with. Unless some of the accidents already referred to occur, the symptoms indeed may be trifling and due only to the pressure or weight of the tumor.

Historically, one of the most interesting cases is that of the first Lord Shaftesbury (Achitopel), who had a tumor below the costal border for many years. It suppurated and was opened by the philosopher John Locke, his physician, who describes with great detail the escape of the bladder-like bodies. Among the Shaftesbury papers in the Record Office are several other cases collected by Locke; the disease may have been more common in England at that period.

Suppuration of the cyst changes the clinical picture into one of pyæmia. There are rigors, sweats, more or less jaundice, and rapid loss of weight. Perforation may occur into the stomach, colon, pleura, bronchi, or externally, and in some instances recovery has taken place. Perforation has occurred into the pericardium and inferior vena cava; in the latter case the daughter cysts have been found in the heart, plugging the tricuspid orifice and the pulmonary artery. Perforation of the bile-passages causes intense jaundice, and may lead to suppurative cholangitis.

An interesting symptom connected with the rupture of hydatid cysts is the occurrence of urticaria, which may also follow aspiration of the cysts.

Brieger has separated a highly toxic material from the fluid, and to it the symptoms of poisoning may be due.

Diagnosis.—Cysts of moderate size may exist without producing symptoms. Large multiple echinococci may cause great enlargement with irregularity of the outline, and such a condition persisting for any time with retention of the health and strength suggests hydatid disease. An irregular, painless enlargement, particularly in the left lobe, or the presence of a large, smooth, fluctuating tumor of the epigastric region is also very suggestive, and in this situation, when accessible to palpation, it gives a sensation of a smooth elastic growth and possibly also the hydatid tremor. When suppuration occurs the clinical picture is really that of abscess, and only the existence of previous enlargement of the liver with good health would point to the fact that the suppuration was associated with hydatids. *Syphilis* may produce irregular enlargement without much disturbance in the health, sometimes also a very definite tumor in the epigastric region, but this is usually firm and not fluctuating. The clinical features may simulate *cancer* very closely. In a case which I reported the liver was greatly enlarged and there were many nodular tumors in the abdomen. The post mortem showed enormous suppurating hydatid cysts in the left lobe of the liver which had perforated the stomach in two places and also the duodenum. The omentum, mesentery, and pelvis also contained numerous cysts. As a rule, the clinical course of the disease would suffice to separate it clearly from cancer. Dilatation of the gall-bladder and hydronephrosis have both been mistaken for hydatid disease. In the former the mobility of the tumor, its shape, and the mucoid character of the contents suffice for the diagnosis. In some instances of hydronephrosis only the exploratory puncture could distinguish between the conditions. More frequent is the mistake of confounding a hydatid cyst of the right lobe pushing up the pleura with pleural effusion of the right side. The heart may be dislocated, the liver depressed, and dulness, feeble breathing, and diminished fremitus are present in both conditions. Frerichs lays stress upon the different character of the line of dulness; in the echinococcus cyst the upper limit presents a curved line, the maximum of which is usually in the scapular region. Suppurative pleurisy may be caused by the perforation of the cyst. If adhesions result, the perforation takes place into the lung, and fragments of the cysts or small daughter cysts may be coughed up. For diagnostic purposes the exploratory puncture should be used. As stated, the fluid is usually perfectly clear or slightly opalescent, the reaction is neutral, and the specific gravity varies from 1.005 to 1.009. It is non-albuminous, but contains chlorides and sometimes traces of sugar. Hooklets may be found either in the clear fluid or in the suppurating cysts. They are sometimes absent, however, as the cyst may be sterile.

2. *Echinococcus of the Respiratory System.*—Of 809 cases of single hydatid cyst collected by Thomas in Australia, the lung was affected in 134 cases. Of 241 American cases, in 16 the pleura or lung was affected. The larvæ may develop primarily in the pleura and attain a large size. The symptoms are at first those of compression of the lung and dislocation of the heart. The physical signs are those of fluid in the pleura. The line of dulness may be quite irregular. As in the echinococcus of the liver, the general

condition of the patient may be excellent in spite of the existence of extensive disease. Pleurisy is rarely excited. The cysts may become inflamed and perforate the chest wall. Cary and Lyon have analyzed 40 cases of primary echinococcus cyst of the pleura; death results in a majority of the cases from the toxæmia following the rupture and the absorption of the fluid or from the sepsis following suppuration.

Echinococci occur more frequently in the lung than in the pleura. If small, they may exist for some time without causing serious symptoms. In their growth they compress the lung and sooner or later lead to inflammatory processes, often to gangrene, and the formation of cavities which connect with the bronchi. Fragments of membrane or small cysts may be expectorated. Hæmorrhage is not infrequent. Perforation into the pleura with empyema is common. A majority of the cases are regarded during life as either phthisis or gangrene, and it is only the detection of the characteristic membranes or the hooklets which leads to the diagnosis. Of a series of 21 cases, 17 recovered; 5 of the cases suppurated (C. H. Fleming, Victoria, personal communication).

3. *Echinococcus of the Kidneys.*—In the collected statistics referred to above the genito-urinary system comes second as the seat of hydatid disease, though here the affection is rare in comparison with that of the liver. Of the 241 American cases, there were 17 in which the kidneys or bladder were involved. The kidney may be converted into an enormous cyst resembling a hydronephrosis.

The diagnosis is only possible by puncture and examination of the fluid. The cyst may perforate into the pelvis of the kidney, and portions of the membrane or cysts may be discharged with the urine, sometimes producing renal colic. I have reported a case in which for many months the patient passed at intervals numbers of small cysts with the urine. The general health was little if at all disturbed, except by the attacks of colic during the passage of the parasites.

4. *Echinococcus of the Nervous System.*—The common cystic disease of the choroidal plexuses has been mistaken for hydatids. Davies Thomas, of Australia, has tabulated 97 cases, including some of the *Cysticercus cellulosæ.* According to his statistics, the cyst is more common on the right than on the left side, and is most frequent in the cerebrum.

The symptoms, very indefinite, as a rule are those of tumor. Persistent headache, convulsions, either limited or general, and gradually developing blindness have been prominent features in many cases.

Multilocular Echinococcus.—This form merits a brief separate description, as it differs so remarkably from the usual type. It has been met with only in Bavaria, Württemberg, the adjacent districts of Switzerland, and in the Tyrol. Possett has reported 13 cases from von Rokitansky's clinic at Innsbruck. In the United States six cases have been described, chiefly in Germans. Delafield and Prudden's patient had lived there five years, and for a year before his death had been jaundiced. A fluctuating tumor was found in the right flank, apparently connected with the liver. This was opened, and death followed from hæmorrhage. In Oertel's case the patient had lived there ten years. He was deeply jaundiced, and had a tumor mass at the right border of the liver, which was enlarged. Bacon resected a cyst from the left lobe of the liver. The primary tumor presents irregularly formed cavities separated from each other by strands of connective tissue, and lined with the echinococcus membrane. The cavities are filled with a gelatinous material, so that the tumor has very much the appearance of an alveolar colloid cancer. It is quite possible that a special form of tænia echinococcus represents the adult type of this peculiar parasite. This form is almost exclusively confined to the liver, and the symptoms resemble more those of tumor or cirrhosis. The liver is, as a rule, enlarged and smooth, not irregular as in presence of the ordinary echinococcus. Jaundice is a common symptom. The spleen is usually enlarged, there is progressive emaciation, and toward the close hæmorrhages are common.

Treatment of Echinococcus Disease.—Medicines are of no avail. Post mortem reports show that in a considerable number of cases the parasite dies and the cyst becomes harmless. Operative measures should be resorted to when the cyst is large or troublesome. The simple aspiration of the contents has been successful in a large number of cases, and may be tried before the more radical procedure of incision and evacuation of the cysts. Suppuration has occasionally followed the puncture. Injections into the sac should not be practiced. With modern methods surgeons now open and evacuate the echinococcus cysts with great boldness, and the Australian records, which are the most numerous and important on this subject, show that recovery is the rule in a large proportion of the cases. Suppurative cysts in the liver should be treated as abscess. Naturally the outlook is less favorable. The practical treatment of hydatid disease has been greatly advanced by Australian surgeons. The works of the Australian physicians, James Graham and Thomas, may be consulted for interesting details in diagnosis and treatment.

Sparganum mansoni is a larval bothriocephalus met with in Japan and China, usually in the subcutaneous tissues, the adult form of which is not known.

III. DISEASES CAUSED BY NEMATODES

1. ASCARIASIS

Ascaris lumbricoides, the most common human parasite, is found chiefly in children. The female is from 7 to 12 inches in length, the male from 4 to 8 inches. In form it is cylindrical, pointed at both ends, with a yellowish-brown, sometimes a slightly reddish color. Four longitudinal bands can be seen, and it is striated transversely. The ova, which are sometimes found in large numbers in the fæces, are small, brownish-red in color, elliptical, and have a very thick covering. They measure 0.075 mm. in length and 0.058 mm. in width. The life history has been demonstrated to be "direct"—*i. e.,* without intermediate host. The parasite occupies the upper portion of the small intestine. Usually not more than one or two are present, but occasionally they occur in enormous numbers. The migrations are peculiar. They may pass into the stomach, whence they may be ejected by vomiting, or they may crawl up the œsophagus and enter the pharynx, from which they may be withdrawn. A child under my care in the smallpox department of the Montreal General Hospital, during convalescence, withdrew in this way more than thirty round worms within a few weeks. In other instances the worm reaches the larynx, and has been known to produce fatal asphyxia, or, passing into the trachea, to cause gangrene of the lung. They may go through the Eustachian tube and appear at the external meatus. The worms have been found in extraordinary numbers in the bile-ducts. Remarkable specimens exist in the Dupuytren, the Wistar-Horner (Philadelphia), and the Netley Museums. Chalmers (Ceylon) and Leys (U. S. N.) have called attention to their importance in causing abscess of the liver. Ebstein reports certain markings, strangulations, on the round worms, as if they had been nipped in the bile-ducts! The bowel may be blocked, or in rare instances an ulcer may be perforated. Even the healthy bowel wall may be penetrated.

A peculiarly irritating substance, often evident to the sense of smell in handling specimens, is formed by the round worms. Peiper and others suggest that the nervous symptoms, sometimes resembling those of meningitis, are due to this poison. Chauffard, Marie, and Tauchon have gone still further, and report a remarkable condition of fever, intestinal symptoms, foul breath, and intermittent diarrhœa in connection with the presence of lumbricoides. They call it typho-lumbricosis. The febrile condition may continue for a month or more. There may be eosinophilia to 25 to 30 per cent., and in some cases a marked anæmia. The question of the toxins produced by intestinal parasites is still an open one.

A few parasites may cause no disturbance. In children there are irritative symptoms usually attributed to worms, such as restlessness, irritability, picking at the nose, grinding of the teeth, twitchings, or convulsions.

Treatment.—Care should be taken to avoid auto-infection by thorough washing after defecation, and those infected should not be allowed to prepare food or serve it to others. It is well to give soft diet on the day previous and give a dose of castor oil the night before treatment. *Santonin* is usually efficient given in the morning in doses of one grain (0.065 gm.) for a small child, and three to five grains (0.2 to 0.3 gm.) for an adult. One to two grains of calomel should be given with it. Three hours later a good dose of saline should be given. This should be done two mornings in succession and repeated in a week if worms or eggs are again passed. The occasional unpleasant effects of santonin (yellow vision, vertigo) should be explained beforehand. If santonin is not effectual male fern or thymol may be given.

Oxyuris vermicularis (Thread-worm; Pin-worm).—This common parasite occupies the rectum and colon. The male measures about 4 mm. in length, the female about 10 mm. They produce great irritation and itching, particularly at night, symptoms which become intensely aggravated by the nocturnal migration of the parasites. The oxyuris may traverse the intestinal wall, and has been found in the peritoneal cavity, where they may form verminous tubercles in Douglas's fossa or peri-rectal abscesses.

The patients become extremely restless and irritable, the sleep is often disturbed, and there may be loss of appetite and anæmia. Though most common in children, the parasite occurs at all ages.

The worm is readily detected in the fæces. Infection probably takes place through the water, or possibly through salads, such as lettuce and cresses. A person the subject of the worms passes ova in large numbers in the fæces, and the possibility of re-infection must be scrupulously guarded against.

Treatment.—Every care should be taken to avoid auto-infection or the infection of others, by care in cleansing the anus and perineum, and thorough washing of the hands after defecation. Auto-infection is often responsible for the persistence of the disease. Treatment must be directed to the removal of the worms both from the small intestine and rectum. Santonin and calomel are useful, given as in ascaris infection, and for several days. Thymol and naphthalein are also used. To remove the worms from the rectum injections are required which should be retained as long as possible; it is well to wash out the bowel before giving them and the injection need not be over six ounces. Cold solutions of salt and water, ice water, vinegar (1 to 40), infusion of quassia (one ounce of quassia chips to a pint of water), lime water, carbolic acid (1 to 500), may be employed and should be used daily for two weeks. For the itching, carbolated vaseline, the gall and opium ointment, or menthol (5 per cent.) in vaseline may be employed.

2. TRICHINIASIS

The *Trichina or Trichinella spiralis* in its adult condition lives in the small intestine. The disease is produced by the embryos, which pass from the intestines and reach the voluntary muscles, where they finally become encapsulated larvæ—muscle trichinæ. It is in the migration of the embryos (possibly from poisons produced by them) that the group of symptoms known as trichiniasis is produced.

The ovoid cysts were described in human muscle by Tiedemann in 1822, and by Hilton in 1832; the parasite was figured and named by Richard Owen. Leidy in 1845 described it in the pig. For a long time the trichina was looked upon as a pathological curiosity; but in 1860 Zenker discovered in a girl in the Dresden Hospital, who had symptoms of typhoid fever, both the intestinal and muscle forms, and established their connection with a serious and often fatal disease.

Description of the Parasites.—(*a*) Adult or intestinal form. The female measures from 3 to 4 mm.; the male, 1.5 mm., and has two little projections from the hinder end.

(*b*) The larva or muscle trichina is from 0.6 to 1 mm. in length and lies coiled in an ovoid capsule, which is at first translucent, but subsequently opaque and infiltrated with lime salts. The worm presents a pointed head and a somewhat rounded tail.

When flesh containing the trichinæ is eaten by man or by any animal in which the development can take place, the capsules are digested and the trichinæ set free. They pass into the small intestine, and about the third day attain their full growth and become sexually mature. Virchow's experiments have shown that on the sixth or seventh day the embryos are fully developed. The young produced by each female trichina have been estimated at several hundred. Leuckart thought that various broods are developed in succession, and that as many as a thousand embryos may be produced by a single worm. The time from the ingestion of the flesh containing the muscle trichinæ to the development of the brood of embryos in the intestines is from seven to nine days. The female worm penetrates the intestinal wall and the embryos are probably discharged directly into the lymph spaces, thence into the venous system, and by the blood stream to the muscles, which constitute their seat of election. J. Y. Graham reviewed the question of the mode of transmission in an exhaustive monograph, and he gives strong arguments in favor of the transmission through the blood stream. They have been found in the blood early in the infection and since the demonstration of their presence by Herrick and Janeway they have been seen by a number of observers. After a preliminary migration in the intermuscular connective tissue they penetrate the primitive muscle-fibres, and in about two weeks develop into the full-grown muscle form. In this process an interstitial myositis is excited and gradually an ovoid capsule develops about the parasite. Two, occasionally three or four, worms may be seen within a single capsule. This process of encapsulation has been estimated to take about six weeks. Within the muscles the parasites do not undergo further change. Gradually the capsule becomes thicker, and ultimately lime salts are deposited within it. This change may take place in man within four or five months. In the hog it may be deferred for many years. The calcification renders the cyst visible, and, since first seen by Tiedemann and Hilton, these small, opaque, oat-shaped bodies have been familiar objects to demonstrators of normal and morbid anatomy. The trichinæ may live within the muscles for an indefinite period. They have been found alive and capable of developing as late as twenty or even twenty-five years after their entrance into the system. In many instances, however, the worms are completely calcified. The trichina has been found or "raised" in twenty-six different species of animals (Stiles). Medical literature abounds in references to its presence in fish, earthworms, etc., but these parasites belong to other genera. In fæcal examinations for the parasite it is well to remember that the "cell body" of the anterior portion of the intestine is a diagnostic criterion of the *T. spiralis*. Experimentally, guinea-pigs and rabbits are readily infected by feeding them with muscle containing the larval form. Dogs are infected with difficulty; cats more readily. Experimentally, animals sometimes die of the disease if large numbers of the parasites have been eaten. In the hog the trichinæ, like the cysticerci, cause few if any symptoms. An animal the muscles of which are swarming with living trichinæ may be well nourished and healthy-looking. An important point also is the fact that in the hog the capsule does not readily become calcified, so that the parasites are not visible as in the human muscles.

The **anatomical changes** are chiefly in the voluntary muscles. The trichinæ enter the primitive muscle bundles, which undergo granular degeneration with marked nuclear proliferation. There is a local myositis, and gradually about the parasite a cyst wall is formed. These changes, as well as the remarkable alterations in the blood, have been described in full by Brown. Cohnheim has described a fatty degeneration of the liver and enlargement of the mesenteric glands. At the time of death, in the fourth or fifth week or later, the adult trichinæ are still found in the intestines.

Incidence.—Man is infected by eating the flesh of trichinous hogs. In Germany, where a thorough and systematic microscopic examination of all swine flesh is made, the proportion of trichinous hogs is about 1 in 1,852. Statistics are not available in England. In America inspections have been made since 1892. The percentage of animals found infected has ranged from 1.04 to 1.95. In 1883, in conjunction with A. W. Clement, I examined 1,000 hogs at the Montreal abattoir, and found only 4 infected.

Modes of Infection.—The danger of infection depends entirely upon the mode of preparation of the flesh. Thorough cooking, so that all parts of the meat reach the boiling point, destroys the parasites; but in large joints the central portions are often not raised to this temperature. The frequency of the disease in different countries depends largely upon the habits of the people in the preparation of pork. In North Germany, where raw ham and *Wurst* are freely eaten, the greatest number of instances have occurred. In South Germany, France, and England cases are rare. In the United States the greatest number of persons attacked have been Germans. Salting and smoking the flesh are not always sufficient, and the Havre experiments showed that animals are readily infected when fed with portions of the pickled or the smoked meat as prepared in America. Carl Fraenkel, however, states that the experiments on this point have been negative, and that it is very doubtful if any cases of trichiniasis in Germany have been caused by American pork. Germany has yet to show a single case of trichiniasis due to pork of unquestioned American origin.

Frequency of Infection.—H. U. Williams, of Buffalo, made a thorough study of the muscle from 505 unselected autopsies, and found 27 cases of trichiniasis, 5.3 per cent. The subjects had all died of causes other than trichiniasis. This important study shows how widespread is the disease, and that in reality we frequently overlook the sporadic form.

The disease occurs in groups or outbreaks in which from a dozen to several hundred individuals are attacked, and in sporadic cases which have been shown of late years to be not infrequent. In the epidemics a large number of persons are infected from one source; in the two famous outbreaks of Hedersleben and Emersleben 337 and 250 individuals were attacked. In the United States Stiles estimates that there have been more than 1,000 small outbreaks. The discovery in my wards at the Johns Hopkins Hospital by T. R. Brown of the eosinophilia in the disease has led to the much more frequent detection of the sporadic cases, and this form of the disease is not at all uncommon in the United States.

Symptoms.—The ingestion of trichinous flesh is not necessarily followed by the disease. When a limited number are eaten only a few embryos pass to the muscles and may cause no symptoms. Well-characterized cases present a gastro-intestinal period and a period of general infection.

In the course of a few days after eating the infected meat there are signs of gastro-intestinal disturbance—pain in the abdomen, loss of appetite, vomiting, and sometimes diarrhœa. The preliminary symptoms, however, are by no means constant, and in some of the large epidemics cases have been observed in which they have been absent. In other instances the gastro-intestinal features have been marked from the outset, and the attack has resembled cholera nostras. Pain in different parts of the body, general debility, and weakness have been noted in some of the epidemics.

The invasion symptoms occur between the seventh and the tenth day.

sometimes not until the end of the second week. There is fever, except in very mild cases. Chills are not common. The thermometer may register 102° or 104°F., and the fever is usually remittent or intermittent. The migration of the parasites into the muscles excites a more or less intense myositis, which is characterized by pain on pressure and movement, and by swelling and tension of the muscles, over which the skin may be œdematous. The limbs are placed in the positions in which the muscles are in least tension. The involvement of the muscles of mastication and of the larynx may cause difficulty in chewing and swallowing. In severe cases the involvement of the diaphragm and intercostal muscles may lead to intense dyspnœa, which sometimes proves fatal. Œdema, a feature of great importance, may be early in the face, particularly about the eyes. Later it occurs in the extremities when the swelling and stiffness of the muscles are at their height. Profuse sweats, tingling and itching of the skin, and in some instances urticaria, have been described.

Blood.—A marked leucocytosis, which may reach above 30,000, is usually present. A special feature is the extraordinary increase in the number of eosinophilic cells, which may comprise more than 50 per cent. of all the leucocytes. There were in four years, in the Johns Hopkins Hospital, 7 cases in which the eosinophilia was most pronounced. In 4 of them the diagnosis was actually suggested by the great increase in the eosinophiles; in 1 case they reached 68 per cent. of the total number of leucocytes.

The general nutrition is much disturbed and the patient becomes emaciated and often anæmic, particularly in the protracted cases. The patellar tendon reflex may be absent. The patients are usually conscious, except in cases of very intense infection, in which the delirium, dry tongue, and tremor give a picture suggesting typhoid fever. In addition to the dyspnœa present in the severer infections, there may be bronchitis, and in the fatal cases pneumonia or pleurisy. In some epidemics polyuria has been a common symptom. Albuminuria is frequent.

The intensity and duration of the symptoms depend entirely upon the grade of infection. In the mild cases recovery is complete in from ten to fourteen days. In the severe forms convalescence is not established for six or eight weeks, and it may be months before the patient recovers the muscular strength. One patient in the Hedersleben epidemic was weak eight years after the attack.

Of 72 fatal cases in the Hedersleben epidemic, the greatest mortality occurred in the fourth and fifth and sixth weeks; namely, 52 cases. Two died in the second week with severe choleraic symptoms.

The mortality has ranged in different outbreaks from 1 or 2 per cent. to 30 per cent. In the Hedersleben epidemic 101 persons died. Among 456 cases reported in the United States there were 122 deaths.

The **prognosis** depends much upon the quantity of infected meat which has been eaten and the number of trichinæ which mature in the intestines. In children the outlook is more favorable. Early diarrhœa and moderately intense gastro-intestinal symptoms are, as a rule, more favorable than constipation.

Diagnosis.—The disease should always be suspected when a large birthday party or *Fest* among Germans is followed by cases of apparent typhoid fever. The parasites may be found in the remnants of the ham or sausages used on the occasion. The worms may be discovered in the stools. The stools should be spread on a glass plate or black background and examined with a low-power lens, when the trichinæ are seen as small, glistening, silvery threads. In doubtful cases the diagnosis may be made by the removal of a small fragment of muscle under cocaine anæsthesia. The disease may be mistaken for rheumatic fever, particularly as the pains are so severe on movement, but there is no special swelling of the joints. The great increase in the eosinophiles in the blood is a most suggestive point in diagnosis. The tenderness is in the muscles both on pressure and on movement. The intensity of the gastro-intestinal symptoms in some cases has led to the diagnosis of cholera. Many of the former epidemics were doubtless described as typhoid fever, which the severer cases, owing to the prolonged fever, the sweats, the delirium, dry tongue, and gastro-intestinal symptoms, somewhat resemble. The pains in the muscles, with tension and swelling, œdema, particularly about the eyes, and shortness of breath, are the most important diagnostic points.

Prophylaxis.—It is not definitely known how swine become diseased. It has been thought that they are infected from rats about slaughter-houses, but it is just as reasonable to believe that the rats are infected by eating portions of the trichinous flesh of swine. The swine should, so far as possible, be grain-fed, and not, as is so common, allowed to eat offal. The most satisfactory prophylaxis is the complete cooking of pork and sausages, and to this custom in England, France, South Germany, and the United States immunity is largely due.

Treatment.—If it has been discovered within twenty-four or thirty-six hours that a large number of persons have eaten infected meat, the indications are to thoroughly evacuate the gastro-intestinal canal. Calomel (gr. ii, 0.13 gm.) should be given at once and repeated in two hours. Four hours after the second dose half an ounce of castor oil or magnesium sulphate should be given and repeated if necessary. An enema should be given unless the bowels move freely. Glycerin has been recommended in large doses, in order that by passing into the intestines it may by its hygroscopic properties destroy the worm. Male fern, kamala, santonin, and thymol have all been recommended in this stage. Turpentine may be tried in full doses. There is no doubt that diarrhœa in the first week or ten days of the infection is distinctly favorable. The indications in the stage of invasion are to relieve the pains, to secure sleep, and to support the patient's strength. There are no medicines which have any influence upon the embryos in their migration through the muscles.

3. ANKYLOSTOMIASIS

(*Hookworm Disease*)

Synonyms.—One of the most important, widespread of all metazoan infections, variously known as uncinariasis; anæmia of miners, bricklayers, tunnel-workers; tropical and Egyptian chlorosis.

History.—For three centuries the disease, but not its nature, was recognized in the tropics under various names. Dubini, in 1838, first described the worms, and gave the name from the curved or bent appearance of the mouth. In 1853 and 1854 Bilhartz and Griesinger recognized the relation of the parasites to the anæmia and dropsy. In South America in 1866 Wucherer called attention to the frequency of the disease in negro slaves. In the "seventies" and "eighties" of the last century the anæmia of brick-workers in Italy and of miners and tunnel diggers was shown to be due to this parasite. Occasional statements were made as to the occurrence of the disease in the United States, but it was not until the extensive investigations of Stiles in 1901, and later, that it was shown that the hookworm was widely prevalent, and that it was responsible for an enormous amount of ill health and anæmia, and that it was directly connected with the old and long-ago described practice of dirt-eating. The studies of Allen J. Smith and others showed how widespread was the disease in the Southern States. Ashford and King studied the disease in Porto Rico, and carried out one of the most successful of modern sanitary campaigns. In 1898 Looss discovered the cardinal fact of the penetration of the skin by the larvæ, and of the route by which they reach the intestine. His great work, one of the most important of recent contributions to helminthology, has just been completed (Part ii, 1911). Special clinical monographs have been published by Dock and Bass, by Ashford and Igaravidez, and by Boycott (all in 1911).

Distribution.—The parasite exists in most parts of the world, and recent studies show that there is scarcely a tropical country in which the disease caused by it does not prevail. In India the infection is from 60 to 80 per cent., in Porto Rico 90 per cent., in the Philippines about 15 per cent. In Europe it is chiefly an affection of miners in Germany, Hungary, France and Belgium. In England there was a small outbreak in Cornwall, but the disease has not extended. The Southern United States are badly infected. Stiles shows that more than 12 per cent. of cotton-mill employees are infected, and the examination of recruits, college students, and school children in different parts of the country gives a percentage of infection of from 20 to 70 or even 80.

Parasites.—There are two chief forms, the *Ankylostoma duodenale,* the old world species, and the *Necator americanus,* the new world species. The Ankylostoma is a small cylindrical nematode, the male about 10 mm. and the female from 10 to 18 mm. in length. The mouth has chitinous plates, and is provided with two pairs of sharp, hook-shaped teeth, with which they pierce the mucosa of the bowel. The male has a prominent, umbrella-like caudal expansion. The new world worm has much the same characters, only it is more slender, the mouth globular, and the arrangement of the teeth quite different. The eggs are from 52 μ to 60 μ by about 34 μ in width in the European form, and from 64 μ to 76 μ by about 36 μ in breadth in the American form. They are very characteristic bodies in the fæces of infected individuals. When laid they are already in process of segmentation. Complete dessication, and direct sunlight, or much water in the fæces kills the eggs; but they are sometimes very tenacious of life, and freezing, followed by a gentle thawing, may be resisted. The rapidity of development depends upon favoring conditions and temperature, and the larvæ after escaping from the eggs may live for months in the mud or water of the mines, and they pass through a series of moults before they reach what is called the ripe stage. They then show a remarkable tenacity of life, and may live in water or slime for many months; and in this, which is the infective stage, they have a great tendency to wander.

Modes of Infection.—An extraordinary number of eggs are passed with each stool of a badly infected person, as many it has been estimated as four millions. They develop most readily in fæces mixed with sand or earth at a temperature of from 70° to 90°. The larvæ become infective when about 4 or 5 days old. Infection takes place either by the mouth directly, which is rare, or by the skin. Looss showed experimentally that the larvæ entering the skin are carried by the veins to the heart, and thence to the lungs, in which they escape from the pulmonary vessels, pass up the bronchi and trachea, and so to the gullet, stomach and intestines. These remarkable observations of Looss have been abundantly confirmed. As C. A. Smith's work has shown, it takes about seven weeks before the ova appear in the stools, and in the process of infection there may be sore throat and fever. It would appear that the skin is the common channel of entrance, and usually shows signs of irritation—ground itch. Larvæ accidentally swallowed may pass through the stomach, and develop in the intestines.

The careless disposition of the fæces permits the pollution of the soil, and in the tropical and sub-tropical districts, and in mines, it is an easy matter to understand how children and others are infected through the skin. Ashford and King give a history of more than 90 per cent. of ground-itch in their cases.

Morbid Anatomy and Pathology.—The worms are chiefly in the jejunum; Sandwith found 1,353 out of 1,524 worms in the first six feet of the bowel. They are also occasionally found in the stomach. A variable number of worms are found attached to the mucosa. Very characteristic lesions are the ecchymoses and small erosions of the mucosa, in the centre of which may be a pale area, slightly raised, to which the worm is attached; it may be almost buried in the mucosa. There are usually more bites or holes than worms. Blood cysts occur in the sub-mucosa, in which, occasionally, worms are found (Whipple). The contents of the bowel are often blood-stained. In long-standing cases the mucosa may show many areas of pigmentation. Other lesions are those of chronic anæmia with fatty degeneration. Much discussion has taken place as to whether the worms live on blood or not. They are certainly built for blood-sucking, and, as Whipple states, when the mucosa is normal the worms feed chiefly on blood, when it is thickened and infiltrated they have to be content with the epithelium and mucosa. The loss of blood is largely direct, but it has been shown by Loeb and A. J. Smith that the head-glands of the worm secrete a substance which retards coagulation, probably a hæmolytic poison, the presence of which Whipple has demonstrated. Another feature of importance is the liability to infection through the bites; and the anæmia may in part, at any rate, be due to poisonous products absorbed through the bowel lesions.

Symptoms.—The hookworm disease presents a very variable picture, nor does the severity of the symptoms seem to depend always upon the number of worms. There have been fatal cases in which only ten or twelve worms were found, while recovery has followed after more than 4,000 worms have been expelled (Dock). In infected districts, as in the Southern States, the hookworm disease causes a widespread degeneration in the community, the children and young adults showing a pallor, under-development, and failure of nutrition. With the infection, too, are associated an apathy and lack of energy, so that the common opinion in the Scuth is that the hookworm is the cause of laziness. There is no question that, as Stiles and others have shown, the widespread infection is responsible for a great deal of ill health and physical incapacity, often without any actual illness. In more severe cases the anæmia is pronounced, the hæmoglobin being from 40 to 50 per cent.; the child is stunted and puberty is long delayed, and the patient may belong to the group of dirt-eaters. The retardation of growth is remarkable, and the individual may continue to grow until he is 25 or 26 years of age. In the severest type of all the anæmia is still more pronounced; the hæmoglobin below 25 or 20 per cent.; œdema occurs, the patient is bedridden, and death occurs from exhaustion, diarrhœa, or some intercurrent affection. The *anæmia* is of a secondary type, averaging from 50 to 60 per cent. of the corpuscles, with, as a rule, a low color index. Leucocytosis is not often present, and the differential count shows nothing unusual except the great increase in the eosinophiles, ranging from 15 to 26 or even 30 per cent.

"Ground-itch," the local lesion through which the parasites enter the system, is most commonly on the feet and legs in children, or on the arms and hands in gardeners and miners. The most common region is between and beneath the toes. The eruption is vesicular at first, and then pustules form with a sticky exudate, and sometimes with much swelling of the skin. The vesicles and pustules gradually dry, and in about eight or ten days heal with exfoliation.

Other general features are the well known circulatory and respiratory features of anæmia. The digestive symptoms are remarkable. In the mild cases there are slight epigastric pain and discomfort; in the severer ones there are anorexia and remarkable perversion of appetite; the patients eat earth, paper, chalk, starch, hair and clay. The dirt-eaters of the Southern States are all subject to the hookworm disease. Mental inertia has already been referred to, and popularly the affection is spoken of as the "lazy disease." With the apathetic, listless expression there is dilatation of the pupils, and Stiles has remarked upon the "dull, blank, almost fish-like or cadaveric stare," which gives a very characteristic appearance to the expression.

Diagnosis.—In tropical and sub-tropical regions slight anæmia and ill health should lead to the examination of the stools, from which a certain diagnosis may be made by finding the eggs. "The combination of anæmia with under-development, weakness, dilated heart, and the history of ground-itch is not likely to be confused with anything else" (Stiles). In badly infected regions a fairly accurate diagnosis may be made on inspection alone, and the diagnosis may be confirmed in the examination of the fæces by the rapid improvement after the administration of thymol. Two or three drachms of fæces suffice; they should be collected in a wide-mouthed bottle. A little practice may be required at first, but the necessary technique is easily acquired. The eggs are characteristic structures, usually containing 4 or 8 segments, sometimes the complete embryo nearly ready to burst its shell. Various estimates have been made of the number of worms based on the number of eggs found. It is to be remembered that the eggs vary greatly in numbers, and the stools may be negative one day and contain many a few days later. Grassi states that 150 eggs per centigram of fæces represent about 1,000 worms. For other special methods of examining the stools the student is referred to the monograph of Dock and Bass.

The presence of eosinophilia is an important diagnostic aid. Boycott and Haldane found that 94 per cent. of infected persons had over 8 per cent. of eosinophiles.

Prophylaxis.—Destruction of the adult worms, removing conditions suitable to the growth of the embryos, and a campaign of sanitary education are the three essentials. The proper disposal of fæces, obtaining a pure water supply, and decreasing the chance of infection by wearing shoes and stockings are important points. The work of the Porto Rico commission, inaugurated by Ashford and King, and carried on by Ashford, Igaravidez and their colleagues, shows what can be done in the tropics, even in the most unfavorable surroundings. The fighting unit in this battle has been the anæmia dispensary, of which 55 were established in Porto Rico, each one with a visiting nurse, and with provisions for the proper examination of the patients. According to the last report, nearly 50,000 patients were treated in 1909-1910. More than 300,000 persons have received specific treatment for the disease since the commission began its work. That the mortality in the island has fallen from 42 per 1,000 in 1899-1900 to 20.9 in 1910 is in great part due to the devoted work of the medical staff and the nurses in dealing with the hookworm disease.

In mines care should be taken to prevent local conditions favoring the growth of the embryos. Oliver has found that cinder and slag are destructive of the larvæ. New workers should be examined and proved not to have the disease before being admitted.

Treatment.—The following directions are given by the Porto Rican commission:

Take one of the two purgatives to-night in water.

Take at 6 o'clock to-morrow morning half of the capsules (thymol).

Take the other half at 8 o'clock the same morning.

Take the other purgative at 10 o'clock.

You should neither drink wine nor any alcoholic liquor during the time you are taking these medicines.

Come for more medicine until the physician says you are cured.

Have a privy in your house. Do not defecate on the surface of the ground, but in the privy.

Do not walk barefooted, so that you may avoid contracting the disease in your feet. Wear shoes and you will never suffer from anæmia.

The purgative preferred is an ordinary saline, and the dose of the thymol is graduated according to the age of the patient, seven grains (0.5 gm.) for children under five, and increasing the dose according to age and strength to sixty grains (4 gm.) for adults. Very few ill effects follow its use, but it sometimes is irritating to the bowels, and occasionally it has been toxic. This treatment should be carried out on one day of each week until the patient is cured. No alcohol or oil should be given at the time of administration of thymol.

Eucalyptus and chloroform may be given as Hermann's mixture (chloroform 3 c. c., oil of eucalyptus 2 c. c., castor oil 40 c. c., taken in two doses at intervals of one hour). Beta-naphthol has been much used in doses of thirty grains (2 gm.) for adults. Male fern has also been given. The anæmia should receive the usual treatment.

4. FILARIASIS

For a full discussion of the zoölogical relations of this important group see Stiles' article in my "System of Medicine," Vol. I.

Under the general term *Filaria sanguinis hominis* three species of nematodes are included:

Filaria bancrofti Cobold, 1877. This is the ordinary blood filaria. The embryos are found in the peripheral circulation only during sleep or at night. The mosquito is the intermediate host. The embryos measure 270 to 340 μ long by 7 to 11 μ broad; tail pointed. The adult male measures 83 mm. long by 0.407 mm. broad; the tail forms two turns of a spiral. The adult female measures 155 mm. long by 0.715 mm. broad; vulva 2.56 mm. from anterior extremity; eggs 38 μ by 14 μ. This is the species to which the hæmatochyluria and elephantiasis are attributed.

Filaria diurna Manson, 1891. The larvæ agree with the preceding, except that Manson indicates the absence of granules in the axis of the body. The worms occur in the peripheral circulation only during the day, or when the patient stays awake. Manson suspects that the *Filaria loa* represents the adult stage.

Filaria perstans Manson, 1891. Only the embryos are known. These are much smaller than the preceding—200 μ long, posterior extremity obtuse, anterior extremity with a sort of retractile rostellum.

Manson is inclined to regard the *Filaria perstans* as the cause of *craw-craw,* a papillo-pustular skin eruption of the west coast of Africa, which is probably the same as Nielly's *dermatose parasitaire,* the parasite of which was called by Blanchard *Rhabditis niellyi.* Manson has shown that in the blood of the aboriginal Indians in British Guiana there are two forms of filarial embryos which differ somewhat from the ordinary types. Daniels and Ozzard have shown the extraordinary prevalence of these parasites in the aborigines—fully 58 per cent. Daniels has found the mature filaria in two subjects in the upper part of the mesentery, near the pancreas and in the subpericardial fat.

The most important of these is the *Filaria bancrofti,* which produces the hæmatochyluria and the lymph-scrotum.

The female produces an extraordinary number of embryos, which enter the blood current through the lymphatics. Each embryo is within its shell, which is elongated, scarcely perceptible, and in no way impedes the movements. They are about the ninetieth part of an inch in length and the diameter of a red blood-corpuscle in thickness, so that they readily pass through the capillaries. They move with the greatest activity, and form very striking and readily recognized objects in a blood-drop under the microscope. A remarkable feature is the periodicity in the occurrence of the embryos in the blood. In the daytime they are almost or entirely absent, whereas at night, in typical cases, they are present in large numbers. If, however, as Stephen Mackenzie has shown, the patient, reversing his habits, sleeps during the day, the periodicity is reversed. In the case reported by Lothrop and Pratt the number of embryos per cubic centimetre of blood was calculated hourly during the night; it rose steadily from four o'clock in the afternoon till midnight, when 2,100 per c. c. were present, then fell, none being found at ten o'clock the following morning. The further development of the embryos is associated with the mosquito, which at night sucks the blood and in this way frees them from the body. After developing a little it was thought that they were set free in the water by the death of the host. S. P. James has found them in the tissues of the proboscis of the mosquito, and the infection is probably direct, as in malaria. The filariæ may be present in the body without causing any symptoms. In the blood of animals filariæ are very common and rarely cause inconvenience. It is only when the adult worms or the ova block the lymph channels that certain definite symptoms occur. Manson suggests that it is the ova (prematurely discharged), which are considerably shorter and thicker than the full-grown embryos, which block the lymph channels and produce the conditions of hæmatochyluria, elephantiasis, and lymph-scrotum.

The parasite is widely distributed, particularly in tropical and sub-tropical countries. Guitéras has shown that the disease prevails extensively in the Southern States, and since his paper appeared contributions have been made by Matas, of New Orleans, Mastin, of Mobile, De Saussure, of Charleston, and Opie.

The effects produced may be described under the following conditions:

1. Hæmatochyluria.—Without any external manifestations, and in many cases without special disturbance of health, the subject from time to time passes urine of an opaque white, milky appearance, or bloody, or a chylous fluid which on settling shows a slightly reddish clot. The condition indicates dilatation and rupture of dilated lymphatics in some part of the urinary tract and obstruction of the thoracic duct. The urine may be normal in quantity or increased. The condition is usually intermittent, and the patient may pass normal urine for weeks or months at a time. Microscopically, the chylous urine contains minute molecular fat granules, and usually red blood-corpuscles in various amounts. The embryos were first discovered by Demarquay at Paris (1863), and in the urine by Wucherer, at Bahia, in 1866. It is remarkable for how long the condition may persist without serious impairment of the health. A patient, sent to me by Dawson, of Charleston, had hæmatochyluria intermittently for eighteen years. The only inconvenience had been in the passage of blood-clots which collected in the bladder. At times he had also uneasy sensations in the lumbar region. The embryos were present in his blood at night in large numbers. Chyluria is not always due to the filaria. The non-parasitic form of the disease is considered elsewhere.

Opportunities for studying the anatomical condition of these cases rarely occur. In the case described by Stephen Mackenzie the renal and peritoneal lymph plexuses were enormously enlarged, extending from the diaphragm to the pelvis. The thoracic duct above the diaphragm was impervious.

2. Elephantiasis is common in all countries in which the filariæ prevail. The parasites are not always found in the blood. The condition is more common in the legs, one or both, beginning below the knee, but grad-

ually involving the entire limb. Next in frequency is *lymph-scrotum* and other forms involving the genitalia. The *scrotal* tumor may reach an enormous size, and 40 to 50 pounds in weight. The onset may be painless and slow, or it may be sudden, with fever and rapid swelling and redness of the part. There may be a series of such attacks, each one leaving the part more swollen.

Sporadic Elephantiasis.—A non-parasitic type may be mentioned here, which is not very uncommon in temperate regions, characterized by progressive enlargement of a limb or portion of the body, due to a hyperplasia of the skin and subcutaneous tissues, due apparently to an obstructive inflammation of the lymph-vessels. It may arise spontaneously without any obvious cause, or it may follow an inflammation of the skin of the part, occasionally removal of the lymph-glands. The legs are most frequently involved, beginning usually in one leg, about the foot or ankle, and gradually extending until the whole leg is greatly enlarged. The skin is usually smooth, but it may be hard and indurated or warty and nodular. Most of the cases I have seen have been in young women, in whom the affection has come on without any obvious cause and progressed slowly until the leg was greatly enlarged. In one case six or eight years elapsed before the other leg became involved, and in another case more than ten years has passed and the disease is still confined to one leg.

Treatment.—So far as I know, no drug destroys the embryos in the blood. In infected districts the drinking-water should be boiled or filtered. In cases of chyluria the patients should use a dry diet and avoid all excess of fat. The chyle may disappear quite rapidly from the urine under these measures, but it does not necessarily indicate that the case is cured. So long as clots and albumin are present the leak in the lymphoid varix is not healed, although the fat, not being supplied to the chyle, may not be present. A single tumblerful of milk will at once give ocular proof of the patency or otherwise of the rupture in the varix (Manson).

Elephantoid fever demands rest, liquid diet, free purgation and sedative applications to painful areas. In *elephantiasis* during periods with acute symptoms the patient should be at rest and the legs firmly bandaged. Good results are reported from the use of fibrolysin.

The surgical treatment of some of these cases is most successful, particularly in the removal of the adult filariæ from the enlarged lymph-glands, especially in the groin. Maitland states that during seven years 25 operations of this kind have been performed without serious symptoms. Surgical measures may be advisable in elephantiasis.

5. DRACONTIASIS

(*Guinea-worm Disease*)

Dracunculus medinensis is a widely spread parasite in parts of Africa and the East Indies. In the United States instances occasionally occur. Jarvis reported a case in a post chaplain who had lived at Fortress Monroe, Va., for thirty years. Van Harlingen's patient, a man aged forty-seven, had never lived out of Philadelphia, so that the worm must be included among the parasites of the United States. A majority of the cases reported in American journals have been imported.

The female develops in the subcutaneous and intermuscular connective tissues and produces vesicles and abscesses. In the large majority of the cases the parasite is found in the leg. Of 181 cases, in 124 the worm was found in the feet, 33 times in the leg, and 11 times in the thigh. It is usually solitary, though there are cases on record in which six or more have been present. It is cylindrical in form, about 2 mm. in diameter, and from 50 to 80 cm. in length. The male has been found by Leiper in a monkey, a very small worm only 22 mm. in length.

The worm gains entrance to the system through the stomach, not through the skin, as was formerly supposed. It is probable that both male and female are ingested; but the former dies and is discharged, while the latter after impregnation penetrates the intestine and attains its full development in the subcutaneous tissues, where it may remain quiescent for a long time and can be felt beneath the skin like a bundle of string. The worm contains an enormous number of living embryos, and to enable them to escape she travels slowly downward head first, and, as mentioned, usually reaches the foot or ankle. The head then penetrates the skin and the epidermis forms a little vesicle, which ruptures, and a small ulcer is left, at the bottom of which the head often protrudes. The distended uterus ruptures and the embryos are discharged in a whitish fluid. After getting rid of them the worm will spontaneously leave her host. In the water the embryos develop in the cyclops—a small crustacean—and it seems likely that man is infected by drinking the water containing these developed larvæ.

When the worm first appears it should not be disturbed, as after parturition it may leave spontaneously. When the worm begins to come out a common procedure is to roll it round a portion of smooth wood and in this way prevent the retraction, and each day wind a little more until the entire worm is withdrawn. It is stated that special care must be taken to prevent tearing of the worm, as disastrous consequences sometimes follow, probably from the irritation caused by the migration of the embryos.

The parasite may be excised entire, or killed by injections of bichloride of mercury (1 to 1,000). It is stated that the leaves of the plant called *amarpattee* are almost a specific in the disease. Asafetida in full doses is said to kill the worm.

6. OTHER NEMATODES

Filariæ.—Among less important filarian worms parasitic in man the following may be mentioned: *Filaria loa,* a cylindrical worm of about 3 cm. in length, whose habitat is beneath the conjunctiva. It has been found on the West African coast, in Brazil, and in the West Indies. *Filaria lentis,* which has been found in a cataract. Three specimens have been found together. *Filaria labialis,* which has been found in a pustule in the upper lip. *Filaria hominis oris,* which was described by Leidy, from the mouth of a child. *Filaria bronchialis,* which has been found occasionally in the trachea and bronchi. This parasite has been seen in a few cases in the bronchioles and in the lungs. There is no evidence that it ever produces an extensive verminous bronchitis similar to that which I have described in dogs. *Filaria immitis*—the common *Filaria sanguinis* of the dog—of which Bowlby has described two cases in man. In one case with hæmaturia female worms were found in the portal vein, and the ova were present in the thickened bladder wall and in the ureters.

Trichocephalus dispar (*Whip-worm*).—This parasite is not infrequently found in the cæcum and large intestine of man. It measures from 4 to 5 cm. in length, the male being somewhat shorter than the female. The worm is readily recognized by the remarkable difference between the anterior and posterior portions. The former, which forms at least three-fifths of the body, is extremely thin and hair-like in contrast to the thick hinder portion of the body, which in the female is conical and pointed, and in the male more obtuse and usually rolled like a spring. The eggs are oval, lemon-shaped, 0.05 mm. in length, and each is provided with a button-like projection.

The number of the worms found is variable, as many as a thousand having been counted. It is a widely spread parasite. In parts of Europe it occurs in from 10 to 30 per cent. of all bodies examined, but in the United States it is not so common. In 285 West Indian workers at Panama Darling found 46 per cent. infected. It is possible, he thinks, that these parasites play a rôle in amœbic dysentery, the lesions of which begin at the exact location of the points of their attachment. The trichocephalus rarely causes symptoms. French and Boycott found ova in 40 of 500 Guy's Hospital patients. They found no etiological relationship of the parasite to appendicitis. Several cases have been reported in which profound anæmia has occurred in connection with this parasite, usually with diarrhœa. Enormous numbers may be present, as in Rudolph's case, without producing any symptoms.

The diagnosis is readily made by the examination of the fæces, which contain, sometimes in great abundance, the characteristic lemon-shaped, hard, dark-brown eggs.

Dicotophyme renale(*Eustrongylus gigas*).—This enormous nematode, the male of which measures about a foot in length and the female about three feet, occurs in very many animals and has occasionally been met with in man. It is usually found in the renal region and may entirely destroy the kidney.

Anguillula aceti.—The Anguillula aceti, or vinegar eel, is sometimes present in the urine (in one case it is said from the bladder). It is most probably a contamination from a dirty bottle in which the urine is collected.

Strongyloides intestinalis.—The parasite was discovered in 1876 by Normand, and is the same as was formerly described as Anguillula stercoralis and Rhabdonema intestinalis. It is a common parasite in tropical diarrhœa, particularly in Cochin China. It is found in about 3 per cent. of the medical patients in the Isthmus of Panama, and in from 20 to 30 per cent. of the patients in the insane division. When in large numbers they cause diarrhœa, but from his studies there Darling concludes that they are not the cause of severe diarrhœa, though they may produce moderate anæmia. The mother worm burrows in the mucous membrane and deposits ova. The parasite is found in the upper parts of the small intestines. They are met with occasionally in the temperate regions. Three cases were reported from my clinic by Thayer.

Acanthocephala (*Thorn-headed Worms.*)—The *Gigantorhynchus* or *Echinorhynchus gigas* is a common parasite in the intestine of the hog and attains a large size. The larvæ develop in cockchafer grubs. The American intermediate host is the June bug (Stiles). Lambl found a small *Echinorhynchus* in the intestine of a boy. Welch's specimen, which was found encysted in the intestine of a soldier at Netley, is stated by Cobbold probably not to have been an *Echinorhynchus.* Recently a case of *Echinorhynchus moniliformis* has been described in Italy by Grassi and Calandruccio.

IV. PARASITIC ARACHNIDA AND TICKS

Pentastomes.—1. LINGUATULA RHINARIA (*Pentastoma tænioides*) has a somewhat lancet-shaped body, the female being from 3 to 4 inches in length, the male about an inch in length. The body is tapering and marked by numerous rings. The adult worm infests the frontal sinuses and nostrils of the dog, more rarely of the horse. The larval form, which is known as the *Linguatula serrata* (*Pentastomum denticulatum*), is seen in the internal organs, particularly the liver, but has also been found in the kidney. The adult worm has been found in the nostril of man, but is very rare and seldom occasions any inconvenience. The larvæ are by no means uncommon, particularly in parts of Germany. The parasite is very rare. Flint refers to a Missouri case in which from 75 to 100 of the parasites were expectorated. The liver was enlarged and the parasites probably occupied this region. In 1869 I saw a specimen which had been passed with the urine by a patient of James H. Richardson, of Toronto.

2. The POROCEPHALUS CONSTRICTUS (*Pentastomum constrictum*), has the length of half an inch, with twenty-three rings on the abdomen. It is found in the Congo district and in parts of Asia. The larvæ, found in cysts in the lungs and liver, cause disease as they wander. The adult form lives in the nasal cavities and lungs of pythons and other snakes and man is infected probably through the drinking water.

Demodex (Acarus) folliculorum (var. hominis).—A minute parasite, from 0.3 mm. to 0.4 mm. in length, which lives in the sebaceous follicles, particularly of the face. It is doubtful whether it produces any symptoms. Possibly when in large numbers they may excite inflammation of the follicles, leading to acne.

Sarcoptes (Acarus) scabiei (*Itch Insect*).—This is the most important of the arachnid parasites, as it produces troublesome and distressing skin eruptions. The male is 0.23 mm. in length and 0.19 mm. in breadth; the female is 0.45 mm. in length and 0.35 mm. in width. The female can be seen readily with the naked eye and has a pearly-white color. It is not so common a parasite in the United States and Canada as in Europe.

The insect lives in a small burrow, about 1 cm. in length, which it makes for itself in the epidermis. At the end of this burrow the female lives. The male is seldom found. The chief seat of the parasite is in the folds where the skin is most delicate, as in the web between the fingers and toes, the backs of the hands, the axilla, and the front of the abdomen. The head and face are rarely involved. The lesions which result from the presence of the itch insect are very numerous and result largely from the irritation of the scratching. The commonest is a papular and vesicular rash, or, in children, an ecthymatous eruption. The irritation and pustulation which follow the scratching may completely destroy the burrows, but in typical cases there is rarely doubt as to the diagnosis.

The *treatment* is simple. It should consist of warm baths with a thorough use of a soft soap, after which the skin should be anointed with sulphur ointment, which in the case of children should be diluted. An ointment of naphthol (drachm to the ounce) is very efficacious.

Leptus autumnalis (*Harvest Bug*).—This reddish-colored parasite, about half a millimetre in size, is often found in large numbers in fields and in gardens. They attach themselves to animals and man with their sharp proboscides, and the hooklets of their legs produce a great deal of irritation. They are most frequently found on the legs. They are readily destroyed by sulphur ointment or corrosive-sublimate lotions.

Ixodiasis (*Tick-fever*).—In South Africa, particularly in the western provinces of the Uganda Protectorate, the western districts of German East Africa and the eastern regions of the Congo Free State, there is a disease known by this name, believed to be transmitted by a tick—the *Ornithodorus* or *Argas monbata*. Christy states that the bite of the *O. savignyi* does not produce any ill effects. The ticks live in old houses, and their habits are very much like those of the common bedbug. This tick transmits the *spirochæta duttoni*, the cause of the African form of relapsing fever already mentioned.

The *Dermacentor occidentalis* is present in the Northwestern States from California to Montana. The bites may cause severe lymphangitis. It appears to be the medium of transmission of the Rocky Mountain spotted fever.

In Arizona and other parts of the Southwestern States a tick—*Ornithodorus megnini*—is occasionally found in the ear and in the nose, causing suppuration and intense suffering.

Several other varieties of ticks are occasionally found on man—the *Ixodes ricinus* and the *Dermacentor americanus*, which are met with in horses and oxen.

V. PARASITIC INSECTS

Pediculi (*Phthiriasis; Pediculosis*).—There are three varieties of the body louse, which are found only in persons of uncleanly habits.

Pediculus capitis.—The male is from 1 to 1.5 mm. in length and the female nearly 2 mm. The color varies somewhat with the different races of men. It is light gray with a black margin in the European, and very much darker in the negro and Chinese. They are oviparous, and the female lays about sixty eggs, which mature in a week. The ova are attached to the hairs, and can be readily seen as white specks, known popularly as nits. The symptoms are irritation and itching of the scalp. When numerous, the insects may excite an eczema or a pustular dermatitis, which causes crusts and scabs, particularly at the back of the head. In the most extreme cases the hair becomes tangled in these crusts and matted together, forming at the occiput a firm mass which is known as *plica polonica,* as it was not infrequent among the Jewish inhabitants of Poland.

PEDICULUS CORPORIS (*vestimentorum*).—This is considerably larger than the head louse. It lives on the clothing, and in sucking the blood causes minute hæmorrhagic specks, which are very common about the neck, back, and abdomen. The irritation of the bites may cause urticaria, and the scratching is usually in linear lines. In long-standing cases, particularly in old dissipated characters, the skin becomes rough and greatly pigmented, a condition which has been termed the vagabond's disease—*morbus errorum* —and which may be mistaken for the bronzing of Addison's disease. The pigmentation in some cases may be extreme and extend to the face and buccal mucosa.

PHTHIRIUS PUBIS differs somewhat from the other forms, and is found in the parts of the body covered with short hairs, as the pubes; more rarely the axilla and eyebrows.

The *taches bleuâtres* or peliomata, excited by the irritation of pediculi, are peculiar subcuticular bluish or slate-colored spots from 5 to 10 mm. in diameter seen about the abdomen and thighs, particularly in febrile cases. They are very well pictured in Murchison's work on Fevers. The spots are more marked on white thin skins. They are stains caused by a pigment in the secretion of the salivary glands of the louse. I have never seen these *maculæ ceruleæ,* as they are also called, without finding the lice or their nits.

TREATMENT.—For the *Pediculus capitis,* when the condition is very bad, the hair should be cut short, as it is very difficult to destroy thoroughly all the nits. Repeated saturations of the hair in coal-oil or in turpentine are usually efficacious, or with lotions of carbolic acid, 1 to 50. Scrupulous cleanliness and care are sufficient to prevent recurrence. In the case of the *Pediculus corporis,* the clothing should be placed for hours in a disinfecting oven. To allay the itching a warm bath containing 4 or 5 ounces of bicarbonate of soda is useful. The skin may be rubbed with a lotion of carbolic acid, 2 drachms to the pint, with 2 ounces of glycerin. For the *Phthirius pubis* white precipitate or ordinary mercurial ointment should be used, and the parts should be thoroughly washed two or three times a day with soft soap and water.

Cimex lectularius (*Common Bedbug*).—The tropical and sub-tropical variety is *Cimex rotundalius* (W. S. Patton). It lives in the crevices of the bedstead and in the cracks in the floor and in the walls. It is nocturnal in its habits. The peculiar odor of the insect is caused by the secretion of a special gland. The parasite possesses a long proboscis, with which it sucks the blood. Individuals differ remarkably in the reaction to the bite of this insect; some are not disturbed in the slightest by them, in others the irritation causes hyperæmia and often intense urticaria. Fumigation with sulphur or scouring with corrosive-sublimate solution or kerosene destroys them. Iron bedsteads should be used.

Pulex irritans (*Common Flea*).—The male is from 2 to 2.5 mm. in length, the female from 3 to 4 mm. The flea is a transient parasite on man. The bite causes a circular red spot of hyperæmia in the centre of which is a little speck where the boring apparatus has entered. The amount of irritation caused by the bite is variable. Many persons suffer intensely and a diffuse erythema or an irritable urticaria develops; others suffer no inconvenience whatever.

The *Pulex penetrans* (*sand-flea, jigger*) is found in tropical countries, particularly in the West Indies and South America. It is much smaller than the common flea, and not only penetrates the skin, but burrows and produces an inflammation with pustular or vesicular swelling. It most frequently attacks the feet. It is readily removed with a needle. Where they exist in large numbers the essential oils are used on the feet as a preventive.

VI. PARASITIC FLIES

(*Myiasis, Myiosis*)

The accidental invasion of the body cavities and of the skin by the larvæ of the diptera is known as myiasis.

The larvæ of the *Lucilia macellaria,* the so-called screw-worm, have been found in the nose, in wounds, and in the vagina after delivery. They can be removed readily with forceps; if there is any difficulty, thorough cleansing and the application of an antiseptic bandage are sufficient to kill them. The ova of the blue-bottle fly may be deposited in the nostrils, the ears, or the conjunctiva—the myiasis narium, aurium, conjunctivæ. This invasion rarely takes place unless these regions are the seat of disease. In the nose and in the ear the larvæ may cause serious inflammation. Even the urethra has not been spared in these dipterous invasions.

Gastro-intestinal myiasis may result from the swallowing of the larvæ of the common house-fly or of species of the genus *Anthomyia.* There are many cases on record in which the larvæ of the *Musca domestica* have been discharged by vomiting. Instances in which dipterous larvæ have been passed in the fæces are less common. Finlayson, of Glasgow, has reported an interesting case in a physician, who, after protracted constipation and pain in the back and sides, passed large numbers of the larvæ of the flower-fly—*Anthomyia canicularis.* Among other forms of larvæ or gentles, as they are sometimes called, which have been found in the fæces are those of the common house-fly, the blue-bottle fly, and the *Techomyza fusca.* The larvæ of other insects are extremely rare. It is stated that the caterpillar of the taby moth has been found in the fæces.

A specimen of the *Homalomyia scalaris,* one of the privy flies, was sent to me by Dr. Hartin, of Kaslo City, British Columbia, the larvæ of which were passed in large numbers in the stools of a man aged twenty-four, a native of Louisiana. They were present in the stools from May 1 to July 15, 1897. There are cases in which the larvæ have been passed for years, in one instance 12 years!

Although no grave results necessarily follow the invasion of the alimentary tract by these larvæ, yet they may be the cause of serious intestinal ulceration manifesting itself by a dysenteric disease with fatal result. Cockayne, who has recently (1912) studied the question, states that there are four deaths on record.

Cutaneous Myiasis.—The most common form of *cutaneous myiasis* is that in which an external wound becomes "living," as it is called. This myiasis vulnerum is caused by the larvæ of either the blue-bottle or the common flesh-fly.

The skin may also be infected by the larvæ of the *Musca vomitoria,* but more commonly by the bot-flies of the ox and sheep which occasionally attack man. This condition is rare in temperate climates. Matas has described a case in which œstrus larvæ were found in the gluteal region. In parts of Central America the eggs of another bot-fly, the *Dermatobia,* are not infrequently deposited in the skin and produce a swelling very like the ordinary boil.

Dermamyiasis linearis migrans œstrosa is a remarkable cutaneous condition, observed particularly in Russia and occasionally in other countries, in which the larva of *Gastrophilus equi* (Samson), the horse bot-fly, makes a slightly raised pale red "line" which travels over the body surface, sometimes with great rapidity. It has been referred to as Larva migrans and as Creeping Eruption. (See Hamburger, Journal of Cutaneous Diseases, 1904.)

In Africa the larvæ of the Cayor fly are not uncommonly found beneath the skin in little boils. In the Congo region Dutton, Todd, and Christy found a troublesome blood-sucking dipterous larva, known as the floor maggot, the fly of which is the *Anchmeromyia luteola.*

Phlebotomous Fever.—In Herzegovina, Malta and Crete and other parts of the Mediterranean there is a fever of two or three days' duration, caused by the bite of the sand-fly, *Phlebotomus papatasii.* The manifestations are those of fever alone, and may be mistaken for abortive typhoid, febricula or mild Malta fever. The disease is known as pappataci fever and on the Dalmatian coast it is severe. The experiments of Doerr and of Birt show that the disease is readily caused by the bite of infected sand-flies.

Caterpillar Rash.—In some districts in Europe the hairs of the procession caterpillar, particularly of the species *Cnethocampa,* cause an intense urticaria, the so-called *U. epidemica.* There are districts in Switzerland which have been rendered uninhabitable in consequence of the skin rashes caused by the caterpillars. Of late years in New England and some other parts of the United States the caterpillar of the brown-tailed moth has caused much discomfort. The hairs are widely distributed by the wind, and the barbs are so arranged that they readily work into the skin. Whole families have been affected by an intense eruption which has been mistaken for that of small-pox. In England, Thresh has called attention to the frequency of these caterpillar rashes due to the yellow-tailed moth, *Porthesia similis.*

Harvest Rash (*Erythema Autumnale*).—In parts of England during the autumn many people are attacked by the harvest bug or harvesters, which may cause a very obstinate and distressing malady. Usually attributed to the harvest spider, it is in reality caused by a mite, parasitic upon it, the hexapod larva of the silky trombidian. It is so small as to be scarcely visible and is brick-red in color. They chiefly attack persons with delicate skins on the ankles and legs, but they may also attack the arms and the neck. The mite attaches itself to the skin by its claws, sucks the blood, and the swollen red abdomen may sometimes be seen as a bright-red dot. A papulo-vesicular, sometimes a pustular, eruption with an intolerable itching is caused by it. So intense may the eruption be, with perhaps an entire family attacked at once, that suspicion of poisoning may be aroused. The parasite is readily killed by benzine.

E. INFECTIOUS DISEASES OF DOUBTFUL OR UNKNOWN ETIOLOGY

I. SMALL-POX (Variola)

Definition.—An acute infectious disease characterized by a cutaneous eruption which passes through the stages of papule, vesicle, pustule, and crust.

History.—The existence of the disease in ancient Egypt is suggested by the eruption on the skin of a mummy of the 20th dynasty—1,200 to 1,100 B. C. (Rüffer and Ferguson). The disease existed in China many centuries before Christ. The *pesta magna* described by Galen (of which Marcus Aurelius died) is believed to have been small-pox. In the sixth century it prevailed, and subsequently, at the time of the Crusades, became widespread. It was brought to America by the Spaniards early in the sixteenth century. The first accurate account was given by Rhazes, an Arabian physician who lived in the ninth century, and whose admirable description is available in Greenhill's translation for the Sydenham Society. In the seventeenth century the illustrious Sydenham differentiated measles from small-pox. Special events in the history of the disease are the introduction of inoculation into Europe, by Lady Mary Wortley Montagu, in 1718, and the discovery of vaccination by Jenner, in 1796.

Etiology.—Small-pox is one of the most virulent of contagious diseases, and persons exposed, if unprotected by vaccination, are almost invariably attacked. Instances of natural immunity are rare. It is said that Diemerbroeck, a celebrated Utrecht professor in the seventeenth century, was not only himself exempt, but likewise many members of his family. One of the nurses in the small-pox department of the Montreal General Hospital stated that she had never been successfully vaccinated, and she certainly had no mark. An attack may not protect for life. There are undoubted cases of a second, reputed instances, indeed, of a third attack.

Age.—Small-pox is common at all ages, but is particularly fatal to young children. Of 3,164 deaths in the Montreal epidemic of 1885-'86, 2,717 were of children under ten years of age. The *fetus in utero* may be attacked, but only if the mother herself is the subject of the disease. The child may be born with the rash out or with the scars. In the case of twins, only one may be attacked; Kaltenbach records an instance of triplets, only two of which were affected (Comby). Children born in a small-pox hospital, if vaccinated immediately, may escape the disease; usually, however, they die early. (See Hunter's works, iv, p. 74.)

Sex.—Males and females are equally affected.

Race.—Among aboriginal races small-pox is terribly fatal. When the disease was first introduced into America the Mexicans died by thousands, and the North American Indians have also been frequently decimated by this plague. It is stated that the negro is especially susceptible, and the mortality is greater—about 42 per cent. in the black, against 29 per cent. in the white (W. M. Welch).

It is claimed that isolation hospitals increase the incidence of the disease in a locality. J. Glaister, who has considered the whole question very carefully, concludes that as a centre of traffic such an institution, through the channels of unavoidable human intercourse, naturally favors the spread of the disease locally, but decides against the aerial conveyance of the disease, in spite of the very strong evidence.

The disease smoulders here and there and when conditions are favorable becomes epidemic. This was well illustrated by the celebrated Montreal outbreak of 1885. For several years there had been no small-pox in the city, and a large unprotected population grew up among the French-Canadians, many of whom were opposed to vaccination. On February 28 a Pullman-car conductor, who had traveled from Chicago, was admitted into the Hôtel-Dieu, the civic small-pox hospital being at the time closed. Isolation was not carried out, and on the 1st of April a servant in the hospital died of small-pox. Following her decease, the authorities of the hospital dismissed all patients presenting no symptoms of contagion who could go home. The disease spread like fire in dry grass, and within nine months 3,164 persons died in the city of small-pox.

Variations in the Virulence of Epidemics.—Sydenham states that "small-pox also has its peculiar kinds, which take one form during one series of years, and another during another"; and not only does what he called the epidemic constitution vary greatly, but one sometimes sees the most extraordinary variations in the intensity of the disease in members of a family all exposed to the same infection. A striking illustration of this variability has been given in the recent epidemics, which have been of so mild a character that in many localities it has been mistaken for chicken-pox; in others, particularly in the United States, the belief prevailed that a new disease had arisen, to which the name "Cuban itch" or "Philippine itch" has been given. Very often a correct diagnosis has not been reached until a fatal case has occurred. As will be mentioned, a small outbreak occurred in one of my wards for colored patients, which we mistook at first for chicken-pox. The same peculiarities have been observed in the Leicester, Nottingham, and Cambridge outbreaks. Even in unvaccinated children the disease has been exceedingly mild. Some of the Leicester cases had only a few pocks (Allan Warner); but this is an old story in the history of the disease. John Mason Good, in commenting on this very point, refers to the great variability in the epidemics, and states that he himself as a child of six (1770) passed through small-pox with "scarcely any disturbance and not more than twenty scattered pustules"!

The disease described in some of the Brazilian states as Alastrin amas, or varioloid varicella, seen also in the West Indies, is probably a mild small-pox.

Recent Prevalence.—In the United States in 1909 there were 24,099 cases with 150 deaths; in 1910, 30,352 cases and 415 deaths. The mild type of the disease continues, but in places there have been virulent outbreaks. In England and Wales there were only 19 deaths from the disease in 1910.

Nature of Contagion.—Protozoön-like bodies were described in the skin lesions by Guarnieri—*the cytoryctes variolæ.* Councilman and his colleagues describe a protozoön with a double cycle and cytoplasmic stage, with small structureless bodies in the lower layer of the epithelial cells. The dried scales constitute by far the most important element, and as a dust-like powder are distributed everywhere in the room during convalescence, becoming attached to clothing and various articles of furniture. The disease is probably contagious from a very early stage, though I think it has not yet been determined whether the contagion is active before the eruption develops. The poison is of unusual tenacity and clings to infected localities. It is conveyed by persons who have been in contact with the sick and by fomites. During epidemics it is no doubt widely spread in street-cars and public conveyances. It must not be forgotten that an unprotected person may contract a very virulent form of the disease from the mild varioloid.

Morbid Anatomy.—The pustules may be seen upon the tongue and the buccal mucosa, and on the palate; sometimes also in the pharynx and the upper part of the œsophagus. In exceptionally rare cases the rash extends down the œsophagus and even into the stomach. Swelling of the Peyer's follicles is not uncommon; the pustules have been seen in the rectum.

In the larynx the eruption may be associated with a fibrinous exudate and sometimes with œdema. Occasionally the inflammation penetrates deeply and involves the cartilages. In the trachea and bronchi there may be ulcerative erosions, but true pocks, such as are seen on the skin, do not occur.

The heart occasionally shows myocardial changes, parenchymatous and fatty; endocarditis and pericarditis are uncommon. French writers have described an endarteritis of the coronary vessels. The spleen is markedly enlarged. Apart from the cloudy swelling and areas of coagulation-necrosis, lesions of the kidneys are not common. Nephritis may occur.

In the hæmorrhagic form extravasations are found on the serous and mucous surfaces, in the parenchyma of organs, in the connective tissues, about the nerve-sheaths and in the muscles. In one instance I found the entire retro-peritoneal tissue infiltrated with a large coagulum, and there were also extensive extravasations in the course of the thoracic aorta. Hæmorrhages in the bone-marrow have also been described. The spleen is firm and hard in hæmorrhagic small-pox, and such was the case in seven instances I examined. In these rapidly fatal forms the liver has been described as fatty, but in 5 of my 7 cases it was of normal size, dense, and firm.

Symptoms.—Three forms of small-pox are described:

(*a*) *Variola vera;* (1) Discrete, (2) Confluent.

(*b*) *Variola hæmorrhagica;* (1) Purpura variolosa or black small-pox; (2) Hæmorrhagic pustular form, variola hæmorrhagica pustulosa.

(*c*) *Varioloid,* or small-pox modified by vaccination.

(*a*) Variola Vera.—The affection may be conveniently described under various stages: *Incubation.*—"From nine to fifteen days; oftenest twelve." I have seen it as early as the eighth day after exposure, and there are well-authenticated instances in which this stage has been prolonged to twenty days. It is unusual for patients to complain of any symptoms.

Invasion.—In adults a chill and in children a convulsion are common initial symptoms. There may be repeated chills within the first twenty-four hours. Intense frontal headache, severe lumbar pains, and vomiting are very constant features. The pains in the back and in the limbs are more severe in the initial stage of this than of any other eruptive fever, and their combination with headache and vomiting is so suggestive that precautionary measures may often be taken several days before the eruption appears. The temperature rises quickly, and may on the first day be 103° or 104°. The pulse is rapid and full, not often dicrotic. In severe cases there may be marked delirium, particularly if the fever is high. The patient is restless and distressed, the face is flushed, and the eyes are bright and clear. The skin is usually dry, though occasionally there are profuse sweats. One cannot judge from the initial symptoms whether a case is likely to be discrete or confluent, as convulsions, severe headache, and high fever may precede a very mild attack.

Initial Rashes.—Two forms can be distinguished: the diffuse, scarlatinal, and the macular or measly form; either of which may be associated with petechiæ and occupy a variable extent of surface. In some instances they are

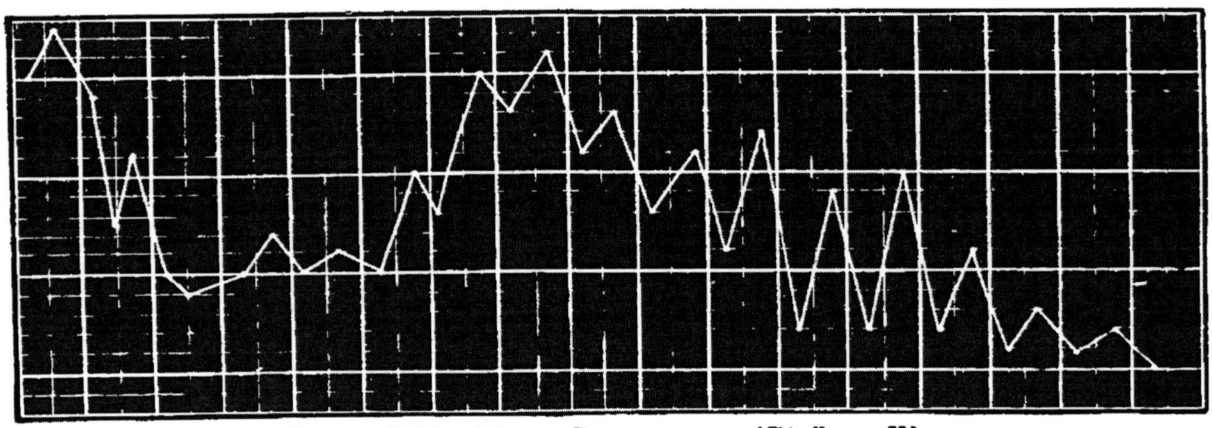

CHART IX.—TRUE SMALL-POX (Strümpell).

general, but as a rule they are limited either to the lower abdominal areas, to the inner surfaces of the thighs, and to the lateral thoracic region, or to the axillæ. Occasionally they are found over the extensor surfaces, particularly in the neighborhood of the knees and elbows. These rashes, usually purpuric, are often associated with an erythematous or erysipelatous blush. The scarlatinal rash may come out as early as the second day, and be as diffuse and vivid as in a true scarlatina. The measly rash may also be diffuse and resemble closely that of measles. Urticaria is only occasionally seen. It was present once in my Montreal cases. The initial rashes are more abundant in some epidemics than in others. They occur in from 10 to 16 per cent. of cases.

Eruption.—(1) In the *discrete form,* usually on the fourth day, macules appear on the forehead, preceded sometimes by an erythematous flush, and on the anterior surfaces of the wrists. Within the first twenty-four hours from their appearance they occur on other parts of the face and on the extremities, and a few are seen on the trunk. The spots are from 2–3 millimetres in diameter, of a bright red color, and disappear completely on pressure. As the rash comes out the temperature falls, the general symptoms subside, and the patient feels comfortable. On the fifth or sixth day the papules change into vesicles with clear summits. Each one is elevated, circular, and presents a little depression or umbilication in the centre. About the eighth day the vesicles change into pustules, the umbilication disappears, the flat top assumes a globular form and becomes grayish-yellow in color, owing to the contained pus. There is an areola of injection about the pustules and the skin between them is swollen. This maturation first takes place on the face, and follows the order of the appearance of the eruption. The temperature now rises—secondary fever—and the general symptoms return. The swelling about the pustules is attended with a good deal of tension and pain in the face; the eyelids become swollen and closed. In the discrete form the temperature of maturation does not usually remain high for more than twenty-four or twenty-six hours, so that on the tenth or eleventh day the fever disappears and the stage of convalescence begins. The pustules rapidly dry, first on the face and then on the other parts, and by the fourteenth or fifteenth day desquamation may be far advanced on the face. The march and distribution of the rash are often most characteristic. The abdomen and groins and the legs are the parts least affected. The rash is often copious on the upper part of the back, scanty on the lower. Vesicles in the mouth, pharynx, and larynx cause soreness and swelling in these parts, with loss of voice. Whether pitting takes place depends a good deal upon the severity of the disease. In a majority of cases Sydenham's statement holds good, that "it is very rarely the case that the distinct small-pox leaves its mark." The odor of a small-pox patient is very distinctive even in the early stages, and I have known it to be a help in the diagnosis of a doubtful case.

(2) *The Confluent Form.*—With the same initial symptoms, though usually of greater severity, the rash appears on the fourth, or, according to Sydenham, on the third day. The more the eruption shows itself before the fourth day the more sure it is to become confluent (Sydenham). The papules at first may be isolated, and it is only later in the stage of maturation that the eruption is confluent. But in severer cases the skin is swollen and hyperæmic and the papules are very close together. On the feet and hands, too, the papules are thickly set; more scattered on the limbs; and quite discrete on the trunk. With the appearance of the eruption the symptoms subside and the fever remits, but not to the same extent as in the discrete form. Occasionally the temperature falls to normal and the patient may be very comfortable. Then, usually on the eighth day, the fever again rises, the vesicles change to pustules, the hyperæmia becomes intense, the swelling of the face and hands increases, and by the tenth day the pustules have fully matured, many of them have coalesced, and the entire skin of the head and extremities is a superficial abscess. The fever rises to 103° or 105°, the pulse is from 110 to 120, and there is often delirium. As pointed out by Sydenham, salivation in adults and diarrhœa in children are common symptoms of this stage. There is usually much thirst. The eruption may also be present in the mouth, and usually the pharynx and larynx are involved and the voice is husky. Great swelling of the cervical lymphatic glands occurs. At this stage the patient presents a terrible picture, unequaled in any other disease and one which fully justifies the horror and fright with which small-pox is associated in the public mind. Even when the rash is confluent on the face, hands, and feet, the pustules remain discrete on the trunk. The danger, as pointed out

by Sydenham, is in proportion to the number upon the face. "If upon the face they are as thick as sand, it is no advantage to have them few and far between on the rest of the body." In fatal cases by the tenth or eleventh day the pulse gets feebler and more rapid, the delirium is marked, there is subsultus, sometimes diarrhœa, and with these symptoms the patient dies. In other instances between the eighth and eleventh day hæmorrhagic features occur. When recovery takes place, the patient enters on the eleventh or twelfth day the period of desiccation.

Desiccation.—The pustules break and the pus exudes or they dry and form crusts. Throughout the third week the desiccation proceeds and in cases of moderate severity the secondary fever subsides; but in others it may persist until the fourth week. The crusts in confluent small-pox adhere for a long time and the process of scarring may take three or four weeks. On the face they fall off singly, but the tough epidermis of the hands and feet may be shed entire.

(*b*) HÆMORRHAGIC SMALL-POX occurs in two forms. In one, the petechial or black small-pox—*purpura variolosa*—the special symptoms appear early and death follows in from two to six days. In the other form the case progresses as one of ordinary variola, and in the vesicular or pustular stage hæmorrhages take place into the pocks or from the mucous membranes—*variola hæmorrhagica pustulosa.*

Purpura variolosa is more common in some epidemics than in others. It is less frequent in children than in adults. Of 27 cases admitted to the small-pox department of the Montreal General Hospital there were 3 under ten years, 4 between fifteen and twenty, 9 between twenty and twenty-five, 7 between twenty-five and thirty-five, 3 between thirty-five and forty-five, and 1 above fifty. Young and vigorous persons seem more liable to this form. Several of my cases were above the average in muscular development. Men are more frequently affected than women; thus in my list there were 21 males and only 6 females. The influence of vaccination is shown in the fact that of the cases 14 were unvaccinated, while not one of the 13 who had scars had been revaccinated. The illness starts with the usual symptoms, but with more intense constitutional disturbance. On the evening of the second or on the third day there is a diffuse hyperæmic rash, particularly in the groins, with small punctiform hæmorrhages. The rash extends, becomes more distinctly hæmorrhagic, and the spots increase in size. Ecchymoses appear on the conjunctivæ, and as early as the third day there may be hæmorrhages from the mucous membranes. Death may take place before the papules appear. In this truly terrible affection the patient may present a frightful appearance. The skin may have a uniformly purplish hue and the unfortunate victim may even look plum-colored. The face is swollen and large conjunctival hæmorrhages with the deeply sunken corneæ give a ghastly appearance to the features. The mind may remain clear to the end. Death occurs from the third to the sixth day; thus in thirteen of my cases it took place between these dates. The earliest death was on the third day and there were no traces of papules. There may be no mucous hæmorrhages; thus in one case of a most virulent character death occurred without bleeding early on the fourth day. Hæmaturia is perhaps most common, next hæmatemesis, and melæna was noticed in a third of the cases. Metrorrhagia was present in one only of the six females on my list. Hæmoptysis occurred in five cases. The pulse in this form of small-pox is rapid and often hard and small. The respirations are greatly increased in frequency and out of all proportion to the intensity of the fever.

In *variola pustulosa hæmorrhagica* the disease progresses as a severe case, and the hæmorrhages do not occur until the vesicular or pustular stage. The first indication is hæmorrhage into the areolæ of the pocks, and later the maturated pustules fill with blood. The earlier the hæmorrhage the greater is the danger. Bleeding from the mucous membranes is also common in this form, and the great majority of the cases prove fatal, usually on the seventh, eighth, or ninth day, but a few cases recover. In patients with the discrete form, if allowed to get up early, hæmorrhage may take place into the pocks on the legs.

Leucocytes.—In variola vera there is a marked leucocytosis, 12–16 thousand, about the eighth day, then a slight decline and a rise again about the twelfth or fourteenth day, sometimes to 18,000 or 20,000. There is an increase in the mononuclear elements, which may be the only marked feature of the mild cases (Magrath, Brinckerhoff, and Bancroft).

(*c*) VARIOLOID.—This term is applied to the modified form which affects persons who have been vaccinated. It may set in with abruptness and severity, the temperature reaching 103°. More commonly it is in every respect milder in its initial symptoms, though the headache and backache may be very distressing. The papules appear on the evening of the third or on the fourth day. They are few in number and may be confined to the face and hands. The fever drops at once and the patient feels perfectly comfortable. The vesiculation and maturation of the pocks take place rapidly, and there is no secondary fever. There is rarely any scarring. As a rule, when small-pox attacks a person who has been vaccinated within five or six years the disease is mild, but it may prove severe, even fatal.

Abortive Types.—As already mentioned, recent epidemics have been characterized by the large number of mild cases. Even in unvaccinated children only a few pustules may appear, and the disease is over in a few days. Even with a thickly set eruption the vesicles at the fifth or sixth day, instead of filling, dry and abort, forming the so-called horn-, crystalline-, or wart-pox. *Variola sine eruptione* is described. I saw no cases of the kind in Montreal. They seem to have been not uncommon in the recent epidemics. Bancroft observed twelve cases in the Boston outbreak, all among physicians and attendants. The symptoms are headache, pain in the back, fever, and vomiting. As already mentioned, the pocks may be very scanty and easily overlooked, even in unvaccinated persons. One of Bancroft's cases was of special interest—a pregnant woman who had slight symptoms after exposure, but no rash. Her child showed a typical eruption when two days old.

Complications.—Considering the severity of many of the cases and the character of the disease, associated with multiple foci of suppuration, the complications in small-pox are remarkably few.

Laryngitis is serious in three ways: it may produce a fatal œdema of the glottis; it is liable to extend and involve the cartilages, producing necrosis; and by diminishing the sensibility of the larynx it may allow irritating particles to reach the lower air-passages, where they excite bronchitis or bronchopneumonia.

Broncho-pneumonia is almost invariably present in fatal cases. *Lobar pneumonia* is rare. *Pleurisy* is common in some epidemics.

The *cardiac* complications are also rare. In the height of the fever a systolic murmur at the apex is not uncommon; but endocarditis, either simple or malignant, is rarely met with. Pericarditis, too, is very uncommon. Myocarditis seems to be more frequent, and may be associated with endarteritis of the coronary vessels.

Of complications in the *digestive* system, parotitis is rare. In severe cases there is extensive pseudo-diphtheritic angina. Vomiting, which is so marked a symptom in the early stage, is rarely persistent. Diarrhœa is not uncommon, as noted by Sydenham, and particularly in children.

Albuminuria is frequent, but true *nephritis* is rare. Inflammation of the testes and of the ovaries may occur.

Among the most interesting and serious complications are those pertaining to the *nervous* system. In children convulsions are common. In adults the delirium of the early stage may persist and become violent, and finally subside into a fatal coma. Post-febrile insanity is occasionally met with during convalescence, and very rarely epilepsy. Many of the old writers spoke of paraplegia in connection with the intense backache of the early stage, but it is probably associated with the severe agonizing lumbar and crural pains and is not a true paraplegia. It must be distinguished from the form occurring in convalescence, which may be due to peripheral neuritis or to a diffuse myelitis (Westphal). The neuritis may, as in diphtheria, involve the pharynx alone, or it may be multiple. Of this nature, in all probability, is the so-called pseudo-tabes, or *ataxie variolique.* Hemiplegia and aphasia have been met with in a few instances, the result of encephalitis.

Among the most constant and troublesome complications are those involving the *skin.* During convalescence boils are very frequent and may be severe. Acne and ecthyma are also met with. Local gangrene in various parts may occur.

Arthritis may occur, usually in the period of desquamation, and may pass on to suppuration. Acute necrosis of the bone is sometimes met with.

A remarkable secondary eruption (recurrent small-pox) occasionally occurs after desquamation.

Special Senses.—The eye affections which were formerly so common and serious are not now so frequent, owing to the care which is given to keeping the conjunctivæ clean. A catarrhal and purulent conjunctivitis is common in severe cases. The secretions cause adhesions of the eyelids, and unless great care is taken a diffuse keratitis is excited, which may go on to ulceration and perforation. Iritis is not very uncommon. Otitis media is an occasional complication, and usually results from an extension of the disease through the Eustachian tubes.

Prognosis.—In unprotected persons small-pox is a very fatal disease, the death-rate ranging from 25 to 35 per cent. In Japan the mortality among unprotected persons has been even higher. In the recent mild epidemic in the United States the mortality has been very slight, e. g., for the five months ending November 24, 1911, 4,852 cases and 35 deaths. At the Municipal Hospital, Philadelphia, of 2,831 cases of variola, 1,534—i. e., 54.18 per cent. —died, while of 2,169 cases of varioloid only 28—i. e., 1.29 per cent.—died

(W. M. Welch). Purpura variolosa is invariably fatal, and a majority of those attacked with the severer confluent forms die. The intemperate and debilitated succumb more readily to the disease. As Sydenham observed, the danger is directly proportionate to the intensity of the disease on the face and hands. "When the fever increases after the appearance of the pustules, it is a bad sign; but if it is lessened on their appearance, that is a good sign" (Rhazes). Very high fever, delirium and subsultus are symptoms of ill omen. The disease is particularly fatal in pregnant women and abortion usually takes place. It is not, however, uniformly so, and I have twice known severe cases to recover after miscarriage. Moreover, abortion is not inevitable. Very severe pharyngitis and laryngitis are fatal complications.

Death results in the early stage from the action of the poison upon the nervous system. In the later stages it usually occurs about the eleventh or twelfth day, at the height of the eruption. In children, and occasionally in adults, the laryngeal and pulmonary complications prove fatal.

Diagnosis.—During an epidemic the initial chill, the headache and back-ache, and the vomiting at once put the physician on his guard.

The initial rashes may lead to error. The scarlatinal rash has rarely the extent and never the persistence of the rash in true scarlet fever. I have known the rash of measles to be mistaken for the initial rash of small-pox. The general condition of the patient, and the presence of coryza, conjunctivitis and Koplik's sign, may be better guides than the rash itself.

Malignant hæmorrhagic small-pox may prove fatal before the characteristic rash appears. Of 27 cases of purpura variolosa, in only one, in which death occurred on the third day, did inspection fail to show the papules. In 3 cases dying on the fourth day the characteristic papular rash was noticed. It may be difficult or impossible to recognize this form of hæmorrhagic small-pox from *hæmorrhagic scarlet fever* or *hæmorrhagic measles,* though in the latter there is rarely so constant involvement of the mucous membranes.

Naturally enough, as they are allied affections, *varicella* is the disease which most frequently leads to error. Particularly has this been the case in the mild epidemic which has prevailed during the past three years. A negro patient was admitted to my wards on the fourth day of the disease. Small-pox was not prevalent at the time, and the case was regarded as one of varicella. Subsequently eight cases appeared, several of exceeding mildness, but our mistake was forcibly brought home to us by the occurrence, in a man who had been exposed in the ward, of a case of confluent small-pox of great severity. The following points are to be borne in mind: first, the experience of the past few years has shown that very mild epidemics of true small-pox may occur; secondly, any large number of cases of a contagious disease with a pustular eruption occurring in adults is strongly in favor of small-pox. The characters of the rash are of less value. Its abundance on the trunk in varicella is important. At the outset the papules have rarely the shotty, hard feel of small-pox. The vesicles are more superficial, the infiltrated areola is not so intense nor so constant, and as a rule the pocks may be seen in the same patient in all stages of development. The longer period of invasion, the prodromal rashes, the great intensity of the onset are also important points in small-pox. But, as I have said, there are mild epidemics in which it must be confessed that the recognition of the nature of the outbreak is sometimes only confirmed by the appearance of a severe case of the confluent or of the hæmorrhagic form.

The disease may be mistaken for *cerebro-spinal fever*, in which purpuric symptoms are not uncommon. A four-year-old child was taken suddenly ill with fever, pains in the back and head, and on the second or third day petechiæ appeared on the skin. There were retraction of the head and marked rigidity of the limbs. The hæmorrhages became more abundant; and finally hæmatemesis occurred and the child died on the sixth day. At the post mortem there were no lesions of cerebro-spinal fever, and in the deeply hæmorrhagic skin the papules could be readily seen. The post mortem diagnosis of small-pox was unhappily confirmed by the mother taking the disease and dying of it.

Pustular Syphilides.—A very copious pustular rash in syphilis may resemble variola, particularly if accompanied by fever, but the history and the distribution, particularly the slight amount on the face, leave no question as to the diagnosis.

Pustular glanders has been mistaken for small-pox. In a remarkable instance of the kind in Montreal there was a widespread pustular eruption, which we thought at first was small-pox, but the subsequent course and the fact that there was glanders among the horses in the stable led to the correct diagnosis. The eruption resembled exactly that described in Rayer's monograph (De la Morve, 1837).

Impetigo contagiosa is stated to have been mistaken for variola.

Prophylaxis.—Thorough vaccination and re-vaccination are the most important preventive measures. All those exposed to infection should be vaccinated at once, as four days after exposure a successful vaccination may protect from the disease. During epidemics general vaccination of the community should be done and special care taken to recognize mild cases. Those who have been exposed should be isolated for sixteen days. Isolation of those with the disease should be rigid and, if possible, they should be placed in a special hospital. The attendants should wear gowns and caps; rubber gloves are an advantage. The linen should be placed in carbolic acid solution (2 per cent.) and boiled afterwards. Dressings should be burned. The patient should not be discharged until all the crusts are removed; a thorough sponging with carbolic solution (2 per cent.) is advisable.

Treatment.—General Considerations.—Segregation in special hospitals is imperative. In the case of local outbreaks temporary barracks or tents may be constructed.

We have no specific treatment. There should be abundance of fresh air; the diet should be liquid and large amounts of water and cold drinks given. A calomel and saline purge is advisable at the onset and later the bowels should be kept open by salines. With severe toxæmia alcohol should be given.

In the early stages two symptoms call for treatment: the pain in the back, which, if not relieved by phenacetine (gr. v, 0.3 gm.), requires opium in some form, as advised by Sydenham; and the vomiting, which is very difficult to check and may be uncontrollable. Nothing should be given except a little ice and champagne, and it usually stops with the appearance of the eruption.

For the fever, cold sponging or the tub bath may be used; when there is much delirium with high fever the latter or the cold pack is preferable. In some cases, particularly with severe toxæmia and marked eruption, the continuous warm bath is advisable.

The treatment of the *eruption* is important. After trying all sorts of remedies, such as puncturing the pustules with nitrate of silver, or treating them with iodine and various ointments, I came to Sydenham's conclusion that in guarding the face against being disfigured by the scars "the only effect of oils, liniments, and the like was to make the white scurfs slower in coming off." The constant application on the face and hands of lint soaked in cold water, to which antiseptics such as carbolic acid (2 per cent.) or bichloride of mercury (1 to 5,000) may be added, is perhaps the most suitable local treatment. It is very pleasant to the patient, and for the face it is well to make a mask of lint, which can then be covered with oiled silk. When the crusts begin to form, the chief point is to keep them thoroughly moist, which may be done with oil or glycerin. This prevents the desiccation and diffusion of the flakes of epidermis. Vaseline is particularly useful, and at this stage may be freely used upon the face. It also relieves the itching. For the odor, which is sometimes so characteristic and disagreeable, the dilute carbolic solutions are probably best. If the eruption is abundant on the scalp, the hair should be cut short to prevent matting and decomposition of the crusts. When suppuration is marked the continuous warm bath (95°) is useful. Boric acid, alum or potassium permanganate may be added to the water.

The papules do not maturate so well when protected from the light, and for centuries attempts have been made to modify the course of the pustules by either excluding the light or by changing its character. In the Middle Ages John of Gaddesden recommended wrapping the patient in red flannel, and treated in this way the son of Edward I. It was an old practice of the Egyptians and Arabians to cover the exposed parts of small-pox patients with gold-leaf. Lutzenberg, a distinguished New Orleans physician, in 1832 treated patients by exclusion of the sunlight. Recently the red-light treatment of the disease has been advocated by Finsen. The statements do not agree as to its value. Nash states that the course of the rash may be modified by the treatment, but Ricketts and Byles could see no influence whatever, even in cases taken at the earliest possible date.

Complications.—If the diarrhœa is severe in children, paregoric may be given. When the pulse becomes feeble and rapid, stimulants may be freely given. The maniacal delirium may require chloroform or morphia, but for less intense nervous symptoms the bath or cold pack is the best. For the severe hæmorrhages of the malignant cases nothing can be done, and it is only cruel to drench the unfortunate patient with iron, ergot, and other drugs. Symptoms of obstruction in the larynx, usually from œdema, may call for tracheotomy. In the late stages of the disease, should the patient be extremely debilitated and the subject of abscesses and bed-sores, he may be placed on a water-bed or treated in the continuous warm bath.

The care of the eyes is most important. The lids should be thoroughly cleansed and the conjunctivæ washed with a warm solution of salt or boracic acid. In the confluent cases the eyelids are much swollen and glued together, and it is only constant watchfulness which prevents keratitis. The edges of the lids should be smeared with vaseline. The mouth and throat should be kept clean, a potassium permanganate or carbolic mouth wash and gargle used, and the treatment of the nose with glycerin or sweet oil should be begun early, as it prevents the formation of hard crusts. Douching the nose with a warm alkaline solution is helpful.

The treatment in the stage of convalescence is important. Frequent bathing helps to soften the crusts, and the skin may be oiled daily. Convalescence should not be considered established until the skin is perfectly smooth and clean and free from any trace of scabs.

II. VACCINIA (Cow-pox)—VACCINATION

Definition.—An eruptive disease of the cow, the virus of which, inoculated into man (vaccination), produces a local pock with constitutional disturbance, which affords protection, more or less permanent, against small-pox.

The vaccine is got either directly from the calf—animal lymph—in which the disease is propagated at regular stations, or is obtained from persons vaccinated (humanized lymph).

History.—For centuries it had been a popular belief among farmer folk that cow-pox protected against small-pox. The notorious Duchess of Cleveland, replying to some joker who suggested that she would lose her occupation if she was disfigured with small-pox, said that she was not afraid of the disease, as she had had a disease that protected her against small-pox. Jesty, a Dorsetshire farmer, had had cow-pox, and in 1774 vaccinated successfully his wife and two sons. Plett, in Holstein, in 1791, also successfully vaccinated three children. When Jenner was a student at Sodbury, a young girl, who came for advice, when small-pox was mentioned, exclaimed, "I cannot take that disease, for I have had cow-pox." Jenner subsequently mentioned the subject to Hunter, who in reply gave the famous advice: "Do not think, but try; be patient, be accurate." As early as 1780 the idea of the protective power of vaccination was firmly impressed on Jenner's mind. The problem which occupied his attention for many years was brought to a practical issue when, on May 14, 1796, he took matter from the hand of a dairy-maid, Sarah Nelmes, who had cow-pox, and inoculated a boy named James Phipps, aged eight years. On July 1st, matter was taken from a small-pox pustule and inserted into the boy, but no disease followed. In 1798 appeared An Inquiry into the Causes and Effects of the Variola Vaccinæ, a Disease discovered in some of the Western Counties of England, particularly Gloucestershire, and known by the Name of Cow-pox (pp. iv, 75, four plates, 4to. London, 1798).

In the United States cow-pox was introduced by Benjamin Waterhouse, Professor of Physic at Harvard, who on July 8, 1800, vaccinated seven of his children. In Boston on August 16, 1802, nineteen boys were inoculated with the cow-pox. On November 9th twelve of them were inoculated with small-pox; nothing followed. A control experiment was made by inoculating two unvaccinated boys with the same small-pox virus; both took the disease. The nineteen children of August 16th were again unsuccessfully inoculated with fresh virus from these two boys. This is one of the most crucial experiments in the history of vaccination, and fully justified the conclusion of the Board of Health—*cow-pox is a complete security against the small-pox.*

Practitioners should familiarize themselves with the literature on vaccination. The centenary number of the British Medical Journal is particularly valuable (1896). The report of the Royal Commission on vaccination (1897), the exhaustive articles in Allbutt and Rolleston's System by T. D. Acland, Copeman and McVail, and Cory's monograph on the subject afford a large body of material. To the public health officials who wish for distribution in handy shape Facts about Small-pox and Vaccination leaflets issued by the British Medical Association will be of the greatest value. The *Vaccination Law* of the German Empire, printed in English (Berlin, B. Paul, 1904), contains important information and statistics.

Nature of Vaccinia.—Is cow-pox a separate independent disease, or is it only small-pox modified by passing through the cow? In spite of a host of observations, this question is not yet settled. The experiments may be divided into two groups. First, those in which the inoculation of the small-pox matter in the heifer produced pocks corresponding in all respects to the vaccine vesicles. Lymph from the first calf inoculated into a second or third produced the characteristic lesions of cow-pox, and from the first, second, or third animal lymph used to vaccinate a child produced a typical localized vaccine vesicle without any of the generalized features of small-pox. The experiments of Ceely, of Babcock, and many other workers seem to leave no question whatever that typical vaccinia may be produced in the calf by the inoculation of variolous matter. A great deal of the vaccine material at one time in use in England was obtained in this way. Secondly, against this are urged Chauveau's Lyons experiments. Seventeen young animals were inoculated with the virus of small-pox. Small reddish papules occurred which disappeared rapidly, but the animals did not acquire cow-pox. Fifteen of the seventeen animals were also vaccinated. Of these only one showed a typical cow-pox eruption. To determine the nature of the original papules one was excised and inoculated into a non-vaccinated child, which developed as a result generalized confluent small-pox. A second child inoculated from the primary pustule of the first child developed discrete small-pox. The French still hold to the Lyons experiments as demonstrating the duality of the diseases.

The weight of evidence favors the view that cow-pox and horse-pox are variola modified by transmission; or, as has been suggested, "small-pox and vaccinia are both of them descended from a common stock—from an ancestor, for instance—which resembled vaccinia far more than it resembled small-pox" (Copeman).

The bodies described by Guarnieri have been very thoroughly studied by Councilman and his colleagues, who regard them as forms of a protozoön—*Cytoryctes vacciniæ*—with a well-characterized development cycle, increasing in size until they undergo segmentation.

Normal Vaccination.—Period of Incubation.—At first there may be a little irritation at the site of inoculation, which subsides.

Period of Eruption.—On the third day, as a rule, a papule is seen surrounded by a reddish zone. This gradually increases, and on the fifth or sixth day shows a definite vesicle, the margins of which are raised while the centre is depressed. By the eighth day the vesicle has attained its maximum size. It is round and distended with a limpid fluid, the margin hard and prominent, and the umbilication is more distinct. By the tenth day the vesicle is still large and is surrounded by an extensive areola. The contents have now become purulent. The skin is also swollen, indurated, and often painful. On the eleventh or twelfth day the hyperæmia diminishes, the lymph becomes more opaque and begins to dry. By the end of the second week the vesicle is converted into a brownish scab, which gradually becomes dry and hard, and in about a week (that is, about the twenty-first or twenty-fifth day from the vaccination) separates and leaves a circular pitted scar. If the points of inoculation have been close together, the vesicles fuse and may form a large combined vesicle. Constitutional symptoms of a more or less marked degree follow the vaccination. Usually on the third or fourth day the temperature rises, and may persist, increasing until the eighth or ninth day. There is a marked leucocytosis. In children it is common to have with the fever restlessness, particularly at night, and irritability; but as a rule these symptoms are trivial. If the inoculation is made on the arm, the axillary glands become large and sore; if on the leg, the inguinal glands. Immunity is not necessarily complete at once after vaccination; it may take as long as three weeks; on the other hand, a person exposed to small-pox and successfully vaccinated at once may escape entirely, or the two diseases may run concurrently, with the small-pox much modified. The duration of the immunity is extremely variable, differing in different individuals. In some instances it is permanent, but a majority of persons within ten or twelve years again become susceptible.

Revaccination should be performed between the tenth and fifteenth year, and whenever small-pox is epidemic. The susceptibility to revaccination is very general. In 1891–'92 vaccination pustules developed in 88.7 per cent. of the newly enrolled troops of the German army, most of whom had been vaccinated twice in their lives before. The vesicle in revaccination is usually smaller, has less induration and hyperæmia, and the resulting scar is less perfect. Particular care should be taken to watch the vesicle of revaccination, as it not infrequently happens that a spurious pock is formed, which reaches its height early and dries to a scab by the eighth or ninth day.

Irregular Vaccination.—(*a*) LOCAL VARIATIONS.—We occasionally meet with instances in which the vesicle develops rapidly with much itching, has not the characteristic flattened appearance, the lymph early becomes opaque, and the crust forms by the seventh or eighth day. The evolution of the pocks may be abnormally slow. In such cases the operation should again be performed with fresh lymph. The contents of the vesicles may be watery and bloody. In the involution the bruising or irritation of the pocks may lead to ulceration and inflammation. A very rare event is the recurrence of the pock in the same place. Sutton reports four such recurrences within six months.

(*b*) GENERALIZED VACCINIA.—It is not uncommon to see vesicles in the vicinity of the primary sore. Less common is a true generalized pustular rash, developing in different parts of the body, often beginning about the wrists and on the back. The secondary pocks may continue to make their appearance for five or six weeks after vaccination. In children the disease may prove fatal. They may be most abundant on the vaccinated limb, and occur usually about the eighth to the tenth day.

(*c*) COMPLICATIONS.—In unhealthy subjects, or as a result of uncleanliness, or sometimes injury, the vesicles inflame and deep excavated ulcers result. Sloughing and deep cellulitis may follow. In debilitated children there may be with this a purpuric rash. Acland thus arranges the dates at which the possible eruptions and complications may be looked for:

1. During the first three days: Erythema; urticaria; vesicular and bullous eruptions; invaccinated erysipelas.

2. After the third day and until the pock reaches maturity: Urticaria; lichen urticatus, erythema multiforme; accidental erysipelas.

3. About the end of the first week: Generalized vaccinia; impetigo; vaccinal ulceration; glandular abscess; septic infections; gangrene.

4. After the involution of the pocks: Invaccinated diseases—for example, syphilis.

(*d*) Transmission of Diseases by Vaccination.—Syphilis has undoubtedly been transmitted by vaccination, but such instances are very rare, and a large number of the cases of alleged vaccino-syphilis must be thrown out. The question has now become really of minor importance since the widespread use of animal lymph. Dr. Cory's sad experiment may here be referred to. He vaccinated himself four times from syphilitic children. With the first vaccination followed, but no syphilis. Two other attempts (negative) were made. The fourth time he was vaccinated from a child the subject of congenital syphilis. The lymph was taken from the child's arm with care, avoiding any contamination with blood. At two of the points of insertion red papules appeared on the twenty-first day. On the thirty-eight day a little ulcer was found, which Sir Jonathan Hutchinson decided was syphilitic. The diseased parts were then removed. By the fiftieth day the constitutional symptoms were well marked.

Among the differences between vaccino-syphilis and vaccination ulcers the most important is perhaps that the chancre never appears before the fifteenth day, usually not until from three to five weeks, whereas the ulceration of ordinary vaccination is present by the twelfth or fifteenth day. The loss of substance in the chancre is usually quite superficial and the induration very parchment-like and specific, with but a slight inflammatory areola. The glandular swelling, too, is constant and indolent, while in the vaccination ulcer it is often absent, or, when present, chiefly inflammatory.

Tuberculosis.—"No undoubted case of invaccinated tubercle was brought before the Royal Commission on Vaccination" (Acland). The risk of transmitting tuberculosis from the calf is so slight that it need not be considered. The transmission of leprosy by vaccination is doubtful.

The observations on the presence of actinomyces in vaccine virus have been confirmed by W. T. Howard, Jr., who found it 24 times in 95 cultures from the virus of five producers in the United States.

Tetanus.—McFarland collected 95 cases, practically all American. Sixty-three occurred in 1901, a majority of which could be traced to one source of supply, in which R. W. Wilson demonstrated the tetanus bacillus. Most of the cases occurred about Philadelphia. Since that date very few cases have been reported. The occurrence of this terrible complication emphasizes the necessity of the most scrupulous care in the preparation of the animal virus, as the tetanus bacillus is almost constantly present in the intestines of cattle.

(*e*) Influence of Vaccination upon Other Diseases.—A quiescent malady may be lighted into activity by vaccination. This has happened with congenital syphilis, occasionally with tuberculosis. An old idea was prevalent that vaccination had a beneficial influence upon existing diseases. Thomas Archer, the first medical graduate in the United States, recommended it in whooping-cough, and said that it had cured six or eight cases in his hands. At the height of the vaccination convulsions may occur and be followed by hemiplegia.

Technique.—That part of the arm about the insertion of the deltoid is usually selected for the operation. Mothers "in society" prefer to have girl babies vaccinated on the leg. The skin should be cleansed and put upon the stretch. Then, with a scalpel, needle, or the ivory point, cross-scratches or superficial incisions should be made in one or more places. Four points of insertion, an inch apart, are best. When glycerin lymph is used the drops may be placed on the skin first and the incisions then made. When the lymph has dried on the points it is best to moisten it in warm water. The clothing of the child should not be adjusted until the spot has dried, and it should be protected for a day or two with lint or a soft handkerchief. When the vesicle forms it can be protected by sterile gauze held in place by strapping. If erysipelas is prevalent, or if there are cases of suppuration in the same house, it is well to apply a pad of antiseptic cotton. Vaccination is usually performed between the fourth and sixth month. If unsuccessful, it should be repeated from time to time. It should be postponed if the child has any ailment or suffers from syphilis or a skin disease. Revaccination should be done at the age of nine years. A person exposed to the contagion of small-pox should always be revaccinated. This, if successful, will usually protect; but not always. The cases in which small-pox is taken within a few years after vaccination are probably instances of spurious vaccination.

The Value of Vaccination.—Sanitation cannot account for the diminution in small-pox and for the low rate of mortality. Isolation, of course, is a useful auxiliary, but it is no substitute. Vaccination is not claimed to be an invariable and permanent preventive of small-pox, but in an immense majority of cases successful inoculation renders the person for many years insusceptible. Communities in which vaccination and revaccination are thoroughly and systematically carried out are those in which small-pox has the fewest victims. The German army since 1874, the date of the stringent laws, has enjoyed practical immunity. On the other hand, communities in which vaccination and revaccination are persistently neglected are those in which epidemics are most prevalent. Owing to a widespread prejudice against vaccination in Montreal, there grew up, between the years 1876 and 1884, a considerable unprotected population, and the materials were ripe for an extensive epidemic. The soil had been prepared with the greatest care, and it only needed the introduction of the seed, which in due time came with the Pullman-car conductor from Chicago, on the 28th of February, 1885. Within the next ten months thousands of persons were stricken with the disease, and 3,164 died. The statistics from Japan, published by Kitasato (1911), show strikingly the efficacy of vaccination in that country. In the Japanese army of more than a million men in a war waged in a country in which small-pox was then endemic there were only 362 cases and 35 deaths. He shows with great clearness the gradual lessening of the intensity of the epidemics in Japan as the system of vaccination has been perfected.

Although the effects of a single vaccination may wear out, as we say, and the individual again become susceptible to small-pox, yet the mortality in such cases is very much lower than in persons who have never been vaccinated. The mortality in persons who have been vaccinated is from 6 to 8 per cent., whereas in the unvaccinated it is at least 35 per cent. There is evidence that the greater the number of marks the greater the protection in relation to small-pox; thus, the English Vaccination Report states that out of 4,754 cases the death-rate with one mark was 7.6 per cent.; with two marks, 7 per cent.; with three marks, 4.2 per cent.; with four marks, 2.4 per cent. W. M. Welch's statistics of 5,000 cases on this point give with good cicatrices 8 per cent.; with fair cicatrices, 14 per cent.; with poor cicatrices, 27 per cent.; post-vaccinal cases, 16 per cent.; unvaccinated cases, 58 per cent.

III. VARICELLA (Chicken-pox)

Definition.—An acute contagious disease, characterized by an eruption of vesicles on the skin.

History.—Ingrassias, a distinguished Neapolitan professor, first recognized the disease as differing from small-pox (1553). Heberden gave it the name chicken-pox (1767).

Etiology.—The disease occurs in epidemics, but sporadic cases are also met with. It may prevail at the same time as small-pox or may follow or precede epidemics of this disease. It is a disease of childhood; a majority of the cases occur between the second and sixth years. Adults who have not had the disease in childhood are very liable to be attacked. The specific germ has not yet been discovered.

Varicella is an affection distinct from variola and without at present any relation whatever to it. An attack of the one does not confer immunity from an attack of the other. A boy, aged five, was admitted to St. Thomas' Hospital with a vesicular eruption, and was isolated in a ward on the same floor as the small-pox ward. The disease was pronounced chicken-pox, however, by Risdon Bennett and Bristowe. The patient was then removed and vaccinated, with a result of four vesicles which ran a pretty normal course. On the eighth day from the vaccination the child became feverish. On the following day the papules appeared and the child had a well-developed attack of small-pox with secondary fever (Sharkey).

Symptoms.—After a period of incubation of ten or fifteen days the child becomes feverish and in some instances has a slight chill. There may be vomiting, and pains in the back and legs. Convulsions are rare. The eruption usually occurs within twenty-four hours. It is first seen upon the trunk, either on the back or on the chest. It may begin on the forehead and face. At first in the form of raised red papules, these are in a few hours transformed into hemispherical vesicles containing a clear or turbid fluid. As a rule there is no umbilication, but in rare instances the pocks are flattened, and a few may even be umbilicated. They are often ovoid in shape and look more superficial than the variolous vesicles. The skin in the neighborhood is not often infiltrated or hyperæmic. At the end of thirty-six or forty-eight hours the contents of the vesicles are purulent. They begin to shrivel, and during the third and fourth days are converted into dark brownish crusts, which fall off and as a rule leave no scar. Fresh crops appear during the first two or three days of the illness, so that on the fourth day one can usually see pocks in all stages of development and decay. They are always discrete, and the number may vary from eight or ten to several hundreds. As in variola, a scarlatinal rash occasionally precedes the development of the eruption. The eruption may occur on the mucous membrane of the mouth, and occasionally in the larynx. In adults the disease may be much more severe, the initial fever high, the rash very widespread, and the constitutional symptoms comparatively severe, so that the diagnosis of variola may be made—the so-called varicella variolaformes. The fever in varicella is slight, but it does not as a rule disappear with the appearance of the rash. The course of the disease is in a large majority of the cases favorable, and no ill effects follow. The disease may recur in the same individual. There are instances in which a person has had three attacks.

There are one or two modifications of the rash which are interesting. The vesicles may become very large and develop into regular bullæ, looking not unlike ecthyma or pemphigus (varicella bullosa). The irritation of the rash may be excessive, and if the child scratches the pocks ulcerating sores may form, which on healing leave ugly scars. Indeed, cicatrices after chicken-pox are more common than after varioloid.

In delicate children, particularly the tuberculous, gangrene (varicella escharotica) may occur about the vesicles, or in other parts, as the scrotum.

Cases have been described of hæmorrhagic varicella with cutaneous ecchymoses and bleeding from the mucous membranes.

Nephritis may occur. Infantile hemiplegia has occurred during an attack of the disease. Death has followed in an uncomplicated case from extensive involvement of the skin.

Diagnosis.—The diagnosis is as a rule easy, particularly if the patient has been seen from the onset. When a case comes under observation for the first time with the rash well out, there may be considerable difficulty. The abundance of the rash on the trunk in varicella is most important. The pocks in varicella are more superficial, more bleb-like, have not so deeply an infiltrated areola about them, and may usually be seen in all stages of development. They rarely at the outset have the hard, shotty feeling of those of small-pox. The general symptoms, the greater intensity of the onset, the prolonged period of invasion, and the more frequent occurrence of prodromal rashes in small-pox are important points in the diagnosis.

Death is very rare, and, unless from the complications, raises a suspicion of the correctness of the diagnosis. Thus of the 116 deaths in England and Wales in 1903 ascribed to chicken-pox, it is probable, as Tatham suggests, that many of these were from unrecognized small-pox.

No special *treatment* is required. If the rash is abundant on the face, great care should be taken to prevent the child from scratching the pustules. A soothing lotion should be applied on lint.

IV. SCARLET FEVER

Definition.—An infectious disease characterized by a diffuse exanthem and an angina of variable intensity.

History.—In the sixteenth century Ingrassias of Naples and Coyttarus of Poitiers recognized the disease; but Sydenham in 1675 gave a full account of it under the name febris scarlatina.

Etiology.—No one of the acute infections varies so greatly in the intensity of the outbreaks, a point to which both Sydenham and Bretonneau called attention. In some years it is mild; in others, with equally widespread epidemics, it is fearfully malignant. It is a widespread affection, occurring in nearly all parts of the globe and attacking all races.

Sporadic cases occur from time to time. The epidemics are most intense in the autumn and winter. There is an extraordinary variability in the severity of the outbreaks, which on the whole appear to be lessening in severity; thus, in Boston from 1894 to 1903 the ratio of cases per ten thousand has ranged from 45.80 to 16.18, and the mortality from 3.94 to .60. In England and Wales the disease is declining. In 1883 there were over 12,000 deaths; in 1903, 4,158; in 1909, 3,215, and in 1910 it was 50 per cent. less than in 1901. Newsholme attributes this in part to the general improvement in sanitation in the home and to hospital isolation, and in part to the striking decline in the severity of the disease.

Seibert's studies in New York show that the disease increases steadily from week to week until the middle of May; the frequency diminishes gradually until the end of June, and gradually increases through October, November, and December. He associates the remarkable drop in July, August, and September with the closure of the schools and the cessation of the daily congregation of infectious material in small areas—school-houses and playgrounds—for so many hours each day.

Age is the most important predisposing factor. Ninety per cent. of the fatal cases are under the tenth year. Sucklings are rarely attacked. The general liability to the disease in childhood is less widespread than in measles. Many escape in childhood; others escape until adult life; some never take it.

Family susceptibility is not infrequently illustrated by the death in rapid succession of four or five members. On the other hand, individual resistance is common, and many physicians constantly exposed escape. An attack as a rule confers subsequent immunity. In rare instances there have been one or even two recurrences.

The natives of India are said to enjoy comparative immunity.

Infectivity.—It is not yet accurately known where in the body the poison is formed. It is probably given off with the secretions of the nose, throat, and respiratory tract. The mild angina of the ambulatory cases may convey the disease, and in this way it is spread in schools, and the "return cases" may find in this way their explanation. Much more attention has been paid of late to this aspect of the scarlatinal infection, and it has even been suggested that the skin is only infective by contamination with the secretions. The general opinion, however, is that the poison is given off chiefly from the skin, particularly when desquamating. Unlike measles, the germ is very resistant and clings tenaciously to clothing, to bedding, the furniture of the room, etc. Even after the most complete disinfection possible, children who have been removed from an infected house may catch the disease on their return. The possibility here of throat and nose infection must be considered. The intractable character of the nasal discharge after scarlet fever is well recognized and this secretion appears to be highly infectious. The chief organisms in it are streptococci. A third person may convey the disease, but undoubted instances are rare. I recall one instance in which I could have been the only possible medium.

The disease is stated to have been conveyed by milk. Of 99 epidemics studied by Kober the disease prevailed in 68 either at the dairy or the milk farm. There appear to be two groups of cases: first, genuine scarlet fever, in which the infection is conveyed through the milk having come in contact with infected persons; and, secondly, outbreaks of an infection resembling scarlet fever, due to disease of the udder of the cows.

By SURGICAL SCARLATINA, first brought to the attention of the profession by Sir James Paget in 1864, is understood an erythematous eruption following an operation or occurring during septic infection. It differs from medical scarlatina in the large number of adults attacked, the shorter incubation, the mildness of the throat symptoms, the starting of the eruption at the wound, and the precocious desquamation. Alice Hamilton, after analyzing 174 cases reported in the literature, concludes that the eruption is most frequently due to septic infection and is not truly scarlatinal, and that in those cases in which the disease was undoubtedly scarlatina there is no convincing evidence that the relation between the wound and the scarlet fever was anything more than one of coincidence.

The SPECIFIC GERM is not known. It is claimed to be only a modified streptococcus infection. The streptococcus pyogenes has often been found in the blood during life and after death, and it is constantly present in the throat in severe cases; but there is no agreement on the subject among the best workers.

Morbid Anatomy.—Except in the hæmorrhagic form, the skin after death shows no traces of the rash. There are no specific lesions. Those which occur in the internal organs are due partly to the fever and partly to infection with pus-organisms.

The anatomical changes in the throat are those of simple inflammation, follicular tonsillitis, and, in extreme grades, of diphtheroid angina. In severe cases there are intense lymphadenitis and much inflammatory œdema of the tissues of the neck, which may go on to suppuration, or even to gangrene. Streptococci are found abundantly in the glands and in the foci of suppuration. The lymph glands and the lymphoid tissue may show hyperplasia and the spleen, liver, and other organs may be the seat of widespread focal necroses.

Endocarditis and pericarditis are not infrequent. Myocardial changes are less common. The renal changes will be considered with the diseases of the kidney.

Affections of the respiratory organs are not frequent. When death results from the pseudo-membranous angina, broncho-pneumonia is not uncommon. Cerebro-spinal changes are rare.

Symptoms.—INCUBATION.—"From one to seven days, oftenest two to four." McCollom considered the usual period to be ten to fourteen days.

INVASION.—The onset is as a rule sudden. It may be preceded by a slight, scarcely noticeable, indisposition. An actual chill is rare. Vomiting is one of the most constant initial symptoms; convulsions are common. The fever is intense; rising rapidly, it may on the first day reach 104° or even 105°. The skin is unusually dry and to the touch gives a sensation of very pungent heat. The tongue is furred, and as early as the first day there may be complaint of dryness of the throat. Cough and catarrhal symptoms are uncommon. The face is often flushed and the patient has all the objective features of an acute fever.

ERUPTION.—Usually on the second day, in some instances within the first twenty-four hours, the rash appears in the form of scattered red points on a deep subcuticular flush; at first on the neck and chest, and spreading so rapidly that by the evening of the second day it may have invaded the entire skin. After persisting for two or three days it gradually fades. At its height the rash has a vivid scarlet hue, quite distinctive and unlike that seen in any other eruptive disease. It is an intense hyperæmia, and the anæmia produced by pressure instantly disappears. There may be fine punctiform hæmorrhages, which do not disappear on pressure. In some cases the rash does not become uniform but remains patchy, and intervals of normal skin separate large hyperæmic areas. Tiny papular elevations may sometimes be seen, but they are not so common as in measles. With each day the rash becomes of a darker color, and there may be in parts even a bluish-red shade. Smooth at the beginning, the skin gradually becomes rougher, and to the touch feels like "goose skin." At the height of the eruption sudaminal vesicles may develop, the fluid of which may become turbid. The entire skin may at the same time be covered with small yellow vesicles on a deep red background—*scarlatina miliaris.* McCollom lays stress upon the appearance of a punctate eruption in the arm-pits, groins, and on the roof of the mouth as positive proof of scarlet fever. Marked transverse lines at the bend of the elbow sometimes occur early.

Occasionally there are petechiæ, which in the malignant type of the disease become widespread and large. The eruption does not always appear upon the face. There may be a good deal of swelling of the skin, which feels uncomfortable and tense. The itching is variable; not as a rule intense at the height of the eruption. By the seventh or eighth day the rash has disappeared. The mucous membrane of the palate, the cheeks, and the tonsils present a vivid red, punctiform appearance. The tongue at first is red at the tip and edges, furred in the centre; and through the white fur are often seen the swollen red papillæ, which give the so-called "strawberry" appearance to the tongue, particularly if the child puts out the tip of the tongue between the lips. In a few days the "fur" desquamates and leaves the surface red and rough, and it is this condition which some writers call the "strawberry," or, better, the "raspberry" tongue. Enlargement of the papillæ was the only constant sign in 1,000 cases (McCollom). The breath often has a very heavy, sweet odor.

The pharyngeal symptoms are:

1. Slight redness, with swelling of the pillars of the fauces and of the

tonsils. 2. A more intense grade of swelling and infiltration of these parts with a follicular tonsillitis. 3. Diphtheroid angina with intense inflammation of all the pharyngeal structures and swelling of the glands below the jaw, and in very severe cases a thick brawny induration of all the tissues of the neck.

The fever, which sets in with such suddenness and intensity, may reach 105° or even 106° F. It persists with slight morning remissions, gradually declining with the disappearance of the rash. In mild cases the temperature may not reach 103° F.; on the other hand, in very severe cases there may be hyperpyrexia, the thermometer registering 108° F., or before death even 109° F.

The pulse ranges from 120 to 150; in severe cases with very high fever from 190 to 200. The respirations show an increase proportionate to the intensity of the fever. A leucocytosis is usually present, which may be high

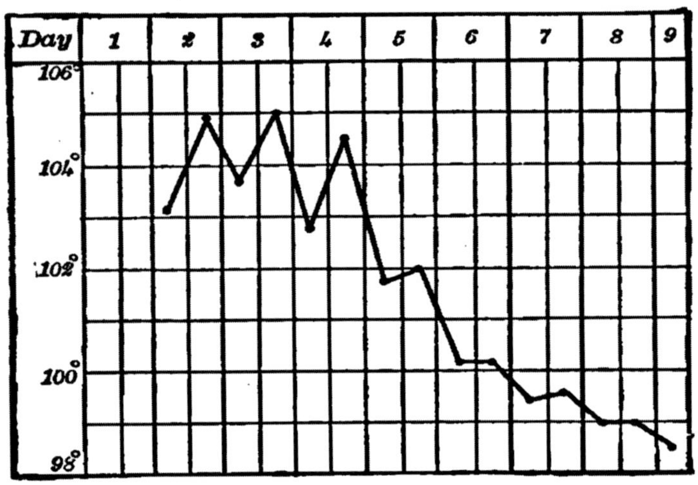

Chart X.—Scarlet Fever.

(30,000 to 50,000 per c. mm.) in the severe cases. The gastrointestinal symptoms are not marked after the initial vomiting, and food is usually well taken. In some instances there are abdominal pains. The edge of the spleen may be palpable. The liver is not often enlarged. With the initial fever nervous symptoms are present in a majority of the cases; but as the rash comes out the headache and the slight nocturnal wandering disappear. The urine has the ordinary febrile characters, being scanty and high colored. Slight albuminuria is by no means infrequent during the stage of eruption. Careful examination of the urine should be made every day. There is no cause for alarm in the trace of albumin which is so often present, not even if it is associated with a few tube casts.

Desquamation.—With the disappearance of the rash and the fever the skin looks somewhat stained, is dry, a little rough, and gradually the upper layer of the cuticle begins to separate. The process usually begins about the neck and chest, and flakes are gradually detached. The degree and character of the desquamation bear some relation to the intensity of the eruption. When the latter has been very vivid and of long standing large flakes may be thrown off. In rare instances the hair and even the nails have been shed. It must not be forgotten that there are cases in which the desquamation has been prolonged, according to Trousseau, even to the seventh or eighth week. The entire process lasts from ten to fifteen or even twenty days.

Atypical Scarlet Fever.—MILD AND ABORTIVE FORMS.—In cases of exceptional mildness the rash may be scarcely perceptible. During epidemics, when several children of a household are affected, one child sickens as if with scarlet fever, and has a sore throat and the "strawberry tongue," but the rash does not appear—*scarlatina sine eruptione*. In school epidemics a third or more of the cases may be without the rash. Desquamation, however, may follow, and in these very mild forms nephritis may occur.

MALIGNANT SCARLET FEVER.—*Fulminant Toxic Variety.*—With all the characteristics of an acute intoxication, the patient is overwhelmed by the intensity of the poison and may die within twenty-four or thirty-six hours. The disease sets in with great severity—high fever, extreme restlessness, headache, and delirium. The temperature may rise to 107° or even 108°, in rare cases even higher. Convulsions may occur and the initial delirium rapidly gives place to coma. The dyspnœa may be urgent; the pulse is very rapid and feeble.

Hæmorrhagic Form.—Hæmorrhages occur into the skin, and there are hæmaturia and epistaxis. In the erythematous rash scattered petechiæ appear, which gradually become more extensive, and ultimately the skin may be universally involved. Death may take place on the second or on the third day. While this form is perhaps more common in enfeebled children, I have twice known it to attack adults apparently in full health.

ANGINOSE FORM.—The throat symptoms appear early and progress rapidly; the fauces and tonsils swell and are covered with a thick membranous exudate, which may extend to the posterior wall of the pharynx, forward into the mouth, and upward into the nostrils. The glands of the neck rapidly enlarge. Necrosis occurs in the tissues of the throat, the fetor is extreme, the constitutional disturbance profound, and the child dies with the clinical picture of a malignant diphtheria. Occasionally the membrane extends into the trachea and the bronchi. The Eustachian tubes and the middle ear are usually involved. When death does not take place rapidly from toxæmia there may be extensive abscess formation in the tissues of the neck and sloughing. In the separation of deep sloughs about the tonsils the carotid artery may be opened, causing fatal hæmorrhage.

SEPTICÆMIC FORM.—In this there is a severe secondary infection and death occurs in the second or third week from severe toxæmia.

Complications and Sequelæ.—ALBUMINURIA.—At the height of the fever there is often a slight trace of albumin in the urine, which is not of special significance. In a majority of cases the kidneys escape without greater damage than occurs in other acute febrile affections.

NEPHRITIS is most common in the second or third week and may follow a very mild attack. It may be delayed until the third or fourth week. As a rule, the earlier it occurs the more severe the attack. It occurs in from 10 to 20 per cent. of the cases. Three grades of cases may be recognized:

1. Acute hæmorrhagic nephritis. There may be suppression of urine or only a small quantity of bloody fluid laden with albumin and tube casts. Vomiting is constant, there are convulsions, and the child dies with the symp-

toms of acute uræmia. In severe epidemics there may be many cases of this sort, and an acute, rapidly fatal, nephritis due to the scarlet fever poison may occur without an exanthem.

2. Less severe cases without serious acute symptoms. There is a puffy appearance of the eyelids, with slight œdema of the feet; the urine is diminished in quantity, smoky, and contains albumin and tube casts. The kidney symptoms then dominate the entire case, the dropsy persists, and there may be effusion into the serous sacs. The condition may drag on and become chronic, or the patient may succumb to uræmic accidents. Fortunately, in a majority of the cases recovery takes place.

3. Cases so mild that they can scarcely be termed nephritis. The urine contains albumin and a few tube casts, but rarely blood. The œdema is extremely slight or transient, and the convalescence is scarcely interrupted. Occasionally, however, serious symptoms may supervene. Œdema of the glottis may prove rapidly fatal, and in one case of the kind a child under my care died of acute effusion into the pleural sacs.

In other cases the œdema disappears and the child improves, though he remains pale, and a slight amount of albumin persists in the urine for months or even for years. Recovery may ultimately take place or a chronic interstitial nephritis may follow.

Occasionally œdema occurs without albuminuria or signs of nephritis. Possibly it may be due to the anæmia; but there are instances in which marked changes have been found in the kidney after death, even when the urine did not show the features characteristic of nephritis.

Arthritis.—There are two forms: first, the severe scarlatinal pyæmia, with suppuration of one or more joints—part of a widespread streptococcus infection. This is an extremely serious and fatal form. Secondly, scarlatinal arthritis, analogous to that occurring in gonorrhœa and other infections. It occurs in the second or third week; many joints are attacked, particularly the small joints of the hands. The heart may be involved. Chorea, subcutaneous fibroid nodules, purpura, and pleurisy may be complications. The outlook is usually good.

Cardiac Complications.—In the severe septic cases a malignant endocarditis, sometimes with purulent pericarditis, closes the scene. Simple endocarditis is not uncommon. It may not be easy to say whether the apex systolic murmur, so often heard, signifies a valvular lesion. The persistence after convalescence, with signs of slight enlargement of the heart, may alone decide that the murmur indicated an organic change. As is the rule, such cases give no symptoms. And, lastly, there may be a severe toxic myocarditis, sometimes leading to acute dilatation and sudden death. It is to be borne in mind that the cardiac complications of the disease are often latent.

Acute bronchitis and broncho-pneumonia are not common. *Empyema* is an insidious and serious complication.

Ear Complications.—Common and serious, due to extension of the inflammation from the throat through the Eustachian tubes, they rank among the most frequent causes of deafness in children. The severe forms of membranous angina are almost always associated with otitis, which goes on to suppuration and to perforation of the drum. The process may extend to the labyrinth and rapidly produce deafness. In other instances there is suppuration in the mastoid cells. In the necrosis which follows the middle-ear disease the facial nerve may be involved and paralysis follow. Later, still more serious complications may follow, such as thrombosis of the lateral sinus, meningitis, or abscess of the brain.

ADENITIS.—In comparatively mild cases of scarlet fever the submaxillary lymph-glands may be swollen. In severer cases the swelling of the neck becomes extreme and extends beyond the limits of the glands. Acute phlegmonous inflammations may occur, leading to widespread destruction of tissue, in which vessels may be eroded and fatal hæmorrhage ensue. The suppurative processes may also involve the retro-pharyngeal tissues.

The swelling of the lymph-glands usually subsides, and within a few weeks even the most extensive enlargement gradually disappears. There are rare instances, however, in which the lymphadenitis becomes chronic, and the neck remains with a glandular collar which almost obliterates its outline. This may prove intractable to all ordinary measures of treatment. A case came under my observation in which, two years after scarlet fever, the neck was enormously enlarged and surrounded by a mass of firm brawny glands.

NERVOUS COMPLICATIONS.—Chorea occasionally complicates the arthritis and endocarditis. Sudden convulsions followed by hemiplegia may occur. In seven of my series of 120 cases of infantile hemiplegia the trouble came on during scarlet fever. Progressive paralysis of the limbs with wasting may present the features of a subacute ascending spinal paralysis. Thrombosis of the cerebral veins may occur. Mental symptoms, mania, and melancholia have been described.

Other rare complications and sequelæ are œdema of the eyelids, without nephritis, symmetrical gangrene, enteritis, noma, and perforation of the soft palate.

The fever may persist for several weeks after the disappearance of the rash, and the child may remain in a septic or typhoid state. This so-called scarlatinal typhoid is usually the result of some chronic suppurative process about the throat or the nose, occasionally the result of a chronic adenitis, and in a few cases nothing whatever can be found to account for the fever.

Measles may be concurrent or follow in the stage of convalescence.

RELAPSE is rare. It was noted in 7 per cent. of 12,000 (Caiger), in 1 per cent. of 1,520 cases (Newsholme), and in 3 per cent. of 5,000 cases (McCollom).

Diagnosis.—The diagnosis of scarlet fever is not difficult, but there are cases in which the true nature of the disease is for a time doubtful. The following are the most common conditions with which it may be confounded:

ACUTE EXFOLIATING DERMATITIS.—This pseudo-exanthem simulates scarlet fever very closely. It has a sudden onset, with fever. The eruption spreads rapidly, is uniform, and after persisting for five or six days begins to fade. Even before it has entirely gone desquamation usually begins. Some of these cases cannot be distinguished from scarlet fever in the stage of eruption. The throat symptoms, however, are usually absent, and the tongue rarely shows the changes which are so marked in scarlet fever. In the desquamation of this affection the hair and nails are commonly affected. It is, too, a disease liable to recur. Some of the instances of second and third attacks of scarlet fever have been cases of this form of dermatitis.

Measles, which is distinguished by the longer period of invasion, the characteristic nature of the prodromes, and the later appearance of the rash. The greater intensity of the measly rash upon the face, the more papular character and the irregular crescentic distribution are distinguishing features in a majority of the cases. Other points are the absence in measles of the sore throat, the peculiar character of the desquamation, the absence of leucocytosis, and the presence of Koplik's sign.

Rötheln.—The rash of rubella is sometimes strikingly like that of scarlet fever, but in the great majority of cases the mistake could not arise. In cases of doubt the general symptoms are our best guide.

Septicæmia.—As already mentioned, the so-called puerperal or surgical scarlatina shows an eruption which may be identical in appearance with that of true scarlet fever.

Diphtheria.—The practitioner may be in doubt whether he is dealing with a case of scarlet fever with intense membranous angina, a true diphtheria with an erythematous rash, or coexisting scarlet fever and diphtheria. In the angina occurring early in and during the course of scarlet fever, though the clinical features may be those of true diphtheria, Löffler's bacilli are rarely found. On the other hand, in the membranous angina occurring during convalescence the bacilli are usually present. The rash in diphtheria is, after all, not so common, is limited usually to the trunk, is not so persistent, and is generally darker than the scarlatinal rash.

Scarlatina and diphtheria may coexist, but in a case presenting widespread erythema and extensive membranous angina with Löffler's bacilli it would puzzle Hippocrates to say whether the two diseases coexisted, or whether it was only an intense scarlatinal rash in diphtheria. Desquamation occurs in either case. The streptococcus angina is not so apt to extend to the larynx, nor are recurrences so common; but it is well to bear in mind that general infection may occur, that the membrane may spread downward with great rapidity, and, lastly, that all the nervous sequelæ of the Klebs-Löffler diphtheria may follow the streptococcus form.

Drug Rashes.—These are partial, and seldom more than a transient hyperæmia of the skin. Occasionally they are diffuse and intense, and in such cases very deceptive. They are not associated, however, with the characteristic symptoms of invasion. There is no fever, and with care the distinction can usually be made. They are most apt to follow the use of belladonna, quinine, and iodide of potassium. The antitoxin erythema is a frequent cause of doubt, particularly in hospitals for infectious diseases.

Coexistence of other Diseases.—Of 48,366 cases of scarlet fever in the Metropolitan Asylum Board Hospitals which were complicated by some other disease, in 1,094 cases the secondary infection was diphtheria, in 899 cases chicken-pox, in 703 measles, in 404 whooping-cough, in 55 erysipelas, in 11 enteric fever, and in 1 typhus fever (F. F. Caiger). Farnarier (1904) could collect only 39 undoubted cases of the coexistence of typhoid and scarlet fever.

How Long Is a Child Infective?—Usually, after desquamation is complete, in four or five weeks the danger is thought to be over, but the occurrence of so-called "return cases" shows that patients remain infective even at this stage. In 1894, with 2,593 patients from the Glasgow fever hospitals sent to their homes convalescent, fresh cases appeared in 70 of the houses (Chalmers). With 15,000 cases submitted to an average period of isolation of forty-nine days or under, the percentage of return cases was 1.86; with an average period of fifty to fifty-six days the percentage was 1.12; where the isolation extended to between fifty-seven and sixty-five days the percentage of return cases was 1 (Neech). This author suggests eight weeks as a minimum and thirteen weeks as a maximum. Special care should be taken of cases with rhinorrhœa and otorrhœa and throat trouble, as the secretions from these parts are probably of greater importance than the skin in the conveyance of the disease.

Prognosis.—As stated, the death-rate has been falling of late years. Epidemics differ remarkably in severity and the mortality is extremely variable. Among the better classes the death-rate is much lower than in hospital practice. There are physicians who have treated consecutively a hundred or more cases without a death. On the other hand, in hospitals and among the poorer classes the death-rate is considerable, ranging from 5 to 10 per cent. in mild epidemics to 20 or 30 per cent. in the very severe. In 1,000 cases reported from the Boston City Hospital by McCollom the death-rate was 9.8 per cent. There is a curious variability in the local mortality from this disease. In England, for example, in some years, certain counties enjoy almost immunity from fatal scarlet fever. The younger the child the greater the danger. In infants under one year the death-rate is very high. The great proportion of fatal cases occurs in children under six years of age. The unfavorable symptoms are very high fever, early mental disturbance with great jactitation, the occurrence of hæmorrhages (cutaneous or visceral), intense diphtheroid angina with cervical bubo, and signs of laryngeal obstruction. Nephritis is always a serious complication, and when setting in with suppression of the urine may quickly prove fatal; a large majority of the cases recover.

Prophylaxis.—Much may be done to prevent the spread of the disease if the physician exercises scrupulous care in each case. Much is to be expected from a rigid system of school inspection, and from the more general recognition of the importance of the latent cases and the persistence of the infection in the secretions of the nose and throat. The attendant in a case of scarlet fever should take the most careful precautions against the conveyance of the disease, wearing a gown in the room and thoroughly washing the hands and face after leaving the room. To the very busy practitioner the minutiæ of proper disinfection are very irksome, but it is his duty to carry out the most rigid disinfection possible, and intelligent people now expect it. The duration of quarantine varies with the attack: six to eight weeks is the average period. Patients with discharge from the ear or nose require longer isolation.

Treatment.—The patient may be treated at home or sent to an isolation hospital. The difficulty in *home treatment* is in securing complete isolation. The risks are well illustrated by the careful studies of Chapin, of Providence, who found that during eight years 26.1 per cent. of the 4,412 persons under twenty-one years of age in infected families took the disease. When practicable, it is better to send the other children out of the house. Chapin's experience on this point is most interesting. In seventeen years, from 652 families infected with scarlet fever, 1,051 children, none of whom had had the disease, were removed. Only 5 per cent. were attacked while away from home. Nineteen who had been sent away from the infected houses were attacked on their return. In Great Britain a very considerable proportion of all patients are removed from their homes. In the segregation hospital groups of patients, from ten to twenty, are treated in separate wards. In the true isolation hospital each patient is in a separate room, and patients with different infectious diseases may be in adjacent rooms.

The disease cannot be cut short. In the presence of the severer forms we are still too often helpless. There is no disease, however, in which the successful issue and the avoidance of complications depend more upon the skilled judgment of the physician and the care with which his instructions are carried out.

The child should be isolated and placed in charge of a competent nurse. The temperature of the room should be constant and the ventilation thorough. The child should wear a light flannel nightgown, and the bedclothing should not be too heavy. The diet should consist of milk, buttermilk, whey, and ice cream; water and fruit juices should be freely given. With the fall of the temperature the diet may be increased and the child may gradually return to ordinary fare. When desquamation begins the child should be thoroughly rubbed every day, or every second day, with sweet oil, or carbolated vaseline, or a 5-per-cent. hydro-naphthol soap, which prevents the drying and the diffusion of the scales. A 5- or 10-per-cent. solution of ichthyol in lanolin may be used. An occasional warm bath may then be given. At any time during the attack the skin may be sponged with warm water. The patient may be allowed to get up after the temperature has been normal for ten days, but for at least three weeks from this time great care should be exercised to prevent exposure to cold. It must not be forgotten, also, that the renal complications are very apt to occur during the convalescence, and after all danger is apparently past. Ordinary cases do not require any medicine, or at the most a simple fever mixture, and during convalescence a bitter tonic. The bowels should be carefully regulated.

Special symptoms in the severe cases call for treatment.

When the fever is above 103° F. the extremities may be sponged with tepid water. In severe cases, with the temperature rapidly rising, this will not suffice, and more thorough measures of hydrotherapy should be practiced. With pronounced delirium and nervous symptoms the cold pack should be used. When the fever is rising rapidly but the child is not delirious, he should be placed in a warm bath, the temperature of which can be gradually lowered. The bath with the water at 80° is beneficial. In giving the cold pack a rubber sheet and a thick layer of blankets should be spread upon a sofa or a bed, and over them a sheet wrung out of cold water. The naked child is then laid upon it and wrapped in the blankets. An intense glow of heat quickly follows the preliminary chilling, and from time to time the blankets may be unfolded and the child sprinkled with cold water. The good effects which follow this plan of treatment are often striking, particularly in allaying the delirium and jactitation, and procuring quiet and refreshing sleep. Parents will object less, as a rule, to the warm bath gradually cooled than to any other form of hydrotherapy. The child may be removed from the warm bath, placed upon a sheet wrung out of tolerably cold water, and then folded in blankets. The ice-cap is very useful and may be kept constantly applied in cases in which there is high fever. Medicinal antipyretics are not of much service in comparison with cold water.

The throat symptoms, if mild, do not require much treatment. If severe, the local measures mentioned under diphtheria should be used. The nose should be kept clean, for which a simple alkaline douche, given gently, is best. Cold applications to the neck are to be preferred to hot, though it is sometimes difficult to get a child to submit to them. If cervical adenitis occurs, an ice bag should be applied, and with the first signs of suppuration an incision made. In connection with the throat, the ears should be specially looked after, and a careful disinfection of the mouth and fauces by suitable antiseptic solutions should be practiced. When the inflammation extends through the tubes to the middle ear, the practitioner should either himself examine daily the condition of the drum, or, when available, a specialist should be called in to assist him in the case. The careful watching of this membrane day by day and the puncturing of it if the tension becomes too great may save the hearing of the child. With the aid of cocaine the drum is readily punctured. The operation may be repeated at intervals if the pain and distention return. No complication of the disease is more serious than this extension of the inflammatory process to the ear.

The nephritis should be dealt with as in ordinary cases; indications for treatment will be found under the appropriate section. It is worth mentioning, however, that Jaccoud insists upon the great value of milk diet in scarlet fever as a preventive of nephritis.

Among other indications for treatment in the disease is cardiac weakness, which is usually the result of the direct action of the poison, and is best met by stimulants.

Serum Treatment.—As a streptococcus infection frequently complicates scarlet fever and is responsible for the secondary infections, the use of antistreptococcus serum seems rational, but it has not proved of great value in the acute stages. More is to be expected from it in the more chronic infections, in which also an autogenous vaccine may be useful. The dosage should be small at first and increased gradually.

V. MEASLES

(*Morbilli*)

Definition.—An acute, highly contagious fever with specific localization in the upper air passages and in the skin.

History.—Rhazes, an Arabian physician, in the ninth century described the disease with small-pox, of which it was believed to be a mild form until Sydenham separated them in the seventeenth century.

Etiology.—As a cause of death measles ranks first among the acute fevers of children. In 1909 there were 12,618 deaths from this disease in England and Wales. The death rate is highest in the second year.

The liability to infection is almost universal in persons unprotected by a previous attack. It is a disease of childhood, but, as shown in the widespread epidemics in the Farroe Islands and in the Fiji Islands, unprotected adults of all ages are attacked. Within the first three months of life there is a relative immunity. Occasionally infants of a month or six weeks take the disease. Intra-uterine cases have been described, and a mother with measles may give birth to a child with the eruption, or the rash may appear in a few days.

The disease is endemic in cities, and becomes epidemic at intervals, prevailing most extensively in the cooler months, though this is by no means a fixed rule.

The germ of the disease is unknown. J. F. Anderson has shown that the blood of a patient inoculated into the Rhesus monkey produces after eight days a fever of short duration with a well-marked slight exanthem. The contagion is present in the blood, the secretions of the mouth and nose, and in the skin. In the eighteenth century Monro and others demonstrated the inoculability of the disease. Direct contagion is the most common. The poison is probably not in the expired air, but in the particles of mucus and in the sputum and the secretions of the mouth and nose, which, dried, are conveyed with the dust. An important point is the contagiousness of the disease in the pre-eruptive stage. A child with only the catarrhal symptoms may be at school and a source of active infection. Indirect contagion by means of fomites is very common. Measles may be thus conveyed by a third person, by clothes, and by infected toys. The germ soon loses its virulence.

Recurrence is rare. Very many cases of the supposed second and third attack represent mistakes in diagnosis. Relapse is occasionally seen, the symptoms recurring at intervals from ten to forty days; but it is not always easy to say in a given case whether there may not have been new infection from without.

Morbid Anatomy.—The catarrhal and inflammatory appearances seen post mortem have nothing characteristic. Fatal cases show, as a rule, broncho-pneumonia and an intense bronchial catarrh. The lymphatic elements all over the body are swollen, the tonsils, the lymph-glands, and the solitary and agminated follicles of the intestines. The spleen is rarely much enlarged. During convalescence latent tuberculous foci are very apt to become active.

Symptoms.—Incubation.—"From seven to eighteen days; oftenest fourteen." The child shows no special changes, but coryza and swelling of the cervical lymph-glands may be present. A leucocytosis has been observed, and the pulse is said to be slow.

Invasion.—In this period, lasting from three to four days, very rarely five or six, the child presents the symptoms of a feverish cold. The onset may be insidious, or it may start with great abruptness, even with a convulsion. There is not often a definite chill. Headache, nausea, and vomiting may usher in the severe cases. The common catarrhal symptoms are sneezing and running at the nose, redness of the eyes and lids, and cough. The fever is slight at first, but gradually there is pungent heat of the skin with turgescence of the face. Prodromal rashes precede the true eruption in a few cases, usually a blotchy erythema or scattered macules. The tongue is furred and the mucous membranes of the mouth and throat are hyperæmic, and frequently show a distinct punctiform rash. The fever of the stage of invasion may rise abruptly; more frequently it takes twenty-four or forty-eight hours to reach the fastigium. The pulse-rate increases with the fever, and may reach 140 or 160 per minute, gradually falling with defervescence.

ERUPTION.—"The symptoms increase till the fourth day. At that period (although sometimes a day later) little red spots, just like flea-bites, begin to come out on the forehead and the rest of the face. These increase both in size and number, group themselves in clusters, and mark the face with largish red spots of different figures. These red spots are formed by small red papules, thick set, and just raised above the level of the skin. The fact that they really protrude can scarcely be determined by the eye. It can, however, be ascertained by feeling the surface with the fingers. From the face—where they first appear—these spots spread downward to the breast and belly; afterward to the thighs and legs" (Sydenham). The papules may feel quite shotty, but do not extend deeply. On the trunk and extremities the swelling of the skin is not so noticeable, the color of the rash not so intense and often

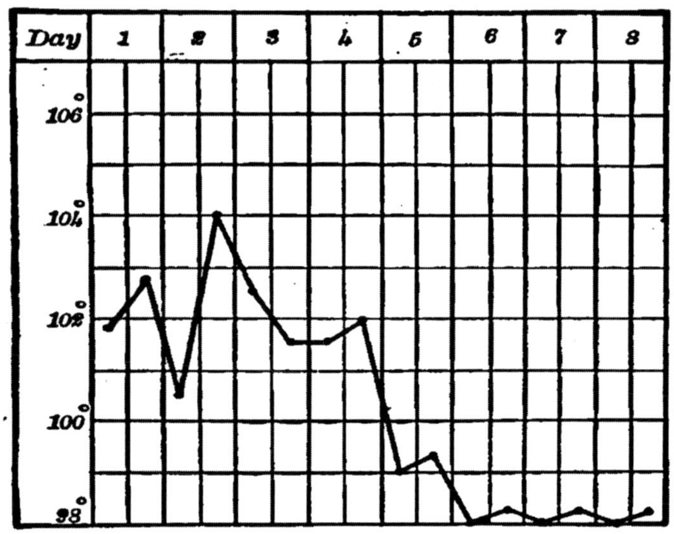

CHART XI.—MEASLES.

less uniform. The mottled, blotchy character is seen most clearly on the chest and the abdomen. It is hyperæmic and disappears on pressure, but in the malignant cases it may become of a deep rose, inclining to purple. These general symptoms do not abate with the occurrence of the eruption, but persist until the end of the fifth or the sixth day, when they lessen. Among peculiarities of the rash may be mentioned the development of numerous miliary vesicles and the occurrence of petechiæ, which are seen occasionally even in cases of moderate severity. Recession of the rash, so much dwelt upon by older writers, is rarely seen. When the "measles sink in suddenly after they have begun to come out, and then the patient is seized with anxiety and a swooning comes on, it is a sign of speedy death" (Rhazes). In reality it is the failing circulation which causes the rash to fade.

BUCCAL SPOTS were described by Filatow in 1895, and by Koplik in 1896. They are seen on a level with the bases of the lower milk molars on either side, or at the line of junction of the molars when the jaws are closed. They are white or bluish-white specks, surrounded by red areolæ. Their importance depends upon the fact of their early appearance and remarkable constancy in the disease—six-sevenths of all cases (Heubner), 97.7 per cent. of 214 cases (Balme).

The fauces may be injected, and there is sometimes an eruption of scattered spots over the entire mucous membrane of the mouth. Ringer was in the habit of calling attention to opaque white spots on the mucous membrane of the lips.

Desquamation.—After the rash fades desquamation begins, usually in the form of fine scales, more rarely in large flakes. It bears a definite relationship to the extent and intensity of the rash. In mild cases desquamation may take only a few days, in severe cases several weeks.

The tonsils and the cervical lymph glands may be slightly swollen and sore; sometimes there is a polyadenitis.

During the course leucocytosis is absent. Its presence generally points to a complication. Myelocytes are often present in small numbers during the eruption (Tileston).

Atypical Measles.—Variations in the course of the disease are not common. There is an *attenuated* form, in which the child may be well by the fourth or fifth day. An *abortive* form, in which the initial symptoms may be present, but no eruption appears—*morbilli sine morbillis.*

Malignant or *black measles* is seen most frequently in the widespread epidemics, but it is also met with in institutions, and occasionally in general practice among children, more rarely in adults. Hæmorrhages occur into the skin and from the mucous membranes; there is very high fever, and all the features of a profound toxæmia, often with cyanosis, dyspnœa, and extreme cardiac weakness. Death may occur from the second to the sixth day.

Complications.—Those of the air passages are the most serious. The *coryza* may become chronic and lead to irritation of the lymphoid tissues of the naso-pharynx, leaving enlarged tonsils and adenoids, and not improbably leaving these parts less able to resist tuberculous invasion. *Epistaxis* may sometimes be serious. *Laryngitis* is not uncommon: the voice becomes husky and the cough croupy in character. Œdema of the glottis and pseudo-membranous inflammation are rare. Ulceration, abscess, and even perichondritis may occur.

Bronchitis and Broncho-pneumonia.—In every case of severe measles the possibility of the existing bronchitis extending to the small tubes and causing lobular pneumonia has to be considered. It is more apt to occur at the height of the eruption or as desquamation begins. The high mortality in institutions is due to this complication, which, as Sydenham remarked, kills more than the small-pox. (For the symptoms, see the section on the subject.)

Lobar pneumonia is less common. *Thrombosis* in veins has been described.

Severe *stomatitis* may follow the slight catarrhal form. In institutions *cancrum oris* or *gangrenous stomatitis* is a terrible complication, attacking sometimes many children. *Parotitis* occasionally occurs. *Intestinal catarrh* and *acute colitis* are special complications of some epidemics.

Nephritis is less rare than is stated. It is not very uncommon to see cases of chronic Bright's disease which date from an attack of measles. Vulvitis may be present as part of the general catarrhal condition.

Endocarditis is rare. *Arthritis* may follow the fever, or come on at its height. It may be general and severe. I saw an instance in which anchylosis of the jaw followed an attack of measles in a child of four years. The conjunctivitis may be followed by *keratitis.* *Otitis media* is not at all uncommon and may lead to perforation of the drum or mastoid disease. *Hemiplegia* is a most serious complication. In 4 of my series of 120 cases the hemiplegia came on during measles. It usually persists. *Paraplegia* due to acute myelitis has been described. *Polyneuritis* may occur with widespread atrophy. Acute mania, *meningitis, abscess of the brain,* and *multiple sclerosis* are among the rare complications or sequelæ. *Scarlet fever* may occur with measles. *Whooping-cough* not infrequently follows measles.

Diagnosis.—During the prevalence of an epidemic the disease is easily recognized. Physicians to isolation hospitals appreciate the practical difficulties. On several occasions I had patients with measles sent to the small-pox hospital, and it is well to bear in mind that in adults the beginning of the eruption on the face, its nodular character, and the isolation of the spots may be suggestive of variola. From scarlet fever measles is distinguished by the longer initial stage with characteristic symptoms, and the blotchy irregular character of the rash, so unlike the diffuse uniform erythema. In measles the mouth (with the early Koplik sign), in scarlet fever the throat, is chiefly affected. Occasionally in measles, when the throat is very sore and the eruption pretty diffuse, there may at first be difficulty in determining which disease is present, but a few days should suffice to make the diagnosis clear. As a rule there is no leucocytosis. It may be extremely difficult to distinguish from rötheln. I have more than once known practitioners of large experience unable to agree upon a diagnosis. The shorter prodromal stage, the absence of oculo-nasal catarrh, and the slighter fever in many cases are perhaps the most important features. It is difficult to speak definitely about the distinctions in the rash, though perhaps the more uniform distribution and the absence of the crescentic arrangement are more constant in rötheln. In Africans the disease is easily recognized; the papules stand out with great plainness, often in groups; the hyperæmia is to be seen on all but the very black skins. The distribution of the rash, the coryza, and the rash in the mouth are important points. Of drug eruptions, that induced by copaiba is very like measles, but is readily distinguished by the absence of fever and catarrh. Antipyrin, chloral, and quinine rashes rarely cause any difficulty in diagnosis. The serum exanthem of a diphtheria antitoxin may be difficult to recognize. In adults the acute malignant measles may resemble typhus fever. Occasionally erythema multiforme may simulate measles.

Prognosis.—The mortality from the disease itself is not high, but the pulmonary complications render it one of the most serious of the diseases of children. In some epidemics, particularly in institutions and in armies, the death-rate may be high, not so much from the fever itself as from the extension of the catarrhal symptoms to the finer bronchial tubes. Imported in 1875 from Sydney by H.M.S. Dido to the Fiji Islands, 40,000 out of 150,000 of the inhabitants died in four months. Panum, the distinguished Danish physician, described the widespread and fatal epidemic which decimated the inhabitants of the Faroe Islands in 1846. In private practice the mortality is from 2 to 3 per cent.; in hospitals from 6 to 8 or 10 per cent.

Prophylaxis.—The difficulty is inherent in the prolonged incubation and the four days of invasion, during which the catarrhal symptoms are marked, and the disease is contagious, and one often finds that the quarantine which has been carried out so efficiently has been in vain. From contact with cases in the stage of invasion and mild cases with scarcely any fever the disease is readily disseminated through schools and conveyed to healthy children in the every-day contact with each other on the streets, in the squares and play-grounds. Once manifested, the child should be carefully quarantined and all possible precautions taken against the spread of the disease in the house. As the germ of measles seems to have a feeble vitality the quarantine need not be so protracted as in scarlet fever, four weeks usually being sufficient.

Treatment.—Confinement to bed in a well-ventilated room and a light diet with abundance of water are the only measures necessary in cases of uncomplicated measles. The fever rarely reaches a dangerous height. If it does it may be lowered by sponging or by the tepid bath gradually reduced. If the rash does not come out well, warm drinks and a hot bath will hasten its maturation. The bowels should be freely opened. If the cough is distressing compresses should be applied to the chest and inhalations of the compound tincture of benzoin given. Small doses of paregoric or codein may be given. The patient should be kept in bed for a few days after the fever subsides. During desquamation the skin should be oiled daily, and warm baths given to facilitate the process. The mouth and nostrils should be carefully cleansed, even in mild cases. The convalescence from measles is the most important stage of the disease. Watchfulness and care may prevent serious pulmonary complications. The frequency with which the mothers of children with simple or tuberculous broncho-pneumonia tell us that "the child caught cold after measles," and the contemplation of the mortality bills, should make us extremely careful in our management of this affection.

VI. RUBELLA

(Rötheln, German Measles)

This exanthem has also the names of *rubeola notha,* or epidemic roseola, and, as it is supposed to present features common to both, has been also known as hybrid measles or hybrid scarlet fever. It is now generally regarded, however, as a separate and distinct affection.

Etiology.—It is propagated by contagion and spreads with great rapidity. It frequently attacks adults, and the occurrence of either measles or scarlet fever in childhood is no protection against it. The epidemics of it are often very extensive.

Symptoms.—These are usually mild, and it is altogether a less serious affection than measles. Very exceptionally, as in the epidemics studied by Cheadle, the symptoms are severe.

The stage of incubation is two weeks or even longer.

In the stage of invasion there are chilliness, headache, pains in the back and legs, and coryza. A macular, rose-red eruption on the throat is a constant symptom, and, indeed, it was on this account that it was originally regarded as a hybrid, having the sore throat of scarlet fever and the rash of measles. There may be very slight fever. In 30 per cent. of Edwards's cases the temperature did not rise above 100°. The duration of this stage is somewhat variable. The rash usually appears on the first day, some writers say on the second, and others again give the duration of the stage of invasion as three days. Griffith places it at two days. The eruption comes out first on the face, then on the chest, and gradually extends so that within twenty-four hours it is scattered over the whole body. It may be the first symptom noted by the mother. The eruption consists of a number of round or oval, slightly raised spots, pinkish-red in color, usually discrete, but sometimes confluent.

The color of the rash is somewhat brighter than in measles. The patches are less distinctly crescentic. After persisting for two or three days (sometimes longer), it gradually fades and there is a slight furfuraceous desquamation. The rash persists as a rule longer than in scarlet fever or measles, and the skin is slightly stained after it. In some cases the rash is scarlatiniform, which may even follow a measly eruption. The lymphatic glands of the neck are frequently swollen, and, when the eruption is very intense and diffuse, the lymph-glands in the other parts of the body.

There are no special complications. The disease usually progresses favorably; but in rare instances, as in those reported by Cheadle, the symptoms are of greater severity. Albuminuria, arthritis, or even nephritis may occur. Pneumonia and colitis have been present in some epidemics. Icterus has been seen.

Diagnosis.—The slightness of the prodromal symptoms, the mildness or the absence of the fever, the more diffuse character of the rash, its rose-red color, and the early enlargement of the cervical glands, are the chief points of distinction between rötheln and measles.

The treatment is that of a simple febrile affection.

"Fourth Disease."—Clement Dukes, in a paper on the confusion of two different diseases under the name rubella, describes what he calls a "fourth disease," in which the body is covered in a few hours with a diffuse exanthem of a bright red color, almost scarlatiniform in appearance. The face may remain quite free. The desquamation is more marked than in rötheln.

Erythema Infectiosum.—Under this term there has been described in Germany, particularly by Escherich, a feebly contagious disease, characterized by a rose-red, maculo-papular rash, appearing chiefly between the ages of four and twelve. It has occurred in epidemic form in the spring and summer. It has followed outbreaks of measles or of rötheln. The most characteristic feature is the morbilliform eruption on the extremities, chiefly on the extensor surfaces. The trunk as a rule remains free.

VII. EPIDEMIC PAROTITIS

(*Mumps*)

Definition.—A specific infectious disease, characterized by swelling of the salivary glands and a special liability to orchitis in males.

Hippocrates described the disease and its peculiarities—an affection of children and young male adults, the absence of suppuration, and the orchitis.

Etiology.—The nature of the virus is unknown.

It is endemic in large centres of population, and at certain seasons, particularly spring and autumn, the cases increase rapidly. It is met most frequently in childhood and adolescence. Very young infants and adults are seldom attacked. Males are somewhat more frequently affected than females. In institutions, barracks, and schools the disease has been known to attack over 90 per cent. of the residents. It may be curiously localized in a city or district, or even in one part of a school or barrack. The disease is contagious and spreads from patient to patient. The infection may persist for as long as six weeks. It may be congenital, and Hale White has reported a case in which the mother and her new-born child were attacked at the same time.

A remarkable idiopathic, non-specific parotitis may follow injury or disease of the abdominal or pelvic organs (see Diseases of the Salivary Glands).

Symptoms.—The period of incubation is from two to three weeks, and there are rarely any symptoms during this stage. The invasion is marked by fever, which is usually slight, rarely rising above 101°, but in exceptionally severe cases reaches 103° or 104°. The child complains of pain just below the ear on one side, where a slight swelling is noticed, which increases gradually, and within forty-eight hours there is great enlargement of the neck and side of the cheek. The swelling passes forward in front of the ear, the lobe of which is lifted, and back beneath the sterno-mastoid muscle. The other side usually becomes affected within a day or two, and the whole neck is surrounded by a collar of doughy infiltration. Only one gland may be involved, or an interval of four or five days may elapse before the other side is involved. The submaxillary and sublingual glands become swollen, though not always; in a few cases they may be alone attacked. The lachrymal glands may be involved. The greatest inconvenience is experienced in taking food, for the patient is unable to open the mouth, and even speech and deglutition become difficult. There may be an increase in the secretion of the saliva, but the reverse is sometimes the case. The mucous membrane of the mouth and throat may be slightly inflamed. There is seldom great pain, but an unpleasant feeling of tension and tightness. There may be earache, even otitis media, and slight impairment of hearing.

After persisting for from seven to ten days, the swelling gradually subsides and the child rapidly regains his strength and health and is none the worse for the attack.

Occasionally the disease is very severe and characterized by high fever, delirium, and great prostration. The patient may even lapse into a typhoid condition.

Relapse is rare, but there may be within a few weeks two or three slight recurrences, in which I have known the cervical glands to enlarge. A second or even a third attack may occur.

Orchitis.—Excessively rare before puberty, it occurs usually about the eighth day, and more particularly if the boy is allowed to leave his bed. One or both testicles may be involved. The swelling may be great, and occasionally effusion takes place into the tunica vaginalis. The orchitis may occur before the parotitis, or in rare instances may be the only manifestation of the infection (*orchitis parotidea*). The inflammation increases for three or four days, and resolution takes place gradually. There may be a muco-purulent discharge from the urethra. In severe cases atrophy may follow, fortunately as a rule only in one organ; occurring in both before puberty the natural development is usually checked. Even when both testicles are atrophied and small, sexual vigor may be retained. The proportion of cases of orchitis varies in different epidemics; 211 cases occurred in 699 cases, and 103 cases of atrophy followed 163 instances of orchitis (Comby). No satisfactory explanation of this remarkable metastasis has been given. Military surgeons, who see so much of the disease in young recruits, have suggested the transference of the virus to the penis with the fingers and its transmission along the urethra.

A vulvo-vaginitis sometimes occurs in girls, and the breasts may become enlarged and tender. Mastitis has been seen in boys. Involvement of the ovaries is rare. The thyroid gland may enlarge in the attack, and there have been features suggestive of acute pancreatitis.

Complications and Sequelæ.—Of these the cerebral affections are perhaps the most serious. As already mentioned, there may be delirium and high fever. In rare instances meningitis has been found. Hemiplegia and coma may also occur. A majority of the fatal cases are associated with meningeal symptoms. These, of course, are very rare in comparison with the frequency of the disease; yet, in the Index Catalogue, under this caption, there are six fatal cases mentioned. In some epidemics the cerebral complications are much more marked than in others. Acute mania has occurred, and there are instances on record of insanity following the disease.

Arthritis, albuminuria, nephritis, with acute uræmia and convulsions, endocarditis, pleurisy, facial paralysis, hemiplegia, and peripheral neuritis are occasional complications.

Suppuration of the gland is an extremely rare complication. Gangrene has occasionally occurred. The special senses may be seriously involved. Deafness may occur, and may be permanent. Affections of the eye are rare, but optic neuritis with atrophy has been described.

Chronic hypertrophy of the gland may follow.

Diagnosis.—The diagnosis of the disease is usually easy. The position of the swelling in front of and below the ear and the elevation of the lobe on the affected side definitely fix the locality of the swelling. In children inflammation of the parotid, apart from ordinary mumps, is excessively rare.

Treatment.—It is well to keep the patient in bed during the height of the disease. The bowels should be freely opened, and the patient given a light liquid diet. No medicine is required unless the fever is high, in which case aconite may be given. Cold compresses may be placed on the gland, but children, as a rule, prefer hot applications. A pad of cotton wadding covered with oil silk is the best application. Suppuration is hardly ever to be dreaded, even though the gland become very tense. Should redness and tenderness develop, leeches may be used. With delirium and head symptoms the ice-cap may be applied. For the orchitis, rest, with support and protection of the swollen gland with cotton-wool, is usually sufficient.

VIII. TYPHUS FEVER

Definition.—An acute infectious disease of unknown origin, highly contagious, characterized by sudden onset, maculated and hæmorrhagic rash, marked nervous symptoms, and a cyclical course terminating by crisis, usually about the end of the second week. Post mortem there are no special lesions other than those associated with fever.

The disease is known by the names of hospital fever, spotted fever, jail fever, camp fever, and ship fever, and in Germany is called *exanthematic* typhus, in contradistinction to *abdominal* typhus. The word signifies "smoke" or "mist" in Greek and was used by Hippocrates to describe any condition with a tendency to stupor. In the eighteenth century the name was given by de Sauvages to the common putrid or pestilential fever, and the general use came in through its adoption by Cullen.

Etiology.—Typhus has been one of the great *epidemics* of the world, whose history, as Hirsch remarks, is written in those dark pages which tell of the grievous visitations of mankind by war, famine, and misery. It now exists in a few endemic areas, where from time to time sporadic cases occur. Ireland was terribly scourged by the disease between the years 1817 and 1819, and again in 1846. It prevailed extensively in all the large cities of Great Britain and the Continent. Its gradual disappearance has been one of the great triumphs of sanitation. In 1875 in England and Wales there were 1,499 deaths from the disease. Of late years the name typhus has rarely appeared in the Registrar-General's report. In the United States and Canada it prevailed extensively in the early years of the nineteenth century, and there were severe epidemics in the wake of the Irish immigrations in '46 and '47. It is endemic in parts of Russia and in the Slav countries, and there have been extensive epidemics in the present war.

Sporadic typhus fever offers peculiarities which are apt to make its recognition difficult. There may be outbreaks of a few cases, the origin of which may be very difficult to trace, though, as Kelsch long ago suggested, tramps may convey the disease, while they themselves are healthy. Two such limited outbreaks came under my observation, one at the House of Refuge, Montreal, in 1877, in which eleven persons were affected, and the second in 1901 at the Johns Hopkins Hospital, where three cases occurred.

A question of interest has arisen as to the relation of typhus fever to the cases of fever, 255 in number, studied by Brill in New York. In all probability it is a sporadic type of typhus, an opinion to which Brill himself leans, and which has been confirmed by the studies of Anderson and Goldberger. Beginning with the usual prodromes, the fever increases rapidly and reaches a maximum about the third or fourth day, where it remains fairly constant between 103° and 104°. On the 5th or 6th day an eruption appears, maculo-papular in type, dull red in color, rarely hæmorrhagic, not appearing in crops, not disappearing on pressure, and neither profuse as in measles nor diffuse as in typical typhus; there may be only a few hundred spots. The rash persists until the crisis and then fades rapidly. The patients are much prostrated, with severe headache, but no abdominal symptoms. Constipation is usually a marked feature. After persisting for 12 to 15 days, the fever declines rapidly, usually with a critical fall, and there is a speedy convalescence. The blood cultures are negative and there is no agglutination with any of the organisms of the typhoid group. The disease does not spread to other patients in the wards or in the home. It is very rarely fatal, and post mortem results show no lesions of the intestines.

The so-called Manchurian type met with in the far East is very similar, and has the same low mortality and slight degree of infectiousness. On the other hand, the typhus fever prevailing in Mexico City, where it is known as Tabardillo, is more severe, and in its study Ricketts of Chicago fell a victim. Neither the Rocky Mountain spotted fever, nor the Flood or River fever of Japan is identical with typhus.

The disease is associated with filth and overcrowding. In epidemics it is one of the most highly contagious of all diseases, and those in attendance upon patients are almost invariably attacked unless special precautions are taken to guard against lice. In a period of twenty-five years in Ireland, among 1,230 physicians attached to institutions, 550 died of this disease. The disease is transmitted by the body louse and possibly by the head louse. Various organisms have been described but none can be regarded as positively established as the cause. Nicole, Anderson and Goldberger have been able to transmit the disease to monkeys, and Nicole has shown that lice fed on the typhus-infected chimpanzee can transmit the disease to monkeys.

Morbid Anatomy.—The anatomical changes are those which result from intense fever. The blood is dark and fluid; the muscles are of a deep red color, and often show a granular degeneration, particularly in the heart; the liver is enlarged and soft and may have a dull clay-like lustre; the kidneys are swollen; there is moderate enlargement of the spleen, and a general hyperplasia of the lymph-follicles. Peyer's glands are not ulcerated. Bronchial catarrh is usually, and hypostatic congestion of the lungs often, present. The skin shows the petechial rash.

Symptoms. —INCUBATION.—This is placed at about twelve days, but it may be less. There may be ill-defined feelings of discomfort. As a rule, however, the *invasion* is abrupt and marked by chills or a single rigor, followed by fever. The chills may recur during the first few days, and there is headache with pains in the back and legs. There is early prostration, and the patient is glad to take to his bed at once. The temperature is high at first, and may attain its maximum on the second or third day. The pulse is full, rapid, and not so frequently dicrotic as in typhoid. The tongue is furred and white, and there is an early tendency to dryness. The face is flushed, the eyes congested, and the expression dull and stupid. Vomiting may be a distressing symptom. In severe cases mental symptoms are present from the outset, either a mild febrile delirium or an excited, active, almost maniacal condition. Bronchial catarrh is common.

STAGE OF ERUPTION.—From the third to the fifth day the eruption appears—first upon the abdomen and upper part of the chest, and then upon the extremities and face; occurring so rapidly that in two or three days it is all out. There are two elements in the eruption: a subcuticular mottling, "a fine, irregular, dusky red mottling, as if below the surface of the skin some little distance, and seen through a semi-opaque medium" (Buchanan); and distinct papular rose-spots which change to petechiæ. In some instances the petechial rash comes out with the rose-spots. Collie describes the rash as consisting of three parts: rose-colored spots which disappear on pressure, dark-red spots which are modified by pressure, and petechiæ upon which pressure produces no effect. In children the rash at first may present a striking resemblance to that of measles and give as a whole a curiously mottled appearance to the skin. The term mulberry rash is sometimes applied to it. In mild cases the eruption is slight, but even then is largely petechial in character. As the rash is hæmorrhagic, it does not disappear after death. Usually the skin is dry, so that sudaminal vesicles are not common. It is stated by some authors that a distinctive odor is present. During the second week the general symptoms are much aggravated. The prostration becomes more marked, the delirium more intense, and the fever rises. The patient lies on his back with a dull, expressionless face, flushed cheeks, injected conjunctivæ, and contracted pupils. The pulse increases in frequency and is feebler; the face

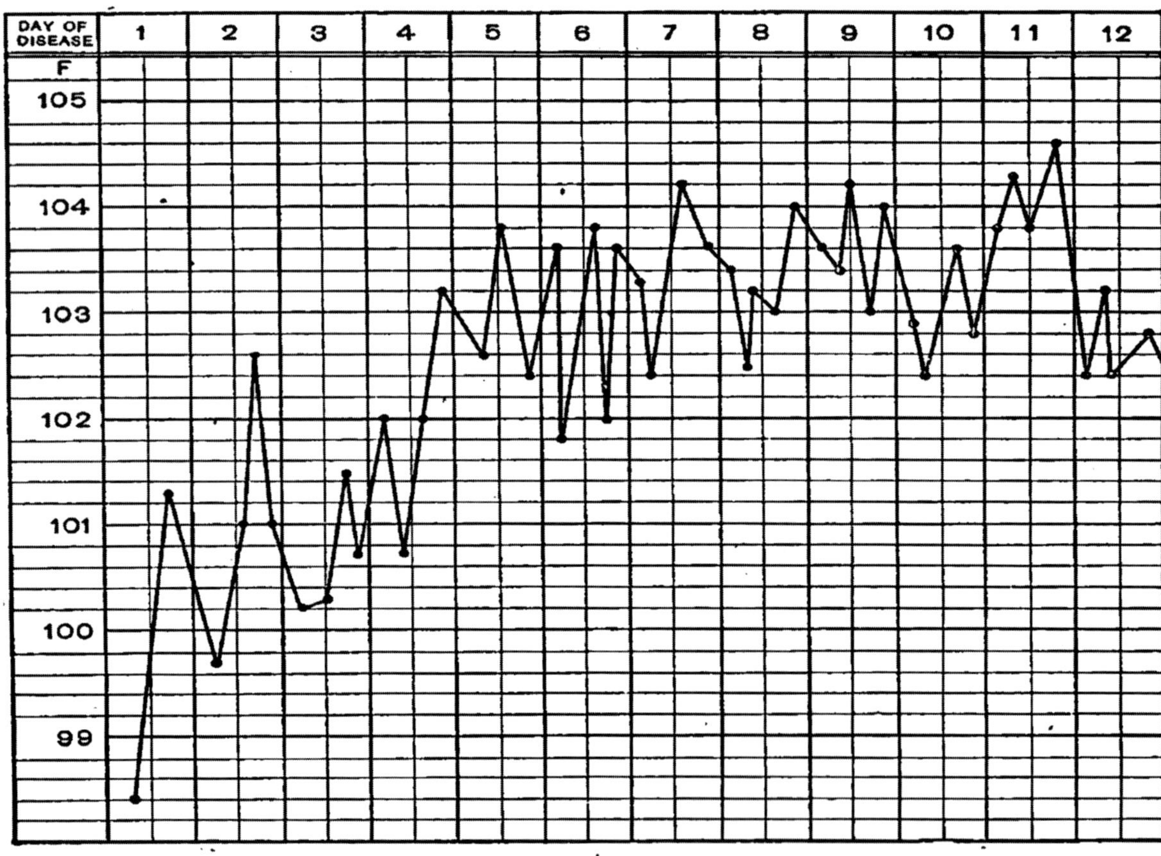

CHART XII.—TYPHUS FEVER (Murchison).

is dusky, and the condition becomes more serious. Retention of urine is common. Coma-vigil is frequent, a condition in which the patient lies with open eyes, but quite unconscious; with it there may be subsultus tendinum and picking at the bedclothes. The tongue is dry, brown, and cracked, and there are sordes on the teeth. Respiration is accelerated, the heart's action becomes more and more enfeebled, and death takes place from exhaustion. In favorable cases about the end of the second week occurs the crisis, in which, often after a deep sleep, the patient awakes feeling much better and with a clear mind. The temperature falls, and although the prostration may be extreme convalescence is rapid and relapse very rare. This abrupt termination by crisis is in striking contrast to the mode of termination in typhoid fever.

FEVER.—The temperature rises steadily during the first four or five days, and the morning remissions are not marked. The maximum is usually attained by the fifth day, when the temperature may be 105°, 106°, or 107° F.

In mild cases it seldom rises above 103° F. After reaching its maximum the fever generally continues with slight morning remissions until the twelfth or fourteenth day, when the crisis occurs, during which the temperature may fall below normal within twelve or twenty-four hours. Preceding a fatal termination, there is usually a rapid rise in the fever to 108° or even 109° F.

The heart may early show signs of weakness. The first sound becomes feeble and almost inaudible, and a systolic murmur at the apex is not infrequent. Hypostatic congestion of the lungs occurs in all severe cases. The brain symptoms are usually more pronounced than in typhoid, and the delirium is more constant. A slight leucocytosis is more common than in typhoid.

The urine in typhus shows the usual febrile increase of urea and uric acid. The chlorides diminish or disappear. Albumin is present in a large proportion of the cases, but nephritis seldom occurs.

Variations in the course of the disease are naturally common. There are malignant cases which rapidly prove fatal within two or three days; the so-called *typhus siderans*. On the other hand, during epidemics there are extremely mild cases in which the fever is slight, the delirium absent, and convalescence is established by the tenth day.

Complications and Sequelæ.—Broncho-pneumonia is perhaps the most common complication. It may pass on to gangrene. In certain epidemics gangrene of the toes, the hands, or the nose, and in children noma or cancrum oris, have occurred. Meningitis is rare. Paralyses, which are probably due to a post-febrile neuritis, are not very uncommon. Septic processes, such as parotitis and abscesses in the subcutaneous tissues and in the joints, are occasionally met with. Nephritis is rare. Hæmatemesis may occur.

Prognosis.—The mortality ranges in different epidemics from 12 to 20 per cent. It is very slight in the young. Children, who are quite as frequently attacked as adults, rarely die. After middle age the mortality is high, in some epidemics 50 per cent. Death usually occurs toward the close of the second week and is due to the toxæmia. In the third week it more commonly results from pneumonia.

Diagnosis.—During an epidemic there is rarely any doubt, for the disease presents distinctive general characters. Isolated cases and the form described by Brill may be very difficult to distinguish from typhoid fever. While in typical instances the eruption in the two affections is very different, yet taken alone it may be deceptive, since in typhoid fever a roseolous rash may be abundant and there may be occasionally a subcuticular mottling and even petechiæ. The difference in the onset, particularly in the temperature, is marked; but cases in which it is important to make an accurate diagnosis are not usually seen until the fourth or fifth day. The suddenness of the onset, the greater frequency of the chill, and the early prostration are the distinctive features in typhus. The brain symptoms, too, are earlier. It is easy to put down on paper elaborate differential distinctions, which are practically useless at the bedside. The Widal reaction and blood cultures are important aids, but in sporadic cases the diagnosis is sometimes extremely difficult. I have seen Murchison himself in doubt, and more than once I have known the diagnosis to be deferred until the *sectio cadaveris*. Severe cerebro-spinal fever may closely simulate typhus at the outset, but the diagnosis is usually clear within a few days. Malignant variola also has certain features in common with severe typhus, but the greater extent of the hæmorrhages and the bleeding from the mucous membranes make the diagnosis clear within a short time. The rash at first resembles that of measles, but in the latter the eruption is brighter red in color, often crescentic or irregular in arrangement, and appears first on the face.

The frequency with which other diseases are mistaken for typhus is shown by the fact that during and following the epidemic of 1881 in New York 108 cases were wrongly diagnosed—one-eighth of the entire number—and sent to the Riverside Hospital (F. W. Chapin).

Treatment.—The general management of the disease is like that of typhoid fever. Hydrotherapy should be thoroughly and systematically employed. Judging from the good results which we have obtained by this method in typhoid cases with nervous symptoms, much may be expected from it. Medicinal antipyretics are even less suitable than in typhoid, as the tendency to heart-weakness is often more pronounced. As a rule, the patients require from the outset a supporting treatment; water should be freely given, and alcohol in suitable doses, according to the condition of the pulse.

The bowels may be kept open by mild aperients. The so-called specific medication, by sulphocarbolates, the sulphides, carbolic acid, etc., is not commended by those who have had the largest experience. The special nervous symptoms and the pulmonary symptoms should be dealt with as in typhoid fever. In epidemics, when the conditions of the climate are suitable, the patients are best treated in tents in the open air.

IX. YELLOW FEVER

Definition.—A fever of tropical and subtropical countries, characterized by a toxæmia of varying intensity, with jaundice, albuminuria, and a marked tendency to hæmorrhage, especially from the stomach, causing the "black vomit." The specific organism has not yet been found, but the disease is capable of being transmitted through the bite of a mosquito, the *Stegomyia fasciata*.

Etiology.—The disease prevails endemically in certain sections of the Spanish Main. Until recently it has existed in Cuba. From these regions it occasionally extended and, under suitable conditions, prevailed epidemically in the Southern States. Now and then it was brought to the large seaports of the Atlantic coast. Formerly it occurred extensively in the United States. In the latter part of the eighteenth century and the beginning of the nineteenth frightful epidemics prevailed in Philadelphia and other Northern cities. The epidemic of 1793, in Philadelphia, so graphically described by Matthew Carey, was the most serious that has ever visited any city of the Middle States. The mortality, as given by Carey, during the months of August, September, October, and November, was 4,041, of whom 3,435 died in the months of September and October. The population of the city at the time was only 40,000. Epidemics occurred in the United States in 1797, 1798, 1799, and in 1802, when the disease prevailed slightly in Boston and extensively in Baltimore. In 1803 and 1805 it again appeared; then for many years the outbreaks were slight and localized. In 1853 the disease raged throughout the Southern States. There were moderately severe epidemics in 1867, 1873, and 1878, and still milder ones in 1897, 1898, and 1899. In July, 1899, a local outbreak occurred in the Soldiers' Home at Hampton, Va. There were 45 cases, with 13 deaths. In September, 1903, yellow fever became epidemic along the Mexican side of the Rio Grande. It crossed into Texas and prevailed in several of the border towns. In Laredo there were 1,014 cases, with 107 deaths. The efficient work of the public health service is shown by the differences between New Laredo on the Mexican border, just across the river, where 50 per cent. of the population contracted the disease, and Laredo, Texas, in which only 10 per cent. out of a population of 10,000 were attacked. In Europe it has occasionally gained a foothold, but there have been no widespread epidemics in the Spanish ports. The disease has existed on the west coast of Africa, and the late Rubert Boyce claimed that it is still widely prevalent. It is sometimes carried to ports in Great Britain and France, but it has never extended into these countries. The *Stegomyia fasciata* exists here, but it is not very abundant and, as Ross points out, yellow fever is a disease in which the parasites live a very short time in the human host, unlike malaria. The infective period in a case lasts only about three days, so that, unless the stegomyia index is high, as in Havana, the disease has no chance to reach epidemic form.

The epidemics in the United States have always been in the summer and autumn months, disappearing rapidly with the onset of cold weather.

Guitéras recognizes three areas of infection: (1) The focal zone in which the disease is never absent, including Vera Cruz, Rio, and other Spanish-American ports. (2) The perifocal zone or regions of periodic epidemics, including the ports of the tropical Atlantic in America and Africa. (3) The zone of accidental epidemics, lying between the 35th and 15th parallels of north latitude.

Mode of Transmission.—No belief has been more strong among the laity than that the disease is transmitted by infected clothing, and quarantine efforts are chiefly directed to the disinfection of fomites of all sorts shipped from infected ports. The remarkable series of experiments carried out by the Yellow Fever Commission of the United States Army, consisting of Drs. Walter Reed, Carroll, Lazear, and Agramonte, have demonstrated conclusively that the disease cannot be conveyed in this way. At Camp Lazear, Cuba, a frame house was so constructed as to shut out the sunlight and fresh air, and the vestibule was thoroughly screened. The average temperature for sixty-three days was kept about 76° F. Boxes filled with sheets, pillow-slips, blankets, etc., contaminated by contact with cases of yellow fever and the discharges, were placed in the house. Dr. R. P. Cooke and two privates of the hospital corps, all non-immunes, entered this building and unpacked the boxes, and for a period of twenty days occupied the room, each morning packing the infected articles in the boxes, and at night unpacking them. In their experiments with the fomites, seven, in all, non-immune subjects during the period of sixty-three days lived in contact with the fomites and remained perfectly well. These experiments, conducted in the most rigid and scientific manner, completely discredit the belief in the transmission of the disease by fomites.

Carlos Finlay, of Havana, in 1881 suggested that the disease was transmitted by mosquitoes. Stimulated by the work of Ross on malaria, the American Commission above named has demonstrated conclusively that yellow fever is transferred by a mosquito, *Stegomyia fasciata,* previously fed on the blood of infected persons. The Commission showed also that in non-immunes the disease could be produced by either the subcutaneous or the intravenous injection of blood taken from patients suffering with the disease.

An interval of about twelve days or more after contamination appears to be necessary before the mosquito is capable of introducing the infection. The bite at an early period after contamination does not confer immunity against a subsequent attack. The period of incubation in 13 cases of experimental yellow fever varied from forty-one hours to five days and seventeen hours.

We must bear testimony to the heroism of the young soldiers who voluntarily, without compensation and purely in the interests of humanity, submitted to the experiments, and also to the zeal with which members of our profession have, at great personal risk, attempted to solve the riddle of this most serious disease. The death of Dr. Lazear, of the American Commission, and of Dr. Myers, of the Liverpool Commission, adds two more names to the already long roll of the martyrs of science.

As Reed pointed out, the mosquito theory fits in with well-recognized facts in connection with the epidemics. After the importation of a case into an uninfected region, a definite period elapses, rarely less than two weeks, before a second case occurs. Like malaria, the disease prevails most during the mosquito season, and disappears with the appearance of frost. Probably, too, as in very malarious districts, the disease is kept up by its prevalence in a very mild form among children. As Guitéras remarks, "the foci of endemicity are essentially maintained by the creole infant population, which is subject to the disease in a very mild form." In all probability the immunity which is acquired by prolonged residence in a locality in which the disease is endemic is due to the occurrence of very slight attacks.

One attack does not always confer immunity. Rosenau reports two attacks within a period of eight years, and Libby two attacks within a period of two years.

The *specific germ* has not yet been discovered.

Morbid Anatomy.—The skin is more or less jaundiced, even though the patient did not appear yellow before death. Cutaneous hæmorrhages may be present. No specific or distinctive internal lesions have been found. The blood-serum may contain hæmoglobin, owing to destruction of the red cells, just as in pernicious malaria. The heart sometimes, not invariably, shows fatty change; the stomach presents more or less hyperæmia of the mucosa with catarrhal swelling. It contains the material which, ejected during life, is known as the *black vomit.* The essential ingredient in this is transformed blood-pigment. There is often general glandular enlargement; the cervical, axillary and mesenteric groups are most involved. The liver is usually of a pale yellow or brownish-yellow color, and the cells are in various stages of fatty degeneration. From the date of Louis' observations at Gibraltar in 1828, the appearances of this organ have been very carefully studied, and some have thought the changes in it to be characteristic. Fatty degeneration and regions of necrosis are present in all cases. The kidneys always show traces of diffuse nephritis. The epithelium of the convoluted tubules is swollen and very granular; there may also be necrotic changes.

Symptoms.—The incubation is usually three or four days; in 13 experimental cases it ranged from forty-one hours to five days, seventeen hours. The onset is sudden, as a rule, without premonitory symptoms, and in the early hours of the morning. Chilly feelings are common, and are usually associated with headache and very severe pains in the back and limbs. The fever rises rapidly and the skin feels very hot and dry. The tongue is furred, but moist; the throat sore. Nausea and vomiting are not constant, and become more intense on the second or third day. The bowels are usually constipated. The following, in detail, are the more important characteristics:

FACIES.—Even as early as the first morning the patient may present a characteristic facies, one of the three distinguishing features of the disease, which Guitéras describes as follows: The face is flushed, more so than in any other acute infectious disease at such an early period. The eyes are injected, the color is a bright red, and there may be a slight tumefaction of the eyelids and of the lips. Even at this early date there is to be noticed in connection with the injection of the superficial capillaries of the face and conjunctivæ a slight icteroid tint, and "the early manifestation of jaundice is undoubtedly the most characteristic feature of the facies of yellow fever."

THE FEVER.—On the morning of the first day the temperature may range from 100° to 106° F., usually it is between 102° and 103° F. During the evening of the first day and the morning of the second day the temperature keeps about the same. There is a slight diurnal variation on the second and third day. In very mild cases the fever may fall on the evening of the second or on the morning of the third day, or in abortive cases even at the end of twenty-four hours. In cases that are to terminate favorably the defervescence takes place by lysis during a period of two or three days. The remission or stage of *calm*, as it has been called, is succeeded by a febrile reaction or secondary fever, which lasts one, two, or three days, and in favorable cases falls by a short lysis. On the other hand, in fatal cases the temperature is continuous, becomes higher than in the initial fever, and death follows shortly.

THE PULSE.—On the first day the pulse is rarely more than 100 or 110. On the second or third day, while the fever still keeps up, the pulse begins to fall, as much perhaps as 20 beats, while the temperature has risen 1.5° or 2°. On the evening of the third day there may be a temperature range of 103° and a pulse of only 75, or "a temperature between 103° and 104° with a pulse running from 70 to 80." This important diagnostic feature was first described by Faget, of New Orleans. During defervescence the pulse may become still lower, down to 50, 48, or 45, or even as low as 30; a slow pulse at this period is not the special circulatory feature of the disease, but *the slowing of the pulse with a steady or even rising temperature.*

ALBUMINURIA.—This, the third characteristic symptom of the disease, occurs as early as the evening of the third day. Guitéras says very truly that it is very rare so early in other fevers except those of an unusually severe type. "Even in the mild cases that do not go to bed—cases of 'walking yellow fever'—on the second, third, or fourth day of the disease albuminuria will show itself." It may be quite transient. In the severer cases the amount of albumin is very large, and there may be numerous tube casts and all the signs of an acute nephritis; or complete suppression may supervene, and death occurs in uræmic convulsions or coma within twenty-four or thirty-six hours.

GASTRIC FEATURES.—*"Black Vomit."*—Irritability of the stomach is present from the very outset, and the vomited matter consists of the contents of the stomach, and subsequently of mucus and a grayish fluid. In the third stage of the disease the vomiting becomes more pronounced and in the severe cases is characterized by the presence of blood. It may be copious and forcible, producing much pain in the abdomen and along the gullet. There is nothing specific in this "black vomit," which consists of altered blood, and it is not necessarily a fatal symptom, though occurring only in the severer forms of the disease. Other hæmorrhagic features may be present—petechiæ on the skin and bleeding from the gums or from other mucous membranes. The bowels are usually constipated, the stools not clay-colored, except late in the disease. They are sometimes tarry from the presence of altered blood.

MENTAL FEATURES.—In very severe cases the onset may be with active delirium. "As a rule, in a majority of cases, even when there is black vomit, there is a peculiar alertness; the patient watches everything going on about him with a peculiar intensity and liveliness. This may be due in part to the terror the disease inspires" (Guitéras).

Relapses occasionally occur. Among the varieties of the disease it is important to recognize the mild cases, characterized by slight fever, continuing for one or two days, and succeeded by a rapid convalescence. In the absence of a prevailing epidemic they would scarcely be recognized as yellow fever. Cases of greater severity have high fever and the features of the disease are well marked—vomiting, extreme prostration, and hæmorrhages. And, lastly, in the malignant form the patient is overwhelmed by the intensity of the fever, and death takes place in two or three days.

In severe cases convalescence may be complicated by parotitis, abscesses in various parts of the body, and diarrhœa.

Diagnosis.—(*a*) FROM DENGUE.—The difficulty in the differential diagnosis of these two diseases lies in their frequent coexistence, as during the epidemic of 1897 in parts of the Southern States. During the autumn of 1897 the profession of Texas was divided on the question of the existence of yellow fever in the State, some claiming that the disease was dengue, others, including Guitéras and West, that yellow fever also existed. In a majority of the cases the three diagnostic points upon which Guitéras lays stress—the facies, the albuminuria, and the slowing of the pulse with maintenance or elevation of the fever—are sufficient for the diagnosis. He states, too, that jaundice, which does sometimes occur in dengue, rarely appears as early as the second or third day of the disease, and on this much stress should be laid. Hæmorrhages are much less common in dengue, but that they do occur has been recognized by authorities ever since the time of Rush.

(*b*) FROM MALARIAL FEVER.—In the early stages of an epidemic cases are very apt to be mistaken for malarial fever. In the Southern States the outbreaks have usually been in the late summer months, the very season in which the æstivo-autumnal fever prevails. Among the points to be specially noted is the absence of early jaundice. Even in the most intense types of malarial infection the color of the skin is rarely changed within four or five days. To the experienced eye the facies would be of considerable help if the case was seen from the outset. Albumin is rarely present in the urine so early as the second day in a malarial infection. Other important points are the marked swelling of the spleen in malaria, while in yellow fever it is not much enlarged. Hæmorrhages, and particularly the black vomit, epistaxis, and bleeding gums are very rare in malarial infection. In the so-called hæmorrhagic malarial fever the patient has usually had previous attacks of malaria. Hæmaturia is a prominent feature, while in yellow fever it is by no means frequent. A special point of greater importance, perhaps, than any of these general symptomatic features is the examination of the blood for malarial parasites. The work of the army surgeons in Cuba showed that in a large proportion of cases there is not much difficulty in recognizing the æstivo-autumnal fever from yellow fever.

Prognosis.—In its graver forms yellow fever is one of the most fatal of epidemic diseases. The mortality has ranged, in various epidemics, from 15 to 85 per cent. In heavy drinkers and those who have been exposed to hardships the death-rate is much higher than among the better classes. In the epidemic of 1878, in New Orleans, while the mortality in hospitals was over 50 per cent. of the white and 21 per cent. of the colored patients, in private practice it was not more than 10 per cent. among the white patients. The death-rate was very low in the epidemic of 1897.

Prophylaxis.—The clearing of Havana by Colonel Gorgas was a direct outcome of the work of Reed and his colleagues. The city, with 250,000 people, had been infected continuously for 130 years. Non-immunes came in at the rate of 20,000 a year, and there were 6,000 children born. The city was divided into districts, each under the charge of an inspector, whose work was arranged under three heads: (1) To prevent the breeding of stegomyia mosquitoes. (2) To destroy those that had become infected. (3) To prevent mosquitoes becoming infected by protecting the sick so that they could not be bitten by mosquitoes.

The work was begun in February, 1901, and the last case of yellow fever occurred in September of that year, since which date, with the exception of a slight return, the city has been free.

At Panama in 1904, the date of the American occupation, the serious problem was how to fight yellow fever. Conditions were such that it took sixteen months before the disease disappeared. There has been no return. It is interesting to note that in the yellow fever wards at Ancon during 1905 all the physicians and nurses were non-immune, but not one of them contracted the disease, as the wards were so screened that no stegomyia mosquitoes could get at the patients to become infected.

Treatment.—Careful nursing and a symptomatic plan of treatment probably give the best results. The patient should be at rest in bed and for the first few days the diet should consist of very simple fluids. Elimination is an important part of treatment. Water should be given as freely as possible, best in the form of cold carbonated alkaline water. The bowels should be opened by a calomel and saline purge and enemata used if necessary. If there is vomiting, fluid should be given by the bowel or by infusion. Ice in small quantities, iced champagne or cocaine (gr. 1/4, 0.016 gm.) may be tried. The fever should be treated by hydrotherapy, sponges, packs or baths being used. The alkaline treatment is favorably regarded, sodium bicarbonate in full doses being given at short intervals and as much alkaline water as possible. For gastric and intestinal hæmorrhage the perchloride of iron or oil of turpentine may be given in doses of 15 minims (1 c. c.). Uræmic symptoms are best treated by the hot baths or packs, the free administration of fluid and hot bowel irrigations. Stimulants, especially strychnine, should be used during the second stage when the heart becomes feeble and rapid.

X. DENGUE

Definition.—An acute infectious disease of tropical and subtropical regions, characterized by febrile paroxysms, pains in the joints and muscles, an initial erythematous and a terminal polymorphous eruption.

It is known as *break-bone* fever from the atrocious character of the pain, and *dandy fever* from the stiff, dandified gait. The word dengue is supposed to be derived from a Spanish, or possibly Hindostanee, equivalent of the word dandy.

History and Geographical Distribution.—The disease was first recognized in 1779 in Cairo and in Java, where Bylon described the outbreak in Batavia. There have been widespread epidemics in India and China. The description by Benjamin Rush of the epidemic in Philadelphia in 1780 is one of the first and one of the very best accounts of the disease. Between 1824 and 1828 it was prevalent at intervals in India and in the Southern States. S. H. Dickson gives a graphic description of the disease as it appeared in Charleston in 1828. Since that date there have been four or five widespread epidemics in tropical countries and on this continent along the Gulf States, the last in the summer of 1897. None of the recent epidemics have extended into the Northern States, but in 1888 it prevailed as far north as Virginia. It has prevailed in the Philippine Islands among the United States troops and among the natives.

Etiology.—The rapidity of diffusion and the pandemic character are the two most important features of dengue. There is no disease, not even influenza, which attacks so large a proportion of the population. In Galveston, in 1897, 20,000 people were attacked within two months. In 1903 Graham showed that the disease could be transmitted to healthy persons by the bite of the mosquito *Culex fatigans,* an observation confirmed by Ashburn and Craig. The specific germ is still undetermined, but is probably ultramicroscopic.

As the disease is rarely fatal, no observations have been made upon its pathological anatomy.

Symptoms.—The period of incubation is from three to five days, during which the patient feels well. The attack sets in suddenly with headache, chilly feelings, and intense aching pains in the joints and muscles. The temperature rises gradually, and may reach 106° or 107°. The pulse is rapid, and there are the other phenomena associated with acute fever—loss of appetite, coated tongue, slight nocturnal delirium, and concentrated urine. The face has a suffused, bloated appearance, the eyes are injected, and the visible mucous membranes are flushed. There is a congested erythematous state of the skin. Rush's description of the pains is worth quoting, as in it the epithet break-bone occurs in the literature for the first time. "The pains which accompanied this fever were exquisitely severe in the head, back, and limbs. The pains in the head were sometimes in the back parts of it, and at other times they occupied only the eyeballs. In some people the pains were so acute in their backs and hips that they could not lie in bed. In others the pains affected the neck and arms, so as to produce in one instance a difficulty of moving the fingers of the right hand. They all complained more or less of a soreness in the seats of these pains, particularly when they occupied the head and eyeballs. A few complained of their flesh being sore to the touch in every part of the body. From these circumstances the disease was sometimes believed to be a rheumatism, but its more general name among all classes of people was the break-bone fever." The large and small joints are affected, sometimes in succession, and become swollen, red, and painful. In some cases cutaneous hyperæsthesia has been noted. Hæmorrhage from the mucous membranes was noted by Rush, and black vomit has also been described.

The fever gradually reaches its maximum by the third or fourth day; the patient then enters upon the apyretic period, which may last from two to four days, and in which he feels prostrated and stiff. A second paroxysm of fever then occurs, and the pains return. In a large number of cases an eruption is common, which, judging from the description, has nothing distinctive, being sometimes macular, like that of measles, sometimes diffuse and scarlatiniform, or papular, or lichen-like. In other instances the rash has been described as urticarial, or even vesicular. The rash may persist for a month after the symptoms have disappeared. Certain writers describe inflammation and hyperæmia of the mucous membrane of the nose, mouth and pharynx. Enlargement of the lymph-glands is not uncommon, and may persist for weeks after the disappearance of the fever. Convalescence is often protracted, and there is a degree of mental and physical prostration out of all proportion to the severity of the primary attack. The pains in the joints or muscles, sometimes very local, may persist for weeks. Rush refers to the former, stating that a young lady after recovery said it should be called break-heart, not break-bone, fever. The average duration of a moderate attack is from seven to eight days. Dengue is very seldom fatal. Dickson saw three deaths in the Charleston epidemic.

Complications are rare. Insomnia and occasionally delirium, resembling somewhat the alcoholic form, have been observed, and convulsions in children. Atrophy of the muscles may occur after the attack. A relapse may occur even as late as two weeks.

Diagnosis.—The diagnosis of the disease, prevailing as it does in epidemic form and attacking all classes indiscriminately, rarely offers any special difficulty. Isolated cases might be mistaken at first for rheumatic fever. The seven-day fever of East Indian ports is believed to be dengue. It is a sporadic fever of the hot weather, attacking a large proportion of Europeans within the first year or two of their arrival. Possibly, as Rogers thinks, it may be a distinct disease, and it is variously known in India as ephemeral fever, mild malaria, or simple continued fever. It is characterized by early and severe pains in the back and limbs, and a fever of six to seven days' duration.

Treatment.—This is entirely symptomatic. Quinine is stated to be a prophylactic, but on insufficient grounds. Hydrotherapy may be employed to reduce the fever. The salicylates or antipyrin may be tried for the pains, which usually, however, require opium. During convalescence iodide of potassium is recommended for the arthritic pains, and tonics are indicated.

XI. ACUTE POLIO-MYELITIS

(*Heine-Medin's Disease*)

Definition.—An acute infection occurring in both epidemic and sporadic forms, characterized anatomically by widespread lesions of the nervous system, with special localization in a majority of the cases in the anterior horns of the gray matter in the spinal cord—hence the common name, polio-myelitis anterior.

History.—In 1840 von Heine separated this type from other forms of paralysis and in 1887 Medin called attention to its occurrence in widespread epidemics, which have been specially studied in Sweden by Wickham, Harbitz, and others. Within the past ten years serious outbreaks have occurred in many parts of the United States and Canada. The incidence of the disease has also slightly increased in Great Britain and on the Continent of Europe, while in Sweden and Norway and parts of Austria the disease has assumed epidemic proportions. In New York City in 1907-8 there were about 2,000 cases, with a mortality of 6 to 7 per cent.; in 1910 throughout the United States there were between eight and nine thousand cases reported.

Etiology.—In its epidemic behavior the disease resembles closely cerebro-spinal fever. Sporadic cases occur in all communities and under at present unknown conditions increase at times to epidemic proportions. It prevails in the late summer and autumn.

Age is a most important predisposing element; a great majority of all cases occur in children in the first dentition. The more prevalent the epidemic form the greater the proportion of young adults attacked. Males and females are about equally attacked. Overexertion, injury, exposure are mentioned as possible factors.

The degree of contagiousness from person to person is slight, and in this the disease resembles cerebro-spinal fever and pneumonia, but the precise mode of transmission has not yet been determined.

The organism has been isolated by Flexner and his co-workers. The colonies consist of globular bodies averaging 0.15 to 0.3 micron in size. Monkeys inoculated with the twentieth generation of the culture developed typical experimental polio-myelitis. The infective agent is present in the brain and spinal cord, in the naso-pharyngeal secretions and in the blood. The disease is inoculable into monkeys and may be transmitted from one animal to another. It has been transmitted also by intracerebral injection of an emulsion made from flies which had fed on the spinal cord of a monkey dead of the disease. An important point is that the virus passes from the central nervous system in the monkey to the nasal mucosa and vice versa, and the application of the virus to this part is a ready means of inoculation. It has also been found in the tonsils and pharyngeal mucosa of children.

So far as we know, the disease is transmitted either directly by contact or possibly by the intervention of healthy carriers. The distribution is more independent of sanitary conditions than in the common children's diseases. The biting flies may convey the virus.

Morbid Anatomy.—One of the most striking results of recent researches has been to demonstrate how widespread the lesions are in the nervous system. We can no longer regard it as an affection limited to the anterior horns of the gray matter of the spinal cord, but a widespread poliomyelo-encephalitis with meningeal complications.

Swelling of the spleen and a marked general hyperplasia of the lymphoid apparatus have been found. The cerebro-spinal fluid is usually increased but clear. The pia mater is hyperæmic and moist, but without exudate. Cases in which the cerebral symptoms have been pronounced show swelling and flattening of the convolutions, with hyperæmia of the gray matter and here and there small hæmorrhages. The changes in the spinal cord are very characteristic. The meninges are moist, the pia is hyperæmic, sometimes with small capillary hæmorrhages. On section the cut surface bulges, the grey matter is hyperæmic, appearing as a reddened H, or the redness is limited to the anterior horns, which may show spots of hæmorrhage. These changes may be localized to the swellings of the cord or extend throughout its entire extent. Microscopically there is small-celled infiltration about the vessels of the meninges, most marked in the lumbar and cervical swellings. The infiltration extends into the fissures of the cord and follows the blood-vessels. The amount of meningeal implication is much more intense than is indicated macroscopically. In the cord itself the smaller blood-vessels are distended, hæmorrhages occur in the gray matter, there is marked perivascular infiltration, chiefly of lymphocytes, which collect about the vessels, forming definite foci. Sometimes the majority of the cells are polynuclear leucocytes. The ganglion cells, usually those of the anterior horns, degenerate and gradually disappear, changes probably secondary to the acute vascular alterations. Foci of infiltration and widespread œdema may be present in the white matter of the cord. In the fatal cases there are changes in the medulla and pons of much the same nature, but the ganglion cells rarely show such widespread destruction.

The path of invasion is apparently by the organism gaining access to the upper respiratory tract. Flexner and Lewis have shown that the infection can travel by the sheath of the sciatic nerve to the cord.

Symptoms.—The incubation period is from 5 to 10 days, during which the patient may complain of headache and pains and stiffness of the limbs. Naso-pharyngeal symptoms are common. Twitchings, even convulsions, and pain in the back and bones may be present. More commonly a child who has gone to bed well awakens in the morning with the paralysis and slight fever. Prodromal symptoms are more common in the epidemic form.

The studies of the past two or three years have shown a number of well-characterized types, of which the following are the most important:

(*a*) Abortive Form.—In epidemics, just as in cerebro-spinal fever, there are cases of illness with the general symptoms of infection, and indications of cerebro-spinal irritation, but without any motor disturbances. The symptoms pass away and the nature of the trouble remains doubtful, nor would suspicion be aroused were it not for the existence of other cases. It is interesting to note that Anderson and Frost have shown the presence of specific immune bodies in the blood of these cases.

(*b*) Common Poliomyelitic or Sporadic Type.—The paralysis is abrupt in its onset, reaches its maximum in a very short time, showing the irregularity and lack of symmetry which is characteristic of the disease. One or both arms may be affected, or one arm and one leg, or both legs, or it may be the right leg and left arm, or vice versa. In the arm the paralysis is rarely complete, the upper-arm muscles may be most affected or the lower-arm group; muscles acting functionally together, with centres near each other in the spinal cord, are paralyzed together. In this type the bladder and rectum are rarely involved.

(*c*) Progressive Ascending Type.—A certain number of cases, particularly in epidemics, run a course similar to Landry's paralysis, with which, no doubt, some of them have been confounded. The disease begins in the legs with the usual initial symptoms, the paralysis extends upward, involving the arms and the trunk, and death may occur with bulbar symptoms from the third to the fifth day. In the Swedish epidemic of 1905 of the 159 cases which died within the first two weeks, 45 presented this type.

(*d*) Bulbar Form.—It has long been known that occasionally in the ordinary spinal paralysis of children the cerebral nerves are involved, but in the epidemic form the disease may begin with paralysis of the ocular, facial, lingual, or pharyngeal muscles. The patient has fever, and the local picture depends upon the extent and distribution of the lesions in the medulla and pons. In the 1905 Swedish epidemic there were 34 cases in which the cerebral nerves were alone involved, and in the New York epidemic this localization was not very uncommon. A fatal result may follow extension of the bulbar symptoms.

(*e*) Meningitic Form.—This is important, as the cases simulate closely and are apt to be mistaken for cerebro-spinal fever. The picture is one of an acute meningitis—headache, pain and stiffness in the neck, vomiting, pain and rigidity in the back, drowsiness and unconsciousness. The disease may begin with the paralytic features and subsequently show the meningeal complications. Convulsions and Kernig's sign may be present. A serious difficulty is that the two diseases may prevail together, and only the careful examination of the cerebro-spinal fluid may give a differential diagnosis.

(*f*) Cerebral Type.—Here the picture is that which we have learned to recognize as the acute encephalitis or polio-encephalitis of children, a description of which we owe to von Strümpell. The disease sets in suddenly, with fever, vomiting and convulsions, followed by paralysis of one side of the body or one limb. Many of the patients die, others recover and present the usual after-picture of the cerebral hemiplegia of children. A large proportion of the cases of this disease probably represent this type of the sporadic form of acute infectious polio-myelo-encephalitis.

(*g*) Polyneuritic Form.—Many cases of the ordinary type, a majority, I should say, of the sporadic form, are painless. It is one of the features of the epidemic form that the patients complain much more of pain. This is particularly the case in a form which stimulates a polyneuritis. There is pain in the affected limbs, particularly on movement, with tenderness on pressure along the nerves and on pressing the muscles; the paralysis may extend like neuritis, involving chiefly the peripheral extensor muscle groups, and be followed by rapid wasting.

Diagnosis.—In the ordinary spinal sporadic cases there is rarely any difficulty. An important point to remember is that in periods of epidemic prevalence the disease presents an extraordinary number of clinical types. Some cases run a course like an acute infection, others have the picture of Landry's paralysis, in others again meningeal symptoms predominate, or there may be hyperæsthesia and pain, with the picture of a polyneuritis.

It seems not improbable that some obscure cases of meningitis are really instances of sporadic poliomyelitis. The same may be said of the acute encephalitis in children causing hemiplegia. The extraordinary complexity of the symptoms makes the diagnosis very difficult, so that we must look for help in the examination of the blood and spinal fluid and the testing the biological reactions of immunity.

If lumbar puncture is done early the cerebro-spinal fluid may be slightly turbid. The fluid contains a large amount of protein and gives a positive reaction to Noguchi's butyric acid test for globulin. This is one of the earliest features and reaches its maximum just before paralysis appears. By this some abortive cases of poliomyelitis have been recognized. In general characters, cytology and in globulin content the spinal fluid of the disease resembles closely that in tuberculous meningitis and in syphilitic myelitis.

Anomalous forms and symptoms are common during the prevalence of an epidemic. The muscles of respiration may be involved early, the diaphragm alone may be paralyzed, or the intercostals or the muscles of the palate and pharynx. Involvement of the facial muscles, usually a slight weakness, may be present, but in 5 out of 90 cases studied by F. R. Fraser the facial muscles alone were involved. In one instance ptosis was the only paralytic symptom on admission. Remarkable types may occur quite unlike the classical picture. In one case there was paralysis of one side of the soft palate with slight fever, the serum of this patient protected a monkey from intra-cerebral injection of the polio-myelitic virus. There may be slight fever with general spasticity of the muscles and tremor or rigidity of the muscles with coma.

The diagnosis from peripheral neuritis may be very difficult; in both the paralysis is of the legs, with wasting, loss of reflexes, and the bladder and rectum may be involved. Loss of the vibrating sensation tested with a large tuning fork is more common in peripheral neuritis, and later the electrical changes and the action of degeneration may be distinctive.

Course.—After the acute features have subsided there is little change for two or three weeks, after which improvement begins. This may continue for two or three months. The atrophy becomes evident in a few weeks from the onset of the attack. The affected limbs show less development as the patient grows older, and the deformity is usually most marked in the leg. The reaction of degeneration is present in the atrophied muscles. Early in the course the muscles lose the faradic response.

Prognosis.—The mortality is low, ranging in different epidemics from 4 to 15 per cent. The fatal cases are usually of the ascending, bulbar and meningeal types. As regards the muscles, complete loss of response to faradism means severe atrophy. If it is never completely lost the outlook is good and even extensive paralyses may disappear.

Prophylaxis.—The disease has been made notifiable. The patient should be isolated, the discharges and articles used by patients and nurses carefully disinfected, and special care should be taken of the nasal and pharyngeal discharges. It does not seem necessary to enforce a quarantine against those who come into relation with the patients, but the throat and nose of such persons should be disinfected with a menthol spray. There is some warrant for the administration of prophylactic doses of hexamine.

Treatment.—Hexamine may be given in doses of gr. v to xv (0.3 to 1 gm.). When the fever is high the general treatment is that of an acute infection. Aspirin and sedatives for the pain may be given. Lumbar puncture has been advised, and if the pressure is found to be high it should be repeated. The affected limb should be wrapped in cotton wool, and, if there is much pain, local sedative applications may be used. In the meningeal type of the disease warm baths and hot packs will be helpful. In the early stages it is well not to attempt to do much to the muscles, but within ten days careful massage may be practiced, using either lanolin or sweet oil. Strychnine hypodermically has been extensively used, but how far it has any influence may be questioned. It should not be given early. Electricity may be used and it has a value in keeping up the nutrition of the muscles. The faradic current should be employed if there is response, if not, the galvanic. The damage always looks to be much worse than it really is, as many of the symptoms depend on meningeal and vascular changes which undergo resolution. A curative serum has not yet been obtained.

The muscle itself as a factor has been emphasized by William MacKenzie of Melbourne (Brit. Med. Jour. 1915, i) as biologically it is all important in treatment. The disease really destroys muscle adjustments, and one of the first things to do is to place the muscle at physiological rest in the zero position, in which it is itself relaxed, and both its own action, and that of its opponent prevented. Massage, he urges, should not be given too early, until, for example, the patient can elevate the upper limb when sitting up, and the heel when lying on the back. Persistent gradual re-education of the muscles yields remarkable results. Passive movements may be used and with toys a child may be encouraged to use the muscles of any group which still act. The treatment of residual deformities is a question of orthopædic surgery.

XII. HYDROPHOBIA

(Lyssa; Rabies)

Definition.—An acute disease of warm-blooded animals, dependent upon a virus which is communicated by inoculation to man.

Distribution.—Rabies is very variously distributed. In Russia it is common. In North Germany it is relatively rare, owing to the wise provision that all dogs must be muzzled. In France it is much more common. In England the muzzling order has been followed by a complete disappearance of the disease and there has been no death from hydrophobia since 1903. In the decennium ending with 1890 the deaths averaged 29 annually (Tatham). In the United States the disease occurs more often than is generally supposed.

Etiology.—Dogs are especially liable to the disease. It also occurs in the wolf, fox, skunk, cat, horse and cow. Most animals are susceptible; and it is communicable by inoculation to the rabbit and pig. The disease is propagated chiefly by the dog. The nature of the poison is as yet unknown. It is contained chiefly in the nervous system and is met with in some of the secretions, particularly in the saliva. Bartarelli has shown that the virus reaches the dog's salivary glands by way of the nerves and not through the blood-vessels.

A variable time elapses between the introduction of the virus and the appearance of the symptoms. Horsley states that this depends upon the following factors: "(*a*) Age. The incubation is shorter in children than in adults. For obvious reasons the former are more frequently attacked. (*b*) Part infected. The rapidity of onset of the symptoms is greatly determined by the part of the body which may happen to have been bitten. Wounds about the face and head are especially dangerous; next in order in degrees of mortality come bites on the hands, then injuries on the other parts of the body. This relative order is, no doubt, greatly dependent upon the fact that the face, head, and hands are usually naked, while the other parts are clothed; it would also appear to depend somewhat upon the richness in nerves of the part. (*c*) The extent and severity of the wound. Puncture wounds are the most dangerous; the lacerations are fatal in proportion to the extent of the surface afforded for absorption of the virus. (*d*) The animal conveying the infection. In order of decreasing severity come: first, the wolf; second, the cat; third, the dog; and fourth, other animals." Only a limited number of those bitten by rabid dogs become affected by the disease; according to Horsley, not more than 15 per cent. On the other hand, the death-rate of those persons bitten by wolves is higher, not less than 40 per cent. Babes gives the mortality as from 60 to 80 per cent.

The incubation period in man is extremely variable. The average is from six weeks to two months. In a few cases it has been under two weeks. It may be prolonged to three months. It is stated that the incubation may be prolonged for a year or even two years, but this has not been definitely settled.

Morbid Anatomy.—The important lesions consist in the accumulation of leucocytes around the blood-vessels and the nerve-cells, particularly the motor ganglion cells, of the central nervous system (rabic tubercles of Babes). Especial importance in the rapid diagnosis of rabies is attached by van Gehuchten and Nelis to the accumulation of lymphoid and endothelioid cells around nerve-cells of the sympathetic and cerebro-spinal ganglia. Negri described in the central nervous system irregular bodies varying from 4 to 10 microns in size, widespread, frequently in the cells of the cerebellum, cerebral cortex and pons, and in the spinal cord. They are probably protozoa, and it is stated that they furnish a rapid and trustworthy means of diagnosis. The inoculation experiments show that the virus is not present in the liver, spleen, or kidneys, but is abundant in the spinal cord, brain, and peripheral nerves.

Symptoms.—Three stages of the disease are recognized:

(*a*) Premonitory stage, in which there may be irritation about the bite, pain, or numbness. The patient is depressed and melancholy; and complains of headache and loss of appetite. He is very irritable and sleepless, and has a constant sense of impending danger. There is often greatly increased sensibility. A bright light or a loud voice is distressing. The larynx may be injected and the first symptoms of difficulty in swallowing are experienced.

The voice also becomes husky. There is a slight rise in the temperature and the pulse.

(*b*) STAGE OF EXCITEMENT.—This is characterized by great excitability and restlessness, and an extreme degree of hyperæsthesia. "Any afferent stimulant—i. e., a sound or a draught of air, or the mere association of a verbal suggestion—will cause a violent reflex spasm. In man this symptom constitutes the most distressing feature of the malady. The spasms, which affect particularly the muscles of the larynx and mouth, are exceedingly painful and are accompanied by an intense sense of dyspnœa, even when the glottis is widely opened or tracheotomy has been performed" (Horsley). Any attempt to take water is followed by an intensely painful spasm of the muscles of the larynx and of the elevators of the hyoid bone. It is this which makes the patient dread the very sight of water and gives the name *hydrophobia* to the disease. These spasmodic attacks may be associated with maniacal symptoms. In the intervals the patient is quiet and the mind unclouded. The temperature in this stage is usually elevated and may reach from 100° to 103°. In some instances the disease is afebrile. The patient rarely attempts to injure his attendants, and in the intense spasms may be particularly anxious to avoid hurting any one. There are, however, occasional fits of furious mania, and the patient may, in the contractions of the muscles of the larynx and pharynx, give utterance to odd sounds. This stage lasts from a day and a half to three days and gradually passes into the—

(*c*) PARALYTIC STAGE.—In rodents the preliminary and furious stages are absent, as a rule, and the paralytic stage may be marked from the outset —the so-called dumb rabies. This stage rarely lasts longer than from six to eighteen hours. The patient then becomes quiet; the spasms no longer occur; unconsciousness gradually supervenes; the heart's action becomes more and more enfeebled, and death occurs by syncope.

Diagnosis.—In man the diagnosis offers no special difficulties. It is advisable, in cases attended with any doubts, as soon as possible after the injury has been inflicted, to secure the medulla oblongata of the supposed rabid animal for the purpose of inoculating rabbits. The subdural inoculation of rabbits with a small quantity of the central nervous system of a rabid animal will be followed by the occurrence of the paralytic form of the disease in from fifteen to twenty days.

Treatment.—Prophylaxis is of the greatest importance, and by a systematic muzzling of dogs the disease can be practically eradicated.

In case of a bite from a suspicious animal, bleeding should be encouraged, the wound freely opened and washed with bichloride of mercury solution (1 to 1,000). Thorough cauterization should be done as soon as possible, for which pure carbolic or nitric acid should be used, being applied to every part of the wound. The wound is washed with a saturated solution of bicarbonate of soda and then with alcohol. When once established the disease is hopelessly incurable. No measures have been found of the slightest avail, consequently the treatment must be palliative. The patient should be kept in a darkened room, in charge of not more than two attendants. To allay the spasm, chloroform may be administered and morphia given hypodermically. It is best to use these powerful remedies from the outset, and not to temporize with chloral, bromide of potassium, and other less potent drugs. By the local application of cocaine, the sensitiveness of the throat may be diminished sufficiently to enable the patient to take liquid nourishment. Sometimes he can swallow readily. Nutrient enemata should be administered.

Preventive Inoculation.—Pasteur found that the virus, when propagated through a series of rabbits, increases in its virulence; so that whereas subdural inoculation of the brain of a mad dog takes from fifteen to twenty days to produce the disease, in successive inoculation in a series of rabbits the incubation period is gradually reduced to seven days (*virus fixe*). The spinal cords of these rabbits contain the virus in great intensity, but when they are preserved in dry air this gradually diminishes. If now dogs are inoculated from cords preserved for from twelve to fifteen days, and then from cords preserved for a shorter period, i. e., with a progressively stronger virus, they gradually acquire immunity against the disease. A dog treated in this way will resist inoculation with the *virus fixe*, which otherwise would inevitably have proved fatal. Relying upon these experiments, Pasteur began inoculations in the human subject, using, on successive days, material from cords in which the virus was of varying degrees of intensity.

In 1910, 410 patients were treated at the Pasteur Institute of Paris without a death; in 1909, 467 cases and one death, in 1908, 524 cases and one death. There has been a progressive decline in the number of cases and in the mortality.

Pseudo-hydrophobia (*Lyssophobia*).—This is a very interesting affection, which may closely resemble hydrophobia, but is really nothing more than a neurotic or hysterical manifestation. A nervous person bitten by a dog, either rabid or supposed to be rabid, has within a few months, or even later, symptoms somewhat resembling the true disease. He is irritable and depressed. He constantly declares his condition to be serious and that he will inevitably become mad. He may have paroxysms in which he says he is unable to drink, grasps at his throat, and becomes emotional. The temperature is not elevated and the disease does not progress. It lasts much longer than the true rabies, and is amenable to treatment. It is not improbable that a majority of the cases of alleged recovery in this disease have been of this hysterical form. Certain cases of acute bulbar paralysis may resemble hydrophobia, and, as already mentioned, there is a form of tetanus with hydrophobic symptoms.

XIII. RHEUMATIC FEVER

Definition.—An acute infection, dependent upon an unknown infective agent, and characterized by multiple arthritis and a marked tendency to inflammation of the endocardium of the valves of the heart.

Etiology.—Distribution and Prevalence.—It prevails in temperate and humid climates. Church has collected interesting statistics on this point. Oddly enough, the two countries with the highest admission in the British army per thousand of strength—Egypt, 7.02, and Canada, 6.26—have climates the most diverse. In the Registrar General's report for England and Wales for 1909 there were 1,970 deaths from the disease, but rheumatic fever has a long arm and no small proportion of the 50,918 deaths from diseases of the heart is to be laid at its door. The disease prevails more in the northern latitudes. In the Montreal General Hospital there were, for the twelve years ending 1903, 2 deaths in 482 cases among 12,044 admissions; at the Royal Victoria Hospital, Montreal, for ten years ending 1903, 3 deaths in 285 cases among 9,286 admissions (John McCrae). At the Johns Hopkins Hospital for the fifteen years ending 1904 there were 360 admissions (330 patients) and 9 deaths (T. McCrae)). The general impression is that the disease prevails more in the British Isles than elsewhere; but, as Church remarks, the returns are very imperfect (this holds good everywhere). In Norway, where cases of rheumatic fever are notified, there were, for the four years 1888-'92, 13,654 cases, with 250 deaths.

Season.—In London the cases reach the maximum in the months of September and October. In the Montreal General Hospital Bell's statistics of 456 cases show that the largest number was admitted in February, March, and April. And the same is true in Baltimore; 55 per cent. of our cases were admitted in the first four months of the year (McCrae). The disease prevails most in the dry years or a succession of such, and is specially prevalent when the subsoil water is abnormally low and the temperature of the earth high (Newsholme).

Age.—Young adults are most frequently affected, but the disease is by no means uncommon in children. In England the incidence in children is very high. In 2,556 examined by Langmead, 133 were definitely rheumatic and in all but 18 the heart was involved. In 43 per cent. of these cases there was some abnormality of the tonsils or pharyngeal mucosa. Sucklings are rarely attacked. Milton Miller has analyzed 19 undoubted cases. The cases have to be distinguished from a totally different affection, the pyogenic arthritis of infants. Of 456 cases admitted to the Montreal General Hospital there were, under fifteen years, 4.38 per cent.; from fifteen to twenty-five years, 48.68 per cent.; from twenty-five to thirty-five years, 25.87 per cent.; from thirty-five to forty-five years, 13.6 per cent.; above forty-five years, 7.4 per cent. Of our 360 admissions, 110 were in the third decade and 65 per cent. below the thirtieth year of age (McCrae). Ten per cent. of the cases had the first attack in the first decade. Of the 655 cases analyzed by Whipham for the Collective Investigation Committee of the British Medical Association, only 32 cases occurred under the tenth year and 80 per cent. between the twentieth and fortieth years. These figures do not give the ratio of cases in children, in whom the milder types of arthritis are very common.

Sex.—If all ages are taken, males are affected oftener than females. Of our patients, 239 were males, 91 females. In the Collective Investigation Report there were 375 males and 279 females. Up to the age of twenty, however, females predominate. Between the ages of ten and fifteen girls are more prone to the disease.

Heredity.—It is a deeply grounded belief with the public and the profession that rheumatism is a family disease, but Church thinks the evidence is still imperfect. In 25 per cent. of our cases there was a history of the disease in the family. The not rare occurrence in several members of the same family is used by those who believe in the infectious origin as an argument in favor of its being a house disease.

Chill.—Exposure to cold, a wetting, or a sudden change of temperature are among the factors in determining the onset of an attack, but they were present in only 12 per cent. of our cases.

Not only does an attack not confer IMMUNITY, but, as in pneumonia, predisposes the subject to the disease.

Rheumatic Fever as an Acute Infectious Disease.—Rheumatic fever, as Newsholme has shown, has epidemic prevalence with irregular periodicity, recurring at intervals of three, four, or six years, and varying much in intensity. A severe epidemic is usually followed by two or three years of slight prevalence.

The disease has many features suggestive of septic infection. As Church points out, the curves of the mortality statistics approximate nearly to those of pyæmia, puerperal fever, and erysipelas. In the character of the fever, the mode of involvement of the joints, the tendency to relapse, the sweats, the anæmia, the leucocytosis, and, above all, in the great liability to endocarditis, and to involvement of the serous membranes. the disease resembles pyæmia very closely.

The nature of the specific germ is still under discussion. Mantle in 1887 obtained a micrococcus from the fluid of the joints and from the blood; since which time many observers have described forms of staphylococci, streptococci and various organisms. The work of Poynton and Payne, Walker, Beattie and others shows that from the joint fluid, the throat and the endocardial vegetations, and sometimes from the blood, organisms may be obtained which, inoculated into animals, cause a condition very similar to that of acute rheumatic fever, with arthritis, endocarditis, and even the fibrous nodules. The difficulty is that the organisms described do not coincide, and Cole in a series of cases in my clinic at the Johns Hopkins Hospital with the strains of streptococci from various sources was able to produce experimentally endocarditis and arthritis. But Beattie claims that the lesions produced by his *Micrococcus rheumaticus* are different. A point of interest is the fact that with his germ Ainley Walker obtained formic acid in the cultures.

The tonsils are culture centres for many septic organisms, particularly of the streptococcus type. The association of rheumatic fever and rheumatic affections generally with infected tonsils is a prevailing view, but it is an old story insisted on by Lasague and other French writers years ago. A not inconsiderable number of cases of rheumatic fever begin with tonsillitis. With organisms isolated from the tonsils experimental arthritis and endocarditis have been caused. The removal of the tonsils has been followed by a complete recovery of sub-acute and chronic forms of arthritis. This is as far as the evidence goes.

There is considerable evidence against the view that it is simply a mild pyogenic infection. Salicylates have no effect on the ordinary streptococcus infections, and the clinical course in the streptococcus arthritis is very different; moreover, rheumatic joints never suppurate. The isolation of streptococci may simply indicate the presence of secondary invaders such as occur in scarlet fever and small-pox.

Morbid Anatomy.—There are no characteristic changes. The affected joints show hyperæmia and swelling of the synovial membranes and of the ligamentous tissues. The fluid in the joint is turbid, albuminous in character, and contains leucocytes and a few fibrin flakes. Rheumatic fever rarely proves fatal, except when there are serious complications, such as pericarditis, endocarditis, myocarditis, pleurisy, or pneumonia. The conditions found show nothing to distinguish them from other forms of inflammation. In death from hyperpyrexia no special changes are found. The blood usually contains an excessive amount of fibrin.

Symptoms.—As a rule, the disease sets in abruptly, but it may be preceded by irregular pains in the joints, slight *malaise,* sore throat, and particularly by tonsillitis. A definite rigor is uncommon; more often there is slight chilliness. The fever rises quickly, and with it one or more of the joints become painful. Within twenty-four hours from the onset the disease is fully manifest. The temperature range is from 102° to 104°. The pulse is frequent, soft, and usually above 100. The tongue is moist, and rapidly becomes covered with a white fur. There are the ordinary symptoms associated with an acute fever, such as loss of appetite, thirst, constipation, and a scanty, highly acid, highly colored urine. In a majority of the cases there are profuse, very acid sweats, of a peculiar sour odor. Sudaminal and miliary vesicles are abundant, the latter usually surrounded by a minute ring of hyperæmia. The mind is clear, except in the cases with hyperpyrexia. The affected joints are painful to move, soon become swollen and hot, and present a reddish flush. The order of frequency of involvement of the joints in our series was knee, ankle, shoulder, wrist, elbow, hip, hand, foot. The joints are not attacked together, but successively. For example, if the knee is first affected, the redness may disappear from it as the wrists become painful and hot. The disease is seldom limited to a single articulation. The amount of swelling is variable. Extensive effusion into a joint is rare, and much of the enlargement is due to the infiltration of the periarticular tissues with serum. The swelling may be limited to the joint proper, but in the wrists and ankles it sometimes involves the sheaths of the tendons and produces great enlargement of the hands and feet. Corresponding joints are often affected. In attacks of great severity every one of the larger joints may be involved. The vertebral, sterno-clavicular, and phalangeal articulations are less often inflamed than in gonorrhœal arthritis. Perhaps no disease is more painful; the inability to change the posture without agonizing pain, the drenching sweats, the prostration and utter helplessness, combine to make it one of the most distressing of febrile affections. A special feature is the tendency of the inflammation to subside in one joint while increasing with great intensity in another.

The temperature range in an ordinary attack is between 102° and 104° F. In only 18 of our cases did the temperature rise above 104° F. In 100 it reached 103° F. or over. It is peculiarly irregular, with marked remissions and exacerbations, and defervescence is usually gradual. The profuse sweats materially influence the temperature curve. If a two-hourly chart is made and observations upon the sweats are noted, the remissions will usually be found coincident with them. The perspiration is sour-smelling and acid at first; but, when persistent, becomes neutral or even alkaline.

The blood is profoundly altered and there is no acute febrile disease in which an anæmia occurs with greater rapidity. The average leucocyte count in our cases was about 12,000 per c. mm.

With the high fever a murmur may often be heard at the apex region. Endocarditis is also a common cause of an apex *bruit*. The heart should be carefully examined at the first visit and subsequently each day.

The urine is, as a rule, reduced in amount, of high density and high color. It is very acid, and, on cooling, deposits urates. The chlorides may be greatly diminished or even absent. Formic acid is present (Walker). Febrile albuminuria is not uncommon.

The so-called *subacute rheumatism* represents a milder form of the disease, in which all the symptoms are less pronounced. The fever rarely rises above 101°; fewer joints are involved; and the arthritis is less intense. The cases may drag on for weeks or months. It should not be forgotten that this mild or subacute form may be associated with endocarditis or pericarditis.

The influence of age on the manifestations of the disease is marked. While the usual description applies to the disease as seen in adults, in young children there may not be any pronounced arthritis, and the discovery of endocarditis often suggests the diagnosis. Endocarditis is as much a feature in children as arthritis in adults.

Complications.—These are important and serious.

(*a*) HYPERPYREXIA.—The temperature may rise rapidly a few days after the onset, and be associated with delirium; but not necessarily, for the temperature may rise to 108° or, as in one of Da Costa's cases, 110°, without cerebral symptoms. Hyperpyrexia is most common in first attacks, 57 of 107 cases (Church). It is most apt to occur during the second week. Delirium may precede or follow its onset. As a rule, with the high fever, the pulse is feeble and frequent, the prostration is extreme, and finally stupor supervenes. In our series there was no instance of hyperpyrexia, which seems rare in the United States.

(*b*) CARDIAC AFFECTIONS.—(1) *Endocarditis,* the most frequent and serious complication, occurs in a considerable percentage of all cases. Of 889 cases, 494 had signs of old or recent endocarditis (Church). The liability to endocarditis diminishes as age advances. The incidence of organic disease in our cases was more than double in patients who had their first attack before the age of twenty years, compared with those with the first attack after twenty years of age. It increases directly with the number of attacks. Of 116 cases, in the first attack 58.1 per cent. had endocarditis, 63 per cent. in the second attack, and 71 per cent. in the third attack (Stephen Mackenzie). Thirty-five per cent. of our cases showed organic valve lesions, in 96 per cent. the mitral was involved, in 27 per cent. the aortic, and in 23 per cent. the lesions were combined. The mitral segments are most frequently involved and the affection is usually of the simple, verrucose variety. Ulcerative endocarditis is very rare. Of 209 cases of this disease which I analyzed, in only 24 did the symptoms of a severe endocarditis arise during the progress of acute or subacute rheumatism. The valvulitis in itself is rarely dangerous, producing few symptoms, and is often overlooked. Unhappily, though the valve at the time may not be seriously damaged, the inflammation starts changes which lead to sclerosis and retraction of the segments, and so to chronic valvular disease. Venous thrombosis is an occasional complication.

(2) *Pericarditis* may occur independently of or together with endocarditis. It may be simple fibrinous, sero-fibrinous, or in children purulent.

Clinically we meet it more frequently in connection with this disease than in any other acute affection. It was present in 20 cases of our series—6 per cent.—in only four of which did effusion occur. The physical signs are very characteristic. The condition will be fully described under its appropriate section. A peculiar form of delirium may accompany rheumatic pericarditis.

(3) *Myocarditis* occurs frequently and especially in connection with endo-pericardial changes. As Sturges insisted, the term *carditis* is applicable to many cases. The anatomical condition is a granular or fatty degeneration of the heart-muscle, which leads to weakening of the walls and to dilatation. S. West has reported instances of acute dilatation of the heart in rheumatic fever, in one of which marked fatty changes were found in the heart-fibres.

(*c*) Pulmonary Affections.—Pneumonia and pleurisy occurred in 9.94 per cent. of 3,433 cases (Stephen Mackenzie). They frequently accompany the cases of endo-pericarditis. According to Howard's analysis of a large number of cases, there were pulmonary complications in only 10.5 per cent. of cases of rheumatic endocarditis; in 58 per cent. of cases of pericarditis; and in 71 per cent. of cases of endo-pericarditis. Congestion of the lung is occasionally found, and in several cases has proved rapidly fatal.

(*d*) Nervous Complications.—These are due, in part, to the hyper-pyrexia and in part to the special action of the toxic agent of the disease. They may be grouped as follows: (*i*) *Cerebral rheumatism,* as it is called, which is characterized by (α) *Delirium,* which is associated with the hyper-pyrexia or the toxæmia, may be active and noisy in character; more rarely it is a low, muttering delirium, passing into stupor and coma. It may be excited by the salicylate of soda, either shortly after its administration, or more commonly a few days later. It was present in only five of our 360 cases, and in four of these we thought the salicylates at fault. A peculiar delirium occurs in connection with rheumatic pericarditis. (β) Coma, which is more serious, may occur without preliminary delirium or convulsions, and may prove rapidly fatal. Certain of these cases are associated with hyperpyrexia; but Southey has reported the case of a girl who, without previous delirium or high fever, became comatose, and died in less than an hour. A certain number of such cases, as those reported by Da Costa, have been associated with marked renal changes and were evidently uræmic. The coma may supervene during the attack, or after convalescence has set in. (γ) *Convulsions* are less common, though they may precede the coma. Of 127 observations cited by Besnier, there were 37 of delirium, only 7 of convulsions, 17 of coma and convulsions, 54 of delirium, coma, and convulsions, and 3 of other varieties (Howard). "Cerebral rheumatism" is a very serious complication; among 107 cases collected by the Clinical Society of London there were 57 deaths. (*ii*) *Chorea.* The relations of this disease and rheumatism will be subsequently discussed. It is sufficient here to say that in only 88 out of 554 cases which I have analyzed from the Infirmary for Diseases of the Nervous System, Philadelphia, were chorea and rheumatism associated. It is most apt to develop in the slighter attacks in childhood. (*iii*) *Meningitis* is extremely rare, though undoubtedly it does occur. It must not be forgotten that in ulcerative endocarditis, which is occasionally associated with rheumatic fever, meningitis is frequent. (*iv*) *Polyneuritis* has been described. I saw a remarkable case which followed hyperpyrexia. Free venesection saved the patient's life. After many months the patient recovered, but with ataxia.

(*e*) Cutaneous Affections.—Sweat-vesicles have already been mentioned as extremely common. A red miliary rash may also develop. Scarlatiniform eruptions are occasionally seen. Purpura, with or without urticaria, may occur, and various forms of erythema. It is doubtful whether the cases of extensive purpura with urticaria and arthritis—peliosis rheumatica—belong truly to rheumatic fever.

(*f*) Rheumatic Nodules.—These curious structures, described originally by Meynet, occur in the form of small subcutaneous nodules attached to the tendons and fasciæ. Barlow and Warner, in England, and T. B. Futcher, in the United States, have paid special attention to their varieties and importance. They vary in size from a small shot to a large pea, and are most numerous on the fingers, hands, and wrists. They also occur about the elbows, knees, the spines of the vertebræ, and the scapulæ. They are not often tender. They are more common after the decline of the fever and in the children with mitral valve disease. In only 5 of our patients were they present during the acute attack. The nodules may grow with great rapidity and usually last for weeks or months. They are more common in children than in adults, and in the former their presence may be regarded as a positive indication of rheumatism. They have been noted particularly in association with chronic rheumatic endocarditis. Subcutaneous nodules occur also in migraine, gout, and arthritis deformans. Histologically they are made up of round and spindle-shaped cells. In addition to these firm, hard nodules, there occur in rheumatism and in chronic vegetative endocarditis remarkable bodies, which have been called by Féréol "nodosités cutanées éphémères."

Course.—The *course* of rheumatic fever is extremely variable. It is, as Austin Flint first showed, a self-limited disease, and it is not probable that medicines have any special influence upon its *duration* or *course.* Gull and Sutton, who likewise studied a series of 62 cases without special treatment, arrived at the same conclusion.

Prognosis.—Rheumatic fever is the most serious of all diseases with a low death-rate. The mortality is rarely above 2 or 3 per cent. Only 9 of our 330 patients died, 2.7 per cent., all with endocarditis and 6 with pericarditis.

Sudden death in rheumatic fever is due most frequently to myocarditis. Herringham has reported a case in which on the fourteenth day there was fatty degeneration and acute inflammation of the myocardium. In a few rare cases it results from embolism. Alarming symptoms of depression sometimes follow excessive doses of the salicylate of soda.

Diagnosis.—Practically, the recognition of rheumatic fever is usually easy; but there are several affections which, in some particulars, closely resemble it.

(*a*) Multiple Secondary Arthritis.—Under this term may be embraced the various forms of arthritis which come on or follow in the course of gonorrhœa, tonsillitis, scarlet fever, dysentery, and cerebro-spinal meningitis.

(*b*) Septic Arthritis, which occurs in the course of pyæmia from any cause, and particularly in puerperal fever. No hard and fast line can be drawn between these and the cases in the first group: but the inflammation rapidly passes on to suppuration and there is more or less destruction of the joints. The conditions under which the arthritis occurs give a clew at once to the nature of the case. Under this section may also be mentioned:

(1) *Acute necrosis* or *acute osteo-myelitis,* occurring in the lower end of the femur, or in the tibia, and which may be mistaken for rheumatic fever Sometimes, too, it is multiple. The greater intensity of the local symptoms, the involvement of the epiphyses rather than the joints, and the more serious constitutional disturbances are points to be considered. The condition is unfortunately often mistaken for acute arthritis, and, as the treatment is essentially surgical, the error may cost the life of the patient.

(2) *The acute arthritis of infants* is usually confined to one joint (the hip or knee), the effusion in which rapidly becomes purulent. The affection is most common in sucklings and undoubtedly pyæmic in character. It may also occur with the gonorrhœal ophthalmia or vaginitis of the new-born, as pointed out by Clement Lucas.

(*c*) GOUT.—While the localization in a single, usually a small, joint, the age, the history, and the mode of onset are features which enable us to recognize acute gout, there are everywhere many cases of acute arthritis, called rheumatic fever, which are in reality gout. The involvement of several of the larger joints is not so infrequent in gout, and unless tophi are present, or unless a very accurate analysis of the urine is made, the diagnosis may be difficult.

(*d*) ACUTE ARTHRITIS DEFORMANS.—In several cases I have mistaken this form for rheumatic fever. It may come on with fever and multiple arthritis, and for weeks there may be no suspicion of the true nature of the disease. Gradually the fever subsides, but the periarticular thickening persists. As a rule, however, in the acute febrile cases the involvement of the smaller joints, the persistence and the early changes in the articulations suggest arthritis deformans.

In children the diagnosis may be very difficult, as arthritis may be slight or entirely absent. The possibility of rheumatic fever should be considered in all febrile attacks in children for which no definite cause can be found. Special care should be given to the examination of the heart.

Treatment.—The main object should be to bring the patient through the attack with an undamaged heart or with as little injury as possible. The first essential is complete rest, which should be begun at once and insisted upon for as long as is necessary. This is especially important for children. The bed should have a smooth, soft, yet elastic, mattress. The patient should wear a flannel nightgown, which may be opened all the way down the front and slit along the outer margin of the sleeves. Three or four of these should be made, so as to facilitate the frequent changes required after the sweats. He may wear also a light flannel cape about the shoulders. He should sleep in blankets, not in sheets, so as to reduce the liability to catch cold and obviate the unpleasant clamminess consequent upon heavy sweating. Chambers insisted that the liability to endocarditis and pericarditis was much reduced when the patients were in blankets.

Milk is the most suitable diet and may be diluted with alkaline mineral waters. Lemonade and oatmeal or barley water should be freely given. The thirst is usually great and may be fully satisfied. There is no objection to broths and soups if the milk is not well borne. As convalescence is established a fuller diet may be allowed, but meat should be used sparingly.

Local treatment is usually necessary. It often suffices to wrap the affected joints in cotton. If the pain is severe, hot cloths may be applied, saturated with Fuller's lotion (carbonate of soda, 6 drachms; laudanum, 1 oz.; glycerine, 2 oz.; and water, 9 oz.) or the lead and opium lotion. Oil of wintergreen is useful, the joint being gently rubbed with it or small amounts sprinkled over flannel, which is then applied. Chloroform liniment is also a good application. Fixation of the joints is of great service in allaying the pain. Splints, padded and bandaged with moderate firmness, will often be found to give comfort. Friction is rarely well borne in an acutely inflamed joint. Cold compresses are much used in Germany. The application of blisters above and below the joint often relieves the pain. This method, which was used so much a few years ago, is not to be compared with the light application of the Paquelin cautery. If there is much effusion, aspiration of the joint is useful.

The drug treatment is still far from satisfactory, though the introduction of the salicyl compounds has been a great boon.

Treatment with the Salicyl Compounds.—Salicin, introduced in 1876 by Maclagan, may be used in doses of 20 grains every hour or two until the pain is relieved. It has the advantage of being less depressing than the salicylate of soda. It is also perhaps the best drug to use for children. Salicylic acid, 15 grains (1 gm.), may be given every two hours in acute cases until the pain is relieved. It is best given in capsules. Salicylate of soda, 15 grain doses every three hours, is perhaps the best for general use in adults. After the pain has been relieved, the drug should be given every four or five hours until the temperature begins to fall. The potassium bicarbonate may be given with it. Oil of wintergreen, 20 minims every two hours in milk, or aspirin (gr. xv, 1 gm.), may be used if the salicylate of soda disagrees. There are many other salicyl compounds, but the best results are obtained from the use of one or the other of the above-named preparations. There can be no question as to their efficacy in relieving the pain. Some observers consider that they also protect the heart, shorten the course, and render relapse less likely.

The Alkaline Treatment.—The urine should be rendered alkaline as soon as possible. Potassium acetate and citrate in doses of 15 grains (1 gm.) each are given every three hours until the urine is alkaline and then often enough to keep it so. Potassium bicarbonate may be given in half-drachm doses every three hours with the salicylic acid or salicin. Fuller's plan was to give a drachm and a half of sodium bicarbonate with half a drachm of potassium acetate in three ounces of water, rendered effervescent at the time of administration by half a drachm of citric acid or an ounce of lemon-juice.

A widespread popular belief attributes marvelous efficacy to bee-stings in all sorts of rheumatism, and a formic-acid treatment has been introduced. A 2½ per cent. solution is injected in the neighborhood of the painful joints. Ainley Walker has collected (B. M. J., October 10, 1908) an interesting literature on the subject.

To allay the pain opium may be given in the form of Dover's powder, or morphia hypodermically. Antipyrin, antifebrin, and phenacetin are useful sometimes for the purpose. During convalescence iron is indicated in full doses, and quinine is a useful tonic. Of the complications, hyperpyrexia should be treated by the cold bath or the cold pack. The treatment of endocarditis and pericarditis and the pulmonary complications will be considered under their respective sections. In all the cardiac complications the importance of prolonged rest must be remembered.

To prevent and arrest endocarditis Caton urges the use of a series of small blisters along the course of the third, fourth, fifth, and sixth intercostal nerves of the left side, applied one at a time and repeated at different points. Potassium or sodium iodide is given in addition to the salicylates. The patients are kept in bed for about six weeks.

TONSILS.—With disease of these and the possibility that they are the portals of entry for the infective agent, the question arises as to their removal. In patients with diseased tonsils in whom rheumatic fever has occurred removal is advisable and should always be complete. In patients with endocarditis and fever this may be done apparently without risk. It is comparable to the removal of any local focus of infection which is causing general symptoms.

XIV. ACUTE TONSILLITIS

Definition.—An acute infection, sporadic or epidemic, involving the structures of the tonsillar ring, usually due to organisms of the streptococcus class.

Etiology.—Acute tonsillitis occurs in sporadic and epidemic forms. The SPORADIC variety, one of the most common of diseases, is met with in young persons particularly at the school age. Infants are rarely attacked. Chronic enlargement of the lymphatic structures of the throat is an important predisposing cause. Exposure to cold and wet may bring on an attack. It is directly communicated from one child to another. A not infrequent precursor of rheumatic fever, Cheadle very properly described it as one link in the rheumatic chain. It may be directly followed by endocarditis, erythema nodosum, chorea, and acute nephritis. In Great Britain it prevails in the autumn months, in the United States in the spring. An old notion held that there was a close relation between the tonsils and the testes and ovaries, and F. J. Shepherd has called attention to the frequency of acute tonsillitis in newly married persons.

EPIDEMIC TONSILLITIS is not infrequent, the cases increasing in the community to epidemic proportions. As a rule it is impossible to trace it to any special cause. There are remarkable localized outbreaks, sometimes in institutions, which have been traced to milk infection. The recent one in Boston (1911) was exceptionally severe, involving more than 1,000 persons, and the connection with the use of the milk from one dairy seems to have been clearly traced. More females than males were attacked, and a large proportion of the cases were adults.

The bacteriology of both forms has been carefully studied. The tonsils, swarming with saprophytic and pathogenic germs, are the main gates through which the invaders try to storm the town. Normally the protecting forces suffice to keep them at bay, but now and again a fiercer battle than usual rages, barricades have to be set up in the shape of exudates and necroses—and a local tonsillitis is the outward and visible sign of the struggle. Too often the enemy gains entrance, and streptococci, staphylococci, pneumococci, etc., pass to distant parts and excite arthritis, endocarditis, and serous membrane inflammations. In the recent Boston epidemic the streptococcus was the common germ, and the same holds good in the sporadic cases.

Morbid Anatomy.—The lacunæ of the tonsils become filled with exudation products, which form cheesy-looking masses, projecting from the orifices of the crypts. Not infrequently the exudations from contiguous lacunæ coalesce. The intervening mucosa is usually swollen, deep red in color, and may present herpetic vesicles, or, in some instances, even membranous exudation, in which case it may be difficult to distinguish the condition from diphtheria. The creamy contents of the crypt are made up of micrococci and epithelial débris.

Symptoms.—Chilly feelings, or even a definite chill, and aching pains in the back and limbs may precede the onset. The fever rises rapidly and in the case of a young child may reach 105° F. on the evening of the first day. The patient complains of soreness of the throat and difficuty in swallowing. On examination the tonsils are seen to be swollen and the crypts present the characteristic creamy exudate. The tongue is furred, the breath is heavy and foul, and the urine is highly colored and loaded with urates. In children the respirations are usually very hurried and the pulse is greatly increased in rapidity. Swallowing is painful and the voice often becomes nasal. Slight swelling of the cervical glands is present.

In epidemic cases the fever may be very high, the secondary enlargement of the glands considerable, and even the deeper tissues may be involved. The complications are very serious: endocarditis, pericarditis, pneumococcic peritonitis, and pneumonia. In the Boston epidemic the clinical sequence was not unlike that seen in rheumatic fever—sore throat, adenitis, multiple arthritis, endocarditis, and pneumonia. Febrile albuminuria is common and in a few cases acute nephritis follows. A diffuse erythema may simulate scarlet fever. Acute otitis media is a frequent complication in children. Relapses are not uncommon and the tonsils may remain enlarged.

In the sporadic and mild epidemic form it is rare to see a fatal case, but in severe outbreaks the mortality from complications may be three or four per cent. There were about 50 deaths in the Boston epidemic.

Occasionally paralyses follow the streptococcus tonsillitis which are identical with those of diphtheria.

Diagnosis.—It may be difficult to distinguish tonsillitis from diphtheria. It would seem, indeed, as if there were intermediate forms between the milder lacunar and the severer pseudo-membranous tonsillitis. In the follicular form, the individual yellowish-gray masses, separated by the reddish tonsillar tissue, are very characteristic; whereas in diphtheria the membrane is ashy-gray and uniform, not patchy. A point of the greatest importance in diphtheria is that the membrane is not limited to the tonsils, but creeps up the pillars of the fauces and appears on the uvula. The diphtheritic membrane, when removed, leaves a bleeding, eroded surface; whereas the exudation of lacunar tonsillitis is easily separated, and there is no erosion beneath it. In all doubtful cases cultures should be made to determine the presence or absence of Löffler's bacillus.

Treatment.—In the follicular form aconite may be given in full doses and it acts very beneficially in children. The salicylates, given freely at the outset, are regarded by some as specific, but I have seen no evidence of such prompt and decisive action. At night a full dose of Dover's powder may be given. The use of guaiacum, in the form of 2-grain lozenges, is warmly recommended. Iron and quinine should be reserved until the fever has subsided. An ice-bag or cold compresses may be applied to the neck. Locally the tonsils may be treated with the dry sodium bicarbonate. The moistened finger-tip is dipped into the soda, which is then rubbed gently on the gland, and this is repeated every hour. Astringent preparations, such as iron and glycerine, alum, zinc, and nitrate of silver, may be tried. To cleanse and disinfect the throat, solutions of borax or thymol in glycerine and water may be used. In severe forms vaccines may be tried, prepared from the throat cultures, or, failing these, the ordinary anti-streptococcic serum.

XV. ACUTE CATARRHAL FEVER

(*Acute Coryza*)

Definition.—An acute infection of the mucous membrane of the upper air passages associated with the presence of the *Micrococcus catarrhalis* alone, or with other organisms.

Etiology.—The micrococcus described by R. Pfeiffer is a diplococcus with close resemblance to the meningococcus and the pneumococcus. It is a normal habitant of the throat and bronchial secretions of many persons. In acute inflammatory conditions of the upper air passages it is found, sometimes in almost pure culture, in the sputum. It is readily cultivated.

Prevailing most extensively in the changeable weather of the spring and early winter, coryza may occur in epidemic form, many cases arising in a community within a few weeks, outbreaks which are very like though less intense than the epidemic influenza. More often it is a local outbreak among the members of a house or of a school.

Symptoms.—The patient feels indisposed, perhaps chilly, has slight headache, and sneezes frequently. In severe cases there are pains in the back and limbs. There is usually slight fever, the temperature rising to 101° F. The pulse is quick, the skin is dry, and there are all the features of a feverish attack. At first the mucous membrane of the nose is swollen, "stuffed up," and the patient has to breathe through the mouth. A thin, clear, irritating secretion flows, and makes the edges of the nostrils sore. The mucous membrane of the tear-ducts is swollen, so that the eyes weep and the conjunctivæ are injected. The sense of smell and, in part, the sense of taste are lost. With the nasal catarrh there is slight soreness of the throat and stiffness of the neck; the pharynx looks red and swollen, and sometimes the act of swallowing is painful. The larynx also may be involved and the voice becomes husky or is even lost. If the inflammation extends to the Eustachian tubes the hearing may be impaired. In more severe cases there are bronchial irritation and cough. Occasionally there is an outbreak of labial or nasal herpes. Usually within thirty-six hours the nasal secretion becomes turbid and more profuse, the swelling of the mucosa subsides, the patient gradually becomes able to breathe through the nostrils, and within four or five days the symptoms disappear, with the exception of the increased discharge from the nose and upper pharynx. There are rarely any bad effects from a simple coryza. When the attacks are frequently repeated the disease may become chronic.

Diagnosis.—The diagnosis is always easy, but caution must be exercised lest the initial catarrh of measles or severe influenza should be mistaken for the simple coryza.

Treatment.—Many attacks are so mild that the patients are able to be about and attend to their work. If there are fever and constitutional disturbance, the patient should be kept in bed and should take a simple fever mixture, and at night a drink of hot lemonade and a full dose of Dover's powder. Many persons find great benefit from the Turkish bath. For the distressing sense of tightness and pain over the frontal sinuses, cocaine is very useful and sometimes gives immediate relief. The 4-per-cent. solution may be injected into the nostrils or cotton wool soaked in it may be inserted into them. Later the snuff recommended by Ferrier is advantageous, composed of morphia (gr. ij), bismuth (ʒ iv), acacia powder (ʒ ij). This may occasionally be blown or snuffed into the nostrils. The fluid extract of hamamelis, "snuffed" from the hand every two or three hours, is much better.

A vaccine treatment has been introduced and may be tried in persons subject to recurring colds.

XVI. FEBRICULA—EPHEMERAL FEVER

Definition.—Fever of slight duration, probably depending upon a variety of causes, some autogenous, others extrinsic and bacterial.

A febrile paroxysm lasting for twenty-four hours and disappearing completely is spoken of as ephemeral fever. If it persists for three, four, or more days without local affection it is referred to as febricula.

The cases may be divided into several groups:

(*a*) Those which represent mild or abortive types of the infectious diseases. It is not very unusual, during an epidemic of typhoid, scarlet fever, or measles, to see patients with some of the prodromal symptoms and slight fever, which persist for two or three days without any distinctive features. Possibly, as Kahler suggests, some of the cases of transient fever are due to the rheumatic poison.

(*b*) In a larger and perhaps more important group of cases the symptoms develop with dyspepsia. In children indigestion and gastro-intestinal catarrh are often accompanied by fever. Possibly some instances of longer duration may be due to the absorption of certain toxic substances. Slight fever has been known to follow the eating of decomposing substances or the drinking of stale beer; but the gastric juice has remarkable antiseptic properties, and the frequency with which persons take from choice articles which are "high" shows that poisoning is not likely to occur unless there is existing gastro-intestinal disturbance.

(*c*) Cases which follow exposure to foul odors or sewer gas. That a febrile paroxysm may follow a prolonged exposure to noxious odors has long been recognized. The cases which have been described under this heading are of two kinds: an acute, severe form with nausea, vomiting, colic, and fever, followed perhaps by a condition of collapse or coma; secondly, a form of low fever with or without chills. A good deal of doubt still exists in the minds of the profession about these cases of so-called sewer-gas poisoning. It is a notorious fact that workers in sewers are remarkably free from disease, and in many of the cases which have been reported the illness may have been only a coincidence. There are instances in which persons have been taken ill with vomiting and slight fever after exposure to the odor of a very offensive post mortem. Whether true or not, the idea is firmly implanted in the minds of the laity that very powerful odors from decomposing matters may produce sickness.

(*d*) Many cases doubtless depend upon slight unrecognized lesions, such as tonsillitis or occasionally an abortive or larval pneumonia. Children are much more frequently affected than adults.

The *symptoms* set in, as a rule, abruptly, though in some instances there may have been preliminary *malaise* and indisposition. Headache, loss of appetite, and furred tongue are present. The urine is scanty and high-colored, the fever ranges from 101° to 103°, sometimes in children it rises higher. The cheeks may be flushed and the patient has the outward manifestations of fever. In children there may be bronchial catarrh with slight cough. Herpes on the lips is a common symptom. Occasionally in children the cerebral symptoms are marked at the outset, and there may be irritation, restlessness, and nocturnal delirium. The fever terminates abruptly by crisis from the second to the fourth day; in some instances it may continue for a week.

The *diagnosis* generally rests upon the absence of local manifestations, particularly the characteristic skin rashes of the eruptive fevers, and, most important of all, the rapid disappearance of the pyrexia. The cases most readily recognized are those with acute gastro-intestinal disturbance.

The *treatment* is that of mild pyrexia—rest in bed, a laxative, and a fever mixture containing nitrate of potassium and sweet spirits of nitre.

XVII. INFECTIOUS JAUNDICE

(*Epidemic Catarrhal Jaundice; Weil's Disease*)

Local and widespread outbreaks of jaundice have been known for years. Three or four cases may occur in one house, or many persons in an institution are attacked, or the disease becomes widespread in a community. In Great Britain this epidemic form is rare. In the United States many outbreaks have occurred. It prevailed extensively in North Carolina in 1899-1900, and a fatal case of that epidemic came under my observation. In Syria, in Greece, in Egypt (Sandwith), in India (S. Anderson), and in South Africa during the Boer war (H. B. Matheas) epidemics have been described. It has prevailed most frequently in the summer months. The symptoms are at first gastric, then fever follows (with the usual concomitants) and jaundice, which may be slight or very intense, and as a rule albuminuria. The liver and spleen enlarge, and in severe forms there are nervous symptoms and hæmorrhages. There is often a secondary fever. The attack lasts from ten days to three weeks. The course is usually favorable; fatal cases are rare in the United States and in India and South Africa, but in the Greek Hospital at Alexandria the death-rate was 32 among 300 cases (Sandwith).

In 1886 Weil described a disease characterized by the features just mentioned, but the cases occurred in groups, and a very large proportion in butchers. It is probable there are several types of acute infectious jaundice. The etiology is unknown. Some epidemics have been associated with paratyphoid bacillus infection. The *proteus* has been described in connection with Weil's disease. In the fatal case from North Carolina the autopsy threw no light on the nature of the disease. The *proteus* was isolated from the liver and kidney, and four other organisms from various parts. It is possible that acute catarrhal jaundice is a mild infection, representing the sporadic form of the disease.

XVIII. MILK-SICKNESS

This remarkable disease prevails in certain districts of the United States, west of the Alleghany Mountains, and is connected with the affection in cattle known as the *trembles.* It prevailed extensively in the early settlements in certain of the Western States and proved very fatal. The general opinion is that it is communicated to man only by eating the flesh or drinking the milk of diseased animals. The butter and cheese are also poisonous. In animals, cattle and the young of horses and sheep are most susceptible. It is stated that cows giving milk do not themselves show marked symptoms unless driven rapidly, and, according to Graff, the secretion may be infective when the disease is latent. When a cow is very ill, food is refused, the eyes are injected, the animal staggers, the entire muscular system trembles, and death occurs in convulsions, sometimes with great suddenness. The disease is most frequent in new settlements.

In man the symptoms are those of a more or less acute intoxication. After a few days of uneasiness and distress the patient is seized with pains in the stomach, nausea and vomiting, fever and intense thirst. There is usually obstinate constipation. The tongue is swollen and tremulous, the breath is extremely foul, and, according to Graff, is as characteristic of the disease as is the odor in small-pox. Cerebral symptoms—restlessness, irritability, coma, and convulsions—are sometimes marked, and there may gradually be produced a typhoid state in which the patient dies.

The duration of the disease is variable. In the most acute form death occurs within two or three days. It may last for ten days, or even for three or four weeks. Graff states that insanity occurred in one case. The poisonous nature of the flesh and of the milk has been demonstrated experimentally. An ounce of butter or cheese, or four ounces of the beef, raw or boiled, given three times a day, will kill a dog within six days. Fortunately, the disease has become rare. No definite pathological lesions are known. Jordan and Harris have studied a New Mexico epidemic (1908) and have found a bacillus (*B. lactimorbi*) with cultures of which the disease may be reproduced in other animals.

XIX. GLANDULAR FEVER

Definition.—An infectious disease of children, developing, as a rule, without premonitory signs, and characterized by slight redness of the throat, high fever, swelling and tenderness of the lymph-glands of the neck, particularly those behind the sterno-cleido-mastoid muscles. The fever is of short duration, but the enlargement of the glands persists for from ten days to three weeks.

In children acute adenitis of the cervical and other glands with fever has been noted by many observers, but Pfeiffer in 1889 called special attention to it under the name of *Druesenfieber*. He described it as an infectious disease of young children between the ages of five and eight years, characterized by the above-mentioned symptoms. Since Pfeiffer's paper a good deal of work has been done in connection with the subject, and in the United States West and Hamill, and in England Dawson Williams, have more particularly emphasized the condition.

Etiology.—It may occur in epidemic form. West, of Bellaire, Ohio, described an epidemic of 96 cases in children between the ages of seven months and thirteen years. Bilateral swelling of the carotid lymph-glands was a most marked feature. In three-fourths of the cases the post-cervical, inguinal, and axillary glands were involved. The mesenteric glands were felt in 37 cases, the spleen was enlarged in 57, and the liver in 87 cases. Coryza was not present, and there were no bronchial or pulmonary symptoms. Cases occurred between the months of October and June. The nature of the infection has not been determined.

Symptoms.—The onset is sudden and the first complaint is of pain on moving the head and neck. There may be nausea and vomiting and abdominal pain. The temperature ranges from 101° to 103°. The tonsils may be a little red and the lymphatic tissues swollen, but the throat symptoms are quite transient and unimportant. On the second or third day the enlarged glands appear, and during the course they vary in size from a pea to a goose-egg. They are painful to the touch, but there is rarely any redness or swelling of the skin, though at times there is some puffiness of the subcutaneous tissues of the neck, and there may be a little difficulty in swallowing. In some instances there has been discomfort in the chest and a paroxysmal cough, indicating involvement of the tracheal and bronchial glands. The swelling of the glands persists for from two to three weeks. Among the serious features of the disease are the termination of the adenitis in suppuration, which seems rare (though Neumann has met with it in 13 cases), and hæmorrhagic nephritis. Acute otitis media and retro-pharyngeal abscess have also been reported.

The outlook is favorable. West suggests the use of small doses of calomel during the height of the trouble.

XX. MILIARY FEVER—SWEATING SICKNESS

The disease is characterized by fever, profuse sweats, and an eruption of miliary vesicles. It prevailed and was very fatal in England in the fifteenth and sixteenth centuries, and was made the subject of an important memoir by Johannes Caius, 1552. Of late years it has been confined entirely to certain districts in France (Picardy) and Italy. An epidemic of some extent occurred in France in 1887. Hirsch gives a chronological account of 194 epidemics between 1718 and 1879, many of which were limited to a single village or to a few localities. Occasionally the disease has become widely spread. Slight epidemics have occurred in Germany and Switzerland. Within the past few years there have been several small outbreaks in Austria. They are usually of short duration, lasting only for three or four weeks—sometimes not more than seven or eight days. As in influenza, a very large number of persons are attacked in rapid succession. In the mild cases there is only slight fever, with loss of appetite, and erythematous eruption, profuse perspiration, and an outbreak of miliary vesicles. The severe cases present the symptoms of intense infection—delirium, high fever, profound prostration, and hæmorrhage. The death-rate at the outset of the disease is usually high, and, as is so graphically described in the account of some of the epidemics of the middle ages, death may occur in a few hours.

XXI. FOOT-AND-MOUTH DISEASE—EPIDEMIC STOMATITIS—APHTHOUS FEVER

Foot-and-mouth disease is an acute infectious disorder met with chiefly in cattle, sheep, and pigs, but attacking other domestic animals. It is of extraordinary activity, and spreads with "lightning rapidity" over vast territories, causing very serious losses. In cattle, after a period of incubation of three or five days, the animal becomes feverish, the mucous membrane of the mouth swells, and little grayish vesicles the size of a hemp seed begin to develop on the edges and lower portion of the tongue, on the gums, and on the mucous membrane of the lips. They contain at first a clear fluid, which becomes turbid, and then they enlarge and gradually become converted into superficial ulcers. There is ptyalism, and the animals lose flesh rapidly. In the cow the disease is also frequently seen about the udder and teats, and the milk becomes yellowish-white in color and of a mucoid consistency.

The transmission to man is by no means uncommon, and several important epidemics have been studied in the neighborhood of Berlin. In Zuill's translation of Friedberger and Fröhner's Pathology and Therapeutics of Domestic Animals (Philadelphia, 1895) the disease is thus described: "In man the symptoms are: fever, digestive troubles, and vesicular eruption upon the lips, the buccal and pharyngeal mucous membranes (angina). The disease does not seem to be transmissible through the meat of diseased animals."

In widespread epidemics there has been sometimes a marked tendency to hæmorrhages. The disease runs, as a rule, a favorable course, but in Siegel's report of an epidemic the mortality was 8 per cent.

When epidemics are prevailing in cattle the milk should be boiled, and the proper prophylactic measures taken to isolate both the cattle and the individuals who come in contact with them.

XXII. PSITTACOSIS

A disease in birds, characterized by loss of appetite, weakness, diarrhœa, convulsions, and death. In Germany, France, and Italy a disease in man characterized by an atypical pneumonia, great weakness and depression, and signs of a profound infection has been ascribed to contagion from birds, particularly parrots. There have usually been house epidemics with a very high rate of mortality. A few cases have been reported in England, and Vickery, of Boston, has reported three probable cases. The bacteriology is still doubtful.

XXIII. ROCKY MOUNTAIN SPOTTED FEVER; TICK FEVER

In the Bitter-root Valley of Montana and in the mountains of Idaho, Nevada, and Wyoming there is an acute infection characterized by chill, fever, pains in back and bones, and a macular rash, becoming hæmorrhagic. It is estimated that seven or eight hundred cases occur annually, with 75 or 80 deaths. It was reported upon occasionally by army surgeons—e. g., Wood—but nothing definite was known until the careful studies of Wilson and Chowning (1902), who described a piroplasma in the blood, and believed the disease to be transmitted by ticks. This latter point has been confirmed, but the existence of the piroplasma is doubtful. The studies of King and Ricketts have demonstrated beyond doubt the transmission of the disease by the tick, *Dermacentor occidentalis,* but the true parasite has not been determined. The tick is widely distributed over the Rocky Mountain regions as far south as New Mexico. It lives on the larger domestic animals, cattle and horses, and is in this way brought into close proximity with human beings. The disease is readily given to the guinea-pig and monkey, and is transmissible from one animal to another by the bite of the tick. Immunity is given by an attack, and in animals this is transmitted to the young. After an incubation of from three to ten days the disease begins with a chill, fever, and severe pains in the limbs. The rash appears from the second to the seventh day, is macular, dark, and becomes hæmorrhagic. Illustrations of it show a rash not unlike that of typhus. The skin is often swollen. Hæmorrhages from the mucous membranes are not uncommon. The temperature range is from 103° to 105° F., and at the height of the disease there is delirium and stupor. Convalescence begins in the fourth week. The death-rate is high for an eruptive fever, reaching 70 per cent. in Montana, but in Idaho it is not more than 2 or 3 per cent. As a prophylactic measure, destruction of the ticks by dipping or scouring the horses and cattle should be carried out. The treatment is that of an acute infection.

XXIV. SWINE FEVER

A few cases have been described from accidental inoculation in the preparation of cultures and in making post mortems upon pigs. In the course of from twelve hours to three days there is swelling of the fingers of the affected hand, which have a blue-red color, and small nodules form. In some of the instances the course has been like that of a painful erythema migrans, with swelling of the lymph-glands. A specific serum has been used with success in several cases.

XXV. RAT-BITE FEVER

A remarkable infection, following rat-bite, characterized by brief febrile paroxysms which may recur at intervals for months.

The disease has been known in China and Japan for several centuries. Attention has been called to it in this country by Horder and in the United States by Proescher. In a recent statistical account from the *Institution for Infectious Diseases* it appears that there have been 49 cases in Japan in the past thirteen years. The features are very unusual. There is a prolonged period of incubation, lasting in some cases for many months. The wound, which has run the ordinary course and perhaps healed, becomes swollen, red, and eroded; an ulcer forms and the regional lymph-glands are involved. The fever sets in suddenly with a chill and lasts three or four days. With its onset there is a skin rash, either erythema or a blotchy eruption somewhat resembling measles. The patient feels very ill, there may be pains in the muscles and joints and sometimes delirium. After persisting for a few days, the temperature falls and the patient feels quite well again. After a varying interval of from a few days to a couple of weeks the attack is repeated, and this may go on for several months or, according to the Japanese reports, for several years. The outlook is favorable; among the 49 Japanese cases only 1 died.

In Horder's last case the boy was bitten on September 15th. From October 6th to 11th, on the 13th, 14th, 17th, 18th, 19th, 23d, 24th, 25th, 28th to 30th, and November 4th, 5th, and 6th, he had attacks of fever, the temperature rising to between 104° and 105° F., and once reaching nearly 106°. Each attack was associated with a rash.

Various organisms have been described. In one of Horder's cases spirilla were seen. Ogata describes a sporozoan parasite, and Proescher a bacillus. Japanese observers have reported spirochætes in two cases. One was treated by mercury and the other by salvarsan; both recovered. Schotmüller, Blake and Tileston each found a streptothrix in their cases. In Tileston's case the organisms were found in fresh smears by dark-field illumination. Blake isolated a streptothrix in a case which at autopsy showed endocarditis, in the vegetations of which the same organism was found.

Treatment.—The wound should be cauterized, salvarsan given intravenously, and the febrile paroxysms treated symptomatically.

SECTION II

DISEASES DUE TO PHYSICAL AGENTS

I. SUNSTROKE; HEAT EXHAUSTION

(*Insolation, Thermic Fever, Siriasis*)

Definition.—Under these terms are comprised certain manifestations following exposure to excessive heat, of which thermic fever, or sunstroke, heat exhaustion, and heat cramps are the common forms.

History.—It is one of the oldest of recognized diseases. The case of the son of the Shunammite woman (2 Kings, IV) is perhaps the oldest on record. The Arabians called the symptoms due to excessive heart "Siriasis," after Sirius the Dog Star. Cardan recognized it in the sixteenth century and thought it was apoplexy due to heat—morbus attonitus. In the eighteenth century Boerhaave regarded it as phrenitis. It was not until the nineteenth century that the Anglo-Indian surgeons and the physicians of the United States gave us a full knowledge of the different affections due to excessive heat. Various classifications have been suggested, but two chief forms are everywhere recognized—heat exhaustion and thermic fever or sunstroke—to which recently Edsall has added the remarkable heat cramps which occur in persons working under very high external temperatures.

Distribution.—Sunstroke occurs in the tropics and in temperate regions during protracted heat waves. It is very common in the Atlantic Coast cities of the United States during the hot spells of summer. In New York and Philadelphia many hundreds of cases may occur daily. It has not been common in Panama. During 1910 no death from it was recorded among nearly 50,000 employees. Heat exhaustion is frequently met with in conditions similar to those in which sunstroke takes place, and it is also a not infrequent affection in the engine-rooms of the large modern steamships, less often in foundries.

Heat Exhaustion.—In the tropics and in temperate regions during protracted heat waves many persons become depressed physically and are unable to work or take nourishment. In children the condition is very often associated with gastro-intestinal disturbances and fever. The true heat syncope is specially seen in persons who have not been in good health or who are intemperate. The heat may be that of the sun or artificial heat, as in the engine-rooms of the large steamers. The symptoms begin with giddiness, nausea, an uncertain, staggering gait; there is pallor, the pulse is small, the heart's action weak, and the patient may quickly become unconscious. Externally the body may be clammy, with sweat, but as a rule the rectal temperature is decreased. In the axilla it may be as low as 95° or 96° F. From slight attacks, such as are seen in the steamships, the patients recover rapidly when brought on deck; in other cases the unconsciousness may end in deep coma and death.

Thermic Fever.—This is more common in men than in women and children, and is principally seen in persons who work in very high external temperatures, and who are too heavily clad, or who are addicted to alcohol. In India regiments on the march are not infrequently attacked. It is more common in Europeans than in the dark races, but in the United States negroes are often attacked.

MORBID ANATOMY AND PATHOLOGY.—Rigor mortis occurs early. Putrefactive changes may come on with great rapidity. The venous engorgement is extreme, particularly in the cerebrum. The left ventricle is contracted (Wood) and the right chamber dilated. The blood is usually fluid; the lungs are intensely congested. Parenchymatous changes occur in the liver and kidneys.

SYMPTOMS.—Many observers have called attention to a fever in the tropics which lasts for a few days, with no special symptoms other than those of pyrexia and weakness. As already mentioned, this may be simply heat exhaustion. It is not uncommon in the Southern States, particularly in Florida and the Carolinas, when it may be mistaken for malaria or mild typhoid fever. John Guitéras, who has unrivalled knowledge of tropical affections, regards these conditions as directly due to prolonged high external temperatures.

The patient may be struck down and die within an hour, with symptoms of heart-failure, dyspnœa, and coma. This form, sometimes known as the asphyxial, occurs chiefly in soldiers and is graphically described by Parkes. Death indeed may be almost instantaneous, the victims falling as if struck upon the head. The more usual form comes on during exposure, with pain in the head, dizziness, a feeling of oppression, and sometimes nausea and vomiting. Visual disturbances are common, and a patient may have colored vision. Diarrhœa or frequent micturition may supervene. Insensibility follows, which may be transient or which deepens into a profound coma. The patients are usually admitted to hospital in an unconscious state, with the face flushed, the skin hot, the pulse rapid and full, and the temperature ranging from 107° to 110° F., or even higher. F. A. Packard states that, of the 31 cases admitted to the Pennsylvania Hospital in the summer of 1887, in a majority of them the temperature was between 110° and 111° F. In one case the temperature was 112° F. The breathing is labored and deep, sometimes stertorous. Usually there is complete relaxation of the muscles, but twitchings, jactitation, or very rarely convulsions may occur. The pupils may at first be dilated, but by the time the patients are admitted to hospital they are (in a majority) extremely contracted. Petechiæ may be present upon the skin. In the fatal cases the coma deepens, the cardiac pulsations become more rapid and feeble, the breathing becomes hurried and shallow and of the Cheyne-Stokes type. The fatal termination may occur within twenty-four or thirty-six hours. Favorable indications are the return of consciousness and a fall in the fever. The recovery in these cases may be complete. In other instances there are remarkable after-effects, the most constant of which is a permanent inability to bear high temperatures. Such patients become very uneasy when the thermometer reaches 80° F. in the shade. Loss of the power of mental concentration and failure of memory are more constant and very troublesome sequelæ. Such patients are always worse in the hot weather. Occasionally there are convulsions, followed by marked mental disturbance. Dercum has described peripheral neuritis as a sequence.

Diagnosis.—It is rarely difficult to distinguish thermic fever from the malignant types of malaria and from the various other forms of coma. The diagnosis in heat exhaustion or thermic fever is readily made. In the one

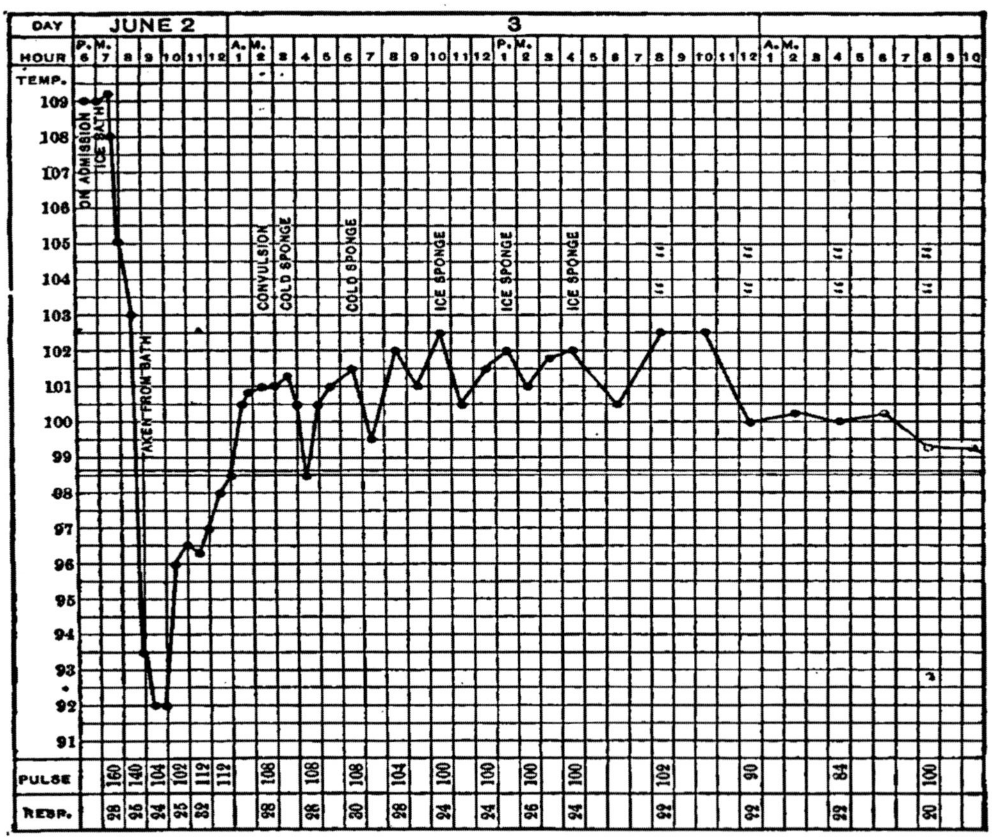

Chart XIII.—Case of Sun-stroke Treated by the Ice-bath; Recovery.

the skin is moist, pale, and cool, the pulse small and soft, and consciousness may remain till near the end; whereas in the other there is high fever with early unconsciousness.

Prognosis.—In the old, the infirm, and in alcoholic subjects the case mortality during a very hot wave may be as high as 30 or 40 per cent. In New York and Philadelphia the death-rate varies very much at different seasons.

Treatment.—In heat exhaustion stimulants should be given freely, and if the temperature is below normal the hot bath should be used. Ammonia may be given if necessary. In thermic fever the indications are to reduce the temperature as rapidly as possible. This may be done by packing the patient in a bath with ice. Rubbing the body with ice was practiced at the New York Hospital by Darrach in 1857, and is an excellent procedure to lower the temperature rapidly. Ice-water enemata may also be employed. At the Pennsylvania Hospital in the summer of 1887 the ice-pack was used with great advantage. Of 31 cases only 12 died, results probably as satisfactory as can be obtained, considering that many of the patients are almost moribund when brought to hospital. They should be compared with Swift's statistics, in which, of 150 cases, 78 died. In the cases in which the symptoms are those of intense asphyxia, and in which death may take place in a few minutes, free bleeding should be practiced, a procedure which saved Weir Mitchell when a young man. For the convulsions, chloroform should be given at once. Of other remedies, the antipyretics have been employed, and may be given when there is any special objection to hydrotherapy, for which, however, they cannot be substituted.

Heat Cramps.—Persons who use the muscles while exposed to a very high temperature are liable to attacks of severe cramp. The condition, which has been described very thoroughly by Edsall, occurs principally in stokers in the furnace-rooms of steamships and in workers in iron foundries. The spasms occur spontaneously, chiefly in the muscles of the calves, the arms, and sometimes in the abdomen; they are often of great intensity and very painful. A movement, pressure, or any stimulus, as electricity, may send the muscle into spasm at once. In addition to ordinary cramps there are sometimes fibrillary contractions. The attacks may last for from 12 to 34 hours and are followed by muscular soreness and sometimes by great weakness.

II. CAISSON DISEASE

(*Compressed Air Disease; Diver's Paralysis*)

Definition.—A disease of caisson workers and divers, due to a saturation of the tissues with N under the increased pressure. If the decompression takes place quickly, a too-rapid escape of the N as bubbles into the blood causes air embolism.

History.—The French writers, Bucquoy, Foley, and Bert, first studied the disease. Leyden recognized the anatomical changes. A. H. Smith and others in the United States contributed important papers, and the recent studies of Haldane, Leonard Hill, and Boycott have thrown light upon the etiology and means of prevention.

Etiology.—The cases are met with chiefly in workers in caissons and tunnels and in divers. "The higher the pressure and the shorter the period of decompression the greater is the risk" (Hill). In caissons the pressure is rarely 30 to 35 pounds, but in the St. Louis bridge the pressure reached as high as 45 to 50 pounds. Divers go down to 20 fathoms with a pressure of 53 pounds; the record depth attained by divers is 210 feet (Hill). The disease may also occur in very deep mines.

In building the St. Louis bridge across the Mississippi, among 352 workers there were 50 cases of paralysis and 14 deaths. In making the Hudson River tunnel the cases were very numerous, and until the conditions were improved there were two or three deaths a month.

Pathology.—To Hoppe-Seyler, Bucquoy, and Paul Bert we owe a rational explanation of the disease as due to gas absorption. During compression the blood passing through the lungs becomes saturated with nitrogen, which is carried to the tissues until the whole body is saturated. "The mass of blood is about 5 per cent. of the body, and the capacity of the tissues to dissolve N is estimated by Boycott as 35 times that of the blood—in a fat man considerably more" (Hill). With active work it does not take long to effect complete saturation. During decompression the process is just the reverse. "The blood gives up N to the alveolar air and returns to the tissues for more. Those organs in which the circulation is rapid will yield up their N quickly, and those with a sluggish circulation slowly . . . . . and at the end of decompression a condition may be set up in which the slow tissues still hold, say 3 per cent. of N, while the blood can dissolve only 1 per cent. Herein we have a danger of bubbles forming" (Hill). They are set free chiefly in the fatty tissues and in the venous blood. Experimentally all the symptoms can be produced in goats, and the spinal cord may contain numerous air emboli. This was the anatomical lesion determined by Leyden, who found fissuring and laceration of the cord, which explains the paraplegia. Pulmonary air embolism also occurs and is responsible for certain features of the disease.

Symptoms.—Within from half an hour to one hour after leaving the caisson, the patient may have headache, giddiness and feel faint, symptoms which may pass off and leave no further trouble. In other instances the patients have severe pains in the extremities, usually the legs and the abdomen, sometimes associated with nausea and vomiting—attacks which the workmen usually speak of as "the bends." The pains may be of the greatest intensity and associated with giddiness and vomiting. The paralysis, usually of the legs, comes on rapidly, and varies in degree from a slight paralysis to complete loss both of motion and sensation. This occurred in 15 per cent. of A. H. Smith's cases and in 61 per cent. of the St. Louis cases. Monoplegia and hemiplegia are rare. In extreme instances the attacks resemble apoplexy; the patient rapidly becomes comatose and death occurs in a few hours. The paraplegia may be permanent, but in slight cases it gradually disappears and recovery may be complete.

Prophylaxis.—The only safeguard is a gradual decompression, which obviates the risk of rapidly setting free the nitrogen from the tissues. Haldane and his colleagues have introduced what they call the "Stage Method," which is now widely adopted with the most beneficial results. For work in very high pressures the shifts should be short, not more than two hours.

Treatment.—The caisson workers found very early that the best remedy for "the bends" was immediate recompression, and Andrew H. Smith of New York introduced a medical air-lock for the Brooklyn bridge workers. The workers should live and sleep not far from the works, where such an air-lock should be provided for immediate treatment. Cases with severe symptoms may be saved by recompression. Hot fomentations, massage and hypodermics of morphia may be necessary for the extreme pains.

III. MOUNTAIN SICKNESS

Definition.—An illness associated with adaptation to low atmospheric pressures, characterized by cyanosis, nausea, headache, intestinal disturbances, hyperpnœa, and sometimes fainting.

Pathology.—The symptoms are directly referable to want of oxygen produced by the diminished pressure of the atmosphere. Haldane, Douglas and Henderson have recently made an exhaustive study of the process of accommodation in a five weeks' residence at the top of Pike's Peak. After acclimatization the symptoms above mentioned disappeared, but dyspnœa, blueness and periodic breathing are apt to follow exertion. The alveolar carbon dioxide pressure was reduced from about 40 mm. to about 27 mm. during rest, which corresponded to an increase of about 50 per cent. in the ventilation of the lung alveoli. As has long been known, this process of accommodation is associated with a remarkable increase in the red blood corpuscles and hæmoglobin to 120 to 150 per cent. These authors conclude that the acclimatization is largely due to increased secretory activity of the alveolar epithelium, to the greater lung ventilation and to the increased hæmoglobin production.

Symptoms.—The symptoms just given, which are the most important, pass away gradually, but may return on exertion. In feeble persons the heart's action may be weak and intermittent, and syncope may follow any effort. Whymper in the ascent of Chimborazo at a height of 16,000 feet had headache, fever, gasping respiration and great weakness. Nausea, vomiting, bleeding at the nose, ringing in the ears and palpitation are not infrequent symptoms.

SECTION III

THE INTOXICATIONS

I. ALCOHOLISM

(a) Acute Alcoholism.—When a large quantity of alcohol is taken, the influence is chiefly on the nervous system, and is manifested in muscular incoordination, mental disturbance, and, finally, narcosis. The individual presents a flushed, sometimes slightly cyanosed face, the pulse is full, respirations deep but rarely stertorous. The pupils are dilated. The temperature is frequently below normal, particularly if the patient has been exposed to cold. Perhaps the lowest reported temperatures have been in cases of this sort. An instance is on record in which the patient on admission to hospital had a temperature of 24° C. (ca. 75° F.), and ten hours later the temperature had not risen to 91° F. The unconsciousness is rarely so deep that the patient cannot be roused to some extent, and in reply to questions he mutters incoherently. Muscular twitchings may occur, but rarely convulsions. The breath has a heavy alcoholic odor. The respirations may be slow; in one case they were only six in the minute.

The diagnosis is not difficult, yet mistakes are frequently made. Persons are brought to a hospital by the police supposed to be drunk when in reality they are dying from apoplexy. Too great care cannot be exercised, and the patient should receive the benefit of the doubt. In some instances the mistake has arisen from the fact that a person who has been drinking heavily has been stricken with apoplexy. In this condition the coma is usually deeper, stertor is present, and there may be evidence of hemiplegia in the greater flaccidity of the limbs on one side. The diagnosis will be considered in the section upon uræmic coma.

Dipsomania is a form of acute alcoholism seen in persons with a strong hereditary tendency to drink. Periodically the victims go "on a spree," but in the intervals they are entirely free from any craving for alcohol.

(b) Chronic Alcoholism.—In moderation, wine, beer, and spirits may be taken throughout a long life without impairing the general health.

The poisonous effects of alcohol are manifested (1) as a functional poison, as in acute narcosis; (2) as a tissue poison, in which its effects are seen on the parenchymatous elements, particularly epithelium and nerve, producing a slow degeneration, and on the blood vessels, causing thickening and ultimately fibroid changes; and (3) as a checker of tissue oxidation, since the alcohol is consumed in place of the fat. This leads to fatty changes and sometimes to a condition of general steatosis.

The chief effects of chronic alcohol poisoning may be thus summarized:

Nervous System.—Functional disturbance is common. Unsteadiness of the muscles in performing any action is a constant feature. The tremor is best seen in the hands and in the tongue. The mental processes may be dull, particularly in the early morning hours, and the patient is unable to transact any business until he has had his accustomed stimulant. Irritability of temper, forgetfulness, and a change in the moral character of the individual gradually come on. The judgment is seriously impaired, the will enfeebled, and in the final stages dementia may supervene. An interesting combination of symptoms in chronic alcoholics is characterized by peripheral neuritis, loss of memory, and pseudo-reminiscences—that is, false notions as to the patient's position in time and space, and fabulous explanations of real occurrences. The peripheral neuritis is not always present; there may be only tremor and jactitation of the lips, and thickness of the speech, with visual hallucinations. The mental condition was described by Jackson and by Wilks. Korsakoff speaks of it as a *psychosis polyneuritica,* and the symptom-complex is sometimes called by his name. The relation of chronic alcoholism to insanity has been much discussed. According to Savage, of 4,000 patients admitted to the Bethlehem Hospital, 133 gave drink as the cause of their insanity. Chronic alcoholism is certainly one of the important elements in the strain which leads to mental breakdown. Epilepsy may result directly from chronic drinking. It is a hopeful form, and may disappear entirely with a return to habits of temperance.

There is a remarkable condition in chronic alcoholism termed "*wet brain,*" in which a heavy drinker, who may perhaps have had attacks of delirium tremens, begins to get drowsy or a little more befuddled than usual; gradually the stupor deepens until he becomes comatose, in which state he may remain for weeks. There may be slight fever, but there are no signs of paralysis, and no optic neuritis. The urine may be normal. The lumbar puncture yields a clear fluid, but under high pressure. In one case, which died at the end of six weeks, there were the anatomical features of a serous meningitis.

No characteristic changes are found in the nervous system. Hæmorrhagic pachymeningitis is not very uncommon. There are opacity and thickening of the pia-arachnoid membranes, with more or less wasting of the convolutions. These are in no way peculiar to chronic alcoholism, but are found in old persons and in chronic wasting diseases. In the very protracted cases there may be chronic encephalo-meningitis with adhesions of the membranes. Finer changes in the nerve-cells, their processes, and the neuroglia have been described. By far the most striking effect of alcohol on the nervous system is the production of the alcoholic neuritis, which will be considered later.

Digestive System.—Catarrh of the stomach is the most common symptom. The toper has a furred tongue, heavy breath, and in the morning a sensation of sinking at the stomach until he has had his dram. The appetite is usually impaired and the bowels are constipated. In beer-drinkers dilatation of the stomach is common.

Alcohol produces definite changes in the liver, leading ultimately to the various forms of cirrhosis, to be described. In Welch's laboratory J. Friedenwald has caused typical cirrhosis in rabbits by the administration of alcohol. The effect is a primary degenerative change in the liver-cells. A special vulnerability of the liver-cells is necessary in the etiology of alcoholic cirrhosis. There are cases in which comparatively moderate drinking for a few years has been followed by cirrhosis; on the other hand, the livers of persons who have been steady drinkers for thirty or forty years may show only a moderate grade of sclerosis. For years before cirrhosis develops heavy drinkers may present an enlarged and tender liver, with at times swelling of the spleen. With the gastric and hepatic disorders the facies often becomes very characteristic. The venules of the cheeks and nose are dilated; the latter becomes enlarged, red, and may present the condition known as *acne rosacea.* The eyes are watery, and conjunctivæ hyperæmic and sometimes bile-tinged.

The *heart and arteries* in chronic topers show degenerative changes, and alcoholism is a factor in causing arterio-sclerosis. Steell has pointed out the frequency of cardiac dilatation in these cases.

Kidneys.—The influence of chronic alcoholism upon these organs is by no means so marked. According to Dickinson the total of renal disease is not greater in the drinking class, and he holds that the effect of alcohol on the kidneys has been much overrated. Formad has directed attention to the fact that in a large proportion of chronic alcoholics the kidneys are increased in size. The Guy's Hospital statistics support this statement, and Pitt notes that in 43 per cent. of the bodies of hard drinkers the kidneys were hypertrophied without showing morbid change. A granular kidney may result indirectly through the arterial changes.

It was formerly thought that alcohol was in some way antagonistic to tuberculous disease, but the observations of late years indicate clearly that the reverse is the case and that chronic drinkers are much more liable to both acute and pulmonary tuberculosis. It is probably altogether a question of altered tissue-soil, the alcohol lowering the vitality and enabling the bacilli more readily to develop and grow.

(c) Delirium tremens (*mania a potu*), an incident in the history of chronic alcoholism, results from the long-continued action of the poison on the brain. The condition was first accurately described early in the 19th century by Sutton, of Greenwich, who had numerous opportunities for studying the different forms among sailors. One of the most careful studies of the disease was made by Ware, of Boston. A spree in a temperate person, no matter how prolonged, is rarely if ever followed by delirium tremens; but in the case of an habitual drinker a temporary excess is apt to bring on an attack. It sometimes follows in consequence of the sudden withdrawal of the alcohol. An accident, a sudden fright or shock, or an acute inflammation, particularly pneumonia, may determine the onset. It is especially apt to occur in drinkers admitted to hospitals for injuries, especially fractures, and, as this seems most likely to occur when the alcohol is withdrawn, it is well to give such patients a moderate amount of alcohol. At the outset of the attack the patient is restless and depressed and sleeps badly, symptoms which cause him to take alcohol more freely. After a day or two the characteristic delirium sets in. The patient talks constantly and incoherently; he is incessantly in motion, and desires to go out and attend to some imaginary business. Hallucinations of sight and hearing develop. He sees objects in the room, such as rats, mice, or snakes, and fancies that they are crawling over his body. The terror inspired by these imaginary objects is great, and has given the popular name "horrors" to the disease. The patients need to be watched constantly, for in their delusions they may jump out of the window or escape. Auditory hallucinations are not so common, but the patient may complain of hearing the roar of animals or the threats of imaginary enemies. There is much muscular tremor; the tongue is covered with a thick white fur, and when protruded is tremulous. The pulse is soft, rapid, and readily compressed. There is usually fever, but the temperature rarely registers above 102° or 103°. In fatal cases it may be higher. Insomnia is a constant feature. On the third or fourth day in favorable cases the restlessness abates, the patient sleeps, and improvement gradually sets in. The tremor persists for some days, the hallucinations gradually disappear, and the appetite returns. In more serious cases the insomnia persists, the delirium is incessant, the pulse becomes more frequent and feeble, the tongue dry, the prostration extreme, and death takes place from gradual heart-failure.

There is a condition termed *acute hallucinosis,* in which auditory hallucinations are marked, orientation is retained, and the mental disturbances are fixed. Ideas of persecution are common. There are intermediate forms between this and the ordinary delirium tremens.

Diagnosis.—The clinical picture of the disease can scarcely be confounded with any other. Cases with fever, however, may be mistaken for meningitis. By far the most common error is to overlook some local disease, such as pneumonia or erysipelas, or an accident, as a fractured rib, which in a chronic drinker may precipitate an attack of delirium tremens. In every instance a careful examination should be made, particularly of the lungs. It is to be remembered that in the severer forms, particularly the febrile cases, congestion of the bases of the lungs is by no means uncommon. Another point to be borne in mind is the fact that pneumonia of the apex is apt to be accompanied by delirium similar to *mania a potu.*

Prognosis.—Recovery takes place in a large proportion of the cases in private practice. In hospital practice, particularly in the large city hospitals to which the debilitated patients are taken, the death-rate is higher. Gerhard states that of 1,241 cases admitted to the Philadelphia Hospital 121 proved fatal. Recurrence is frequent, almost, indeed, the rule, if the drinking is kept up.

Treatment.—Acute alcoholism rarely requires any special measures, as the patient sleeps off the effects of the debauch. In the case of profound alcoholic coma it may be advisable to wash out the stomach, and if collapse symptoms occur the limbs should be rubbed and hot applications made to the body. Should convulsions supervene, chloroform may be carefully administered. In the acute, violent alcoholic mania the hypodermic injection of apomorphia, one-eighth or one-sixth of a grain, is usually very effectual, causing nausea and vomiting, and rapid disappearance of the maniacal symptoms.

Chronic alcoholism is a condition very difficult to treat, and once fully established the habit is rarely abandoned. The most obstinate cases are those with marked hereditary tendency. Withdrawal of the alcohol is the first essential. This is most effectually accomplished by placing the patient in an institution, in which he can be carefully watched during the trying period of the first week or ten days of abstention. The absence of temptation in institution life is of special advantage. For the sleeplessness the bromides or hyoscine may be employed. Quinine and strychnine in tonic doses may be given. Cocaine or the fluid extract of coca has been recommended as a substitute for alcohol, but it is not of much service. Prolonged seclusion in a suitable institution is in reality the only effectual means of cure. When an hereditary tendency exists a lapse into the drinking habit is almost inevitable.

In delirium tremens the patient should be confined to bed and carefully watched night and day. The danger of escape in these cases is very great, as the patient imagines himself pursued by enemies or demons. Flint mentions the case of a man who escaped in his nightclothes and ran barefooted for fifteen miles on the frozen ground before he was overtaken. The patient should not be strapped in bed, as this aggravates the delirium; sometimes, however, it may be necessary, in which case a sheet tied across the bed may be sufficient, and this is certainly better than violent restraint by three or four men. Alcohol should be withdrawn at once unless the pulse is feeble.

Delirium tremens is a disease which, in a large majority of cases, runs a course very slightly influenced by medicine. The indications for treatment are to procure sleep and to support the strength. In mild cases half a drachm (2 gm.) of bromide of potassium combined with tincture of capsicum may be given every three hours. Chloral is often of great service, and may be given without hesitation unless the heart's action is feeble. Good results sometimes follow the hypodermic use of hyoscine, one one-hundredth of a grain. Opium must be used cautiously. A special merit of Ware's work was the demonstration that on a rational or expectant plan of treatment the percentage of recoveries was greater than with the indiscriminate use of sedatives, which had been in vogue for many years. When opium is indicated it should be given as morphia, hypodermically. The effect should be carefully watched, and, if after three or four quarter-grain doses have been given the patient is still restless and excited, it is best not to push it farther. Repeated doses of trional (grs. xv-xx) every four hours may be tried. Lambert advises ergotin hypodermically in both the acute and chronic alcoholism. When fever is present the tranquilizing effects of a cold douche or cold bath may be tried, or the cold or warm packs. The large doses of digitalis formerly employed are not advisable.

Careful feeding is the most important element in the treatment of these cases. Milk and concentrated broths should be given at stated intervals. If the pulse becomes rapid and shows signs of flagging, alcohol may be given in combination with the aromatic spirits of ammonia.

II. MORPHIA HABIT

(*Morphinomania; Morphinism*)

Taken at first to allay pain, a craving for the drug is gradually engendered, and the habit in this way acquired. The effects of the constant use of opium vary very much. In the East, where opium-smoking is as common as tobacco-smoking with us, the ill effects are, according to good observers, not very striking. Taken as morphia and hypodermically, as is the rule, it is very injurious, but a moderate amount may be taken for years without serious damage.

The habit is particularly prevalent among women and physicians who use the hypodermic syringe for the alleviation of pain, as in neuralgia or sciatica. The acquisition of the habit as a pure luxury is rare.

Symptoms.—The symptoms at first are slight and for months there may be no disturbance of health. There are exceptional instances in which for a period of years excessive amounts have been taken without deterioration of the mental or bodily functions. As a rule, the dose necessary to obtain the desired sensation has gradually to be increased. As the effects wear off the victim experiences sensations of lassitude and mental depression, accompanied often with slight nausea and epigastric distress, or even recurring colic, which may be mistaken for appendicitis. The confirmed opium-eater usually has a sallow, pasty complexion, is emaciated, and becomes prematurely gray. He is restless, irritable, and unable to remain quiet for any time. Itching is a common symptom. The sleep is disturbed, the appetite and digestion are deranged, and except when directly under the influence of the drug the mental condition is one of depression. Occasionally there are profuse sweats, which may be preceded by chills. The pupils, except when under the direct influence of the drug, are dilated, sometimes unequal. In one case there was a persistent œdema of the legs without sufficient renal changes or anæmia to account for it. Persons addicted to morphia are inveterate liars, and no reliance whatever can be placed upon their statements. In many instances this is not confined to matters relating to the vice. In women the symptoms may be associated with those of pronounced hysteria or neurasthenia. The practice may be continued for an indefinite time, usually requiring increase in the dose until ultimately enormous quantities may be needed to obtain the desired effect. Finally a condition of asthenia is induced, in which the victim takes little or no food and dies from the extreme bodily debility. An increase in the dose is not always necessary, and there are *habitués* who reach the point of satisfaction with a daily amount of 2 or 3 grains of morphia, and who are able to carry on successfully for many years the ordinary business of life. They may remain in good physical condition, and indeed often look ruddy.

Treatment.—The treatment of the morphia habit is extremely difficult, and can rarely be successfully carried out by the general practitioner. Isolation, systematic feeding, and gradual withdrawal of the drug are the essential elements. As a rule, the patients must be under control in an institution and should be in bed for the first ten days. It is best in a majority of cases to reduce the morphia gradually. The diet should consist of beef-juice, milk, and egg-white, which should be given at short intervals. The sufferings of the patients are usually very great, more particularly the abdominal pains, sometimes nausea and vomiting, and the distressing restlessness. Usually within a week or ten days the opium may be entirely withdrawn. In all cases the pulse should be carefully watched and, if feeble, stimulants should be given, with the aromatic spirit of ammonia and digitalis. For the extreme restlessness a hot bath is serviceable. The sleeplessness is the most distressing symptom, and various drugs may have to be resorted to, particularly hyoscine and sulphonal and sometimes, if the insomnia persists, morphia itself.

It is essential in the treatment of a case to be certain that the patient has no means of obtaining morphia. Even under the favorable circumstances of seclusion in an institution, and constant watching by a night and a day nurse,

I have known a patient to practice deception for a period of three months. After an apparent cure the patients are only too apt to lapse into the habit.

The condition is one which has become so common, and is so much on the increase, that physicians should exercise the utmost caution in prescribing morphia, particularly to female patients. Under no circumstances should a patient be allowed to use the hypodermic syringe, and it is even safer not to intrust this dangerous instrument to the hands of the nurse.

III. LEAD POISONING

(Plumbism, Saturnism)

Etiology.—The disease is widespread, particularly in the lead industries and among plumbers, painters, and glaziers. For the ten years ending 1909, 8,973 cases with 667 deaths were reported to the Home Office (England) as occurring in 18 industries, but Legge points out there has been in this period a reduction of more than 50 per cent. of cases. In the United States it is not easy to get accurate statistics. Alice Hamilton reports 358 cases with 16 deaths in 23 white lead factories during the 16 months to May 1, 1911. In New York State in 1909 and 1910, 60 deaths were certified from lead poisoning. The metal is introduced into the system in many forms. Miners usually escape, but those engaged in the smelting of lead-ores are often attacked. Animals in the neighborhood of smelting furnaces have suffered with the disease, and even the birds that feed on the berries in the neighborhood may be affected. Men engaged in the white-lead factories are particularly prone to plumbism. Accidental poisoning may come in many ways; most commonly by drinking water which has passed through lead pipes or been stored in lead-lined cisterns. Wines and cider which contain acids quickly become contaminated in contact with lead. It was the frequency of colic in certain of the cider districts of Devonshire which gave the name of Devonshire colic, as the frequency of it in Poitou gave the name *colica Pictonum.* Among the innumerable sources of accidental poisoning may be mentioned milk, various sorts of beverages, hair dyes, false teeth, and thread. A few cases have followed the retention of lead bullets in gun-shot wounds. Given medicinally, lead rarely causes poisoning, but we had in the Johns Hopkins Hospital four cases following the use of lead and opium pills for dysentery, of which cause Miller has collected many cases from the literature. It has also followed the use of Emplastrum Diachylon to produce abortion, and there is a case reported in an infant from the application of lead-water on the mother's nipples. One grain every three hours for three days, and two grains every three hours for one day, have caused signs of poisoning. A serious outbreak of lead-poisoning, investigated by David D. Stewart, occurred in Philadelphia, owing to adulteration of a baking-powder with chromate of lead, which was used to give a yellow tint to the cakes.

All ages are attacked, but children are relatively less liable. The largest number of cases occur between thirty and forty. According to Oliver, females are more susceptible than males. They are much more quickly brought under its influence, and in a recent epidemic in which a thousand cases were involved the proportion of females to males was four to one. Miscarriage is common, and it is rare for a woman working in lead to carry a child to term. It also destroys the reproductive power in man.

The lead gains entrance to the system through the lungs, the digestive organs, or the skin. Poisoning may follow the use of cosmetics containing lead. Through the lungs it is freely absorbed. The chief channel, according to Oliver, is the digestive system. It is rapidly eliminated by the kidneys and skin, and is present in the urine of lead-workers. The susceptibility is remarkably varied. The symptoms may be manifest within a month of exposure. On the other hand, Tanquerel (des Planches) met with a case in a man who had been a lead-worker for fifty-two years.

Morbid Anatomy.—Small quantities of lead occur in the body in health. J. J. Putnam's reports show that of 150 persons not presenting symptoms of lead-poisoning traces of lead occurred in the urine of 25 per cent. Of 264 deaths in persons subjects of plumbism 32 were due to an encephalopathy, 43 to Bright's disease, 47 to cerebral hæmorrhage, 43 to paralysis, 44 to lead poisoning, 38 to phthisis, and 40 to various maladies, pneumonia, heart disease, aneurism, etc. (Legge).

In chronic poisoning lead is found in the various organs. The affected muscles are yellow, fatty, and fibroid. The nerves present the features of a peripheral degenerative neuritis. The cord and the nerve-roots are, as a rule, uninvolved. In the primary atrophic form the ganglion cells of the anterior horns are probably implicated. In the acute fatal cases there may be the most intense entero-colitis.

Symptoms.—ACUTE FORM.—We do not refer here to the accidental or suicidal cases, which present vomiting, pain in the abdomen, and collapse symptoms. In workers in lead there are several manifestations which follow a short time after exposure and set in acutely. There may be, in the first place, a rapidly developing anæmia. Acute neuritis has been described, and convulsions, epilepsy, and a delirium, which may be not unlike that produced by alcohol. There are also cases in which the gastro-intestinal symptoms are most intense and rapidly prove fatal. These acute forms occur more frequently in persons recently exposed, and are more frequent in winter than in summer. Da Costa has reported the onset of hemiplegia after three days' exposure to the poison.

CHRONIC POISONING.—(*a*) *Blood Changes.*—A moderate grade of *anæmia,* the so-called saturnine cachexia, is usually present. The corpuscles do not often fall below 50 per cent. Many of the red cells show a remarkable granular, *basophilic degeneration* when stained with Jenner's stain, or with polychrome methylene blue. Grawitz first demonstrated their presence in cases of pernicious anæmia, and Pepper (tertius) and White showed that they were constantly present in lead-poisoning. Further observations by Vaughan and others have shown that such granulations are found in the blood in a great variety of conditions, even in normal blood, but that they are most numerous in lead-poisoning, in which their occurrence in very large numbers is of considerable value in diagnosis. Cadwalader has shown the constant presence of *nucleated red blood-corpuscles* even when the anæmia is of very slight grade.

(*b*) *Blue line* on the gums, which is a valuable indication, but not invariably present. Two lines must be distinguished: one, at the margin between the gums and teeth, is on, not in the gums, and is readily removed by rinsing the mouth and cleansing the teeth. The other is the well-known characteristic blue-black line at the margin of the gum. The color is not uniform, but being in the papillæ of the gums the line is, as seen with a magnifying-glass, interrupted. The lead is absorbed and converted in the tissues into a black sulphide by the action of sulphuretted hydrogen from the tartar of the teeth. The line may form in a few days after exposure (Oliver) and disappear within a few weeks, or may persist for many months. Philipson has noted the occurrence of a black line in miners, due to the deposition of carbon.

The most important symptoms of chronic lead-poisoning are colic, lead-palsy, and the encephalopathy. Of these, the colic is the most frequent. Of Tanquerel's cases, there were 1,217 of colic, 101 of paralysis, and 72 of encephalopathy.

(*c*) *Colic* is the most common symptom of chronic lead-poisoning. It is often preceded by gastric or intestinal symptoms, particularly constipation. The pain is over the whole abdomen. The colic is usually paroxysmal, like true colic, and is relieved by pressure. There is often, in addition, between the paroxysms a dull, heavy pain. There may be vomiting. During the attack, as Riegel noted, the pulse is increased in tension and the heart's action is retarded. Attacks of pain with acute diarrhœa may recur for weeks or even for three or four years.

Certain of the cases with colic may present the features of an acute intra-abdominal inflammatory condition. A case may be admitted to the surgical wards with a diagnosis of appendicitis, or simulate intestinal obstruction. Localized pain, slight fever, and moderate leucocytosis may be present. The history, the presence of a blue line on the gums, and the blood changes are of importance in differential diagnosis.

(*d*) *Lead-palsy.*—This is rarely a primary manifestation. Among 54 cases of lead-poisoning treated in the J. H. H. and dispensary there were 30 cases of lead-paralysis (H. M. Thomas). The upper limbs are most frequently affected. In 26 cases the arms alone were affected, and 18 of these showed the typical double wrist-drop. In 7 the right arm alone was involved, and in one the left. In 4 cases both arms and legs were attacked. The onset may be acute, subacute, or chronic. It usually occurs without fever. In its distribution it may be partial, limited to a muscle or to certain muscle groups, or generalized, involving in a short time the muscles of the extremities and the trunk. Madame Déjerine-Klumpke recognizes the following *localized forms:* (1) Antebrachial type, paralysis of the extensors of the fingers and of the wrist. In this the musculo-spiral nerve is involved, causing the characteristic wrist-drop. The supinator longus usually escapes. In the long-continued flexion of the carpus there may be slight displacement backward of the bones, with distention of the synovial sheaths, so that there is a prominent swelling over the wrist known as Gruebler's tumor. (2) Brachial type, which involves the deltoid, the biceps, the brachialis anticus, and the supinator longus, rarely the pectorals. The atrophy is of the scapulo-humeral form. It is bilateral, and sometimes follows the first form, but it may be primary. (3) The Aran-Duchenne type, in which the small muscles of the hand and of the thenar and hypothenar eminences are involved. The atrophy is marked, and may be the first manifestation of the lead-palsy. Möbius has shown that this form is particularly marked in tailors. (4) The peroneal type. According to Tanquerel, the lower limbs are involved in the proportion of 13 to 100 of the upper limbs. The lateral peroneal muscles, the extensor communis of the toes, and the extensor proprius of the big toe are involved, producing the *steppage* gait. (5) Laryngeal form. Adductor paralysis has been noted by Morell Mackenzie and others in lead-palsy.

Generalized Palsies.—There may be a slow, chronic paralysis, gradually involving the extremities, beginning with the classical picture of wrist-drop. More frequently there is a rapid generalization, producing complete paralysis in all the muscles of the parts in a few days. It may pursue a course like an ascending paralysis, associated with rapid wasting of all four limbs. Such cases, however, are very rare. Death has occurred by involvement of the diaphragm. Oliver reports a case of Philipson's in which complete paralysis supervened. A patient with generalized paralysis was admitted in the winter of 1904 in whom the paralysis began in the legs after but two weeks' work as an enameler. It spread rapidly, so that in a little over a week he was bedridden, and on admission to the hospital nearly every muscle below the neck was involved. The diaphragm was completely paralyzed. He was walking about when he left the hospital, though there was still some weakness remaining. Déjerine-Klumpke also recognizes a febrile form of general paralysis in lead-poisoning, which may closely resemble the subacute spinal paralysis of Duchenne.

There is also a primary saturnine muscular atrophy in which the weakness and wasting come on together. It is this form, according to Gowers, which most frequently assumes the Aran-Duchenne type.

The electrical reactions are those of lesions of the lower motor segment. The reaction of degeneration in its different grades may be present, depending upon the severity of the disease. Usually with the onset of the paralysis there are pains in the legs and joints, the so-called saturnine arthralgias. Sensation may, however, be unaffected.

(*e*) The *cerebral symptoms* are numerous. Seven of our cases showed marked cerebral involvement. One had delusions and maniacal excitement and had to be removed to an asylum. In other cases there occurred transient delirium, attacks of unconsciousness, and in one case convulsions. Optic neuritis or neuro-retinitis may occur. Hysterical symptoms occasionally occur in girls. Convulsions are not uncommon, and in an adult the possibility of lead-poisoning should always be considered. True epilepsy may follow the convulsions. An acute delirium may occur with hallucinations. The patients may have trance-like attacks, which follow or alternate with convulsions. A few cases of lead encephalopathy finally drift into lunatic asylums. Tremor is one of the commonest manifestations of lead-poisoning.

(*f*) *Arterio-sclerosis.*—Lead-workers are notoriously subject to arterio-sclerosis with contracted kidneys and hypertrophy of the heart. The cases usually show distinct gouty deposits, particularly in the big-toe joint; but in the United States acute gout in lead-workers is rare. According to Sir William Roberts, the lead favors the precipitation of the crystalline urates of the tissues.

Prognosis.—In the minor manifestations this is good. According to Gowers, the outlook is bad in the primary atrophic form of paralysis. Convulsions are, as a rule, serious, and the mental symptoms which succeed may be permanent. Occasionally the wrist-drop persists.

Treatment.—Prophylactic measures should be taken at all lead-works, but, unless employees are careful, poisoning is apt to occur even under the most favorable conditions. Cleanliness of the hands and of the finger-nails, frequent bathing, and the use of respirators when necessary should be insisted upon. When the lead is in the system the iodide of potassium should be given in from 5- to 10-grain (0.3-0.6 gm.) doses three times a day. For the colic local applications and, if severe, morphia may be used. An occasional morning purge of magnesium sulphate may be given. For the anæmia iron should be used. In the very acute cases it is well not to give the iodide, as, according to some writers, the liberation of the lead which has been deposited in the tissues may increase the severity of the symptoms. For the local palsies massage and the constant current should be used. Bulletin No. 95 (1911) of the Bureau of Labor, Washington, contains an elaborate study of industrial lead-poisoning in Europe by Oliver, and of the conditions in the United States by Alice Hamilton and John B. Andrews.

IV. ARSENICAL POISONING

Acute poisoning by arsenic is common, particularly by Paris green and such mixtures as "Rough on Rats," which are used to destroy vermin and insects. The chief symptoms are intense pain in the stomach, vomiting, and, later, colic, with diarrhœa and tenesmus; occasionally the symptoms are those of collapse. If recovery takes place, paralysis may follow. The treatment should be similar to that of other irritant poisons—rapid removal with the stomach pump, the promotion of vomiting, and the use of milk and eggs. If the poison has been taken in solution, dialyzed iron may be used in doses of from 6 to 8 drachms.

Chronic Arsenical Poisoning.—Arsenic is used extensively in the arts, particularly in the manufacture of colored papers, artificial flowers, and in many of the fabrics employed as clothing. The glazed green and red papers used in kindergartens also contain arsenic. It is present, too, in many wall-papers and carpets. Much attention has been paid to this question of late years, as instances of poisoning have been thought to depend upon wall-papers and other household fabrics. The arsenic compounds may be either in the form of solid particles detached from the paper or as gaseous volatile bodies formed from arsenical organic matter by the action of several moulds, notably *Penicilium brevicaule, Mucor mucedo,* etc. (Gosio). In moisture, and at a temperature of from 60° to 95° F., a volatile compound is set free, probably "an organic derivative of arsenic pentoxide" (Sanger). The chronic poisoning from fabrics and wall-papers may be due, according to this author, to the ingestion of minute continued doses of this derivative. Contaminated glucose, used in manufacturing beer, caused a widespread epidemic of poisoning at Manchester. The associated presence of selenium compounds may have played a part in the production of the poisoning (Tunnicliffe and Rosenheim). Arsenic is eliminated in all the secretions, and has been found in the milk. J. J. Putnam, it should be remembered, has shown that it is not uncommon to find traces of arsenic in the urine of many persons in apparent health. The effects of moderate quantities of arsenic are not infrequently seen in medical practice. In chorea and in pernicious anæmia steadily increasing doses are often given until the patient takes from 15 to 20 drops of Fowler's solution three times a day. Flushing and hyperæmia of the skin, puffiness of the eyelids or above the eyebrows, nausea, vomiting, and diarrhœa are the most common symptoms. Redness and sometimes bleeding of the gums and salivation occur. In the protracted administration of arsenic patients may complain of numbness and tingling in the fingers. Cutaneous pigmentation and keratosis are very characteristic, and, as a late rare sequence of the latter, epithelioma. In chorea neuritis has occurred, and a patient of mine with Hodgkin's disease had multiple neuritis after taking ℥ iv ʒ j of Fowler's solution in seventy-five days, during which time there were fourteen days on which the drug was omitted.

In the Manchester epidemic nearly all cases presented signs of neuritis and lesions of the skin. In some the sensory disturbances predominated, in others the motor, the individuals being unable to walk or to use their hands. In a certain number there was muscular incoördination, resembling that of locomotor ataxia. Rapid muscular atrophy characterized some cases. In not a few patients a condition of erythromelalgia was present. Occasionally a catarrh of the respiratory and alimentary tracts was the chief feature. Pigmentation, keratosis, and herpes were the most characteristic cutaneous manifestations.

How far similar symptoms are to be attributed to the small quantities of arsenic absorbed from wall-papers and fabrics is by some considered doubtful. That children and adults may take with impunity large doses for months without unpleasant effects, and the fact of the gradual establishment of a toleration which enables Styrian peasants to take as much as 8 grains of arsenious acid in a day, speak strongly against it. On the other hand, as Sanger states, we do not know accurately the effects of many of the compounds in minute and long-continued doses, notably the arsenates.

Arsenical paralysis has the same characteristics as lead-palsy, but the legs are more affected than the arms, particularly the extensors and peroneal group, so that the patient has the characteristic *steppage* gait of peripheral neuritis.

The electrical reaction in the muscles may be disturbed before there is any loss of power, and when the patient is asked to extend the wrist fully and to spread the fingers slight weakness may be detected early.

V. FOOD POISONING

There may be "death in the pot" from many causes. Food poisons may be *endogenous* or *exogenous*. Those articles in which the poison is of endogenous origin can scarcely be designated as foods. The poisonous mushroom, for example, is often mistaken for the edible form. The former is injurious because it normally produces a highly poisonous alkaloid, muscarine. Certain fish also produce normal physiological but toxic products. When eaten by mistake, as frequently occurs in the West Indies and Japan, these fish may cause poisonous symptoms. The exogenous origin of food poisons is by far the commonest. Under this head come those foods which are rendered poisonous by accidental contamination from outside sources. Food may contain the specific organisms of disease, as of tuberculosis or trichinosis; milk and other foods may become infected with typhoid bacilli, and so convey the disease.

Animals (or insects, as bees) may feed on substances which cause their flesh or products to be poisonous to man.

The grains used as food may be infected with fungi and cause the epidemics of ergotism, etc.

Foods of all sorts may become contaminated with the bacteria of putrefaction, the products of which may be highly poisonous.

The term "ptomaine poisoning" has been popularized to such an extent that it is used synonymously with food poisoning. The term *ptomaine* was introduced by the Italian chemist, Selmi, to designate basic alkaloidal products formed in putrefaction. It is largely through the labors of Brieger that our knowledge of ptomaines was gained. Mytilotoxin, found in poisonous mussels, is of this class, and is by far the most poisonous of the known ptomaines.

Among the more common forms are the following:

Meat Poisoning.—Outbreaks of disease due to poisons of bacterial origin or due to chemical changes in meat are not uncommon. Several groups of cases have been recognized.

(*a*) From the colon bacillus or the typho-coli group of organisms, which occupy a position intermediate between the typhoid and colon bacillus. In severe forms symptoms come on a few hours after eating the meat; violent vomiting, purging, pains in the abdomen and collapse and death may occur within twenty-four hours. Individuals react very differently, as shown in the remarkable outbreak investigated by McWeeney in the Industrial School, Limerick. Among 73 cases every grade of severity was seen, from severe cholera nostras to headache with slight fever. Indeed, there were cases without symptoms, but with the typhoid blood reaction.

Some of these cases have a close resemblance to the paratyphoid infection, and, as Durham pointed out, the bacilli are divisible into two groups: The Gaertner type (*B. enteritidis*) and the Aertryk type.

The important matter in connection with this type of poisoning is the unaltered appearance of the meat. The danger seems greatest from beef and veal, and in Germany has particularly followed the use of meat from cattle ill with some septic or diarrhœal condition. Pork is a not infrequent cause in England, and severe attacks have followed the eating of pork pies.

(*b*) Meat poisoning associated with putrefaction. Here alterations of appearance, of smell and taste are usually present. The products are those of protein hydrolysis, various aromatic compounds, but more particularly the bodies known as putrescine, cadaverine and sepsin. How far these bodies themselves are responsible for the symptoms, how far they are due to infection with associated organisms, particularly the proteus and the colon bacilli, has not yet been definitely settled. Many cases of food poisoning have been reported as due to proteus and its toxins. A point of interest is the fact that this organism was found to be the cause of a severe outbreak due to eating potato salad.

(*c*) Meat poisoning due to *Bacillus botulinus.* This is a rare form, the organism of which was discovered by van Ermengem in a ham, the eating of which had given rise to 50 cases of botulism. The symptoms resemble those of atropine poisoning—dryness of the throat, dilatation of the pupil, deafness, facial and cardio-respiratory paralysis.

Certain game birds, particularly the grouse, are poisonous in special districts and at certain seasons. It is interesting to note that mutton and lamb have thus far not been implicated as a cause of food poisoning.

Poisoning by Meat Products.—(*a*) The poisonous effects which follow the drinking of milk infected with saprophytic bacteria are considered in the section on the diarrhœa of infants.

(*b*) *Cheese Poisoning.*—Various milk products, ice cream, custard, and cheese, may prove highly poisonous. Among the poisons Vaughan now states that the tyrotoxicon "is not the one most frequently present, nor is it the most active one." In one epidemic he and Novy have isolated from cheese a substance belonging to the poisonous albumins, and in an extensive ice-cream epidemic Vaughan and Perkins found in the ice cream a highly pathogenic bacillus, but its toxin has not been separated. The symptoms are those of acute gastro-intestinal irritation.

Poisoning by Shell-fish and Fish.—(*a*) *Mussel Poisoning.*—Brieger has separated a ptomaine—mytilotoxin—which exists chiefly in the liver of the mussel. The observations of Schmidtmann and Cameron have shown that the mussel from the open sea only becomes poisonous when placed in filthy waters, as at Wilhelmshafen.

Dangerous, even fatal, effects may follow the eating of either raw or cooked mussels. The symptoms are those of an acute poisoning with profound action on the nervous system, and without gastro-intestinal manifestations. There are numbness and coldness, no fever, dilated pupils, and rapid pulse; death occurs sometimes within two hours with collapse symptoms. In an epidemic at Wilhelmshafen, Germany, in 1885, nineteen persons were attacked, four of whom died. Salkowski and Brieger isolated the *mytilotoxin* from specimens of the mussels. Poisoning occasionally follows the eating of oysters which are stale or decomposed. The symptoms are usually gastro-intestinal.

(*b*) *Fish Poisoning.*—There are two distinct varieties; in one the poison is a physiological product of certain glands of the fish, in the other it is a product of bacterial growth. The salted sturgeon used in parts of Russia has sometimes proved fatal to large numbers of persons. In the middle parts of Europe the barb is stated to be sometimes poisonous, producing the so-called "*barben cholera.*" In China and Japan various species of the *tetrodon* are also toxic, sometimes causing death within an hour, with symptoms of intense disturbance of the nervous system.

Grain and Vegetable Food Poisoning.—(*a*) *Ergotism.*—The prolonged use of meal made from grains contaminated with the ergot fungus (*claviceps purpurea*) causes a series of symptoms known as ergotism, epidemics of which have prevailed in different parts of Europe. Two forms of this chronic ergotism are described—the one, gangrenous, is believed to be due to the sphacelinic acid, the other, convulsive or spasmodic, is due to the cornutin. In the former mortification affects the extremities—usually the toes and fingers, less commonly the ears and nose. Preceding the onset of the gangrene there are usually anæsthesia, tingling, pains, spasmodic movements of the muscles, and gradual blood stasis in certain vascular territories.

The nervous manifestations are very remarkable. After a prodromal stage of ten to fourteen days, in which the patient complains of weakness, headache, and tingling sensations in different parts of the body, perhaps accompanied with slight fever, symptoms of spasm develop, producing cramps in the muscles and contractures. The arms are flexed and the legs and toes extended. These spasms may last from a few hours to many days and relapses are frequent. In severer cases epilepsy develops and the patient may die in convulsions. Mental symptoms are common, manifested sometimes in a preliminary delirium, but more commonly, in the chronic poisoning, as melancholia or dementia. Posterior spinal sclerosis occurs in chronic ergotism. In the interesting group of 29 cases studied by Tuczek and Siemens 9 died at various periods after the infection, and four post mortems showed degeneration of the posterior columns. A condition similar to tabes dorsalis is gradually produced by this slow degeneration in the spinal cord.

(*b*) *Lathyrism* (Lupinosis).—An affection produced by the use of meal from varieties of vetches, chiefly the *Lathyrus sativus* and *L. cicera.* The grain is popularly known as the chick-pea. The grains are usually powdered and mixed with the meal from other cereals in the preparation of bread. As early as the seventeenth century it was noticed that the use of flour with which the seeds of the *Lathyrus* were mixed caused stiffness of the legs. The subject did not, however, attract much attention before the studies of James Irving, in India, who between 1859 and 1868 published several important communications, describing a form of spastic paraplegia affecting large numbers of the inhabitants in certain regions of India and due to the use of meal made from the *Lathyrus* seeds. It also produces a spastic paraplegia in animals. The Italian observers describe a similar form of paraplegia, and it has been observed in Algiers by the French physicians. The condition is that of a spastic paralysis, involving chiefly the legs, which may proceed to complete paraplegia. The arms are rarely, if ever, affected. It is evidently a slow sclerosis induced under the influence of this toxic agent. The precise anatomical condition, so far as I can ascertain, has not yet been determined.

(*c*) *Potato-poisoning.*—It has long been known that potatoes contain normally a very small amount (about 0.06 per cent.) of the poisonous principle solanin, but it is only quite recently that it has been discovered that, under certain circumstances, they may contain the poison in amounts sufficient to cause grave disturbance of the system. The increase is due to the action of at least two species of bacteria, *Bacterium solaniferum non-colorabile* and *Bacterium solaniferum colorabile,* and occurs in those tubers which, during growth, have lain partially exposed above ground, and in those which, during storage, have become well sprouted. The most extensive outbreak of potato-poisoning recorded occurred in 1899 in a German regiment, fifty-six members of which, after eating sprouted potatoes, were seized with chills, fever, headache, vomiting, diarrhœa, colic, and great prostration. Many were jaundiced and several collapsed, but all recovered. Samples of the remaining potatoes yielded 0.38 per cent. of solanin, and this would indicate that a full portion must have contained about 5 grains.

Treatment.—The source of the infection must be ascertained and the offending food destroyed. The stomach should be washed out and the bowels evacuated by a brisk saline purge. Saline infusions, hypodermic or intravenous, may promote the elimination of the toxins.

VI. PELLAGRA

Definition.—A disorder of metabolism, with periodical manifestations characterized by gastro-intestinal disturbances, skin lesions, and a tendency to changes in the nervous system.

Historical.—The disease appears to have been endemic in Spain by 1735 and the first description is by Cazal (1762), who named it *mal de la rosa.* It existed in Italy in 1750 and was described in 1771 by Frapolli, who gave it the name of pellagra (rough skin). By the eighteenth century it had spread over northern Italy and had appeared in France and Roumania. It is quite probable that there have been sporadic cases in the United States for the last fifty years.

Distribution.—The disease is prevalent in parts of southern Europe, particularly in Italy and Roumania. There are probably 100,000 cases in Italy and 50,000 in Roumania. It exists in Spain, Portugal, France, Egypt and the United States, in the southern part of which country the disease has spread with extraordinary rapidity in the last few years. Better diagnosis can hardly explain the frequency, as the disease is so striking in its manifestations that many cases could hardly be overlooked. There is evidence that the disease is to some extent one of particular localities, as beri-beri; it is also a disease of the country more than of the cities. This applies particularly to Europe, but in the United States many of the small towns and villages show a number of cases. As regards the influence of place, the number of cases in the asylums of the United States is significant. A few cases have occurred in England.

Etiology.—There are two main views, one that it is due to a defect in the diet, in other words, a deficiency disease, and the other that it is due to infection of some kind. If the latter be the case the infectious agent is apparently not conveyed directly from person to person, and Sambon suggested that it may be a protozoal disease, carried by sand flies of the genus *Simulium.* There is absence of proof that the disease is communicated from one person to another. In the Italian institutions, where a large number of pellagrins are treated, no attendant has contracted the disease. If due to food intoxication, the accused article is corn (maize), comparable to the part thought to be played by rice in beri-beri. The experiments of Goldberger and Wheeler support the dietetic view. Eleven prisoners were kept on ordinary diet from February 4 to April 19, 1915, from which date until October 31, 1915, they received a restricted diet lacking meat, eggs, milk, beans, peas and other proteins. The food was chiefly maize, rice, sweet potatoes, brown gravy, syrup, sugar and coffee—all of the best quality. Within five months, six of the eleven volunteers had dermatitis said by experts to be pellagra.

Age.—The disease occurs at any age, but the majority of cases are between twenty and forty years. As regards races, the negro is more susceptible than the white, and, in reference to sex, women are apparently slightly more susceptible than men.

OCCUPATION.—In Europe the disease is almost confined to laborers of the poorer classes, but this is not true of the United States.

SEASON.—The effect of this is very striking and the disease occurs particularly in the spring and sometimes in the autumn, both in its onset and recurrences.

Pathology.—There is nothing characteristic in the morbid anatomy. In the acute cases there may be atrophy of the walls of the intestines, fatty degeneration of the internal organs and changes in the nervous system. The alterations in the cord are fairly constant. There is degeneration of the lateral columns in the dorsal region and of the posterior columns in the cervical and dorsal regions. In the brains of patients with mental deterioration atrophy of the cerebrum is found. As regards the *pathogenesis* there are two views, one that it is a chronic disease with recurring exacerbations, the other that it is due to repeated poisoning.

Symptoms.—These vary markedly in severity, usually appearing in the spring and sometimes in the autumn. There is always a tendency to recurrence, and with each succeeding attack more damage is done, particularly to the nervous system. The onset is usually in the spring with indefinite symptoms, such as weakness, headache, and depression.

DIGESTIVE TRACT.—Disturbance of the alimentary tract is usually an early symptom. In the mouth there may be sensations of heat, with loss of taste. Stomatitis is common, the mucous membrane is very red, ulcers may appear and the epithelium is stripped off, leaving a raw surface so that chewing is painful. Anorexia, nausea, vomiting and dyspeptic symptoms are common; there is also diarrhœa, often severe and accompanied by pain, the stools being serous or bloody. It may alternate with constipation.

SKIN.—The erythema usually begins on the backs of the hands and at first resembles an ordinary sunburn. There may be puffy swelling. The affected areas are symmetrical and sharply defined as a rule, extending above the wrist and down to the last finger joint. The face, neck and feet may be affected in the same way. The process may not advance any further, the skin becomes darker and desquamates, after which some pigmentation remains. In other cases vesicles and bullæ form, containing serum or pus. These dry gradually, with the production of fissures. After drying and desquamation the skin may have a dry appearance and a deep red color. With repeated attacks the skin may become indurated, thickened and dark in color; later atrophy and thinning may follow. Exposure to the sun may have an influence on the eruption, but is not the cause. The erythema occurs sometimes on protected parts.

NERVOUS SYSTEM.—Headache and vertigo are common. Mental features are often marked, among which are confusion, dullness, lassitude, irritability, feelings of anxiety and depression, change in the disposition, and hallucinations of sight and hearing. These may progress to profound depression and ultimately to dementia. Mania occurs sometimes and suicidal tendencies are not uncommon. The symptoms due to changes in the *cord* vary with the lesion. A spastic condition, disturbances of sensation, paralysis of the sphincters, or loss of the reflexes of the legs may be found.

The blood shows no special features beyond those of a secondary anæmia. The temperature is usually normal except in the acute cases in which fever occurs.

Clinical Forms.—The disease occurs in two main forms, an acute and a chronic recurrent form. In the acute form there are fever, marked prostration, severe diarrhœa, delirium or stupor and a rapid downward course. Death may occur in a few weeks from the onset. These cases seem to be more frequent in the United States than in Europe. In the chronic form the manifestations are not severe, but tend to recur each year, and each attack leaves the patient in a worse condition. There is always the tendency to mental deterioration which occurs in fully 10 per cent. of the cases. Death occurs from exhaustion and cachexia, or some intercurrent disease. Fortunately, succeeding attacks are not necessarily more severe than the preceding ones. There are instances of this form persisting for twenty-five years. Cases without the skin lesions—pellagra sine pellagra—have been described.

Diagnosis.—A typical case offers no difficulties, but in the absence of the skin lesions considerable difficulty may be experienced. Scurvy might give difficulty, but the absence of the other features of pellagra should be conclusive. Skin lesions of the nature of erythema might cause confusion, but the absence of the general features removes doubt. Sprue may be difficult to separate; in fact, some consider it a form of pellagra. The psychical features might suggest general paresis, but the skin lesions and digestive disturbance should make the diagnosis clear. The acute cases might be mistaken for various infections, but the erythema and gastro-intestinal features should prevent this.

Prognosis.—In the United States the outlook is regarded as serious, if not as regards death, certainly as regards ultimate recovery. In Europe, where the disease has existed for a long time, the prognosis is more favorable, and in Italy in some years the mortality was only 4 per cent. In cases with acute features or fever the prognosis is grave and signs of severe toxæmia or of mental involvement are ominous. Erythema of a moist character is regarded as a grave sign. Any complications should be regarded seriously. The prognosis is best in the chronic cases without mental features. The outlook is serious in asylum cases.

Prophylaxis.—"Peasant life, poverty, and polenta (corn)" have been given as the causal factors. Improvement in the living conditions and good sanitation are important points in the prevention. Too much corn or maize should not be used, particularly in institutions. The experiments noted above suggest that it is a deficiency disease which may possibly be eradicated by a proper protein diet, as has been the case with beri-beri.

Treatment.—The patient should be placed in the best general conditions and a change of diet and climate is advisable. Rest in bed is necessary while the symptoms are acute. The diet should be as nutritious as possible and the diarrhœa need not interfere with taking sufficient nourishment. Salt should be given freely. There is no proof that we have any remedy with a specific influence. Arsenic has been given by the mouth or by injection. Atoxyl and salvarsan have been used in ordinary dosage, but arsenic by mouth, as Fowler's solution, is apparently more useful than the newer preparations given by injection. Transfusion of blood, both from healthy individuals and those who have recovered from the disease, has been done apparently with good results in some cases. Symptomatic treatment, on the whole, seems to have been as successful as any special measure and should be carried out as demanded by the conditions in each patient.

VII. BERI-BERI

(Kakke, Endemic Multiple Neuritis)

Definition.—A deficiency disease due to the absence of certain elements of the food, the so-called vitamines, and characterized clinically by multiple neuritis, anasarca, and muscular atrophy.

History.—The disease is believed to be of great antiquity in China, and is possibly mentioned in the oldest known medical treatise. In the early years of the nineteenth century it attracted much attention among the Anglo-Indian surgeons, and we may date the modern scientific study of the disease from Malcolmson's monograph, published at Madras in 1835. The opening of Japan gave an opportunity to the European physicians holding university positions, particularly Anderson, Baelz, Scheube, and more recently Grimm, to investigate the disease. The studies of the native Japanese physicians, particularly Miura and Takagi, and of the Dutch physicians in the East, have contributed much to our knowledge. The recent studies of Schaumann, Fraser, Stanton, and others and the dietetic experiments in the Philippines have confirmed the older views that it is a disorder depending upon an imperfect dietary.

Distribution.—It is specially prevalent among the Malays, Chinese and Japanese, and during the Russian war more than 50,000 cases occurred in the Japanese army. It prevails excessively in the Philippines. In India it is less common. Localized outbreaks have occurred in Australia. It prevails in parts of South America, and in the West Indies. It is met with among the fishermen of Norway and of the Newfoundland Banks. It occurs also in asylums, in which there have been severe outbreaks in the United States, and in the Richmond Asylum, Dublin, in the years 1894, 1896 and 1897 under conditions of over-crowding.

Etiology.—Two main views have prevailed: That it is an acute infection and that it is a disorder of metabolism. Numerous bacteriological studies have not determined the presence of any definite organism. On the other hand, the work of the past few years has confirmed the food theory widely held in Japan.

Studies in the Far East leave no doubt that the disease is there due to a diet of rice from which the pericarp has been removed, in what is called "polishing" or "milling." This is an old story, as the Dutch knew of the association of the disease with rice, and it was by modifying the rice diet of the sailors that Takagi eradicated beri-beri from the Japanese navy. Braddon, too, showed the importance of the retention of the pericarp for the prevention of the disease.

Schaumann's experiments, which have been amply confirmed by Fraser and Stanton, leave no question that beri-beri is associated with a diet freed from the materials existing in the pericarp. Whether these are the phosphorus compounds, as Schaumann believes, or unknown substances, the so-called vitamines, as Fraser and Stanton hold, has not yet been settled.

That beri-beri occurs in ships and in institutions may be explained by the fact that in the dietary, though it may not be of rice, similar compounds are lacking. On the other hand, certain French workers in the East hold that white rice alone does not produce the disease, and that there must be some other factor, since the great majority of rice-eaters in the East are immune.

Other factors are overcrowding, as in ships, jails and asylums, hot and moist seasons, and exposure to wet. Males are more subject to the disease than females. Under good hygienic conditions Europeans rarely contract the disease.

Symptoms.—The incubation period is unknown, but it probably extends over several months. The following forms of the disease are recognized by Scheube:

(*a*) The incomplete or rudimentary form which often sets in with catarrhal symptoms, followed by pains and weakness in the limbs and a lowering of the sensibility in the legs, with the occurrence of paræsthesia. Slight œdema sometimes appears. After a time paræsthesia is felt in other parts of the body, and the patient may complain of palpitation of the heart, uneasy sensations in the abdomen, and sometimes shortness of breath. There may be weakness and tenderness of the muscles. After lasting from a few days to many months, these symptoms all disappear, but with the return of the warm weather there may be a recurrence. One of Scheube's patients suffered in this way for twenty years.

(*b*) The atrophic form sets in with much the same symptoms, but the loss of power in the limbs progresses more rapidly, and very soon the patient is no longer able to walk or to move the arms. The atrophy, which is associated with a good deal of pain, may extend to the muscles of the face. The œdematous symptoms and heart troubles play a minor rôle in this form, which is known as the dry or paralytic variety.

(*c*) The Wet or Dropsical Form.—Setting in as in the rudimentary variety, the œdema soon becomes the most marked feature, extending over the whole subcutaneous tissue, and associated with effusions into the serous sacs. The atrophy of the muscles and disturbance of sensation are not such prominent symptoms. On the other hand, palpitation and rapid action of the heart and dyspnœa are common. The wasting may not be apparent until the dropsy disappears.

(*d*) The acute, pernicious, or cardiac form is characterized by threatenings of an acute cardiac failure, coming on rapidly after the existence of slight symptoms, such as occur in the rudimentary form. Death may follow within twenty-four hours; more commonly the symptoms extend over several weeks. Widespread paralysis with anæsthesia may be present.

The mortality of the disease varies greatly, from 2 or 3 per cent. to 40 or 50 per cent. among the coolies in certain of the settlements of the Malay Archipelago.

Morbid Anatomy.—The most constant and striking features are changes in the peripheral nerves and degenerative inflammation involving the axis cylinder and medullary sheaths. In the acute cases this is found not only in the peripheral nerves, but also in the pneumogastric and in the phrenic. The fibres of the voluntary muscles, as well as of the myocardium, are also much degenerated.

Diagnosis.—In tropical countries there is rarely any difficulty in the diagnosis. In cases of peripheral neuritis, associated with œdema, coming from tropical ports, the possibility of this disease should be remembered.

The peculiar epidemic dropsy of Calcutta and Bengal is probably beri-beri. Greig has shown it to be a nutritional disorder associated with the use of polished rice.

Prophylaxis.—Much has been done to prevent the disease, particularly in Japan. There has been no more remarkable triumph of modern hygiene than Takagi's dietetic reforms in the Japanese navy. Everywhere in the East a change in the diet has been followed by the disappearance of the disease. In the Straits Settlements a group of men took No. 1 polished white Siam rice, and developed beri-beri within sixty days. A group that took unpolished rice remained free from the disease. By exchange of clothing, contact, living together, the disease was not conveyed from one group to the other. Then the group that had partaken of the unpolished rice was fed with polished rice, and within two months developed beri-beri.

The change of diet in the Philippine Scouts instituted on September 30th, 1909, has been followed by remarkable results. Instead of 20 ounces of highly milled rice, the amount was limited to 16 ounces of unpolished rice. The number of admissions for the disease in 1908 and 1909 in a strength of men of 5,000 was 619 and 558. In 1910 there were 50 cases, and in the first five months of 1911 only one case. Chamberlain, from whose report I quote, states that the Philippine experiments bear out at every point the polished rice theory of the production of the disease. After having been continuously present for five years at the Culion Leper Colony in the Philippines, beri-beri disappeared entirely in nine months after the use of unpolished rice was enforced (Heiser).

Treatment.—It is a very chronic and obstinate malady. A nutritious diet, without much rice, rest in bed, purgation for the dropsy, cardiac stimulants, and the usual measures for the neuritis are the important factors in the treatment. Salicylates and saline laxatives are used in Japan. When the œdema has subsided massage, passive movements, and electricity may be used for the atrophic muscles.

SECTION IV

DISEASES OF METABOLISM

I. GOUT

(*Podagra*)

Definition.—A disorder of metabolism associated with retention of uric acid and of other purin bodies in the body, characterized clinically by attacks of acute arthritis, the deposition of sodium-biurate in and about the joints, and by the occurrence of irregular constitutional symptoms.

Etiology.—The purin bodies, adenin, guanin, hypoxanthin, xanthin, and uric acid, result from the transformation of the nucleo-proteins of the food and of the tissues by ferments or enzymes, each one of which has its own specific action. Among the proteolytic enzymes nuclease has a universal distribution, and, no matter what the source of the nucleo-protein, it sets free adenin and guanin. Specific enzymes also liberate uric acid from the nucleo-proteins of the tissues and from the purins of the food. Once formed, the difficulty is to get rid of uric acid from the system, and this appears to be one essential factor in the etiology of gout. Birds and serpents, unable to oxidize it, excrete large quantities. "All mammals, with the important exception of man, are able to destroy uric acid rapidly and in considerable quantities. This destruction is an oxidation accomplished by a specific enzyme called uricase, and the reaction seems to consist of the removal of one of the carbon atoms from the uric acid, thus converting it into the more readily soluble allantoin" (Wells). These transforming enzymes are very variously distributed in the body; nuclease is present in all cells, adenase and the xanthin enzyme are not so widely distributed. Uricase, on which the uricolytic power of the different tissues depends, is present chiefly in the liver and kidneys of mammals, and to a less degree in the muscles. Man alone seems to have a difficulty in oxidizing uric acid. Even on a purin-free diet he excretes daily a certain amount, and purin-rich food is at once followed by a rise. In other mammals it is readily oxydized into allantoin, of which human urine never contains more than a trace.

Gout, then, cannot be regarded as loss of the power of a given individual to destroy uric acid, since this does not appear to be an active function in the human body. Loss of power to eliminate favors the deposition of uric acid, and individuals who cannot get rid easily of their purins, endogenous or exogenous, may be said to be gouty.

There is a form of gout in swine, characterized by a deposit of guanin in the muscles—the chalky flakes which are so often seen in old Virginia and Westphalian hams—and it has been found that the pig's liver is deficient in the enzyme guanase, which in other animals oxidizes this purin body. We cannot say yet how great is the part played by uric acid in human gout and how much by the other purin bodies, but recent work favors the view that imperfect elimination rather than imperfect oxidation of the purin bodies is the chief factor in the disease.

The normal daily output of uric acid is from 0.04 to 1.0 gm., and it is greater by day than by night. The amount from the intake of the exogenous oxy-purins varies from 40 to 60 per cent. of the total purin content. The more active the functions of the body the greater the discharge. Severe exertion, fever and exposure to cold increase the output. The amount is greatly influenced by food, particularly when rich in purin bases. For example, after a meal containing sweetbread the amount may be doubled. In gouty persons the output is low, and I have had cases of tophaceous gout in which, in the intervals between the attacks, the excretion was nil (Futcher). With the onset of an attack the output rises, and the phosphoric acid is also greatly increased, as shown in Chart XIV.

PREDISPOSING FACTORS.—Heredity is important. In from 50 per cent. to 60 per cent. of all cases the disease existed in the parents or grandparents, and the transmission is more marked on the male side. Males are more subject than females. It is rarely seen before the thirtieth year, though cases have occurred before puberty, and even in infants at the breast.

Alcohol is an important factor in the etiology. Fermented liquors are more apt to cause it than distilled spirits, and the disease is much more common in England and in Germany, the countries which consume the largest amount of beer *per capita*. The disease is common in the United States, and is perhaps on the increase. As Futcher pointed out, gout is only one-third less frequent at the Johns Hopkins Hospital than at St. Bartholomew's Hospital, London. Among 18,000 patients in my wards there were 59 cases of gout; all but three in whites, and all in males but two (Futcher).

Food plays a rôle of importance equal to alcohol. Overeating without active exercise is a special predisposing cause. But the disease is by no means confined to the well-to-do. A combination of poor food, defective hygiene and the excessive consumption of malt liquors makes "poor man's gout" not infrequent.

Occupation is of great importance, and the disease is much more common in workers in breweries, and in persons who deal in any way with alcohol.

It is not uncommon in persons of great mental and bodily vigor. Among distinguished members of our profession who have been terrible sufferers were the elder Scaliger, Jerome Cardan and Sydenham. The statement of the latter, however, that "more wise men than fools are victims" of the affection, does not hold good to-day. The celebrated Pirckheimer wrote a famous "Apology for Gout" (1521), and there is much truth in what Podagra says: "For I take no pleasure in those hard, rough, rusticke, agresticke kind of people, who never are at rest, but always exercise their bodies with hard labors, are ever moyling and toyling, do seldom or never give themselves to pleasure, do endure hunger, which are content with a slender diet." (English Edition, 1617.)

Among the directly EXCITING CAUSES of an attack may be mentioned a meal with large quantities of rich food and too much to drink; worry, or a sudden mental shock, and in sensitive persons a slight injury or accident may be followed by acute arthritis.

Morbid Anatomy.—The *blood* contains an excess of uric acid. The average amount in 156 non-gouty patients was 1.7 mgs. per 100 gm. of blood with variations from 0.7 to 4.5 mgs. (Adler and Ragle). Pratt's studies in 16

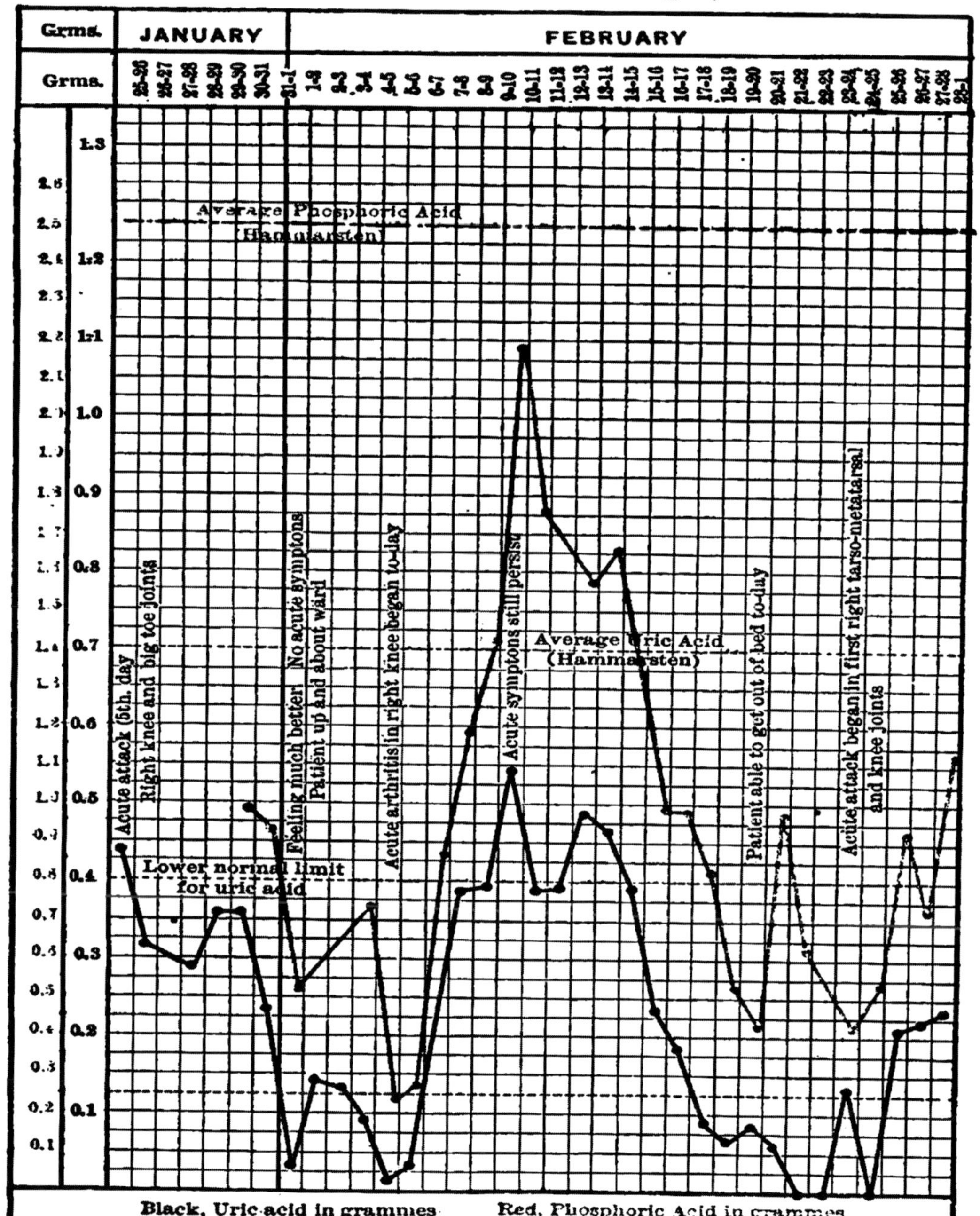

Chart XIV.—Uric Acid and Phosphoric Acid Output in Case of Acute Gout.

gouty patients showed an average of 3.7 mgs. per 100 gm. of blood. The high uric acid content is generally constant in gout and the amount is apparently greater during an attack than in the intervals. This excess, also, is not peculiar to gout, but occurs in leukæmia and chlorosis. The red cells in the "lead-gout" cases may show basophilic granular staining.

The important changes are in the articular tissues. The first joint of the great toe is most frequently involved; then the ankles, knees, and the small joints of the hands and wrists. The deposits may be in all the joints of the lower limbs and absent from those of the upper limbs (Norman Moore). If death takes place during an acute paroxysm, there are signs of inflammation, hyperæmia, swelling of the ligamentous tissues, and of effusion into the joint. The primary change, according to Ebstein, is a local necrosis, due to the presence of an excess of urates in the blood. This is seen in the cartilage and other articular tissues in which the nutritional currents are slow. In these areas of coagulation necrosis the reaction is always acid and the neutral urates are deposited in crystalline form, as insoluble acid urate. The articular cartilages are first involved. The gouty deposit may be uniform, or in small areas. Though it looks superficial, the deposit is invariably interstitial and covered by a thin lamina of cartilage. The deposit is thickest at the part most distant from the circulation. The ligaments and fibro-cartilage ultimately become involved and are infiltrated with biurate deposits, the so-called chalk-stones, or tophi. These are usually covered by skin; but in some cases, particularly in the metacarpo-phalangeal articulations, this ulcerates and the chalk-stones appear externally. The synovial fluid may also contain crystals. In very long-standing cases, owing to an excessive deposit, the joint becomes immobile. The marginal outgrowths in gouty arthritis are true exostoses (Wynne). The cartilage of the ear may contain tophi, which are seen as whitish nodules at the margin of the helix. The cartilages of the nose, eyelids, and larynx are less frequently affected.

Of changes in the internal organs those in the renal and vascular systems are the most important. The kidney changes believed to be characteristic of gout are: (*a*) A deposit of urates chiefly in the region of the papillæ. This, however, is less common than is usually supposed. Norman Moore found it in only 12 out of 80 cases. The apices of the pyramids show lines of whitish deposit: Ebstein has described and figured areas of necrosis in both cortex and medulla, in the interior of which were crystalline deposits of urate of soda. (*b*) An interstitial nephritis, either the ordinary "contracted kidney" or the arterio-sclerotic form, neither of which is in any way distinctive.

The metatarso-phalangeal joint of the big toe should be carefully examined, as it may show typical lesions of gout without any outward token of arthritis.

Arterio-sclerosis and cardiac hypertrophy are very constant lesions. Concretions of urate of soda may occur on the valves. Myocarditis is common.

Changes in the respiratory system are rare. Deposits have been found in the vocal cords, and uric-acid crystals have been found in the sputum of a gouty patient (J. W. Moore).

Symptoms.—Gout is usually divided into acute, chronic, and irregular forms.

ACUTE GOUT.—Premonitory symptoms are common—twinges of pain in the small joints of the hands or feet, nocturnal restlessness, irritability of temper, and dyspepsia. The urine is acid, scanty, and high-colored. It deposits urates on cooling, and there may be transient albuminuria. There may be traces of sugar (gouty glycosuria). Before an attack the output of uric acid is low and is also diminished in the early part of the paroxysm. The relation of uric and phosphoric acids to the acute attacks is well represented in Chart XIV, prepared by Futcher. Both are extremely low in the intervals, but reach normal limits shortly after the onset of the acute symptoms. The phosphoric acid and uric acid show almost parallel curves. The patient was on a very light fixed diet at the time the determinations were made. In some instances the throat is sore, and there may be asthmatic symptoms. The attack sets in usually in the early morning hours. The patient is aroused by a severe pain in the metatarso-phalangeal articulation of the big toe, and more commonly on the right than on the left side. The pain is agonizing, and, as Sydenham says, "insinuates itself with the most exquisite cruelty among the numerous small bones of the tarsus and metatarsus, in the ligaments of which it is lurking." The joint swells rapidly, and becomes hot, tense, and shiny. The sensitiveness is extreme, and the pain makes the patient feel as if the joint were being pressed in a vice. There is fever, and the temperature may rise to 102° to 103° F. Toward morning the severity of the symptoms subsides, and, although the joint remains swollen, the day may be passed in comparative comfort. The symptoms recur the next night, and the fit, as it is called, usually lasts for from five to eight days, the severity of the symptoms gradually abating. There is usually a moderate leucocytosis during the acute manifestations. Occasionally other joints are involved, particularly the big toe of the opposite foot. The inflammation, however intense, never goes on to suppuration. With the subsidence of the swelling the skin desquamates. The tarsus alone may be involved and so obstinate may be the inflammation that the question of surgical interference may be raised in the belief that it is tuberculous or suppurative. After the attack the general health may be much improved. As Aretæus remarks, a person in the interval has won the race at the Olympian games. Recurrences are frequent. Some patients have three or four attacks in a year; others suffer at longer intervals.

The term *retrocedent* or *suppressed* gout is applied to serious internal symptoms, coincident with a rapid disappearance or improvement of the local signs. Very remarkable manifestations may occur under these circumstances. The patient may have severe gastro-intestinal symptoms—pain, vomiting, diarrhœa, and great depression—and death may occur during such an attack. Or there may be cardiac manifestations—dyspnœa, pain, and irregular action of the heart. In some instances, in which the gout is said to attack the heart, an acute pericarditis proves fatal. So, too, there may be marked cerebral manifestations—delirium or coma, and even apoplexy—but in a majority of these instances the symptoms are, in all probability, uræmic.

Chronic Gout.—With increased frequency in the attacks, the articular symptoms persist for a longer time, and gradually many joints become affected. Deposits of urates take place, at first in the articular cartilages and then in the ligaments and capsular tissues; so that in the course of years the joints become swollen, irregular, and deformed. The feet are usually first affected, then the hands. In severe cases there may be extensive concretions about the elbows and knees and along the tendons and in the bursæ. The tophi appear in the ears. Finally, a unique clinical picture is produced which can not be mistaken for that of any other affection. The skin over the tophi may rupture or ulcerate, and about the knuckles the chalk-stones may be freely exposed. Patients with chronic gout are usually dyspeptic, often of a sallow complexion, and show signs of arterio-sclerosis. The pulse tension is increased, the vessels are stiff, and the left ventricle is hypertrophied. The urine is increased in amount, is of low specific gravity, and usually contains a slight amount of albumin, with a few hyaline casts. Severe cramps involving the calf, abdominal, and thoracic muscles are common. Intercurrent attacks of acute polyarthritis may occur, in which the joints become inflamed, and the temperature ranges from 101° to 103° F. There may be pain, redness, and swelling of several joints without fever. Uræmia, pleurisy, pericarditis, peritonitis, and meningitis are common terminal affections.

Irregular Gout.—This is a motley, ill-defined group of symptoms, manifestations of a condition of disordered nutrition, to which the terms *gouty diathesis* or *lithœmic state* have been given. Cases are seen in members of gouty families, who may never themselves have suffered from the acute disease, and in persons who have lived not wisely but too well, who have eaten and drunk largely, lived sedentary lives, and yet have been fortunate enough to escape an acute attack. It is interesting to note the various manifestations of the disease in a family with marked hereditary disposition. The daughters often escape, while one son may have gouty attacks of great severity, even though he lives a temperate life and tries in every way to avoid the conditions favoring the disorder. Another son has, perhaps, only the irregular manifestations and never the acute articular affection. While the irregular features are perhaps more often met with in the hereditary affection, they are by no means infrequent in persons who appear to have acquired the disease. The tendency in some families is to call every affection gouty. Even infantile complaints, such as scald-head, naso-pharyngeal vegetations, and enuresis, are often regarded, without sufficient grounds, as evidences of the family ailment. Among the commonest manifestations of irregular gout are the following:

(*a*) *Cutaneous Eruptions.*—Garrod and others have called special attention to the frequent association of eczema with the gouty habit.

(*b*) *Gastro-intestinal Disorders.*—Attacks of what is termed biliousness, in which the tongue is furred, the breath foul, the bowels constipated, and the action of the liver torpid, are not uncommon in gouty persons. A gouty parotitis is described.

(*c*) *Cardio-vascular Symptoms.*—With gout arterio-sclerosis is frequently associated. The blood tension is persistently high, the vessel walls become stiff, and cardiac and renal changes gradually occur. In this condition the symptoms may be renal, as when the albuminuria becomes more marked, or dropsical symptoms supervene. The manifestations may be cardiac, when the hypertrophy of the left ventricle fails and there are palpitation, irregular action, and ultimately a condition of asystole. Or, finally, the manifestations may be vascular, and thrombosis of the coronary arteries may cause sudden death, or, as most frequently happens, a blood-vessel gives away in the brain, and the patient dies of apoplexy. It makes but little difference whether we regard this condition as primarily an arterio-sclerosis or as a gouty nephritis; the point to be remembered is that the nutritional disorder with which an excess of uric acid is associated induces in time increased tension, arterio-sclerosis, chronic interstitial nephritis, and changes in the myocardium. Pericarditis is not an infrequent terminal complication of gout. Phlebitis is a troublesome and not very uncommon complication. It may arise in connection with varicose veins of the legs or it may occur in many venous districts in succession or simultaneously.

(*d*) *Nervous Manifestations.*—Headache and migraine attacks are not infrequent. Neuralgias, sciatica, and paræsthesias are not uncommon. A common gouty manifestation, upon which Duckworth has laid stress, is the occurrence of hot or itching feet at night. Plutarch mentions that Strabo called this symptom "the lisping of the gout." Cramps in the legs may also be very troublesome. Hutchinson has called attention to hot and itching eyeballs. Associated or alternating with this symptom there may be attacks of episcleral congestion. Apoplexy is a common termination of gout. Meningitis may occur, usually basilar.

(*e*) *Urinary Disorders.*—The urine is highly acid and high-colored, and may deposit on standing crystals of uric acid. Transient and temporary increase in this ingredient cannot be regarded as serious. In many cases of chronic gout the amount may be diminished, and increased only at certain periods, forming the so-called uric-acid showers. A sediment of uric acid in a urine does not necessarily mean an excess. It is often dependent on the inability of the urine to hold it in solution. Sugar is found intermittently in the urine of gouty persons—gouty glycosuria. It may pass into true diabetes, but is usually very amenable to treatment. Oxaluria may also be present. Gouty persons are specially prone to calculi, Jerome Cardan to the contrary, who reckoned freedom from stone among the chief of the *dona podagræ.* Minute quantities of albumin are very common in persons of gouty dyscrasia, and, when the renal changes are well established, tube-casts. Urethritis, with a purulent discharge, may arise, so it is stated, usually at the end of an attack. It may occur spontaneously, or follow a pure connection.

(*f*) *Pulmonary Disorders.*—There are no characteristic changes, but chronic bronchitis occurs with great frequency in persons of a gouty habit.

(*g*) Of eye affections, iritis, glaucoma, hæmorrhagic retinitis, and suppurative panophthalmitis have been described.

Diagnosis.—Recurring attacks of arthritis, limited to the big toe or to the tarsus, occurring in a member of a gouty family, or in a man who has lived too well, leave no question as to the nature of the trouble. There are many cases of gout, however, in which the feet do not suffer most severely. After an attack or two in one toe, other joints may be affected, and it is just in such cases of polyarthritis that the difficulty in diagnosis is apt to arise. I have had cases admitted for the third or fourth time with involvement of three or more of the larger joints. The presence of tophi has settled the nature of a trouble which in the previous attacks had been regarded as rheumatic. The following are suggestive points in such cases: (1) The patient's habits and occupation. In the United States the brewery men and barkeepers are often affected. (2) The presence of tophi. The ears should always be inspected in a case of polyarthritis. The diagnosis may rest with a small tophus. The student should learn to recognize, on the ear margin, Woolner's tip, fibroid nodules, and small sebaceous tumors. The last are easily recognized microscopically. The needle-shaped sodium biurate crystals are distinctive of the tophi. (3) The condition of the urine. As shown in Chart

XIV, the uric-acid output is usually very low during the intervals of the paroxysm. At the height of the attack the elimination, as a rule, is greatly increased. The ratio of the uric acid to the urea excretion is disturbed in gouty cases, and may fall as low as 1 to 100 or 1 to 150. (4) The gouty polyarthritis may be afebrile. A patient with three or four joints red, swollen, and painful in rheumatic fever has pyrexia, and, while it may be present and often is in gout, its absence is, I think, a valuable diagnostic sign. Many cases go a-begging for a diagnosis. A careful study of the patient's habits as to beer drinking, of the location of the initial arthritic attacks, and the examination for tophi in the ears will prevent many cases being mistaken for rheumatic fever or arthritis deformans. Lastly, in these doubtful forms of arthritis a careful study of the purin metabolism will give important information.

Prognosis.—"Once gouty, always gouty" is usually true, but by care the frequency and intensity of attacks can be much reduced. As regards the duration of life, the state of the circulation and kidneys is the most important factor.

Treatment.—Hygienic.—Individuals who have inherited a tendency to gout, or who have shown any manifestations of it, should live temperately, abstain from alcohol, and eat moderately. An open-air life, with plenty of exercise and regular hours, does much to counteract an inborn tendency to the disease. The skin should be kept active: if the patient is robust, by the morning cold bath with friction after it; but if he is weak or debilitated the evening warm bath should be substituted. An occasional Turkish bath with active shampooing is very advantageous. The patient should dress warmly, avoid rapid alterations in temperature, and be careful not to have the skin suddenly chilled.

Dietetic.—With few exceptions, persons over forty eat too much, and the first injunction to a gouty person is to keep his appetite within reasonable bounds, to eat at stated hours, and to take plenty of time at his meals. In the matter of food, quantity is a factor of more importance than quality with many gouty persons. As Sir William Roberts well says, "Nowhere perhaps is it more necessary than in gout to consider the man as well as the ailment, and very often more the man than the ailment."

The weight of opinion leans to the use of a modified nitrogenous diet, without excess in starchy and saccharine articles of food. Animal foods rich in nuclear material, such as sweetbreads, liver, kidneys, and brain, should be avoided. Beef extracts are injurious, owing to their richness in extractives belonging to the xanthin group. Milk and eggs are particularly useful, owing to their not containing any nuclein. Fresh vegetables and fruits may be used freely, but among the latter strawberries and bananas should be avoided.

Ebstein urges strongly the use of fat in the form of good fresh butter, from 2½ to 3½ ounces in the day. He says that stout gouty subjects not only do not increase in weight with plenty of fat in the food, but that they acutally become thin and the general condition improves very much. Hot bread of all sorts and the various articles of food prepared from Indian corn should, as a rule, be avoided. Roberts advised gouty patients to restrict as far as practicable the use of common salt with their meals, since the sodium biurate very readily crystallizes out in tissues with a high percentage of sodium salts.

In this matter of diet each individual case must receive separate consideration.

There are very few conditions in the gouty in which stimulants of any sort are required. Whenever indicated, whisky will be found perhaps the most serviceable. While all are injurious to these patients, some are much more so than others, particularly malted liquors, champagne, port, and a very large proportion of all the light wines.

MINERAL WATERS.—All forms may be said to be beneficial in gout, as the main element is the water, and the ingredients are usually indifferent. Much of the humbuggery in the profession still lingers about mineral waters, more particularly about the so-called lithia waters.

The question of the utility of alkalies in the treatment of gout is closely connected with this subject of mineral waters. This deep-rooted belief in the profession was rudely shaken a few years ago by Sir William Roberts, who claimed to have shown conclusively that alkalescence as such has no influence whatever on the sodium biurate. The sodium salts are believed by this author to be particularly harmful, but, in spite of all the theoretical denunciation of the use of the sodium salts in gout, the gouty from all parts of the world flock to those very Continental springs in which these salts are most predominant.

Of the mineral springs best suited for the gouty may be mentioned, in the United States, those of Saratoga, Bedford, and the White Sulphur; Buxton and Bath, in England; in France, Aix-les-Bains and Contrexeville; and in Germany, Carlsbad, Wildbad, Homburg, and Marienbad. Excellent results are claimed for these mineral waters with special radio-active properties.

The efficacy in reality is in the water, in the way it is taken, on an empty stomach, and in large quantities; and, as every one knows, the important accessories in the modified diet, proper hours, regular exercises, with baths, douches, etc., play a very important rôle in the "cure."

MEDICAL TREATMENT.—In an acute attack the limb should be elevated and the affected joint wrapped in cotton-wool. Warm fomentations, or Fuller's lotion, may be used. The local hot-air or passive hyperæmia treatment may be tried. A brisk mercurial purge is always advantageous at the outset. The wine or tincture of colchicum, in doses of 20 to 30 minims (1.2 to 2 c. c.) may be given every four hours in combination with the citrate of potash or the citrate of lithium. The action of the colchicum should be carefully watched; its effect is most marked when free purgation follows. It has in a majority of the cases a powerful influence over the symptoms—relieving the pain, and reducing, sometimes with great rapidity, the swelling and redness. It should be promptly stopped so soon as it has relieved the pain. In cases in which the pain and sleeplessness are distressing and do not yield to colchicum morphia is necessary. The patient should be placed on a diet chiefly of milk and barley-water, but if there is any debility, strong broths or eggs may be given. It is occasionally necessary to give small quantities of stimulants. During convalescence meats and fish and game may be taken, and gradually the patient may resume the diet previously laid down.

In some of the subacute intercurrent attacks of arthritis sodium salicylate or aspirin is occasionally useful.

The chronic and irregular forms of gout are best treated by the dietetic and hygienic measures already referred to. Potassium iodide is sometimes useful, and preparations of guaiacum, quinine, and the bitter tonics combined with alkalies are undoubtedly of benefit.

Piperazin has been much lauded as an efficient aid in the solution of uric acid. The clinical results, however, are very discordant. It may be employed in doses of from 15 to 30 grains in the day, and is conveniently given in aërated water containing 5 grains to the tumblerful. Piperazin, as a uric acid solvent, was rapidly followed by lysidin, urotropin, urea, and urol among others—a sure indication of their therapeutic worthlessness.

Albu speaks favorably of lemon-juice as a remedy. The vegetable acids are converted in the system into alkaline carbonates, thus enabling the blood to keep the uric acid compounds in solution, and consequently facilitating their elimination by the kidneys.

Where the arthritic attacks are confined to one joint, such as the great-toe joint, surgical interference may be considered. Riedel reports two successful cases in which he removed the entire joint capsule of the big-toe joint, with permanent relief.

II. DIABETES MELLITUS

(Disturbances of the Carbohydrate Metabolism)

Definition.—A syndrome due to disturbance in the carbohydrate metabolism from various causes, in which sugar appears in the urine, either as a slight and transient condition (Glycosuria), or as a more severe form associated with thirst, polyuria, wasting and imperfect oxidation of the fats (Diabetes).

History.—The disease was known to Celsus. Aretæus first used the term diabetes, calling it a wonderful affection "melting down the flesh and limbs into urine." He suggested that the disease got its name from the Greek word signifying a syphon. Willis in the seventeenth century gave a good description and recognized the sweetness of the urine "as if there has been sugar and honey in it." Dobson in 1776 demonstrated the presence of sugar, and Rollo in 1797 wrote an admirable account and recommended the use of a meat diet. The modern study of the disease dates from Claude Bernard's demonstration of the glycogenic function of the liver in 1857.

Etiology.—The enzymes of the intestinal mucosa convert the starches and sugars of the food into monosaccharides—dextrose, galactose and levulose—which pass into the portal circulation, but the major portion remains in the liver, where it is converted into glycogen. The percentage of sugar in the systemic blood remains constant—0.05 to 0.15 per cent. Part of the sugar passes to the muscles, where it is stored as glycogen. The total storage capacity of the liver is estimated at about one-tenth of its weight, *i. e.*, about 150 gms. for an ordinary organ weighing 1,500 gms. Not all of the glycogen comes from the carbohydrates, a small part in health is derived from the proteins and fats. This treble process of transformation, storage and re-transformation of the sugars is effected by special enzymes, which are furnished by internal secretions, chiefly of the pancreas and hypophysis, and are directly influenced by the nervous system. According to Claude Bernard the sugar is simply warehoused on demand in the liver, and given out to the muscles which need it in their work. On the other hand, Pavy maintained that the glycogen was not converted into sugar, but into fat, and also helped to build up the proteins. In any case, the sugar, one of the chief fuels of the body, is burned up, supplying energy to the muscles, and is eliminated as CO_2 and water. The nature of the intermediate stages of the transformation is still under discussion.

The following are the conditions which influence the appearance of sugar in the urine:

(*a*) Excess of Carbohydrate Intake.—As mentioned, in a normal state the sugar in the blood is never above 0.15 per cent. Once past this point, the hyperglycæmia is immediately manifested by the appearance of sugar in the urine. The healthy person has a definite limit of carbohydrate assimilation; the total storage capacity for glycogen is estimated at about 300 gms. Following the ingestion of enormous amounts of carbohydrates the liver and the muscles may not be equal to the task of storing it; the blood content of sugar passes beyond the 0.15 or 0.2 per cent. limit and the cells of the renal epithelium immediately begin to get rid of the surplus. Like the balance at the Mint, which is sensitive to the correct weight of the gold coins passing over it, they only react at a certain point of saturation. Fortunately excessive quantities of pure sugar itself are not taken. The carbohydrates are chiefly in the form of starch, the digestion and absorption of which take place slowly, so that this so-called alimentary glycosuria very rarely occurs, though enormous quantities may be taken. The assimilation limit of a normal fasting individual for sugar itself is about 250 gms. of grape sugar, and considerably less of cane and milk sugar. Clinically one meets with many cases in which glycosuria is present as a result of excessive ingestion of carbohydrates, particularly in stout persons and heavy feeders—so-called lipogenic diabetes—a form very readily controlled.

(*b*) Disturbances in the Nervous System.—Bernard shows that there was a centre in the medulla—the diabetic centre—puncture of which is followed by hyperglycæmia due to an increased outflow of sugar from the liver warehouse. He demonstrated that the efferent path of this influence was through the splanchnic nerves and the afferent through the vagi. The exact location of this centre has never been determined, and its precise rôle in the carbohydrate metabolism is obscure. Clinically, however, it has long been known that many lesions of the nervous system cause glycosuria—tumors, particularly those in the neighborhood of the medulla, injuries both to the brain and to the upper part of the spinal cord, meningitis, and hæmorrhage. Some of these may disturb Claude Bernard's centre in the medulla, but, as will be mentioned later, a great many of them disturb the internal secretion of the hypophysis. Clinically, glycosuria arising from disturbances in the nervous system is not a very important variety.

(*c*) Disturbances of the Internal Secretions.—The part played in the carbohydrate metabolism by the ductless glands is of the first importance. Though not yet fully understood, the following are the chief points, so far as they bear on clinical work:

(1) *Pancreatic Secretion.*—Extirpation of the pancreas in a dog is followed by hyperglycæmia and prolonged glycosuria, which is not relieved by feeding pancreas to the animal, but which is checked if experimentally a portion of healthy organ from another dog is inserted into the portal circulation. The pancreas contains structures known as "the islands of Langerhans," which, from the work of Opie and others, are believed to furnish an internal secretion necessary to normal carbohydrate metabolism. A portion of the organ separated from the rest, and its duct ligated, atrophies, but a tissue remains composed of enlarged islands of Langerhans. If the remainder of the pancreas be removed, this atrophied portion is able to ward off glycosuria; but if this is removed glycosuria appears immediately (W. G. MacCallum). In some way the secretion furnished by this organ is essential to the proper preparation of the sugars. Cohnheim suggests a correlation of this internal secretion with a muscle enzyme, to which it acts as an ambocepter, and that it is by the combined action of these two glycolytic bodies that the sugars are normally burned up in the muscles. Many diseases of the pancreas are associated with glycosuria, some with permanent diabetes. Hæmorrhagic pancreatitis, cancer, calculus, chronic interstitial pancreatitis, catarrh of the ducts may all be associated with a profound disturbance in the metabolism of the sugars. In fact, there is no one organ the disease of which is more constantly associated with glycosuria, and the studies of Opie warrant the belief that the essential factor is a disturbance of the function of the internal secretion provided by the islands of Langerhans.

(2) *Hypophysis.*—It was long known that glycosuria occurred in tumors of the region of the hypophysis, particularly in acromegaly, and it follows fractures of the base of the skull. Experimentally, Cushing and his students have shown that the posterior lobe of the pituitary gland has an important influence in carbohydrate metabolism. The secretion of this portion of the gland is discharged into the third ventricle, and any operative disturbance of it, or of the infundibulum, is at once followed by glycosuria, and by a remarkable lowering of the assimilation limit for sugars. On the other hand, a deficiency of this secretion, or the removal of this portion of the gland alone, is followed by a remarkable increased tolerance for carbo-hydrates.

Clinically, this sequence is not infrequently seen. A tumor which at first irritates the gland, as in the early stages of acromegaly, may cause glycosuria, but later, as the posterior lobe of the gland is destroyed, there is an extraordinarily high assimilation limit for sugars, and associated with it a great increase in the deposition of fat in the body, a syndrome to be referred to later. Intravenous or subcutaneous injection of the extract of the posterior lobe promptly lowers this high assimilation limit for carbohydrates.

(3) *Adrenals and Thyroids.*—We have less positive information about the relation of carbohydrate metabolism to the internal secretions of these glands. Glycosuria does not necessarily follow lesions of the adrenals, but experimentally it has been shown that adrenalin has a powerful influence on the carbohydrate metabolism, and glycosuria may be readily produced in animals by subcutaneous injection, and by the local application of adrenalin to the pancreas. Clinically, we know practically nothing of an adrenal glycosuria. It does not occur in Addison's disease. It has occasionally been noticed in the prolonged therapeutic use of adrenalin. In disturbances of the

thyroid gland glycosuria is not uncommon. There is a lowered tolerance for sugar in Graves' disease which is sometimes associated with a true diabetes, and in the remarkable instances of acute myxœdema the amount of sugar in the urine may be large. The use of thyroid extract is occasionally followed by glycosuria. On the other hand, patients may take the extract continuously for many years without the appearance of sugar in the urine.

Possibly the glycosuria associated with pregnancy is due to a disturbance in the internal secretions at this period. It is a transient condition, usually disappearing with parturition, and rarely leads to diabetes. I have known it to recur in successive pregnancies.

(*d*) Disturbances in the Function of the Liver.—One of the most remarkable features in carbohydrate metabolism is that the great warehouse of the sugars may be damaged to any degree without causing hyperglycæmia or glycosuria. Whether or not there is a type of disease to which the name of "liver diabetes" may be given is doubtful. There are cases of cirrhosis of the liver and of gallstones—particularly those associated with enlargement of the organ—in which glycosuria is present, but they are probably all associated with coincident affections of the pancreas. In the "bronze diabetes," which is accompanied by great hypertrophy of the liver, the glycosuria is probably pancreatic.

(*e*) Disturbances in the Kidney Functions.—Disease of the kidneys is rarely associated with glycosuria. Occasionally one finds it in chronic Bright's disease, but the existence of a true diabetes depending upon changes in the kidneys has not been proved. There is a remarkable experimental diabetes of great interest in connection with carbohydrate metabolism. If phloridzin, a glucoside prepared from the bark of the apple-tree, is given by mouth or subcutaneously to man or animals glycosuria results, and even continues on a nitrogenous diet, and in man when fasting. The amount of sugar excreted may be large, yet there is no hyperglycæmia. It seems that the sugar is directly manufactured by the kidney epithelium, and largely from the proteins.

(*f*) Miscellaneous Disturbances.—The carbohydrate metabolism may be upset in acute fevers, in many of which a transient glycosuria is present. It is not uncommon after the administration of ether, less so after chloroform. Metabolic disturbances in gout are not infrequently associated with glycosuria, and cachexias and profound anæmias may be accompanied by transient glycosuria. A mental shock, a severe nervous strain and worry precede many cases. Patients suffocated by smoke, or poisoned by coal gas, may have sugar in the urine.

Incidence.—According to statistics diabetes appears to be about as frequent in the United States as in European countries. In England and Wales the death-rate from diabetes is about 9 per 100,000 of population. The disease is on the increase in the United States. The statistics for 1870 gave 2.1; for 1880, 2.8; for 1890, 3.8; for 1900, 9.3; and for 1914, 16.2 deaths to the 100,000 population. This apparent increase may be in part due to more accurate vital statistics records. Among 27,618 patients admitted to the medical wards of the Johns Hopkins Hospital in twenty-two years there were 276 cases of diabetes, or one per cent.

Hereditary influences play an important rôle and cases are on record of its occurrence in many members of the same family. Morton, who calls the disease *hydrops ad matulam* (Phthisiologia, 1689), records a remarkable family in which four children were affected, one of which recovered on a milk diet and diascordium. An analysis of the cases in my series gave only 6 cases with a history of diabetes in relatives (Pleasants). Naunyn obtained a family history of diabetes in 35 out of 201 private cases, but in only 7 of 157 hospital cases. There are instances of the coexistence of the disease in man and wife. Among 516 married pairs collected by Senator, in which either husband or wife was diabetic, in 18 cases the second partner had become diabetic. It is not easy to explain this conjugal diabetes. The suggestion of contagion seems scarcely tenable.

SEX.—Men are more frequently affected than women, the ratio being about three to two. Of the 276 cases of diabetes above referred to 179 were in males and 97 in females (Futcher). It is a disease of adult life; a majority of the cases occur from the third to the sixth decade. Of the 276 cases, the largest number—70, or 25 per cent.—occurred between fifty and sixty years of age.

DIABETES IN CHILDREN.—Stern has analyzed 117 cases in children. They usually occur among the better classes. Six were under one year of age. Hereditary influences were marked. The course of the disease is, as a rule, much more rapid than in adults. The shortest duration was two days, and in 7 cases it did not last a month. One case is mentioned of a child apparently born with glycosuria, who recovered in eight months.

In the above series there were 2 cases in the first hemi-decade, 5 in the second, and 24 in the second decade.

Persons of a neurotic *temperament* are often affected. It is a disease of the higher classes. Van Noorden states that the statistics for London and Berlin show that the number of cases in the upper ten thousand exceeds that in the lower hundred thousand inhabitants.

RACE.—Hebrews seem especially prone to it; one-fourth of Frerichs' patients were of the Semitic race. I have been much impressed with the frequency of the disease among them. Diabetes is comparatively rare in the colored race, but not so uncommon as was formerly supposed. Of the series of 276 cases, 29, or 10.6 per cent., were in negroes.

Metabolism in Diabetes.—Glycosuria, neurotic, dietetic or toxic, may be a matter of simple overflow, but the essence of true diabetes is a waste of the carbohydrates, which hurry through the body, in great part never warehoused as glycogen. Why this should be, whether the liver and muscles are at fault in refusing to transform the carbohydrate, or whether the defect is the enzymes of the ductless glands, are problems awaiting solution. Naunyn held that hyperglycæmia is due to a failure of the liver and muscles to store up glycogen as in health. On the other hand, Lépine, Opie, and others support the view that the glycolitic ferments are lacking—the former may depend on the latter. In either case the result is a failure of the normal oxidation of the carbohydrates. Hyperglycæmia is responsible for the thirst and the polyuria, and there is a very considerable daily loss of energy in warming the liquids taken to the temperature of the body, according to Benedict and Joslin nearly 6 per cent. of the total heat of the day; and it is this excess of sugar in the system that renders the body so favorable a culture medium for pus organisms. There is loss of energy with the steady waste of sugar fuel; practically every gram of sugar excreted in the urine results in a loss of 4.1 calories, consequently a diabetic patient excreting 100 grams of sugar and 20 grams of β-oxybutyric acid loses 500 calories in this way, so that the patients are apt to be underfed, unless this loss is made up by a full amount of other food (Benedict and Joslin). Studies upon the respiratory quotient—which is the ratio between the CO_2 given out and the O taken in by a healthy individual on a mixed diet (expressed by the fraction 0.9)—favor the view that there is failure in the proper combustion of the carbohydrates. Benedict and Joslin conclude that a respiratory quotient above 0.74 indicates a fairly liberal supply of glycogen stored in the body; while a respiratory quotient of 0.70, or below that, indicates that the patient has no available carbohydrates, and has lost in a measure the power of storing them. And here comes the special danger; as the carbohydrates pass through the body unburned, the energy must be provided from the proteins and fats. The metabolism of the former does not appear to be seriously disturbed, and the carbohydrate portion of the protein molecule is well tolerated and in part supplies the place of the lost sugars. The danger is in the metabolism of the fats. The carbohydrates are not used as fuel; the proteins are easily utilized, but apparently it takes so much draught to burn them that not enough is left to consume the fats completely; and the products of incomplete combustion accumulate in the system and suffocate the patient as effectually as does the CO of a charcoal stove. The chief product of this incomplete combustion of the fats is the β-oxybutyric acid, which itself is the source of the diacetic acid and acetone, and the special danger of the disease is now recognized to be the production of an acidosis in consequence of this imperfect fat metabolism. One of the most valuable advances in our knowledge of the metabolism of the disease has been the work of Beddard, Pembrey and Spriggs and more recently of Poulton, who have shown that the amount of CO_2 in the alveolar air may be taken as a measure of the acidosis. The acetone bodies in the urine indicate a large production in the body but this may have been completely compensated. The blood examination is more important to determine the degree of accumulation and with even slight degrees there are changes in the alveolar air.

Morbid Anatomy.—The *nervous system* shows no constant lesions. In a few instances there have been tumors or sclerosis in the medulla, or a cysticercus has pressed on the floor. A secondary multiple neuritis is not rare, and to it the so-called diabetic tabes is probably due, and changes occur in the posterior columns of the cord similar to those which have been found in pernicious anæmia. In the sympathetic system the ganglia have been enlarged and in some instances sclerosed. The *heart* is hypertrophied in some cases. Endocarditis is very rare. Arterio-sclerosis is common. The *lungs* show important changes. Acute broncho-pneumonia or croupous pneumonia (either of which may terminate in gangrene) and tuberculosis are common. The so-called diabetic phthisis is always tuberculous and results from a caseating broncho-pneumonia. In rare cases there is a chronic interstitial pneumonia, non-tuberculous. Fat embolism of the pulmonary vessels may occur in connection with diabetic coma.

The *liver* is usually enlarged; fatty degeneration is common. In the so-called diabetic cirrhosis—the *cirrhosis pigmentaire*—the liver is enlarged and sclerotic, and cachexia develops with melanoderma. Dilatation of the stomach with enlargement of the duodenum and colonic stasis are common.

Pancreas.—Of 15 autopsies in 27 fatal cases, in 9 the pancreas was found atrophic. In one of these fat necroses were present, in another calculi. Hyaline degeneration of the islands of Langerhans has been described by Opie and is a special feature in certain cases. Chronic interstitial pancreatitis is common.

The *kidneys* show a diffuse nephritis with fatty degeneration. Hyaline change is often found in the tubal epithelium, particularly of the descending limb of the loop of Henle, and in the Malphigian tufts.

Symptoms.—*Acute* and *chronic* forms are recognized, but there is no essential difference between them, except that in the former the patients are younger, the course is more rapid, and the emaciation more marked. I have twice seen acute diabetes in the aged.

The *onset* of the disease is gradual, and either frequent micturition or inordinate thirst first attracts attention. Very rarely it sets in rapidly, after a sudden emotion, an injury, or after a severe chill. When fully established the disease is characterized by great thirst, the passage of large quantities of saccharine urine, a voracious appetite, and, as a rule, progressive emaciation.

Among the GENERAL SYMPTOMS of the disease *thirst* is one of the most distressing. Large quantities of water are required to keep the sugar in solution and for its excretion in the urine. The amount of fluid consumed will be found to bear a definite ratio to the quantity excreted. Instances, however, are not uncommon of pronounced diabetes in which the thirst is not excessive; but in such cases the amount of urine passed is never large. The thirst is most intense an hour or two after meals. As a rule, the digestion is good and the appetite inordinate. The condition is sometimes termed *bulimia* or *polyphagia.* Lumbar pain is common.

The tongue is usually dry, red, and glazed, and the saliva scanty. The gums may become swollen, and in the later stages aphthous stomatitis is common. Constipation is the rule.

In spite of the enormous amount of food consumed a patient may become rapidly emaciated. This loss of flesh bears some ratio to the polyuria, and when, under suitable diet, the sugar is reduced, the patient may quickly gain in flesh. The skin is dry and harsh, and sweating rarely occurs, except when phthisis coexists. Drenching sweats have been known to alternate with excessive polyuria. General pruritus or pruritus pudendi may be very distressing, and occasionally is one of the earliest symptoms. The temperature is often subnormal; the pulse is usually frequent, and the tension increased. Many diabetics do not show marked emaciation. Patients past the middle period of life may have the disease for years without much disturbance of the health, and may remain well nourished. These are the cases of the *diabète gras* in contradistinction to *diabète maigre.*

THE URINE.—The amount varies from 3 to 4 litres in mild cases to 15 to 20 litres in very severe cases. In rare instances the quantity of urine is not much increased. Under strict diet the amount is much lessened, and in intercurrent febrile affections it may be reduced to normal. The specific gravity is high, ranging from 1.025 to 1.045; but in exceptional cases it may be low, 1.013 to 1.020. The highest specific gravity recorded, so far as I know, is by Trousseau—1.074. Very high specific gravities—1.070 + —suggest fraud. The urine is pale in color, almost like water, and has a sweetish odor and a distinctly sweetish taste. The reaction is acid. Sugar is present in varying amounts. In mild cases it does not exceed 1½ or 2 per cent., but it may reach from 5 to 10 per cent. The total amount excreted in the twenty-four hours may range from 10 to 20 ounces (320 to 640 grams) and in exceptional cases from 1 to 2 pounds.

Ketonuria.—The ketone bodies, acetone, diacetic acid and β-oxybutyric acid are present, sometimes in small amounts in mild cases but increasing with the severity of the disease; and are indications of acidosis. In coma the excretion of β-oxybutyric acid may be as much as 100 gm. or more a day.

Glycogen has also been found in the urine, and in rare instances sugars other than glucose occur, lactose, levulose, and pentose, and to these conditions the term *melituria* is sometimes applied. *Albumin* is not infrequent.

Pneumaturia, gas in the urine, due to fermentation in the bladder, is occasionally met with. Cammidge's reaction may be present. Fat may be passed in the urine in the form of a fine emulsion (lipuria).

Blood in Diabetes.—The water content is lower than normal. Polycythæmia may be present to 6 or 8 millions of red cells per cmm. Towards the end and with complications there may be a leucocytosis and the leucocytes may contain glycogen. Hyperglycæmia is present to 0.3 or even 0.8 per cent., instead of the normal 0.1 to 0.15 per cent. The increase in the blood sugar may persist after glycosuria has disappeared. Recent studies have shown the great importance of estimating the sugar content of the blood.

The alkalinity is lessened and the specific gravity reduced. Lipæmia is present in many cases and may be readily recognized by the presence of dancing particles among the red cells in a slide of fresh blood. In a centrifugalized specimen the serum is creamy. Normally the blood contains about 1 per cent. of lipoid substances; in severe acidosis the content may rise to 15 per cent. Serous exudates may be turbid with fat. Lipæmia may be present without acidosis and is sometimes due to surcharging of the blood stream with the products of fatty digestion as in the normal lipæmia of sucklings.

Complications.—(*a*) Coma.—There are three groups of cases:

(1) Typical dyspnœic coma, the air-hunger of Kussmaul, in which with loud and deep in- and expirations, the pulse grows weak, and the patient gradually fails and dies, sometimes within twenty-four hours. The breath very often has the fruity odor of acetone. It may come on without any premonition and the patient may waken out of sleep in dyspnœa. An acyanotic dyspnœa is one of the best indications of acidosis. (2) Cases in which, without any previous dyspnœa or distress, the patient is attacked with headache, a feeling of intoxication, thick speech and a staggering gait, and gradually falls into deep coma. (3) Cases in which, particularly after exertion, the patient is attacked suddenly with weakness, giddiness and fainting; the hands and feet are cold and livid, the pulse small, respiration rapid; the patient becomes drowsy, and death occurs within a few hours. Dyspepsia, constipation, abdominal pain, marked irritability and restlessness may precede the onset of coma and should suggest its possibility.

(*b*) Cutaneous.—Boils and carbuncles are extremely common. Painful onychia may occur. Eczema is also met with, and at times an intolerable itching. In women the irritation of the urine may cause the most intense pruritus pudendi, and in men a balanitis. Rarer affections are xanthoma and purpura. Gangrene is not uncommon, and is associated usually with arterio-sclerosis. Perforating ulcer of the foot occurred in 7 of 276 cases. Bronzing of the skin (*diabète bronzé*) occurs in certain cases in which the diabetes arises as a late event in the disease known as hæmochromatosis, which is further characterized by pigmentary cirrhosis of the liver and pancreas. With the onset of severe complications the tolerance of the carbohydrates is much increased. Profuse sweats may occur.

(*c*) Pulmonary.—The patients are not infrequently carried off by *acute pneumonia,* which may be lobar or lobular. *Gangrene* is very apt to supervene, but the breath does not necessarily have the foul odor of ordinary gangrene. Abscess following lobar pneumonia occurred in one of my cases. *Tuberculous broncho-pneumonia* is very common and may run a very rapid course.

(*d*) Renal.—*Albuminuria* is a tolerably frequent complication. The amount varies greatly, and, when slight, does not seem to be of much moment. Œdema of the feet and ankles is not an infrequent symptom. General anasarca is rare, however, owing to the marked polyuria. It is sometimes associated with arterio-sclerosis. It occasionally precedes the occurrence of the diabetic coma. Occasionally cystitis is a troublesome symptom.

(*e*) Nervous System.—*Peripheral Neuritis.*—Neuralgia, numbness and tingling, uncommon symptoms in diabetes, are probably minor neuritic manifestations. The involvement may be general of the upper and lower extremities. Sometimes it is unilateral, or the neuritis may be in a single nerve—the sciatic or the third nerve. Herpes zoster may occur.

Diabetic Tabes (so-called).—This is a peripheral neuritis, characterized by lightning pains in the legs, loss of knee-jerk—which may occur without the other symptoms—and a loss of power in the extensors of the feet. The gait is the characteristic *steppage,* as in arsenical, alcoholic, and other forms of neuritic paralysis. Charcot states that there may be atrophy of the optic nerves. Changes in the posterior columns of the cord have been found by Williamson and others.

Diabetic Paraplegia.—This is also in all probability due to neuritis. There are cases in which power has been lost in both arms and legs.

Mental Symptoms.—The patients are often morose, and there is a strong tendency to become hypochondriacal. General paralysis has been met with. Some patients display an extraordinary degree of restlessness and anxiety.

(*f*) Special Senses.—Cataract is liable to occur, and with rapidity in young persons. Diabetic retinitis closely resembles the albuminuric form. Hæmorrhages are common. Sudden amaurosis, similar to that which occurs in uræmia, may occur. Paralysis of the muscles of accommodation may be present; and, lastly, atrophy of the optic nerves. Aural symptoms may come on with great rapidity, either an otitis media, or in some instances inflammation of the mastoid cells. Ocular tension may be lowered in coma.

(*g*) Sexual Function.—Impotence is common, and may be an early symptom. Conception is rare; if it occurs, abortion is apt to follow. A diabetic mother may bear a healthy child; there is no known instance of a diabetic mother bearing a diabetic child. The course of the disease is usually aggravated after delivery.

Diagnosis.—There is no difficulty in determining the presence of sugar in the urine if the proper tests are applied. Alcapton may prove very deceptive, and in one case of ochronosis which I reported a diagnosis of diabetes was made by four or five of the leading physicians in Europe, one of whom was an authority on diabetes. Deception may be practiced. A young girl under my care had urine with a specific gravity of 1.065, but the reactions were for cane sugar; and there is a case in the literature in which, when the cane sugar fraud was detected, the woman bought grape sugar and put it into her bladder.

To determine whether the case is one of simple glycosuria or of true diabetes is not always easy, as the one readily merges into the other. The younger the individual the greater the probability that the case is one of true diabetes. It is well always to test the assimilation limit; 100 grams of glucose given in solution two hours after a breakfast of a roll and butter with coffee should not give glycosuria. To do so indicates a deficiency in the capacity to store carbohydrates and a possibility that true diabetes may follow. Transient glycosuria occurs in a great many conditions already mentioned. For practical purposes the common form is that met with in persons above 50 years of age, who eat and drink too much and tend to grow stout. The detection of a little sugar in the urine may have the great advantage of frightening the patient into a more rational mode of life. The forms following anæsthesia, accidents, business worries, fright and that which occurs in pregnancy are, as a rule, readily controlled.

Prognosis.—The younger the patient the less likely is recovery. In children the disease may run a very rapid course, and death may occur within a few weeks, or, indeed, a child may die in coma before the condition has been recognized. The case referred to by Morton, in which one recovered of four children in a family affected, is one of the few instances on record. Personally I have not known an instance of recovery in a child. On the other hand, in persons over fifty sugar may be present in the urine for years without any impairment of strength or health. The outlook is good in the fat, bad in the lean. It is particularly good in the stout, active, business man, whose glycosuria has come on as a result of worry, work, and excess in food and drink.

The following steps should be taken to estimate the gravity of a case. The carbohydrate tolerance should be estimated in exact figures and the presence of acetone and diacetic acid determined, as they usually indicate a serious disturbance in the metabolism of the fats. It is well to remember, however, that the acetone bodies may be only temporarily present, and it is not necessary to sign the patient's death warrant so soon as they appear. A patient may live for many years with traces, and they may disappear after having been present for months.

Treatment.—In families with a marked predisposition to the disease the use of starchy and saccharine articles of diet should be restricted.

The personal hygiene of a diabetic patient is of the first importance. Sources of worry should be avoided, and he should lead an even, quiet life, if possible in an equable climate. The heat waste should be prevented by wearing warm clothes and avoiding cold. A warm, or, if tolerably robust, a cold, bath should be taken every day. An occasional Turkish bath is useful. Systematic, moderate exercise should be taken. When this is not feasible, massage should be given. It is well to study accurately the dietetic capabilities of each patient, for no two can be treated alike. The weight should be recorded weekly. A patient who is glycosuric and losing weight on a non-carbohydrate diet must be regarded as doing badly, but as a result of the fasting treatment we have learned that some patients are better after a moderate loss of weight.

Diet.—Keep the patient for three or four days on an ordinary diet, containing moderate amounts of carbohydrates—to ascertain the amount of sugar excretion. For two days more the starches are gradually cut off. Then place him on the following non-carbohydrate diet, modified according to the patient's age and weight, and arranged from a list recommended by von Noorden:

Breakfast: 7:30, 200 c. c. (℥ vi) of tea or coffee: 150 grams (℥ iv) of beefsteak, mutton-chops without bone, or boiled ham; one or two eggs.

Lunch: 12:30, 200 grams (℥ vi) cold roast beef; 60 grams (℥ ij) celery, fresh cucumbers or tomatoes with vinegar, olive oil, pepper and salt to taste; 20 c. c. (ʒ v) whisky with 400 c. c. (℥ xiij) water; 60 c. c. (℥ ij) coffee, without milk or sugar.

Dinner: 6 P. M., 200 c. c. clear bouillon; 250 grams (℥ viiss) roast beef; 10 grams (ʒ iiss) butter; 80 grams (℥ ij) green salad, with 10 grams (ʒ iiss) vinegar and 20 grams (ʒ v) olive oil, or three tablespoonfuls of some well-cooked green vegetable, three sardines à l'huile; 20 c. c. (ʒ v) whisky, with 400 c. c. (℥ xiij) water.

Supper: 9 P. M., two eggs (raw or cooked); 400 c. c. (℥ xiij) water.

This diet contains about 200 grams of albumin and about 135 grams of fat. The effect of the diet on the sugar excretion is remarkable. In many cases there is an entire disappearance of the sugar from the urine in three or four days. In cases in which the urine becomes free from sugar gradually increasing quantities of starch up to 20, 50, and 100 grams are added daily. White bread contains fifty-five per cent. of starch. The effect of the non-carbohydrate diet is to improve the metabolic functions so that the system can warehouse considerable quantities of carbohydrates without sugar appearing in the urine.

In cases in which a standard diet is not ordered it is well to begin cutting off article by article until the sugar disappears from the urine. Within a month or two the patient may be allowed a more liberal diet, testing the different kinds of food.

The *oatmeal diet,* introduced by von Noorden, is most excellent, particularly in the severer forms. Two hundred and fifty grams of oatmeal, the same amount of butter and the whites of six or eight eggs constitute the day's food. The oatmeal is cooked for two hours, and the butter and albumin stirred in. It may be taken in four portions during the day. Coffee, tea, or whisky and water may be taken with it.

Fasting Treatment.—From Naunyn to Nellis Foster authors have recognized the value of fasting days, but, based on careful and elaborate experiments, F. M. Allen has introduced prolonged fasting followed by a low diet, as a systematic treatment. Control and education of the patient are essential factors. So far the reports are favorable: of 42 patients treated by Allen, all severe forms and many young, 7 died; of 55 cases treated by Joslin, 6 died. Great enthusiasm is expressed. "At one stroke the patient is delivered from medicines, patent and otherwise, sham kinds of treatment, gluten breads, and in 99 cases out of 100 of alkalis" (Joslin). As a rule the patients stand the fasting well.

The patient is put to bed, the treatment explained, a note-book and a diet-card given, and he is taught to test the urine. The following are the steps in the treatment, which I take from the papers of Allen and of Joslin.

(1) Determine the glycosuria and ketonuria on an ordinary diet for two days.

(2) Fasting, the patient should be in bed in charge of an intelligent nurse; no food is given until the urine is sugar-free and acid-free. The time ranges from two to five days. Water is given freely, and tea and coffee. Alcohol in small doses may be taken every three hours. If after two days fasting the sugar persists give 300 c.c. of clear meat broth in divided doses. Once the urine is sugar-free and acid-free the second part of the treatment is begun, to determine the lowest grade of nutrition at which the patient can live in comfort without glycosuria and ketonuria. Here the intelligent co-operation of the patient is essential.

(3) Carbohydrate tolerance. When a 24-hour specimen of the urine is free, give 150 grams of the 5 per cent. vegetables (see annexed list) and continue to add 5 grams of carbohydrate daily up to 20 grams; and then 5 grams every other day, passing through the 5, 10 and 15 per cent. vegetables, and 5, 10 and 15 per cent. fruits (see list). Of the more starchy foods, potatoes, or oatmeal may be used, and then bread, if sugar does not reappear.

(4) Protein tolerance. When the urine is sugar-free for two days add 20 grams of protein—3 eggs—and then five grams of meat daily until the patient is getting 1 gram of protein per kilogram of body weight. It may even be raised to 1.5 gram per kilo of weight.

(5) Fat tolerance. A small amount of fat is in the meat and eggs. Later add 25 grams daily until the patient ceases to lose weight. Bacon, butter and oil may be used.

(6) Re-appearance of sugar calls for a fasting day and a return to the low diet.

(7) Days of Reduced Diet. In every case it is well to restrict the diet on one day a week. When the tolerance is less than 20 grams of carbohydrates daily the patient should fast one day in seven. In mild cases the carbohydrate should be reduced to one-half or one-third of the usual amount. A day when only eggs and 5 per cent. vegetables are taken is an advantage, or a day on which nothing but broth is allowed. The lower the carbohydrate tolerance the greater the importance of a fast day.

Each case must be dealt with separately, and the number of calories given is to be gauged by the absence of glycosuria and ketonuria, not by the state of the nutrition which has often to be kept permanently low. Alkalis may be given for the first few days of the fast, particularly if coma seems imminent, but under the fasting treatment there is not the same necessity for their administration. The patient is encouraged to feel that the treatment is largely in his own hands.

Medicinal Treatment.—Opium alone stands the test of experience as a remedy capable of limiting the progress of the disease. Codeia is less constipating than morphia. A patient may begin with half a grain three times

QUANTITY OF FOOD Required by a Severe Diabetic Patient Weighing 60 kilograms. (Joslin.)

Food	Quantity Grams	Calories per Gram	Total Calories
Carbohydrate	10	4	40
Protein	75	4	300
Fat	150	9	1,350
Alcohol	15	7	105
			1,795

STRICT DIET. (Foods without sugar.) Meats, Poultry, Game, Fish, Clear Soups, Gelatine, Eggs, Butter, Olive Oil, Coffee, Tea and Cracked Cocoa.

Foods Arranged Approximately According to Content of Carbohydrates

	5% ±	10% ±	15% ±	20% ±
VEGETABLES	Lettuce Spinach Sauerkraut String Beans Celery Asparagus Cucumbers Brussels Sprouts Sorrel Endive Dandelion Greens Swiss Chard Vegetable Marrow Cauliflower Tomatoes Rhubarb Egg Plant Leeks Beet Greens Water Cress Cabbage Radishes Pumpkin Kohl-Rabi Sea Kale	Onions Squash Turnip Carrots Okra Mushrooms Beets	Green Peas Artichokes Parsnips Canned Lima Beans	Potatoes Shell Beans Baked Beans Green Corn Boiled Rice Boiled Macaroni
FRUITS	Ripe Olives (20 per cent. fat) Grape Fruit	Lemons Oranges Cranberries Strawberries Blackberries Gooseberries Peaches Pineapples Watermelon	Apples Pears Apricots Blueberries Cherries Currants Raspberries Huckleberries	Plums Bananas
NUTS	Butternuts Pignolias	Brazil Nuts Black Walnuts Hickory Pecans Filberts	Almonds Walnuts (Eng.) Beechnuts Pistachios Pine Nuts	Peanuts **40%** Chestnuts
MISCELLANEOUS	Unsweetened and Unspiced Pickle Clams Scallops Fish Roe Oysters Liver			

30 grams (1 oz.) contain approximately	Protein	Fat	Carbohydrates	Calories
	Grams			
Oatmeal	5	2	20	110
Meat (uncooked)	6	2	0	40
" (cooked)	8	3	0	60
Potato	1	0	6	25
Bacon	5	15	0	155
Cream, 40%	1	12	1	120
" 20%	1	6	1	60
Milk	1	1	2	20
Bread	3	0	13	90
Rice	3	0	21	110
Butter	0	25	0	230
Egg (one)	6	5	0	75
Brazil Nuts	5	20	2	210
Orange (one)	0	0	10	40
Grape Fruit (one)	0	0	10	40
Vegetables from 5–6% groups	0.5	0	1	6

1 gram protein contains 4 calories.
1 " carbohydrate contains 4 calories.
1 " fat contains 9 calories.
1 " alcohol contains 7 calories.

1 kilogram — 2.2 pounds.
6.25 grams protein contain 1 gram nitrogen.
A patient "at rest" requires 30 calories per kilogram body weight.

Chart XV.—Diabetic Food Tables. (Joslin.)

a day, which may be gradually increased to 6 or 8 grains in the twenty-four hours. Not much effect is noticed unless the patient is on a rigid diet. When the sugar is reduced to a minimum, or is absent, the opium should be gradually withdrawn. The patients not only bear well these large doses of the drug, but they stand its gradual reduction.

Glycerine extracts of the pancreas and glycolytic ferments have been used but without satisfactory results. The worst vagaries of hormonic therapy have of late been in connection with the treatment of diabetes.

Of the complications, the *pruritus* and *eczema* are best treated by cooling lotions of boric acid or hyposulphite of soda (1 ounce; water, 1 quart), or the use of ichthyol and lanolin ointment.

The bowels should be kept open and the urine tested at short intervals for acetone and diacetic acid—the derivatives of β-oxybutyric acid.

Coma.—The presence of acetone and diacetic acid is a sign for reduction in the diet, especially carbohydrates and fats. If sugar is present fasting is usually indicated. If signs of coma are present fasting should be begun at once, as outlined above. The use of bicarbonate of soda in very large doses is recommended to neutralize the acid intoxication. It may be used intravenously; as much as 80 grams have been injected. The solution used for intravenous injection is a 1 to 2 per cent. solution of sodium bicarbonate in normal salt solution, made from freshly distilled water. A litre may be injected slowly into a vein every six hours in desperate cases. In the less serious cases administration should be by mouth, or mouth and rectum. The sodium bicarbonate should be pushed until the urine is alkaline, and as much as 100 grams given daily. All diabetics with a marked diacetic acid reaction in the urine should be placed on sodium bicarbonate. By the "Murphy drip" method large amounts of alkali and fluid may be introduced. The bowels of a diabetic patient should be kept acting freely, as constipation is believed to predispose to the development of coma.

III. DIABETES INSIPIDUS

Definition.—A chronic affection characterized by the passage of large quantities of normal urine of low specific gravity.

The condition is to be distinguished from diuresis or polyuria, which is a frequent symptom in hysteria, in Bright's disease, and occasionally in cerebral or other affections. Willis in 1674 first recognized the distinction between a saccharine and non-saccharine form of diabetes.

Etiology.—The disease is most common in young persons. Of the 85 cases collected by Strauss, 9 were under five years; 12 between five and ten years; 36 between ten and twenty-five years. Males are more frequently attacked than females. The affection may be congenital. A hereditary tendency has been noted in many instances, the most extraordinary of which has been reported by Weil. Of 91 members in four generations, 23 had persistent polyuria without any deterioration in health.

Clinical Classification.—There are two forms: primary or idiopathic, in which there is no evident organic basis, and secondary or symptomatic, in which there is evidence of disease in the brain or elsewhere. Of 9 cases reported from my clinic by Futcher, 4 belonged to the former and 5 to the latter group. Trousseau stated that the parents of children with diabetes insipidus frequently have glycosuria or albuminuria. The disease has followed rapidly the copious drinking of cold water, or a drinking bout, or has set in during the convalescence from an acute disease.

The secondary or symptomatic form is almost always associated with injury or disease of the nervous system, traumatism to the head or, in some cases, to the trunk. It occurs in 30 per cent. of the cases, according to Stoermer. Tumors of the brain, lesions of the medulla and of the hypophysis (with dystrophia adiposo-genitalis) and hæmorrhage are found, but above all syphilis, present in 5 of 9 cases in my clinic. The lesion is usually at the base, and meningitic. Hemianopsia is present in a number of these cases; it occurred in 2 of Futcher's series. It is not necessary that the lesions should involve the medulla. It has been met with in spinal cord lesions. In tumors and aneurisms in the abdomen, in tuberculous peritonitis, and in carcinoma there may be excessive polyuria. The condition of the pituitary gland should be studied in the so-called idiopathic cases.

The most reasonable view of the production of the polyuria is that it results from a vasomotor disturbance of the renal vessels, due either to local irritation, as in a case of abdominal tumor, to central disturbance in cases of brain-lesion, or to functional irritation of the centre in the medulla, giving rise to continuous renal congestion. In some cases the functional capacity of the kidney to eliminate salt and urea is diminished.

Morbid Anatomy.—There are no constant anatomical lesions. The *kidneys* have been found enlarged and congested. The *bladder* has been found hypertrophied. Dilatation of the ureters and of the pelves of the kidneys has been present. Death has not infrequently resulted from chronic pulmonary disease. Very varied lesions have been met with in the nervous system.

Symptoms.—The disease may come on rapidly, as after a fright or an injury; more commonly it is gradual. A copious secretion of urine, with increased thirst, is the prominent feature of the disease. The amount of urine in the twenty-four hours may range from 20 to 40 pints, or even more. Trousseau speaks of a patient who consumed 50 pints of fluid daily and passed about 56 pints of urine in the twenty-four hours. In two of our cases the amount passed was greater than that ingested in liquids and solids. The specific gravity is low, 1.001 to 1.005; the color is extremely pale and watery. The total solid constituents may not be reduced. The amount of urea has sometimes been found in excess. Abnormal ingredients are rare. Muscle-sugar, inosite, has been occasionally found. Albumin is rare. Traces of sugar have been met with. Naturally, with the passage of such enormous quantities of urine, there is a proportionate thirst, and the only inconvenience of the disease is the necessity for frequent micturition and frequent drinking. The appetite is usually good, rarely excessive as in diabetes mellitus; but Trousseau tells of the terror inspired by one of his patients in the keepers of those eating-houses where bread was allowed without extra charge to the extent of each customer's wishes, and says that the man was paid to stay away. The patients may be well nourished and healthy-looking. The disease in many instances does not appear to interfere in any way with the general health. The perspiration is naturally slight and the skin is harsh. The amount of saliva is small and the mouth usually dry. The tolerance of alcohol is remarkable, and patients have been known to take a couple of pints of brandy, or a dozen or more bottles of wine, in the day.

Course.—The course depends entirely upon the nature of the primary trouble. Sometimes, with organic disease, either cerebral or abdominal, the general health is much impaired; the patient becomes thin, and rapidly loses strength. In the essential or idiopathic cases good health may be maintained for an indefinite period, and the affection has been known to persist for fifty years. Death usually results from some intercurrent affection. Spontaneous cure may take place.

Diagnosis.—A low specific gravity and the absence of sugar in the urine distinguish the disease from diabetes mellitus. Hysterical polyuria may sometimes simulate it very closely. The amount of urine excreted may be enormous, and only the development of other hysterical manifestations may enable the diagnosis to be made. This condition is, however, always transitory.

In certain cases of chronic Bright's disease a very large amount of urine of low specific gravity may be passed, but the presence of albumin and of hyaline casts and the existence of heightened arterial tension, stiff vessels, and hypertrophied left ventricle make the diagnosis easy.

Treatment.—The treatment is not satisfactory. No attempt should be made to reduce the amount of liquid. In some cases gradual reduction of the protein and salt intake is useful. This should be done gradually. Opium is highly recommended, but is of doubtful service. The preparations of valerian may be tried; either the powdered root, beginning with 5 grains (0.3 gm.) three times a day, and increasing until 2 drachms (8 gm.) are taken in the day, or the valerianate of zinc, in 15-grain (1 gm.) doses, gradually increased to 30 grains (2 gm.), three times a day. Theocin is sometimes useful in doses of 5 grains (0.3 gm.) three times a day. Antisyphilitic treatment should be thoroughly tried in patients with a suspicious history or a positive Wassermann reaction. Electricity may be used.

IV. RICKETS (RHACHITIS)

Definition.—A disease of infants, characterized by impaired nutrition of the entire body and alterations in the growing bones.

Glisson, the anatomist of the liver, accurately described the disease in 1650. The name is derived from the old English word *wrickken,* to twist. Glisson suggested to change the name to rhachitis, from the Greek, *ῥάχις*, the spine, as it was one of the first parts affected, and also from the similarity in the sound to rickets.

Etiology.—Rickets exists in all parts of the world, but is particularly marked among the poor of the larger cities, who are badly housed and ill fed. It is much more common in Europe than in America. In Vienna and London from 50 to 80 per cent. of all the children at the clinics present signs of rickets. It is a comparatively rare disease in Canada. In the cities of the United States it is very prevalent, particularly among the children of the negro and of the Italian races. Want of sunlight, impure air, confinement, and lack of exercise are important factors. Prolonged lactation and suckling the child during pregnancy are accessory influences in some cases.

30

There is no evidence that the disease is hereditary.

Rickets affects male and female children equally. It is a disease of the first and second years of life, rarely beginning before the sixth month. Jenner has described a late rickets, in which form the disease may not appear until the ninth or even until the twelfth year, or later (the osteomalacia of puberty). A faulty diet is a factor in the production of the disease. Like scurvy, rickets may be found in the families of the wealthy under perfect hygienic conditions. It is most common in children fed on condensed milk, the various proprietary foods, cow's milk, and food rich in starches. "An analysis of the foods on which rickets is most frequently and certainly produced shows invariably a deficiency in two of the chief elements so plentiful in the standard food of young animals—namely, animal fat and proteid" (Cheadle). Bland Sutton's interesting experiment with the lion's cubs at the "Zoo" illustrates this point. When milk, pounded bones, and cod-liver oil were added to the meat diet the rickets disappeared, and for the first time in the history of the society the cubs were reared. Associated with the defect in food is a lack of proper assimilation of the lime salts.

Morbid Anatomy.—Glisson's original description of the external appearances of the body of a rickety child is remarkably complete; indeed, the entire monograph is an enduring monument to the skill and powers of observation of this great physician. "(1) An irregular or unusual proportion of its parts. The head is evidently larger than normal, and the face fatter in respect to the other parts. . . . (2) The external members and muscles of the whole body are seen to be delicate and emaciated, as though consumed by atrophy or tabes, and this (so far as we know) is always observed in those dead of this affection. (3) The whole skin, both the true and the fleshy and fatty layers, is flaccid and rather pendulous, like a loose glove, so that you think it could hold much more flesh. (4) About the joints, especially in the wrists and ankles, there are certain protuberances which, if opened, are seen to arise, not in the fleshy or membranous parts, but in the ends of the bones themselves, especially in their epiphyses. (5) The joints, limbs, and habitus of all these external parts are less firm and rigid, less inflexible than in other dead bodies, and the neck scarcely becomes rigid, *a frigore,* post mortem, or to a less extent than in other cadavers. (6) The chest externally is thin and much narrowed, especially beneath the scapulæ, as though compressed from the sides, and the sternum accuminated like the keel of a ship or the breast of a fowl. (7) The ends of the ribs which join with the cartilages of the sternum are nodular, like the ends of the wrists and ankles."

He also describes the prominent abdomen, the enlarged liver, and the changes in the mesenteric glands.

The bones show the most important changes, particularly the ends of the long bones and the ribs. Between the shaft and epiphyses a slight bulging is apparent, and on section the zone of proliferation, which normally is represented by two narrow bands, is greatly thickened, bluish in color, more irregular in outline, and very much softer. The width of this cushion of cartilage varies from 5 to 15 mm. The line of ossification is also irregular and more spongy and vascular than normal. The periosteum strips off very readily from the shaft, and beneath it there may be a spongy tissue not unlike decalcified bone. The practical outcome of these changes is an imperfect ossification, so that the bone has neither the natural rate of growth nor the normal firmness. In the cranium there may be large areas, particularly in the parieto-occipital region, in which the ossification is delayed, producing the so-called cranio-tabes, so that the bone yields readily to pressure with the finger. There are localized depressed spots of atrophy, which, on pressure, give the so-called "parchment crackling." Flat hyperostoses arise on the outer table, particularly on the frontal and parietal bones, producing the characteristic broad forehead with prominent frontal eminences, a condition sometimes mistaken for hydrocephalus.

Kassowitz, the leading authority on the anatomy of rickets, regards the hyperæmia of the periosteum, the marrow, the cartilage, and of the bone itself as the primary lesion, out of which all the others arise. It is interesting to note that Glisson attributed rickets to disturbed nutrition by arterial blood, and believed the changes in the long bones to be due to excessive vascularity.

The chemical analysis of rickety bones shows a marked diminution in the calcareous salts, which may be as low as 25 or 35 per cent.

The liver and spleen are usually enlarged, and sometimes the mesenteric glands. As Gee suggested, these conditions probably result from the general state of the health associated with rickets. Beneke has described a relative increase in the size of the arteries in rickets.

Symptoms.—The disease comes on insidiously about the period of dentition, before the child begins to walk. Mild grades of it are often overlooked. In many cases digestive disturbances precede the appearance of the characteristic lesions, and the nutrition of the child is markedly impaired. There is usually slight fever, the child is irritable and restless, and sleeps badly. If he has already walked, he now shows a marked disinclination to do so, and seems feeble and unsteady in his gait. Sir William Jenner called attention to three general symptoms of great importance: First, a diffuse soreness of the body, so that the child cries when an attempt is made to move it, and prefers to keep perfectly still. Secondly, slight fever (100° to 101.5° F.), with nocturnal restlessness, and a tendency to throw off the bedclothes. This may be partly due to the fact that the general sensitiveness is such that even their weight may be distressing. And, thirdly, profuse sweating, particularly about the head and neck, so that in the morning the pillow is found soaked with perspiration.

The tissues become soft and flabby; the skin is pale; and from a healthy, plump condition the child becomes puny and feeble. The muscular weakness may be marked, particularly in the legs, and paralysis may be suspected. This so-called pseudo-paresis of rickets results in part from the flabby, weak condition of the legs and in part from the pain associated with the movements. Coincident with, or following closely upon, the general symptoms the characteristic skeletal lesions are observed. Among the first of these to appear are the changes in the ribs, at the junction of the bone with the cartilage, forming the so-called rickety rosary. When the child is thin these nodules may be distinctly seen, and in any case can be easily made out by touch. They very rarely appear before the third month. They may increase in size up to the second year, and are rarely seen after the fifth year. The thorax undergoes important changes. Just outside the junction of the cartilages with the ribs there is an oblique, shallow depression extending downward and outward.

A transverse curve, sometimes called Harrison's groove, passes outward from the level of the ensiform cartilage toward the axilla, and may be deepened at each inspiration. It is rendered more prominent by the eversion and prominence of the costal border. The sternum projects, particularly in its lower half, forming the so-called pigeon or chicken breast. These changes in the thorax are not peculiar, however, to rickets, and are much more commonly associated with hypertrophy of the tonsils, or any trouble which interferes with the free entrance of air into the lungs. The spine is often curved posteriorly, the processes are prominent; lateral curvature is not so common.

The head of a rickety child usually looks large in proportion both to the body and the face, and the fontanelles remain open for a long time. There are areas, particularly in the parieto-occipital regions, in which ossification is imperfect; and the bone may yield to the pressure of the finger, a condition to which the term *cranio-tabes* has been given. Coincidently with this, hyperplasia proceeds in the frontal and parietal eminences, so that these portions of the skull increase in thickness, and may form irregular bosses. In one type the skull may be large and elongated, with the top considerably flattened. In another, and perhaps more common, case the shape of the skull, when seen from above, is rectangular—the *caput quadratum.* The skull looks large in proportion to the face. The forehead is broad and square, and the frontal eminences marked. The anterior fontanelle is late in closing, and may remain open until the third or fourth year. The skin is thin, the veins are full and prominent, and the hair is often rubbed from the back of the skull.

On placing the ear over the anterior fontanelle, or in the temporal region, a systolic murmur may frequently be heard. This condition, first described by John D. Fisher, of Boston, in 1833, is heard with the greatest frequency in rickets, but its presence and persistence in perfectly healthy infants have been amply demonstrated. The murmur is rarely present after the fifth year. A knowledge of the existence of this systolic brain murmur may prevent errors. A case has been reported as an instance of tumor of the brain.

Changes occur in the bones of the face, chiefly in the maxillæ, which are reduced in size. The normal process of dentition is much disturbed; indeed, late teething is one of the marked features in rickets. The teeth which appear may be small and badly formed.

In the upper limbs changes in the scapulæ are not common. The clavicle may be thickened at the sternal end, and there may be thickening near the attachment of the sterno-cleido muscle. The most noticeable changes are at the lower ends of the radius and ulna. The enlargement is at the junction-area of the shaft and epiphysis. Less evident enlargements may occur at the lower end of the humerus. In severe cases the natural shape of the bones of the arm may be much altered, since they have had to support the weight of the child in crawling on the floor. The changes in the pelvis are of special importance, particularly in female children, as in extreme cases they lead to great deformity, with narrowing. In the legs, the lower end of the tibia first becomes enlarged; and in slight cases it may alone be affected. In the severe forms the upper end of the bone, the corresponding parts of the fibula, and the lower end of the femur become greatly thickened. If the child walks, slight bowing of the tibiæ inevitably results. In more advanced cases the tibiæ, and even the femora, may be arched forward. In other instances the condition of knock-knee occurs. Unquestionably the chief cause of these deformities is the weight of the body in walking, but muscular action takes part in it. The green-stick fracture is not uncommon in the soft bones of rickets.

These changes in the skeleton proceed slowly, and the general symptoms vary a good deal with their progress. The child becomes more or less emaciated, though "fat rickets" is by no means uncommon, and a child may be well nourished but "pasty" and flabby. Fever is not constant, but in actively progressing changes in the bone there is usually a slight pyrexia. The abdomen is large, "pot-bellied," due partly to flatulent distention, partly to enlargement of the liver, and in severe cases to diminution of the volume of the thorax. The spleen is often enlarged and readily palpable. The urine is stated to contain an excess of lime salts. There is usually slight anæmia, the hæmoglobin is absolutely and relatively decreased; a leucocytosis may or may not be present; it is more common with enlargement of the spleen (Morse). Many rickety children show marked nervous symptoms; irritability, peevishness, and sleeplessness are constantly present. Jenner called attention to the close relationship which existed between rickets and infantile convulsions, particularly to the fits which occur after the sixth month. Tetany is by no means uncommon. It involves most frequently the arms and hands; occasionally the legs as well. Laryngismus stridulus is a common complication, and though not, as some state, invariably associated, yet it is certainly much more frequent in rickety than in other children. Severe rickets interferes seriously with the growth of a child. Extreme examples of rickety dwarfs are not uncommon. Acute rickets, so-called, is in reality a manifestation of scurvy and will be described with that disease.

Prognosis.—The disease is never in itself fatal, but the condition of the child is such that it is readily carried off by intercurrent affections. particularly those of the respiratory organs. Spasm of the larynx and convulsions occasionally cause death. In females the deformity of the pelvis is serious, as it may lead to difficulties in parturition.

Treatment.—The better the condition of the mother during pregnancy the less likelihood is there of the development of rickets in the child. Rapidly repeated pregnancies and suckling of a child during pregnancy seem important factors in the production of the disease. Of the general treatment, attention to the feeding of the child is the first consideration. If the mother is unhealthy, or cannot from any cause nurse the child, a suitable wet-nurse should be provided, or the child must be artificially fed, in which case cow's milk, diluted according to the age of the child, should constitute the chief food. Care should be taken to examine the condition of the stools, and if curds are present the child is taking too much, or it is not sufficiently diluted. Barley-water and carefully strained and well-boiled oatmeal gruel form excellent additions to the milk.

The child should be warmly clad and should be in the fresh air and sunshine the greater part of the day. The child should be bathed daily in warm water. Careful friction with sweet oil is very advantageous, and, if properly performed, allays rather than aggravates the sensitiveness. Special care should be taken to prevent deformity. The child should not be allowed to walk, and for this purpose splints applied so as to extend beyond the feet are very effective. Of medicines, phosphorus has been warmly recommended by Kassowitz, and its use is also advised by Jacobi. The child may be given gr. 1/120 two or three times a day, dissolved in olive oil. The best preparation in such cases is the elixir phosphori, six to ten or twelve minims three times a day (Jacobi). Cod-liver oil, in doses of from a half to one teaspoonful, is very advantageous. The syrup of the iodide of iron may be given with the oil. The digestive disturbances, together with the respiratory and nervous complications, should receive appropriate treatment.

V. SCURVY

(*Scorbutus*)

Definition.—A disorder of metabolism of unknown origin, characterized by great debility, with anæmia, a spongy condition of the gums, and a tendency to hæmorrhages.

Etiology.—The disease has been known from the earliest times, and has prevailed particularly in armies in the field and among sailors on long voyages. It has been well called "the calamity of sailors."

From the early part of the last century, owing largely to the efforts of Lind and to a knowledge of the conditions upon which the disease depends, scurvy has gradually disappeared from the naval service. In the mercantile marine cases still occasionally occur, owing to the lack of proper and suitable food.

In parts of Russia scurvy is endemic. In the United States scurvy is not a very rare disease. To the hospitals in the seaport towns sailors are now and then admitted with it. In large almshouses outbreaks occasionally occur. A very great increase of foreign population of a low grade has in certain districts made the disease not at all uncommon. In the mining districts of Pennsylvania the Hungarian, Bohemian, and Italian settlers are not infrequently attacked. McGrew has reported 42 cases in Chicago, limited entirely to Poles. He ascertained that in a large proportion of the cases the diet was composed of bread, strong coffee, and meat. Occasionally one meets with scurvy among quite well-to-do people. Some years ago scurvy was not infrequent in the large lumbering camps in the Ottawa Valley. In Great Britain and Ireland it has become very rare; only 302 cases were admitted to the Seaman's Hospital in the twenty-two years ending 1896 (Johnson Smith). It is not uncommon in the South African natives.

The cause is unknown; there are three theories of the disease:

(*a*) That it is the result of an absence of those ingredients in the food which are supplied by fresh vegetables. What these constituents are has not yet been definitely determined, whether the potassium salts or the absence of the organic salts present in fruits and vegetables. Wright has brought forward evidence which suggests that it may be an acid intoxication. That it is not due to an absence of fresh vegetables or the salts of fruits and vegetables seems to have been settled by Nansen and his comrades, who, living for months under the most unfavorable hygienic surroundings, but eating fresh bear's meat and bear's blood, escaped scurvy.

(*b*) That it is due to toxic materials in the food—some unknown organic poison the product of decomposition. Holst and Frölich oppose this toxic view, and maintain that the disease is due to the lack in the food of nutrient constituents which so far have not been identified.

(*c*) In opposition to these chemical views it is urged that the disease depends upon a specific (as yet unknown) micro-organism.

Other factors play an important part, particularly physical and moral influences—overcrowding, dwelling in cold, damp quarters, and prolonged fatigue under depressing influences, as during the retreat of an army. Among prisoners, mental depression plays an important rôle. It is stated that epidemics of the disease have broken out in the French convict ships *en route* to New Caledonia even when the diet was amply sufficient. Nostalgia is sometimes an important element. It is an interesting fact that prolonged starvation in itself does not necessarily cause scurvy. Not one of the professional fasters of late years has displayed any scorbutic symptom. The disease attacks all ages, but the old are more susceptible to it. Sex has no special influence, but during the siege of Paris it was noted that the males attacked were greatly in excess of the females.

Morbid Anatomy.—The anatomical changes are marked, though by no means specific, and are chiefly those associated with hæmorrhage. The blood is dark and fluid. The microscopic alterations are those of a severe anæmia, without leucocytosis. The skin shows the ecchymoses evident during life. There are hæmorrhages into the muscles, and occasionally about or even into the joints. Hæmorrhages occur in the internal organs, particularly on the serous membranes and in the kidneys and bladder. The gums are swollen and sometimes ulcerated, so that in advanced cases the teeth are loose and have even fallen out. Ulcers are occasionally met with in the ileum and colon. Hæmorrhages into the mucous membranes are extremely common. The spleen is enlarged and soft. Parenchymatous changes are constant in the liver, kidneys, and heart.

Symptoms.—The disease is insidious in its onset. Early symptoms are loss in weight, progressive weakness, and pallor. Very soon the gums are noticed to be swollen and spongy, to bleed easily, and in extreme cases to present a fungous appearance. These changes, regarded as characteristic, are sometimes absent. The teeth may become loose and even fall out. Actual necrosis of the jaw is not common. The breath is excessively foul. The tongue is swollen, but may be red and not much furred. The salivary glands are occasionally enlarged. Hæmorrhages beneath the mucous membranes of the mouth are common. The skin becomes dry and rough, and ecchymoses soon appear, first on the legs and then on the arms and trunk, and particularly into and about the hair-follicles. They are petechial, but may become larger, and when subcutaneous may cause distinct swellings. In severe cases, particularly in the legs, there may be effusion between the periosteum and the bone, forming irregular nodes, which may break down and form foul-looking sores. The slightest bruise or injury causes hæmorrhages into the injured part. Œdema about the ankles is common. The "scurvy sclerosis," seen oftenest in the legs, is a remarkable infiltration of the subcutaneous tissues and muscles, forming a brawny induration, the skin over which may be blood-stained. Hæmorrhages from the mucous membranes are less constant symptoms; epistaxis is, however, frequent. Hæmoptysis and hæmatemesis are uncommon. Hæmaturia and bleeding from the bowels may be present in very severe cases.

Palpitation of the heart and feebleness and irregularity of the impulse are prominent symptoms. A hæmic murmur can usually be heard at the base. Hæmorrhagic infarction of the lungs and spleen has been described. Respiratory symptoms are not common. The appetite is impaired, and owing to the soreness of the gums the patient is unable to chew the food. Constipation is more frequent than diarrhœa. The urine is often albuminous. The changes in its composition are not constant; the specific gravity is high; the color is deeper. The statements with reference to the inorganic constituents are contradictory. Some authorities have found the phosphates and potassium salts to be deficient; others hold that they are increased.

There are mental depression, indifference, in some cases headache, and in the later stages delirium. Cases of convulsions, or hemiplegia, and of meningeal hæmorrhage have been described. Remarkable ocular symptoms are occasionally met with, such as night-blindness or day-blindness.

In advanced cases necrosis of the bones may occur, and in young persons even separation of the epiphyses. There are instances in which the cartilages have separated from the sternum. The callus of a recently repaired fracture has been known to undergo destruction. Fever is not present, except in the later stages, or when secondary inflammations in the internal organs appear. The temperature may, indeed, be sometimes below normal. Acute arthritis is an occasional complication.

Diagnosis.—No difficulty is met in the recognition of scurvy when a number of persons are affected together. In isolated cases, however, the disease is distinguished with difficulty from certain forms of purpura. The association with manifest insufficiency in diet, and the rapid amelioration with suitable food, are points by which the diagnosis can be readily settled.

Prognosis.—The outlook is good, unless the disease is far advanced and the conditions persist which lead to its occurrence. The mortality now is rarely great. Death results from gradual heart-failure, occasionally from sudden syncope. Meningeal hæmorrhage, extravasation into the serous cavities, entero-colitis, and other intercurrent affections may prove fatal.

Prophylaxis.—The regulations of the Board of Trade require that a sufficient supply of antiscorbutic articles of diet be taken on each ship; so that now, except as the result of accident, the occurrence of scurvy is rare in sailors.

Treatment.—The juice of two or three lemons daily and a diet of plenty of meat and fresh vegetables suffice to cure all cases of scurvy, unless far advanced. When the stomach is much disordered, small quantities of scraped meat and milk should be given at short intervals, and the lemon-juice in gradually increasing quantities. As the patient gains in strength the diet may be more liberal, and he may eat freely of potatoes, cabbage, water-cresses, and lettuce. The stomatitis is the symptom which causes the greatest distress. A permanganate of potash or dilute carbolic acid solution forms the best mouth-wash. Penciling the swollen gums with a tolerably strong solution of nitrate of silver is very useful. The solution is better than the solid stick, as it reaches to the crevices between the granulations. The constipation which is so common is best treated with large enemata. For other conditions, such as hæmorrhages and ulcerations, suitable measures must be employed.

INFANTILE SCURVY

(*Barlow's Disease*)

A special form of scurvy occurs in children in consequence of imperfect food supply.

W. B. Cheadle and Gee, in London, described in very young children a cachexia associated with hæmorrhage. Cheadle regarded the cases as scurvy ingrafted on a rickety stock. Gee called his cases periosteal cachexia. Cases had previously been regarded as acute rickets.

A few years later Barlow made an exhaustive study of the condition with careful anatomical observations. The affection is now recognized as infantile scurvy, and is called Barlow's disease. The American Pædiatric Society collected 379 cases in 1898 in the United States. Of these, the hygienic surroundings were good in 303. A majority of the patients were under twelve months. The proprietary foods, particularly malted milk and condensed milk, seem to be the most important factors in producing the disease. There are instances in which it has developed in breast-fed infants, and in others fed on the carefully prepared milk of the Walker-Gordon laboratories.

The following clinical summary is taken from Barlow's description:

"So long as it is left alone the child is tolerably quiet; the lower limbs are kept drawn up and still; but when placed in its bath or otherwise moved there is continuous crying, and it soon becomes clear that the pain is connected with the lower limbs. At this period the upper limbs may be touched with impunity, but any attempt to move the legs or thighs gives rise to screams. Next, some obscure swelling may be detected, first on one lower limb, then on the other, though it is not absolutely symmetrical. . . . The swelling is ill-defined, but is suggestive of thickening round the shafts of the bones, beginning above the epiphyseal junctions. Gradually the bulk of the limbs affected becomes visibly increased. . . . The position of the limbs becomes somewhat different from what it was at the outset. Instead of being flexed they lie everted and immobile, in a state of pseudo-paralysis. . . . About this time, if not before, great weakness of the back becomes manifest. A little swelling of one or both scapulæ may appear, and the upper limbs may show changes. These are rarely so considerable as the alterations in the lower limbs. There may be swelling above the wrists, extending for a short distance up the forearm, and some swelling in the neighborhood of the epiphyses of the humerus. There is symmetry of lesions, but it is not absolute; and the limb affection is generally consecutive, though the involvement of one limb follows very close upon another. The joints are free. In severe cases another symptom may now be found—namely, crepitus in the regions adjacent to the junctions of the shafts with the epiphyses. The upper and lower extremities of the femur, and the upper extremity of the tibia, are the common sites of such fractures; but the upper end of the humerus may also be so affected. . . . A very startling appearance may be observed at this period in the front of the chest. The sternum, with the adjacent costal cartilages and a small portion of the contiguous ribs, seems to have sunk bodily back, *en bloc,* as though it had been subjected to some violence which had fractured several ribs in the front and driven them back. Occasionally thickenings of varying extent may be found on the exterior of the vault of the skull, or even on some of the bones of the face. . . . Here also must be mentioned a remarkable eye phenomenon. There develops a rather sudden proptosis of one eyeball, with puffiness and very slight staining of the upper lid. Within a day or two the other eye presents similar appearances, though they may be of less severity. The ocular conjunctiva may show a little ecchymosis, or may be quite free. With respect to the constitutional symptoms accompanying the above series of events the most important feature is the profound anæmia which is developed. . . . The anæmia is proportional to the amount of limb involvement. As the case proceeds there is a certain earthy-colored or sallow tint, which is noteworthy in severe cases, and when once this is established bruise-like ecchymoses may appear, and more rarely small purpura. Emaciation is not a marked feature, but asthenia is extreme and suggestive of muscular failure. The temperature is very erratic; it is often raised for a day or two, when successive limbs are involved, especially during the tense stage, but is rarely above 101° or 102° F. At other times it may be normal or subnormal." If the teeth have appeared the gums may be spongy.

In young children with difficulty in moving the lower limbs, or in whom paralysis is suspected, the condition should always be looked for. What is known sometimes as Parrot's disease, or syphilitic pseudo-paralysis, may be confounded with it. In it the loss of motion is more or less sudden in the upper or lower limbs, or in both, due to a solution of continuity and separation of the cartilage at the end of the diaphysis. There are usually crepitation and much pain on movement.

The essential lesion is a subperiosteal blood extravasation, which causes the thickening and tenderness in the shafts of the bones. In some instances there is hæmorrhage in the intramuscular tissue.

The prophylaxis is most important. The various proprietary forms of condensed milk and preserved foods for infants should not be used. The fresh cow's milk should be substituted, and a teaspoonful of meat-juice or gravy may be given with a little mashed potato. Orange-juice or lemon-juice should be given three or four times a day. Recovery is usually prompt and satisfactory.

VI. OBESITY

Definition.—A disorder of metabolism characterized by excessive deposit of fat in the body.

Etiology.—Corpulence, an overgrowth of the bodily fat, an "oily dropsy," as Byron termed it, is a common condition which may be a source of great bodily and mental distress. Primarily it results from inadequate oxidation of the food stuffs, associated either with excessive absorption of the materials which produce fat, or with incomplete combustion. Both factors probably take part. It is not always due to excessive intake of food; many stout persons are light eaters. On the other hand, there are cases in which the increase in weight is directly due to an excessive consumption of food. There is a marked hereditary tendency. Certain races are prone to obesity, and women are more often affected than men.

Fat metabolism is as yet imperfectly understood; it is under the control of the internal secretions. We see the deposition of fat in connection with many processes with which the internal secretions are concerned. At puberty there is a great increase in the fat deposits, particularly of the skin. Following castration there is an increase in the amount of subcutaneous fat. Eunuchs as a rule are very stout. At the menopause increase in weight is common, and during both pregnancy and lactation the subcutaneous fat may be greatly increased.

In only one point have we positive knowledge as to the internal secretions controlling fat metabolism. It has been known that tumors of the pituitary gland or in its neighborhood may be associated with general adiposity and sexual infantilism (Frölich's syndrome). The studies of Cushing and his students have shown that the pituitary body controls carbohydrate metabolism, and that with the removal of the posterior lobe there is a great increase in the body weight. There seems to be a definite hypophysial syndrome of increased tolerance for carbohydrates with adiposity. It is not unlikely that many of the cases of extreme obesity in young persons are due to hypopituitarism. The remarkable acute obesity, in which as much as 70 pounds in weight may be gained in six months, probably depends upon perversions of some internal secretions.

Symptoms.—Inconvenience caused by the bulk, and loss of good looks in women, are the features for which we are usually consulted. While fat is no sign of health, the great bulk may be consistent with remarkable vigor and activity. Shortness of breath, embarrassed cardiac action, difficulty in walking are the most common complaints. In children obesity is very often associated with careless habits in eating and lack of proper control on the part of parents. The condition is increasing, particularly in the United States, where one sees an extraordinary number of very stout children. A remarkable phenomenon associated with excessive fat in young persons is an uncontrollable tendency to sleep—like the fat boy in Pickwick. It is quite possible that this narcolepsy is also a manifestation of disturbed internal secretions.

Treatment.—In women obesity is a very distressing state, accompanied with all sorts of inconveniences and discomforts. With a marked hereditary tendency not much can be expected. The famous George Cheyne, who was a man of enormous bulk, reduced himself by dieting from thirty-two stones (448 pounds) to proper dimensions. One of his aphorisms says: "Every wise man after Fifty ought to begin and lessen at least the quantity of his Aliment, and if he would continue free from great and dangerous Distempers and preserve his Senses and Faculties clear to the last, he ought every seven years to go on abating gradually and sensibly, and at last descend out of life as he ascended into it, even into a Child's Diet." Put in other words, it reads —We eat too much after forty years of age.

In the case of children very much may be done by regulating the diet, reducing the starches and fats in the food, not allowing them to eat sweets, and encouraging systematic exercises. In the case of women who tend to grow stout after child-bearing or at the climacteric, in addition to systematic exercises, they should be told to avoid taking too much food, and particularly to reduce the starches and sugars. There are a number of methods or systems in vogue at present. In the celebrated one of Banting the carbohydrates and fats were excluded and the amount of food was greatly reduced.

Oertel's method is given under the treatment of fatty heart. He reduces the amount of liquid taken, and this is practically, too, the so-called Schweninger cure, in which liquids are allowed only two hours after the food.

Von Noorden's dietary is as follows: Eight o'clock, 80 grams of lean, cold meat, 25 grams of bread, one cup of tea, with a spoonful of milk, no sugar. Ten o'clock, one egg. Twelve o'clock, a cup of strong meat broth. One o'clock, a small plate of meat soup flavored with vegetables, 150 grams of lean meat of one or two sorts, partly fish, partly flesh, 100 grams of potatoes with salad, 100 grams of fresh fruit, or compote without sugar. Three o'clock, a cup of black coffee. Four o'clock, 200 grams of fresh fruit. Six o'clock, a quarter of a litre of milk, if desired, with tea. Eight o'clock, 125 grams of cold meat, or 180 grams of meat weighed raw and grilled, and eaten with pickles or radishes and salad, 30 grams of Graham bread, and two or three spoonfuls of cooked fruit without sugar. He believes it more satisfactory to give in addition to the three meals smaller quantities of food at shorter intervals, so as to obviate the tendency to weakness which these patients often experience. In addition he allows twice in the day a glass of wine. The use of mineral water, weak tea, or lemonade is not limited at the meal times or in the intervals. An occasional "hunger-day" is given.

In the treatment of extreme obesity it is very much better that the patient should be in hospital, or under the care of a nurse, who will undertake the proper weighing and administration of the food. The amount of fluid ingested should not be reduced below one litre a day. Many of these patients are anæmic, even with a florid appearance, and for them iron in full doses is advisable.

The thyroid extract should be used only in a systematic "cure." Five grains three times a day is a sufficient dose. In conjunction with the diet and exercises it is useful, but it should not be ordered indiscriminately to fat persons. Pituitary gland extracts have also been used.

VII. THE LIPOMATOSES

Various forms of localized deposits of fat may be considered here, and I follow the division in Lyon's thorough study of these conditions (*Archives of Internal Medicine,* VI, 1).

I. Adiposis Dolorosa (*Dercum's Disease*).—In the words of the original description this is a disorder characterized by irregular symmetrical deposits of fatty masses in various portions of the body, preceded or attended by pain, and associated sometimes with asthenia and psychical changes.

The lipomatous masses are diffuse and symmetrical, involving the abdomen, chest, arms or legs; or localized on the limbs or trunk. The hands, face and feet are usually spared. The pain is sometimes spontaneous and is easily excited by pressure. Asthenia, not always present, may be a marked feature. The patients are often irritable, and the French writers have described cases with mental changes. Sometimes the skin over the areas of infiltration is markedly hyperæsthetic. The affection is more common in females. Nine or ten autopsies have been made, none of which threw clear light on the pathology. Quite possibly it is a disturbance of the internal secretions.

II. Nodular Circumscribed Lipomatosis.—The cases are common. The lipomata are distributed in various localities and vary in size from small encapsulated nodules to large circumscribed tumors, solitary or multiple, sometimes symmetrically placed. They may be painful, and Lyon calls attention to the fact that the accessory features of asthenia and psychical changes may also be present.

III. Diffuse Symmetrical Lipomatosis of the Neck.—This remarkable affection, also called adeno-lipomatosis, is characterized by symmetrical fatty infiltrations, either simple or lobulated, of the subcutaneous tissues, forming a huge collar about the neck. It may occur in this part alone, or other limited lipomata are found elsewhere. Males are much more frequently attacked than females. The tumors interfere but little with health, but as they increase the condition becomes very disfiguring. There are sometimes constitutional symptoms. The name "*adeno*-lipomatosis" has been given because scattered throughout the diffuse fatty masses there are small firm nodules of lymphatic tissue—sometimes hæmo-lymph glands.

IV. Cerebral Adiposity (*Dystrophia Adiposo-Genitalis, Frölich*).—As already mentioned, a condition of obesity may occur in connection with tumors of the hypophysis, or adjacent parts, associated with a hypoplasia of the genital organs and a condition of infantilism. The condition will be further discussed in the section on internal secretions, as it would appear from the researches of Cushing to be associated with the perversion of the function of the pituitary gland.

V. Pseudo-Lipoma.—Sydenham made the keen observation that in hysterical patients there were sometimes swellings, which neither yielded to the impress of the finger nor left a mark. Charcot described the condition as "hysterical œdema," of which there is both a blue and a white variety.

Many of these subcutaneous infiltrations, just as in the soft, supraclavicular pad, so common in stout women, are due to fat, and French writers describe all grades of transition from a pseudo-œdema to a true lipoma.

Treatment.—This is not satisfactory. A trial of thyroid extract in small doses is advisable, but it is well to suspend its use for a week in every month. Extracts of other glands may also be tried. In patients with signs of tumor of the hypophysis surgical measures should be considered.

VIII. HÆMOCHROMATOSIS

Definition.—A disorder of metabolism characterized by a deposition of an iron containing pigment in the glandular organs, and by an increase in the normal pigmentation with which is associated a progressive sclerosis of various organs, and, in a large proportion of the cases, diabetes. The disease was first described by von Recklinghausen.

Etiology.—There are about 60 cases on record (1911), all, with the exception of about a dozen, with diabetes. Only one occurred in a woman. In the majority of the patients, middle-aged men, there seemed to be no marked predisposing causes, though Blumer in a recent study maintains that alcohol plays an important part.

Pathology.—On autopsy the ochre or bronze color of the organs is the striking feature. The liver is large and sclerotic; the spleen also enlarged, and the pancreas either small and atrophic or fatty and fibroid. The lymph nodes are also pigmented. The pigment is hæmosiderin or iron-reacting. It is chiefly in the cells of the glands, in the muscle cells of the heart, and in the lymph nodes. The amount in the various organs is enormous, a hundred times the normal in the liver, for example. The hæmofuscin, the non-iron-reacting pigment, varies in different amounts, and it has a yellow tint, and is found chiefly in the connective tissue cells. The blood shows no special changes.

The pathogenesis of the disease is obscure, and Sprunt, whose recent study (*Archives of Internal Medicine,* July, 1911) contains an admirable summary of our knowledge, concludes that there is no evidence of abnormal blood destruction, and that it is a primary disorder of metabolism, "implicating many of the body tissues, and manifested by a change in the chromogenic groups of the proteid molecule with the deposition of pigments."

Clinical Features.—There are two groups of cases, the larger one in which diabetes is present, and the smaller in which there is no sugar in the urine. The former group is spoken of by the French as *diabète bronzé,* which has the features of a severe diabetes with weakness, progressive pigmentation of the skin, and an enlarged liver. The pigmentation of the skin which is the feature that attracts attention varies in color from a dark brown to a leaden or bluish black. Dr. Maude Abbott's case was known as *Blue Mary.* The liver is in a state of hypertrophic cirrhosis, a smooth and uniform enlargement. The spleen may be enlarged secondarily. It was very large in two of my cases. The diabetes is usually severe, and runs a rapid course. Prior to the onset of diabetes the disease may last for years.

There is no special treatment beyond measures for the general health; in the patients with diabetes the usual treatment for that disease should be carried out.

IX. OCHRONOSIS

Definition.—A rare disorder of metabolism associated with blackening of the cartilages and fibrous tissues and pigmentation of the skin, and the presence of dark urine due to alcapton or to derivatives of carbolic acid.

Etiology.—There are two groups of cases:

(*a*) There is a congenital life-long chemical malformation, sometimes a family affection, in which there is a failure to complete the catabolism of certain aromatic compounds, with the result that peculiar bodies, homogenistic acid and uroleucic acid are excreted in the urine, which blackens on exposure to air—alcaptonuria. The anomaly may be present in three generations.

(*b*) In the other group the dark urine and the blackening of the tissues are due to the prolonged use of carbolic acid, usually the application of strong solutions externally to ulcers. There may possibly be other causes.

Symptoms.—When well developed, ochronosis presents a very striking picture. The discoloration of the fibrous tissues is best seen about the knuckles, and in thin persons the tendons of the hands and feet show a bluish-gray appearance. The cartilage of the ear has a bluish tint, and there may be symmetrical black patches on the sclerotics. Widespread pigmentation of the skin has been observed. In one of my patients there was a coal-black discoloration of the skin over the nose and cheeks, and the same was beginning in the hands. This may occur also in the carboluria group, as well shown in the colored illustration of Dr. Pope's patient. Several of the reported cases had arthritis, and the two brothers in the Maryland family had a curious anterior inclination of the trunk, and a peculiar waddling gait. There are few symptoms directly due to the chemical malformation. The patients enjoy good health, but the disfigurement may be very great. Post mortem, the appearance is remarkable, as pictured in Virchow's original case; the cartilages, ligaments and fibrous structures are everywhere of a brown-black color.

SECTION V

DISEASES OF THE DIGESTIVE SYSTEM

A. DISEASES OF THE MOUTH

STOMATITIS

Acute Stomatitis.—Simple or erythematous stomatitis, the commonest form, results from the action of irritants of various sorts. Frequent at all ages, in children it is usually associated with dentition and with gastro-intestinal disturbance, particularly in ill-nourished, unhealthy subjects; in adults it may follow the abuse of tobacco, or the use of too hot or too highly seasoned food; it is a concomitant of indigestion, or of the specific fevers.

The affection may be limited to the gums and lips or may extend over the whole surface of the mouth and include the tongue. There are at first superficial redness and dryness of the membrane, followed by increased secretion and swelling of the tongue, which is furred, and indented by the teeth. There is rarely any constitutional disturbance, but in children there may be slight elevation of temperature. The condition causes considerable discomfort, sometimes amounting to actual distress and pain, particularly in mastication.

In infants the mouth should be carefully sponged after each feeding. A mouth-wash of borax or glycerin and borax may be used, and in severe cases, which tend to become chronic, a dilute solution of nitrate of silver (3 or 4 grains to the ounce) may be applied.

Aphthous Stomatitis.—This form, also known as *follicular* or *vesicular* stomatitis, is characterized by the presence of small, slightly raised spots, from 2 to 4 mm. in diameter, surrounded by reddened areolæ. The spots appear first as vesicles, which rupture, leaving small ulcers with grayish bases and bright-red margins. They are seen most frequently on the inner surfaces of the lips, the edges of the tongue, and the cheeks. They are seldom present on the mucous membrane of the pharynx. This form is met with most often in children under three years, either as an independent affection or in association with one of the febrile diseases of childhood or with an attack of indigestion. The vesicles come out with great rapidity and the little ulcers may be fully formed within twenty-four hours. The child complains of soreness of the mouth and takes food with reluctance. The buccal secretions are increased and the breath is heavy, but not foul. The constitutional symptoms are usually those of the disease with which the aphthæ are associated. The disease must not be confounded with thrush. No special parasite has been found in connection with it. It is not a serious condition, and heals rapidly with the improvement of the constitutional state. In severe cases it may extend to the pillars of the fauces and to the pharynx, and produce ulcers which are irritating and difficult to heal.

Each ulcer should be touched with nitrate of silver and the mouth should be thoroughly cleansed after taking food. A wash of chlorate of potassium, or of borax and glycerin, may be used. The constitutional symptoms should receive careful attention.

A curious affection occurs in southern Italy sometimes in epidemic form, characterized by a pearly-colored membrane with induration, immediately beneath the tongue on the frænum (Riga's disease). There may be much induration and ultimately ulceration. It occurs in both healthy and cachectic children, usually about the time of the eruption of the first teeth.

Ulcerative Stomatitis.—This form, which is also known by the names of *fetid stomatitis*, or *putrid sore mouth*, occurs particularly in children after the first dentition. It may prevail as a widespread epidemic in institutions in which the sanitary conditions are defective. It has been met with in jails and camps. Insufficient and unwholesome food, improper ventilation, and prolonged damp, cold weather seem to be special predisposing causes. Lack of cleanliness of the mouth, the presence of carious teeth, and the collection of tartar around them favor the occurrence of the disease. The affection spreads like a specific disease, but the microbe has not yet been isolated. It has been held that the disease is the same as the foot-and-mouth disease of cattle, and that it is conveyed by the milk, but there is no positive evidence on these points.

The morbid process begins at the margin of the gums, which become swollen and red, and bleed readily. Ulcers form, the bases of which are covered with a grayish-white, firmly adherent membrane. In severe cases the teeth may become loosened and necrosis of the alveolar process may occur. The ulcers extend along the gum-line of the upper and lower jaws; the tongue, lips, and mucosa of the cheeks are usually swollen, but rarely ulcerated. There is salivation, the breath is foul, and mastication is painful. The submaxillary lymph-glands are enlarged. An exanthem may appear and be mistaken for measles. The constitutional symptoms are often severe, and in debilitated children death sometimes occurs.

In the treatment of this form of stomatitis chlorate of potassium has been found to be almost specific. It should be given in doses of 10 grains (0.6 gm.), three times a day, to a child, and to an adult double that amount. Locally it may be used as a mouth-wash, or the powdered salt may be applied directly to the ulcerated surfaces. When there is much fetor, a solution of potassium permanganate may be used as a wash, and an application of nitrate of silver made to the ulcers.

A *variety* of ulcerative sore mouth, which differs entirely from this form, is common in nursing women, and is usually seen on the mucous membrane of the lips and cheeks. The ulcers arise from the mucous follicles, and are from 3 to 5 mm. in diameter. They may cause little or no inconvenience; but in some instances they are very painful and interfere seriously with the taking of food and its mastication. As a rule they heal readily after the application of nitrate of silver, and the condition is an indication for tonics, fresh air, and a better diet.

Recurring outbreaks of an *herpetic,* even *pemphigoid,* stomatitis are seen in neurotic individuals (*stomatitis neurotica chronica,* Jacobi). It may precede or accompany the fatal form of *pemphigus vegetans.*

Parrot describes the occasional appearance in new-born, debilitated children of small ulcers symmetrically placed on the hard palate on either side of the middle line. They rarely heal, but tend to increase in size, and may involve the bone.

Bednar's aphthæ consist of small patches and ulcers on the hard palate, caused as a rule in young infants by the artificial nipple or the nurse's finger.

Parasitic Stomatitis (*Thrush; Soor; Muguet*).—This affection, most commonly seen in children, is dependent upon a fungus, *Saccharomyces albicans,* called by Robin *Oïdium albicans.* It belongs to the order of yeast fungi, and consists of branching filaments, from the ends of which ovoid torula cells develop. The disease does not arise apparently in a normal mucosa. The use of an improper diet, uncleanliness of the mouth, the acid fermentation of remnants of food, or the occurrence, from any cause, of catarrhal stomatitis predispose to the growth. In institutions it is frequently transmitted by unclean feeding-bottles, spoons, etc. It is not confined to children, but is met with in adults in the final stages of fever, in chronic tuberculosis, diabetes, and in cachectic states. The parasite grows in the upper layers of the mucosa, and the filaments form a dense felt-work among the epithelial cells. The disease begins on the tongue and is seen in the form of slightly raised, pearly-white spots, which increase in size and gradually coalesce. The membrane thus formed can be readily scraped off, leaving an intact mucosa, or, if the process extends deeply, a bleeding, slightly ulcerated surface. The disease spreads to the cheeks, lips, and hard palate, and may involve the tonsils and pharynx. In very severe cases the entire buccal mucosa is covered by the grayish-white membrane. It may even extend into the œsophagus and to the stomach and cæcum. It is occasionally met with on the vocal cords. Robust, well-nourished children are sometimes affected, but it is usually met with in enfeebled, emaciated infants with digestive or intestinal troubles. In such cases the disease may persist for months.

The affection is readily recognized, and must not be confounded with aphthous stomatitis, in which the ulcers, preceded by the formation of vesicles, are perfectly distinctive. In thrush the microscopic examination shows the presence of the characteristic fungus throughout the membrane. In this condition, too, the mouth is usually dry—a striking contrast to the salivation accompanying aphthæ.

Thrush is more readily prevented than removed. The child's mouth should be kept scrupulously clean, and, if artificially fed, the bottles should be thoroughly sterilized. Lime-water or any other alkaline fluid, such as the bicarbonate of soda (a drachm to a tumbler of water), may be employed. When the patches are present these alkaline mouth-washes may be continued after each feeding. A spray of borax or of sulphite of soda (a drachm to the ounce) or the black wash with glycerine may be employed. The permanganate of potassium is also useful. The constitutional treatment is of equal importance, and it will often be found that the thrush persists, in spite of all local measures, until the general health of the infant is improved by change of air or the relief of the diarrhœa, or, in obstinate cases, the substitution of a natural for the artificial diet.

Gangrenous Stomatitis (*Cancrum Oris; Noma*).—An affection characterized by a rapidly progressing gangrene, starting on the gums or cheeks, and leading to extensive sloughing and destruction. This terrible, but fortunately rare, disease is seen only in children under very insanitary conditions or during convalescence from the acute fevers. It is more common in girls than in boys. It is met with between the ages of two and five years. In at least one-half of the cases the disease has occurred during convalescence from measles. Cases have been seen also after scarlet fever and typhoid. The mucous membrane is first affected, usually of the gums or of one cheek. The process begins insidiously, and when first seen there is a sloughing ulcer of the mucous membrane, which spreads rapidly and leads to brawny induration of the skin and adjacent parts. The sloughing extends, and in severe cases the cheek is perforated. The disease may spread to the tongue and chin; it may invade the bones of the jaws and even involve the eyelids and ears. In mild cases an ulcer forms on the inner surface of the cheek, which heals or may perforate and leave a fistulous opening. Naturally in such a severe affection the constitutional disturbance is very great, the pulse is rapid, the prostration extreme, and death usually takes place within a week or ten days. The temperature may reach 103° or 104° F. Diarrhœa is usually present, and aspiration pneumonia is a common complication. No specific organism has been found.

In many cases the onset is so insidious that there is an extensive sloughing sore when the case first comes under observation. Destruction of the sore by the Paquelin cautery or fuming nitric acid is the most effectual. Antiseptic applications should be made to destroy the fetor. The child should be carefully nourished and stimulants given freely.

Mercurial Stomatitis (*Ptyalism*).—It occurs in persons with a special susceptibility, rarely now as a result of the excessive use of the drug, and also in those whose occupation necessitates the constant handling of mercury. It may follow the administration of repeated small doses. Thus, a patient with heart-disease who was ordered an eighth of a grain of calomel every three hours for diuretic purposes had, after taking eight or ten doses, a severe stomatitis, which persisted for several weeks. I have known it to follow the administration of small doses of gray powder. The patient complains first of a metallic taste in the mouth, the gums become swollen, red, and sore, mastication is difficult, the salivary glands become enlarged and painful, and there is a great increase in their secretion. The tongue is swollen, the breath has a foul odor, and, if the affection progresses, there may be ulceration of the mucosa, and, in rare instances, necrosis of the jaw. Although troublesome and distressing, the disease is rarely serious, and recovery usually takes place in a couple of weeks. Instances in which the teeth become loosened or detached or in which the inflammation extends to the pharynx and Eustachian tubes are rarely seen now.

The administration of mercury should be suspended so soon as the gums are "touched." Mild cases of the affection subside within a few days and require only a simple mouth-wash. In severer cases the chlorate of potassium may be given internally, and used to rinse the mouth. The bowels should be freely opened; the patient should take a hot bath every evening and should drink plentifully of alkaline mineral waters. Atropine is sometimes serviceable, and may be given in doses of 1/100 of a grain twice a day. Iodine is also recommended. When the salivation is severe and protracted the patient becomes much debilitated and anæmic, so that a supporting treatment is indicated. The diet is necessarily liquid, for the patient finds the chief difficulty in taking food. If the pain is severe Dover's powder may be given at night.

Here may be appropriately mentioned the influence of stomatitis, particularly the mercurial form, upon the developing teeth of children. The condition known as *erosion,* in which the teeth are honeycombed or pitted owing to defective formation of enamel, is indicative, as a rule, of infantile stomatitis. Such teeth must be distinguished carefully from those of congenital syphilis, which may, of course, coexist, but the two conditions are distinct. The honeycombing is frequently seen on the incisors; but, according to Jonathan Hutchinson, the test teeth of infantile stomatitis are the first permanent molars, then the incisors, "which are almost as constantly pitted, eroded, and of bad color, often showing the transverse furrow which crosses all the teeth at the same level." Magitot regards these transverse furrows as the result of infantile convulsions or of severe illness during early life. He thinks they are analogous to the furrows on the nails which so often follow a serious disease.

Geographical Tongue (*Eczema of the Tongue*).—A remarkable desquamation of the superficial epithelium of the tongue in circinate patches, which spread while the central portions heal. Fusion of patches leads to areas with sinuous outlines. When extensive the tongue may be covered with these areas, like a geographical map. The affection causes a good deal of itching and heat, and it may be a source of much mental worry to the patients, who often dread lest it may be a commencing cancer.

The etiology of the disease is unknown. It occurs in infants and children, and it is not very infrequent in adults. It has been regarded as a gouty manifestation, and transient attacks may accompany indigestion. It is very liable to relapse. In adults it may prove very obstinate, and I know of one instance in which the disease persisted in spite of all treatment for more than two years. Solutions of nitrate of silver give the most satisfactory results in relieving the intense burning.

There is a superficial glossitis, limited usually to the border and point of the tongue, which presents irregular reddish spots, looking as if the epithelium was removed, and the papillæ are reddened and swollen. The condition is sometimes known as Möller's glossitis. Local treatment with nitrate of silver as a rule gives relief.

Leukoplakia Buccalis.—Samuel Plumbe described the condition as *icthyosis lingualis.* It has also been called *buccal psoriasis* and *leuco-keratosis mucosæ oris.* The following forms occur: (*a*) Small white spots upon the tongue, slightly raised, even papillomatous—lingual corns. (*b*) Diffuse thickening of the epithelial coating of the tongue, either a thin, bluish-white color or opaque white, depending upon the thickness. It is patchy, and more often upon the dorsum and sides. (*c*) Diffuse oral leukoplakia, a remarkable condition in which the roof of the mouth, the gums, lips, and cheeks are covered with an opaque white, sometimes smooth, sometimes fissured, rugose layer.

In this widespread form the tongue may be spared. The visible mucosa of the lips may be involved, and occasionally the genital mucosa.

While appearing spontaneously, the condition is most common in heavy smokers, and has been called smoker's tongue. Epithelioma occasionally starts from the localized patches. A majority of the patients have had syphilis, but the condition does not yield, as a rule, to specific treatment.

Leukoplakia is a very obstinate affection. All irritants, such as smoke and very hot food, should be avoided. Local treatment with one-half-per-cent. corrosive sublimate or a one-per-cent. chromic-acid solution has been recommended. The propriety of active local treatment is doubtful. Papillomatous outgrowths should be cut off. The X-rays may be tried. The most extensive form may disappear spontaneously.

The *glossy flat atrophy* of the posterior part of the tongue, described by Virchow, is in a majority of instances of syphilitic origin. Scars may give an irregular appearance to the surface. Symmers found this smooth atrophy in 55 of 75 post mortems in syphilitic subjects.

Fetor Oris.—The practitioner is frequently consulted for foul breath, and is daily made aware of its widespread prevalence. All unconscious, he is himself too often subject of the condition, to the disgust of his patients, with whom he has to come into such close contact. It is impossible to give even a list of all the causes mentioned. The following are a few of the more important: (*a*) In connection with indigestion and the associated catarrhal disturbances in the mouth, pharynx, and stomach. The breath is "heavy," as the mothers say. A simple mouth-wash and a mercurial purge suffice to remove it. In a more serious disease of the stomach the breath may be foul, and occasionally, in sloughing cancer, horribly stinking. (*b*) Local conditions in the mouth: (1) All the forms of stomatitis. Smokers should remember that, apart altogether from the smell of tobacco, their breath in the morning is usually, to say the least, "heavy." (2) Pyorrhœa alveolaris. This is the most common cause of foul breath in adults, and is almost constantly present after middle life, causing a perfectly distinctive odor only too well known to all of us. To test for the presence draw a bit of stout thread or the edge of a sheet of paper high up between the teeth and the gums and then smell it. Scrupulous treatment of the gums by a dentist is needed, and daily scouring, etc. (*c*) The tonsillar diseases. In the crypts of the tonsils the epithelial débris accumulates, and, invaded by micro-organisms, gradually forms the little round or triangular bodies which can be squeezed out of the lacunæ, and when pressed between the fingers smell like Limburger cheese. The fetor oris from this cause is quite distinctive. To test the presence in child or adult, smell the finger after it has been rubbed firmly upon the tonsil. Local treatment is needed. (*d*) Decayed teeth, the foul odor of which is quite distinct from that of pyorrhœa or chronic tonsillitis. (*e*) Respiratory. Many diseases of the nose, larynx, bronchi, and lungs are associated with foul breath. (*f*) Hæmic. The halitus—the expired air from the lung—may be impregnated with odors from the blood. Of this there are many well-known instances.

For practical purposes it is to be remembered that pyorrhœa alveolaris and what is called chronic lacunar tonsillitis are the two most common causes of foul breath.

Oral Sepsis.—To William Hunter, of Charing Cross Hospital, is due the credit of insisting upon the importance of the mouth as the chief channel of entrance of the pyogenic organisms, and as itself the seat of septic processes. Necrosed teeth, pyorrhœa alveolaris, gingivitis, alveolar abscess, etc., are present in a great many people. A systemic infection may follow or the general health may be lowered by the continuous production of pus. In extensive pyorrhœa alveolaris the daily amount of pus must be considerable, and there can be no question that it has a debilitating influence on the general health and is sometimes associated with a moderate anæmia and with a pasty complexion. Hunter describes septic gastritis and septic enteritis as common sequences; indeed, he regards appendicular, pleuritic, gall-bladder and pyelitic inflammations as forms of "medical sepsis" due largely to infection from the mouth. One form of pernicious anæmia—infective hæmolytic anæmia—he believes to be due to oral sepsis, or an infective glossitis. Certain types of nephritis and forms of arthritis are believed to be due to oral infection.

There is no question of the importance of the subject, and we should insist upon scrupulous cleanliness of the mouth and teeth, particularly clearing away the tartar and the pockets of pus. An adult should have his teeth cleansed in this way by a dentist once a month. We should, too, have less delicacy in telling our friends in whom the odor of the breath reveals the presence of pyorrhœa. It is a very difficult condition to cure. Locally much may be done to keep it under control. Vaccines have been used extensively, sometimes, but not always, with success. If possible, the patient should be referred to a dentist who is specially competent to deal with it. The tartar should be removed from the teeth and antiseptic mouth washes, such as carbolic acid (1 per cent.), used frequently. Hydrogen peroxide may be applied locally.

Affections of the mucous glands are not very common. In catarrhal troubles in children and in measles they may be swollen. They are enlarged and very prominent in Mikulicz's disease, with chronic symmetrical enlargement of the salivary and lachrymal glands. There is a singular affection of the mucous glands of the lips, chiefly of the lower, with much swelling and infiltration. It was described by Volkmann, and has been called Bälz's disease. The mucous glands are enlarged, the ducts much dilated, and on pressure a mucoid or muco-purulent secretion may exude. The skin over the lips may be reddened and swollen.

B. DISEASES OF THE SALIVARY GLANDS

Supersecretion (*Ptyalism*).—The normal amount of saliva varies from 2 to 3 pints in the twenty-four hours. The secretion is increased during the taking of food and in the physiological processes of dentition. A great increase, to which the term *ptyalism* is applied, is met with (1) occasionally in mental and nervous affections and in rabies; (2) occasionally in the acute fevers, particularly in small-pox; (3) sometimes with disease of the pancreas; (4) during gestation, usually early, though it may persist through the entire course; (5) occasionally at each menstrual period; and, lastly, it is a common effect of certain drugs—mercury, gold, copper, the iodine compounds, and (among vegetable remedies) jaborandi, muscarin, and tobacco excite the salivary secretion. Of these we most frequently see the effect of mercury in producing ptyalism. The salivation may be present without any inflammation of the mouth. For treatment atropine or the bromides may be given in small doses at first and the effect watched until the most efficient dosage is found.

Xerostomia (*Arrest of the Salivary and Buccal Secretions; Dry Mouth*).—In this condition, first described by Jonathan Hutchinson, the secretions of the mouth and salivary glands are suppressed. The tongue is red, sometimes cracked, and quite dry; the mucous membrane of the cheeks and of the palate is smooth, shining, and dry; and mastication, deglutition, and articulation are very difficult. A majority of the cases are in women, and in several instances have been associated with nervous phenomena. The general health, as a rule, is unimpaired. It may be due to involvement of some centre which controls the secretion of the salivary and buccal glands. The free use of glycerin locally is sometimes of value and jaborandi or pilocarpine can be given cautiously.

Inflammation of the Salivary Glands.

(*a*) *Specific Parotitis.* (See Mumps.)

(*b*) *Symptomatic parotitis* or *parotid bubo* occurs:

(1) In the course of the infectious fevers—typhus, typhoid, pneumonia, pyæmia, etc. In ordinary practice it occurs oftenest, perhaps, in typhoid fever. It is the result either of septic infection through the blood, or the inflammation, in many cases, passes up the salivary duct, and so reaches the gland. The process is usually very intense and leads rapidly to suppuration. It is, as a rule, an unfavorable indication in the course of a fever. Parotitis may occur in secondary syphilis.

(2) In connection with injury or disease of the abdomen or pelvis, a condition to which Stephen Paget has called special attention. Of 101 cases of this kind, "10 followed injury or disease of the urinary tract, 18 were due to injury or disease of the alimentary canal, and 23 were due to injury or disease of the abdominal wall, the peritoneum, or the pelvic cellular tissue. The remaining 50 were due to injury, disease, or temporary derangement of the genital organs." By temporary derangement is meant slight injuries or natural processes—a slight blow on the testis, the introduction of a pessary, menstruation, or pregnancy. Bucknell has brought forward strong evidence to show that in all these cases infection takes place through the duct.

(3) In association with facial paralysis, as in a case of fatal peripheral neuritis described by Gowers; in diabetes and chronic metallic poisoning.

In the infectious diseases rigid cleanliness is an important preventive measure. In the treatment of parotitis the application of half a dozen leeches will sometimes reduce the inflammation and promote resolution. An ice bag often aids, or hot fomentations may be applied. A free incision should be made *early* if there are signs of suppuration.

(*c*) *Chronic parotitis,* a condition in which the glands are enlarged, rarely painful, may follow inflammation of the throat or mumps. Salivation may be present. It may be due to lead, mercury, or potassium iodide. It occurs also in chronic Bright's disease and in secondary syphilis. Symmetrical enlargement of the parotids of moderate extent is not very uncommon among hospital patients. The cases at the Johns Hopkins clinic have been reported by C. P. Howard (*Internat. Clinics.*, xix, 1). It may be associated with xerostomia. The parotid and submaxillary glands are affected with equal frequency. In one case the swelling recurred over a period of 20 years (Greig).

(*d*) *Mikulicz's Disease.*—In this remarkable affection, described in 1888 the salivary and lachrymal glands are enlarged simultaneously. The condition is painless and chronic, lasting sometimes for several years, and of unknown etiology. The gland substance itself may not be disturbed, but there is a great infiltration of the interstitial connective tissue. In my case the lachrymal glands were replaced by fibrous tissue. The cases so far reported in America have been in negroes. The enlargement may subside after an acute fever. Good results have followed the use of arsenic.

(*e*) *Gaseous Tumors of Steno's Duct and of the Parotid Gland.*—In glass-blowers and musicians Steno's duct may become inflated with air and form a tumor the size of a nut or of an egg. Some have contained a mixture of air, saliva, and pus. In rare cases there are gaseous tumors of the glands, which give a sensation of crepitation on palpation.

C. DISEASES OF THE PHARYNX

Circulatory Disturbances.—(*a*) *Hyperæmia* is common in acute and chronic affections of the throat, and is frequently seen as a result of the irritation of tobacco smoke, and from the constant use of the voice. Venous stasis is seen in valvular disease of the heart, and in mechanical obstruction of the superior vena cava by tumor or aneurism. In aortic insufficiency the capillary pulse may sometimes be seen, and the intense throbbing of the internal carotid may be mistaken for aneurism.

(*b*) *Hæmorrhage* is found in association with bleeding from other mucous surfaces, or it is due to local causes—granulations, varicosities, or vegetations. It may be mistaken for hæmorrhage from the lungs or stomach. Sometimes the patient finds the pillow stained in the morning with bloody secretion. The condition is rarely serious, and requires only suitable local treatment. Occasionally a hæmorrhage takes place into the mucosa, producing a pharyngeal hæmatoma. I have thrice seen a condition of the uvula resembling hæmorrhagic infarction. One was in a patient with rheumatic fever, to whom large doses of salicylic acid had been given; the other two were instances of peliosis rheumatica, in both of which partial sloughing of the uvula took place.

(*c*) *Œdema.*—An infiltrated œdematous condition of the uvula and adjacent parts is not very uncommon in conditions of debility, in profound anæmia, and in Bright's disease. The uvula is sometimes enormously enlarged from this cause, whence may arise difficulty in swallowing or in breathing.

Acute Pharyngitis (*Sore Throat; Angina Simplex*).—The entire pharyngeal structures, often with the tonsils, are involved. The condition may follow cold or exposure. In other instances it is associated with constitutional states, such as gout, or with digestive disorders. The patient complains of uneasiness and soreness in swallowing, of a feeling of tickling and dryness in the throat, together with a constant desire to hawk and cough. Frequently the inflammation extends into the larynx and produces hoarseness. Not uncommonly it is only part of a general naso-pharyngeal catarrh. The process may pass into the Eustachian tubes and cause slight deafness. There is stiffness of the neck, the lymph-glands of which may be enlarged and painful. The constitutional symptoms are rarely severe. The disease sets in with a chilly feeling and slight fever; the pulse is increased in frequency. Occasionally the febrile symptoms are more severe, particularly if the tonsils are specially involved. The examination of the throat shows general congestion of the mucous membrane, which is dry and glistening, and in places covered with sticky secretion. The uvula may be much swollen.

Acute pharyngitis lasts only a few days and requires mild measures. Cold compresses or an ice bag may be applied to the neck. If the tonsils are involved and the fever is high, aconite or sodium salicylate may be given. Guaiacum also is beneficial; but in a majority of the cases a calomel purge or a saline aperient and simple inhalations meet the indications.

Chronic Pharyngitis.—This may follow repeated acute attacks. It is very common in persons who smoke or drink to excess, and in those who use the voice very much, such as clergymen, hucksters, and others. It is frequently associated with chronic nasal catarrh. The naso-pharynx and the posterior wall are the parts most frequently affected. The mucous membrane is relaxed, the venules are dilated, and roundish bodies, from 2 to 4 mm. in diameter, reddish in color, project to a variable distance beyond the mucous membrane. These represent the proliferations of lymph tissue about the mucous glands. They may be very abundant, forming elongated rows in the lateral walls of the pharynx. With this there may be a dry glistening state of the pharyngeal mucosa, sometimes known as *pharyngitis sicca*. The pillars of the fauces and the uvula are often much relaxed. The secretion forms at the back of the pharynx and the patient may feel it drop down from the vault, or it is tenacious and adherent, and is only removed by repeated efforts at hawking.

In the *treatment* special attention must be paid to the general health. If possible, the cause should be ascertained. The condition is almost constant in smokers, and cannot be cured without stopping the use of tobacco. The use of food either too hot or too much spiced should be forbidden. When it depends upon excessive exercise of the voice, rest should be enjoined. In many of these cases change of air and tonics help very much. In the local treatment of the throat, gargles, washes, and pastilles of various sorts give temporary relief, but when the hypertrophic condition is marked the spots should be thoroughly destroyed by the galvano-cautery. In many instances this affords great and permanent relief, but in others the condition persists, and, as it is not unbearable, the patient gives up all hope of permanent relief.

Ulceration of the Pharynx.—(*a*) *Follicular.*—The ulcers are usually small, superficial, and generally associated with chronic catarrh.

(*b*) *Syphilitic.*—Most frequently painless and situated on the posterior wall of the pharynx, they occur in the secondary stage as small, shallow excavations with the mucous patches. In the tertiary stage they are due to erosion of gummata, and in healing they leave whitish cicatrices.

(*c*) *Tuberculous.*—Not very uncommon in advanced cases of phthisis, if extensive, they form one of the most distressing features of the disease. The ulcers are irregular, with ill-defined edges and grayish-yellow bases. The posterior wall of the pharynx may have an eroded, worm-eaten appearance. These ulcers are, as a rule, intensely painful. Occasionally the primary disease is about the tonsils and the pillars of the fauces.

(*d*) *Ulcers* occur in connection with pseudo-membranous inflammation, particularly the diphtheritic. In cancer and in lupus ulcers are also present.

(*e*) Ulcers are met with in certain of the fevers, particularly in typhoid.

In many instances the diagnosis of the nature of pharyngeal ulcers is very difficult. The tuberculous and cancerous varieties are readily recognized, but it happens not infrequently that a doubt arises as to the syphilitic character of an ulcer. In many instances the local conditions may be uncertain. Then other evidences of syphilis should be sought for, and the patient should be placed on mercury and iodide of potassium, under which remedies specific ulcers usually heal with great rapidity.

Acute Infectious Phlegmon of the Pharynx.—Under this term Senator has described cases in which, along with difficulty in swallowing, soreness of the throat, and sometimes hoarseness, the neck enlarges, the pharyngeal mucosa becomes swollen and injected, the fever is high, the constitutional symptoms are severe, and the inflammation passes on rapidly to suppuration. The symptoms are very intense. The swelling of the pharyngeal tissues early reaches such a grade as to impede respiration. Similar symptoms may be produced by foreign bodies in the pharynx.

Retro-pharyngeal abscess occurs: (*a*) In healthy children between six months and two years of age. The child becomes restless, the voice changes; it becomes nasal or metallic in tone, and there are pain and difficulty in swallowing. Inspection of the pharynx reveals a projecting tumor in the middle line, or, if it be not visible, it is readily felt, on palpation, projecting from the posterior wall. (*b*) As a not infrequent sequel of the fevers, particularly of scarlet fever and diphtheria. (*c*) In caries of the bodies of the cervical vertebræ.

The diagnosis is readily made, as the projecting tumor can be seen, or felt with the finger on the posterior wall of the pharynx.

Angina Ludovici (*Ludwig's Angina; Cellulitis of the Neck*).—In medical practice this is seen as a secondary inflammation in the specific fevers, particularly diphtheria and scarlet fever. It may, however, occur idiopathically or result from trauma. It is probably always a streptococcus infection which spreads rapidly from the glands. The swelling at first is most marked in the submaxillary region of one side. The symptoms are, as a rule, intense, and, unless early and thorough surgical measures are employed, there is great risk of systemic infection. The various acute septic inflammations of the throat —acute œdema of the larynx, phlegmon of the pharynx and larynx, and angina Ludovici—"represent degrees varying in virulence of one and the same process" (Semon). Treatment is surgical, and free incisions should be made.

D. DISEASES OF THE TONSILS

I. SUPPURATIVE TONSILLITIS

Etiology.—Acute suppuration of the tonsillar tissues is met with most frequently in young persons, with chronic enlargement of the glands, sometimes as a sequence of the acute follicular form already described among the infectious diseases, sometimes as a result of exposure to cold or wet.

Symptoms.—The constitutional disturbance is very great. The temperature rises to 104° or 105° F., and the pulse ranges from 110 to 130. Nocturnal delirium is not uncommon. The prostration may be extreme. There is no local disease of similar extent which so rapidly exhausts the strength of a patient. Soreness and dryness of the throat, with pain in swallowing, are the symptoms of which the patient first complains. One or both tonsils may be involved. They are enlarged, firm to the touch, dusky red and œdematous, and the contiguous parts are also much swollen. The swelling of the glands may be so great that they meet in the middle line, or one tonsil may even push the uvula aside and almost touch the other gland. The salivary and buccal secretions are increased. The glands of the neck enlarge, the lower jaw is fixed, and the patient is unable to open his mouth. In from two to four days the enlarged gland becomes softer, and fluctuation can be distinctly felt by placing one finger on the tonsil and the other at the angle of the jaw. The abscess points usually toward the mouth, but in some cases toward the pharynx. It may burst spontaneously, affording instant and great relief. Suffocation has followed the rupture of a large abscess and the entrance of the pus into the larynx. When the suppuration is peritonsillar and extensive, the internal carotid artery may be opened; but these are, fortunately, very rare accidents.

Occasionally a small focus of deep-seated suppuration is the cause of a fever lasting for weeks or months.

Treatment.—Hot applications in the form of poultices and fomentations are more comfortable and better than the ice-bag. The gland should be felt —it cannot always be seen—from time to time, and should be opened when fluctuation is distinct. The progress of the disease may be shortened and the patient spared several days of great suffering if an incision is made early. The curved bistoury, guarded nearly to the point with plaster or cotton, is the most satisfactory instrument. The incision should be made from above downward, parallel with the anterior pillar. There are cases in which, before suppuration takes place, the parenchymatous swelling is so great that the patient is threatened with suffocation. In such instances either the tonsil must be excised or tracheotomy performed. Delavan refers to two cases in which he states that tracheotomy would, under these circumstances, have saved life. Patients with this affection require a nourishing liquid diet, and during convalescence iron in full doses.

Early removal of the tonsils should be practiced when a child suffers with recurring attacks, and thorough local treatment should be given to the nasopharynx. Particular care should be taken of the child's mouth and throat.

II. CHRONIC TONSILLITIS

(Chronic Naso-pharyngeal Obstruction; Adenoids; Mouth-breathing; Aprosexia)

Under this heading will be considered also hypertrophy of the adenoid tissue in the vault of the pharynx, sometimes known as the pharyngeal tonsil, as the affection usually involves both the tonsils proper and this tissue, and the symptoms are not to be differentiated.

Chronic enlargement of the tissues of the tonsillar ring is an affection of great importance, and may influence in an extraordinary way the mental and bodily development of children.

Etiology.—"Adenoids" have become recognized as one of the most common and important affections of childhood, occurring most frequently between the fifth and tenth years. The introduction of the systematic inspection of school children has done more than anything else to force upon the profession and the public the recognition of the condition as one influencing seriously the bodily and mental growth, disturbing hearing and furnishing a focus for the development of pathogenic organisms. Few children escape altogether. In many it is a trifling affair, easily remedied; in others it is a serious and obstinate trouble, taxing the skill and judgment of the specialist. It is not easy to say why the disease has become so prevalent. In the United States it is attributed to the dry, hot air of the houses, in England to the cold, damp climate. In winter nearly all the school children in England have the "snuffles," and a considerable proportion of them adenoids. Interested in the subject ever since reading Meyer's original paper, I thought American children especially prone, but the disease seems to be even more prevalent in England.

Adenoids may be associated with slight enlargement of the lymph-glands, thymus and spleen in the condition of lymphatism.

Morbid Anatomy.—The tonsils are enlarged, due to multiplication of all the constituents of the glands. The lymphoid elements may be chiefly involved without much development of the stroma. In other instances the fibrous matrix is increased, and the organ is then harder, smaller, firmer, and is cut with much greater difficulty.

The adenoids, which spring from the vault of the pharynx, form masses varying in size from a small pea to an almond. They may be sessile, with broad bases, or pedunculated. They are reddish in color, of moderate firmness, and contain numerous blood-vessels. "Abundant, as a rule, over the vault, on a line with the fossa of the Eustachian tube, the growths may lie posterior to the fossa—namely, in the depression known as the fossa of Rosenmüller, or upon the parts which are parallel to the posterior wall of the pharynx. The growths appear to spring in the main from the mucous membrane covering the localities where the connective tissue fills in the inequalities of the base of the skull" (Harrison Allen). The growths are most frequently papillomatous with a lymphoid parenchyma. Hypertrophy of the pharyngeal adenoid tissue may be present without great enlargement of the tonsils proper. Chronic catarrh of the nose usually coexists.

Symptoms.—The direct effect of adenoids is the establishment of mouth-breathing. The indirect effects are deformation of the thorax, changes in the facial expression, sometimes marked alteration in the mental condition, in certain cases stunting of the growth, and in a great many subjects deafness. Woods Hutchinson has suggested that the embryological relation of these structures and the pituitary body may account for the interference with development. The establishment of mouth-breathing is the symptom which first attracts the attention. It is not so noticeable by day, although the child may present the vacant expression characteristic of this condition. At night the child's sleep is greatly disturbed; the respirations are loud and snorting, and there are sometimes prolonged pauses, followed by deep, noisy inspirations. The pulse may vary strangely during these attacks, and in the prolonged intervals may be slow, to increase greatly with the forced inspirations. The alæ nasi should be observed during the sleep of the child, as they are sometimes much retracted during inspiration, due to a laxity of the walls, a condition readily remedied by the use of a soft wire dilator. Night terrors are common. The child may wake up in a paroxysm of shortness of breath. Sometimes these attacks are of great severity and the dyspnœa, or rather orthopnœa, may suggest pressure of enlarged glands on the trachea. Sometimes there is a nocturnal paroxysmal cough of a very troublesome character (Balne's cough), usually excited by lying down. The attacks may occur through the day.

When the mouth-breathing has persisted for a long time definite changes are brought about in the face, mouth, and chest. The facies is so peculiar and distinctive that the condition may be evident at a glance. The expression is dull, heavy, and apathetic, due in part to the fact that the mouth is habitually left open. In long-standing cases the child is very stupid-looking, responds slowly to questions, and may be sullen and cross. The lips are thick, the nasal orifices small and pinched-in-looking, the superior dental arch is narrowed and the roof of the mouth considerably raised.

The remarkable alterations in the shape of the chest in connection with enlarged tonsils were first carefully studied by Dupuytren (1828), who evidently fully appreciated the great importance of the condition. He noted "a lateral depression of the parietes of the chest consisting of a depression, more or less great, of the ribs on each side, and a proportionate protrusion of the sternum in front." J. Mason Warren (Medical Examiner, 1839) gave an admirable description of the constitutional symptoms and the thoracic deformities induced by enlarged tonsils. These, with the memoir of Lambron (1861), constitute the most important contributions to our knowledge on the subject. Three types of deformity may be recognized:

(*a*) The pigeon or chicken breast, by far the most common form, in which the sternum is prominent and there is a circular depression in the lateral zone (Harrison's groove), corresponding to the attachment of the diaphragm. The ribs are prominent anteriorly and the sternum is angulated forward at the manubrio-gladiolar junction. As a mouth-breather is watched during sleep one can see the lower and lateral thoracic regions retracted during inspiration by the action of the diaphragm.

(*b*) Barrel Chest.—Some children, the subject of chronic naso-pharyngeal obstruction, have recurring attacks of asthma, and the chest may be gradually deformed, becoming rounded and barrel-shaped, the neck short, and the shoulders and back bowed. A child of ten or eleven may have the thoracic conformation of an old man with emphysema.

(*c*) THE FUNNEL BREAST (*Trichterbrust*).—This remarkable deformity, in which there is a deep depression at the lower sternum, has excited much controversy as to its mode of origin. In some instances, at least, it is due to the obstructed breathing in connection with adenoid vegetations. I have seen two cases in children, in which the condition was in process of formation. During inspiration the lower sternum was forcibly retracted, so much so that at the height the depression corresponded to that of a well-marked "*Trichterbrust.*" While in repose, the lower sternal region was distinctly excavated.

The voice is altered and acquires a nasal quality. The pronunciation of certain letters is changed, and there is inability to pronounce the nasal consonants *n* and *m*. Bloch lays great stress upon the association of mouth-breathing with stuttering.

The hearing is impaired, usually owing to the extension of inflammation along the Eustachian tubes and the obstruction with mucus or the narrowing of their orifices by pressure of the adenoid vegetations. In some instances it may be due to retraction of the drums, as the upper pharynx is insufficiently supplied with air. Naturally the senses of taste and smell are much impaired. With these symptoms there may be little or no nasal catarrh or discharge, but the pharyngeal secretion of mucus is always increased. Children, however, do not notice this, as the mucus is usually swallowed, but older persons expectorate it with difficulty.

Among other symptoms may be mentioned headache, which is by no means uncommon, general listlessness, and an indisposition for physical or mental exertion. Habit-spasm of the face has been described in connection with it. I have known several instances in which permanent relief has been afforded by the removal of the adenoid vegetations. Enuresis is occasionally an associated symptom. The influence upon the mental development is striking. Mouth-breathers are usually dull, stupid, and backward. It is impossible for them to fix the attention for long at a time, and to this impairment of the mental function Guye, of Amsterdam, has given the name *aprosexia*. Headaches, forgetfulness, inability to study without discomfort are frequent symptoms of this condition in students. There is more than a grain of truth in the aphorism *shut your mouth and save your life*, which is found on the title-page of Captain Catlin's celebrated pamphlet on mouth-breathing (1861), to which cause he attributed all the ills of civilization.

A symptom specially associated with enlarged tonsils is fetor of the breath. In the tonsillar crypts the inspissated secretion undergoes decomposition and an odor not unlike that of Limburger cheese is produced. The little cheesy masses may sometimes be squeezed from the crypts of the tonsils. Though the odor may not apparently be very strong, yet if the mass be squeezed between the fingers its intensity will at once be appreciated. In some cases of chronic enlargement the cheesy masses may be deep in the tonsillar crypts; and if they remain for a prolonged period lime salts are deposited and a tonsillar calculus is in this way produced.

Children with adenoids are especially prone to take cold and to recurring attacks of follicular disease. They are also more liable to diphtheria, and in them the anginal features in scarlet fever are always more serious. The ultimate results of untreated adenoid hypertrophy are important. In some cases the vegetations disappear, leaving an atrophic condition of the vault of the pharynx. Neglect may also lead to the so-called Thornwaldt's disease, in which there is a cystic condition of the pharyngeal tonsil and constant secretion of muco-pus.

Diagnosis.—The facial aspect is usually distinctive. Enlarged tonsils are readily seen on inspection of the pharynx. There may be no great enlargement of the tonsils and nothing apparent at the back of the throat even when the naso-pharynx is completely blocked with adenoid vegetations. In children the rhinoscopic examination is rarely practicable. Digital examination is the most satisfactory. The growths can then be felt either as small, flat bodies or, if extensive, as velvety, grape-like papillomata.

Treatment.—If the tonsils are large and the general state is evidently influenced by them they should be at once removed. Applications of iodine and iron, or penciling the crypts with nitrate of silver, are of service in the milder grades, but it is waste of time to apply them to very enlarged glands. There is a condition in which the tonsils are not much enlarged, but the crypts are constantly filled with cheesy secretions and cause a very bad odor in the breath. In such instances the removal of the secretion and thorough penciling of the crypts with chromic acid may be practiced. The galvano-cautery is of great service in many cases of enlarged tonsils when there is any objection to the more radical surgical procedure.

The treatment of the adenoid growths in the pharynx is of the greatest importance, and should be thoroughly carried out. Parents should be frankly told that the affection is serious, one which impairs the mental not less than the bodily development of the child. In spite of the thorough ventilation of this subject by specialists, practitioners do not appear to have grasped as yet the full importance of this disease. They are far too apt to temporize and unnecessarily to postpone radical measures. The child must be anæsthetized. Severe hæmorrhage has followed in a few cases. Special examination should be made of the thymus and lymph glands, as if they are enlarged the operation should be postponed. In this state of lymphatism death during anæsthesia has occurred. The good effects of the operation are often apparent within a few days, and the child begins to breathe through the nose. In some instances the habit of mouth-breathing persists. As soon as the child goes to sleep the lower jaw drops and the air is drawn into the mouth. In these cases a chin strap can be readily adjusted, which the child may wear at night. In severe cases it may take months of careful training before the child can speak properly. An all-important point in the treatment of lesions of the naso-pharynx (and, indeed, in the prevention of this unfortunate condition) is to increase the breathing capacity of the chest by making the child perform systematic exercises, which cause the air to be driven freely and forcibly in and out through the naso-pharynx. I cannot too strongly commend this suggestion of Mr. Arbuthnot Lane.

Throughout the entire treatment attention should be paid to hygiene and diet, and cod-liver oil and the iodide of iron may be administered with benefit.

E. DISEASES OF THE ŒSOPHAGUS

I. ACUTE ŒSOPHAGITIS

Etiology.—Acute inflammation occurs (*a*) in the catarrhal processes of the specific fevers; more rarely as an extension from catarrh of the pharynx. (*b*) As a result of intense mechanical or chemical irritation, produced by foreign bodies, by very hot liquids, or by strong corrosives. (*c*) In the form of pseudo-membranous inflammation in diphtheria, and occasionally in pneumonia, typhoid fever, and pyæmia. (*d*) As a pustular inflammation in small-pox, and, according to Laennec, as a result of a prolonged administration of tartar emetic. (*e*) In connection with local disease, particularly cancer either of the tube itself or extension to it from without. And, lastly, acute œsophagitis, occasionally with ulceration, may occur spontaneously in sucklings.

Morbid Anatomy.—It is extremely rare to see redness of the mucosa, except when chemical irritants have been swallowed. More commonly the epithelium is thickened and has desquamated, so that the surface is covered with a fine granular substance. The mucous follicles are swollen and occasionally there may be seen small erosions. In the pseudo-membranous inflammation there is a grayish croupous exudate, usually limited in extent, at the upper portion of the gullet. The pustular disease is very rare in small-pox. In the phlegmonous inflammation the mucous membrane is greatly swollen, and there is purulent infiltration in the submucosa. It may even extend throughout a large part of the gullet. Gangrene occasionally supervenes. There is a remarkable fibrinous or membranous œsophagitis, most frequently met with in the fevers, sometimes also in hysteria, in which long casts of the tube may be vomited.

Symptoms.—Pain in deglutition is always present in severe inflammation of the œsophagus. A dull pain beneath the sternum is also present. In the milder forms of catarrhal inflammation there are usually no symptoms. The presence of a foreign body is indicated by dysphagia and spasm with the regurgitation of portions of the food. Later, blood and pus may be ejected. It is surprising how extensive the disease may be in the œsophagus without producing much pain or great discomfort, except in swallowing. The intense inflammation which follows the swallowing of corrosives, when not fatal, gradually subsides, and often leads to cicatricial contraction and stricture. In the cases in which there is danger of contraction œsophageal bougies should be passed before this is marked. The patient should swallow some oil before the passage of the bougie, the size of which should be gradually increased. Dilatation should be done every few days at first.

Treatment.—The treatment of acute inflammation of the œsophagus is extremely unsatisfactory, particularly in the severer forms. The slight catarrhal cases require no special treatment. When the dysphagia is intense it is best not to give food by the mouth, but to feed entirely by enemata. Fragments of ice may be given, and as the pain and distress subside, demulcent drinks. External applications of cold often give relief.

A *chronic* form of œsophagitis is described, but this results usually from the prolonged action of the causes which produce the acute form.

Catarrhal Ulceration.—Follicular ulcers are not uncommon. Tuberculous and syphilitic ulcers are rare. Very prominent varicose veins and small erosions are not uncommon. The other forms are the carcinomatous, the erosion due to aneurism, and the ulcerative action of corrosive substances. There are two other important varieties—the ulcers in acute infectious diseases, diphtheria, scarlet fever, and pneumonia; and the peptic ulcer, first described by Albers in 1839. Tileston has collected forty cases of peptic ulcer in the œsophagus. The pain, dysphagia, vomiting, and hæmorrhage have been the most important symptoms. Perforation occurred in six cases, in one instance into the aorta. Treatment is difficult; in severe cases gastrostomy should be done.

Œsophageal Varices.—Associated with chronic heart-disease and more frequently with the senile and the cirrhotic liver, the œsophageal veins may become distended and varicose. The mucous membrane is in a state of chronic catarrh, and the patient has frequent eructations of mucus. Rupture of these varices is one of the commonest causes of hæmatemesis in cirrhosis of the liver and in enlarged spleen. The blood may pass per rectum alone.

II. SPASM OF THE ŒSOPHAGUS

(*Œsophagismus*)

This so-called spasmodic stricture of the gullet is met with in hysterical patients and hypochrondriacs, also in chorea, epilepsy, and especially hydrophobia. It is sometimes associated also with the lodgment of foreign bodies, or with cases in which a patient has swallowed a foreign body and thinks it has stuck. For weeks there may be spasm, due perhaps to autosuggestion, though the bougie passes freely. The idiopathic form is found in females of a marked neurotic habit, but may also occur in elderly men. It may be present only during pregnancy. The patient complains of inability to swallow solid food, and in extreme instances even liquids are rejected. The attack may come on abruptly, and be associated with emotional disturbances and with substernal pain. The bougie, when passed, may be arrested temporarily at the seat of the spasm, which gradually yields, or it may slip through without the slightest effort. The condition is rarely serious, though it may persist for years. Spasm of the lower end of the gullet, associated with cardio-spasm, may be the cause of a remarkable fusiform dilatation of the œsophagus.

The *diagnosis* is not difficult, particularly in young persons with marked nervous manifestations. In elderly persons œsophagismus is almost always connected with hypochondriasis, but great care must be taken to exclude cancer.

In some cases a cure is at once effected by the passage of a bougie. The general neurotic condition also requires special attention.

Paralysis of the œsophagus scarcely demands separate consideration. It is a very rare condition, due most often to central disease, particularly bulbar paralysis. It may be peripheral in origin, as in diphtheritic paralysis. Occasionally it occurs also in hysteria. The essential symptom is dysphagia.

III. STRICTURE OF THE ŒSOPHAGUS

This results from: (*a*) Congenital stenosis of the œsophagus.—There are two groups of cases, one in which there is complete occlusion, and the middle of the tube is converted into a fibrous cord; the other, the more common, in which the lower part opens into the trachea or one of the bronchi. There are some 19 cases on record (William Thomas). (*b*) The cicatricial contraction of healed ulcers, usually due to corrosive poisons, occasionally to syphilis, and in rare instances after the fevers. (*c*) The growth of tumors in the walls, as in the so-called cancerous stricture. Eighty-five per cent. of the cases are of this nature. (*d*) External pressure by aneurism, enlarged lymph-glands, enlarged thyroid, other tumors, and sometimes by pericardial effusion.

The cicatricial stricture may occur anywhere in the gullet, and in extreme cases may, indeed, involve the whole tube, but in a majority of instances it is found either high up near the pharynx or low down toward the stomach. The narrowing may be extreme, so that only small quantities of food can trickle through, or the obstruction may be quite slight. When the stricture is low down the œsophagus is dilated and the walls are usually much hypertrophied. When the obstruction is high in the gullet, the food is usually rejected at once, whereas, if it is low, it may be retained and a considerable quantity collects before it is regurgitated. Any doubt as to its having reached the stomach is removed by the alkalinity of the material ejected and the absence of the characteristic gastric odor. Auscultation of the œsophagus may be practiced and is sometimes of service. The patient takes a mouthful of water and the auscultator listens along the left of the spine. The normal œsophageal *bruit* may be heard later than seven seconds, the normal time, or there may be heard a loud splashing, gurgling sound. The secondary murmur, heard as the fluid enters the stomach, may be absent. The bismuth meal and the fluoroscope now make the diagnosis very easy. The passage of the œsophageal bougie will determine accurately the locality. Conical bougies attached to a flexible whalebone stem are the most satisfactory, but the gum-elastic stomach tube may be used; a large one should be tried first. The patient should be placed on a low chair with the head well thrown back. The index finger of the left hand is passed far into the pharynx, and in some instances this procedure alone may determine the presence of a new growth. The bougie is passed beside the finger until it touches the posterior wall of the pharynx, then along it, more to one side than in the middle line, and so gradually pushed into the gullet. It is to be borne in mind that in passing the cricoid cartilage there is often a slight obstruction. Great gentleness should be used, as it has happened more than once that the bougie has been passed through a cancerous ulcer into the mediastinum or through a diverticulum. It is well always, as a precautionary measure before passing the bougie, to examine carefully for aneurism, which may produce all the symptoms of organic stricture. In cases in which the narrowing is extreme there is always emaciation. For treatment, surgical works must be consulted.

IV. CANCER OF THE ŒSOPHAGUS

This is usually epithelioma. It is not a common disease; there were only 38 cases in the medical wards of the Johns Hopkins Hospital in twenty-three years. It may occur in quite young persons, and is more frequent in males than in females. The middle and lower thirds are most often affected. At first confined to the mucous membrane, the cancer gradually increases and soon ulcerates. The lumen of the tube is narrowed, but when ulceration is extensive in the later stages the stricture may be less marked. Dilatation of the tube and hypertrophy of the walls usually take place above the cancer. The ulcer may perforate the trachea or a bronchus, the lung, the pleura, the mediastinum, the aorta or one of its larger branches, the pericardium, or it may erode the vertebral column. The recurrent laryngeal nerves are not infrequently implicated. Perforation of the lung produces, as a rule, local gangrene.

Symptoms.—The earliest symptom is dysphagia, which is progressive and may become extreme, so that the patient emaciates rapidly. Regurgitation may take place at once; or, if the cancer is situated near the stomach, it may be deferred for ten or fifteen minutes, or even longer if the tube is much dilated. The rejected materials may be mixed with blood and may contain cancerous fragments. In persons over fifty years of age persistent difficulty in swallowing accompanied by rapid emaciation usually indicates œsophageal cancer. The cervical lymph-glands are frequently enlarged and may give early indication of the nature of the trouble. Pain may be persistent or be present only when food is taken. In certain instances the pain is very great. The latent cases are very rare. Bronchitis and broncho-pneumonia are common terminal events.

Diagnosis.—The bismuth meal and the Röntgen-ray picture give information as to the position of the stricture, and a very dense growth may throw a shadow. In the diagnosis of the condition it is important, in the first place, to exclude pressure from without, as by aneurism or other tumor. The history enables us to exclude cicatricial stricture and foreign bodies. The sound may be passed and the presence of the stricture determined. As mentioned above, great care should be exercised. Fragments of carcinomatous tissue may in some instances be removed with the tube. On auscultation along the left side of the spine the primary œsophageal murmur may be much altered in quality.

Treatment.—In most cases milk and liquids can be swallowed, but supplementary nourishment should be given by the rectum. It may be advisable in some instances to pass a tube into the stomach and introduce food in this way. When there is difficulty in feeding the patient it is very much better to have gastrostomy performed at once, as it gives the greatest comfort and ease, and prolongs the patient's life.

V. RUPTURE OF THE ŒSOPHAGUS

(*a*) Rupture may occur in a healthy organ as a result of prolonged vomiting after a full meal, or when intoxicated. Eight cases are on record (Virchow's Archiv, vol. 162). Boerhaave described the first case in Baron Wassennar, who "broke asunder the tube of the œsophagus near the diaphragm, so that, after the most excruciating pain, the elements which he swallowed passed, together with the air, into the cavity of the thorax, and he expired in twenty-four hours."

(*b*) In a few cases the rupture has occurred in a diseased and weakened tube, near the scar of an ulcer, for example.

(*c*) Post mortem softening—œsophago-malacia—a not very uncommon condition, must not be mistaken for it. In spontaneous rupture the rent is clean-cut and circumferential; in malacia it is rounded and often cribriform, and the margins are softened. The contents of the stomach may be in the left pleura.

VI. DILATATIONS AND DIVERTICULA

Stenosis of the gullet is followed by secondary dilatation of the tube above the constriction and great hypertrophy of the walls. Primary dilatation, which is extremely rare, appears to be associated with spasm of the lower end of the gullet and of the cardiac orifice. The tube may attain extraordinary dimensions, as in the specimen presented in 1904 to the Association of American Physicians by Kinnicutt. Regurgitation of food is the most common symptom. There may also be difficulty in breathing from pressure.

Diverticula are of two forms: (*a*) Pressure diverticula, which are most common at the junction of the pharynx and gullet, on the posterior wall. Owing to weakness of the muscles at this spot, local bulging occurs, which is gradually increased by the pressure of food, and finally forms a saccular pouch. (*b*) The traction diverticula situated on the anterior wall near the bifurcation of the trachea result, as a rule, from the extension of inflammation from the lymph-glands with adhesion and subsequent cicatricial contraction, by which the wall of the gullet is drawn out. The diagnosis of these forms is now readily made with the bismuth meal and X-rays. Diverticula have been successfully extirpated.

A rare and remarkable condition, of which a case has been recorded by MacLachlan, and of which a second was in attendance at my clinic, is the œsophago-pleuro-cutaneous fistula. In my patient fluids were discharged at intervals through a fistula in the right infra-clavicular region, which communicated with a cavity in the upper part of the pleura or lung. The condition had persisted for more than twenty-five years.

F. DISEASES OF THE STOMACH

I. ACUTE GASTRITIS

(*Simple Gastritis; Acute Gastric Catarrh; Acute Dyspepsia*)

Etiology.—Acute gastric catarrh, one of the most common of complaints, occurs at all ages, and is usually traceable to errors in diet. It may follow the ingestion of more food than the stomach can digest, or it may result from taking unsuitable articles, which either themselves irritate the mucosa or, remaining undigested, decompose, and so excite an acute dyspepsia. A frequent cause is the taking of food which has begun to decompose, particularly in hot weather. In children these fermentative processes are very apt to excite acute catarrh of the bowels as well. Another very common cause is the abuse of alcohol, and the acute gastritis which follows a drinking-bout is one of the most typical forms of the disease. The tendency to acute indigestion varies very much in different individuals, and, indeed, in families. We recognize this in using the expressions a "delicate stomach" and a "strong stomach." Gouty persons are generally thought to be more disposed to acute dyspepsia than others. Acute catarrh of the stomach occurs at the outset of many of the infectious fevers.

Morbid Anatomy.—Beaumont's study of St. Martin's stomach showed that in acute catarrh the mucous membrane is reddened and swollen, less gastric juice is secreted, and mucus covers the surface. Slight hæmorrhages may occur or even small erosions. The submucosa may be somewhat œdematous. Microscopically the changes are chiefly noticeable in the mucous and peptic cells, which are swollen and more granular, and there is an infiltration of the intertubular tissue with leucocytes.

Symptoms.—In mild cases the symptoms are those of slight "indigestion" —an uncomfortable feeling in the abdomen, headache, depression, nausea, eructations, and vomiting, which usually gives relief. The tongue is heavily coated and the saliva is increased. In children there are intestinal symptoms —diarrhœa and colicky pains and often slight fever. The duration is rarely more than twenty-four hours. In the severer forms the attack may set in with a chill and febrile reaction, in which the temperature rises to 102° or 103° F. The tongue is furred, the breath heavy, and vomiting is frequent. The ejected substances, at first mixed with food, subsequently contain much mucus and bile-stained fluids. There may be constipation, but very often there is diarrhœa. The urine presents the usual febrile characteristics, and there is a heavy deposit of urates. The abdomen may be somewhat distended and slightly tender in the epigastric region. Herpes may appear on the lips. The attack may last from one to three days, and occasionally longer. The examination of the vomitus shows, as a rule, absence of hydrochloric acid, the presence of lactic and fatty acids, and marked increase in the mucus.

Diagnosis.—The ordinary afebrile gastric catarrh is readily recognized. The acute febrile form is so similar to the initial symptoms of many of the infectious diseases that it is impossible for a day or two to make a diagnosis, particularly in the cases which have come on, so to speak, spontaneously and independently of an error in diet. Some of these resemble closely an acute infection; the symptoms may be very intense, and if, as sometimes happens, the attack sets in with severe headache and delirium, the case may be mistaken for meningitis. When the abdominal pains are intense the attack may be confounded with gallstone colic. It is a very common error to class under "gastric fever" the mild forms of the various infectious disorders. The gastric crises in locomotor ataxia have in many instances been confounded with a simple acute gastritis, and it is always wise in adults to test the knee-jerks and pupillary reactions.

Treatment.—Mild cases recover spontaneously in twenty-four hours, and require no treatment other than a dose of castor oil in children or of blue mass in adults. In the severer forms, if there is much distress in the region of the stomach, the vomiting should be promoted by warm water, or the stomach tube may be employed for some patients. A dose of calomel, 2 to 3 grains (0.13 to 0.2 gm.), should be given, and followed, after some hours, by a saline cathartic. If there is eructation of acid fluid, bicarbonate of soda and bismuth may be given. The stomach should have, if possible, absolute rest, and it is a good plan in the case of strong persons, particularly in those addicted to alcohol, to cut off all food for a day or two. The patient may be allowed soda water and ice freely. It is well not to attempt to check the vomiting unless it is excessive and protracted. Recovery is usually complete, though repeated attacks may lead to subacute gastritis or to the establishment of chronic dyspepsia.

Phlegmonous Gastritis; Acute Suppurative Gastritis.—The disease is due to infection of the submucosa, probably through a minute abrasion. Males are more frequently affected than females, and most of the cases are in comparatively young people. In a majority of the instances in which the examination has been made streptococci have been present, but the pneumococcus has been found in a few cases. The disease is rare; Leith was able to collect only 85 cases. There is a widespread suppurative infiltration of the submucosa, with great thickening of the walls. Sometimes there is a localized abscess formation, with tumor, which may burst into the stomach, or into the peritoneum. I have seen three instances of this condition, all in connection with cancer of the stomach.

The important symptoms are pain, high fever, vomiting, dry tongue, all the features of a severe infection, and sometimes jaundice. A diagnosis is rarely made; occasionally there is a large tumor mass to be felt. The cases are uniformly fatal unless one counts the one reported by Bovee, in which he cut down and opened an acute abscess, the size of a man's fist, in the anterior wall of the pyloric region.

Toxic Gastritis.—This most intense form of inflammation of the stomach is excited by the swallowing of concentrated mineral acids or strong alkalies, or by such poisons as phosphorus, corrosive sublimate, ammonia, arsenic, etc. In the non-corrosive poisons, such as phosphorus, arsenic, and antimony, the process consists of an acute degeneration of the glandular elements, and hæmorrhage. With the powerful concentrated poisons the mucous membrane is extensively destroyed, and may be converted into a brownish-black eschar. In the less severe grades there may be areas of necrosis surrounded by inflammatory reaction, while the submucosa is hæmorrhagic and infiltrated. The process is of course more intense at the fundus, but the active peristalsis may drive the poison through the pylorus into the intestine.

Symptoms.—The symptoms are intense pain in the mouth, throat, and stomach, salivation, great difficulty in swallowing, and constant vomiting, the vomited materials being bloody and sometimes containing portions of the mucous membrane. The abdomen is tender, distended, and painful on pressure. In the most acute cases symptoms of collapse supervene; the pulse is weak, the skin pale and covered with sweat; there is restlessness, and sometimes convulsions. There may be albumin or blood in the urine, and petechiæ may occur on the skin. When the poison is less intense, the sloughs may separate, leaving ulcers, which too often lead, in the œsophagus to stricture, in the stomach to chronic atrophy, and finally to death from exhaustion.

Diagnosis.—The diagnosis of toxic gastritis is usually easy, as inspection of the mouth and pharynx shows, in many instances, corrosive effects, while the examination of the vomit may indicate the nature of the poison.

In poisoning by acids, magnesia should be administered in milk or with egg albumen. When strong alkalies have been taken, the dilute acids should be administered. If the case is seen early, lavage should be used. For the severe inflammation which follows the swallowing of the stronger poisons palliative treatment is alone available, and morphia may be freely employed to allay the pain.

Diphtheritic or Membranous Gastritis.—This condition is met with occasionally in diphtheria, but more commonly as a secondary process in typhus or typhoid fever, pneumonia, pyæmia, small-pox, and occasionally in debilitated children. The exudation may be extensive and uniform or in patches. The condition is not recognizable during life, unless the membranes are vomited.

Mycotic and Parasitic Gastritis.—It occasionally happens that fungi grow in the stomach and excite inflammation. One of the most remarkable cases of the kind is that reported by Kundrat, in which the favus fungus occurred in the stomach and intestine.

In cancer and in dilatation of the stomach the sarcinæ and yeast fungi probably aid in maintaining the chronic gastritis. As a rule, the gastric juice is capable of killing the ordinary bacteria. Orth states that the anthrax bacilli, in certain cases, produce swelling of the mucosa and ulceration. Eug. Fraenkel has reported a case of acute emphysematous gastritis probably of mycotic origin. The larvæ of certain insects may excite gastritis, as in the cases reported by Gerhardt, Meschede, and others.

II. CHRONIC GASTRITIS

(*Chronic Catarrh of the Stomach; Chronic Dyspepsia*)

Definition.—A condition of disturbed digestion associated with increased mucous formation, qualitative or quantitative changes in the gastric juice, enfeeblement of the muscular coats, so that the food is retained for an abnormal time in the stomach; and, finally, with alterations in the structure of the mucosa.

Etiology.—The causes of chronic gastritis may be classified as follows: (*a*) *Dietetic.* Unsuitable or improperly prepared food, and the persistent use of certain articles of diet, such as very fat substances or foods containing too much of the carbohydrates. The use in excessive quantity of hot bread, hot cakes, and pie is a fruitful cause, particularly in the United States. The use in excess of tea or coffee, and, above all, of alcohol in its various forms. Under this heading, too, may be mentioned the habits of eating at irregular hours or too rapidly and imperfectly chewing the food. Excess in eating does more damage than excess in drinking. The platter kills more than the sword. A common cause of chronic catarrh is drinking too freely of ice-water during meals, a practice which plays no small part in the prevalence of dyspepsia in America. Another frequent cause is the abuse of tobacco, particularly chewing. (*b*) *Constitutional causes.* Anæmia, chlorosis, chronic tuberculosis, gout, diabetes, and Bright's disease are often associated with chronic gastric catarrh. (*c*) *Local conditions:* (1) of the stomach, as in cancer, ulcer, and dilatation, which are invariably accompanied by catarrh; (2) conditions of the portal circulation, causing chronic engorgement of the mucous membrane, as in cirrhosis, chronic heart-disease, and certain chronic lung affections.

Morbid Anatomy.—In simple chronic gastritis the organ is usually enlarged, the mucous membrane pale gray in color, and covered with closely adherent, tenacious mucus. The veins are large, patches of ecchymosis are not infrequently seen, and in the chronic catarrh of portal obstruction and of chronic heart-disease small hæmorrhagic erosions. Toward the pylorus the mucosa is not infrequently irregularly pigmented, and presents a rough, wrinkled, mammilated surface, the *état mameloné* of the French, a condition which may sometimes be so prominent that writers have described it as *gastritis polyposa.* The membrane may be thinner than normal, and much firmer, tearing less readily with the finger-nail. The minute anatomy shows the picture of a parenchymatous and an interstitial inflammation. The mucous membrane may undergo complete atrophy and be represented by a smooth cuticular membrane resembling that of the cardiac portion of the horse's stomach. This was the condition in a case of profound anæmia reported by F. P. Henry and myself. The mucularis mucosa was hypertrophied, but with no great general thickening of the stomach walls.

Symptoms.—The affection persists for an indefinite period, and, as is the case with most chronic diseases, changes from time to time. The appetite is variable, sometimes greatly impaired, at others very good. Among early symptoms are feelings of distress or oppression after eating, which may become aggravated and amount to actual pain. When the stomach is empty there may also be a painful feeling. The pain differs in different cases, and may be trifling or of extreme severity. When localized and felt beneath the sternum or in the præcordial region it is known as heart-burn or sometimes cardialgia. There is pain on pressure over the stomach, usually diffuse and not severe. The tongue is coated, and the patient complains of a bad taste in the mouth. The tip and margin of the tongue are very often red. Associated with this catarrhal stomatitis there may be an increase in the salivary and pharyngeal secretions. Nausea is an early symptom, and is particularly apt to occur in the morning hours. It is not, however, nearly so constant a symptom in chronic gastritis as in cancer of the stomach, and in mild grades of the affection it may not occur at all. Eructation of gas, which may continue for some hours after taking food, is a very prominent feature in cases of so-called flatulent dyspepsia, and there may be marked distention of the intestines. With the gas, bitter fluids may be brought up. Vomiting, which is not very frequent, occurs either immediately after eating or an hour or two later. In the chronic catarrh of old topers a bout of morning vomiting is common, in which a slimy mucus is brought up. The vomitus consists of food in various stages of digestion and slimy mucus, and the chemical examination shows the presence of abnormal acids, such as butyric, or even acetic, in addition to lactic acid, while the hydrochloric acid, if present, is much reduced in quantity. The digestion may be much delayed, and, on washing out the stomach as late as seven hours after eating, portions of food are still present. The prolonged retention favors decomposition, the stomach becomes distended with gas, and this, with the chronic catarrh, may induce gradually an atony of the muscular walls, but the motor function of the stomach is not usually much impaired. The absorption is slow, and iodide of potassium, given in capsules, which should normally reach the saliva within fifteen minutes, may not be evident for more than half an hour.

Constipation is usually present, but in some instances there is diarrhœa, and undigested food passes rapidly through the bowels. The urine is often scanty, high-colored, and deposits a heavy sediment of urates.

Of other symptoms headache is common, and the patient feels constantly out of sorts, indisposed for exertion, and low-spirited. In aggravated cases melancholia may occur. Trousseau called attention to the occurrence of vertigo, a marked feature in certain cases. The pulse is small, sometimes slow, and there may be palpitation of the heart. Fever does not occur. Cough is sometimes present, but the so-called stomach cough of chronic dyspeptics is in all probability dependent upon pharyngeal irritation. J. T. Pilcher has called attention to the frequency with which absence of free hydrochloric acid is found with the presence of occult blood in chronic gastritis. In very many of these the stomach condition appears to be secondary to local disease elsewhere in the abdomen, particularly the appendix, gall-bladder or the pancreas. The bleeding comes from small erosions, and is always of the so-called occult variety. Many varieties of pathogenic organisms are almost constantly found, of which the streptococci are the most important.

The Gastric Contents.—The fasting stomach may be empty or it may contain much mucus—*gastritis mucipara* of Boas. In the test breakfast, withdrawn in an hour, the HCl is usually diminished, though it may be normal—*gastritis acida.* In other cases the free HCl may be absent—*gastritis anacida.* While in the advanced forms of atrophy of the mucosa there may be neither acids nor ferments—*gastritis atrophicans.*

The symptoms of atrophy of the mucous membrane of the stomach, without contraction of the organ, are very complex, and cannot be said to present a uniform picture. The majority of the cases present the symptoms of an aggravated chronic dyspepsia, often of such severity that cancer is suspected. In one of the cases which I examined the persistent distress after eating, the vomiting, and the gradual loss of flesh and strength very naturally led to this diagnosis, but the duration of the disease far exceeded that of ordinary carcinoma. The clinical picture may be that of a severe anæmia. As early as 1860 Flint called attention to this connection between atrophy of the gastric tubules and anæmia, an observation which Fenwick and others have amply confirmed.

Diagnosis.—Ewald distinguishes three forms of chronic gastritis: (1) Simple gastritis; (2) mucous (*schleimige*) gastritis; (3) atrophic gastritis.

In (1) the fasting stomach contains only a small quantity of a slimy fluid, while after the test breakfast the HCl is diminished in quantity or may be absent. Lactic acid and the fatty acids may be present. After Boas's more rigid test meal the organic acids are rarely found. The pepsin and rennin are always present.

In (2) the acidity is always slight and the condition is distinguished from (1) chiefly by the large amount of mucus present.

In (3) the fasting stomach is generally empty, while after the test breakfast HCl, pepsin, and rennin are wholly wanting.

The diagnosis of cancer of the stomach from chronic gastritis may be very difficult when a tumor is not present. The cases require most careful study, and it is important to decide whether the stomach is primarily at fault, or whether the chronic gastritis is associated with disease of the other organs—liver, gall-bladder, appendix or pancreas.

Treatment.—When possible the cause in each case should be ascertained and an attempt made to determine the special form of indigestion. Usually there is no difficulty in differentiating the ordinary catarrhal and the nervous varieties. A careful study of the phenomena of digestion, though not essential in every instance, should certainly be carried out in the more obstinate and obscure forms. Two important questions should be asked of every dyspeptic—first, as to the time taken at his meals; and, second, as to the quantity he eats. Practically a large majority of all cases of disturbed digestion come from hasty and imperfect mastication of the food and from overeating. Especial stress should be laid upon the former point. In some instances it will alone suffice to cure dyspepsia if the patient will count a certain number before swallowing each mouthful. The second point is of even greater importance. People habitually eat too much, and it is probably true that a greater number of maladies arise from excess in eating than from excess in drinking. Chittenden's researches have shown that we require much less nitrogenous food to maintain a standard of perfect health—a lesson that the Hindoos and Japanese have also taught us. George Cheyne's thirteenth aphorism, already quoted under the section on Obesity, contains a volume of dietetic wisdom.

(*a*) General and Dietetic.—A careful and systematically arranged dietary is the first, sometimes the only, essential in the treatment of a case of chronic dyspepsia. It is impossible to lay down rules applicable to all cases. Individuals differ extraordinarily in their capability of digesting different articles of food, and there is much truth in the old adage, "One man's food is another man's poison." The individual preferences for different articles of food should be permitted in the milder forms. Physicians have probably been too arbitrary in this direction, and have not yielded sufficiently to the intimations given by the appetite and desires of the patient.

A rigid milk diet may be tried. "Milk and sweet sound Blood differ in nothing but in Color: *Milk* is *Blood*" (George Cheyne). In the forms associated with Bright's disease and chronic portal congestion, as well as in many instances in which the dyspepsia is part of a neurasthenic or hysterical trouble, this plan in conjunction with rest is most efficacious. If milk is not digested well it may be diluted one-third with soda water or Vichy, or 5 to 10 grains of carbonate of soda, or a pinch of salt may be added to each tumblerful. In many cases the milk from which the cream has been taken is better borne. Buttermilk is particularly suitable, but can rarely be taken for so long a time alone, as patients tire of it much more readily than [illegible] do of ordinary milk. Not only can the general nutrition be maintained on this diet, but patients sometimes increase in weight, and the unpleasant gastric symptoms disappear entirely. It should be given at fixed hours and in definite quantities. A patient may take 6 or 8 ounces every three hours. The amount necessary varies a good deal, but at least 3 to 5 pints should be given in the twenty-four hours. This form of diet is not, as a rule, well borne when there is a tendency to dilatation of the stomach. The milk may be previously peptonized, but it is impossible to feed a chronic dyspeptic in this way. The stools should be carefully watched, and if more milk is taken than can be digested it is well to supplement the diet with eggs and dry toast or biscuits.

In a large proportion of the cases of chronic indigestion it is not necessary to annoy the patient with such strict dietaries. It may be quite sufficient to cut off certain articles of food. Thus, if there are acid eructations or flatulency the farinaceous foods should be restricted, particularly potatoes and the coarser vegetables. A fruitful source of indigestion is the hot bread which, in different forms, is regarded as an essential part of an American breakfast. This, as well as the various forms of pancakes, pies and tarts, with heavy pastry, and fried articles of all sorts, should be strictly forbidden. As a rule, white bread, toasted, is more readily digested than bread made from the whole meal. Persons, however, differ very much in this respect, and the Graham or brown bread is most digestible for many people. Sugar and very sweet articles of food should be taken in great moderation or avoided altogether by persons with chronic dyspepsia. Many instances of aggravated indigestion have come to my notice due to the prevalent practice of eating largely of ice-cream. One of the most powerful enemies of the American stomach in the present day is the soda-water fountain, which has usurped so important a place in the apothecary shop.

Fats, with the exception of a moderate amount of good butter, very fat meats, and thick, greasy soups should be avoided. Ripe fruit in moderation is often advantageous, particularly when cooked. Bananas are not, as a rule, well borne. Strawberries are to many persons a cause of an annual attack of indigestion and sore throat.

As stated, in the matter of special articles of food it is impossible to lay down rigid rules, and it is the common experience that one patient with indigestion will take with impunity the very articles which cause the greatest distress to another.

Another detail of importance which may be mentioned in this connection is the general hygienic management of dyspeptics. These patients are often introspective, dwelling in a morbid manner on their symptoms, and much inclined to take a despondent view of their condition. Very little progress can be made unless the physician gains their confidence from the outset. Their fears and whims should not be made too light of or ridiculed. Systematic exercise, carefully regulated, particularly when, as at watering places, it is combined with a restricted diet, is of special service. Change of air and occupation, a prolonged sea voyage, or a summer in the mountains will sometimes cure the most obstinate dyspepsia.

(*b*) Medicinal.—The special therapeutic measures may be divided into those which attempt to replace in the digestive juices important elements which are lacking and those which stimulate the weakened action of the organ.

In the first group come the hydrochloric acid and ferments, which are so freely employed in dyspepsia. The former is the most important. It is the ingredient in the gastric juice most commonly deficient. It is not only necessary for its own important actions, but its presence is intimately associated with that of the pepsin, as it is only in the presence of a sufficient quantity that the pepsinogen is converted into the active digestive ferment. It is best given as the dilute acid taken in somewhat larger quantities than are usually advised. Ewald recommends large doses—of from 90 to 100 drops—at intervals of fifteen minutes after the meals. Leube and Riegel advise smaller doses. Probably from 15 to 20 drops is sufficient. The prolonged use of it does not appear to be in any way hurtful. The use, however, should be restricted to cases of neurosis and atrophy of the mucous membrane. In actual gastritis its value is doubtful.

Nitrate of silver is a good remedy in some cases, used in solution in the lavage (1 to 1,500 or 1 to 2,000), or in pill form, one-eighth to one-fourth of a grain three times a day. For many years Pepper advocated the more extended use of this drug in chronic gastritis. I have seen an instance of argyria after its protracted use.

The digestive ferments are extensively employed to strengthen the weakened gastric and intestinal secretions. The use of pepsin, according to Ewald, may be limited to the cases of advanced mucous catarrh and the instances of atrophy of the stomach, in which it should be given, in doses of from 10 to 15 grains, with dilute hydrochloric acid a quarter of an hour after meals. Pancreatin is of equal or even greater value than pepsin, but pains should be taken to use a good article. It should be given in doses of from 15 to 20 grains, in combination with bicarbonate of soda. It is conveniently administered in tablets, each of which contains 5 grains of the pancreatin and the soda, and of these two or three may be taken fifteen or twenty minutes after each meal. Ptyalin and diatase are particularly indicated when the acid is excessive. The action of the former continues in the stomach during normal digestion. The malt diastase is often very serviceable given with alkalies.

Of measures which stimulate the glandular activity in chronic dyspepsia lavage is by far the most important, particularly in the forms characterized by the secretion of a large quantity of mucus. Lukewarm water should be used, or, if there is much mucus, a 1-per-cent. salt solution, or a 3- to 5-per-cent. solution of bicarbonate of soda. If there is much fermentation the 3-per-cent. solution of boric acid may be used. It is best employed in the morning on an empty stomach, or in the evening some hours after the last meal in those cases in which there is much nocturnal distress and flatulency. Once a day is, as a rule, sufficient, or, in the case of delicate persons, every second day. The irrigation may be continued until the water which comes away is quite clear. It is not necessary to remove all the fluid after the irrigation. While perhaps in some hands this measure has been carried to extremes, it is one of such extraordinary value in certain cases that it should be more widely employed. When there is an insuperable objection to lavage a substitute may be used in the form of warm alkaline drinks, taken slowly in the early morning or the last thing at night.

Of medicines which stimulate the gastric secretion the most important are the bitter tonics, such as nux vomica, quassia, gentian, calumba, and cardamom. These are probably of more value in chronic gastritis than the hydrochloric acid. Of these nux vomica is the most powerful, though none of them have probably any very great stimulating action on the secretion, and influence rather the appetite than the digestion. Of stomachics which are believed to favorably influence digestion the most important are alcohol and common salt. The former would appear to act in moderate quantities by increasing the acid in the gastric juice, and with it probably the pepsin formation. Others hold that it is not so much the secretory as the motor function of the stomach which the alcohol stimulates. In moderate quantities it has certainly no directly injurious influence on the digestive processes. Special care should be taken, however, in ordering alcohol to dyspeptics. If a patient has been in the habit of taking beer or light wines or stimulants with his meals, the practice may be continued if moderate quantities are taken. Beer, as a rule, is not well borne. A dry sherry or a glass of claret is preferable. In the case of women with any form of dyspepsia stimulants should be employed with the greatest caution, and the practitioner should know his patient well before ordering alcohol.

The importance of salt in gastric digestion rests upon the fact that its presence is essential in the formation of the hydrochloric acid. An increase in its use may be advised in all cases of chronic dyspepsia in which the acid is defective.

(*c*) Treatment of Special Conditions.—*Fermentation and Flatulency.*—When the digestion is slow or imperfect, fermentation goes on in the contents, with the formation of gas and the production of lactic, butyric, and acetic acids. For the treatment of this condition careful dieting may suffice, particularly forbidding such articles as tea, pastry, and the coarser vegetables. It is usually combined with pyrosis, in which the acid fluids are brought into the mouth. Bismuth and carbonate of soda sometimes suffice to relieve the condition. Thymol, creasote, and carbolic acid may be employed. For acid dyspepsia Sir William Roberts recommended the bismuth lozenge of the British Pharmacopœia, the antacid properties of which depend on chalk and bicarbonate of soda. It should be taken an hour or two after meals, and only when the pain and uneasiness are present. The burnt magnesia is also a good remedy. Glycerin in from 20- to 60-minim doses, the essential oils, animal charcoal alone or in combination with compound cinnamon powder may be tried. If there is much pain, chloroform in 20-minim doses or a teaspoonful of Hoffman's anodyne may be used. In obstinate cases lavage is indicated and is sometimes striking in its effects. Alkaline solutions may be used.

Vomiting is not a feature which often calls for treatment in chronic dyspepsia; sometimes in children it is a persistent symptom. Creasote and carbolic acid in drop doses, a few drops of chloroform or of dilute hydrocyanic acid, cocaine, bismuth, and oxalate of cerium may be used. If obstinate, the stomach should be washed out daily.

Constipation is a frequent and troublesome feature of most forms of indigestion. Occasionally small doses of mercury, podophyllin, the laxative mineral waters, sulphur, and cascara may be employed. Glycerin suppositories and the injection of from half a teaspoonful to a teaspoonful of glycerin are very efficacious.

Many cases of chronic dyspepsia are greatly benefited by the use of mineral waters, particularly a residence at the springs with a careful supervision of the diet and systematic exercise.

III. CIRRHOSIS VENTRICULI

(*Plastic Linitis*)

Brinton described under the term linitis plastica a condition of diffuse sclerosis of the stomach with thickening of the walls and reduction of the lumen.

It may be localized, but more commonly involves the whole organ, and a similar condition has been found in the colon, small bowel, and rectum. In the first case I saw, a patient of Dr. Drake's, Montreal, the stomach was no bigger than a cucumber, and the cæcum and part of the ascending colon showed the same thickening. The special lesion is an enormous hypertrophy of the submucosa, with atrophy of the gland elements and hypertrophy of the muscular layers, so that the wall is six to eight times the normal thickness; but, as Brinton remarks, the layers remain distinct. There are two forms, benign and malignant, which are not easy to separate without the most careful microscopic examination. Lyle has collected 118 cases from the literature, more than half of which were the true plastic linitis of Brinton.

The *symptoms* are at first indefinite, but when well established vomiting becomes marked and there is inability to retain even small amounts of food. The presence of a sausage-shaped tumor in the epigastrium is important. Hæmorrhage may be present. The X-ray picture should be of great help. In the only case in which I made a diagnosis the protracted history, the restriction in capacity of the stomach, and the tumor seemed characteristic. Nothing could be done at operation; and in a more recent case the walls were so hard and the stomach so small that it was impossible to make a gastroenterostomy, of which Lyle has reported a successful case. Total gastrectomy has been performed in three cases.

IV. DILATATION OF THE STOMACH

(*Gastrectasis*)

Etiology.—Acute dilatation is a very serious condition, described by Hilton Fagge, characterized by sudden onset, vomiting of enormous quantities of fluid, and symptoms of collapse. Of 102 cases collected by Lewis A. Conner 42 followed operation with general anæsthesia. The next largest group occurs in the course of severe diseases, or during convalescence. Cases have followed injuries, particularly of the head and spine. In 9 cases the symptoms came on after a single large meal; 6 cases were associated with spinal disease, in 3 while the patients were in a plaster of Paris jacket, and in a few cases it has come on in persons in good health. There were 74 deaths. In 69 autopsies the duodenum was found dilated in 38 cases. In a majority of cases it is due to a constriction of the lower end of the duodenum by traction on the mesenteric root, which is particularly apt to occur when there is a long mesentery and when the coil of small bowel is empty and falls into the true pelvis. The diagnosis is usually easy—repeated vomiting of large quantities of bilious non-fæcal fluid, with subnormal temperature, pain, collapse symptoms, and distended abdomen are the common features. The treatment consists in repeated emptying of the stomach with the tube; change in posture from the dorsal to the belly position or the knee-elbow position has been followed by prompt relief. Operation has not proved very satisfactory.

CHRONIC DILATATION results from: (*a*) *Pyloric obstruction* due to narrowing of the orifice or of the duodenum by the cicatrization of an ulcer, hypertrophic stenosis of the pylorus (whether cancerous or simple) congenital stricture, or occasionally by pressure from without of a tumor or of a floating kidney. The pylorus may be tilted up by adhesions to the liver or gall-bladder, or the stomach may be so dilated that the pylorus is dragged down and kinked. Adhesions about the gall-bladder may extend along the adjacent parts of the stomach and hitch up the pylorus into the hilus of the liver, forming a very acute kink. (*b*) *Relative or absolute insufficiency of the muscular power* of the stomach, due on the one hand to repeated overfilling of the organ with food and drink, and on the other to atony of the coats induced by chronic inflammation or the degeneration of impaired nutrition, the result of constitutional affections.

The most extreme forms are met with as a sequence of the cicatricial contraction of an ulcer. There may be considerable stenosis without much dilatation, the obstruction being compensated by hypertrophy of the muscular coats.

In the second group, due to atony of the muscular coats, we must distinguish between instances in which the stomach is simply enlarged and those with actual dilatation, conditions characterized by Ewald as *megalogastria* and *gastrectasis* respectively. The size of the stomach varies greatly in different individuals, and the maximum capacity of a normal organ Ewald places at about 1,600 c. c. Measurements above this point indicate absolute dilatation.

Atonic dilatation of the stomach may result from weakness of the coats, due to repeated overdistention or to chronic catarrh of the mucous membrane, or to the general muscular debility which is associated with chronic wasting disorders of all sorts. The combination of chronic gastric catarrh with over-feeding and excessive drinking is one of the most fruitful sources of atonic dilatation, as pointed out by Naunyn. The condition is frequently seen in diabetics, in the insane, and in beer-drinkers. In Germany this form is very common in men employed in the breweries. Possibly muscular weakness of the coats may result in some cases from disturbed innervation. Dilatation of the stomach is most frequent in middle-aged or elderly persons, but the condition is not uncommon in children, especially in association with rickets.

Symptoms.—In *atonic dilatation* there may be no symptoms whatever, even with a very greatly enlarged organ; more frequently there are the associated features of neurasthenia, enteroptosis, and nervous dyspepsia; while in a third group there may be all the symptoms of pyloric obstruction—vomiting of enormous quantities, etc. There is no limit to the capacity of the organ in this condition. Gould and Pyle mention an instance in which the stomach held 70 pints!

The features of *pyloric obstruction,* from whatever cause, are usually very evident. Dyspepsia is present in nearly all cases, and there are feelings of distress and uneasiness in the region of the stomach. The patient may complain much of hunger and thirst and eat and drink freely. The most characteristic symptom is the vomiting at intervals of enormous quantities of liquid and of food, amounting sometimes to four or more litres. The material is often of a dark-grayish color, with a characteristic sour odor due to the organic acids present, and contains mucus and remnants of food. On standing it separates into three layers, the lowest consisting of food, the middle of a turbid, dark-gray fluid, and the uppermost of a brownish froth. The microscopic examination shows a large variety of bacteria, yeast fungi, and the sarcina ventriculi. There may also be cherry stones, plum stones, and grape seeds.

The hydrochloric acid may be absent, diminished, normal, or in excess, depending upon the cause of the dilatation. The fermentation produces lactic, butyric, and, possibly, acetic acid and various gases.

In consequence of the small amount of fluid which passes from the stomach or is absorbed there are constipation, scanty urine, and extreme dryness of the skin. The general nutrition of the patient suffers greatly; there is loss of flesh and strength, and in some cases the most extreme emaciation. The gastric tetany will be considered in the section on that disease.

Physical Signs.—*Inspection.*—The abdomen may be large and prominent, the greatest projection occurring below the navel in the standing posture. In some instances the outline of the distended stomach can be plainly seen, the small curvature a couple of inches below the ensiform cartilage, and the greater curvature passing obliquely from the tip of the tenth rib on the left side, toward the pubes, and then curving upward to the right costal margin. Too much stress can not be laid on the importance of inspection. Very often the diagnosis may be made *de visu.* Active peristalsis may be seen in the dilated organ, the waves passing from left to right. Occasionally anti-peristalsis may be seen. In cases of stricture, particularly of hypertrophic stenosis, as the peristaltic wave reaches the pylorus, the tumor-like thickening can sometimes be distinctly seen through the thin abdominal wall. To stimulate the peristalsis the abdomen may be flipped with a wet towel. Inflation may be practiced with carbonic-acid gas. A small teaspoonful of tartaric acid dissolved in an ounce of water is first given, then a rather larger quantity of bicarbonate of soda. In many cases, particularly in thin persons, the outline of the dilated stomach stands out with great distinctness, and waves of peristalsis are seen in it.

Palpation.—The peristalsis may be felt, and usually in stenosis a tumor is evident at the pylorus. The resistance of a dilated stomach is peculiar, and has been aptly compared to that of an air cushion. Bimanual palpation elicits a splashing sound—*clapotage*—which is, of course, not distinctive, as it can be obtained whenever there is much liquid and air in the organ. The splashing may be very loud, and the patient may produce it himself by suddenly depressing the diaphragm, or it may be readily obtained by shaking him. The gurgling of gas through the pylorus may be felt.

Percussion.—The note is tympanitic over the greater portion of a dilated stomach; in the dependent part the note is flat. In the upright position the percussion should be made from above downward, in the left parasternal line, until a change in resonance is reached. The line of this should be marked, and the patient examined in the recumbent position, when it will be found to have altered its level. When this is on a line with the navel or below it, dilatation of the stomach may generally be assumed to exist. The fluid may be withdrawn from the stomach with a tube, and the dulness so made to disappear, or it may be increased by pouring in more fluid. In cases of doubt the organ should be artificially distended with carbonic-acid gas in the manner described above, or the stomach is inflated through a stomach-tube with a Davidson's syringe.

Auscultation.—The *clapotage* or succussion can be obtained readily. Frequently a curious sizzling sound is present, not unlike that heard when the ear is placed over a soda-water bottle when first opened. It can be heard naturally, and is usually evident when the artificial gas is being generated. The heart sounds may sometimes be transmitted with great clearness and with a metallic quality.

Mensuration may be used by passing a hard sound into the stomach until the greater curvature is reached. Normally it rarely passes more than 60 cm., measured from the teeth, but in cases of dilatation it may pass as much as 70 cm.

Diagnosis.—This can usually be made without much difficulty. I would like to emphasize again the great value of inspection, particularly in combination with inflation of the stomach. Curious errors, however, are on record, one of the most remarkable of which was the confounding of dilated stomach with an ovarian cyst; even after tapping and the removal of portions of food and fruit seeds, abdominal section was performed and the dilated stomach opened. The diagnosis of ascites has been made and the abdomen opened. The *prognosis* depends upon the cause; it is good in simple atony, bad in cancerous stricture, fairly good in simple stricture, from whatever cause.

Treatment.—In the cases due to atony careful regulation of the diet and proper treatment of the associated catarrh will suffice to effect a cure. Strychnine, ergot, and iron are recommended. Washing out the stomach is of great service, though we do not see such striking and immediate results in this form. In cases of mechanical obstruction the stomach should be emptied and thoroughly washed, either with warm water or with an antiseptic solution. We accomplish in this way three important things: We remove the weight, which helps to distend the organ; we remove the mucus and the stagnating and fermenting material which irritates and inflames the stomach and impedes digestion; and we cleanse the inner surface of the organ by the application of water and medicinal substances. The patient can usually be taught to wash out his own stomach, and in a case of dilatation from simple stricture I have known the practice to be followed daily for three years with great benefit. The rapid reduction in the size of the stomach is often remarkable, the vomiting ceases, food is taken readily, and in many cases the general nutrition improves rapidly. As a rule, once a day is sufficient, and it may be practiced either the first thing in the morning or before going to bed. So soon as the fermentative processes have been checked lukewarm water alone should be used.

The food should be taken in small quantities at frequent intervals, and should consist of scraped beef, Leube's beef solution, and tender meats of all sorts. Fatty and starchy articles of diet are to be avoided. Liquids should be taken sparingly.

Surgery should be resorted to early in cases of organic stricture; in atonic dilatation after all other measures have been given a thorough trial, gastro-enterostomy may be practiced.

V. THE PEPTIC ULCER, GASTRIC AND DUODENAL

The round, perforating, simple or peptic ulcer is usually single, and occurs in the stomach and in the duodenum as far as the papilla. Post mortem statistics show a great preponderance of the gastric ulcer, but the enormous experience of surgeons has taught us that in more than fifty per cent. of the clinical cases the ulcer is outside the pyloric ring.

Erosions.—Small abrasions of the mucosa—2 to 4 mm.—usually multiple, are common, extending half way or quite through the layer. They are often called hæmorrhagic erosions from their blood-stained appearance. They are met with in the new-born, in cachectic states in children, in chronic heart and arterial disease, in cirrhosis of the liver, etc. Of no clinical importance, as a rule, occasionally an acute hæmorrhagic erosion of quite small size opens a large artery, and the patient bleeds to death. There is no difference between this condition and the acute form of the gastric ulcer.

In many cases of chronic dyspepsia small fragments of the mucosa are washed out by the stomach tube, and Einhorn thinks that this may be a special form characterized by pains, dyspepsia, and weakness.

In certain acute infections with the pneumococcus (Dieulafoy) and septic organisms there may be hæmorrhagic erosions, which occasionally prove fatal by hæmatemesis.

And, lastly, it is probable that the post-operative hæmatemesis, slight or grave, may be due to these erosions. The French have described them as if peculiar to operations for appendicitis (*vomito-negro appendiculaire*), but cases occur after all sorts of abdominal operations. It is probable that the slight gastric hæmorrhages which occur in connection with the throbbing aorta in neurotic women are due to these erosions.

Etiology of Peptic Ulcer.—INCIDENCE.—The disease is much more common than medical and pathological statistics indicate. The surgical work of the Mayo clinic and of Moynihan of Leeds has taught us that the peptic ulcer exists in many cases which we had regarded as simple hyperchlorhydria. In two points surgical experience has completely changed our medical standpoint, viz.: the incidence of ulcer in the male is greater than in the female, and the duodenal is much more common than the gastric ulcer. Perhaps nothing illustrates more forcibly the frequency of duodenal ulcer than the fact that in the month of July, 1910, 17 cases were operated upon at the Mayo clinic, 5 of which had perforated, and in the same period only three cases of ulcer of the stomach came to operation. The surgical statistics, now amounting to many hundreds of cases, have sent our medical statistics to the scrap heap. The incidence of the disease appears to vary in different localities, and post mortem figures from the United States and Canada show a much lower percentage of cases (1.32) than on the continent of Europe (5 per cent.), and in London, 4.2 per cent. (C. P. Howard).

Sex.—Of 1,699 cases collected from hospital statistics by W. H. Welch and examined post mortem, 40 per cent. were in males and 60 per cent. were in females. In 82 cases (J. H. H.) there were 48 males and 28 females—in striking contrast to the Massachusetts General Hospital figures, 5 females to 1 male. Recent surgical statistics show an enormous preponderance of males.

Age.—In females the largest number of cases occurred between fifteen and twenty-five; in males between forty and fifty, in our series. It may occur in old people. E. G. Cutler has studied a series of 29 cases in children. In 6 the symptoms came on immediately after birth. There were 8 cases under seven years of age, and 9 between eight and thirteen.

Heredity appears to play a part in some cases (Dreschfeld).

Occupation.—It was impossible in our series to say that occupation had any influence. Among women, chlorotic, dyspeptic servant girls seem very prone. Shoemakers are thought to be specially liable. It appears relatively more common in the hospital classes.

Trauma.—Ulcers have been known to follow a blow in the region of the stomach. There was a history of injury in 7 cases in our series.

Associated Diseases.—Anæmia and chlorosis predispose strongly to gastric ulcer, particularly in women and in association with menstrual disorders. A very considerable number of all cases of gastric ulcer occur in chlorotic girls. It has been found also in connection with disease of the heart, arteriosclerosis, and disease of the liver. The tuberculous and syphilitic ulcers of the stomach have already been considered.

Burns.—The duodenal ulcer may follow large superficial burns. Perry and Shaw found it in five of one hundred and forty-nine autopsies in cases of burns of the skin.

Morbid Anatomy and Pathology.—Ninety per cent. of gastric ulcers are to be found at the pyloric end; nearly all duodenal ulcers are in the first or ascending portion, and more than one-half extend up to or within three-fourths of an inch of the pylorus, while twenty per cent. involve the margin of the pyloric ring (Mayo). It may not be easy on the operating table to distinguish between an ulcer of the duodenum and that of the stomach, but Mayo says that the position of the pyloric vein gives the exact location. Multiple ulcers may occur, 8.2 per cent. in Mayo's series. From 5 to 34 have been found. In the stomach, post mortem statistics (Welch) give, in 793 cases, 288 on the lesser curvature, 235 on the posterior wall, 69 on the anterior wall, 95 at the pylorus, 50 at the cardia, 29 at the fundus, and 27 on the greater curvature.

The acute ulcer is usually small, punched out, the edges clean-cut, the floor smooth, and the peritoneal surface not thickened. The chronic ulcer is of larger size, the margins are no longer sharp, the edges are indurated, and the border is sinuous. It may reach an enormous size, as in the one reported by Peabody, which measured 19 by 10 cm. and involved all of the lesser curvature and spread over a large part of the anterior and posterior walls. The sides are often terraced. The floor is formed either by the submucosa, by the muscular layers, or, not infrequently, by the neighboring organs, to which the stomach has become attached. In the healing of the ulcer, if the mucosa is alone involved, the granulation tissue grows from the edges and the floor and the newly formed tissue gradually contracts and unites the margins, leaving a smooth scar. In larger ulcers which have become deep and involved the muscular coat the cicatricial contraction may cause serious changes, the most important of which is narrowing of the pyloric orifice and consequent dilatation of the stomach. In the case of a girdle ulcer hour-glass contraction of the stomach may be produced. Large ulcers persist for years without any attempt at healing.

Among the more serious changes which may proceed in an ulcer are the following:

PERFORATION.—This occurred in 28.1 per cent. of 1,871 cases collected by Musser. In some series (Mayo's) duodenal perforation is the more common. Of 272 cases of duodenal ulcer in Mayo's series (to June 1, 1908), perforation was found sixty-six times, 16 acute, 13 subacute with abscess, and 37 chronic and protected. Perforation of the anterior wall of the stomach usually excites an acute peritonitis. On the posterior wall the ulcer penetrates directly into the lesser peritoneal cavity, in which case it may produce an air-containing abscess with the symptoms of the condition known as subphrenic pyopneumothorax. In rare instances adhesions and a gastrocutaneous fistula form, usually in the umbilical region. Fistulous communication with the colon may also occur, or a gastroduodenal fistula. The pericardium may be perforated, and even the left ventricle. Perforation into the pleura may also occur. It is to be noted that general emphysema of the subcutaneous tissues occasionally follows perforation of a gastric ulcer.

EROSION OF BLOOD-VESSELS.—In both forms of ulcer hæmorrhage occurs, in 8.1 per cent. of Musser's series of 1,871 cases. In Moynihan's 114 cases of duodenal ulcer, hæmorrhage occurred in 41. It is more common in the chronic form. Ulcers on the posterior wall may erode the splenic artery, but perhaps more frequently the bleeding proceeds from the artery of the lesser curvature. In the case of duodenal ulcer the pancreaticoduodenal artery may be eroded, or (as in one of my cases) fatal hæmorrhage may result from the opening of the hepatic artery, or more rarely the portal vein. Interesting changes occur in the vessels. Embolism of the artery supplying the ulcerated region has been met with in several cases; in others diffuse endarteritis. Small aneurisms have been found in the floor of the ulcers by Douglas Powell, Welch, and others. A rare event is emphysema of the sub-peritoneal tissue, which may be very extensive and even pass on to the posterior mediastinum. Jurgensen ascribes it to entrance of air into the veins, but Welch thinks it represents an invasion with the gas bacillus.

CICATRIZATION.—Superficial ulcers often heal without leaving any serious damage. Stenosis of the pyloric orifice not infrequently follows the healing of an ulcer in its neighborhood. In other instances the large annular ulcer may cause in its cicatrization an hour-glass contraction of the stomach. The adhesion of the ulcer to neighboring parts may subsequently be the cause of much pain. The parts of the mucosa in the neighborhood of the ulcer frequently show signs of chronic gastritis.

PERIGASTRIC ADHESIONS.—The condition is common, as high as 5 per cent. of post mortem records. It follows ulcer, lesions of the gall-bladder, pancreatic disease, syphilitic disease of the liver, and chronic tuberculosis. In some instances the lesions are quite extensive, and the condition has been called plastic perigastritis. It may be associated, too, with hypertrophic thickening of the coats of the stomach and with chronic plastic peritonitis. In some instances the pylorus may be narrowed as a result of the adhesions, or a sort of hour-glass stomach may be produced, or the motility of the organ is interfered with. Pain is the most constant feature, and may simulate that of gastric ulcer or of hyperacidity, and may be present constantly or at intervals. It is much influenced by posture and usually relieved by pressure. Local tenderness is present in a majority of instances. The cases are chronic, the general health is but slightly interfered with, and there are not, as a rule, signs of gastric dilatation. A definite tumor may be present about the region of the pylorus.

Carcinoma and Ulcer.—The observations at the Mayo clinic by Wilson and MacCarty show a much closer relationship between these conditions than we had previously supposed. The latter author, who has made a study of 216 resections of the stomach for ulcer or cancer, concludes that 71 per cent. of the resected specimens of cancer were associated with ulcer, and that 68 per cent. of the resected gastric ulcers were associated with cancer.

Mode of Origin.—The mode of origin is unknown. The anatomical basis is an interference with the blood supply in a limited area of the mucosa, attributed to embolism, thrombosis, or spasm of the arteries. As they are not end vessels, simple obstruction can not account for it. Trophic influences, bacterial necrosis of the mucosa, spasm of the muscular coat in limited areas, etc., are among the hypotheses which have been advanced. The erosion is effected by the gastric juice, and the healing is probably retarded by its high grade of acidity.

A few cases of acute duodenal ulcer have a curious relation with superficial burns. Bardeen's researches upon the necroses in the viscera following extensive burns throw an important light upon these cases, showing especially how the gastro-intestinal mucous membrane is implicated in the toxic effects.

Jejunal Peptic Ulcer.—This may occur after gastrojejunostomy, but in many cases the ulcer involves both stomach and jejunum. The condition is rare, as after 1,141 gastrojejunostomies at the Mayo clinic not one developed an ulcer.

Symptoms.—The condition may be latent and only met with accidentally, post mortem. The first symptoms may be those of perforation. In other cases again, for months and years, the patient has had dyspepsia, and the ulcer may not have been suspected until the occurrence of a sudden hæmorrhage.

Dyspepsia may be slight and trifling or of a most aggravated character. In a considerable proportion of all cases nausea and *vomiting* occur, the latter not for two or more hours after eating. The vomitus usually contains a large amount of hydrochloric acid.

Hæmorrhage is present in at least one-third of all cases. It may be latent (occult). A patient may feel faint and turn pale and sweat; the next day the stools may be tarry from the blood that has passed into the small bowel. These concealed hæmorrhages are more often small, and the blood is not readily seen in the vomitus or stools. Weber's test may be tried; the fluid to be examined is mixed with 2 or 3 c. c. of glacial acetic acid, and then shaken with sulphuric ether. If blood be present the ethereal extract has a Tokay wine-like color. Meat should not be eaten for a few days before the test is made. These small, latent hæmorrhages may cause a slowly progressive anæmia. More commonly the bleeding is profuse, and the blood may be in such quantities and brought up so quickly that it is fluid, bright red in color, and quite unaltered. When it remains for some time in the stomach and is mixed with food it may be greatly changed, but the vomiting of a large quantity of unaltered blood is very characteristic of ulcer. As a rule, there are only one or two attacks; in our series 7 cases had one hæmorrhage, 7 two, 11 three, 1 four, and 15 many (Howard). Profuse bleedings may occur at intervals for many years. Death may follow directly. From 16 to 18 per cent. of the fatal cases are due to it (S. and W. Fenwick).

The immediate effect of the hæmorrhage is a severe anæmia, from which it may take months to rally; slight fever is common. Rare and untoward effects are convulsions, sometimes only the usual convulsions of extreme cerebral anæmia from which recovery takes place, or they may precede a hemiplegia, due probably to thrombosis.

Amaurosis may follow the hæmorrhage, and unfortunately may be permanent, due to degeneration of the retinal ganglion cells, or to a thrombosis of the cerebral arteries or veins.

Pain is perhaps the most constant and distinctive feature of ulcer. It varies greatly in character; it may be only a gnawing or burning sensation, which is particularly felt when the stomach is empty, and is relieved by taking food, but the more characteristic form comes on in paroxysms, in which the pain is not only felt in the epigastrium, but radiates to the back and to the sides. In many cases the two points of epigastric pain and dorsal pain, about the level of the tenth dorsal vertebra, are very well marked. These attacks are most frequently induced by taking food, and they may recur at a variable period after eating, sometimes within fifteen or twenty minutes, at others as late as two or three hours. It is usually stated that when the ulcer is near the cardia the pain is apt to set in earlier, but there is no certainty on this point. In some cases it comes on in the early morning hours. The attacks may occur at intervals with great intensity for weeks or months at a time, so that the patient constantly requires morphia, then again they may disappear entirely for a prolonged period. In the attack the patient is usually bent forward, and finds relief from pressure over the epigastric region; one patient during the attack would lean over the back of a chair; another would lie flat on the floor, with a hard pillow under the abdomen. Pressure is, as a rule, grateful. It has been thought that the posture assumed during the attack would indicate the site of the ulcer, but this is very doubtful.

Tenderness on pressure is a common symptom in ulcer, and patients wear the waist-band very low. Pressure should be made with great care, as rupture of an ulcer is said to have been induced by careless manipulation.

In old ulcers with thickened bases an indurated mass may be felt in the neighborhood of the pylorus.

Of general symptoms, *loss of weight* results from the prolonged dyspepsia, but it rarely, except in association with cicatricial stenosis of the pylorus, reaches the high grade met with in cancer. The *anæmia* may be extreme, and in one case of duodenal ulcer, which I examined, the blood-count was as low as 700,000 per c. mm. Of 44 cases in my wards in which blood-counts were made, the lowest was 1,902,000 per c. mm. There are instances, such as the one reported by Pepper and Griffith, in which the extreme anæmia can not be explained by the occurrence of hæmorrhage. In a few instances polycythæmia is present, even after a hæmorrhage, due to concentration of the blood and possibly associated dilatation of the stomach. In a few cases *parotitis* occurs, with the perforation sometimes, or after a hæmorrhage. In one of my cases there was a remarkable *pigmentation* of the face and of the axillary folds.

Perforation.—This occurred in 28.1 per cent. of Musser's series. The acute, perforating form is much more common in women than in men. The symptoms are those of perforative peritonitis. Particular attention must be given to this accident, since it has come so succesfully within the sphere of the surgeon. As already mentioned, perforation may take place either into the lesser peritoneum or into the general peritoneal cavity, in both of which cases operation is indicated; in rare instances the ulcer may perforate the pericardium. This was the case in 10 of 28 cases in which the diaphragm was perforated (Pick).

Localized, more frequently subphrenic, abscess may follow perforation.

Urine.—Albumin is occasionally present; in 14 of our series with dilatation of the stomach. Indican may be present. Acetone and diacetic acid (with syncopal attacks) have been described by Dreschfeld.

Hour-glass stomach most frequently results from the cicatrization of an ulcer. In a few cases it is congenital. The symptoms, fairly characteristic, are thus given by Moynihan:

(*a*) In washing out the stomach part of the fluid is lost. (*b*) If the stomach is washed clean, a sudden reappearance of stomach contents may take place. (*c*) "Paradoxical dilatation"; when the stomach has apparently been emptied, a splashing sound may be elicited by palpation of the pyloric segment. (*d*) After distending the stomach, a change in the position of the distention tumor may be seen in some cases. (*e*) Gushing, bubbling, or sizzling sounds are heard on dilatation with carbon dioxide at a point distinct from the pylorus. (*f*) In some cases, when both parts are dilated, two tumors with a notch or sulcus between are apparent to sight or touch. To these may now be added (*g*) a most characteristic X-ray picture.

Prognosis.—In all statistics the acute and chronic ulcer have been considered together. The former is more amenable to medical treatment, but grave complications may occur even before the digestive symptoms have been very pronounced. The chronic ulcer may last for years—twelve, eighteen, or even twenty—with intervals of good health. The all-important point in the prognosis relates to the question of medical or surgical treatment—which gives the best results? So far as figures count, the exhaustive study of Musser favors the former, 12.4 per cent. mortality against 20 per cent. for the latter. This for simple cases including complications. In private practice many series of cases have not a mortality above 6 per cent. The mortality of the chronic peptic ulcer in the hands of such experts as the Mayos and Moynihan is very low. In 311 gastrojejunostomies for ulcer of the stomach and duodenum the mortality was less than 1 per cent., and only three patients required a secondary operation (Mayo's). In Moynihan's cases of duodenal ulcer, 114 in number (exclusive of perforation), there were only two deaths. The end results of gastro-enterostomy for the chronic ulcer appear to be excellent.

Diagnosis.—The acute non-indurated ulcer may cause very few symptoms—nothing beyond ordinary dyspepsia with pain. Examination of the stomach contents shows an increase in the free HCl. Hæmatemesis may be the first symptom of moment. This group of cases is seen chiefly in young girls, and appears to be much more common in England than in the United States. A condition which may be confounded with it is *gastrostaxis,* described by Hale White. The stomach symptoms are marked, the bleeding may be profuse, but post mortem or at operation no ulcer is found. Of course very careful inspection must be made, as fatal bleeding may come from a very small erosion. The symptoms of non-indurated mucous ulcer yield to a few months' medical treatment.

In the chronic cases the nutrition at first may remain good, and the patient looks well. The whole complaint is of the stomach, of pain and distress, with belching and nausea or vomiting from two to four hours after meals. This special feature of the recurrence of the pain some hours after taking food, its extraordinary regularity, persisting day by day for months or even years, and the relief afforded by taking food clearly separate the dyspeptic features of ulcer from other types.

Einhorn has introduced an ingenious *thread test.* A perforated olive with a long white thread attached is swallowed and remains in the stomach for 10 or 12 hours. If an ulcer, gastric or duodenal, is present, there is a stain corresponding to the part of the thread that has lain in contact with the ulcer, and the position on the thread gives an idea of the distance of the ulcer from the cardia.

Treatment.—Post mortem observations show that a very large number of ulcers heal completely, but the process is slow and tedious, often requiring months, or, in severe cases, years. The following are the important points in treatment:

(*a*) Absolute rest in bed.

(*b*) A carefully and systematically regulated diet. While theoretically it is better to give the stomach complete rest by rectal feeding, yet in practice this strict limitation is not found satisfactory. The food should be bland, easily digested, and given at stated intervals. The following dietary will be found useful: At 8 a. m. give 200 c. c. of Leube's beef solution; at 12 m., 300 c. c. of milk gruel or peptonized milk. The gruel should be made with ordinary flour or arrowroot, and is mixed with an equal quantity of milk. If necessary it may be peptonized. Buttermilk is very well borne by these patients. At 4 p. m. the beef solution again, and at 8 p. m. the milk gruel or buttermilk. Feeding by the duodenal tube is often successful.

The stomach in some cases is so irritable that the smallest amount of food is not well borne. In such cases lavage may be practiced, if necessary, every morning, with mildly alkaline water, after which the beef solution is given and the feeding supplemented by the rectal injections. Ill effects rarely follow the careful use of the stomach tube in gastric ulcer. There are some patients who do well from the outset on a milk diet, given at regular intervals,

3 or 4 ounces every two hours. When milk is not well borne egg albumen may be substituted, or the whites of eight eggs may be alternated with Leube's beef solution. At the end of a month, if the condition has improved, the patient may be allowed scraped beef or young chicken, perfectly fresh sweetbread, and farinaceous puddings made with milk and eggs. Local applications, such as warm fomentations, over the abdomen are very useful. The patient should be told that the treatment will take at least three months, and for the greater portion of the time he should be in bed.

(*c*) Medicinal measures are of very little value in gastric ulcer, and the remedies employed probably do not benefit the ulcer, but the gastric catarrh. The Carlsbad salts are warmly recommended by von Ziemssen. The artificial preparation (sulphate of sodium, 50 parts; bicarbonate of sodium, 6; chloride of sodium, 3) may be substituted, of which a teaspoonful is taken every morning. Bismuth, in doses of 30 to 60 grains (2 to 4 gm.) three times a day, and nitrate of silver may be given, but they influence the associated conditions rather than the ulcer.

The pain, if severe, requires opium. Unless the gastralgia is intense morphia should not be given hypodermically, as there is a very serious danger in these cases of establishing the morphia habit. Doses of an eighth of a grain, with the bicarbonate of soda and bismuth, will allay the mild attacks, but the very severe ones require the hypodermic injection of a quarter or often half a grain. Antipyrin and antifebrin may be tried, but, as a rule, are quite ineffectual. In the milder attacks Hoffman's anodyne, or 20 or 30 drops of spirit of chloroform, or the spirits of camphor, will give relief. Counter-irritation over the stomach with mustard or cantharides is often useful.

When the stomach is irritable, the patient should be fed per rectum. He will sometimes retain food which is passed into the stomach through the tube, and Leube's beef solution or milk may be given in this way. Cracked ice, chloroform, oxalate of cerium, and bismuth may be tried. When hæmorrhage occurs the patient should be put under the influence of opium as rapidly as possible. No attempt should be made to check the hæmorrhage by administering medicines by the mouth; as the profuse bleeding is always from an eroded artery, frequently from one of considerable size, it is doubtful if acetate of lead, tannic and gallic acids, and the usual remedies have the slightest influence. The essential point is to give rest, which is best obtained by opium. Nothing should be given by the mouth except small quantities of ice. In profuse bleeding the extremities may be tightly bandaged. Not infrequently the loss of blood is so great that the patient faints. A fatal result is not, however, very common from hæmorrhage. Transfusion, direct from artery to vein by Crile's method, or the subcutaneous infusion of saline solution, may be necessary.

The patients usually recover rapidly from the hæmorrhage and require iron in full doses, which may, if necessary, be given hypodermically.

Surgical interference is indicated: (1) For perforation; (2) in the chronic indurated ulcer. Experience has shown that after gastro-enterostomy the ulcer heals rapidly, and in some cases the ulcer itself may be located; (3) in all cases when the ulcer has caused mechanical interference with the passage of the gastric contents; (4) in all cases associated with recurring hæmorrhages. In young girls the single severe attack of hæmatemesis may be a simple gastrorrhexis, or from a simple ulcer that heals readily, but in men severe hæmatemesis is almost always from the chronic ulcer; (5) in the perigastric adhesions after chronic ulcer operation is sometimes helpful; (6) in chronic cases in which medical treatment fails to give relief.

In the present state of our knowledge it is not easy to determine the limits of medical and surgical practice in the treatment of peptic ulcer. The old statistics are not of much avail, since it is quite clear that scores of cases have been masquerading under the names of hyperchlorhydria, acid dyspepsia, and so forth. The simple non-indurated ulcer is, in the majority of cases, a medical disease. A chronic indurated form is best treated surgically.

VI. CANCER OF THE STOMACH

Etiology.—INCIDENCE.—In an analysis of 30,000 cases of cancer, W. H. Welch found the stomach involved in 21.4 per cent., this organ thus standing next to the uterus in order of frequency. Among 8,464 cases admitted to my wards, there were 150 cases of cancer of the stomach. There were 39 cases among the first 1,000 autopsies in the post mortem room of the Johns Hopkins Hospital. The disease is more common in some countries. Figures indicate that cancer of the stomach, as of other organs, is increasing in frequency.

SEX.—In 150 cases from my wards there were 126 males and 24 females (McCrae). Welch gives the ratio as 5 to 4.

AGE.—Of our 150 cases the ages were as follows: Between twenty and thirty, 6; from thirty to forty, 17; forty to fifty, 38; fifty to sixty, 49; sixty to seventy, 36; seventy to eighty, 4. Fifty-eight per cent. occurred between the ages of forty and sixty. Of the 6 cases occurring under the thirtieth year, the youngest was twenty-two. Of the large number of cases analyzed by Welch, three-fourths occurred between the fortieth and seventieth years. Congenital cancer of the stomach has been described, and cases have been met with in children.

RACE.—Among our 150 cases, 131 were white; 19 were negroes.

HEREDITY.—Of the 150 cases in only 11 was there a positive history of cancer in the family. In some families, as the Bonapartes, the disease seems to prevail. In our series a very much larger number—38—had a family history of tuberculosis.

PREVIOUS DISEASES, HABITS, ETC.—A history of dyspepsia was present in only 33 cases; of these, 17 had had attacks at intervals, 11 had had chronic stomach trouble, and 5 had had dyspepsia for one or two years before the symptoms of cancer developed. Napoleon, discussing this interesting point with his physician Antommarchi, said that he had always had a stomach of iron and felt no inconvenience until the onset of what proved to be his fatal illness.

ALCOHOL.—Seventy-seven of our patients had used it regularly, 65 of these moderately (?), 8 excessively.

TRAUMA.—Only one case gave a positive history. In one case the cancer followed rapidly upon a blow on the stomach, and the patient lost sixty pounds in weight in three months.

Gastric Ulcer.—The relation to this condition is in dispute—the physicians are against, the surgeons are in favor. In only 4 cases in my series was there a history pointing to ulcer. On the other hand, in the Mayo clinic nearly 75 per cent. of the cancers are believed to originate in ulcer.

Morbid Anatomy.—The most common varieties of gastric cancer are the cylindrical-celled adeno-carcinoma and the encephaloid or medullary carcinoma; next in frequency is scirrhous, and then colloid cancer. With reference to the situation of the tumor, Welch analyzed 1,300 cases, in which the distribution was as follows: Pyloric region, 791; lesser curvature, 148; cardia, 104; posterior wall, 68; the whole or greater part of the stomach, 61; multiple tumors, 45; greater curvature, 34; anterior wall, 30; fundus, 19.

The medullary cancer occurs in soft masses, which involve all the coats of the stomach and usually ulcerate early. The tumor may form villous projections or cauliflower-like outgrowths. It is soft, grayish-white in color, and contains much blood. The cylindrical-celled epithelioma may also form large irregular masses, but the consistence is usually firmer, particularly at the edges of the cancerous ulcers. Cysts are not uncommon in this form. The scirrhous variety is characterized by great hardness, due to the abundance of the stroma and the limited amount of alveolar structures. It is seen most frequently at the pylorus, where it is a common cause of stenosis. It may be combined with the medullary form. It may be diffuse, involving all parts of the organ, and leading to a condition which can not be recognized macroscopically from cirrhosis. This form has also been seen in the stomach secondary to cancer of the ovaries. In connection with the diffuse carcinomatosis there may be simultaneous involvement of the small and large intestines. The colloid cancer is peculiar in its wide-spread invasion of all the coats. It also spreads with greater frequency to the neighboring parts, and it occasionally causes extensive secondary growths of the same nature in other organs. The appearance on section is very distinctive, and even with the naked eye large alveoli can be seen filled with the translucent colloid material. The term alveolar cancer is often applied to this form. Ulceration is not constantly present, and there are instances in which, with most extensive disease, digestion has been but slightly disturbed. There is a specimen in the Warren Museum, at the Harvard Medical School, of the most widespread colloid cancer, in which the stomach contained after death large pieces of undigested beef-steak.

Secondary Cancer of the Stomach.—Of 37 cases collected by Welch, 17 were secondary to cancer of the breast. Among the first 1,000 autopsies at the Johns Hopkins Hospital there were 3 cases of secondary cancer.

Changes in the Stomach.—Cancer at the cardia is usually associated with wasting of the organ and reduction in its size. The œsophagus above the obstruction may be greatly dilated. On the other hand, annular cancer at the pylorus causes stenosis with great dilatation of the organ. In a few rare instances the pylorus has been extremely narrowed without any increase in the size of the stomach. In diffuse scirrhous cancer the stomach may be very greatly thickened and contracted. It may be displaced or altered in shape by the weight of the tumor, particularly in cancer of the pylorus; in such cases it has been found in every region of the abdomen, and even in the true pelvis. The mobility of the tumors is at times extraordinary and very deceptive, and they may be pushed into the right hypochondrium or into the splenic region, entirely beneath the ribs. Adhesions very frequently occur, particularly to the colon, the liver, and the anterior abdominal wall.

Secondary cancerous growths in other organs are very frequent, as shown by the following analysis by Welch of 1,574 cases: Metastasis occurred in the lymphatic glands in 551; in the liver in 475; in the peritoneum, omentum, and intestine in 357; in the pancreas in 122; in the pleura and lung in 98; in the spleen in 26; in the brain and meninges in 9; in other parts in 92. The lymph glands affected are usually those of the abdomen, but the cervical and inguinal glands are not infrequently attacked, and give an important clue in diagnosis. Secondary metastatic growths occur subcutaneously, either at the navel or beneath the skin in the vicinity, and are of great value in diagnosis.

PERFORATION.—This occurred into the peritoneum in 17 of the 507 cases of cancer of the stomach collected by Brinton. In our series perforation occurred in 4 cases. When adhesions form, the most extensive destruction of the walls may take place without perforation into the peritoneal cavity. In one instance which came under my observation a large portion of the left lobe of the liver lay within the stomach. Occasionally a gastro-cutaneous fistula is established. Perforation may occur into the colon, the small bowel, the pleura, the lung, or into the pericardium.

Symptoms.—LATENT CARCINOMA.—The cases are not very infrequent. There may be no symptoms pointing to the stomach, and the tumor may be discovered accidentally after death. In a second group the symptoms of carcinoma are present, not of the stomach, but of the liver or some other organ, or there are subcutaneous nodules, or, as in one of our cases, secondary masses on the ribs and vertebræ. In a third group, seen particularly in elderly persons in institutions, there is gradual asthenia, without nausea, vomiting, or other local symptoms.

FEATURES OF ONSET.—Of the 150 cases in our series, 48 complained of pain, 44 of dyspepsia, 21 of vomiting, 13 of loss in weight, 3 of difficulty in swallowing, 1 of tumor. In 7 the features of onset suggested pernicious anæmia. In 37 cases there was a history of sudden onset.

GENERAL SYMPTOMS.—*Loss of Weight.*—Progressive emaciation is one of the most constant features of the disease. In 79 of our cases in which exact figures were taken: To 30 pounds, 32 cases; 30 to 50 pounds, 36 cases; 50 to 60 pounds, 5 cases; 60 to 70 pounds, 4; over 70 pounds, 1; 100 pounds, a case of cancer at the cardiac end with obstruction to swallowing. The loss in weight is not always progressive. We see increase in weight under three conditions: (*a*) Proper dieting, with treatment of the associated catarrh of the stomach; (*b*) in cases of cancer of the pylorus after relief of the dilatation of the organ by lavage, etc.; (*c*) after a profound mental impression. I have known a gain of ten pounds to follow the visit of an optimistic consultant. In Keen and D. D. Stewart's case there was a gain of seventy pounds after an exploratory operation!

Loss in strength is usually proportionate to the loss in weight. One sees sometimes remarkable vigor almost to the close, but this is exceptional.

Anæmia is present in a large proportion of all cases, and with the emaciation gives the picture of cachexia. There is often a yellow or lemon tint of the skin. In 59 cases careful blood-counts were made; in 3 the red corpuscles were above 6,000,000 per c. mm. This occurs in the concentrated condition of the blood in certain cases of cancer of the pylorus with dilatation of the stomach. The average count in the 59 cases was 3,712,186 per c. mm. In only 8 cases was the count below 2,000,000, and in none below 1,000,000. The average of the hæmoglobin was 44.9 per cent. In only 9 was it below 30 per cent. In 62 cases in which the leucocytes were counted there were only 18 cases in which they were above 12,000 per c. mm.; in only 3 cases were they above 20,000. The features of onset may suggest a primary anæmia.

Among other general symptoms may be mentioned *fever,* which was present at some time in 74 of our 150 cases. In only 13 of these did the temperature rise above 101°. In 2 it was above 103°. Fifteen presented fairly constant elevation of temperature. Eight presented sudden rises. Two cases had *chill,* with elevation to 103° and 104°. Chills may be associated with suppuration at the base of the cancer.

Urine.—There may be no changes throughout; in 65 of our cases there were no alterations, in 36 albumin was found, and in 34 albumin with tube-casts. Glycosuria, peptonuria, and acetonuria have been described. Indican is common.

Œdema.—Swelling of the ankles is of frequent occurrence toward the close. In some cases there is even early a general anasarca, usually in combination with extreme anæmia. The cancer is usually overlooked.

The *bowels* are often constipated. In only 12 cases in our series was diarrhœa present. In 2 cases blood was passed per rectum. There are no special *cardiac symptoms;* the pulse becomes progressively weaker. Thrombosis of one femoral vein may occur, or, as in one of our cases, wide-spread thrombosis in the superficial veins of the body.

Symptoms on the part of the nervous system are rare; consciousness is often retained to the end. *Coma* may occur similar to that seen in diabetes, and is believed to be due to an acid intoxication.

Functional Disturbances.—*Anorexia,* loss of desire for food, is a frequent and valuable symptom, more constant perhaps than any other. *Nausea* is a striking feature in many cases; there is often a sudden repulsion at the sight of food. In exceptional cases the appetite is retained throughout.

Vomiting may come on early, or only after the dyspepsia has persisted for some time. It occurred in 128 cases in our series. At first it is at long intervals, but subsequently it is more frequent, and may recur several times in the day. There are cases in which it comes on in paroxysms and then subsides; in other cases it sets in early, persists with great violence, and may cause a fatal termination within a few weeks. Vomiting is more frequent when the cancer involves the orifices, particularly the pylorus, in which case it is usually delayed for an hour or more after taking the food. When the cardiac orifice is involved it may follow at a shorter interval. Extensive disease of the fundus or of the anterior or posterior wall may be present without the occurrence of vomiting. The food is sometimes very little changed, even after it has remained in the stomach for twenty-four hours.

Hæmorrhage occurred in 36 of our 150 cases; in 32 the blood was dark and altered, in 3 it was bright red. In 2 cases vomiting of blood was the first symptom. The bleeding is rarely profuse; more commonly there is slight oozing, and the blood is mixed with, or altered by, the secretions, and, when vomited, the material is dark brown or black, the so-called "coffee-ground" vomit. The blood can be recognized by the microscope as shadows of the red blood-corpuscles and irregular masses of altered blood pigment. Occult blood may be found in the fæces.

Pain, an early and important symptom, was present in 130 of our cases. It is very variable in situation and, while most common in the epigastrium, it may be referred to the shoulders, the back, or the loins. The pain is described as dragging, burning, or gnawing in character, and very rarely occurs in severe paroxysms, as in gastric ulcer. As a rule, the pain is aggravated by taking food. There is usually marked tenderness on pressure in the epigastric region. The areas of skin tenderness are referred, as Head has shown, to the region between the nipple and the umbilicus in front and behind from the fifth to the twelfth thoracic spine.

THE STOMACH CONTENTS.—The finding of pus and blood in the empty stomach and pus, blood and mucus two hours after the test meal is suggestive. Diminished motility may be an early finding in pyloric cancer. There is often a downward trend in the curve of acid secretion. The protein curve often shows a marked divergence from the acid curve which increases as digestion goes on and is most marked in cases of subacidity or achylia. The test for soluble albumin (Wolff-Junghans) is of value, especially two hours after the test meal. The tryptophan test and ereptic reaction are of doubtful value owing to frequent regurgitation of duodenal contents. Bacteria in large numbers occur, one, the Oppler-Boas bacillus—an unusually long non-motile form—is supposed to be of diagnostic value, and to be largely responsible for the formation of lactic acid. Blood is a most important ingredient; the persistent presence microscopically of red corpuscles in the early morning washings is always very suspicious. Later, when coffee-ground vomiting takes place, the macroscopic evidence is sufficient. Fragments of the new growth may be vomited or may appear in the washings.

Examination of the Test Breakfast.—The Ewald test meal, consisting of a slice of stale bread and a large cup of weak tea without cream or sugar, is given at 7 a. m. and withdrawn at 8 a. m. The Boas test meal, consisting of a gruel made of a tablespoonful of oatmeal flour in a litre of water, is used in the estimation of lactic acid. As an outcome of the enormous number of observations made of late years, it may be said that free HCl is absent in a large proportion of all cases of cancer of the stomach. Of 94 cases in which the contents were examined in 84 free HCl was absent. In 5 undoubted cases the reaction was good; in 2 of these the history suggested previous ulcer. HCl may be absent in chronic gastritis and in atrophy of the gastric mucosa. The presence of lactic acid after Boas' test meal is regarded as a valuable sign.

PHYSICAL EXAMINATION.—*Inspection.*—After a preliminary survey, embracing the facies, state of nutrition, etc., particular attention is given to the abdomen. An all-important matter is to have the patient in a good light. Fullness in the epigastric region, inequality in the infracostal grooves, the existence of peristalsis, a wide area of aortic pulsation, the presence of subcutaneous nodules or small masses about the navel, and, lastly, a well-defined tumor mass—these, together or singly, may be seen on careful inspection.

I can not emphasize too strongly the value of this method of examination. In 62 of the 150 cases a positive tumor could be seen. In 52 the tumor descended with inspiration; in 36 peristalsis was visible; in 3 cases movements were visible in the tumor itself. In 10 cases with visible peristalsis no tumor was seen, but could be felt on palpation. Inflation with carbonic-acid gas may be tried, except when hæmorrhage has been profuse or the cancer is very extensive. The dilatation often renders evident the peristalsis or may bring a tumor into view. The presence of subcutaneous and umbilical nodules is sometimes a very great help. They were found in 5 of our series.

Palpation.—In 115 cases a tumor could be felt; in 48 in the epigastric region, in 25 in the umbilical, in 18 in the left hypochondriac, in 17 in the right hypochondriac region, while in 7 cases a mass descended in deep inspiration from beneath the left costal margin. These figures illustrate in how large a proportion of the cases the tumor is in evidence. In rare cases examination in the knee-elbow position is of value. *Mobility* in gastric tumor is a point of much importance. First, the change with respiration, already referred to; a mass may descend 3 or 4 inches in deep inspiration; secondly, the communicated pulsation from the aorta, which is often in its extent suggestive; thirdly, the intrinsic movements in the hypertrophied muscularis in the neighborhood of the cancer. This may give a remarkable character to the mass, causing it to appear and disappear, lifting the abdominal wall in the epigastric region; and, fourthly, mechanical movements, with inflation, with change of posture, or communicated with the hand. Tumors of the pylorus are the most movable, and in extreme cases can be displaced to either hypochondrium or pushed far down below the navel (see illustrative cases in my Lectures on the Diagnosis of Abdominal Tumors). Pain on palpation is common; the mass is usually hard, sometimes nodular. Gas can at times be felt gurgling through the tumor at the pyloric region.

Percussion gives less important indications—the note over a tumor is rarely flat, more often a flat tympany. *Auscultation* may reveal the gurgling through the pylorus; sometimes a systolic bruit is transmitted from the aorta, and when a local peritonitis exists a friction may be heard.

Complications.—*Secondary growths* are common. In 44 autopsies in our series there were metastases in 38; in 29 the lymph-glands were involved; in 23 the liver, in 11 the peritoneum, in 8 the pancreas, in 8 the bowel, in 4 the lung, in 3 the pleura, in 4 the kidneys, and in 2 the spleen. In 8 no deposits were found.

Perforation may lead to peritonitis, but in 3 of our 4 cases there was no general involvement. Cancerous ascites is not very uncommon. Dock has called attention to the value of the examination of the fluid in such cases as a help to diagnosis. The cells show mitoses and are very characteristic. Secondary cancer of the *liver* is very common; the enlargement may be very great, and such cases are not infrequently mistaken for primary cancer of the organ. Involvement of the *lymph-glands* may give valuable indications. There may be early enlargement of a gland at the posterior border of the left sterno-cleido-mastoid muscle; later adjacent glands may become affected. This occurs also in uterine cancer.

A very remarkable picture is presented when the cancer *sloughs* or becomes gangrenous; the vomitus has a foul odor, often of a penetrating nature, to be perceived throughout the room. In cases in which the ulcer perforates the colon the vomiting may be fæcal. I have, however, met with the fæcal odor in a case with incessant vomiting in which there was no perforation of the colon at autopsy.

Course.—While usually *chronic* and lasting from a year to eighteen months, *acute* cancer of the stomach is by no means infrequent. Of the 69 cases in which we could determine accurately the duration, 15 lasted under three months, 16 from three to six months, 14 from six to twelve months—a total of 45 under one year. Four cases lasted for two years or over. One case lived for at least two years and a half.

Diagnosis.—In 115 of our 150 cases a tumor existed, and with this the recognition is rarely in doubt. The chief difficulty is in cases with gastric symptoms or anæmia, or both, without the presence of tumor. In the one a chronic gastritis is suspected; in the other a primary anæmia. In *chronic gastritis* the history of long-standing dyspepsia, the absence of cachexia, the absence of lactic acid in the test meal, and the less striking blood changes are the important points for consideration. The cases with grave *anæmia* without tumor offer the greatest difficulty. The blood-count is rarely so low as in pernicious anæmia, a point on which F. P. Henry has laid special stress. In only 8 of our 59 cases with careful blood examination was the number below 2,000,000 per c. mm. The lower color index, as in secondary anæmia, the absence of megaloblasts, and a leucocytosis speak for cancer. With metastases in the bone marrow the blood picture may be that of pernicious anæmia (Harrington and Teacher). Some lay stress on the differential count of the leucocytes, but there is not evidence enough to enable us to speak positively on this point. The chemical findings are of greater value. From a recent careful study at the London Hospital Panton and Tidy conclude that in carcinoma the Günsberg reaction is always negative and the average total acidity is 26, while in ulcer the reaction is positive, the average free hydrochloric acid is above normal, and the total acidity 58.

From *ulcer of the stomach* malignant disease is, as a rule, readily recognized. The *ulcus carcinomatosum* usually presents a well-marked history of ulcer for years. The greatest difficulty is offered when there is ulcer with tumor due to cicatricial contraction about the pylorus. In 3 such cases we mistook the mass for cancer, and even at operation it may (as in one of them) be impossible to say whether a neoplasm is present. The persistent hyperchlorhydria is the most important single feature of ulcer, and, taken with the gastralgic attacks and the hæmorrhages, rarely leaves doubt as to the condition. The X-rays are sometimes an aid.

Nowadays, when exploratory laparotomy may be advised with such safety, the surgeon often makes the diagnosis.

The practitioner should recognize the fact that there are cases of cancer of the stomach in which a positive diagnosis can not be reached for weeks or months by any known means at our command except exploration.

Treatment.—In early surgical treatment lies the only hope, but there is great difficulty in the diagnosis. Operated upon early, complete removal is sometimes possible. In a majority of cases the operation is only palliative. In suitable cases early exploration should be advised; the operation *per se* is sometimes beneficial and the patient is rarely the worse for it. To January

27th, 1910, 627 cases were operated upon at the Mayo clinic, of which 206 were in a hopeless condition. In 169 gastrostomy was performed, in 266 a tumor was resected, and among these there were 34 deaths. The after-results are given as far as possible: in 39 cases whose condition was known, who had been operated upon over 5 years before, 7 were alive; of 64, condition known, over 4 years, 13 alive; of 88, condition known, over 3 years, 18 alive and well.

The diet should consist of readily digested substances of all sorts. Many patients do best on milk alone. Washing out the stomach, which may be done with a soft tube without any risk, is particularly advantageous when there is obstruction at the pylorus, and is by far the most satisfactory means of combating the vomiting. The excessive fermentation is also best treated by lavage. When the pain becomes severe, particularly if it disturbs the rest at night, morphia must be given. One-eighth of a grain, combined with carbonate of soda (gr. v), bismuth (gr. v-x), usually gives prompt relief, and the dose does not always require to be increased. Creasote (♏ j-ij) and carbolic acid are very useful. The bleeding in gastric cancer is rarely amenable to treatment.

Other Forms of Tumor.—*Non-cancerous tumors* of the stomach rarely cause inconvenience. *Polypi* (polyadenomata) are common and they may be numerous; as many as 150 have been reported in one case. There is a form in which the adenoma exists as an extensive area slightly raised above the level of the mucosa—*polyadénome en nappe* of the French. An extraordinary multiple adenoma associated with multiple tumors throughout the intestines and subcutaneous hæmangio-endotheliomata has been described by Winternitz. H. B. Anderson has described a case of remarkable multiple *cysts* in the walls of the stomach and small intestine. *Sarcomata* are very rare. *Fibromata* and *lipomata* have been described. External polypoid tumors, myo- or fibro-sarcomata may grow from the peritoneal surface, usually the posterior, of which Sherran has collected 18 cases.

Foreign bodies occasionally produce remarkable tumors of the stomach. The most extraordinary is the *hair tumor,* of which there are many cases in the literature. The cases occur in hysterical women who have been in the habit of eating their own hair. A specimen in the medical museum of McGill University is in two sections, which form an exact mold of the stomach. The tumors are large, very puzzling, and are usually mistaken for cancer. Of 7 cases operated upon, 6 recovered; in 9 cases the condition was found post mortem (Schulten).

VII. HYPERTROPHIC STENOSIS OF THE PYLORUS

In Adults.—Microscopically, the condition is found to be very largely hypertrophy of the muscularis and submucosa of the pylorus. It was well described by the older writers. The symptoms are those of dilatation of the stomach. The question is whether some of these cases may not really be congenital, as there have been instances reported in girls as early as the twelfth and sixteenth years.

Congenital.—This remarkable affection, first recognized by Beardsley of Connecticut, has been thoroughly studied of late years by Hirschsprung, John Thomson, and others.

Etiology.—Whether congenital or not is much discussed; certainly in a majority of cases there are no symptoms at first. It is much more common in boys than in girls, and fully one-third of the cases are in first children. The causation is unknown. Two views prevail: (*a*) that it is a congenital hypertrophy, and (*b*) that in the early days of life spasm of the pylorus occurs with consecutive hypertrophy and stenosis. The association with an early acid dyspepsia is very doubtful. In any case the part played by spasm must be considerable, as the degree of obstruction varies; many patients recover permanently, and the condition of hypertrophy may exist long after the symptoms have disappeared.

Symptoms.—Vomiting of food and wasting are constantly present; the former begins, as a rule, during the second or third week, and in a few instances at birth; it occurs usually two or three times a day, or it may be much more frequent. It is often of the expulsive type; the wasting becomes extreme, there are marked constipation, great weakness, sometimes terminal diarrhœa, or a sudden fatal syncope.

Physical Signs.—These are distinctive—visible peristalsis and palpable tumor. The peristalsis is best seen after feeding, when the waves pass at intervals, in characteristic form, from left to right above the navel; two or three waves may be seen at once. The pyloric tumor may be felt as a firm, hard, freely movable body, which varies in size and consistency, and through which gas may sometimes be felt to gurgle. When in doubt the X-ray examination with bismuth may be made.

Treatment.—Whether this should be medical or surgical is under discussion, but the former appears to have given the best results. The collected statistics of Hutchinson, Heubner, Starck, and Bendix give 85 cases with 80 recoveries (Semon); while the surgical mortality was as high as 50 per cent. it has been greatly reduced. The hospital cases admitted late do badly; of 64 cases at Great Ormond Street Hospital treated medically 78 per cent. died. Careful feeding and lavage are the important measures. The bottle-fed baby may recover with a wet-nurse. Feedings of an ounce an hour with lavage morning and evening, and occasional rectal feeding or saline injections, should be given a trial before operation.

VIII. HÆMORRHAGE FROM THE STOMACH

(*Hæmatemesis*)

Etiology.—*Gastrorrhagia,* as this symptom is called, may result from many conditions, local or general. (*a*) In local disease: (1) cancer; (2) ulcer; (3) disease of the blood-vessels, such as miliary aneurisms and occasionally varicose veins; (4) acute congestion, as in gastritis, and possibly in vicarious hæmorrhage; (5) following operations in the abdomen, particularly when the omentum is wounded, erosions of the gastric mucosa may occur, from which hæmorrhage takes place. Many cases have followed operation for appendicitis. It is a very fatal complication, as it is usually associated with peritonitis (Richardson).

(*b*) Passive congestion due to obstruction in the portal system. This may be either (1) hepatic, as in cirrhosis of the liver, thrombosis of the portal vein, or pressure upon the portal vein by tumor, and secondarily in cases of chronic disease of the heart and lungs. (2) Splenic. Gastrorrhagia is by no means an uncommon symptom in enlarged spleen, and is explained by the intimate relations which exist between the vasa brevia and the splenic circulation.

(*c*) Toxic: (1) The poisons of the specific fevers, small-pox, measles, yellow fever; (2) poisons of unknown origin, as in acute yellow atrophy and in purpura; (3) phosphorus.

(*d*) Traumatism: (1) Mechanical injuries, such as blows and wounds, and occasionally by the stomach-tube; (2) the result of severe corrosive poisons.

(*e*) Certain constitutional diseases: (1) Hæmophilia; (2) profound anæmias, whether idiopathic or due to splenic enlargements or to malaria; (3) cholæmia.

(*f*) In certain nervous affections, particularly hysteria, and occasionally in progressive paralysis of the insane and epilepsy.

(*g*) The blood may not always come primarily from the stomach. Thus it may belong to the nose or the pharynx. In hæmoptysis some of the blood may find its way into the stomach. Again, in bleeding from the œsophagus blood may trickle into the stomach, from which it is ejected. This occurs in the case of rupture of aneurism and of the œsophageal varices. A child may draw blood with the milk from the mother's breast even in considerable quantities and then vomit it.

(*h*) Gastrostaxis.—Under this name Hale White describes cases of hæmorrhage from the stomach in young girls without any lesion of the mucosa. They are often mistaken for ulcer. He has collected 29 cases. Surgeons have taught us that the condition is by no means uncommon. At operation the blood has been seen oozing from points in the mucosa. There may be no pain or any of the ordinary features of ulcer.

(*i*) Miscellaneous causes: Aneurism of the aorta or of its branches may rupture into the stomach. There are instances in which a patient has vomited blood once without ever having a recurrence or without developing symptoms pointing to disease of the stomach.

In new-born infants hæmatemesis may occur alone or in connection with bleeding from other mucous membranes.

In medical practice, hæmorrhage from the stomach occurs most frequently in connection with cirrhosis of the liver and ulcer of the stomach.

Morbid Anatomy.—When death has occurred from the hæmatemesis there are signs of intense anæmia. The lesion is evident in cancer and in ulcer of the stomach. It is to be borne in mind that fatal hæmorrhage may come from a small miliary aneurism communicating with the surface by a pinhole perforation, or the bleeding may be due to the rupture of a submucous vein and the erosion in the mucosa may be small and readily overlooked. It may require a careful and prolonged search to avoid overlooking such lesions. In the large group associated with portal obstruction, whether due to hepatic or splenic disease, the mucosa is usually pale, smooth, and shows no trace of any lesion. In cirrhosis, fatal by hæmorrhage, one may sometimes search in vain for any focal lesion to account for the gastrorrhagia, and we must conclude that it is possible for even the most profuse bleeding to occur by diapedesis. The stomach may be distended with blood and yet the source of the hæmorrhage be not apparent either in the stomach or in the portal system. In such cases the œsophagus should be examined, as the bleeding may come from that source. In toxic cases there are invariably hæmorrhages in the mucous membrane itself.

Symptoms.—In rare instances fatal syncope may occur without any vomiting. In a case of the kind, in which the woman had fallen over and died in a few minutes, the stomach contained between three and four pounds of blood. The sudden profuse bleedings rapidly lead to profound anæmia. When due to ulcer or cirrhosis the bleeding usually recurs for several days. Fatal hæmorrhage from the stomach is met with in ulcer, cirrhosis, enlargement of the spleen, and in instances in which an aneurism ruptures into the stomach or œsophagus. Gastrorrhagia may occur in splenic anæmia or in leukæmia before the condition has aroused attention.

The vomited blood may be fluid or clotted; it is usually dark in color, but in the basin the outer part rapidly becomes red from the action of the air. The longer blood remains in the stomach the more altered is it when ejected.

The amount of blood lost is very variable, and in the course of a day the patient may bring up three or four pounds, or even more. In a case under the care of George Ross, in the Montreal General Hospital, the patient lost during seven days ten pounds, by weight, of blood. The usual symptoms of anæmia develop rapidly, and there may be slight fever, and subsequently œdema may occur. Syncope, convulsions, and occasionally hemiplegia occur after very profuse hæmorrhage. Blindness may follow, the result either of thrombosis of the retinal arteries or veins, or an acute degeneration of the ganglion cells of the retina.

Diagnosis.—In a majority of instances there is no question as to the origin of the blood. Occasionally it is difficult, particularly if the case has not been seen during the attack. Examination of the vomit readily determines whether blood is present or not. The materials vomited may be stained by wine, the juice of strawberries, raspberries, or cranberries, which give a color very closely resembling that of fresh blood, while iron and bismuth and bile may produce the blackish color of altered blood. In such cases the microscope will show clearly the presence of the shadowy outlines of the red blood-corpuscles, and, if necessary, spectroscopic and chemical tests may be applied.

Deception is sometimes practiced by hysterical patients, who swallow and then vomit blood or colored liquids. With a little care such cases can usually be detected. The cases must be excluded in which the blood passes from the nose or pharynx, or in which infants swallow it with the milk.

There is not often difficulty in distinguishing between hæmoptysis and hæmatemesis, though the coughing and the vomiting are not infrequently combined. The following are points to be borne in mind in the diagnosis:

HÆMATEMESIS	HÆMOPTYSIS
1. Previous history points to gastric, hepatic, or splenic disease.	1. Cough or signs of some pulmonary or cardiac disease precedes, in many cases, the hæmorrhage.

2. The blood is brought up by vomiting, prior to which the patient may experience a feeling of giddiness or faintness.	2. The blood is coughed up, and is usually preceded by a sensation of tickling in the throat. If vomiting occurs, it follows the coughing.
3. The blood is usually clotted, mixed with particles of food, and has an acid reaction. It may be dark, grumous, and fluid.	3. The blood is frothy, bright red in color, alkaline in reaction. If clotted, rarely in such large coagula, and muco-pus may be mixed with it.
4. Subsequent to the attack the patient passes tarry stools, and signs of disease of the abdominal viscera may be detected.	4. The cough persists, physical signs of local disease in the chest may usually be detected, and the sputum may be blood-stained for many days.

Prognosis.—Except in the case of rupture of an aneurism or of large veins, hæmatemesis rarely proves fatal. In my experience death has followed more frequently in cases of cirrhosis and splenic enlargement than in ulcer or cancer. In ulcer it is to be remembered that in the chronic hæmorrhagic form the bleeding may recur for years. The treatment of hæmatemesis is considered under gastric ulcer.

IX. NEUROSES OF THE STOMACH

(*Nervous Dyspepsia*)

Serious functional disturbances of the stomach may occur without any discoverable anatomical basis. The cases are met with most frequently in those who have either inherited a nervous constitution or who have gradually, through indiscretions, brought about a condition of nervous prostration. Not infrequently, however, the gastric symptoms stand so far in the foreground that the general neuropathic character of the patient quite escapes notice. Sometimes the gastric manifestations have apparently a reflex origin depending on organic disturbances in other parts, such as the appendix or gall-bladder.

The nervous derangements of the stomach may be divided into motor, secretory, and sensory neuroses. These disturbances rarely occur singly; they are usually met with in combined forms. The clinical picture resulting from such a complex of gastric neuroses is known as *nervous dyspepsia*. As Leube has pointed out, the sensory disturbances usually play the more important part.

The sufferer from nervous dyspepsia presents a varying picture. All grades occur, from the emaciated skeleton-like patient with anorexia nervosa to the well-nourished, healthy-looking, fresh-complexioned individual whose only complaint is distress and uneasiness after eating.

Motor Neuroses.—(*a*) Hyperkinesis or Supermotility.—An increase in the normal motor activity of the stomach results in too early a discharge of the ingesta into the intestine. It is more commonly a secondary neurosis dependent upon superacidity or supersecretion of the gastric juice; but it may occur primarily, possibly from reflex causes. The diagnosis is to be reached only by means of the stomach-tube. It gives rise to no characteristic clinical symptoms.

(*b*) Peristaltic Unrest.—This condition, as described by Kussmaul, is an extremely common and distressing symptom. Shortly after eating the peristaltic movements of the stomach are increased, and borborygmi and gurgling may be heard, even at a distance. The subjective sensations are most annoying, and it would appear as if in the hyperæsthetic condition of the nervous system the patient felt normal peristalsis, just as in these states the usual beating of the heart may be perceptible to him. A further analogy is afforded by the fact that emotion increases this peristalsis. It may extend to the intestines, particularly to the duodenum, and on palpation over this region the gurgling is most marked. The movement may be anti-peristalsis, in which the wave passes from right to left, a condition which may also extend to the intestines. There are cases on record in which colored enemata or even scybala have been discharged from the mouth.

(*c*) Nervous Eructations.—*Aerophagia.*—In this condition severe attacks of noisy eructations, following one another often in rapid succession, occur. When violent they last for hours or days. At other times they occur in paroxysms, depending often upon mental excitement. They are more commonly observed in hysterical women and neurasthenics, but also, not infrequently, in children. The hysterical nature of the affection is sometimes testified to by the occurrence, especially in children, of several instances in one household. The expelled gas in these cases is atmospheric air, which is swallowed or aspirated from without. Sometimes the whole process may be clearly observed, but in other instances the act of swallowing may be almost or quite imperceptible.

(*d*) Nervous Vomiting.—A condition which is not associated with anatomical changes in the stomach or with any state of the contents, but is due to nervous influences acting either directly or indirectly upon the centres presiding over the act of vomiting. The patients are, as a rule, women—usually brunettes—and the subject of more or less marked hysterical manifestations. A special feature of this form is the absence of the preliminary nausea and of the straining efforts of the ordinary act of vomiting. It is rather a regurgitation, and without visible effort and without gagging the mouth is filled with the contents of the stomach, which are then spat out. It comes on, as a rule, after eating, but may occur at irregular intervals. In some cases the nutrition is not impaired, a feature which may give a clew to the true nature of the disease, as there may be no other hysterical manifestation present. As noted by Tuckwell, it may occur in children, and Edsall suggests that this recurring vomiting is an acid intoxication, as in some cases acetone and diacetic acid have been found in the urine. Treatment with full doses of bicarbonate of soda every two hours has been found to relieve it. Nervous vomiting may be a very serious condition. We have had at least two fatal cases. In some instances, after persisting for weeks or months at home, the patient gets well in a few days in hospital. In other instances the course is protracted, and the cases are among the most trying we are called upon to treat.

A type of vomiting is that associated with certain diseases of the nervous system—particularly locomotor ataxia—forming part of the gastric crises. Leyden has reported cases of primary periodic vomiting, which he regards as a neurosis.

(*e*) Rumination; Merycismus.—In this remarkable and rare condition the patients regurgitate and chew the cud like ruminants. It occurs in neurasthenic or hysterical persons, epileptics, and idiots. In some patients it is hereditary. There is an instance in which a governess taught it to two children. The habit may persist for years, and does not necessarily impair the health.

(*f*) Spasm of the Cardia.—Spasmodic, usually painful, contraction of the circular muscle fibres at the cardiac orifice may follow the introduction of a sound, hasty eating, or the taking of too hot or too cold food. It may occur in tetanus and also in hysterical and neurasthenic individuals, especially in air swallowers, in whom, if it be combined with pyloric spasm, it may result in painful gastric distention—"pneumatosis." Here the spasm may be of considerable duration. The condition is rare and practically not of much moment.

(*g*) Pyloric Spasm.—This is usually a secondary occurrence, following superacidity, supersecretion, ulcer, or the introduction into the stomach of irritating substances. The spasm often causes pain in the region of the pylorus and increased gastric peristalsis. In cases where the spasm is combined with superacidity and supersecretion marked dilatation with atony may follow. Sometimes the pylorus may be felt as an oval, hard tumor, which relaxes under the fingers as gas passes through it. It is not easy to distinguish organic stricture and pylorospasm, but Einhorn's duodenal bucket will pass the latter, and the thread next it is bile-stained.

(*h*) Atony of the Stomach.—Motor insufficiency of the stomach is generally due to injudicious feeding, to organic disease of the stomach itself, or to general wasting processes. In some otherwise normal individuals of neurotic temperaments an atony may, however, occur which possibly deserves to be classed among the neuroses. The symptoms are usually those of a moderate dilatation, and are often associated with marked sensory disturbances—feelings of weight and pressure, distention, eructations, and so forth.

Great care must be taken in the diagnosis to rule out all other possible causes.

(*i*) Insufficiency or Incontinence of the Pylorus.—This condition was described first by de Séré and later by Ebstein. It may be recognized by the rapid passing of gas from the stomach into the bowel on attempts at inflation of the former, as well as by the presence of bile and intestinal contents in the stomach. There are no distinctive clinical symptoms.

(*j*) Insufficiency of the Cardia.—This condition is only recognized by the occurrence of eructations or in rumination.

Secretory Neuroses.—(*a*) Hyperacidity; Superacidity; Hyperchlorhydria.—In nervous dyspepsia with hyperacidity of the gastric juices the symptoms depend upon the secretion of an abnormally acid gastric juice at the time of digestion. This is a common form of dyspepsia in young and neurotic individuals, and in chlorotic girls. The symptoms are very variable. They do not, as a rule, immediately follow the ingestion of food, but occur one to three hours later, at the height of digestion. There is a sense of weight and pressure, sometimes of burning in the epigastrium, commonly associated with acid eructations. If vomiting occurs, the pain is relieved. The patient is usually relatively well nourished, and the appetite is often good, though the sufferer may be afraid to eat on account of the anticipated pain. Its association with ulcer has been referred to. There is commonly constipation.

(*b*) SUPERSECRETION, INTERMITTENT AND CONTINUOUS.—This is a form of dyspepsia which has been long recognized, but specially studied by Reichmann and others. The increased flow of the gastric juice may be intermittent or continuous. The secretion under such circumstances is usually superacid, though this is not always the case. The periodical form—the *gastroxynsis* of Rossbach—may be quite independent of the time of digestion. Great quantities of highly acid gastric juice may be secreted in a very small space of time. Such cases are rare, and are especially associated either with profound neurasthenia or with locomotor ataxia. The attack may last for several days. It usually sets in with a gnawing, unpleasant sensation in the stomach, severe headache, and shortly after the patient vomits a clear, watery secretion of such acidity that the throat is irritated and made raw and sore. As mentioned, the attacks may be quite independent of food. *Continuous supersecretion* is more common. The constant presence of fluid in the stomach, together with the pyloric spasm, which commonly results from the irritation of the overacid gastric juice, are followed by a more or less extensive dilatation. Digestion of the starches is retarded, and there are eructations of acid fluid and gastric distress. This secretion of highly acid gastric juice may continue when the stomach is free from food. In these cases pain, burning acid eructations, and even vomiting, occurring during the night and early in the morning, are rather characteristic.

(*c*) NERVOUS SUBACIDITY OR ANACIDITY; ACHYLIA GASTRICA NERVOSA.—Lack of the normal amount of acid is found in chronic catarrh, and particularly in cancer. As Leube has shown, a reduction in the normal amount of acid may exist with the most pronounced symptoms of nervous dyspepsia and yet the stomach will be free from food within the regular time. A condition in which free acid is absent in the gastric juice may occur in cancer, in extreme sclerosis of the mucous membrane, as a nervous manifestation, and occasionally in tabes. In most of these cases, though there be no free acid, yet the other digestive ferments—pepsin and the curdling ferments—or their zymogens are to be demonstrated in the gastric juice. There may, however, be a complete absence of the gastric secretion. To these cases Einhorn has given the name of *achylia gastrica*. This condition was at first thought to occur only in cases of total atrophy of the gastric mucosa, but recent observations have shown that it may occur as a neurosis. In a case of Einhorn's the gastric secretions returned after five years of total *achylia gastrica*.

The symptoms of subacidity, or even of *achylia gastrica*, vary greatly in intensity; they may be almost or quite absent in cases of advanced atrophy of the mucosa, and, as a rule, are not marked so long as the motor activity of the stomach remains good. If atony, however, occurs and abnormal fermentative processes arise, severe gastric and intestinal symptoms may follow. In the cases associated with hysteria and neurasthenia, even though the food may be well taken care of by the intestines, there are very commonly grave sensory disturbances in the region of the stomach, in addition to the general nervous symptoms.

Sensory Neuroses.—(*a*) HYPERÆSTHESIA.—In this condition the patients complain of fullness, pressure, weight, burning, and so forth, during digestion, just such symptoms as accompany a variety of organic diseases of the stomach, and yet in all other respects the gastric functions appear quite normal. Sometimes these distressing sensations are present even when the stomach is empty. These symptoms are usually associated with other manifestations of hysteria and neurasthenia. The pain often follows particular articles of food. An hysterical patient may apparently suffer excruciating pain after taking the smallest amount of food of any sort, while anything prescribed as a medicine may be well borne. In severe cases the patient may be reduced to an extreme degree by starvation.

(*b*) GASTRALGIA; GASTRODYNIA.—Severe pains in the epigastrium, paroxysmal in character, occur (1) as a manifestation of a functional neurosis, independent of organic disease, and usually associated with other nervous symptoms (it is this form which will here be described); (2) in chronic disease of the nervous system, forming the so-called gastric crises; and (3) in organic disease of the stomach, such as ulcer or cancer.

The functional neurosis occurs chiefly in women, very commonly in connection with disturbed menstrual function or with pronounced nervous symptoms. The affection may set in as early as puberty, but it is more common at the menopause. Anæmic, constipated women who have worries and anxieties at home are most prone to the affection. It is more frequent in brunettes than in blondes. Attacks of it sometimes occur in robust, healthy men. More often it is only one feature in a condition of general neurasthenia or a manifestation of that form of nervous dyspepsia in which the gastric juice or hydrochloric acid is secreted in excess. I am very skeptical as to the existence of a gastralgia of purely malarial origin.

The *symptoms* are very characteristic; the patient is suddenly seized with severe pains in the epigastrium, which pass toward the back and around the lower ribs. The attack is usually independent of the taking of food, and may recur at definite intervals, a periodicity which has given rise to the supposition in some cases that the affection is due to malaria. The most marked periodicity, however, may be in the gastralgic attacks of ulcer. They frequently come on at night. Vomiting is rare; more commonly the taking of food relieves the pain. To this, however, there are striking exceptions. Pressure upon the epigastrium commonly gives relief, but deep pressure may be painful. It seems scarcely necessary to separate the forms, as some have done, into irritative and depressive, as the cases insensibly merge into each other. Stress has been laid upon the occurrence of painful points, but they are so common in neurasthenia that very little importance can be attributed to them.

The *diagnosis* offers many difficulties. Organic disease either of the stomach or of the nervous system, particularly the gastric crises of locomotor ataxia, must be excluded. In the case of ulcer or cancer this is not always easy. The fact that the pain is most marked when the stomach is empty and is relieved by the taking of food is sometimes regarded as pathognomonic of simple gastralgia, but to this there are many exceptions, and in ulcer the pains may be relieved on eating. The prolonged intervals between the attacks and their independence of diet are important features in simple gastralgia; but in many instances it is less the local than the general symptoms of the case which enable us to make the diagnosis. In gall-stone colic jaundice is frequently absent, and in any long-standing case of gastralgia, in which the attacks recur at intervals for years, the question of cholelithiasis should be considered. There may be hyperacidity associated with gastric atony. Such a case may be treated for months as one of nervous dyspepsia until a more severe attack than usual is followed by jaundice.

(*c*) Anomalies of the Sense of Hunger and Repletion; Bulimia.—Abnormally excessive hunger coming on often in paroxysmal attacks, which cause the patient to commit extraordinary excesses in eating. This condition may occur in diabetes mellitus and sometimes in gastric disorders, particularly those associated with supersecretion. It is, however, more commonly seen in hysteria and in psychoses. It may occur in cerebral tumors, in Graves' disease, and in epilepsy.

The attacks often begin suddenly at night, the patient waking with a feeling of faintness and pain, and an uncontrollable desire for food. Sometimes such attacks occur immediately after a large meal. The attack may be relieved by a small amount of food, while at other times enormous quantities may be taken. In obstinate cases gastritis, atony, and dilatation frequently result from the abuse of the stomach.

Akoria.—An absence of the sense of satiety. This condition is commonly associated with bulimia and polyphagia, but not always. The patient always feels "empty." There are usually other well-marked manifestations of hysteria or neurasthenia.

Anorexia Nervosa.—This condition, which is a manifestation of a neurotic temperament, is discussed subsequently under the general heading of Hysteria.

Treatment of Neuroses of the Stomach.—The most important part of the treatment of nervous dyspepsia is often that directed toward the improvement of the general physical and mental condition of the patient. The possibility that the symptoms may be of reflex origin should be borne in mind. The possibility of eye-strain, cholelithiasis, or chronic appendicitis should be considered. A large proportion of cases of nervous dyspepsia are dependent upon mental and physical exhaustion or worry, and a vacation or a change of scene will often accomplish what years of treatment at home have failed to do. The manner of life of the patient should be investigated and a proper amount of physical exercise in the open air and systematic hydrotherapy insisted upon. This alone will in some cases be sufficient to cause the disappearance of the symptoms.

Many cases of nervous dyspepsia with marked neurasthenic or hysterical symptoms do well on the Weir Mitchell treatment, and in obstinate forms it should be given a thorough trial. The most striking results are perhaps seen in the case of anorexia nervosa, which will be referred to subsequently. It is also of value in nervous vomiting.

In *cardiac spasm* care should be taken to eat slowly, to avoid swallowing too large morsels or irritating substances. The methodical introduction of thick sounds may be of value.

The treatment in *atony* of the stomach should be similar to that adopted in moderate dilatation—the administration of small quantities of food at frequent intervals; the limitation of the fluids, which should also be taken in small amounts at a time; lavage. Strychnine in full doses may be of value.

In the distressing cases of *hyperacidity,* in addition to the treatment of the general neurotic condition, alkalies must be employed either in the form of magnesia or bicarbonate of soda. These should be given in large doses and at the *height of digestion.* The burning acid eructations may be relieved in this way. In hyperacidity and hypersecretion the use of atropine frequently gives relief. It should be given before food and in small doses at first, beginning with 1/150 grain (0.0004 gm.) and gradually increasing. The combination of bromide and codeia is sometimes useful. The diet should be mainly albuminous, and should be administered in a non-irritating form. Stimulating condiments and alcohol should be avoided. Starches should be sparingly allowed, and only in most digestible forms. Fats are fairly well borne.

Limiting the patient to a strictly meat diet is a valuable procedure in many cases of dyspepsia associated with hyperacidity. The meat should be taken either raw or, if an insuperable objection exists to this, very slightly cooked. It is best given finely minced or grated on stale bread. An ample dietary is 3¼ ounces (100 grams) of meat, two medium slices of stale bread, and an ounce (30 grams) of butter. This may be taken three times a day with a glass of Apollinaris water, soda water, or, what is just as satisfactory, spring water. The fluid should not be taken too cold. The use of fats, as cream, butter, and olive oil, is often of value. Special care should be taken in the examination of the meat to guard against tape-worm infection, but suitable instructions on this point can be given. This is sufficient for an adult man, and many obstinate cases yield satisfactorily to a month or six weeks of this treatment, after which time the less readily digested articles of food may be gradually added to the dietary.

In *supersecretion* the use of the stomach-tube is of the greatest value. In the periodical form it should be used as soon as the attack begins. The stomach may be washed with alkaline solutions or solutions of nitrate of silver, 1 to 1,000, may be used. Where this is impracticable the taking of albuminous food may give relief. One of my patients used to have by his bedside two hard-boiled eggs, by the eating of which nocturnal attacks were alleviated. Alkalies in large doses are also indicated.

In cases of *continued supersecretion* there are usually atony and dilatation. The diet here should be much as in superacidity, but should be administered in smaller quantities at frequent intervals. Lavage with alkaline solutions or with nitrate of silver is of great value. To relieve pain large quantities of bicarbonate of soda or magnesia should be given at the height of digestion.

In *subacidity* a carefully regulated, easily digestible mixed diet, not too rich in albuminoids, is advisable. Bitter tonics before meals are sometimes of value. In *achylia gastrica* the use of predigested foods and of hydrochloric acid in full doses may be of assistance.

In marked *hyperæsthesia,* beside the treatment of the general condition, nitrate of silver in doses of gr. ¼-½ (0.016 to 0.032 gm.), taken in three or four ounces of water on an empty stomach, is advised by Rosenheim. In some instances rectal feeding may have to be resorted to.

For pain large doses of alkalies should be given, of which the light magnesia and bicarbonate of soda are the best. A teaspoonful of either or of a mixture of equal parts may be given after food and when required. A combination of potassium bromide (gr. xv, 1 gm.) with codeia (gr. 1/3, 0.02 gm.) is sometimes useful. Opium is rarely necessary, but, if used, should be given by mouth.

Chloroform in small doses or Hoffman's anodyne will sometimes allay the severe pains. The general condition should receive careful attention, and in many cases the attacks recur until the health is restored by change of air with the prolonged use of arsenic. If there is anæmia iron may be given freely. Nitrate of silver in doses of gr. ¼ to ½ in a large claret-glass of water taken on an empty stomach is useful in some cases.

There are forms of nervous dyspepsia occurring in women who are often well nourished and with a good color, yet who suffer—particularly at night—with flatulency and abdominal distress. The sleep may be quiet and undisturbed for two or three hours, after which they are aroused with painful sensations in the abdomen and eructations. The appetite and digestion may appear to be normal. Constipation is, however, usually present. In many of these patients the condition seems rather intestinal dyspepsia, and the distress is due to the accumulation of gases, the result of excessive putrefaction. The fats, starches, and sugars should be restricted. A diastase ferment is sometimes useful. The flatulency may be treated by the methods above mentioned. Naphthalin, salicylate of bismuth, and salol have been recommended. Some of these cases obtain relief from thorough irrigation of the colon at bedtime.

In all forms of gastric neurosis special care should be taken to prevent constipation.

G. DISEASES OF THE INTESTINES

I. DISEASES OF THE INTESTINES ASSOCIATED WITH DIARRHŒA

CATARRHAL ENTERITIS; DIARRHŒA

In the classification of catarrhal enteritis the anatomical divisions of the bowel have been too closely followed, and a duodenitis, jejunitis, ileitis, typhlitis, colitis, and proctitis have been recognized; whereas in a majority of cases the entire intestinal tract, to a greater or lesser extent, is involved, sometimes the small most intensely, sometimes the large bowel; but during life it may be quite impossible to say which portion is specially affected.

Etiology.—The causes may be either *primary* or *secondary*. Among the causes of *primary* catarrhal enteritis are: (*a*) Improper food, one of the most frequent, especially in children, in whom it follows overeating, or the ingestion of unripe fruit. In some individuals special articles of diet will always produce a slight diarrhœa, which may not be due to a catarrh of the mucosa, but to increased peristalsis induced by the offending material. (*b*) Various toxic substances. Many of the organic poisons, such as those produced in the decomposition of milk and articles of food, excite the most intense intestinal catarrh. Certain inorganic substances, as arsenic and mercury, act in the same way. (*c*) Changes in the weather. A fall in the temperature of from twenty to thirty degrees, particularly in the spring or autumn, may induce—how, it is difficult to say—an acute diarrhœa. We speak of this as a catarrhal process, the result of cold or of chill. On the other hand, the diarrhœal diseases of children are associated in a very special way with the excessive heat of summer months. (*d*) Changes in the constitution of the intestinal secretions. We know too little about the *succus entericus* to be able to speak of influences induced by change in its quantity or quality. It has long been held that an increase in the amount of bile poured into the bowel might excite a diarrhœa; hence the term bilious diarrhœa, so frequently used by the older writers. Possibly there are conditions in which an excessive amount of bile is poured into the intestine, increasing the peristalsis, and hurrying on the contents; but the opposite state, a scanty secretion, by favoring the natural fermentative processes, much more commonly causes an intestinal catarrh. Absence of the pancreatic secretion from the intestine has been associated in certain cases with a fatty diarrhœa. (*e*) Nervous influences. It is by no means clear how mental states act upon the bowels, and yet it is an old and trustworthy observation, which every-day experience confirms, that the mental state may profoundly affect the intestinal canal. These influences should not properly be considered under catarrhal processes, as they result simply from increased peristalsis or increased secretion, and are usually described under the heading *nervous diarrhœa*. In children it frequently follows fright. It is common, too, in adults as a result of emotional disturbances. Canstatt mentions a surgeon who always, before an important operation, had watery diarrhœa. In hysterical women it is seen as an occasional occurrence, due to transient excitement, or as a chronic, protracted diarrhœa, which may last for months or even years.

Among the *secondary* causes of intestinal catarrh may be mentioned: (*a*) Infectious diseases. Dysentery, cholera, typhoid fever, pyæmia, septicæmia, tuberculosis, and pneumonia are occasionally associated with intestinal catarrh. In dysentery and typhoid fever the ulceration is in part responsible for the catarrhal condition, but in cholera it is probably a direct influence of the bacilli or of the toxic materials produced by them. (*b*) The extension of inflammatory processes from adjacent parts. Thus, in peritonitis, catarrhal swelling and increased secretion are always present in the mucosa. In cases of invagination, hernia, tuberculosis, or cancerous ulceration catarrhal processes are common. (*c*) Circulatory disturbances cause a catarrhal enteritis, usually of a very chronic character. This is common in diseases of the liver, such as cirrhosis, and in chronic affections of the heart and lungs—all conditions, in fact, which produce engorgement of the terminal branches of the portal vessels. (*d*) In the cachectic conditions met with in cancer, profound anæmia, Addison's disease, and Bright's disease intestinal catarrh may occur as a terminal event.

Morbid Anatomy.—It is rare to see the mucous membrane injected; more commonly it is pale and covered with mucus. In the upper part of the small intestine the tips of the valvulæ conniventes may be deeply injected. Even in extreme grades of portal obstruction intense hyperæmia is not often seen. The entire mucosa may be softened and infiltrated, the lining epithelium swollen, or even shed, and appearing as large flakes among the intestinal contents. This is, no doubt, a post mortem change. The lymph follicles are almost always swollen, particularly in children. The Peyer's patches may be prominent and the solitary follicles in the large and small bowel may stand out with distinctness and present in the centres little erosions, the so-called follicular ulcers. This may be a striking feature in the intestine in all forms of catarrhal enteritis in children, quite irrespective of the intensity of the diarrhœa.

When the process is more chronic the mucosa is firmer, in some instances thickened, in others distinctly thinned, and the villi and follicles present a slaty pigmentation.

Symptoms.—Acute and chronic forms may be recognized. The important symptom of both is diarrhœa, which, in the majority of instances, is the sole indication of this condition. It is not to be supposed that diarrhœa is invariably caused by, or associated with, catarrhal enteritis, as it may be produced by nervous and other influences. It is probable that catarrh of the jejunum may exist without any diarrhœa; indeed, it is a very common circumstance to find post mortem a catarrhal state of the small bowel in persons who have not had diarrhœa during life. The stools vary extremely in character. The color depends upon the amount of bile with which they are mixed, and they may be of a dark or blackish brown, or of a light yellow, or even of a grayish-white tint. The consistence is usually very thin and watery, but in some instances the stools are pultaceous like thin gruel. Portions of undigested food can often be seen (lienteric diarrhœa), and flakes of yellowish-brown mucus. Microscopically there are innumerable micro-organisms, epithelium and mucous cells, crystals of phosphate of lime, oxalate of lime, and occasionally cholesterin and Charcot's crystals.

Pain in the abdomen is usually present in the acute catarrhal enteritis, particularly when due to food. It is of a colicky character, and when the colon is involved there may be tenesmus. More or less tympanites exists, and there are gurgling noises or borborygmi, due to the rapid passage of fluid and gas from one part to another. In the very acute attacks there may be vomiting. Fever is not, as a rule, present, but there may be a slight elevation of one or two degrees. The appetite is lost, there is intense thirst, and the tongue is dry and coated. In very acute cases, when the quantity of fluid lost is great and the pain excessive, there may be collapse symptoms. The number of evacuations varies from four or five to twenty or more in the course of the day. The attack lasts for two or three days, or may be prolonged for a week or ten days.

Chronic catarrh of the bowels may follow the acute form, or may come on gradually as an independent affection or as a sequence of obstruction in the portal circulation. It is characterized by diarrhœa, with or without colic. The dejections vary; when the small bowel is chiefly involved the diarrhœa is of a lienteric character, and when the colon is affected the stools are thin and mixed with much mucus. A special form of mucous diarrhœa will be subsequently described. The general nutrition in these chronic cases is greatly disturbed; there may be much loss of flesh and great pallor. The patients are inclined to suffer from low spirits, or hypochondriasis may develop.

Diagnosis.—It is important, in the first place, to determine, if possible, whether the large or small bowel is chiefly affected. In catarrh of the small bowel the diarrhœa is less marked, the pains are of a colicky character, borborygmi are not so frequent, the fæces usually contain portions of food, and are more yellowish-green or grayish-yellow and flocculent and do not contain much mucus. When the large intestine is at fault there may be no pain whatever, as in the catarrh of the large intestine associated with tuberculosis and Bright's disease. When present, the pains are most intense, and, if the lower portion of the bowel is involved, there may be marked tenesmus. The stools have a uniform soupy consistence; they are grayish in color and granular throughout, with here and there flakes of mucus, or they may contain very large quantities of mucus.

There are no positive symptoms by which the diagnosis of duodenitis can be made. It is usually associated with acute gastritis and, if the process extends into the bile-duct, with jaundice. Neither jejunitis nor ileitis can be separated from general intestinal catarrh.

The Cœliac Affection.—Under this heading Gee has described an intestinal disorder, most commonly met with in children between the ages of one and five, characterized by the occurrence of pale, loose stools, not unlike gruel or oatmeal porridge. They are bulky, not watery, yeasty, frothy, and extremely offensive. The affection has received various names, such as *diarrhœa alba* or *diarrhœa chylosa*. It is not associated with tuberculosis or other hereditary disease. It begins insidiously and there are progressive wasting, weakness, and pallor. The belly becomes doughy and inelastic. There is often flatulency. Fever is usually absent. The disease is lingering and a fatal termination is common. So far nothing is known of the pathology of the disease. Ulceration of the intestines has been met with, but it is not constant.

Sprue or Psilosis.—A remarkable disease of the tropics, characterized by "a peculiar, inflamed, superficially ulcerated, exceedingly sensitive condition of the mucous membrane of the tongue and mouth; great wasting and anæmia; pale, copious, and often loose, frequent, and frothy fermenting stools; very generally by more or less diarrhœa; and also by a marked tendency to relapse" (Manson). It is very prevalent in India, China, and Java. Nothing definite is known as to its cause.

When fully established the chief symptoms are a disturbed condition of the bowels, pale, yeasty-looking stools, a raw, bare, sore condition of the tongue, mouth, and gullet, sometimes with actual superficial ulceration. With these gastro-intestinal symptoms there are associated anæmia and general wasting. It is very chronic with numerous relapses. There are no characteristic anatomical changes. There are usually ulcers in the colon, and the French think it is a form of dysentery.

Manson recommends rest and a milk diet as curative in a large proportion of the cases. The monograph by Thin and the article by Manson in Allbutt and Rolleston's System give very full descriptions of the disease.

DIPHTHEROID OR CROUPOUS ENTERITIS

A croupous or diphtheroid inflammation of the mucosa of the small and large intestines occurs (*a*) most frequently as a secondary process in the infectious diseases—pneumonia, pyæmia in its various forms, and typhoid fever; (*b*) as a terminal process in many chronic affections, such as Bright's disease, cirrhosis of the liver, or cancer; and (*c*) as an effect of certain poisons —mercury, lead, and arsenic.

There are three different anatomical pictures. In one group of cases the mucosa presents on the top of the folds a thin grayish-yellow diphtheroid exudate situated upon a deeply congested base. In some cases all grades may be seen between the thinnest film of superficial necrosis and involvement of the entire thickness of the mucosa. In the colon similar transversely arranged areas of necrosis are seen situated upon hyperæmic patches, and it may be here much more extensive and involve a large portion of the membrane. There may be most extensive inflammation without any involvement of the solitary follicles of the large or small bowel.

In a second group of cases the membrane has rather a croupous character. It is grayish-white in color, more flake-like and extensive, limited, perhaps, to the cæcum or to a portion of the colon; thus, in several cases of pneumonia I found this flaky adherent false membrane, in one instance forming patches 1 to 2 cm. in diameter, which in form were not unlike rupia crusts.

In a third group the affection is really a follicular enteritis, involving the solitary glands, which are swollen and capped with an area of diphtheroid necrosis or are in a state of suppuration. Follicular ulcers are common in this form. The disease may run its course without any symptoms, and the condition is unexpectedly met with post mortem. In other instances there are diarrhœa, pain, but not often tenesmus or the passage of blood-stained mucus. In the toxic cases the intestinal symptoms may be very marked, but in the terminal colitis of the fevers and of constitutional affections the symptoms are often trifling.

The ulcerative colitis of chronic disease may be only a terminal event in these diphtheroid processes.

PHLEGMONOUS ENTERITIS

As an independent affection this is excessively rare, even less frequent than its counterpart in the stomach. It is seen occasionally in connection with intussusception, strangulated hernia, and chronic obstruction. Apart from these conditions it occurs most frequently in the duodenum, and leads to suppuration in the submucosa and abscess formation. Except when associated with hernia or intussusception the affection can not be diagnosed. The symptoms usually resemble those of peritonitis.

ULCERATIVE ENTERITIS

In addition to the specific ulcers of tuberculosis, syphilis, and typhoid fever, the following forms of ulceration occur in the bowels:

Follicular Ulceration.—As previously mentioned, this is met with very commonly in the diarrhœal diseases of children, and also in the secondary or terminal inflammations in many fevers and constitutional disorders. The ulcers are small, punched-out, with sharply cut edges, and they are usually limited to the follicles. With this form may be placed the catarrhal ulcers of some writers.

Stercoral ulcers, which occur in long-standing cases of constipation. Very remarkable indeed are the cases in which the sacculi of the colon become filled with rounded small scybala, some of which produce distinct ulcers in the mucous membrane. The fæcal masses may have lime salts deposited in them, and thus form little enteroliths.

Simple Ulcerative Colitis.—Simple idiopathic or innominate ulcerative colitis has been differentiated from amœbic and bacillary dysentery by Hale White and others. It is a disease of adults, of unknown origin. The sexes are equally affected; of 177 cases collected by Eric Smith, 89 were in males. Some patients have had previous bowel trouble; sometimes there have been intermittent attacks of diarrhœa and constipation. When established, the main features are:

(*a*) Diarrhœa: the motions very frequent in the day, up to 20 or 30, usually small, bile-stained, with mucus and blood, sometimes mixed with the motion or separate. There may be clotted lumps of blood, or the blood is uniformly mixed, and the motions look like anchovy sauce. The pain, while severe, is usually diffuse, abdominal, and colicky, and, not so frequently, in the rectum. Many of the motions pass without pain.

(*b*) Fever, which occurs in the majority of the cases, though severe forms may be free throughout.

(*c*) Wasting, debility, and progressive anæmia.

The disease may run a very acute course, but most frequently it is chronic, lasting from eight weeks to three or four months. Transient improvement may follow, and a relapse. Death is most commonly from exhaustion, occasionally from hæmorrhage, and in a few instances from perforation. Post mortem, the colon is dilated, often without hypertrophied walls; the ulceration, as a rule, limited to it and very extensive, the ulcers ranging in size from a pin's head to large areas, with infiltrated, rarely undermined, edges. The Shiga bacillus is not present; the colon bacilli are found in various forms, but no one organism has apparently any definite relation to the disease.

Ulceration from External Perforation.—This may result from the erosion of new growths or, more commonly, from localized peritonitis with abscess formation and perforation of the bowel. This is met with most frequently in tuberculous peritonitis, but it may occur in the abscess which follows perforation of the appendix or suppurative or gangrenous pancreatitis. Fatal hæmorrhage may result from the perforation.

Cancerous Ulcers.—In very rare instances of multiple cancer or sarcoma the submucous nodules break down and ulcerate. In one case the ileum contained eight or ten sarcomatous ulcers secondary to an extensive sarcoma in the neighborhood of the shoulder-joint.

Solitary Ulcer.—Occasionally a solitary ulcer is met with in the cæcum or colon, which may lead to perforation. Two instances of ulcer of the cæcum, both with perforation, have come under my observation, and in one instance a simple ulcer of the colon perforated and led to fatal peritonitis.

Diagnosis of Intestinal Ulcers.—As a rule, diarrhœa is present in all cases, but exceptionally there may be extensive ulceration, particularly in the small bowel, without diarrhœa. Very limited ulceration in the colon may be associated with frequent stools. The character of the dejections is of great importance. Pus, shreds of tissue, and blood are the most valuable indications. Pus occurs most frequently in connection with ulcers in the large intestine, but when the bowel alone is involved the amount is rarely great, and the passage of any quantity of pure pus is an indication that it has come from without, most commonly from the rupture of a pericæcal abscess, or in women of an abscess of the broad ligament. Pus may also be present in cancer of the bowel, or it may be due to local disease in the rectum. A purulent mucus may be present in the stools in cases of ulcer, but it has not the same diagnostic value. The swollen, sago-like masses of mucus which are believed by some to indicate follicular ulceration are met with also in mucous colitis. Hæmorrhage is an important and valuable symptom of ulcer in the bowel, particularly if profuse. It occurs under so many conditions that taken alone it may not be specially significant, but with other coexisting circumstances it may be the most important indication of all.

Fragments of tissue are occasionally found in the stools in ulcer, particularly in the extensive and rapid sloughing in dysenteric processes. Definite portions of mucosa, shreds of connective tissue, and even bits of the muscular coat may be found. Pain occurs in many cases, either of a diffuse, colicky character, or sometimes, in the ulcer of the colon, very limited and well defined.

Perforation is an accident liable to happen when the ulcer extends deeply. In the small bowel it leads to a localized or general peritonitis. In the large intestine, too, a fatal peritonitis may result, or, if perforation takes place in the posterior wall of the ascending or descending colon, the production of a large abscess cavity in the retro-peritoneum.

Treatment of the Previous Conditions

Acute Dyspeptic Diarrhœa.—All solid food should be withheld. If vomiting is present ice may be given, and small quantities of milk and soda water may be taken. If the attack has followed the eating of large quantities of indigestible material, castor oil or calomel is advisable, but is not necessary if the patient has been freely purged. If the pain is severe, 20 drops (1.3 c. c.) of laudanum and a drachm (4 c. c.) of spirit of chloroform may be given, or, if the colic is very intense, a hypodermic of a quarter of a grain (0.016 gm.) of morphia. It is not well to check the diarrhœa unless it is profuse, as it usually stops spontaneously within forty-eight hours. If persistent, the aromatic chalk powder or large doses of bismuth (30 to 40 grains, 2 gm.) may be given. A small enema of starch (2 ounces, 60 c. c.), with 20 drops (1.3 c. c.) of laudanum, every six hours, is a most valuable remedy.

Chronic diarrhœa, including chronic catarrh and ulcerative enteritis. It is important, in the first place, to ascertain, if possible, the cause and whether ulceration is present or not. So much in treatment depends upon the careful examination of the stools—as to the amount of mucus, the presence of pus, the occurrence of parasites, and, above all, the state of digestion of the food—that the practitioner should pay special attention to them. Many patients simply require rest in bed and a restricted diet. Chronic diarrhœa of many months' or even of several years' duration may be sometimes cured by strict confinement to bed and a diet of boiled milk and albumen water.

In that form in which immediately after eating there is a tendency to loose evacuations it is usually found that some one article of diet is at fault. The patient should rest for an hour or more after meals. Sometimes this alone is sufficient to prevent the occurrence of the diarrhœa. In those forms which depend upon abnormal conditions in the small intestine, either too rapid peristalsis or faulty fermentative processes, bismuth is indicated. It must be given in large doses—from half a drachm to a drachm (2 to 4 gm.) three times a day. The smaller doses are of little use. Naphthalin preparations here do much good, given in doses of from 10 to 15 grains (1 gm.) four or five times a day. Larger doses may be needed. Salol and the salicylate of bismuth may be tried.

An extremely obstinate and intractable form is the diarrhœa of hysterical women. A systematic rest cure will be found most advantageous, and if a milk diet is not well borne the patient may be fed exclusively on egg albumen. The condition seems to be associated in some cases with increased peristalsis, and in such the bromides may do good, or preparations of opium may be necessary. There are instances which prove most obstinate and resist all forms of treatment, and the patient may be greatly reduced. A change of air and surroundings may do more than medicines.

In a large group of the chronic diarrhœas the mischief is seated in the colon and is due to ulceration. Medicines by the mouth are here of little value. The stools should be carefully watched and a diet arranged which shall leave the smallest possible residue. Boiled or peptonized milk may be given, but the stools should be examined to see whether there is an excess of food or of curds. Meat is, as a rule, badly borne in these cases. The diarrhœa is best treated by enemata. The starch and laudanum should be tried, but when ulceration is present it is better to use astringent injections. From 2 to 4 pints of warm water, containing from half a drachm to a drachm (2 to 4 gm.) of nitrate of silver, may be used. In the chronic diarrhœa which follows dysentery this is particularly advantageous. In giving large injections the patient should be in the dorsal position, with the hips elevated, and it is best to allow the injection to flow in gradually from a siphon bag. In this way the entire colon can be irrigated and the patient can retain the injection for some time. The silver injections may be very painful, but they are invaluable in all forms of ulcerative colitis. Acetate of lead, boracic acid, sulphate of copper, sulphate of zinc, and salicylic acid may be used in 1 per cent. solutions. In obstinate cases appendicostomy should be done and the bowel irrigated through the opening.

In the intense forms of choleraic diarrhœa in adults associated with constant vomiting and frequent watery discharges the patient should be given at once a hypodermic of a quarter of a grain of morphia, which should be repeated in an hour if the pains return or the purging persists. This gives prompt relief, and is often the only medicine needed in the attack. The patient should be given stimulants, and, when the vomiting is allayed by suitable remedies, small quantities of milk and lime water.

II. DIARRHŒAL DISEASES IN CHILDREN

Children are particularly susceptible to disorders of the alimentary tract. Although several forms are recognized, they so often merge the one into the other that a sharp differentiation is impossible.

General Etiology.—Certain factors predispose to diarrhœa. AGE.—The largest number of cases occur just after the nursing period; the highest mortality is in the second half of the first year, when this period falls in the hot weather; hence the dread of the "second summer."

DIET.—Diarrhœa is most frequent in artificially fed babies. Of nineteen hundred and forty-three fatal cases collected by Holt, only 3 per cent. were breast-fed. The recent agitation for pure milk in the large cities has decreased materially the number of diarrhœa cases among bottle-fed infants.

Among the poor the bowel complaint comes with artificial feeding, and is due either to milk ill-suited in quantity or poor in quality, or to indigestible articles of diet. Very many of the fatal cases have been fed upon condensed milk.

TEMPERATURE.—The relation of the atmospheric temperature to the prevalence of the disease in children has long been recognized. The mortality curve begins to rise in May, increases in June, reaching the maximum in July, and gradually sinks through August and September. The maximum corresponds closely with the highest mean temperature, yet we can not regard the heat itself as the direct agent, but only as one of several factors. Thus the mean temperature of June is only four or five degrees lower than that of July, and yet the mortality is not more than one-third. Seibert, who has carefully analyzed the mortality and the temperature month by month in New York for ten years, fails to find a constant relation between the degrees of heat and the number of cases of diarrhœa. Neither barometric pressure nor humidity appears to have any influence.

BACTERIOLOGY.—The discovery by Duvall and Bassett, working at the Thomas Wilson Sanitarium, in the dejecta of children suffering from summer diarrhœa, of a bacillus apparently identical with the organism shown by Shiga to be the cause of epidemic dysentery in Japan, has awakened renewed interest in the relation of bacteria to these disorders in children.

The Rockefeller Institute research showed that this organism was present in a large number of cases of so-called "summer diarrhœa." No instances of cholera infantum were studied. The laboratory studies of Martini and Lentz, Flexner, Hiss, Parke, and others indicate that there is a group of closely allied forms of bacilli differing slightly from the original Shiga bacillus in their action on certain sugars and in agglutinating properties.

The type of organisms most frequently associated with the diarrhœas of children belongs to the so-called "acid type," and, unlike the Shiga cultures, ferments mannite with acid production.

The causal connection of this group of bacteria with all the diarrhœal diseases of children has not been proved. In the hands of some workers they have been found in the fæces of a large proportion of all cases examined, and also less frequently in the sporadic diarrhœas occurring throughout the year. These organisms are often found in comparatively small numbers, and are more easily isolated from mucus or blood-stained stools. They occur in the acute primary intestinal infection in children, in subacute infection without previous symptoms coincident with or following other acute diseases such as measles, pneumonia, etc., and in the terminal intestinal infection following malnutrition or marasmus. They have been found in breast-fed infants as well as bottle-babies.

The mode of entrance of the organism has not been determined. Simultaneous outbreaks of many cases in remote parts of a community where there can be no common milk supply, and occurrence of the disease in breast- and condensed-milk-fed babies, indicate that cow's milk is not the only conveyor of the infection, and point to some common cause, possibly to the water, as a means of contamination, although dysentery bacilli have not yet been isolated from city water.

The importance of other organisms must not be overlooked. The observations of Escherich showed the remarkable simplicity of bacterial flora in the intestines of healthy milk-fed children, *Bacterium lactis ærogenes* being present in the upper portion of the bowel and *Bacterium coli commune* in the lower bowel, each almost in pure culture.

When diarrhœa is set up the number and varieties of bacteria are greatly increased, although heretofore no forms had been found to bear a constant or specific relationship to the diarrhœal fæces.

Certain diarrhœas in children are apparently induced by the lactic acid organisms in milk, others by *colon* or *proteus bacilli*, and others, again, by the *pyogenic cocci* and other forms; all these bacteria may be associated with the dysentery bacilli.

There is considerable evidence to support the view that the destructive lesions of the intestines may be produced by the *Streptococcus pyogenes* after an initial infection with a member of the dysentery group.

Morbid Anatomy.—In mild cases there may be only a slight catarrhal swelling of the mucosa of both small and large bowel, with enlargement of the lymph follicles. The mucous membrane may be irregularly congested; often this is most marked at the summit of the folds. The submucosa is usually infiltrated with serum and small round cells. In more severe cases ulceration may take place. The loss of substance begins, usually, in the mucosa, over swollen lymph follicles. About the ulcer there is a more or less distinctly marked inflammatory zone. The destruction of the tissue is limited to the region of the follicles and becomes progressive by the union of several adjoining ulcers. This process is usually confined to the lower bowel, and may be so extensive as to leave only ribbons of intact mucosa. The ulcers never perforate. Rarely there is a croupous or pseudo-membranous enteritis affecting the lower ilium, colon, and rectum. The constant features are the increased secretion of mucus and the lymphoid hyperplasia. The mesenteric glands are enlarged.

The changes in the other organs are neither numerous nor characteristic. Broncho-pneumonia occurs in many cases. The liver is often fatty, the spleen may be swollen. Brain lesions are rare; the membranes and substance are often anæmic, but meningitis or thrombosis is very uncommon.

Clinical Forms.—ACUTE INTESTINAL INDIGESTION.—This form occurs in children of all ages, and is associated with improper food. The symptoms often begin abruptly with nausea and vomiting, or, especially in stronger children, several hours or a day or two after the disturbing diet. The local symptoms are colicky pains, moderate tympanites, and diarrhœa. The stools are four to ten in twenty-four hours; at first fæcal, then fluid, with more or less mucus and particles from undigested material. There is no blood. The usual intestinal bacteria are found. Occasionally, when there is mucus, dysentery bacilli are present. There is always fever. It is rarely very high, and never continues. The pulse may be rapid and the prostration marked in very young or weak children. These symptoms usually subside shortly after the emptying of the bowel.

In weakened infants, or when the treatment has been delayed or the diet remains unchanged, this disturbance may lead to more serious conditions. Attacks of intestinal indigestion tend to recur.

ACUTE DYSPEPSIA, OR FERMENTATIVE DIARRHŒA.—This form is characterized by more severe constitutional symptoms. It may begin after an intestinal indigestion of several days in which the stools are fluid and offensive, and contain undigested food and curds. In other cases the disease sets in abruptly with vomiting, griping pains, and fever, which may rapidly reach 104°-105°F.

Nervous symptoms are usually prominent. The child is irritable and sleeps poorly. Convulsions may usher in the acute symptoms or occur later. An increasing drowsiness, ending in coma, has been noted in many cases. The stools, which vary from four to twenty in twenty-four hours, soon lose their fæcal character and become fluid. Later they consist largely of green or translucent mucus. An occasional fleck of blood is noticed in the mucus, but this is never present in large amounts.

Microscopically, besides the food residue and mucous strands are a moderate number of leucocytes and red blood-corpuscles. Epithelial cells are found with numerous bacteria.

The acute symptoms generally pass away in a few days with judicious treatment. Relapses are frequent, following any indiscretion. The attack may be the beginning of severe ileo-colitis.

These gastro-intestinal intoxications are largely confined to the summer months and form an important group of the summer diarrhœas of children.

CHOLERA INFANTUM.—This term should be reserved for the fulminating form of gastro-intestinal intoxication. The typical cases are rare and form only a very small proportion of the diarrhœal diseases of infants. The disease sets in with vomiting, which is incessant and is excited by an attempt to take food or drink. The stools are profuse and frequent; at first fæcal in character, brown or yellow in color, and finally thin, serous, and watery. The stools first passed are very offensive; subsequently they are odorless. The thin, serous stools are alkaline. There is fever, but the axillary temperature may register three or more degrees below that of the rectum. From the outset there is marked prostration; the eyes are sunken, the features pinched.

the fontanelles depressed, and the skin has a peculiar ashy pallor. At first restless and excited, the child subsequently becomes heavy, dull, and listless. The tongue is coated at the onset, but subsequently becomes red and dry. As in all choleraic conditions, the thirst is insatiable; the pulse is rapid and feeble, and toward the end becomes irregular and imperceptible. Death may occur within twenty-four hours, with symptoms of collapse and great elevation of the internal temperature. Before the end the diarrhœa and vomiting may cease. In other instances the intense symptoms subside, but the child remains torpid and semi-comatose, with fingers clutched, and there may be convulsions. The head may be retracted and the respirations interrupted, irregular, and of the Cheyne-Stokes type. The child may remain in this condition for some days without any signs of improvement. It was to this group of symptoms in infantile diarrhœa that Marshall Hall gave the term "hydrencephaloid," or spurious hydrocephalus. As a rule, no changes in the brain or other organs are found. The condition of sclerema is described as a sequel of cholera infantum. The skin and subcutaneous tissue becomes hard and firm, and the appearance has been compared to that of a half-frozen cadaver.

No constant organism has been found in these cases. Baginsky considers the disease the result of the action on the system of the poisonous products of decomposition encouraged by the various bacteria present—a *Fäulniss* disease. The clinical picture is that produced by an acute bacterial infection, as in Asiatic cholera.

Diagnosis.—The diagnosis is readily made. There is no other intestinal affection in children for which it can be mistaken. The constant vomiting, the frequent watery discharges, the collapse symptoms, and the elevated temperature make an unmistakable clinical picture. The outlook in the majority of cases is bad, particularly in children artificially fed. Hyperpyrexia, extreme collapse, and incessant vomiting are the most serious symptoms.

ILEO-COLITIS (*Entero-colitis, Inflammatory Diarrhœa*).—In this form there is evidence of an inflammatory alteration of the intestinal wall, usually of the lower ileum and large intestine. Several sub-varieties are recognized according to the nature and site of the lesions. Many of the cases are grafted on the simple forms above described. The mucous discharges continue, mingled with food residue and often streaked with blood. Pus cells are numerous under the microscope. The temperature remains elevated or may be remittent. After two or three weeks the symptoms gradually subside, the stools become fewer in number, and the fæcal character returns.

In other instances the severe involvement of the intestines seems evident within a few hours of the onset, with abdominal pain, vomiting, and fever. Blood and pus may be present in nearly every stool. Tenesmus is frequent and prolapsus ani is not uncommon. In severe attacks the prostration is marked, the tongue is dry, the mouth covered with sordes, and death may ensue in a few days from profound sepsis, or, if the acute stage is survived, the patient may continue desperately ill for weeks, gradually recover, or die from asthenia.

Hæmorrhage of large amounts of blood is extremely rare. The appearance of bright red stains on the napkin indicates, usually, ulceration of the lower bowel or rectum. When the blood is dark brown the lesion is in the ileum or near the valve. The extent of the ulceration can not be accurately determined by the quantity of the blood passed.

Membranous-colitis is usually only to be distinguished by the discovery of the membrane in the rectum through a speculum or in prolapsus, or by the passage of a fragment of the membrane in the stools.

Inflammation of the colon often occurs in marantic infants. It may consist of a catarrhal or follicular inflammation of the lower bowel without destructive lesion, and is frequently a terminal infection.

Ileo-colitis may become chronic and persist for months. The signs of active inflammation subside; there is little pain or fever, but more or less mucus remains in the stools. The general condition of the child suffers. There is a continuous loss in weight; the skin is dry and hangs in folds; nervous symptoms are always present. There may be stiffness and contraction of the extremities, with opisthotonos. The progress of the disease is irregular, marked by short periods of improvement. Death is often due to a relapse, to asthenia, or to broncho-pneumonia. In many of these cases, both acute and chronic, the dysentery bacilli have been found in association with other organisms.

Prevention.—Unquestionably, most of the intestinal disorders of children can be prevented. In many of our large cities the mortality from the summer diarrhœas has been greatly reduced by prophylactic measures.

The infant should have abundance of air-space in the home, with plenty of sunlight and fresh air. In hot weather it may be well for him to sleep out of doors, day and night. His clothing must not be too heavy in midsummer; often only a binder and thin dress. This clothing should be altered with every change of the temperature. The greatest cleanliness should surround the life of the baby, and the nursing-bottles and nipples are to be boiled each day and kept scrupulously clean. Breast-feeding is continued whenever possible.

With bottle-babies, in warm weather, the diet should be reduced in strength—i. e., weaker milk mixtures used and more water given. In all crowded communities the milk should be sterilized or pasteurized during the summer months, and all the water given the baby, either with or between the nourishment, boiled. It is better that a child should be in the country during the hot weather, but when this is impossible the various parks in our large cities afford much relief.

Treatment.—Hygienic Management.—Even after the illness has begun, much can be done by hygienic measures to diminish the severity. Change of air to seashore or mountain is often followed by a marked improvement in the child's condition. The patient must not be too warmly clad. The temperature may be lowered and nervous symptoms allayed by hydrotherapy. Baths, warm and cool, are helpful. Colon irrigations serve the double purpose of flushing the bowel and stimulating the nervous system. They should be given cool when there is much fever.

Medicinal.—In all cases of diarrhœa there are more or less congestion of the intestinal mucosa, hypersecretion of mucus, and increased peristalsis due in part to the irritant action of improper food. In certain forms toxic symptoms from the absorption of poisons from the intestinal tract are early noticed. In other instances inflammatory lesions in the wall of the bowel are present. The keynote, then, of the treatment is promptness. Nature's effort to remove the disturbing cause should be assisted, not checked, and care must be taken to introduce food that will afford the least pabulum for the disturbing bacteria.

Castor oil and calomel are to be preferred as purgatives, especially for infants. A drachm (4 c. c.) of the former, repeated, if necessary, will usually sweep the intestinal tract and relieve the irritation. Where there is much nausea or intestinal fermentation, calomel is indicated. It may be given in divided doses at short intervals until one or two grains (0.065 or 0.13 gm.) have been taken, or until the characteristic green stools appear. Very early in the attack, if nausea is a marked symptom, nothing relieves so quickly as gastric lavage with warm water, or a weak soda solution when there is much acidity. In older children a large draught of boiled water may be substituted. In many cases irrigation of the lower bowel with large quantities of salt solution flushes the colon, removing the irritating material, and diminishes the absorption of toxins. It also reduces the temperature and allays nervous symptoms. The irrigating fluid should be cool when there is much fever. The infant is placed in the dorsal position or turned a little to the left, with hips elevated, and the fluid from a fountain syringe, about three feet above the patient, is allowed to flow into the rectum through a large soft rubber catheter. Usually about a pint can be retained before expulsion. If desired, the catheter can be gently pushed into the bowel as it becomes distended with fluid. Two or three quarts should be used at one irrigation, which may be repeated several times in twenty-four hours if it is beneficial.

Where there is ulceration of the lower bowel various astringents, such as alum, witch hazel (one or two teaspoonfuls to one quart), silver nitrate, 1-4,000, or a weak solution of permanganate of potassium, may be used as the irrigating fluid.

When there is much loss of fluid from the body or when toxic symptoms are marked infusion of normal salt solution under the skin may be tried. One to three hundred c. c. of the solution can be readily introduced. This procedure is not so permanently helpful as it was thought to be some years ago. There is rarely any necessity to transfuse.

Of the many drugs vaunted as intestinal astringents and antiseptics, bismuth, either as subgallate or subnitrate, has proven most serviceable. It should not be given until the disturbing material has been removed and the temperature is falling; then it should be administered in large doses, 5 to 10 grains (0.3 to 0.6 gm.) every hour, until there is discoloration of the stools. In some cases this may be hastened by lac sulphur in grain doses. Opium should be very sparingly used, and then only for a specific purpose, to check excessive peristalsis, violent colic, or very numerous passages. It may be given to an infant as Dover's powder, ¼-1 grain (0.016 to 0.065 gm.); or paregoric, 5-10 minims (0.3 to 0.6 c. c.) every four hours; or morphia, hypodermically, 1/200-1/50 grain (0.00032 to 0.0013 gm.), when prompt action is desired. Occasionally it is well to combine it with atropia, 1/1,000-1/250 grain. The bowels should not be locked when the stools are foul or the temperature is high.

In all cases where there is prostration stimulants are indicated. Alcohol, such as brandy or whisky, ½ to 1 ounce in twenty-four hours in frequent doses, diluted six to ten times with water, or, where there is much nausea, champagne with cracked ice, is most helpful. Strychnine, 1/200-1/100 grain (0.0003 to 0.0006 gm.), or digitalin in similar doses, may be indicated. Camphor is also an excellent stimulant.

SERUM THERAPY.—Thus far the results of serum therapy have been disappointing. Of 83 cases collected during the summer of 1903 by the Rockefeller Institute, there were no cures which could be certainly ascribed to the serum, nor was the mortality, as compared with previous years, appreciably lowered by serum prepared from either the so-called acid or alkaline type of organism. In nearly all instances, however, in which the serum was given several days had elapsed after the onset of the illness. It was only in the very early cases that any improvement at all was noticed. It may be that an earlier trial will be followed by better results.

Certainly the marked reduction in the mortality in adult dysentery in Japan, reported by Shiga, should encourage the further trial of this treatment in the epidemic diarrhœa, as no ill effects whatever have been ascribed to its use. It is given in 10-40 c. c. doses, hypodermically.

DIET.—The dietetic management is of the utmost importance. In acute cases with fever the milk, whether breast or cow's milk, and all its modifications, must be stopped at once. It is best to give the infant nothing but water for several hours, it may be for two or three days, or until the acute symptoms subside; a cereal water may then be substituted, preferably dextrinized, to which may be added egg albumen, broth, or beef juice. Preparations of broth and beef juice, and occasionally a weak tea, may be given. The time at which it is safe to return to a milk diet varies with each case, and no definite rules can be laid down. It is usually better to defer milk until the temperature is nearly normal.

If the stools are offensive from proteid decomposition, a diet consisting largely of carbohydrates—i. e., barley water—is indicated; whereas proteid diet, such as beef juice and egg albumen, is more helpful when the stools are strongly acid.

Experience has shown that the ingredient in the milk that is not well borne is the fat; hence skimmed milk, diluted or partially digested, can often be safely given before diluted whole milk. Whey is often helpful. In Germany buttermilk has been widely used in convalescence from intestinal disturbances. The various proprietary foods, or condensed milk mixed with water, although not to be given over long periods, may be found serviceable in the gradual return of the child to a normal diet.

In children from three to seven years of age these acute derangements are rarely serious, and usually respond promptly after purgation and restricted diet, consisting largely of boiled milk.

It must be borne in mind that injudicious treatment, either in diet or medication, may interrupt what otherwise would be a prompt recovery and bring on the most serious intestinal lesions. The chronic cases, both in infants and older children, especially those with ileo-colitis and ulceration, present unusual difficulties. Each case must be studied by itself. Food which is digested in the upper portion of the intestinal tract is preferable. Milk, properly modified with cereal water or predigested, if intelligently prescribed, offers the best chance of success. The so-called percentage system of milk modification, which enables the physician to alter at will the proportion of fat or carbohydrate present in the milk mixture, is of great service in feeding these long-standing cases.

Care must be taken not to over-feed, although occasionally, when there is persistent anorexia, gavage may be necessary. This is best accomplished through a nasal tube. Some infants will retain food given through a catheter when they will vomit the same mixture taken from a bottle. Beef juice or one of the beef-peptone preparations is frequently useful. They should always be given with considerable fluid. In a large majority of instances ulceration is confined to the large intestine, and can be reached by local treatment. Irrigations which flush the injured surface are of service. They should be discontinued if much exhaustion follows, but this is rare.

No very definite results have followed the various astringent preparations recommended. Probably warm salt or weak soda solutions are as useful. Silver nitrate is stimulating and healing where the ulcerations are in the rectum. In great local irritation and tenesmus, enemata (2 ounces, 60 c. c.) of flaxseed or starch, with 2 to 5 drops (0.12 to 0.3 c. c.) of laudanum, are soothing and beneficial.

Treatment of Cholera Infantum.—In cholera infantum serious symptoms may occur with great rapidity, and here the incessant vomiting and frequent purging render the administration of remedies extremely difficult. Irrigation of the stomach and large bowel is of great service, and when the fever is high ice-water injections may be used, or a graduated bath. As in the acute choleraic diarrhœa of adults, morphia hypodermically is the remedy which gives greatest relief, and in the conditions of extreme vomiting and purging, with restlessness and collapse symptoms, this drug alone commands the situation. A child of one year may be given from 1/100 to 1/80 of a grain (0.00065 to 0.0008 gm.) to be repeated in an hour, and again if not better.

In all cases of diarrhœa convalescence requires very careful management. An infant which has suffered from a severe attack should be especially watched throughout the remainder of the hot weather. During this time it is rarely safe to return to a full diet.

III. APPENDICITIS

Inflammation of the vermiform appendix is the most important of acute intestinal disorders. Formerly the "iliac phlegmon" was thought to be due to disease of the cæcum—typhlitis—or of the peritoneum covering it—perityphlitis; but we now know that with rare exceptions the cæcum itself is not affected, and even the condition formerly described as stercoral typhlitis is in reality appendicitis. The contribution of Fitz in 1886 served to put the whole question on a rational basis. For historical and special details the reader is referred to the monograph of Kelly and Hurdon.

Etiology.—The exciting causes of appendicitis are not always evident. An infection is the essential factor. The lumen of the appendix forms a sort of test-tube, in which the fæces lodge and are with difficulty discharged, so that the mucosa is liable to injury from retention of the secretions or from the presence of inspissated fæces or occasionally foreign bodies. In some instances the appendicitis is a local expression of a general infection. The causes of the undoubted increase of the disease are not known; some have attributed it to the prevalence of influenza. By others the poison of rheumatic fever is believed to be a cause, and just as it may excite tonsillitis, so it may cause inflammation of the lymphatic tissues of the appendix. It is remarkable, too, that there may be two or three cases of appendicitis at the same time in one family. The acute catarrhal form may be associated with pneumonia or typhoid fever or any of the acute infections. Direct injury, as in straining and heavy lifting, is an occasional exciting cause.

The BACTERIOLOGY of the disease is most varied. The *Bacillus coli* is present in a large number of cases, and the pyogenic organisms, particularly the *Streptococcus pyogenes*. The disease may be produced experimentally in rabbits by the intravenous injection of pneumococci and other organisms; Poynton and Paine have caused it with the organism isolated from rheumatic cases.

AGE.—Appendicitis is a disease of young persons, 50 per cent. of the cases occurring before the twentieth year. It has been met with as early as the seventh week, but it is rarely seen prior to the fifth year. Of 1,223 cases at the Johns Hopkins Hospital only 9 cases were under 5 years, 59 in children under 10, 140 between 11 and 15, 199 between 16 and 20, and 255 between 21 and 25 (Churchman).

SEX.—It is about equally common in males and in females.

OCCUPATION.—Persons whose work necessitates the lifting of heavy weights seem more prone to the disease. Trauma plays a very definite rôle, and in a number of cases the symptoms have followed very closely a fall or a blow.

Indiscretions in diet are very prone to bring on an attack, particularly in the recurring form of the disease, in which pain in the appendix region not infrequently follows the eating of indigestible articles of food.

Varieties.—McCarty from a study of 5,000 appendices removed at the Mayo clinic makes the following classification:

(*a*) APPENDICITIS CATARRHALIS ACUTA, a condition in which the mucosa is infiltrated with leucocytes and congested with inflammatory reaction in the lymph follicles and lymphatic tissues of the submucosa.

(*b*) APPENDICITIS CATARRHALIS CHRONICA, following repeated mild or severe acute catarrh, marked by increase of scar tissue, and distortion of the normal regularity of the structure. Blood pigment is often present.

(*c*) APPENDICITIS PURULENTA NECROTICA, an advanced stage of the acute catarrhal condition, plus the formation of intramural abscesses, necrosis, and perforation.

(*d*) PERI-APPENDICITIS ACUTA, an extension to the peritoneum of the conditions just described.

(*e*) OBLITERATION, a condition of the lumen, the result of destruction of the mucosa and the formation of scar tissue, occurring in about 24 per cent. of all cases, and an inflammatory, not an involutionary, process.

There are cases, too, in which the appendix becomes sphacelated *en masse*, and may slough off.

Fæcal Concretions.—The lumen of the appendix may contain a mould of fæces, which can readily be squeezed out. Even while soft the contents of the tube may be moulded in two or three sections with rounded ends. Concretions—enteroliths, coproliths—are also common. Of 700 cases of foreign bodies there were 45 per cent. of fæcal concretions (J. F. Mitchell). The enteroliths often resemble date stones in shape. The importance of these concretions is shown by the great frequency with which they are found in all acute inflammations of the appendix.

Foreign Bodies.—Of 1,400 cases of appendicitis collected by J. F. Mitchell these were present in 7 per cent.; in 28 cases pins were found. It is well to bear in mind that some of the concretions bear a very striking resemblance to cherry and date stones.

Symptoms.—In a large proportion of all cases of acute appendicitis the following symptoms are present: (*a*) Sudden pain in the abdomen, usually referred to the right iliac fossa; (*b*) fever, often of moderate grade; (*c*) gastro-intestinal disturbance—nausea, vomiting, and frequently constipation; (*d*) tenderness or pain on pressure in the appendix region.

Pain.—A sudden, violent pain in the abdomen is, according to Fitz, the most constant, first, decided symptom of perforating inflammation of the appendix, and occurred in 84 per cent. of the cases analyzed by him. In fully half of the cases it is localized in the right iliac fossa, but it may be central, diffuse, but usually in the right half of the abdomen. Even in the cases in which the pain is at first not in the appendix region it is usually felt here within thirty-six or forty-eight hours. It may extend toward the perineum or testicle. It is sometimes very sharp and colic-like, and cases have been mistaken for nephritic or for biliary colic. Some patients speak of it as a sharp, intense pain—serous-membrane pain; others as a dull ache—connective-tissue pain. While a very valuable symptom, pain is at the same time one of the most misleading. Some of the forms of recurring pain in the appendix region Talamon has called appendicular colic. The condition is believed to be due to partial occlusion of the lumen, leading to violent and irregular peristaltic action of the circular and longitudinal muscles in the expulsion of the mucus.

Fever.—Fever is always present in the early stage, even in the mildest forms, and is a most important feature. J. B. Murphy states that he would not operate on a case in which he was confident that no fever had been present in the first thirty-six hours of the disease. An initial chill is very rare. The fever may be moderate, from 100° to 102°; sometimes in children at the very outset the thermometer may register above 103.5°. The thermometer is one of the most trustworthy guides in the diagnosis of acute appendicitis. Appendicular colic of great severity may occur without fever. When a localized abscess has formed, and in some very virulent cases of general peritonitis, the temperature may be normal, but at this stage there are other symptoms which indicate the gravity of the situation. The pulse is quickened in proportion to the fever.

Gastro-intestinal Disturbance.—The tongue is usually furred and moist, seldom dry. Nausea and vomiting are symptoms which may be absent, but which are commonly present in the acute perforative cases. The vomiting rarely persists beyond the second day in favorable cases. Constipation is the rule, but the attack may set in with diarrhœa, particularly in children.

Local Signs.—Inspection of the abdomen is at first negative; there is no distention, and the iliac fossæ look alike. On palpation there are usually from the outset two important signs—namely, great tension of the right rectus muscle, and tenderness or actual pain on deep pressure. The muscular rigidity may be so great that a satisfactory examination can not be made without an anæsthetic. McBurney has called attention to the value of a localized point of tenderness on deep pressure, which is situated at the intersection of a line drawn from the navel to the anterior-superior spine of the ilium, with a second, vertically placed, corresponding to the outer edge of the right rectus muscle. Firm, deep, continuous pressure with one finger at this spot causes pain, often of the most exquisite character. In addition to the tenderness, rigidity, and actual pain on deep pressure, there is to be felt, in a majority of the cases, an induration or swelling. In some cases this is a boggy, ill-defined mass in the situation of the cæcum; more commonly the swelling is circumscribed and definite, situated in the iliac fossa, two or three fingers' breadth above Poupart's ligament. Some have been able to feel and roll beneath the fingers the thickened appendix. The later the case comes under observation the greater the probability of the existence of a well-marked tumor mass. It is not to be forgotten that there may be neither tumor mass nor induration to be felt in some of the most intensely virulent cases of perforative appendicitis. The pain may be mistaken for that of hip joint disease.

In addition may be mentioned great irritability of the bladder, which may be a very early symptom. The urine is scanty and often contains albumin and indican. The attitude is somewhat suggestive, the decubitus is dorsal, and the right leg is semi-flexed. Examination *per rectum* in the early stages rarely gives any information of value. The symptoms may be entirely pelvic when the appendix dips over the brim and the inflamed area is in direct contact with the uterine adnexa.

Leucocytosis.—The blood picture is of value equal to the pulse and temperature. As a rule, in acute attacks there is a leucocytosis of 12,000 to 15,000, chiefly of the polynuclears. In mild catarrhal cases there may be no increase. Usually the degree is an expression of the peritoneal irritation. A low leucocytosis or a leucopenia with increase in the mononuclear neutrophiles, what is called Arnette's blood picture, is an indication of a virulent infection.

Albuminuria is common. Sometimes there is an acute nephritis, and Dieulafoy has described an acute toxic form. He thinks that the kidneys are not infrequently damaged in the disease.

There are three possibilities in any case: (1) Gradual recovery, (2) the formation of a local abscess, and (3) general peritonitis.

Recovery is the rule in the mild catarrhal cases. The pain lessens at the end of the second or third day, the temperature falls, the tongue becomes cleaner, the vomiting ceases, the local tenderness is less marked, and the bowels are moved. By the end of a week the acute symptoms have subsided. So liable is the attack to recur that relapsing appendicitis is spoken of.

Local Abscess Formation.—As a result of ulceration and perforation, sometimes following the necrosis, by the end of the fourth or fifth day there is an extensive area of induration in the right iliac fossa, with great tenderness, and operations have shown that even at this very early date an abscess cavity may have formed. Though as a rule the fever becomes aggravated with the onset of suppuration, this is not always the case. The two most important elements in the diagnosis of abscess formation are the gradual increase of the local tumor and the aggravation of the general symptoms. Nowadays, when operation is so frequent, we have opportunities of seeing the abscess in various stages of development. Quite early the pus may lie between the cæcum and the coils of the ileum, with the general peritoneum shut off by fibrin, or there is a sero-fibrinous exudate with a slight amount of pus between the lower coils of the ileum. The abscess cavity may be small and lie on the psoas muscle, or at the edge of the promontory of the sacrum, and never reach a palpable size. The sac, when larger, may be roofed in by the small bowel and present irregular processes and pockets leading in different directions. In larger collections in the iliac fossa the roof is generally formed by the abdominal wall. Some of the most important of the localized abscesses are those which are situated entirely within the pelvis. The various directions and positions into which the abscess may pass or perforate have already been referred to under morbid anatomy, but it may be here mentioned again that, left alone, it may discharge externally, or burrow in various directions, or be emptied through the rectum, vagina, or bladder. Death may be caused by septicæmia, by perforation into an artery or vein, or by pylephlebitis.

General Peritonitis.—This may be caused by direct perforation of the appendix and general infection of the peritoneum before any delimiting inflammation is excited. In a second group of cases there has been an attempt at localizing the infective process, but it fails, and the general peritoneum becomes involved. In a third group of cases a localized focus of suppuration exists about an inflamed appendix, and from this perforation takes place.

Death in appendicitis is due usually to general peritonitis.

The gravity of appendix disease lies in the fact that from the very onset the peritoneum may be infected; the initial symptoms of pain, with nausea and vomiting, fever, and local tenderness, present in all cases, may indicate a wide-spread infection of this membrane. The onset is usually sudden, the pain diffuse, not always localized in the right iliac fossa, but it is not so much the character as the greater intensity of the symptoms from the outset that makes one suspicious of a general peritonitis. Abdominal distention, diffuse tenderness, and absence of abdominal movements are the most trustworthy local signs, but they are not really so trustworthy as the general symptoms. The initial nausea and vomiting persist, the pulse becomes more rapid, the tongue is dry, the urine scanty. In very acute cases, by the end of twenty-four hours the abdomen may be distended. By the third and fourth days the classical picture of a general peritonitis is well established—a distended and motionless abdomen, a rapid pulse, a dry tongue, dorsal decubitus with the knees drawn up, and an anxious, pinched, Hippocratic facies. The picture may be that of septicopyæmia or sapræmia; high fever, chills, sweats, without local reaction. These are generally acute, gangrenous cases with anomalous position of the appendix, behind the colon, or deep in the pelvis. Even when looked for carefully there may be no local indications.

Sometimes there have been gastro-intestinal symptoms for a few days before, to which no attention has been paid by the family. In one case, seen by the family physician at 2 p. m. for the first time, by me at 4.30 p. m., at 7 p. m. by a surgeon who refused to operate, death occurred within 12 hours after the physician was first called.

Remote Effects.—The remote effects of perforative appendicitis are interesting. Hæmorrhage may occur. In one of my cases the appendix was adherent to the promontory of the sacrum, and the abscess cavity had perforated in two places into the ileum. Death resulted from profuse hæmorrhage. Cases are on record in which the internal iliac artery or the deep circumflex iliac artery has been opened. Suppurative pylephlebitis may result from inflammation of the mesenteric veins near the perforated appendix. The appendix may perforate in a hernial sac. Many instances of this have been recorded.

After operation, thrombosis of the iliac or femoral veins is not uncommon, and sudden death from pulmonary embolism has followed. The leg may be permanently enlarged. Hernia may occur in the wound. Strangulation of the bowel is an occasional sequence. Recurrence of the symptoms after operation has been noted, due in some cases to incomplete removal.

Diagnosis.—Appendicitis is by far the most common inflammatory condition, not only in the cæcal region, but in the abdomen generally in persons under thirty. The surgeons have taught us that, almost without exception, sudden pain in the right iliac fossa, with fever and localized tenderness, with or without tumor, means appendix disease. There are certain diseases of the abdominal organs characterized by pain which are apt to be confounded with appendicitis. Biliary colic, kidney colic, and the colicky pains at the menstrual period in women have in some cases to be most carefully considered.

Diseases of the tubes and pelvic peritonitis may simulate appendicitis very closely, but the history and the local examination under ether should in most cases enable the practitioner to reach a diagnosis. I have seen several cases supposed to be recurring appendicitis which proved to be tubo-ovarian disease.

The Dietl's crises in floating kidney have been mistaken for appendicitis.

Acute hæmorrhagic pancreatitis may also produce symptoms very like those of appendicitis with general peritonitis. The relation of typhoid fever and appendicitis is interesting. The gastro-intestinal symptoms, particularly the pain and the fever, may at the onset suggest appendicitis. Operations have been comparatively frequent. In the second and third weeks of typhoid fever perforation of the appendix may occur, and occasionally late in the convalescence perforation of an unhealed ulcer of the appendix.

In a great many patients with chronic appendicitis stomach symptoms predominate, and an appendicular dyspepsia has been recognized particularly by the French writers and by surgeons. Many of the patients are neurotic. The dyspeptic symptoms are irregular, and food rarely gives relief, as in ulcer. Pain is the prevailing symptom, often caused by food, and more abdominal than epigastric, without radiation, and there are frequently pain and tenderness at McBurney's point. Vomiting is rare, but there is usually much flatulency. Without being seriously ill, the patient's condition is constantly below par, and he may go the rounds of physicians for years. In an analysis of 100 cases of this type at the Mayo clinic by Graham and Guthrie, reported on a year after operation, 77 per cent. were cured by the removal of the appendix. As a majority of these patients are neurotic, it is not easy to say how far the good results have been due directly to the removal of the appendix, the pathological condition of which, as reported upon by Graham and Guthrie, did not seem to differ much from that which is met with, according to Aschoff, in a majority of individuals in the fourth decade. I can testify that in a certain number of these patients the relief after removal of the appendix has not been permanent.

There is a well-marked appendicular hypochondriasis. Through the pernicious influence of the daily press, appendicitis has become a sort of fad, and the physician has often to deal with patients who have almost a fixed idea that they have the disease. The worst cases of this class which I have seen have been in members of our profession, and I know of at least one instance in which a perfectly normal appendix was removed. The question really has its ludicrous side. A well-known physician in a Western city having one night a bellyache, and feeling convinced that his appendix had perforated, summoned a surgeon, who quickly removed the supposed offender!

Hysteria may of course simulate appendicitis very closely, and it may require a very keen judgment to make a diagnosis. Mucous colitis with enteralgia in nervous women is sometimes mistaken for appendicitis.

Perinephritic and pericæcal abscess from perforation of ulcer, either simple or cancerous, and circumscribed peritonitis in this region from other causes, can rarely be differentiated until an exploratory incision is made.

Chronic obliterative appendicitis can not always be differentiated from the perforative form, and in intensity of pain, severity of symptoms, and, in rare instances, even in the production of peritonitis, the two may be identical.

Briefly stated, localized pain in the right iliac fossa, with or without induration or tumor, the existence of McBurney's tender point, fever, furred tongue, vomiting, with constipation or diarrhœa, indicate appendicitis. The occurrence of general peritonitis is suggested by increase and diffusion of the abdominal pain, tympanites (as a rule), marked aggravation of the constitutional symptoms, particularly elevation of fever and increased rapidity of the pulse. Obliteration of hepatic dulness is rarely present, as the peritoneum in these cases does not often contain gas.

Appendicitis and Pregnancy.—The association is not uncommon. Of 103 perforative or gangrenous cases 89 were operated upon, with 36 deaths. Of 14 cases not operated upon all died. Of the 103 cases 80 aborted before or after operation. Of 104 non-perforative cases 50 were operated upon with 1 death; of the remaining 54, 4 died; 13 of these non-perforative cases aborted (Babler). Mild cases recover; in the severer forms it is safer to operate at once.

Prognosis.—*There would be no percentage of deaths from appendicitis if every case commencing with acute pain and developing tenderness and rigidity of the abdomen and quickening of the pulse were operated upon within twelve hours* (Rutherford Morison).

Treatment.—Gradually the profession has learned to recognize that appendicitis is a surgical disease. In hospital practice the cases should be admitted directly to the surgical wards. Many lives are lost by temporizing. The general practitioner does well to remember—whether his leanings be toward the conservative or the radical methods of treatment—that the surgeon is often called too late, never too early.

There is no medicinal treatment of appendicitis. There are remedies which will allay the pain, but there are none capable in any way of controlling the course of the disease. Rest in bed, a light diet, measures directly to allay the vomiting—upon these all are agreed. The practice of giving opium in some form in appendicitis and peritonitis is decreasing, but is still too common. Surgeons almost unanimously condemn the practice, as obscuring the clinical picture and tending to give a false sense of security; and since they control the situation, we should not give opium, and trust to the persistent use of ice locally to relieve the pain. General opinion among the best surgeons is, I believe, opposed to the use of saline purges.

Operation is indicated in all cases of acute inflammatory trouble in the cæcal region, whether tumor is present or not, when the general symptoms are severe, and *when at the end of twelve hours, or even earlier, the features of the case point to a progressive lesion.* The mortality from early operation under these circumstances is very slight.

In recurring appendicitis, when the attacks are of such severity and frequency as seriously to interrupt the patient's occupation, the mortality in the hands of capable operators is very small.

IV. INTESTINAL OBSTRUCTION

Intestinal obstruction may be caused by strangulation, intussusception, twists and knots, strictures and tumors, by abnormal contents, and by paralysis of the muscular coat of the bowel.

Etiology and Pathology.—(*a*) STRANGULATION.—This is the most frequent cause of acute obstruction, and occurred in 34 per cent. of the 295 cases analyzed by Fitz, and in 35 per cent. of the 1,134 cases of Leichtenstern. Of the 101 cases of strangulation in Fitz's table, which has the special value of having been carefully selected from the literature since 1880, the following were the causes: Adhesions, 63; vitelline remains, 21; adherent appendix, 6; mesenteric and omental slits, 6; peritoneal pouches and openings, 3; adherent tube, 1; peduncular tumor, 1. The bands and adhesions result, in a majority of cases, from former peritonitis. A number of instances have been reported following operations upon the pelvic organs in women. The strangulation may be recent and due to adhesion of the bowel to the abdominal wound or a coil may be caught between the pedicle of a tumor and the pelvic wall. Such cases are only too common. Late occlusion after recovery from the operation is due to bands and adhesions.

The vitelline remains are represented by Meckel's diverticulum, which forms a finger-like projection from the ileum, usually within eighteen inches of the ileo-cæcal valve. It is a remnant of the omphalo-mesenteric duct, through which, in the early embryo, the intestine communicated with the yolk-sac. The end, though commonly free, may be attached to the abdominal wall near the navel, or to the mesentery, and a ring is thus formed through which the gut may pass.

Seventy per cent. of the cases of obstruction from strangulation occur in males; 40 per cent. of all the cases occur between the ages of fifteen and thirty years. In 90 per cent. of the cases of obstruction from these causes the site of the trouble is in the small bowel; the position of the strangulated portion was in the right iliac fossa in 67 per cent. of the cases, and in the lower abdomen in 83 per cent.

(*b*) INTUSSUSCEPTION.—In this condition one portion of the intestine slips into an adjacent portion, forming an invagination or intussusception. The two portions make a cylindrical tumor, which varies in length from a half inch to a foot or more. The condition is always a descending intussusception, and, as the process proceeds, the middle and inner layers increase at the expense of the outer layer. An intussusception consists of three layers of bowel: the outermost, known as the intussuscipiens, or receiving layer; a middle or returning layer; and the innermost or entering layer. The student can obtain a clear idea of the arrangement by making the end of a glove-finger pass into the lower portion. The actual condition can be very clearly studied in the post mortem invaginations which are so common in the small bowel of children. In the statistics of Fitz, 93 of 295 cases of acute intestinal obstruction were due to this cause. Of these, 52 were in males and 27 in females. The cases are most common in early life, 34 per cent. under one year and 56 per cent. under the tenth year. Of 103 cases in children, nearly 50 per cent. occurred in the fourth, fifth, and sixth months (Wiggin). No definite causes could be assigned in 42 of the cases; in the others diarrhœa or habitual constipation had existed.

The site of the invagination varies. We may recognize (1) an *ileo-cæcal,* when the ileo-cæcal valve descends into the colon. There are cases in which this is so extensive that the valve has been felt *per rectum.* This form occurred in 75 per cent. of the cases; in 89 per cent. of Wiggin's collected cases. In the *ileo-colic* the lower part of the ileum passes through the ileo-cæcal valve. (2) The *ileal,* in which the ileum is alone involved. (3) The *colic,* in which it is confined to the large intestine. (4) *Colico-rectal,* in which the colon and rectum are involved. (5) Intussusception of the appendix is rare, but there are about 30 cases on record, most of them in children.

Irregular peristalsis is the essential cause of intussusception. Nothnagel found in the localized peristalsis caused by the faradic current that it was not the descent of one portion into the other, but the drawing up of the receiving layer by contraction of the longitudinal coat. Invagination may follow any limited, sudden, and severe peristalsis.

In the post mortem examination, in a case of death from intussusception, the condition is very characteristic. Peritonitis may be present or an acute injection of the serous membrane. When death occurs early, as it may do from shock, there is little to be seen. The portion of bowel affected is large and thick, and forms an elongated tumor with a curved outline. The parts are swollen and congested, owing to the constriction of the mesentery between the layers. The entire mass may be of a deep livid-red color. In very recent processes there is only congestion, and perhaps a thin layer of lymph, and the intussusception can be reduced, but when it has lasted for a few days, lymph is thrown out, the layers are glued together, and the entering portion of the gut can not be withdrawn.

The anatomical condition accounts for the presence of the tumor, which exists in two-thirds of all cases; and the engorgement, which results from the compression of the mesenteric vessels, explains the frequent occurrence of blood in the discharges, which has so important a diagnostic value. If the patient survives, necrosis and sloughing of the invaginated portion may occur, and, if union has taken place between the inner and outer layers, the calibre of the gut may be restored and a cure in this way effected. Many cases of the kind are on record. In the Museum of the Medical Faculty of the McGill University are 17 inches of small intestine, which were passed by a lad who had symptoms of internal strangulation, and who made a complete recovery.

(*c*) Twists, Knots, and Traction Kinks.—Volvulus or twist occurred in 42 of the 295 cases (Fitz). Sixty-eight per cent. were in males. It is most frequent between the ages of thirty and forty. In the great majority of all cases the twist is axial and associated with an unusually long mesentery. In 50 per cent. of the cases it was in the sigmoid flexure. The next most common situation is about the cæcum, which may be twisted upon its axis or bent upon itself. As a rule, in volvulus the loop of bowel is simply twisted upon its long axis, and the portions at the end of the loop cross each other and so cause the strangulation. It occasionally happens that one portion of the bowel is twisted about another.

Traction kinks occur at three regions—the third portion of the duodenum, the last part of the ileum, and the sigmoid flexure. What is known as gastro-mesenteric ileus is caused by compression of the lower portion of the duodenum by the root of the mesentery with its contained blood-vessels. The condition has been described under acute dilatation of the stomach.

The *ileum kink* occurs within a few inches of the cæcum. This portion has a short tight mesentery and a large loose cæcum sags over the brim of the pelvis and may cause a definite kink of the ileum with constipation, pain in the right iliac fossa, and symptoms which simulate appendicitis.

Traction of a very full sigmoid flexure may, without any special twist, compress and obstruct a neighboring coil of the colon.

(*d*) Strictures and Tumors.—These are very much less important causes of acute obstruction, as may be judged by the fact that there are only 15 instances out of the 295 cases, in 14 of which the obstruction occurred in the large intestine (Fitz). On the other hand, they are common causes of chronic obstruction.

Lipoma may occur, growing from the submucosa, and cause intussusception. In a number of cases the tumor has been passed *per rectum.* S. B. Ward has collected 9 cases.

The obstruction may result from: (1) *Congenital stricture.* These are exceedingly rare. Much more commonly the condition is that of complete occlusion, either forming the imperforate anus or the congenital defect by which the duodenum is not united to the pylorus. (2) *Simple cicatricial stenosis,* which results from ulceration, tuberculous or syphilitic, more rarely from dysentery, and most rarely of all from typhoid ulceration. (3) *New growths.* The malignant strictures are due chiefly to cylindrical epithelioma, which forms an annular tumor, most commonly met with in the large bowel, about the sigmoid flexure, or the descending colon. Of benign growths, papillomata, adenomata, lipomata, and fibromata occasionally induce obstruction. (4) *Compression and traction.* Tumors of neighboring organs, particularly of the pelvic viscera, may cause obstruction by adhesion and traction. In the healing of tuberculous peritonitis the contraction of the thick exudate may cause compression and narrowing of the coils.

(*e*) Abnormal Contents.—Foreign bodies, such as fruit stones, coins, pins, needles, or false teeth, are occasionally swallowed accidentally, or by lunatics on purpose. Round worms may become rolled into a tangled mass and cause obstruction. In reality, however, the majority of foreign bodies, such as coins, buttons, and pins, swallowed by children, cause no inconvenience whatever, but in a day or two are found in the stools. Occasionally such a foreign body as a pin will pass through the œsophagus and will be found lodged in some adjacent organ, as in the heart (Peabody), or a barley ear may reach the liver (Dock).

Medicines, such as magnesia or bismuth, have been known to accumulate in the bowels and produce obstruction, but in the great majority of the cases the condition is caused by fæces, gall-stones, or enteroliths. Of 44 cases, in 23 the obstruction was by gall-stones, in 19 by fæces, and in 2 by enteroliths. Obstruction by fæces may happen at any period of life. As mentioned when speaking of dilatation of the colon, it may occur in young children and persist for weeks. In fæcal accumulation the large bowel may reach an enormous size and the contents become very hard. The retained masses may be channeled, and small quantities of fæcal matter are passed until a mass too large enters the lumen and causes obstruction. There may be very few symptoms, as the condition may be borne for weeks or even for months.

Obstruction by gall-stones is not very infrequent, as may be gathered from the fact that 23 cases were reported in the literature in eight years. Eighteen of these were in women and 5 in men. In six-sevenths of the cases it occurred about the fiftieth year. The obstruction is usually in the ileo-cæcal region, but it may be in the duodenum. These large solitary gall-stones ulcerate through the gall-bladder, usually into the small intestine, occasionally into the colon. In the latter case they rarely cause obstruction. Courvoisier has collected 131 cases in the literature.

Enteroliths may be formed of masses of hair, more commonly of the phosphates of lime and magnesia, with a nucleus formed of a foreign body or of hardened fæces. Nearly every museum possesses specimens of this kind. They are not so common in men as in ruminants, and, as indicated in Fitz's statistics, are very rare causes of obstruction.

(*f*) Paralytic Ileus.—Without any obstruction in the lumen, in a localized area or in a wide section of the bowel, the muscular walls may be so paralyzed that no movement of the contents occurs, causing a condition which virtually amounts to obstruction. The best illustrations of local paralytic ileus are seen in the embolic and thrombotic processes in the mesenteric arteries, when the corresponding portions of the intestinal wall are in a state of infarct. This is the condition which occurs in the verminous aneurism in a horse, and is associated with the common intestinal colic. It is more common in the small than in the large bowel, but I saw an instance of paralytic ileus due to localized involvement of about eight inches of the wall of the transverse colon without, so far as one could discover, any affection of the blood-vessels, and the symptoms were those of acute obstruction.

Following operations, particularly on the abdomen, after injuries, following paracentesis in ascites, in pneumonia, pleurisy, and occasionally in heart disease, a paralytic state of the bowel may occur, with cessation of peristalsis, distention of the abdomen, vomiting, and other signs of obstruction. There are remarkable cases of hysteria with symptoms of chronic obstruction of the bowels and fæcal vomiting—the so-called ileus hystericus.

Symptoms.—(*a*) Acute Obstruction.—Constipation, pain in the abdomen, and vomiting are the three important symptoms. Pain sets in early and may come on abruptly while the patient is walking, or, more commonly, during the performance of some action. It is at first colicky in character, but subsequently it becomes continuous and very intense. Vomiting follows quickly and is a constant and most distressing symptom. At first the contents of the stomach are voided, and then greenish, bile-stained material, and soon, in cases of acute and permanent obstruction, the material vomited is a brownish-black liquid, with a distinctly fæcal odor. This sequence of gastric, bilious, and, finally, stercoraceous vomiting is perhaps the most important diagnostic feature of acute obstruction. The constipation may be absolute, without the discharge of either fæces or gas. Very often the contents of the bowel below the stricture are discharged. Distention of the abdomen usually occurs, and, when the large bowel is involved, it is extreme. On the other hand, if the obstruction is high up in the small intestine, there may be very slight tympany. At first the abdomen is not painful, but subsequently it may become acutely tender.

The constitutional symptoms from the outset are severe. The face is pallid and anxious, and finally collapse symptoms supervene. The eyes become sunken, the features pinched, and the skin is covered with a cold, clammy sweat. The pulse becomes rapid and feeble. There may be no fever; the axillary temperature is often subnormal. The tongue is dry and parched and the thirst is incessant. The urine is high-colored, scanty, and there may be suppression, particularly when the obstruction is high up in the bowel. This is probably due to the constant vomiting and the small amount of liquid which is absorbed. The case terminates, as a rule, in from three to six days. In some instances the patient dies from shock or sinks into coma. A leucocytosis of 75,000 or 80,000 per c. mm. may be present.

(*b*) Symptoms of Chronic Obstruction.—When due to fæcal impaction, there is a history of long-standing constipation. There may have been discharge of mucus, or, in some instances, the fæcal masses have been channeled, and so have allowed the contents of the upper portion of the bowel to pass through. In elderly persons this is not infrequent; but examination, either *per rectum* or externally, in the course of the colon, will reveal the presence of hard scybalous masses. There may be retention of fæces for weeks without exciting serious symptoms. In other instances there are vomiting, pain in the abdomen, gradual distention, and finally the ejecta become fæcal. The hardened masses may excite an intense colitis or even peritonitis.

In stricture, whether cicatricial or cancerous, the symptoms of obstruction are very diverse. Constipation gradually comes on, is extremely variable, and it may be months or even years before there is complete obstruction. There are transient attacks, in which from some cause the fæces accumulate above the stricture, the intestine becomes greatly distended, and in the swollen abdomen the coils can be seen in active peristalsis. In such attacks there may be vomiting, but it is very rarely of a fæcal character. In the majority of these cases the general health is seriously impaired; the patient gradually becomes anæmic and emaciated, and, finally, in an attack in which the obstruction is complete, death occurs with all the features of acute occlusion, or the case may be prolonged for ten or twelve days.

Diagnosis.—(*a*) The Situation of the Obstruction.—Hernia must be excluded, which is by no means always easy, as fatal obstruction may occur from the involvement of a very limited portion of the gut in the external ring or in the obturator foramen. A thorough rectal and, in women, a vaginal examination should be made, which will give important information as to the condition of the pelvic and rectal contents, particularly in cases of intussusception, in which the descending bowel can sometimes be felt. In cases of obstruction high up the empty coils sink into the pelvis and can there be detected. Rectal exploration with the entire hand is of doubtful value. In the inspection of the abdomen there are important indications, as the special prominence in certain regions, the occurrence of well-defined masses, and the presence of hypertrophied coils in active peristalsis. John Wyllie has called attention to the great value in diagnosis of the "patterns of abdominal tumidity." In obstruction of the lower end of the large intestine not only may the horseshoe of the colon stand out plainly, when the bowel is in rigid spasm, but even the pouches of the gut may be seen. When the cæcum or lower end of the ileum is obstructed the tumidity is in the lower central region, and during spasm the coils of the small bowel may stand out prominently, one above the other, either obliquely or transversely placed—the so-called "ladder pattern." In obstruction of the duodenum or jejunum there may only be slight distention of the upper part of the abdomen, associated usually with rapid collapse and anuria.

In the ileum and cæcum the distention is more in the central portion of the abdomen; the vomiting is distinctly fæcal and occurs early. In obstruction of the colon tympanites is much more extensive and general. Tenesmus is more common, with the passage of mucus and blood. The course is not so quick, the collapse does not supervene so rapidly, and the urinary secretion is not so much reduced.

In obstruction from stricture or tumor the situation can in some cases be accurately localized, but in others it is very uncertain. Digital examination of the rectum should first be made. The rectal tube may then be passed, but it is impossible to get beyond the sigmoid flexure. In the use of the rigid tube there is danger of perforation of the bowel in the neighborhood of a stricture. The quantity of fluid which can be passed into the large intestine should be estimated. The capacity of the large bowel is about six quarts. Wiggin advises about a pint and a half from a height of three feet for an infant. To thoroughly irrigate the bowel the patient should be chloroformed and should lie on the back or on the side—best on the back, with the hips elevated. Treves suggests that the cæcal region should be auscultated during the passage of the fluid. For diagnostic purposes the rectum may be inflated, either by the bellows or by the use of bicarbonate of soda and tartaric acid. In certain cases these measures give important indications as to the situation of the obstruction in the large bowel.

(*b*) Nature of the Obstruction.—This is often difficult, not infrequently impossible, to determine. *Strangulation* is not common in very early life. In many instances there have been previous attacks of abdominal pain, or there are etiological factors which give a clew, such as old peritonitis or operation on the pelvic viscera. Neither the onset nor the character of the pain gives us any information. In rare instances nausea and vomiting may be absent. The vomiting usually becomes fæcal from the third to the fifth day. A tumor is not common in strangulation, and was present in only one-fifth of the cases. Fever is not of diagnostic value.

Intussusception is an affection of childhood, and is of all forms of internal obstruction the one most readily diagnosed. The presence of tumor, bloody stools, and tenesmus are the important factors. The tumor is usually sausage-shaped and felt in the region of the transverse colon. It existed in 66 of 93 cases. It became evident the first day in more than one-third of the cases, on the second day in more than one-fourth, and on the third day in more than one-fifth. Blood in the stools occurs in at least three-fifths of the cases, either spontaneously or following the use of an enema. The blood may be mixed with mucus. Tenesmus is present in one-third of the cases. Fæcal vomiting is not very common and was present in only 12 of the 93 instances. Abdominal tympany is a symptom of slight importance, occurring in only one-third of the cases.

Volvulus can rarely be diagnosed. The frequency with which it involves the sigmoid flexure is to be borne in mind. The passage of a flexible tube or injecting fluids might in these cases give valuable indications.

In fæcal obstruction the condition is usually clear, as the fæces can be felt *per rectum* and also in the distended colon. Fæcal vomiting, tympany, abdominal pain, nausea, and vomiting are late and are not so constant. In obstruction by gall-stone a few of the cases gave a previous history of gall-stone colic. Jaundice was present in only 2 of the 23 cases. Pain and vomiting, as a rule, occur early and are severe, and fæcal vomiting is present in two-thirds of the cases. A tumor is rarely evident.

(*c*) Diagnosis from Other Conditions.—Acute enteritis with great relaxation of the intestinal coils, vomiting, and pain may be mistaken for obstruction. Of late years many instances have been reported in which peritonitis following disease of the appendix has been mistaken for acute obstruction. The intense vomiting, the general tympany and abdominal tenderness, and, in some instances, the suddenness of the onset are very deceptive. In appendix disease the temperature is more frequently elevated, the vomiting is never fæcal, and in many cases there is a history of previous attacks in the cæcal region. Acute hæmorrhagic pancreatitis may produce symptoms which simulate closely intestinal obstruction.

Treatment.—Purgatives should not be given. For the pain hypodermic injections of morphia are indicated. To allay the distressing vomiting, the stomach should be washed out. Not only is this directly beneficial, but Kussmaul claims that the abdominal distention is relieved, the pressure in the bowel above the seat of obstruction is lessened, and the violent peristalsis is diminished. It may be practiced three or four times a day, and in some instances has proved beneficial; in others curative. Thorough irrigation of the large bowel with injections should be practiced, the warm fluid being allowed to flow in from a fountain syringe, and the amount carefully estimated.

Inflation may also be tried, by forcing the air into the rectum with the bellows or with a Davidson's syringe. It is a measure not without risk, as instances of rupture of the bowel have been reported. Of 39 cases in children treated by inflation or enemata 16 recovered (Wiggin). In cases of acute obstruction surgical measures should be resorted to early.

For the tympanites turpentine stupes and hot applications may be applied. In cases of chronic obstruction the diet must be carefully regulated, and opium and belladonna are useful for the paroxysmal pains. Enemata should be employed, and, if the obstruction becomes complete, resort must be had to surgical measures.

V. CONSTIPATION

(*Costiveness*)

Definition.—Retention of fæces from any cause.

Constipation in Adults.—The causes are varied and may be classed as general and local.

General Causes.—(*a*) Constitutional peculiarities: Torpidity of the bowels is often a family complaint and is found more often in dark than in fair persons. (*b*) Sedentary habits, particularly in persons who eat too much and neglect the calls of nature. (*c*) Certain diseases, such as anæmia, neurasthenia, and hysteria, chronic affections of the liver, stomach, and intestines, and the acute fevers. Under this heading may appropriately be placed that most injurious of all habits, *drug-taking*. (*d*) Either a coarse diet, which leaves too much residue, or a diet which leaves too little.

Local Causes.—Weakness of the abdominal muscles in obesity or from overdistention in repeated pregnancies. Atony of the large bowel from chronic disease of the mucosa; the presence of tumors, physiological or pathological, pressing upon the bowel; enteritis; foreign bodies, large masses of scybala, and strictures of all kinds. An important local cause is atony of the colon, particularly of the muscles of the sigmoid flexure by which the fæces are propelled into the rectum. An obstinate form is that associated with a contracted state of the bowel, sometimes spoken of as spasmodic constipation. This is met with—first, as a sequence of chronic dysentery or ulcerative colitis; secondly, in protracted cases of hysteria and neurasthenia in women, particularly in association with uterine disease; and, thirdly, in very old persons often without any definite cause. It may be that the sigmoid flexure and lower colon are in a condition of contraction and spasm, while the transverse and ascending parts are in a state of atony and dilatation. The most characteristic sign of this variety is the presence of hard, globular masses, or, more rarely, small and sausage-like fæces.

Radiography has taught us much of the conditions favoring intestinal stasis. The upward position in man favors visceroptosis, with which we find associated many of the most obstinate cases of constipation. Arbuthnot Lane has emphasized the fact of this dropping or dragging of the intestines, particularly at certain points—e. g., the third part of the duodenum, at the end of which there may be an abrupt kink associated with a considerable dilatation of the duodenum itself. This is of course relieved immediately when the patient lies down. The second is the ileal kink, already spoken of, caused by a dropping of the cæcum, and the lower coil of the ileum itself. The obstruction may result in considerable dilatation of the end of the ileum, with delay in the passage of the fluid fæces. A third point is the fixed splenic flexure of the colon, and the X-ray may show an ascending colon as low as the level of the iliac crest, and the transverse in the pelvis necessarily causing delay in the passage of the fæces past this angle. The sigmoid loop seems specially designed to promote stasis; the rectum may also present an elongated S-shaped loop, and, finally, there is the sharp pelvi-rectal flexure, above which the fæces accumulate.

The studies of Hertz, Jordan, and others have shown how accurately the rate of the passage of the fæces through the large bowel may be estimated with the X-rays. After a bismuth meal the cæcum is reached in about four hours, the hepatic flexure two hours later, the splenic flexure three hours after that, and the beginning of the pelvic colon twelve hours after the commencement of the meal. The fæces do not pass beyond the pelvi-rectal flexure until just before defæcation.

Hertz divides all cases of constipation into two main groups. In one the delay occurs in the passage through the colon, particularly in the distal half; in the other the passage as far as the pelvic colon is normal, but defæcation is not properly performed. Every case of chronic constipation ought to be carefully studied with the X-rays.

Symptoms.—The most persistent constipation for weeks or even months may exist with fair health. Debility, lassitude, and a mental depression are frequent symptoms in constipation, particularly in persons of a nervous temperament. Headache, loss of appetite, a furred tongue, and foul breath may also occur. In girls the skin is "muddy," acne is common, chlorosis may follow, and there is a flabby state of the system generally. Lane claims that chronic mastitis, chronic pancreatitis and gall-stones may follow intestinal stasis.

When persistent, the accumulation of fæces leads to unpleasant, sometimes serious, local symptoms, such as piles, ulceration of the colon, distention of the sacculi, perforation, enteritis, and occlusion. In women pressure may cause pain at the time of menstruation and a sensation of fullness and distention in the pelvic organs. Neuralgia of the sacral nerves may be caused by an overloaded sigmoid flexure. The fæces collect chiefly in the colon. Even in extreme grades of constipation it is rare to find dry fæces in the cæcum. The fæces may form large tumors at the hepatic or splenic flexures, or a sausage-like, doughy mass above the navel, or an irregular lumpy tumor in the left inguinal region. In old persons the sacculi of the colon become distended and the scybala may remain in them and undergo calcification, forming enteroliths.

In cases with prolonged retention the fæcal masses become channeled and diarrhœa may occur for days before the true condition is discovered by rectal or external examination. In women who have been habitually constipated attacks of diarrhœa with nausea and vomiting should excite suspicion and lead to a thorough examination of the large bowel. Fever may occur in these cases, and Meigs has reported an instance in which the condition simulated typhoid fever.

Captivated by the theories of Metchnikoff we have been for some years on the crest of a colonic wave, and intestinal toxæmia has been held responsible for many of the worst of the ills that flesh is heir to, more particularly arterio-sclerosis and old age. The seniles and preseniles of two continents have been taking sour milk and lacto-bacillary compounds, to the great benefit of the manufacturing chemists! But the fad is passing, not, I hope, to be replaced by one even more serious, in which operation is advised for every case of severe intestinal stasis.

Constipation in infants is a common and troublesome disorder. The causes are congenital, dietetic, and local. There are instances in which the child is constipated from birth and may not have a natural movement for years, and yet thrive and develop. There are cases of enormous dilatation of the large bowel with persistent constipation. The condition appears sometimes to be a congenital defect. In some of these patients there may be constricting bands, or, as in a case of Cheever's, a congenital stricture.

Dietetic causes are more common. In sucklings it often arises from an unnatural dryness of the small residue which passes into the colon, and it may be very difficult to decide whether the fault is in the mother's milk or in the digestion of the child. Most probably it is in the latter, as some babies may be persistently costive on natural or artificial foods. Deficiency of fat in the milk is believed by some writers to be the cause. In older children it is of the greatest importance that regular habits should be enjoined. Carelessness on the part of the mother in this matter often lays the foundation of troublesome constipation in after life. Impairment of the contractility of the intestinal wall in consequence of inflammation, disturbance in the normal intestinal secretions, and mechanical obstruction by tumors, twists, and intussusception are the chief local causes.

Treatment.—Much may be done by systematic habits, particularly in the young. The patient should go to stool at a fixed hour every day, whether there is desire or not, and the desire should always be granted. Exercise in moderation is helpful. In stout persons and in women with pendulous abdomens the muscles should have the support of a bandage. Friction or regularly applied massage is invaluable in the more chronic cases. A good substitute is a metal ball weighing from four to six pounds, which may be rolled over the abdomen every morning for five or ten minutes. The diet should be light, with plenty of fruit and vegetables, particularly salads and tomatoes. Oatmeal is usually laxative, though not to all; brown bread is better than that made from fine white flour. Of liquids, water and aërated mineral waters may be taken freely. A tumblerful of hot or cold water on rising, taken slowly, is efficacious in many cases. A glass of hot water at night may also be tried alone. A pipe or a cigar after breakfast is with many men an infallible remedy.

When the condition is not very obstinate it is well to try to relieve it by hygienic and dietetic measures. If drugs must be used they should be the milder saline laxatives or the compound liquorice powder. Enemata are often necessary, and it is much preferable to employ them early than to constantly use purgative pills. Glycerine either in the form of suppository or as a small injection is very valuable. Half a drachm of boric acid placed within the rectum is sometimes efficacious. The injections of tepid water, with or without soap, may be used for a prolonged period with good effect and without damage. The patient should be in the dorsal position with the hips elevated, and it is best to let the fluid flow in slowly from a fountain syringe.

The usual remedies employed are often useless in the constipation associated with contracted bowel. A very satisfactory measure is the olive or cotton seed oil injection, as recommended by Kussmaul. The patient lies on the back with the hips elevated, and with a cannula and tube from 15 to 20 ounces of pure oil are allowed to flow slowly (or are injected) into the bowel. The operation should take at least fifteen minutes. This may be repeated every day until the intestine is cleared, and subsequently a smaller injection every few days will suffice. In the cases with a spastic colon the injection of oil at bedtime, which is retained during the night, is often effectual.

There are various drugs which are of special service, particularly the combination of ipecacuanha, nux vomica, or belladonna, with aloes, or podophyllin. Cascara sagrada, phenolphthalein, and agar agar are useful. Persistent effort should be made to reduce the dosage by attention to hygienic measures. In anæmia and chlorosis, a sulphur confection taken in the morning, and a pill of iron, rhubarb, and aloes throughout the day, are very serviceable. Certain very severe cases are benefited by "short-circuiting," the lower end of the ileum being joined to the lower end of the colon.

In children the indications should be met, as far as possible, by hygienic and dietetic measures. In the constipation of sucklings a change in the diet of the mother may be tried, or from one to three teaspoonfuls of cream may be given before each nursing. In artificially fed children the top milk with the cream should be used. Drinking of water, barley water, or oatmeal water will sometimes obviate the difficulty. If laxatives are required, simple syrup, manna, or olive oil may be sufficient. The conical piece of soap, so often seen in nurseries, is sometimes efficacious. Massage along the colon may be tried. Small injections of cold water may be used. Large injections should be avoided, if possible. If it is necessary to give a laxative by the mouth, castor oil or the fluid magnesia is the best. The saline purgatives appear to act by increasing the muscular and glandular activity of the bowel. If there are signs of gastro-intestinal irritation, rhubarb and soda or gray powder may be given. In older children the diet should be carefully regulated.

VI. ENTEROPTOSIS

(*Glénard's Disease*)

Definition.—"Dropping of the viscera," visceroptosis, is not a disease, but a symptom group characterized by looseness of the mesenteric and peritoneal attachments, so that the stomach, the intestines, particularly the transverse colon, the liver, the kidneys, and the spleen occupy an abnormally low position in the abdominal cavity.

Symptoms and Physical Signs.—It is important to recognize two groups of cases. In one the splanchnoptosis follows the loss of normal support of the abdominal wall in consequence of repeated pregnancies or recurring ascites. The condition may be extreme without the slightest distress on the part of the patient.

The second and more important group occurs usually in young persons, who present, with splanchnoptosis, the features of more or less marked neurasthenia.

In the first group inspection of the abdomen shows a very relaxed abdominal wall, and, as a rule, the lineæ albicantes of recurring pregnancies. Peristalsis of the intestines may be seen, and in extreme cases the outlines of the stomach itself with its waves of peristalsis. On inflating the stomach with carbonic-acid gas the organ stands out with great prominence, and the lesser and greater curvatures are seen, the latter extending perhaps a hand's breadth below the level of the navel. The waves of peristalsis are feeble and without the vigor and force of those seen in the stomach dilated from stricture of the pylorus. The condition of descensus ventriculi with atony is best studied in this group of cases. An important point to remember is that it may exist in an extreme grade without symptoms.

In the other group is embraced a somewhat motley series of cases, in which, with a pronounced nervous or, as we call it now, neurasthenic basis, there are displacements of the viscera *with symptoms*. The patients are usually young, more frequently women than men, and of spare habit. The condition may follow an acute illness with wasting. They complain, as a rule, of dyspepsia, throbbing in the abdomen, and dragging pains or weakness in the back, and inability to perform the usual duties of life. A very considerable proportion of all the cases of neurasthenia present the local features of enteroptosis. When preparing for the examination one notices usually an erythematous flushing of the skin; the scratch of the nail is followed instantly by a line of hyperæmia, less often of marked pallor. The pulsation of the abdominal aorta is readily seen.

Radiography has given much information of the position of the viscera and the patients should be examined carefully after a bismuth meal. The stomach is vertically placed and reaches far below the navel; its motility may be normal, but there may be stasis from associated pyloric spasm or from kinking of the duodenum. Inflated with gas the outlines may be seen through the thin skin. Clapotâge or splashing is usually distinct.

Nephroptosis, or displacement of the kidney, is one of the most constant phenomena in enteroptosis. It is well, perhaps, to distinguish between the kidney which one can just touch on deep inspiration—palpable kidney—one which is freely movable, and which on deep inspiration descends so that one can put the fingers of the palpating hand above it and hold it down, and, thirdly, a floating kidney, which is entirely outside the costal arch, is easily grasped in the hand, readily moved to the middle line, and low down toward the right iliac fossa. It is held by some that the designation floating kidney should be restricted to the cases in which there is a meso-nephron, but this is excessively rare, while extreme grades of renal mobility are common. Some of the more serious sequences of movable kidney, namely, Dietl's crises and intermittent hypdronephrosis, will be considered with diseases of the kidney.

Displacement of the liver is very much less common. In thin women who have laced, the organ is often tilted forward, so that a very large surface of the lobes comes in contact with the abdominal wall; it is a very common mistake under these circumstances to think that the organ is enlarged. Dislocation of the liver itself will be considered later.

Mobility of the spleen is sometimes very marked in enteroptosis. In an extreme grade it may be found in almost any region of the abdomen. It is very frequently mistaken for a fibroid or ovarian tumor. A considerable proportion of the cases come first under the care of the gynecologist.

There is usually much relaxation of the mesentery and of the peritoneal folds which support the intestines. The colon is displaced downward (coloptosis), with consequent kinking at the flexures. The descent may be so low that the transverse colon is at the brim of or even in the pelvis. It may indeed be fixed or bent in the form of a V. It is frequently to be felt, as Glénard states, as a firm cord crossing the abdomen at or below the level of the navel. This kinking may take place not only in the colon, but at the pylorus, where the duodenum passes into the jejunum, and where the ileum enters the cæcum.

The explanation of the phenomena accompanying enteroptosis is by no means easy. It has been suggested by Glénard and others that overfilling of the splanchnic vessels in consequence of displacements and kinking accounts for the feelings of exhaustion and general nervousness. In a large proportion of the cases, however, no symptoms occur until after an illness or some protracted nervous strain.

Treatment.—In a majority of all cases four indications are present: To treat the existing neurasthenia, to relieve the nervous dyspepsia, to overcome the constipation, and to afford mechanical support to the organs. Three of these are considered under their appropriate sections. In cases in which the enteroptosis has followed loss in weight after an acute illness or worries and cares an important indication is to fatten the patient.

A well-adapted abdominal bandage is one of the most important measures in enteroptosis. In many of the milder grades it alone suffices. I know of no single simple measure which affords relief to distressing symptoms in so many cases as the abdominal bandage. It is best made of linen, should fit snugly, and should be arranged with straps so that it can not ride up over the hips. A special form must be used, as will be mentioned later, for movable kidney. In some cases support may be given by the use of adhesive strapping. Some of the more aggravated types of enteroptosis are combined with such features of neurasthenia that a rigid Weir Mitchell treatment is indicated. In a few very refractory cases surgical interference may be called for.

And, lastly, the physician must be careful in dealing with the subjects of enteroptosis not to lay too much stress on the disorder. It is well never to tell the patient that a kidney is movable; the symptoms may date from a knowledge of the existence of the condition.

VII. MISCELLANEOUS AFFECTIONS

I. MUCOUS COLITIS

Known by various names, such as *membranous enteritis, tubular diarrhœa, mucous colic,* and *myxoneurosis intestinalis,* this remarkable disease has been recognized for several centuries. An exhaustive description of it is given by Woodward in vol. ii of the Medical and Surgical Reports of the Civil War. The passage of mucus in large quantities from the bowel is met with, *first,* in catarrh of the intestine, due to various causes. It is not uncommon in children, and may be associated with disturbances of digestion and slight colic. *Secondly,* in local disease or irritation of the bowel, in cancer of the colon and of the rectum. In tubo-ovarian disease much mucus and slime may be passed. *Thirdly,* true mucous colitis, a secretion neurosis of the large intestine met with particularly in nervous and hysterical patients. It is more common in women than in men. It has increased greatly of late years, and has become the fashionable complaint, displacing neuritis to a great extent. There is an abnormal secretion of a tenacious mucus, which may be slimy and gelatinous, like frog-spawn, or it is passed in strings or strips, more rarely as a continuous tubular membrane. I have twice seen this membrane *in situ,* closely adherent to the mucosa, but capable of separation without any lesion of the surface. Microscopically the casts are mucoid, of a uniform granular ground substance through which there are remnants of cells, some of which have undergone a definite hyaline transformation. Triple phosphate, cholesterin, and fatty crystals are present, and occasionally fine, sand-like concretions. The epithelium of the mucosa seems to be intact.

Symptoms.—In a large proportion of all the cases the subjects are nervous in greater or less degree. Some cases have had hysterical outbreaks, and there may be hypochondriasis or melancholia. The patients are self-centred and often much worried about the mucous stools. Some of the cases are among the most distressing with which we have to deal, invalids of from ten to twenty years' standing, neurasthenic to an extreme degree, with recurring attacks of pain and the passage of large quantities of mucus or even of intestinal casts.

In many cases the attacks may come on in paroxysms, associated with colicky pains, or occasionally crises of the greatest severity, so that appendicitis may be suspected. Emotional disturbances, worry of all sorts, or an error in diet may bring on an attack. Constipation is a special feature in many cases. Sometimes there are attacks of nervous diarrhœa.

While the disease is obstinate and distressing, it is rarely serious, though Herringham states that he knew of three cases of mucous colitis in which death occurred suddenly, in all with great pain in the left side of the abdomen. The abdomen itself is rarely distended. There is often a very painful spot just between the navel and the left costal border, tender on pressure, and sometimes the paroxysms of pain seem centred in this region. A spastic condition of the colon frequently exists and is easily recognized by palpation.

Diagnosis.—The diagnosis is rarely doubtful, but it is important not to mistake the membranes for other substances; thus, the external cuticle of asparagus and undigested portions of meat or sausage-skins sometimes assume forms not unlike mucous casts, but microscopic examination will quickly differentiate them. Mucous colitis with severe pain may be mistaken for appendicitis.

Treatment.—Drugs are of little value. It is quite useless to give bismuth and so-called intestinal remedies. First the basic neurasthenic state is to be dealt with, and this may suffice for a cure. Secondly, daily irrigations of the colon through a long tube—one to two pints of warm alkaline fluid. At Plombières, Harrogate, and other spas this treatment is most successfully carried out. The injection of olive oil at bedtime is sometimes helpful. It should be retained during the night. Thirdly, the coarser sorts of food which leave a large residue should be eaten, and, lastly, should these measures fail, the question of opening the colon or irrigating through the appendix may be considered.

II. DILATATION OF THE COLON

There are four groups of cases. In the first the distention is entirely gaseous, and occurs not infrequently as a transient condition. In many cases it has an important influence, inasmuch as it may be extreme, pushing up the diaphragm and seriously impairing the action of the heart and lungs. It is an occasional cause of sudden heart-failure. In pneumonia and other acute diseases this inflation of the colon may be extreme.

In the second group are the cases in which the distention of the colon is caused by solid substances, as fæcal matter, occasionally by foreign bodies introduced from without, and more rarely by gall-stones. In institutions, particularly in insane asylums, it is not infrequent to find the aged with great distention of the colon.

When, thirdly, the dilatation is due to an organic obstruction in front of the dilated gut, the colon may reach a very large size. These cases are common enough in malignant tumors and sometimes in volvulus. Dilatation of the sigmoid flexure occurs particularly when this portion of the bowel is congenitally very long. In such cases the bowel may be so distended that it occupies the greater part of the abdomen, pushing up the liver and the diaphragm. An acute condition is sometimes caused by a twist in the meso-colon. And, fourthly—

Idiopathic Dilatation.—Hirschsprung's disease. The cases are not uncommon, occurring in children and in young adults. The sigmoid flexure alone or the entire colon is involved, and the size may be colossal. In Formad's case the circumference of the colon was from fifteen to thirty inches, and the weight of the contents forty-seven pounds. The origin is obscure. In some the condition is congenital, and the dilatation and hypertrophy increase progressively; in others there is an unusually long sigmoid flexure; in others again narrowing of the terminal portion of the descending colon or a valve-like structure has been found. The *symptoms* are very definite—constipation, an enlarged abdomen, attacks of pain with increasing distention, and then diarrhœa, either natural or induced, with relief. Such attacks may occur from birth and continue to the twentieth or thirtieth year. The abdominal picture is distinctive—the great enlargement of the upper half of the abdomen, the spreading of the costal arch, the remarkable length from the ensiform cartilage to the navel, and in the attacks the coils of the colon stand out prominently, and even the longitudinal bands may be seen.

The outlook is uncertain. Medical treatment is of little avail. I have seen one case in a young child in which scrupulous care of the bowels seemed to check the progress; but, as a rule, it is a progressive malady for which surgery alone offers complete relief. Resection of the enlarged colon has now been done in a good many cases with success. Colotomy gives relief; colostomy has also been successful. Of 44 cases treated surgically, 15 were completely cured and 7 were improved (Finney).

III. INTESTINAL SAND

"Sable Intestinal."—There are two groups of cases in which sand-like material is passed with the stools. The *false,* in which it is made up of the remains of vegetable food and fruits which have resisted digestion or which have become encrusted with earthy salts. *True* intestinal sand of animal origin, gritty fine particles, usually gray or colorless, sometimes dark, is formed in the bowel and is made up largely of lime salts. In mucous colitis this material may be passed at intervals for months.

IV. DIVERTICULITIS—PERISIGMOIDITIS

In the lower part of the descending colon and in the sigmoid flexure diverticula occur, sometimes congenital, sometimes acquired, most commonly in women and in association with constipation. Of 81 cases collected by Telling, 53 were in males. They are prone to form at the site of the appendices epiploicæ. Intestinal obstruction, acute gangrene, perforation with the formation of abscess, peritonitis, vesico-colic fistula, and metastatic suppuration are occasional complications. In acute cases left-sided appendicitis is diagnosed, while in the chronic cases the mimicry of cancer is very close. The cases are more common than we have heretofore supposed. Resection of the affected portion of the colon has been successfully performed.

V. AFFECTIONS OF THE MESENTERY

Hæmorrhage (*Hæmatoma*).—Instances in which the bleeding is confined to the mesenteric tissues are rare; more commonly the condition is associated with hæmorrhagic infiltration of the pancreas and with retroperitoneal hæmorrhage. It occurs in rupture of aneurisms, either of the abdominal aorta or of the superior mesenteric artery, in malignant forms of the infectious fevers, small-pox, and, lastly, in individuals in whom no predisposing conditions exist.

Affections of the Mesenteric Vessels.—(*a*) ANEURISM (see under Arteries).

(*b*) EMBOLISM AND THROMBOSIS.—*Infarction of the Bowel.*—When the mesenteric vessels are blocked by emboli or thrombi the condition of infarction follows in the territory supplied, which may pass on to gangrene or to perforation and peritonitis. If the superior mesenteric artery is blocked the result is fatal. In the veins the thrombosis may be primary, following infective processes in the intestines, particularly about the appendix, or it occurs in cachectic states. Secondary thrombosis is met with in cirrhosis of the liver, syphilis, and pylephlebitis, or may result from the stasis caused by arterial emboli. Jackson, Porter, and Quimby have made an exhaustive study of 30 Boston cases, and have collected 214 cases. They recognize two groups—acute and chronic. In the former the onset is sudden, with colic, nausea, vomiting, and a bloody diarrhœa, so that the picture is one of acute obstruction. The abdomen becomes distended and death occurs in collapse within a few days. In the chronic cases the onset is insidious, and there may be no symptoms referable to the abdomen. Of the 214 cases, 64 per cent. were in men. The diagnosis is extremely difficult, and the acute cases are usually regarded as obstruction. Exploratory operation has been made in 47 cases, 4 of which have recovered. In J. W. Elliot's successful case 48 inches of the bowel were resected. In the horse, infarction of the intestine, commonly in connection with the verminous aneurisms of the mesenteric arteries, is the usual cause of colic.

Diseases of the Mesenteric Veins.—Dilatation and sclerosis occur in cirrhosis of the liver. In instances of prolonged obstruction there may be large saccular dilatations with calcification of the intima, as in a case of obliteration of the venæ portæ described by me. Suppuration of the mesenteric veins is not rare, and occurs usually in connection with pylephlebitis. The mesentery may be much swollen and is like a bag of pus, and it is only on careful dissection that one sees that the pus is really within channels representing extremely dilated mesenteric veins.

Disorders of the Chyle Vessels.—Varicose, cavernous, and cystic chylangiomata are met with in the mucosa and submucosa of the small intestine, occasionally of the stomach. Extravasation of chyle into the mesenteric tissue is sometimes seen. Chylous cysts are found. I saw one the size of an egg at the root of the mesentery. Bramann records a case in a man aged sixty-three, in which a cyst of this kind the size of a child's head was healed by operation. There is an instance on record of a congenital malformation of the thoracic duct, in which the receptaculum formed a flattened cyst which discharged into the peritoneum, and a chylous ascitic fluid was withdrawn on several occasions. Homans reported the case of a girl who, from the third to the thirteenth year, had an enlarged abdomen. Laparotomy showed a series of cysts containing clear fluid. They were supposed to be dilated lymph vessels connected with the intestines.

Cysts of the Mesentery.—They may be either dermoid, hydatid, serous, sanguineous, or chylous. They occur at any portion of the mesentery, and range from a few inches in diameter to large masses occupying the entire abdomen. They are frequently adherent to the neighboring organs, to the liver, spleen, uterus, and sigmoid flexure.

The symptoms usually are those of a progressively enlarging tumor in the abdomen. Sometimes a mass develops rapidly, particularly in the hæmorrhagic forms. Colic and constipation are present in some cases. The general health, as a rule, is well maintained in spite of the progressive enlargement of the abdomen, which is most prominent in the umbilical region. Mesenteric cysts may persist for many years, even ten or twenty.

The diagnosis is extremely uncertain, and no single feature is in any way distinctive. The important signs are: the great mobility, the situation in the middle line, and the zone of tympany in front of the tumor. Of these, the second is the only one which is at all constant, as when the tumors are large the mobility disappears, and at this stage the intestines, too, are pushed to one side. It is most frequently mistaken for ovarian tumor. Movable kidney, hydronephrosis, and cysts of the omentum have also been confused with it. In certain instances puncture may be made for diagnostic purposes, but it is better to advise laparotomy for the purpose of drainage, or, if possible, enucleation may be practiced.

H. DISEASES OF THE LIVER

I. JAUNDICE

(*Icterus*)

Definition.—Jaundice or icterus is a condition characterized by coloration of the skin, mucous membranes, and fluids of the body by the bile-pigment.

Like albuminuria, jaundice is a symptom and not a disease, and is met with in a variety of conditions.

1. OBSTRUCTIVE JAUNDICE

The chief causes of obstructive jaundice are: (1) Obstruction by foreign bodies within the ducts, as gall-stones and parasites; (2) by inflammatory tumefaction of the duodenum or of the lining membrane of the duct; (3) by stricture or obliteration of the duct; (4) by tumors closing the orifice of the duct or growing in its interior; (5) by pressure on the duct from without, as by tumors of the liver itself, of the stomach, pancreas, kidney, or omentum; by pressure of enlarged glands in the fissures of the liver, and, more rarely, of abdominal aneurism, fæcal accumulation, or the pregnant uterus.

In these case of extra-hepatic or obstructive jaundice the pressure within the biliary capillaries, usually low, becomes increased and the bile is absorbed by the lymphatics of the liver and not by the blood capillaries. To these causes some add lowering of the blood pressure in the portal system so that the tension in the smaller bile-ducts is greater than in the blood-vessels. For this view, however, there is no positive evidence. In this class may perhaps be placed the cases of jaundice from mental shock or depressed emotions, which "may conceivably cause spasm and reversed peristalsis of the bile-duct" (W. Hunter).

General Symptoms of Obstructive Jaundice.—(*a*) *Icterus, or tinting of the skin and conjunctivæ.* The color ranges from a lemon-yellow in catarrhal jaundice to a deep olive-green or bronzed hue in permanent obstruction. In some instances the color of the skin is greenish black, the so-called "black jaundice." Except the central nervous system, all of the tissues are stained.

(*b*) In the more chronic forms *pruritus* is a most distressing symptom. There is a curious preicteric itching, which Riessman thinks is suggestive of cancer, but I have seen it most marked in gall-stone cases. Sweating is common, and may be curiously localized to the abdomen or to the palms of the hands. Lichen, urticaria, and boils may occur. *Xanthoma multiplex* is rare. Only two cases have occurred under my observation. Usually in the flat form, rarely nodular, they are most common in the eyelids and on the hands and feet. They may be very numerous over the whole body. Occasionally the tumors are found in the bile duct. After persisting for years they may disappear. In very chronic cases telangiectases develop in the skin, sometimes in large numbers over the body and face, occasionally on the mucous membrane of the tongue and lips, forming patches of a bright red color from 1 to 2 cm. in breadth.

(*c*) The *secretions* are colored with bile-pigment. The sweat tinges the linen; the tears and saliva and milk are rarely stained. The expectoration is not often tinted unless there is inflammation, as when pneumonia coexists with jaundice. The urine may contain the pigment before it is apparent in the skin or conjunctiva. The color varies from light greenish yellow to a deep black-green. In cases of jaundice of long standing or great intensity the urine usually contains albumin and always bile-stained tube-casts.

(*d*) *No bile passes into the intestine.* The stools therefore are of a pale drab or slate-gray color, and usually very fetid and pasty. The "clay-color" of the stools is also in part due to the presence of undigested fat which, according to Müller, may be increased from 7 to 10 per cent., which is normal, to 55 or 78.5 per cent. There may be constipation; in many instances, owing to decomposition, there is diarrhœa.

(*e*) *Slow pulse.* The heart's action may fall to 40, 30, or even to 20 per minute. It is particularly noticeable in the cases of catarrhal and recent jaundice, and is not as a rule an unfavorable symptom. Whether this is due to interrupted conductivity or to direct poisoning of the auriculo-ventricular bundle has not been determined. It occurs only in the early stages of jaundice. At this time bile acids pass into the blood, but are produced in very small quantities when jaundice is established. The respirations may fall to 10 or even to 7 per minute. Xanthopsia, or yellow vision, may occur.

(*f*) *Hæmorrhage.* The tendency to bleeding in chronic icterus is a serious feature. It has been shown that the blood-coagulation time may be much retarded, and instead of from three minutes and a half to four minutes and a half we have found it in some cases as late as eleven or twelve minutes. This is a point which should be taken account of by surgeons, inasmuch as incontrollable hæmorrhage is a well-recognized accident in operating upon patients with chronic obstructive jaundice. Purpura, large subcutaneous extravasations, more rarely hæmorrhages from the mucous membranes, occur in protracted jaundice, and in the more severe forms.

(*g*) *Cerebral symptoms.* Irritability, great depression of spirits, or even melancholia may be present. In any case of persistent jaundice special nervous phenomena may develop and rapidly prove fatal—such as sudden coma, acute delirium, or convulsions. Usually the patient has a rapid pulse, slight fever, and a dry tongue, and he passes into the so-called "typhoid state." These features are not nearly so common in obstructive as in febrile jaundice, but they not infrequently terminate a chronic icterus in whatever way produced. The group of symptoms has been termed *cholæmia,* or, on the supposition that cholesterin is the poison, *cholesteræmia;* but its true nature has not yet been determined. In some of the cases the symptoms may be due to uræmia.

2. TOXÆMIC AND HÆMOLYTIC JAUNDICE

The term hæmatogenous jaundice was formerly applied to this group in contradistinction to the hepatogenous jaundice, associated with manifest obstructive changes in the bile-passages. The toxic jaundice cases are essentially obstructive in origin, and it is doubtful whether there are any true non-obstructive cases. The manner in which the jaundice is produced in these cases has been experimentally worked out by Stadelmann and Afanassiew. The obstruction is due to the extreme viscidity of the bile associated with a mild angiocolitis. The sequence of events is as follows: Destruction of blood by hæmolysis; liberation of hæmoglobin with increased formation and excretion of bile pigments (polychromia); increased viscidity of the bile, which, at the low pressure at which the bile is excreted, causes a temporary obstruction, with reabsorption of the bile and jaundice; finally the bile loses its viscid character, the flow is reëstablished, and the jaundice disappears. Stadelmann found that a similar explanation applies to other varieties of jaundice associated with increased blood destruction. For this type the name "hæmohepatogenous" jaundice has been suggested. Rolleston refers to them as cases of "intrahepatic" jaundice. Hunter groups the causes as follows: 1. Jaundice produced by the action of poisons, such as toluylendiamin, phosphorus, arsenic, snake-venom. 2. Jaundice met with in various specific fevers and conditions, such as yellow fever, malaria (remittent and intermittent), pyæmia, relapsing fever, typhus, enteric fever, scarlatina. 3. Jaundice met with in various conditions of unknown but more or less obscure infective nature, and variously designated as epidemic, infectious, febrile, malignant jaundice, icterus gravis, Weil's disease, acute yellow atrophy.

The symptoms are not nearly so striking as in the obstructive variety. The bile is present in the stools. The skin has in many cases only a slight lemon tint. The urine may contain no bile-pigment, but the urinary pigments are considerably increased. In the severer forms, as in acute yellow atrophy, the color may be more intense, but in malaria and pernicious anæmia the tint is usually light. The constitutional disturbance may be very profound, with high fever, delirium, convulsions, suppression of urine, black vomit, and cutaneous hæmorrhages. In certain cases of hæmolytic jaundice the fragility of the red corpuscles is greatly increased and they may be smaller than normal (Widal, Chauffard) and show granular degeneration. This is particularly the case in the group of congenital icterus with enlarged spleen.

3. HEREDITARY ICTERUS

A family form of icterus has long been known. We must recognize, indeed, several groups. First, icterus neonatorum, as in the remarkable instance described by Glaister (Lancet, March, 1879), in which a woman had eight children, six of whom died of jaundice shortly after birth; one of the cases had stenosis of the common duct, which, as John Thomson has shown, is, with angiocholitis, a common lesion in this affection. Still more remarkable is it that the mother of this woman had twelve children, all of whom were icteric after birth, but the jaundice gradually disappeared. A brother of the woman had several children who also were jaundiced at birth. Glaister states that all of the children of Morgagni, fifteen in number, had icterus neonatorum. Secondly, the congenital acholuric icterus. Minkowski reported eight cases in three generations. The jaundice is slight, the stools are not clay colored, the urine has no bile pigment but contains urobilin, the general health is little if at all disturbed. Splenic enlargement is a marked feature. Many cases have now been reported of this Minkowski type, nearly all in family groups, but Chauffard has met with a case without hereditary basis and I have seen at least one case of the kind. No special changes have been found in the liver or bile passages. Thirdly, a group of cases with enlargement of the spleen and liver and marked constitutional disturbances, anæmia, dwarfing of stature, infantilism, and slight jaundice. Cases which have been described as Hanot's cirrhosis have occurred in two or three members of a family, and the jaundice has dated from early childhood.

Jaundice has been described in connection with the various fevers, malaria, yellow fever, and Weil's disease. Two special affections may here receive consideration, the icterus of the new-born and acute yellow atrophy.

II. ICTERUS NEONATORUM

New-born infants are liable to jaundice, which in some instances rapidly proves fatal. A mild and a severe form may be recognized.

The *mild or physiological icterus* of the new-born is a common disease in foundling hospitals, and is not very infrequent in private practice. In 900 consecutive births at the Sloane Maternity icterus was noted in 300 cases (Holt). The discoloration appears early, usually on the first or second day, and is of moderate intensity. The urine may be bile-stained and the fæces colorless. The nutrition of the child is not usually disturbed, and in the majority of cases the jaundice disappears within two weeks. This form is never fatal. The cause of this jaundice is not at all clear. Some have attributed it to stasis in the smaller bile-ducts, which are compressed by the distended radicals of the portal vein. Others hold that the jaundice is due to the destruction of a large number of red blood-corpuscles during the first few days after birth.

The *severe form* of icterus in the new-born may depend upon (*a*) congenital absence of the common or hepatic duct, of which there are many instances on record; (*b*) congenital syphilitic hepatitis; and (*c*) septic poisoning, associated with phlebitis of the umbilical vein. This is a severe and fatal form, in which also hæmorrhage from the cord may occur.

Curiously enough, in contradistinction to other forms, the brain and cord may be stained yellow in icterus neonatorum, sometimes diffusely, more rarely in definite foci corresponding to the ganglion cells which have become deeply stained (Schmorl).

III. ACUTE YELLOW ATROPHY

(Malignant Jaundice; Icterus Gravis)

Definition.—An acute widespread autolytic necrosis of the liver cells of unknown origin, characterized by jaundice, toxæmia and a reduction in the volume of the liver.

Etiology.—The first authentic account was given by the famous old Paris doctor Ballonius—sometimes called the French Hippocrates (1538-1616). Bright gave a good description in 1836. It is a rare disease, as among 28,000 medical cases admitted to the Johns Hopkins Hospital in nearly twenty-three years there were only three cases. It varies in frequency in different countries, and seems to be more rare in the United States than in Germany and England. The majority of cases occur between the tenth and the fortieth year. Rolleston has collected 22 cases occurring within the first ten years of life.

Recent studies have thrown a good deal of light upon the subject; we now know that acute necrosis of the liver occurs under many conditions: (*a*) In the infections, syphilis, typhoid fever, diphtheria, septicæmia, these necroses may be widespread. (*b*) Non-bacterial poisons. The remarkable delayed chloroform poisoning is a hepatic necrosis resembling very closely acute yellow atrophy. Phosphorus produces a similar condition, and possibly mercury. (*c*) Autogenous poisons, produced in connection with pregnancy and parturition. The ordinary necrotic foci of the liver in pregnancy are the same kind but less in degree than those of acute yellow atrophy.

An exaggeration of any of these types may lead to a clinical condition which we call acute yellow atrophy. Its association with pregnancy is remarkable. More than one-half of the cases occur in women, and in a large proportion of these during the middle or latter half of pregnancy. The disease has followed a profound shock, or mental emotion. It occurs occasionally in syphilis and other acute infections, and there are cases of cirrhosis of the liver, particularly of the hypertrophic form, associated with diffuse necrosis, intense jaundice and toxæmia. We are as yet ignorant of the conditions under which the poisons, bacterial or metabolic, cause this widespread necrosis.

Morbid Anatomy.—The liver is greatly reduced in size, looks thin and flattened, and sometimes does not reach more than one-half or even one-third of its normal weight. It is flabby and the capsule is wrinkled. Externally the organ has a greenish-yellow color. On section the color may be yellowish-brown, yellowish-red, or mottled, and the outlines of the lobules are indistinct. The yellow and dark-red portions represent different stages of the same process—the yellow an earlier, the red a more advanced stage. The organ may cut with considerable firmness. Microscopically the liver-cells are seen in all stages of necrosis, and in spots appear to have undergone complete destruction, leaving a fatty, granular *débris* with pigment grains and crystals of leucin and tyrosin. Hæmorrhages occur between the liver-cells. There is a cholangitis of the smaller bile-ducts. Marchand, MacCallum, and others have described regenerative changes in the cases which do not run an acute course.

The other organs show extensive bile-staining, and there are numerous hæmorrhages. The kidneys may show marked granular degeneration of the epithelium, and usually there is fatty degeneration of the heart. In a majority of the cases the spleen is enlarged.

Symptoms.—In the initial stage there is gastro-duodenal catarrh, and at first the jaundice is thought to be of a simple nature. In some instances this lasts only a few days, in others two or three weeks. Then severe symptoms set in—headache, delirium, trembling of the muscles, and, in some instances, convulsions. Vomiting is a constant symptom, and blood may be brought up. Hæmorrhages occur into the skin or from the mucous surfaces; in pregnant women abortion may occur. The jaundice usually increases, coma sets in and gradually deepens until death. The body temperature is variable; in a majority of the cases the disease runs an afebrile course, though sometimes just before death there is an elevation. In some instances, however, there has been marked pyrexia. The pulse is usually rapid, the tongue coated and dry, and the patient is in a "typhoid state." There may be complete obliteration of the liver dulness. This is due to the flabby organ falling away from the abdominal walls and allowing the intestinal coils to take its place.

The urine is bile-stained and often contains tube-casts. Frequently albuminuria and occasionally albumosuria occur. Urea is markedly diminished. There is a corresponding increase in the percentage of nitrogen present as ammonia. Herter finds it may be increased from the normal 2 to 5 per cent. up to 17 per cent. The diminution in urea is probably partly due to the liver-cells failing to manufacture urea from ammonia, but it may also be in part due to organic acids seizing on the ammonia, and thus preventing the formation of urea out of the basic ammonia. Leucin and tyrosin are not constantly present; of 23 cases collected by Hunter, in 9 neither was found; in 10 both were present; in 3 tyrosin only; in 1 leucin only. The present view is that the leucin and tyrosin are derived from the liver-cells themselves as a result of their extensive destruction. In the majority of cases no bile enters the intestines, and the stools are clay-colored. The disease is almost invariably fatal. In a few instances recovery has been noted. I saw in Leube's clinic, at Würzburg, a case which was convalescent.

The duration and the type of the disease depend upon the extent and the rapidity of progress of the necrosis. Cases have lasted as long as forty days, while death has occurred as early as the second day. A sub-acute form has been described by Milne, a slow necrosis lasting many months, associated with jaundice—a protracted stage from which recovery is possible by regeneration of liver tissue, but consecutive cirrhosis is the rule.

Diagnosis.—Jaundice with vomiting, diminution of the liver volume, delirium, and the presence of leucin and tyrosin in the urine, form a characteristic and unmistakable group of symptoms. Leucin and tyrosin are not, however, distinctive. They may be present in cases of afebrile jaundice with slight enlargement of the liver.

It is not to be forgotten that any severe jaundice may be associated with intense cerebral symptoms. The clinical features in certain cases of hypertrophic cirrhosis are almost identical, but the enlargement of the liver, the more constant occurrence of fever, and the absence of leucin and tyrosin are distinguishing signs. Phosphorus poisoning may closely simulate acute yellow atrophy, particularly in the hæmorrhages, jaundice, and the diminution in the liver volume, but the gastric symptoms are usually more marked, and leucin and tyrosin are stated not to occur in the urine.

Treatment.—No known remedies have any influence on the course of the disease. Theoretically, efforts should be made to eliminate the toxins before they produce their degenerative effects by free purgation and the use of subcutaneous and intravenous saline injections. Gastric sedatives may be used to allay the distressing vomiting.

IV. AFFECTIONS OF THE BLOOD-VESSELS OF THE LIVER

Anæmia.—On the post mortem table, when the liver looks anæmic, as in the fatty or amyloid organ, the blood-vessels, which during life were probably well filled, can be readily injected. There are no symptoms indicative of this condition.

Hyperæmia.—This occurs in two forms.

(*a*) Active Hyperæmia.—After each meal the rapid absorption by the portal vessels induces transient congestion of the organ, which, however, is entirely physiological; but it is quite possible that in persons who persistently eat and drink too much this active hyperæmia may lead to functional disturbance, or, in the case of drinking too freely of alcohol, to organic change. In the fevers an acute hyperæmia may be present.

The *symptoms* of active hyperæmia are indefinite. Possibly the sense of distress or fullness in the right hypochondrium, so often metioned by dyspeptics and by those who eat and drink freely, may be due to this cause. There are probably diurnal variations in the volume of the liver. In cirrhosis with enlargement the rapid reduction in volume after a copious hæmorrhage indicates the important part which hyperæmia plays even in organic troubles. It is stated that suppression of the menses or suppression of a hæmorrhoidal flow is followed by hyperæmia of the liver. Andrew H. Smith has described a case of periodical enlargement of the liver.

(*b*) Passive Congestion.—This is much more common and results from an increase of pressure in the efferent vessels or sub-lobular branches of the hepatic veins. Every condition leading to venous stasis in the right heart at once affects these veins.

In chronic valvular disease, in emphysema, cirrhosis of the lung, and in intrathoracic tumors mechanical congestion occurs and finally leads to very definite changes. The liver is enlarged, firm, and of a deep-red color; the hepatic vessels are greatly engorged, particularly the central vein in each lobule and its adjacent capillaries. On section the organ presents a peculiar mottled appearance, owing to the deeply congested hepatic and the anæmic portal territories; hence the term *nutmeg* which has been given to this condition. Gradually the distention of the central capillaries reaches such a grade that atrophy of the intervening liver-cells is induced. Brown pigment is deposited about the centre of the lobules and the connective tissue is greatly increased. In this cyanotic induration or cardiac liver the organ is large in the early stage, but later it may become contracted. Occasionally in this form the connective tissue is increased about the lobules as well, but the process usually extends from the sub-lobular and central veins.

The symptoms of this form are not always to be separated from those of the associated conditions. Gastro-intestinal catarrh is usually present and hæmatemesis may occur. The portal obstruction in advanced cases leads to ascites, which may precede the development of general dropsy. There is often slight jaundice, the stools may be clay-colored, and the urine contains bile-pigment.

On examination the organ is found to be increased in size. It may be a full hand's breadth below the costal margin and tender on pressure. It is in this condition particularly that we meet with pulsation of the liver. We must distinguish the communicated throbbing of the heart, which is very common, from the heaving, diffuse impulse due to regurgitation into the hepatic veins, in which, when one hand is upon the ensiform cartilage and the other upon the right side at the margin of the ribs, the whole liver can be felt to dilate with each impulse.

The indications for *treatment* in passive hyperæmia are to restore the balance of the circulation and to unload the engorged portal vessels. In cases of intense hyperæmia 18 or 20 ounces of blood may be directly aspirated from the liver, as advised by George Harley and practiced by many Anglo-Indian physicians. Good results sometimes follow this hepato-phlebotomy. The prompt relief and marked reduction in the volume of the organ which follow an attack of hæmatemesis or bleeding from piles suggest this practice. Salts administered by Matthew Hay's method deplete the portal system freely and thoroughly. As a rule, the treatment must be that of the condition with which it is associated.

Diseases of the Portal Vein.—(*a*) THROMBOSIS; ADHESIVE PYLEPHLEBITIS.—Coagulation of blood in the portal vein is met with in cirrhosis, in syphilis of the liver, invasion of the vein by cancer, proliferative peritonitis involving the gastro-hepatic omentum, perforation of the vein by gall-stones, and occasionally follows sclerosis of the walls of the portal vein or of its branches. In rare instances a complete collateral circulation is established, the thrombus undergoes the usual change, and ultimately the vein is represented by a fibrous cord, a condition which has been called *pylephlebitis adhesiva*. In a case of this kind which I dissected the portal vein was represented by a narrow fibrous cord; the collateral circulation, which must have been completely established for years, ultimately failed, ascites and hæmatemesis supervened and rapidly proved fatal. The diagnosis of obstruction of the portal vein can rarely be made. A suggestive symptom, however, is a *sudden* onset of the most intense engorgement of the branches of the portal system, leading to hæmatemesis, melæna, ascites, and swelling of the spleen.

Infarcts are not common in the liver and may be either anæmic or hæmorrhagic. They are met with in obstruction of the portal vessels, or of the portal and hepatic veins at the same time, occasionally in disease of the hepatic artery.

(*b*) SUPPURATIVE PYLEPHLEBITIS will be considered in the section on abscess.

Affections of the hepatic vein are extremely rare. Dilatation occurs in cases of chronic enlargement of the right heart, from whatever cause produced. Emboli occasionally pass from the right auricle into the hepatic veins.

Stenosis of the orifices of the hepatic veins may occur as a primary lesion with a special syndrome which has been described by Craven Moore—a progressive enlargement of the liver, signs of involvement of the inferior vena cava, and ascites.

Hepatic Artery.—Enlargement of this vessel is seen in cases of cirrhosis of the liver. It may be the seat of extensive sclerosis. Aneurism of the hepatic artery is rare, but instances are on record, and will be referred to in the section on arteries.

V. DISEASES OF THE BILE-PASSAGES AND GALL-BLADDER

I. ACUTE CATARRH OF THE BILE-DUCTS

(*Catarrhal Jaundice*)

Definition.—Jaundice due to swelling and obstruction of the terminal portion of the common duct.

Etiology.—General catarrhal inflammation of the bile-ducts is usually associated with gall-stones. The catarrhal process now under consideration is probably always an extension of a gastro-duodenal catarrh, and the process is most intense in the *pars intestinalis* of the duct, which projects into the duodenum. The mucous membrane is swollen, and a plug of inspissated mucus fills the diverticulum of Vater, and the narrower portion just at the orifice, completely obstructing the outflow of bile. It is not known how widespread this catarrh is in the bile-passages, and whether it really passes up the ducts. It would, of course, be possible to have a catarrh of the finer ducts within the liver, which some French writers think may initiate the attack, but the evidence for this is not strong, and it seems more likely that the terminal portion of the duct is always first involved. In the only instance which I have had an opportunity to examine post mortem the orifice was plugged with inspissated mucus, the common and hepatic ducts were slightly distended and contained a bile-tinged, not a clear, mucus, and there were no observable changes in the mucosa of the ducts.

This catarrhal or simple jaundice results from the following causes: (*a*) Duodenal catarrh, in whatever way produced, most commonly following an attack of indigestion. It is most frequently met with in young persons, but may occur at any age, and may follow not only errors in diet, but also cold, exposure, and malaria, as well as the conditions associated with portal obstruction, chronic heart-disease, and Bright's disease. (*b*) Emotional disturbances may be followed by jaundice, which is believed to be due to catarrhal swelling. Cases of this kind are rare and the anatomical condition is unknown. (*c*) Simple or catarrhal jaundice may occur in epidemic form. (*d*) Catarrhal jaundice is occasionally seen in the infectious fevers, such as pneumonia and typhoid fever. The nature of acute catarrhal jaundice is still unknown. It may possibly be an acute infection. In favor of this view are the occurrence in epidemic form and the presence of slight fever. The spleen, however, is not often enlarged. In only 4 out of 23 cases was it palpable.

Symptoms.—There may be neither pain nor distress, and the patient's friends may first notice the yellow tint, or the patient himself may observe it in the looking-glass. In other instances there are dyspeptic symptoms and uneasy sensations in the hepatic region or pains in the back and limbs. In the epidemic form the onset may be more severe, with headache, chill, and vomiting. Fever is rarely present, though the temperature may reach 101 degrees, sometimes 102 degrees. All the signs of obstructive jaundice already mentioned are present, the stools are clay-colored, and the urine contains bile-pigment. The skin has a bright-yellow tint; the greenish, bronzed color is never seen in the simple form. I have once seen spider angiomata on the face in catarrhal jaundice. They disappeared in a few months. The pulse may be normal, but occasionally it is remarkably slow, and may fall to 40 or 30 beats in the minute, and the respirations to as low as 8 per minute. Sleepiness, too, may be present. The liver may be normal in size, but is usually slightly enlarged, and the edge can be felt below the costal margin. Occasionally the enlargement is more marked. As a rule the gall-bladder can not be felt. The spleen may be increased in size. The duration of the disease is from four to eight weeks. There are mild cases in which the jaundice disappears within two weeks; on the other hand, it may persist for three months or even longer. The stools should be carefully watched, for they give the first intimation of removal of the obstruction.

Diagnosis.—This is rarely difficult. The onset in young, comparatively healthy persons, the moderate grade of icterus, the absence of emaciation or of evidences of cirrhosis or cancer usually make the diagnosis easy. Cases which persist for two or three months cause uneasiness, as the suspicion is aroused that it may be more than simple catarrh. The absence of pain, the negative character of the physical examination, and the maintenance of the general nutrition are the points in favor of simple jaundice. There are instances in which time alone can determine the true nature of the case. The possibility of Weil's disease must be borne in mind in anomalous types.

Treatment.—The diet should be simple and the fats restricted. Measures should be used to allay the gastric catarrh, if it is present. A dose of calomel may be given, and the bowels kept open subsequently by salines. The patient should not be violently purged. Bismuth and bicarbonate of soda may be given, and the patient should drink freely of the alkaline mineral waters, of which Vichy is the best. Irrigation of the large bowel with cold water may be practiced. The cold is supposed to excite peristalsis of the gall-bladder and ducts, and thus aid in the expulsion of the mucus.

II. CHRONIC CATARRHAL ANGIOCHOLITIS

This may possibly occur also as a sequel of the acute catarrh. I have never met with an instance, however, in which a chronic, persistent jaundice could be attributed to this cause. A chronic catarrh always accompanies obstruction in the common duct, whether by gall-stones, malignant disease, stricture, or external pressure. There are two groups of cases:

With Complete Obstruction of the Common Duct.—In this form the bile-passages are greatly dilated, the common duct may reach the size of the thumb or larger, there is usually dilatation of the gall-bladder and of the ducts within the liver. The contents of the ducts and of the gall-bladder are a clear, colorless mucus. The mucosa may be everywhere smooth and not swollen. The clear mucus is usually sterile. The patients are the subjects of chronic jaundice, usually without fever.

With Incomplete Obstruction of the Duct.—There is pressure on the duct or there are gall-stones, single or multiple, in the common duct or in the diverticulum of Vater. The bile-passages are not so much dilated, and the contents are a bile-stained, turbid mucus. The gall-bladder is rarely much dilated. In a majority of all cases stones are found in it.

The symptoms of this type of catarrhal angiocholitis are sometimes very distinctive. With it is associated most frequently the so-called hepatic intermittent fever, recurring attacks of chills, fever, and sweats. It is most important to bear in mind that the chills, fever, and sweats do not necessarily mean suppuration.

III. SUPPURATIVE AND ULCERATIVE ANGIOCHOLITIS

The condition is a diffuse, purulent angiocholitis involving the larger and smaller ducts. In a large proportion of all cases there is associated suppurative disease of the gall-bladder.

Etiology.—It is the most serious of the sequels of gall-stones. Occasionally a diffuse suppurative angiocholitis follows the acute infectious cholecystitis; this, however, is rare, since fortunately in the latter condition the cystic duct is usually occluded. Cancer of the duct, or foreign bodies, such as lumbricoids or fish bones, are occasional causes. There may be extension from a suppurative pylephlebitis. In rare instances suppurative cholangitis occurs in the acute infections, as pneumonia and influenza.

The common duct is greatly dilated and may reach the size of the index finger or the thumb; the walls are thickened, and there may be fistulous communications with the stomach, colon, or duodenum. The hepatic ducts and their extensions in the liver are dilated and contain pus mixed with bile. On section of the liver small abscesses are seen, which correspond to the dilated suppurating ducts. The gall-bladder is usually distended, full of pus, and with adhesions to the neighboring parts, or it may have perforated.

Symptoms.—The symptoms of suppurative cholangitis are usually very severe. A previous history of gall-stones, the development of a septic fever, the swelling and tenderness of the liver, the enlargement of the gall-bladder, and the leucocytosis are suggestive features. Jaundice is always present, but is variable. In some cases it is very intense, in others it is slight. There may be very little pain. There are progressive emaciation and loss of strength. In a recent case parotitis developed on the left side, which subsided without suppuration.

Ulceration, stricture, perforation, and fistulæ of the bile-passages will be considered with gall-stones.

IV. ACUTE INFECTIOUS CHOLECYSTITIS

Etiology.—Acute inflammation of the gall-bladder is usually due to bacterial invasion, with or without the presence of gall-stones. Three varieties or grades may be recognized: the catarrhal, the suppurative, and the phlegmonous. The condition is very serious, difficult to diagnose, often fatal, and may require for its relief prompt surgical intervention.

Acute non-calculous cholecystitis is a result of bacterial invasion. The colon bacillus, the typhoid bacillus, the pneumococcus and staphylococci and streptococci have been the organisms most often found. The frequency of gall-bladder infection in the fevers is a point already referred to, particularly in typhoid fever.

The association of appendix lesions with cholecystitis is interesting, fully 69 per cent. at the Mayo clinic; but this is not surprising in view of studies which show a normal appendix to be a rarity. There are indications, however, that chronic changes in this organ may reflexly disturb the mechanism of the secretion, storage, and outflow of bile.

Condition of the Gall-bladder.—The organ is usually distended and the walls tense. Adhesions may have formed with the colon or the omentum. In the acute stage the mucous membrane is swollen and the amount of mucin increased. As the process continues the mucosa becomes thickened, the epithelium desquamates, there are areas of necrosis, and the villi may be much hypertrophied and stand out, giving a strawberry appearance. With the obstruction of the duct and pyogenic infection there may be acute necrotic cholecystitis, with rapid perforation, or a more chronic purulent cholecystitis —empyema of the gall-bladder.

Symptoms.—Severe paroxysmal pain is, as a rule, the first indication, most commonly in the right side of the abdomen in the region of the liver. It may be in the epigastrium or low down in the region of the appendix. "Nausea, vomiting, rise of pulse and temperature, prostration, distention of the abdomen, rigidity, general tenderness becoming localized" usually follow (Richardson). In this form, without gall-stones, jaundice is not often present. The local tenderness is extreme, but it may be deceptive in its situation. Associated probably with the adhesion and inflammatory processes between the gall-bladder and the bowel are the intestinal symptoms, and there may be complete stoppage of gas and fæces; indeed, the operation for acute obstruction has been performed in several cases. The distended gall-bladder may sometimes be felt. As a sequel there may be purulent distention or empyema.

Diagnosis.—The diagnosis is by no means easy. The symptoms may not indicate the section of the abdomen involved. Appendicitis may be diagnosed; or acute intestinal obstruction. The history of the cases is often a valuable guide. Occurring during the convalescence from typhoid fever, after pneumonia, or in a patient with previous cholecystitis, such a group of symptoms as mentioned would be highly suggestive. The differentiation of the variety of the cholecystitis can not be made. In the acute suppurative and phlegmonous forms the symptoms are usually more severe, perforation is very apt to occur, with local or general peritonitis, and unless operative measures are undertaken death ensues.

There is an acute cholecystitis, probably an infective form, in which the patient has recurring attacks of pain in the region of the gall-bladder. The diagnosis of gall-stones is made, but an operation shows simply an enlarged gall-bladder filled with mucus and bile, and the mucous membrane perhaps swollen and inflamed. In some of these cases gall-stones may have been present and have passed before the operation.

Treatment.—In the milder catarrhal forms the inflammation subsides spontaneously; in severer form operation is indicated and the results are excellent. Of 675 cholecystectomies at the Mayo clinic there were only seventeen deaths.

V. CANCER OF THE BILE-PASSAGES

Incidence.—Of 3,908 operations on the gall-bladder and biliary passages, in 85 or 2.1 per cent. cancer was found (Mayo). It is more common in women, 3 to 1 (Musser), and in three-fourths of the cases gall-stones are or have been present. The fundus of the bladder is usually attacked first.

Symptoms.—When the disease involves the *gall-bladder,* a tumor can be detected extending diagonally downward and inward toward the navel, variable in size, occasionally very large, due either to great distention of the gall-bladder or to involvement of contiguous parts. It is usually very firm and hard.

Among the important symptoms are jaundice, which was present in 69 per cent. of Musser's cases; pain, often of great severity and paroxysmal in character. The pain and tenderness on pressure persist in the intervals between the paroxysmal attacks. There is loss of weight, sometimes fever and sweats. When the liver becomes involved the picture is that of carcinoma of the organ.

Primary malignant disease in the *bile-ducts* is less common, and rarely forms tumors that can be felt externally. The tumor is usually in the common duct, 57 of 80 cases collected by Rolleston. There is usually an early, intense, and persistent jaundice. The gall-bladder is usually enlarged in obstruction of the common duct by malignant disease. The dilated gall-bladder may rupture. At best the diagnosis is very doubtful, unless cleared up by an exploratory operation. A very interesting form of malignant disease of the ducts is that which involves the diverticulum of Vater. Rolleston has collected 16 cases.

VI. STENOSIS AND OBSTRUCTION OF THE BILE-DUCTS

Stenosis.—Stenosis or complete occlusion may follow ulceration, most commonly after the passage of a gall-stone. In these instances the obstruction is usually situated low down in the common duct. Instances are extremely rare. Foreign bodies, such as the seeds of various fruits, may enter the duct, and occasionally round worms crawl into it. Liver-flukes and echinococci are rare causes of obstruction in man.

Obstruction.—Obstruction by *pressure* from without is more frequent. Cancer of the head of the pancreas, less often a chronic interstitial inflammation, may compress the terminal portion of the duct; rarely, cancer of the pylorus. Secondary involvement of the lymph-glands of the liver is a common cause of occlusion of the duct, and is met with in many cases of cancer of the stomach and other abdominal organs. Rare causes of obstruction are aneurism of a branch of the cœliac axis of the aorta, and pressure of very large abdominal tumors.

Symptoms.—The symptoms produced are those of chronic obstructive jaundice. At first, the liver is enlarged, but in chronic cases it may be reduced in size, and be found of a deeply bronzed color. The hepatic intermittent fever is not often associated with complete occlusion of the duct from any cause, but it is most frequently met with in chronic obstruction by gall-stones. Permanent occlusion of the duct terminates in death. In a majority of the cases the conditions which lead to the obstruction are in themselves fatal. The liver, which is not necessarily enlarged, presents a moderate grade of cirrhosis. Cases of cicatricial occlusion may last for years.

DIAGNOSIS.—A history of colic, jaundice of varying intensity, paroxysms of pain, and intermittent fever point to gall-stones. In cancerous obstruction the tumor mass can sometimes be felt in the epigastric region. In cases in which the lymph-glands in the transverse fissure are cancerous the primary disease may be in the pelvic organs or the rectum, or there may be a limited cancer of the stomach, which has not given any symptoms. In these cases the examination of the other lymphatic glands may be of value. Involvement of the clavicular groups of lymph-glands may also be serviceable in diagnosis. The gall-bladder is usually enlarged in obstruction of the common duct, except in the cases of gall-stones (Courvoisier's law). Great and progressive enlargement of the liver with jaundice and moderate continued fever is more commonly met with in cancer.

Congenital Obliteration of the Ducts.—John Thomson, in 1892, collected 49 cases and studied the condition thoroughly. C. P. Howard and Wolbach, reviewing the recent literature, bring the cases up to 76, exclusive of those associated with syphilis. Jaundice sets in early, but may be delayed for ten or twelve days, and is progressive and deep. Hæmorrhages in the skin, from the gastro-intestinal tract, and from the umbilical cord have occurred in fully 50 per cent. Nearly one-half of the cases die within the first month, a few live on for five or six months, but rarely as long as the tenth or twelfth.

Thomson regards congenital malformation as the chief cause, others are due to cholangitis and a few to congenital cirrhosis of the liver.

VI. CHOLELITHIASIS

No chapter in medicine is more interesting than that which deals with the question of gall-stones. Few affections present so many points for study—chemical, bacteriological, pathological, and clinical. The past few years have seen a great advance in our knowledge in two directions: First, as to the mode of formation of the stones, and, secondly, as to the surgical treatment of the cases.

Origin of Gall-stones.—Two important points with reference to the formation of calculi in the bile-passages were brought out by Naunyn: (*a*) The origin of the cholesterin of the bile, as well as of the lime salts from the mucous membrane of the biliary passages, particularly when inflamed; and (*b*) the remarkable association of micro-organisms with gall-stones. It is stated that Bristowe first noticed the origin of cholesterin in the gall-bladder itself, but Naunyn's observations showed that both the cholesterin and the lime were in great part a production of the mucosa of the gall-bladder and of the bile-ducts, particularly when in a condition of catarrhal inflammation excited by the presence of microbes. According to the views of this author, the lithogenous catarrh (which, by the way, is quite an old idea) modifies materially the chemical constitution of the bile and favors the deposition about epithelial *débris* and bacteria of the insoluble salts of lime in combination with the bilirubin. Welch and others have demonstrated the presence of micro-organisms in the centre of gall-stones. Three additional points of interest may be referred to:

First, the demonstration that the gall-bladder is a peculiarly favorable habitat for micro-organisms. The colon bacilli, staphylococci, streptococci, pneumococci, and the typhoid bacilli have all been found here under varying conditions of the bile. A remarkable fact is the length of time that they may live in the gall-bladder, as was first demonstrated by Blachstein in Welch's laboratory. The typhoid bacillus has been isolated in pure culture 20 or 30 years after an attack.

Secondly, the experimental production of gall-stones has been successfully accomplished by Gilbert and Fournier by injecting micro-organisms into the gall-bladder of animals.

Thirdly, the association of gall-stones with the specific fevers. Bernheim, in 1889, first called attention to the frequency of gall-stone attacks after typhoid.

While it is probable that a lithogenous catarrh, induced by micro-organisms, is the most important single factor, there are other accessory causes of great moment.

Country.—Gall-stones are less frequent in the United States than in Germany, 6.94 to 12 per cent. (Mosher). They are less common in England than on the Continent.

Age.—Nearly 50 per cent. of all the cases occur in persons above forty years of age. They are rare under twenty-five. They have been met with in the new-born, and in infants (John Thomson).

Sex.—Three-fourths of the cases occur in women. Pregnancy has an important influence. Naunyn states that 90 per cent. of women with gall-stones have borne children.

All conditions which favor *stagnation of bile* in the gall-bladder predispose to the formation of stones. Among these may be mentioned corset-wearing, enteroptosis, nephroptosis, and occupations requiring a "leaning forward" position. Lack of exercise, sedentary occupations, particularly when combined with over-indulgence in food, constipation, and depressing mental emotions are also to be regarded as favoring circumstances. The belief prevailed formerly that there was a lithiac diathesis closely allied to that of gout.

Physical Characters of Gall-stones.—They may be single, in which case the stone is usually ovoid and may attain a very large size. Instances are on record of gall-stones measuring more than 5 inches in length. They may be extremely numerous, ranging from a score to several hundreds or even several thousands, in which case the stones are very small. When moderately numerous, they show signs of mutual pressure and have a polygonal form, with smooth facets; occasionally, however, five or six gall-stones of medium size are met with in the bladder which are round or ovoid and without facets. They are sometimes mulberry-shaped and very dark, consisting largely of bile-pigments. Again there are small, black calculi, rough and irregular in shape, and varying in size from grains of sand to small shot. These are sometimes known as gall-sand. On section, a calculus contains a nucleus, which consists of bile-pigment, rarely a foreign body. The greater portion of the stone is made up of cholesterin, which may form the entire calculus and is arranged in concentric laminæ showing also radiating lines. Salts of lime and magnesia, bile acids, fatty acids, and traces of iron and copper are also found in them. Most gall-stones consist of from 70 to 80 per cent. of cholesterin, in either the amorphous or the crystalline form. As above stated, it is sometimes pure, but more commonly it is mixed with the bile-pigment. The outer layer of the stone is usually harder and brownish in color.

Seat of Formation.—Within the liver itself calculi are occasionally found, but are here usually small and not abundant, and in the form of ovcid, greenish-black grains. A large majority of all calculi are formed within the gall-bladder. The stones in the larger ducts have usually had their origin in the gall-bladder.

Symptoms.—In a number of cases gall-stones cause no symptoms. The gall-bladder will tolerate the presence of large numbers for an indefinite period of time, and post mortem examinations show that they are present in 25 per cent. of all women over sixty years of age (Naunyn). Moynihan claims that in most cases there are early symptoms—a sense of fullness, weight, and oppression in the epigastrium; a catch in the breath, a feeling of faintness or nausea, and a chilliness after eating. Attacks of indigestion are common, and it is important to remember that persistent gastric symptoms are often due to gall-stones. I have seen two cases with obstinate attacks of urticaria.

The main symptoms of cholelithiasis may be divided into (1) the aseptic, mechanical accidents in consequence of migration of the stone or of obstruction, either in the ducts or in the intestines; (2) the septic, infectious accidents, either local (the angiocholitis and cholecystitis with empyema of the gall-bladder, and the fistulæ and abscess of the liver and infection of the neighboring parts) or general, the biliary fever and the secondary visceral lesions.

Biliary Colic.—Gall-stones may become engaged in the cystic or the common duct without producing pain or severe symptoms. More commonly the passage of a stone excites the violent symptoms known as biliary colic. The attack sets in abruptly with agonizing pain in the right hypochondriac region, which radiates to the shoulder, or is very intense in the epigastric and in the lower thoracic regions. It is often associated with a rigor and a rise in temperature from 102 degrees to 103 degrees. The pain is usually so intense that the patient rolls about in agony. There are vomiting, profuse sweating, and great depression of the circulation. There may be marked tenderness in the region of the liver, which may be enlarged, and the gall-bladder may become palpable and very tender. In other cases the fever is more marked. The spleen is enlarged (Naunyn) and the urine contains albumin with red blood-corpuscles. Ortner holds that *cholecystitis acuta,* occurring in connection with gall-stones, is a septic (bacterial) infection of the bile-passages. The symptoms of acute infectious cholecystitis and those of what we call gall-stone colic are very similar, and surgeons have frequently performed cholecystotomy for the former condition, believing calculi were present. In a large number of the cases jaundice occurs, but it is not a necessary symptom. Of course it does not happen during the passage of the stone through the cystic duct, but only when it becomes lodged in the common duct. The pain is due (*a*) to the slow progress in the cystic duct, in which the stone takes a rotary course owing to the arrangement of the Heisterian valve; the cystic duct is poor in muscle fibres but rich in nerves and ganglia; (*b*) to the acute inflammation which usually accompanies an attack; (*c*) to the stretching and distention of the gall-bladder by retained secretions.

The attack varies in duration. It may last for a few hours, several days, or even a week or more. If the stone becomes impacted in the orifice of the common duct, the jaundice becomes intense; much more commonly it is a slight transient icterus. The attack of colic may be repeated at intervals for some time, but finally the stone passes and the symptoms disappear.

Occasionally accidents occur, such as rupture of the duct with fatal peritonitis. Fatal syncope during an attack and the occurrence of repeated convulsive seizures have come under my observation. These are, however, rare events. Palpitation and distress about the heart may be present, and occasionally a mitral murmur occurs during the paroxysm, but the cardiac conditions described by some writers as coming on acutely in biliary colic are possibly preëxistent in these patients.

The *diagnosis* of acute hepatic colic is generally easy. The pain is in the upper abdominal and thoracic regions, whereas the pain in nephritic colic is in the lower abdomen. A chill, with fever, is much more frequent in biliary colic than in gastralgia, with which it is liable, at times, to be confounded. A history of previous attacks is an important guide, and the occurrence of jaundice, however slight, determines the diagnosis. To look for the gall-stones, the stools should be thoroughly mixed with water and carefully filtered through a narrow-meshed sieve. Pseudo-biliary colic is not infrequently met with in nervous women, and the diagnosis of gall-stones made. This nervous hepatic colic may be periodical; the pain may be in the right side and radiating; sometimes associated with other nervous phenomena, often excited by emotion, fatigue or excesses. The liver may be tender, but there are neither icterus nor inflammatory conditions. The combination of colic and jaundice, so distinctive of gall-stones, is not always present. The pains may not be colicky, but more constant and dragging in character. A remarkable xanthoma of the bile-passages has been found in association with hepatic colic. Many patients with gall-stones have stomach symptoms—flatulency, regurgitation, and distress after eating. Sometimes the pain may be much increased by food or on exertion. In chronic gall-bladder cases, with adhesions and perforation, the clinical picture may resemble closely that of ulcer.

Obstruction of the Cystic Duct.—The effects may be thus enumerated:

(*a*) *Dilatation* of the gall-bladder—hydrops vesicæ felleæ. In acute obstruction the contents are bile mixed with much mucus or muco-purulent material. In chronic obstruction the bile is replaced by a clear fluid mucus. This is an important point in diagnosis, particularly as a dropsical gall-bladder may form a very large tumor. The reaction is not always constant. It is either alkaline or neutral; the consistence is thin and mucoid. Albumin is usually present. A dilated gall-bladder may reach an enormous size, and in one instance Tait found it occupying the greater part of the abdomen. In such cases, as is not unnatural, it has been mistaken for an ovarian tumor. I have described a case in which it was attached to the right broad ligament. The dilated gall-bladder can usually be felt below the edge of the liver, and in many instances it has a characteristic outline like a gourd. An enlarged and relaxed organ may not be palpable, and in acute cases the distention may be upward toward the hilus of the liver. The dilated gall-bladder usually projects directly downward, rarely to one side or the other, though occasionally toward the middle line. It may reach below the navel, and in persons with thin walls the outline can be accurately defined. Riedel has called attention to a tongue-like projection of the anterior margin of the right lobe in connection with enlarged gall-bladder. It is to be remembered that distention of the gall-bladder may occur without jaundice; indeed, the greatest enlargement has been met with in such cases.

Gall-stone crepitus may be felt when the bladder is very full of stones and its walls not very tense. It is rarely well felt unless the abdominal walls are much relaxed. It may be found in patients who have never had any symptoms of cholelithiasis.

(*b*) *Acute cholecystitis.* The simple form is common, and to it are due probably very many of the symptoms of the gall-stone attack. Phlegmonous cholecystitis is rare. Perforation may occur with fatal peritonitis.

(*c*) *Suppurative cholecystitis,* empyema of the gall-bladder, is much more common, and in the great majority of cases is associated with gall-stones. There may be enormous dilatation, and over a litre of pus has been found. Perforation and the formation of abscesses in the neighborhood are not uncommon.

(*d*) *Calcification* of the gall-bladder is commonly a termination of the previous condition. There are two separate forms: incrustation of the mucosa with lime salts and the true infiltration of the wall with lime, the so-called ossification.

(*e*) *Atrophy* of the gall-bladder. This is by no means uncommon. The organ shrinks into a small fibroid mass, not larger, perhaps, than a good-sized pea or walnut, or even has the form of a narrow fibrous string; more commonly the gall-bladder tightly embraces a stone. This condition is usually preceded by hydrops of the bladder.

Occasionally the gall-bladder presents diverticula, which may be cut off from the main portion, and usually contain calculi.

Obstruction of the Common Duct.—There may be a single stone tightly wedged in the duct in any part of its course, or a series of stones, sometimes extending into both hepatic and cystic ducts, or a stone lies in the diverticulum of Vater. There are three groups of cases: (*a*) In rare instances a stone tightly corks the common duct, causing *permanent occlusion;* or it may partly rest in the cystic duct, and may have caused thickening of the junction of the ducts; or a big stone may compress the hepatic or upper part of the common duct. The jaundice is deep and enduring, and there are no septic features. The pains, the previous attacks of colic, and the absence of enlarged gall-bladder help to separate the condition from obstruction by new growths, although it cannot be differentiated with certainty. The ducts are usually much dilated and everywhere contain a clear mucoid fluid.

(*b*) *Incomplete obstruction, with infective cholangitis.* There may be a series of stones in the common duct, a single stone which is freely movable, or a stone (ball-valve stone) in the diverticulum of Vater. These conditions may be met with at autopsy, without the subjects having had symptoms pointing to gall-stones; but in a majority of cases there are very characteristic features.

The common duct may be as large as the thumb; the hepatic duct and its branches through the liver may be greatly dilated, and the distention may be even apparent beneath the liver capsule. Great enlargement of the gall-bladder is rarer. The mucous membrane of the ducts is usually smooth and clear, and the contents consist of a thin, slightly turbid bile-stained mucus.

Naunyn has given the following as the distinguishing signs of stone in the common duct: "(1) The continuous or occasional presence of bile in the fæces; (2) distinct variations in the intensity of the jaundice; (3) normal size or only slight enlargement of the liver; (4) absence of distention of the gall-bladder; (5) enlargement of the spleen; (6) absence of ascites; (7) presence of febrile disturbance; and (8) duration of the jaundice for more than a year."

In connection with the ball-valve stone, which is most commonly found in the diverticulum of Vater, though it may be in the common duct itself, there is a special symptom group: (*a*) Ague-like paroxysms, chills, fever, and sweating; the *hepatic intermittent fever* of Charcot; (*b*) jaundice of varying intensity, which persists for months or even years, and deepens after each paroxysm; (*c*) at the time of the paroxysm, pains in the region of the liver with gastric disturbance. These symptoms may continue on and off for three or four years, without the development of suppurative cholangitis. The condition has lasted from eight months to three years. The rigors are of intense severity, and the temperature rises to 103° or 105° F. The chills may recur daily for weeks, and present a tertian or quartan type, so that they are often attributed to malaria, with which, however, they have no connection. The jaundice is variable, and deepens after each paroxysm. The itching may be most intense. Pain, which is sometimes severe and colicky, does not always occur. There may be marked vomiting and nausea. As a rule there is no progressive deterioration of health. In the intervals between the attacks the temperature is normal.

The clinical history and the post mortem examinations show conclusively that this condition may persist for years without a trace of suppuration within the ducts. It is probable that the toxic symptoms develop only when a certain grade of tension is reached. An interesting and valuable diagnostic point is the absence of dilatation of the gall-bladder in cases of obstruction from stone—Courvoisier's rule.

(*c*) *Incomplete obstruction, with suppurative cholangitis.* When suppurative cholangitis exists the mucosa is thickened, often eroded or ulcerated; there may be extensive suppuration in the ducts throughout the liver, and even empyema of the gall-bladder. Occasionally the suppuration extends beyond the ducts, and there is localized liver abscess, or there is perforation of the gall-bladder with the formation of abscess between the liver and stomach.

Clinically it is characterized by a fever which may be intermittent, but more commonly is remittent and without prolonged intervals of apyrexia. The jaundice is rarely so intense, nor do we see the deepening of the color after the paroxysms. There is usually greater enlargement of the liver, and tenderness and more definite signs of septicæmia. The cases run a shorter course, and recovery never takes place.

THE MORE REMOTE EFFECTS OF GALL-STONES.—(*a*) *Biliary Fistulæ.*—(1) *Cutaneous.*—The external fistula is the most common, 184 out of 384 cases (Naunyn). A majority occur in the region of the navel, to which part the falciform ligament directs the suppuration. The number of stones discharged varies from one or two to many hundreds. Of the 184 cases in Courvoisier's statistics recovery took place in 78. In rare instances the fistula is in the right iliac fossa, or even in the thigh.

(2) *Gastro-intestinal Fistulæ.*—The duodenal is the most frequent, 108 of 384 cases (Naunyn). Usually the opening is between the fundus of the gall-bladder and the first part of the duodenum. A big stone may ulcerate through, leaving little or no damage. In other instances the cicatrization leads to obstruction. Communication with the ileum and jejunum is rare. Fistulæ between the common duct and the duodenum occurred in 15 cases in Naunyn's series. Biliary gastric fistulæ are rare. The vomiting of gall-stones is not necessarily proof of the perforation, but in the majority of such cases the stones probably pass up through the pylorus.

(3) *Broncho-biliary Fistulæ.*—Of J. E. Graham's collected series of 35 cases, 19 were due to gall-stones; 11 to hydatids; 2 to round-worms; and in 2 the cause was doubtful. In a great many cases the amœbic abscess perforating into the lung is followed by a permanent biliary fistula.

(4) Perforation may occur into the *portal vein*, of which there are 3 or 4 cases on record, one of which, according to tradition, was the famous Ignatius Loyola.

(5) Perforation into the *hepatic artery* or one of its branches is exceedingly rare. Either an erosion from the common duct, or an hepatic aneurism may rupture into the gall-bladder.

(6) Fistula into the *urinary passages* may be with the pelvis of the kidney in which the gall-stone has been found, or into the urinary bladder, of which there are few cases on record.

(7) Lastly, the communication between the *pericardium* and the biliary tract is referred to by Naunyn in a single case.

(*b*) *Perforation into the Peritoneum.*—Of 119 cases (Courvoisier) in 70 the rupture occurred directly into the peritoneal cavity; in 49 an encapsulated abscess formed. As a rule, the condition is due to an acute cholecystitis.

(*c*) *Obstruction of the Bowel by Gall-stones.*—Reference has already been made to this; its frequency appears from the fact that of 295 cases of obstruction, occurring during eight years, analyzed by Fitz, 23 were by gall-stones. Courvoisier's statistics give a total number of 131 cases, in 6 of which the calculi had a peculiar situation, as in a diverticulum or in the appendix. Of the remaining 125 cases, in 70 the stone was spontaneously passed, usually with severe symptoms. The post mortem reports show that in some of these cases even very large stones have passed *per viam naturalem*, as the gall-duct has been enormously distended, its orifice admitting the finger freely. This, however, is extremely rare. The stones have been found most commonly in the ileum.

Treatment of Gall-stones and Their Effects.—GENERAL TREATMENT.—In an attack of biliary colic the patient should be kept under morphia, given hypodermically, in quarter-grain doses. In an agonizing paroxysm it is well to give a whiff or two of chloroform until the morphia has had time to act. Great relief is experienced from the hot bath and from fomentations in the region of the liver. The patient should be given laxatives and should drink copiously of alkaline mineral waters. Olive oil has proved useless in my hands. When taken in large quantities, fatty concretions are passed with the stools, which have been regarded as calculi; and concretions due to eating pears have been also mistaken, particularly when associated with colic attacks. Since the days of Durande, whose mixture of ether with turpentine is still largely used in France, various remedies have been advised to dissolve the stones within the gall-bladder, none of which are efficacious.

The diet should be regulated, the patient should take regular exercise and avoid, as much as possible, the starchy and saccharine foods. The soda salts recommended by Prout are believed to prevent the concentration of the bile and the formation of gall-stones. Either the sulphate or the phosphate may be taken in doses of from 1 to 2 drachms daily. For the intolerable itching McCall Anderson's dusting powder may be used: starch, an ounce; camphor, a drachm and a half; and oxide of zinc, half an ounce. Some of this should be finely dusted over the skin with a powder-puff. Powdering with starch, strong alkaline baths (hot), pilocarpin hypodermically (gr. 1/8–1/6, 0.008–0.01 gm.), and antipyrin (gr. v, 0.3 gm.), may be tried. Ichthyol and lanolin ointment sometimes gives relief.

Surgical Treatment.—The indications for operation are: (*a*) Repeated attacks of gall-stone colic. The patient is much safer in the hands of a surgeon than when left to Nature, with the feeble assistance of drugs and mineral waters. (*b*) The presence of a distended gall-bladder, associated with attacks of pain or with fever. (*c*) When a gall-stone is permanently lodged in the common duct, and the group of symptoms above described are present, the question, then, of advising operation depends largely upon the personal methods and success of the surgeon who is available.

Of 4,000 operations performed by the Mayo brothers to February 20th, 1911, the mortality was 2.57 per cent. Of 2,920 cases in which the gall-bladder alone was involved the mortality was 1.8 per cent. Of 492 cases in which the common duct was involved the mortality was 8 per cent. In 2.25 per cent. there was the complication of malignant disease.

The question comes up as to the re-formation of stones, but the possibility of this is very slight. In the Mayo series there were but 3 cases and it is probable that in the majority of instances the stones had not re-formed, but were incompletely removed.

VII. THE CIRRHOSES OF THE LIVER

General Considerations.—The many forms of cirrhoses of the liver have one feature in common—an increase in the connective tissue of the organ. In fact, we use the term cirrhosis (by which Laennec characterized the tawny, yellow color of the common atrophic form) to indicate similar changes in other organs.

Etiology.—There are five types of primary lesion, any one of which may lead to cirrhosis.

1. *Toxic Cirrhosis.*—This is the only acute type and it is seen post partum, in chloroform narcosis and sometimes as a terminal lesion in any form of disease. There is a central necrosis about the hepatic vein which may be slight in amount, or in some cases an acute yellow atrophy, very extensive so that the liver is rapidly reduced in size. Into the necrotic areas leucocytes migrate, the dead liver cells are quickly removed and there is an apparent increase of the connective tissue. Great regeneration of the liver cells is possible. Clinically this type can scarcely be spoken of as cirrhosis.

2. *Infectious Cirrhosis.*—Adami and his school hold that in many cases the colon bacilli from the bowel pass to the liver and there gradually excite a slow proliferation of connective tissue, regarding it as a kind of sub-infection. Mallory, whose classification I am following, thinks that the only type of true infectious cirrhosis is through the bile ducts, usually when there is bile stasis or gall-stones or other obstructions are present. Cases are described in which invasion occurs along apparently normal bile ducts and the organisms cause necrosis of the liver cells, proliferation of the fibroblasts, and thickening of the walls of the smaller bile ducts which may be dilated and tortuous.

Clinically this type is rare, and characterized by a chronic jaundice and enlargement of the liver.

3. *Pigment Cirrhosis.*—This may be an external pigment as in anthracosis in which the irritation of the coal particles reaching the liver through the lymphatics may excite a moderate grade of cirrhosis. The endogenous pigment is a transformation of hæmoglobin either as in malaria or as in the remarkable affection known as hæmochromatosis.

4. *Syphilitic Cirrhosis.*—Whether congenital or acquired, the essential lesion is produced by the *Treponema pallidum,* either a diffuse proliferation of fibroblasts, or a more localized lesion, the gumma.

5. *Alcoholic Cirrhosis.*—As a result of the toxic action of the alcohol, the liver cells, singly or in groups, undergo a slow necrosis, following which there is a multiplication of the fibroblasts with a hyalin degeneration of some cells and multiplication of others and an increase in the smaller bile ducts. Fatty infiltration is common, so that the organ may be enlarged.

Of these types the toxic and one form of the alcoholic are associated with shrinkage, the infectious, the pigmentary and the fatty cirrhosis with enlargement of the organ. Clinically we may consider four forms, the portal, the hypertrophic (of Hanot), the syphilitic, and the capsular.

1. PORTAL CIRRHOSIS

Etiology.—The disease occurs most frequently in middle-aged males who have been addicted to drink. Whisky, gin, and brandy are more potent to cause cirrhosis than beer. It is more common in countries in which strong spirits are used than in those in which malt liquors are taken. Among 1,000 autopsies in my colleague Welch's department of the Johns Hopkins Hospital there were 63 cases of small atrophic liver, and 8 cases of the fatty cirrhotic organ. Lancereaux claims that the *vin ordinaire* of France is a common cause of cirrhosis. Of 210 cases, excess in wine alone was present in 68 cases.

He thinks it is the sulphate of potash in the plaster of Paris used to give the "dry" flavor which damages the liver.

Cirrhosis of the liver in young children is not very rare. In a certain number of the cases there is an alcoholic history, in others syphilis has been present, while a third group, due to the poisons of the infectious diseases, embraces a certain number of the cases of Hanot's hypertrophic cirrhosis.

Morbid Anatomy.—Practically on the post mortem table we see alcoholic cirrhosis in two well-characterized forms:

THE ATROPHIC CIRRHOSIS OF LAENNEC.—The organ is greatly reduced in size and may be deformed. The weight is sometimes not more than a pound or a pound and a half. It presents numerous granulations on the surface; is firm, hard, and cuts with great resistance. The substance is seen to be made up of greenish-yellow islands surrounded by grayish-white connective tissue. W. G. MacCallum has shown that regenerative changes in the cells are almost constantly present. This yellow appearance of the liver induced Laennec to give to the condition the name of cirrhosis.

THE FATTY CIRRHOTIC LIVER.—Even in the atrophic form the fat is increased, but in typical examples of this variety the organ is not reduced in size, but is enlarged, smooth or very slightly granular, anæmic, yellowish-white in color, and resembles an ordinary fatty liver. It is, however, firm, cuts with resistance, and microscopically shows a great increase in the connective tissue. This form occurs most frequently in beer-drinkers.

The two essential elements in cirrhosis are destruction of liver-cells and obstruction to the portal circulation.

In an autopsy on a case of atrophic cirrhosis the peritoneum is usually found to contain a large quantity of fluid, the membrane is opaque, and there is chronic catarrh of the stomach and of the small intestines. The spleen is enlarged, in part, at least, from the chronic congestion, possibly due in part to a toxic influence (Parkes Weber). The pancreas frequently shows interstitial changes. The kidneys are sometimes cirrhotic, the bases of the lungs may be much compressed by the ascitic fluid, the heart often shows marked degeneration, and arterio-sclerosis is usually present. A remarkable feature is the association of acute tuberculosis with cirrhosis. In seven cases of my series the patients died with either acute tuberculous peritonitis or acute tuberculous pleurisy. Rolleston has found that tuberculosis was present in 28 per cent. of 706 fatal cases of cirrhosis. Peritoneal tuberculosis was found in 9 per cent. of a series of 584 cases.

The compensatory circulation is usually readily demonstrated. It is carried out by the following set of vessels: (1) The accessory portal system of Sappey, of which important branches pass in the round and suspensory ligaments and unite with the epigastric and mammary systems. These vessels are numerous and small. Occasionally a large single vein, which may attain the size of the little finger, passes from the hilus of the liver, follows the round ligament, and joins the epigastric veins at the navel. Although this has the position of the umbilical vein, it is usually, as Sappey showed, a para-umbilical vein—that is, an enlarged vein by the side of the obliterated umbilical vessel. There may be produced about the navel a large bunch of varices, the so-called caput Medusæ. Other branches of this system occur in the gastro-epiploic omentum, about the gall-bladder, and, most important of all, in the suspensory ligament. These latter form large branches, which anastomose freely with the diaphragmatic veins, and so unite with the vena axygos. (2) By the anastomosis between the œsophageal and gastric veins. The veins at the lower end of the œsophagus may be enormously enlarged, producing varices which project on the mucous membrane. (3) The communications between the hæmorrhoidal and the inferior mesenteric veins. The freedom of communication in this direction is very variable, and in some instances the hæmorrhoidal veins are not much enlarged. (4) The veins of Retzius, which unite the radicles of the portal branches in the intestines and mesentery with the inferior vena cava and its branches. To this system belong the whole group of retroperitoneal veins, which are in most instances enormously enlarged, particularly about the kidneys, and which serve to carry off a considerable proportion of the portal blood.

Symptoms.—The most extreme grade of atrophic cirrhosis may exist without symptoms. *So long as the compensatory circulation is maintained* the patient may suffer little or no inconvenience. The remarkable efficiency of this collateral circulation is well seen in those rare instances of permanent obliteration of the portal vein. The symptoms may be divided into two groups—obstructive and toxic.

Obstructive.—The overfilling of the blood-vessels of the stomach and intestine leads to chronic catarrh, and the patients suffer with nausea and vomiting, particularly in the morning; the tongue is furred and the bowels are irregular. Hæmorrhage from the stomach may be an early symptom; it is often profuse and liable to recur. It seldom proves fatal. The amount vomited may be remarkable as in a case already referred to, in which ten pounds were ejected in seven days. Following the hæmatemesis melæna is common; but hæmorrhages from the bowels may occur for several years without hæmatemesis. The bleeding very often comes from œsophageal varices. Very frequently epistaxis occurs. Enlargement of the spleen may, as Parkes Weber suggests, be due to a toxæmia. The organ can usually be felt. Evidences of the establishment of the collateral circulation are seen in the enlarged epigastric and mammary veins, more rarely in the presence of the caput Medusæ and in the development of hæmorrhoids. The distended venules in the lower thoracic zone along the line of attachment of the diaphragm are not specially marked in cirrhosis. The most striking feature of failure in the compensatory circulation is ascites, the effusion of serous fluid into the peritoneal cavity, which may appear suddenly. The conditions under which this occurs are still obscure. In some cases it is due more to chronic peritonitis than to the cirrhosis. The abdomen gradually distends, may reach a large size, and contain as much as 15 to 20 litres. Œdema of the feet may precede or develop with the ascites. The dropsy is rarely general.

Jaundice is usually slight, and was present in 107 of 293 cases of cirrhosis collected by Rolleston. The skin has frequently a sallow, slightly icteroid tint. The urine is often reduced in amount, contains urates in abundance, often a slight amount of albumin, and, if jaundice is intense, tube-casts. The disease may be afebrile throughout, but in many cases, as shown by Carrington, there is slight fever, from 100° to 102.5° F.

Examination at any early stage of the disease may show an enlarged and painful liver. In very many of the cases of alcoholic cirrhosis the organ is "enlarged at all stages of the disease, and, whether enlarged or contracted, the clinical symptoms and course are much the same" (Foxwell). The patient may first come under observation for dyspepsia, hæmatemesis, slight jaundice, or nervous symptoms. Later in the disease the patient has an unmistakable hepatic facies; he is thin, the eyes are sunken, the conjunctivæ watery, the nose and cheeks show distended venules, and the complexion is muddy or icteroid. On the enlarged abdomen the vessels are distended, and a bunch of dilated veins may surround the navel. A venous hum, sometimes accompanied by a thrill, may be present in the epigastrium or over varicosities. Nævi of a remarkable character may appear on the skin, either localized stellate varices—spider angiomata—usually on the face, neck, and back, and also "mat" nævi, as I have called them—areas of skin of a reddish or purplish color due to the uniform distention of small venules. When much fluid is in the peritoneum it is impossible to make a satisfactory examination, but after withdrawal the area of liver dulness is found to be diminished, particularly in the middle line, and on deep pressure the edge of the liver can be detected, and occasionally the hard, firm, and even granular surface. The spleen can be felt in the left hypochondriac region. Examination of the anus may reveal the presence of hæmorrhoids.

Toxic Symptoms.—At any stage of atrophic cirrhosis the patient may have cerebral symptoms, either a noisy, joyous delirium, or stupor, coma, or even convulsions. The condition is not infrequently mistaken for uræmia. The nature of the toxic agent is not yet settled. Without jaundice, and not attributable to cholæmia, the symptoms may come on in hospital when the patient has not had alcohol for weeks.

The fatty cirrhotic liver may produce symptoms similar to those of the atrophic form, but more frequently it is latent and is found accidentally in topers who have died from various diseases. The greater number of the cases clinically diagnosed as cirrhosis with enlargement come in this division.

Diagnosis.—With ascites, a well-marked history of alcoholism, the hepatic facies, and hæmorrhage from the stomach or bowels, the diagnosis is rarely doubtful. If, after withdrawal of the fluid, the spleen is found to be enlarged and the liver either not palpable or, if it is enlarged, hard and regular, the probabilities in favor of cirrhosis are very great. In the early stages of the disease, when the liver is increased in size, it may be impossible to say whether it is a cirrhotic or a fatty liver. The differential diagnosis between common and syphilitic cirrhosis can sometimes be made. A marked history of syphilis or the existence of other syphilitic lesions, with great irregularity in the surface or at the edge of the liver, are the points in favor of the latter. Thrombosis or obliteration of the portal vein can rarely be differentiated. In a case of fibroid transformation of the portal vein which came under my observation, the collateral circulation had been established for years, and the symptoms were simply those of extreme portal obstruction, such as occur in cirrhosis. Thrombosis of the portal vein may occur in cirrhosis and be characterized by a rapidly developing ascites.

Prognosis.—The outlook is bad. When the collateral circulation is fully established the patient may have no symptoms whatever. There are instances of enlargement of the liver, slight jaundice, cerebral symptoms, and even hæmatemesis, in which the liver becomes reduced in size, the symptoms disappear, and the patient may live in comparative comfort for many years. There are cases, too, possibly syphilitic, in which, after one or two tappings, the symptoms have disappeared and the patients have apparently recovered. Ascites is a very serious event, especially if due to the cirrhosis and not to an associated peritonitis. Of 34 cases with ascites 10 died before tapping was necessary; 14 were tapped, and the average duration of life after the swelling was first noticed was only eight weeks; of 10 cases the diagnosis was wrong in 4, and in the remaining 6, who were tapped oftener than once, chronic peritonitis and perihepatitis were present (Hale White).

2. HYPERTROPHIC BILIARY CIRRHOSIS (*Hanot*)

This well-characterized form was first described by Requin in 1846, but our accurate knowledge of the condition dates from the work of Hanot (1875), whose name in France it bears—*maladie de Hanot.*

Cirrhosis with enlargement occurs in the early stage of atrophic cirrhosis; there is an enlarged fatty and cirrhotic liver of alcoholics, a pigmentary form occurs in hæmochromatosis, and in association with syphilis the organ is often very large. The hypertrophic cirrhosis of Hanot is easily distinguished from these forms.

Etiology.—Males are more often affected than females—in 22 of Schachmann's 26 cases. The subjects are young; some of the cases in children probably belong to this form. Alcohol plays a minor part, and not one of my patients had been a heavy drinker. The absence of all known etiological factors is a remarkable feature.

Morbid Anatomy.—The organ is enlarged, weighing from 2,000 to 4,000 grams. The form is maintained, the surface is smooth, or presents small granulations; the color in advanced cases is of a dark olive green; the consistence is greatly increased. The section is uniform, greenish yellow in color, and the liver nodules may be seen separated by connective tissue. The bile-passages present nothing abnormal. The cirrhosis is mono- or multilobular, with a connective tissue rich in round cells. The bile-vessels are the seat of an angiocholitis, catarrhal and productive, and there is an extraordinary development of new biliary canaliculi. The liver-cells are neither fatty nor pigmented, and may be increased in size and show karyokinetic figures. From the supposed origin about the bile-vessels it has been called biliary cirrhosis, but the histological details have not yet been worked out fully, and the separation of this as a distinct form should, for the present at least, rest upon clinical rather than anatomical grounds. The spleen is greatly enlarged and may weigh 600 or more grams.

Symptoms.—As previously stated, the cases occur in young persons; there is not, as a rule, an alcoholic history, and males are usually affected. The features are: (*a*) A remarkably chronic course of from four to six, or even ten years. (*b*) Jaundice, usually slight, often not more than a lemon tint, or a tinging of the conjunctivæ. At any time during the course an *icterus gravis,* with high fever and delirium, may develop. There is bile in the urine; the stools are not clay-colored as in obstructive jaundice, but may be very dark and "bilious." (*c*) Attacks of pain in the region of the liver, which may be severe and associated with nausea and vomiting. The pain may be slight and dragging, and in some cases is not at all a prominent symptom. The jaundice may deepen after attacks of pain. (*d*) Enlarged liver. A fullness in the upper abdominal zone may be the first complaint. On inspection the enlargement may be very marked. In one of my cases the left lobe was unusually prominent and stood out almost like a tumor. An exploratory operation showed only an enlarged, smooth organ without adhesions. On palpation the hypertrophy is uniform, the consistence is increased, and the edge distinct and hard. The gall-bladder is not enlarged. The vertical flatness is much increased and may extend from the sixth rib to the level of the navel. (*e*) The spleen is enlarged, easily palpable, and very hard. (*f*) Certain negative features are of moment—the usual absence of ascites and of dilatation of the subcutaneous veins of the abdomen. Among other symptoms may be mentioned hæmorrhages. One of my patients had bleeding at the gums for a year; another had had for years most remarkable attacks of purpura with urticaria. Pruritus, xanthoma, lichen, and telangiectasis may be present in the skin. In one of my patients the skin became very bronzed, almost as deeply as in Addison's disease. Slight fever may be present, which increases during the crises of pain. There may be a marked leucocytosis. A curious attitude of the body has been seen, in which the right shoulder and right side appear dragged down. The patients die with the symptoms of icterus gravis, from hæmorrhage, from an intercurrent infection, or in a profound cachexia. Certain of the cases of cirrhosis of the liver in children are of this type; the enlargement of the spleen may be very pronounced.

3. SYPHILITIC CIRRHOSIS

This is considered in the section on syphilis (p. 273). I refer to it again to emphasize (1) its frequency; (2) the great importance of its differentiation from the alcoholic form; (3) its curability in many cases; and (4) the tumor formations in connection with it.

4. CAPSULAR CIRRHOSIS—PERIHEPATITIS

Local capsulitis is common in many conditions of the liver. The form of disease here described is characterized by an enormous thickening of the entire capsule, with great contraction of the liver, but not necessarily with special increase in the connective tissue of the organ itself. Our chief knowledge of the disease we owe to the Guy's Hospital physicians, particularly to Hilton Fagge and to Hale White, who collected 22 cases from the records. The liver substance itself was "never markedly cirrhotic; its tissue was nearly always soft." Chronic capsulitis of the spleen and a chronic proliferative peritonitis are almost invariably present. In 19 of the 22 cases the kidneys were granular. Hale White regards it as a sequel of interstitial nephritis. The youngest case in his series was twenty-nine. The symptoms are those of atrophic cirrhosis—ascites, often recurring and requiring many tappings. Jaundice is not often present. I have met with two groups of cases—the one in adults usually with ascites and regarded as ordinary cirrhosis. I have never made a diagnosis in such a case. Signs of interstitial nephritis, recurring ascites, and absence of jaundice are regarded by Hale White as important diagnostic points. In the second group of cases the perihepatitis, perisplenitis, and proliferative peritonitis are associated with adherent pericardium and chronic mediastinitis. In one such case the diagnosis of capsular hepatitis was very clear, as the liver could be grasped in the hand and formed a rounded, smooth organ resembling the spleen. The child was tapped 121 times (Archives of Pædiatrics, 1896).

TREATMENT OF THE CIRRHOSES

The portal function of the liver may be put out of action without much damage to the body. There may be an extreme grade of cirrhotic atrophy without symptoms; the portal vein may be obliterated, or, experimentally, the portal vein may be anastomosed with the cava. So long as there is an active compensatory circulation a patient with atrophic cirrhosis may remain well. In the hypertrophic form toxæmia is the special danger. In the hypertrophic cirrhosis we have no means of arresting the progress of the disease. In the alcoholic form it is too late, as a rule, to do much after symptoms have occurred. In a few cases an attack of jaundice or hæmatemesis may prove the salvation of the patient, who may afterward take to a temperate life. The diet should be very simple and large amounts of water taken to aid elimination. The bowels should be kept open, for which the use of the salines is generally best. An occasional course of potassium iodide may be given. With the advent of ascites the critical stage is reached. Restriction of fluid intake and free purgation may relieve a small exudate, rarely a large one, and it is best to tap early, or to advise Talma's operation. In the syphilitic cirrhosis much more can be done, and a majority of the cases of cure after ascites are of this variety. Iodide of potassium in moderate doses, 15 to 30 drops of the saturated solution, and the Addison pill save a number of cases even after repeated tapping. The diagnosis may be reached only after removal of the fluid, but in every case with a history of syphilis, a positive Wassermann reaction, or with irregularity of the liver this treatment should be tried.

SURGICAL TREATMENT.—(*a*) *Tapping.*—When the ascites increases it is better to tap early. As Hale White remarks, a case of cirrhosis of the liver which is tapped rarely recovers, but there are instances in which early and repeated paracentesis is followed by cure. Accidents are rare; hæmorrhage, acute peritonitis, or erysipelas at the point of puncture occasionally follow; collapse may occur during the operation, to guard against which Mead advised the use of the abdominal binder. Continuous drainage with Southey's tubes is not often practicable and has no special advantages. (*b*) *Laparotomy,* with complete removal of the fluid, and freshening or rubbing the peritoneal surfaces, to stimulate the formation of adhesions. (*c*) *Omentopexy,* the stitching of the omentum to the abdominal wall, and the establishment of collateral circulation in this way between the portal and the systemic vessels. This operation is sometimes very successful, and may be recommended. In 224 cases there were 84 deaths and 129 recoveries; 11 cases doubtful. Among the 129 successful cases, in 25 the ascites recurred; 70 appeared to have completely recovered. (*d*) *Fistula of Eck.* The porto-caval anastomosis has been performed once in man in cirrhosis of the liver (Widal, *La Semaine Médicale,* 1903). The patient lived for three months.

VIII. ABSCESS OF THE LIVER

Etiology.—Suppuration within the liver, either in the parenchyma or in the blood or bile passages, occurs under the following conditions:

(*a*) The *tropical abscess*, also called the *solitary*, commonly follows amœbic dysentery. It frequently occurs among Europeans in India, particularly those who drink alcohol freely and are exposed to great heat. Cases may occur without a history of previous dysentery, and there have been fatal cases without any affection of the large bowel. In the United States the large solitary abscess is not very infrequent. The relation of this form of abscess to the *Amœba dysenteriæ* has been considered.

(*b*) *Traumatism* is an occasional cause. The injury is generally in the hepatic region. Two instances of it have come under my notice in trainmen who were injured while coupling cars. Injury to the head is not infrequently followed by liver abscess.

(*c*) *Embolic* or *pyæmic abscesses* are the most numerous, occurring in a general pyæmia or following foci of suppuration in the territory of the portal vessels. The infective agents may reach the liver through the hepatic artery, as in those cases in which the original focus of infection is in the area of the systemic circulation; though it may happen occasionally that the infective agent, instead of passing through the lungs, reaches the liver through the inferior vena cava and the hepatic veins. A remarkable instance of multiple abscesses of arterial origin was afforded by the case of aneurism of the hepatic artery reported by Ross and myself. Infection through the portal vein is much more common. It results from dysentery and other ulcerative affections of the bowels, appendicitis, occasionally after typhoid fever, in rectal affections, and in abscesses in the pelvis. In these cases the abscesses are multiple and, as a rule, within the branches of the portal vein—suppurative pylephlebitis.

(*d*) A not uncommon cause of suppuration is *inflammation of the bile-passages* caused by gall-stones, more rarely by parasites—suppurative cholangitis.

In some instances of tuberculosis of the liver the affection is chiefly of the bile-ducts, with the formation of multiple tuberculous abscesses containing a bile-stained pus

(*e*) *Foreign bodies and parasites.* In rare instances foreign bodies, such as a needle, may pass from the stomach or gullet, lodge in the liver, and excite an abscess, or, as in several instances which have been reported, a foreign body, such as a needle or a fish-bone, has perforated a branch or the portal vein itself and induced pylephlebitis. Echinococcus cysts frequently cause suppuration, the penetration of round worms into the liver less commonly, and most rarely of all the liver-fluke.

Morbid Anatomy.—(*a*) Of the Solitary or Tropical Abscess.—This has been described under amœbic dysentery.

(*b*) Of Septic and Pyæmic Abscesses.—These are usually multiple, though occasionally, following injury, there may be a large solitary collection of pus.

In suppurative pylephlebitis the liver is uniformly enlarged. The capsule may be smooth and the external surface of the organ of normal appearance. In other instances, numerous yellowish-white points appear beneath the capsule. On section there are isolated pockets of pus, either having a round outline or in some places distinctly dendritic, and from these the pus may be squeezed. They look like small, solitary abscesses, but, on probing, are found to communicate with the portal vein and to represent its branches, distended and suppurating. The entire portal system within the liver may be involved; sometimes territories are cut off by thrombi. The suppuration may extend into the main branch or even into the mesenteric and gastric veins. The pus may be fetid and is often bile-stained; it may, however, be thick and tenacious. In suppurative cholangitis there is usually obstruction by gallstones, the ducts are greatly distended, the gall-bladder enlarged and full of pus, and the branches within the liver are extremely distended, so that on section there is an appearance not unlike that described in pylephlebitis. An abscess may have a sponge-like appearance due to the fusion of numerous points of suppuration.

Suppuration about the echinococcus cysts may be very extensive, forming enormous abscesses, the characters of which are at once recognized by the remnants of the cysts.

Symptoms.—(*a*) Of the Large Solitary Abscess.—The abscess may be latent and run a course without definite symptoms; death may occur suddenly from rupture.

Fever, pain, enlargement of the liver, and a septic condition are the important symptoms of hepatic abscess. The temperature is elevated at the outset and is of an intermittent or septic type. It is irregular, and may remain normal or even subnormal for a few days; then the patient has a rigor and the temperature rises to 103° F. or higher. Owing to this intermittent character of the fever the disease is often mistaken for malaria. The fever may rise every afternoon without a rigor. Profuse sweating is common, particularly when the patient falls asleep. In chronic cases there may be little or no fever. One of my patients, with a liver abscess which had perforated the lung, coughed up pus after his temperature had been normal for weeks. The pain is variable, and is usually referred to the back or shoulder; or there is a dull aching sensation in the right hypochondrium. When turned on the left side, the patient often complains of a heavy, dragging sensation, so that he usually prefers to lie on the right side; at least, this has been the case in a majority of the instances which have come under my observation. Pain on pressure over the liver is usually present, particularly on deep pressure at the costal margin in the nipple line.

The enlargement of the liver is most marked in the right lobe, and, as the abscess cavity is usually situated more toward the upper than the under surface, the increase in volume is upward and to the right, not downward, as in cancer and the other affections producing enlargement. Percussion in the mid-sternal and parasternal lines may show a normal limit. At the nipple-line the curve of liver dulness begins to rise, and in the mid-axillary it may reach the fifth rib, while behind, near the spine, the area of dulness may be almost on a level with the angle of the scapula. Of course there are instances in which this characteristic feature is not present, as when the abscess occupies the left lobe. The enlargement of the liver may be so great as to cause bulging of the right side, and the edge may project a hand's-breadth or more below the costal margin. In such instances the surface is smooth. Palpation is painful, and there may be fremitus on deep inspiration. In some instances fluctuation may be detected. Adhesions may form to the abdominal wall and the abscess may point below the margin of the ribs, or even in the epigastric region. In many cases the appearance of the patient is suggestive. The skin has a sallow, slightly icteroid tint, the face is pale, the complexion muddy, the conjunctivæ are infiltrated, and often slightly bile-tinged. There is in the facies and in the general appearance of the patient a strong suggestion of the existence of abscess. There is no internal affection associated with suppuration which gives, I think, just the same hue as certain instances of abscess of the liver. Marked jaundice is rare. Diarrhœa may be present and may give an important clew to the nature of the case, particularly if amœbæ are found in the stools. Constipation may occur.

Perforation of the lung occurred in 9 of the 27 cases in my series. The symptoms are most characteristic. The extension may occur through the diaphragm, without actual rupture, and with the production of a purulent pleurisy and invasion of the lung. With cough of an aggravated and convulsive character, there are signs of involvement at the base of the right lung, defective resonance, feeble tubular breathing, and increase in the tactile fremitus; but the most characteristic feature is the presence of a reddish-brown expectoration of a brick-dust color, resembling anchovy sauce. This, which was noted originally by Budd, was present in our cases, and in addition Reese and Lafleur found the *amœbæ coli* identical with those which exist in the liver abscess and in the stools. They are present in variable numbers and display active amœboid movements. The brownish tint of the expectoration is due to blood-pigment and blood-corpuscles, and there may be orange-red crystals of hæmatoidin.

The abscess may perforate externally, as mentioned already, or into the stomach or bowel; occasionally into the pericardium. The duration of this form is very variable. It may run its course and prove fatal in six or eight weeks or may persist for several years.

The prognosis is serious, as the mortality is more than 50 per cent. The death-rate has been lowered of late years, owing to the great fearlessness with which the surgeons now attack these cases.

(*b*) Of the Pyæmic Abscess and Suppurative Pylephlebitis.—Clinically these conditions cannot be separated. Occurring in a general pyæmia, no special features may be added to the case. When there is suppuration within the portal vein the liver is uniformly enlarged and tender, though pain may not be a marked feature. There is an irregular, septic fever, and the complexion is muddy, sometimes distinctly icteroid. The features are indeed those of pyæmia, plus a slight icteroid tinge, and an enlarged and painful liver. The latter features alone are peculiar. The sweats, chills, prostration, and fever have nothing distinctive.

Diagnosis.—Abscess of the liver may be confounded with intermittent fever, a common mistake in malarial regions. Practically an intermittent fever which resists quinine is not malarial. Laveran's organisms are also absent from the blood. When the abscess bursts into the pleura a right-sided empyema is produced and perforation of the lung usually follows. When the liver abscess has been latent and dysenteric symptoms have not been marked, the condition may be considered empyema or abscess of the lung. In such cases the anchovy-sauce-like color of the pus and the presence of the amœbæ will enable one to make a definite diagnosis. Perforation externally is readily recognized, and yet in an abscess cavity in the epigastric region it may be difficult to say whether it has proceeded from the liver or is in the abdominal wall. When the abscess is large, and the adhesions are so firm that the liver does not descend during inspiration, the exploratory needle does not make an up-and-down movement during aspiration. The diagnosis of suppurating echinococcus cyst is rarely possible, except in Australia and Iceland, where hydatids are so common.

Perhaps the most important affection from which suppuration within the liver is to be separated is the intermittent hepatic fever associated with gall-stones. Of the cases reported a majority have been considered due to suppuration, and in two of my cases the liver had been repeatedly aspirated. Post mortem examinations have shown conclusively that the high fever and chills may recur at intervals for years without suppuration in the ducts. The distinctive features of this condition are paroxysms of fever with rigors and sweats—which may occur with great regularity, but which more often are separated by long intervals—the deepening of the jaundice after the paroxysms, the entire apyrexia in the intervals, and the maintenance of the general nutrition. The time element also is important, as in some of these cases the disease has lasted for several years. Finally, it is to be remembered that abscess of the liver, in temperate climates at least, is invariably secondary, and the primary source must be carefully sought for, either in dysentery, slight ulceration of the rectum, suppurating hæmorrhoids, ulcer of the stomach, or in suppurative disease of other parts of the body, particularly within the skull or in the bones.

Leucocytosis may be absent in the amœbic abscess of the liver; in septic cases it may be very high.

In suspected cases, whether the liver is enlarged or not, exploratory aspiration may be performed. The needle may be entered in the anterior axillary line in the lowest interspace, or in the seventh interspace in the mid-axillary line, or over the centre of the area of dulness behind. The patient should be placed under ether, for it may be necessary to make several deep punctures. It is not well to use too small an aspirator. No ill effects follow this procedure, even though blood may leak into the peritoneal cavity. Extensive suppuration may exist, and yet be missed in the aspiration, particularly when the branches of the portal vein are distended with pus.

Treatment.—Pyæmic abscess and suppurative pylephlebitis are invariably fatal. Treves, however, reports a case of pyæmic abscess following appendicitis in which the patient recovered after an exploratory operation. Surgical measures are not justified in these cases, unless an abscess shows signs of pointing. As the abscesses associated with dysentery are often single, they afford a reasonable hope of benefit from operation. If, however, the patient is expectorating the pus, if the general condition is good and the hectic fever not marked, it is best to defer operation, as many of these instances recover spontaneously. The large single abscesses are the most favorable for operation. The general medical treatment of the cases is that of ordinary septicæmia.

IX. NEW GROWTHS IN THE LIVER

These may be cancer, either primary or secondary, sarcoma, or angioma.

Etiology.—Cancer of the liver is third in order of frequency of internal cancer. It is rarely primary, usually secondary to cancer in other organs. It is a disease of late adult life. According to Leichtenstern, over 50 per cent. of the cases occur between the fortieth and the sixtieth years. It occasionally occurs in children. Women are attacked less frequently than men. It is stated by some authors that secondary cancer is more common in women, owing to the frequency of cancer of the uterus. Heredity is believed to have an influence in from 15 to 20 per cent.

In many cases trauma is an antecedent, and cancer of the bile-passages is associated in many instances with gall-stones. Cancer is stated to be less common in the tropics.

Morbid Anatomy.—The following forms of new growths occur in the liver and have a clinical importance:

CANCER.—*Primary Cancer.*—This is rare. Of 163 cases collected by Eggel, 63.3 per cent. were in males. There are several varieties. Nodular forms, in which there are scattered growths throughout the organ; the massive form in which the solitary tumor occupies a large area, either a lobe or the greater part of it; and small metastatic nodules. A very important form is that in which the liver is diffusely infiltrated with small growths, with much hyperplasia of the connective tissue—the so-called cancer with cirrhosis. The course of the disease is rapid, jaundice often occurs, splenic enlargement is not infrequent, ascites and œdema are common and toxic features are frequent toward the close.

Secondary Cancer.—The organ may reach an enormous size, 30½ pounds (Osler), 33 pounds (Christian). The cancerous nodules project beneath the capsule, and can be felt during life or even seen through the thin abdominal walls. They are usually disseminated equally, though in rare instances they may be confined to one lobe. The consistence of the nodules varies; in some cases they are firm and hard and those on the surface show a distinct umbilication, due to the shrinking of the fibrous tissue in the centre. These superficial cancerous masses are still sometimes spoken of as "Farre's tubercles." More frequently the masses are on section grayish-white in color, or hæmorrhagic. Rupture of blood-vessels is not uncommon in these cases. In one specimen there was an enormous clot beneath the capsule of the liver, together with hæmorrhage into the gall-bladder and into the peritoneum. The secondary cancer shows the same structure as the initial lesion, and is usually either an alveolar or cylindrical carcinoma. Degeneration is common in these secondary growths; thus the hyaline transformation may convert large areas into a dense, dry, grayish-yellow mass. Extensive areas of fatty degeneration may occur, sclerosis is not uncommon, and hæmorrhages are frequent. Suppuration sometimes follows.

Cancer of the bile-passages which has been already considered.

Sarcoma.—Of primary sarcoma of the liver very few cases have been reported. Secondary sarcoma is more frequent, and many examples of lympho-sarcoma and myxo-sarcoma are on record, less frequently glio-sarcoma or the smooth or striped myoma.

The most important form is the melano-sarcoma, secondary to sarcoma of the eye or of the skin. Very rarely melano-sarcoma occurs primarily in the liver. In this form the liver is greatly enlarged, is either uniformly infiltrated with the growth, which gives the cut surface the appearance of dark granite, or there are large nodular masses of a deep black or marbled color. There are usually extensive metastases, and in some instances every organ of the body is involved. Nodules of melano-sarcoma of the skin may give a clew to the diagnosis.

Other Forms of Liver Tumor.—One of the commonest tumors in the liver is the angioma, which occurs as a small, reddish body the size of a walnut, and consists simply of a series of dilated vessels. Occasionally in children angiomata grow and produce large tumors.

Cysts are occasionally found in the liver, either single, which is not very uncommon, or multiple, when they usually coexist with congenital cystic kidneys.

Symptoms.—It is often impossible to differentiate primary and secondary cancer of the liver unless the primary seat of the disease is evident, as in the case of scirrhus of the breast, or cancer of the rectum, or of a tumor in the stomach, which can be felt. As a rule, cancer of the liver is associated with progressive enlargement; but in some cases of primary nodular cancer and in the cancer with cirrhosis the organ may not be enlarged. Gastric disturbance, loss of appetite, nausea, and vomiting are frequent. Progressive loss of flesh and strength may be the first symptoms. Pain or a sensation of uneasiness in the right hypochondriac region may be present, but enormous enlargement of the liver may occur without the slightest pain. Jaundice, which is present in at least half of the cases, is usually of moderate extent, unless the common duct is occluded. Ascites is rare, except in the form of cancer with cirrhosis, in which the clinical picture is that of the atrophic form. Pressure by nodules on the portal vein or extension of the cancer to the peritoneum may also induce ascites.

Inspection shows the abdomen to be distended, particularly in the upper zone. In late stages of the disease, when emaciation is marked, the cancerous nodules can be plainly seen beneath the skin, and in rare instances even the umbilications. The superficial veins are enlarged. On palpation the liver is felt, a hand's-breadth or more below the costal margin, descending with each inspiration. The surface is usually irregular, and may present large masses or smaller nodular bodies, either rounded or with central depressions. In instances of diffuse infiltration the liver may be greatly enlarged and present a perfectly smooth surface. The growth is progressive, and the edge of the liver may ultimately extend below the level of the navel. Although generally uniform and producing enlargement of the whole organ, occasionally the tumor in the left lobe forms a solid mass occupying the epigastric region. By percussion the outline can be accurately limited and the progressive growth of the tumor estimated. The spleen is rarely enlarged. Pyrexia is present in many cases, usually a continuous fever, ranging from 100° to 102° F.; it may be intermittent, with rigors. This may be associated with the cancer alone, or, as in one of my cases, with suppuration. Œdema of the feet, from anæmia, usually supervenes. Cancer of the liver kills in from three to fifteen months. One of my patients lived for more than two years.

Diagnosis.—The diagnosis is easy when the liver is greatly enlarged and the surface nodular. The smoother forms of diffuse carcinoma may at first be mistaken for fatty or amyloid liver, but the presence of jaundice, the rapid enlargement, and the more marked cachexia will usually suffice to differentiate it. Perhaps the most puzzling conditions occur in the rare cases of enlarged amyloid liver with irregular gummata. The large echinococcus liver may present a striking similarity to carcinoma, but the projecting nodules are usually softer, the disease lasts much longer, and the cachexia is not marked.

Hypertrophic cirrhosis may at first be mistaken for carcinoma, as the jaundice is usually deep and the liver very large; but the absence of a marked cachexia and wasting and the painless, smooth character of the enlargement are points against cancer. In large, rapidly growing secondary cancers the superficial rounded masses may almost fluctuate and these soft tumor-like projections may contain blood. The form of cancer with cirrhosis can scarcely be separated from atrophic cirrhosis itself. Perhaps the wasting is more extreme and more rapid, but the jaundice and the ascites are identical. Melano-sarcoma causes great enlargement of the organ. There are frequently symptoms of involvement of other viscera, as the lungs, kidneys, or spleen. Secondary tumors may occur in the skin. A very important symptom, not present in all cases, is melanuria, the passage of a very dark-colored urine, which may, however, when first voided, be quite normal in color. The existence of a melano-sarcoma of the eye, or the history of blindness in one eye, with subsequent extirpation, may indicate at once the true nature of the hepatic enlargement.

There are several conditions in which the liver itself, or portions of it, may be mistaken for tumor. (*a*) In a progressive cirrhosis with enlargement the left lobe may increase out of all proportion to the right, and form a prominent mass in the epigastrium. (*b*) Riedel's tongue-like lobe projecting from the edge in the neighborhood of the gall-bladder, and often associated with distention of this organ. (*c*) The extreme left portion of the organ may be almost separated by a broad, flat band, containing little or no liver tissue. In a very thin person this section may feel like a separate tumor mass, as in an instance reported by J. P. Inglis (Polyclinic, Jan., 1911). A small portion of the liver lay directly over the cœliac axis, connected with the left lobe by a mesentery. The tumor was palpable. Lastly, the contracted, deformed organ in perihepatitis may form a visible, freely movable tumor in the upper portion of the abdomen, without a semblance of the normal liver. Such an instance I figure in my lectures on *Abdominal Tumors*.

Treatment.—The treatment must be entirely symptomatic. The question of surgical interference may be discussed. Keen has collected reports of 76 cases of resection of tumors of the liver, 63 of which recovered.

X. FATTY LIVER

Two different forms of this condition are recognized—the fatty infiltration and fatty degeneration.

Fatty infiltration occurs, to a certain extent, in normal livers, since the cells always contain minute globules of oil.

In fatty degeneration, which is a much less common condition, the protoplasm of the liver-cells is destroyed and the fat takes its place, as seen in cases of malignant jaundice and in phosphorus poisoning.

Fatty liver occurs under the following conditions: (*a*) In association with general obesity, in which case the liver appears to be one of the storehouses of the excessive fat. (*b*) In conditions in which the oxidation processes are interfered with, as in cachexia, profound anæmia, and in phthisis. The fatty infiltration of the liver in heavy drinkers is to be attributed to the excessive demand made by the alcohol upon the oxygen. (*c*) Certain poisons, of which phosphorus is the most characteristic, produce an intense fatty degeneration with necrosis of the liver-cells. The poison of acute yellow atrophy, whatever its nature, acts in the same way.

The fatty liver is uniformly increased in size. The edge may reach below the level of the navel. It is smooth, looks pale and bloodless; on section it is dry, and renders the surface of the knife greasy. The liver may weigh many pounds, and yet the specific gravity is so low that the entire organ floats in water.

The symptoms of fatty liver are not definite. Jaundice is never present; the stools may be light colored, but even in the most advanced grades the bile is still formed. Signs of portal obstruction are rare. Hæmorrhoids are not very infrequent. Altogether, the symptoms are ill defined, and are chiefly those of the disease with which the degeneration is associated. In cases of great obesity the physical examination is uncertain; but in phthisis and cachectic conditions the organ can be felt to be greatly enlarged, though smooth and painless. Fatty livers are among the largest met with at the bedside.

XI. AMYLOID LIVER

The waxy, lardaceous, or amyloid liver occurs as part of a general degeneration, associated with cachexias, particularly when the result of long-standing suppuration.

In practice, it is found oftenest in the prolonged suppuration of tuberculous disease, either of the lungs or of the bones. Next in order of frequency are the cases associated with syphilis. Here there may be ulceration of the rectum, with which it is often connected, or chronic disease of the bone, or it may be present when there are no suppurative changes. It is found occasionally in rickets, in prolonged convalescence from the infectious fevers, and in the cachexia of cancer.

The amyloid liver is large, and may attain dimensions equalled only by those of the cancerous organ. Wilks speaks of a liver weighing fourteen pounds. It is solid, firm, resistant, on section anæmic, and has a semitranslucent, infiltrated appearance. Stained with a dilute solution of iodine, the areas infiltrated with the amyloid matter assume a rich mahogany-brown color.

There are no characteristic *symptoms* of this condition. Jaundice does not occur; the stools may be light-colored, but the secretion of bile persists. The physical examination shows the organ to be uniformly enlarged and painless, the surface smooth, the edge rounded, and the consistence greatly increased. Sometimes the edge, even in very great enlargement, is sharp and hard. The spleen also may be involved, but there are no evidences of portal obstruction.

The *diagnosis* of the condition is, as a rule, easy. Progressive and great enlargement in connection with suppuration of long standing or with syphilis is almost always of this nature. In rare instances, however, the amyloid liver is reduced in size.

In *leukæmia* the liver may attain considerable size and be smooth and uniform, resembling, on physical examination, the fatty organ. The blood condition at once indicates the true nature of the case.

XII. ANOMALIES IN FORM AND POSITION OF THE LIVER

In transposition of the viscera the right lobe of the organ may occupy the left side. A common and important anomaly is the tilting forward of the organ, so that the antero-posterior axis becomes vertical, not horizontal. Instead of the edge of the right lobe presenting just below the costal margin, a considerable portion of the surface of the lobe is in contact with the abdominal parietes, and the edge may be felt as low, perhaps, as the navel. This anteversion is apt to be mistaken for enlargement of the organ.

The "lacing" liver is met with in two chief types. In one the anterior portion, chiefly of the right lobe, is greatly prolonged, and may reach the transverse navel line, or even lower. A shallow transverse groove separates the thin extension from the main portion of the organ. The peritoneal coating of this groove may be fibroid, and in rare instances the deformed portion is connected with the organ by an almost tendinous membrane. The liver may be compressed laterally and have a pyramidal shape, and the extreme left border and the hinder margin of the left lobe may be much folded and incurved. The projecting portion of the liver, extending low in the right flank, may be mistaken for a tumor, or more frequently for a movable right kidney. Its continuity with the liver itself may not be evident on palpation or on percussion, as coils of intestine may lie in front. It descends, however, with inspiration, and usually the margin can be traced continuously with that of the left lobe of the liver. The greatest difficulty arises when this anomalous lappet of the liver is either naturally very thick and united to the liver by a very thin membrane, or when it is swollen in conditions of great congestion of the organ.

The other principal type of lacing liver is quite different in shape. It is thick, broader above than below, and lies almost entirely above the transverse line of the cartilages. There is a narrow groove just above the anterior border, which is placed more transversely than normal.

Movable Liver.—This rare condition has received much attention, and J. E. Graham collected 70 reported cases from the literature. In a very considerable number of these there has been a mistaken diagnosis. A slight grade of mobility of the organ is found in the pendulous abdomen of enteroptosis, and after repeated ascites.

The organ is so connected at its posterior margin with the inferior vena cava and diaphragm that any great mobility from this point is impossible, except on the theory of a meso-hepar or congenital ligamentous union between these structures. The ligaments, however, may show an extreme grade of relaxation (the suspensory 7.5 cm., and the triangular ligament 4 cm., in one of Leube's cases) ; and when the patient is in the erect posture the organ may drop down so far that its upper surface is entirely below the costal margin. The condition is rarely met with in men; 56 of the cases were in women.

I. DISEASES OF THE PANCREAS

I. PANCREATIC INSUFFICIENCY

Failure of the internal secretion is followed by disturbance in the carbohydrate metabolism, of the external secretion by disturbances of digestion, or by the injurious effects of the retained secretion. The low sugar tolerance, the chief sign of impairment of the internal secretion, has been considered under diabetes. Insufficiency of the external secretion is indicated by:

Changes in the Character of the Stools.—(*a*) STEATORRHŒA.—The proportion of fat in the fæces varies; above 30 per cent. of the dried weight suggests pancreatic insufficiency. The stools are either oily like butter, or gray like asbestos. The ability to digest fat differs greatly and there are healthy persons who constantly have a high percentage of fat in the stools. Steatorrhœa may last for many years without impairment of health. There is also a disturbance in the normal ratio between the neutral fats and the fatty acids. Cammidge gives the following average figures: Normal per cent., total fats 21, neutral fats 11, fatty acids 10; malignant disease, total fats 77, neutral fats 50, fatty acids 27; chronic pancreatitis, total fats 50, neutral fats 32, fatty acids 18.

(*b*) AZOTORRHŒA, the presence of undigested proteid materials in the stools, has long been known as an association of pancreatic disease. Normally only 5 or 6 per cent. of the undigested proteids appears in the fæces, but in pancreatic disease as much as 30 or 40 per cent. may be recovered. Schmidt claims that the nuclear material of meat is digested by the pancreatic juice alone and that persistence of the nuclei of the meat fibres in the stools indicates defective tryptic digestion.

In jaundice due to malignant disease of the head of the pancreas stercobilin is absent; in that due to chronic pancreatitis or gall-stones it is either absent or present only in traces.

Cammidge's Pancreatic Reaction.—For details of the reaction the student must consult special manuals. It is claimed that the reaction is positive in all cases of active inflammatory changes in the pancreas, and that by this means acute forms of pancreatitis can be differentiated from intestinal obstruction, and that by it chronic pancreatitis causing blocking of the common duct can be diagnosed from gall-stones. In malignant disease the reaction is negative in about three-fourths of the cases. It is unfortunate that Cammidge's work lacks confirmation. The studies (1911) at the Mayo clinic under Wilson's direction lead to the conclusion that "if knowledge of the clinical histories and other factors of the personal equation be eliminated, the end results, judged by Cammidge's own criteria, must be considered, as a means of diagnosing disease of the pancreas, as both valueless and misleading." From observations of Whipple and others it seems that rapid disintegration of any of the body cells, particularly the polynuclear leucocytes, may give rise to the reaction.

II. PANCREATIC NECROSIS

The entire series of pancreatic lesions, from hæmorrhage to gangrene, and from fat necrosis to pancreatic cyst, may result from tryptic auto-digestion (Chiari). This is met with under four conditions: (*a*) Trauma, as in gunshot wounds, blows, or perforation of a peptic ulcer. (*b*) Primary thrombosis in the venous radicles of the glands. (*c*) Obstruction of the free flow of secretion in the duct. (*d*) Entrance of the bile into the ducts.

In the mildest forms there are only a few small hæmorrhages or circumscribed areas of necrosis of the gland tissue with fat necrosis in the neighborhood; in severer forms groups of acini or the whole gland may be involved.

Fat necrosis occurs whenever the pancreatic juice, obstructed from any cause and dammed back on the gland, infiltrates its tissues, or escaping by the lymph spaces finds its way to structures at some distance from the gland. The necrosis is due to the fat-splitting ferment in the secretion (Opie).

Balser first called attention to this remarkable change which is found in the interlobular pancreatic tissue, in the mesentery, in the omentum, in the abdominal fatty tissue generally, and occasionally in the pericardial and subcutaneous fat. The necroses are most frequent in the acute and necrotic forms of pancreatitis, less common in the suppurative. In the pancreas the lobules are seen to be separated by a dead white necrotic tissue, which gives a remarkable appearance to the section. In the abdominal fat the areas are usually not larger than a pin's head; they at once attract attention, and may be mistaken, on superficial examination, for miliary tubercles or neoplasms. They may be larger; instances have been reported in which they were the size of a hen's egg. On section they have a soft tallowy consistence, and the substance is a combination of lime with certain fatty acids. The necroses may be crusted with lime, and in a man aged 80, who died of nephritis, I found the lobules of the pancreas entirely isolated by areas of fat necrosis with extensive deposition of lime salts.

III. HÆMORRHAGE

Both Spiess (1866) and Zenker (1874) were acquainted with hæmorrhage into the pancreas as a cause of sudden death, but the great medico-legal importance of the subject was first fully recognized by F. W. Draper, of Boston, whose townsmen, Harris, Fitz, Whitney, and others, have contributed additional studies. In 4,000 autopsies Draper met with 19 cases of pancreatic hæmorrhage, in 9 or 10 of which no other cause of death was found. When the bleeding is extensive the entire tissue of the gland is destroyed and the blood invades the retro-peritoneal tissue. In other instances the peritoneal covering is broken and the blood fills the lesser peritoneum (see hæmoperitoneum). The hæmorrhage may be in connection with an acute pancreatitis or with necrotic inflammation of the gland.

The *symptoms* are thus briefly summarized by Prince: "The patient, who has previously been perfectly well, is suddenly taken with the illness which terminates his life. . . . When the hæmorrhage occurs the patient may be quietly resting or pursuing his usual occupation. The pain which ushers in the attack is usually very severe and located in the upper part of the abdomen. It steadily increases in severity, is sharp or perhaps colicky in character. It is almost from the first accompanied by nausea and vomiting; the latter becomes frequent and obstinate, but gives no relief. The patient soon becomes anxious, restless, and depressed; he tosses about, and only with difficulty can he be restrained in bed. The surface is cold and the forehead is covered with a cold sweat. The pulse is weak, rapid, and sooner or later imperceptible. The abdomen becomes tender, the tenderness being located in the upper part of the abdomen or epigastrium. Tympanites is sometimes marked. The temperature is usually normal or subnormal. The bowels are constipated."

IV. ACUTE PANCREATITIS

Acute Hæmorrhagic Pancreatitis.—In this form the inflammation is combined with hæmorrhage, and it is difficult to separate clearly the two processes.

Etiology.—A large majority of the cases occur in adult males. McPhedran has reported one in a nine months' old child. Many of the patients had been addicted to alcohol; others had suffered occasionally with severe pains and vomiting or with gall-stone colic. Peiser found that 8 out of 121 collected cases of acute pancreatitis were associated with parturition. He suggests that the changes bringing about the pancreatitis in these cases may be analogous to those occurring in the liver, kidneys, and other organs in eclampsia.

The pancreas is found enlarged, and the interlobular tissue infiltrated with blood, and perhaps with clots. The relation of gall-stones to the condition has been demonstrated by Opie, and they were present in four of five cases at the Johns Hopkins Hospital. The calculus may be very small, and situated in the diverticulum of Vater. Bile finding its way into the pancreas may cause hæmorrhagic inflammation. Injection of bile into the pancreatic ducts of dogs reproduces the lesion. The anatomical appearances are very characteristic. The tissues about the gland are infiltrated with blood and there may be fluid in the lesser peritoneum. Areas of fat necrosis are seen in the retroperitoneal fat, the mesocolon and mesentery. The gland itself is swollen and in section the stroma has a mottled dark brown appearance and the outlines of the acini may be lost. In a case which I have reported the semilunar ganglia were swollen, the nerve-cells indistinct, and there was an interstitial infiltration of round cells. The Pacinian corpuscles in the neighborhood of the pancreas were enormously swollen and œdematous.

SYMPTOMS.—One of the most characteristic features is the suddenness of the onset, usually with violent colicky pain in the upper part of the abdomen. Nausea and vomiting follow, with collapse symptoms, more or less severe according to the intensity of the attack. The abdomen becomes swollen and tense and there is constipation. The temperature at first may be low; subsequently fever sets in, sometimes initiated by a chill. There may be early delirium. Collapse symptoms supervene, and death occurs usually from the second to the fourth day, or even earlier. The swelling and infiltration in the region of the pancreas necessarily involve the cœliac plexus, and the stretching of the nerves may account for the agonizing pain and the sudden collapse. Deep pressure on the upper part of the abdomen may give evidence of circumscribed resistance.

DIAGNOSIS.—Intestinal obstruction or acute perforating peritonitis is usually suspected. Now that the condition has become better known, the diagnosis *intra vitam* has been made. "Acute pancreatitis is to be suspected when a previously healthy person or a sufferer from occasional attacks of indigestion is suddenly seized with a violent pain in the epigastrium followed by vomiting and collapse, and in the course of twenty-four hours by a circumscribed epigastric swelling, tympanitic or resistant, with slight elevation of temperature. Circumscribed tenderness in the course of the pancreas and tender spots throughout the abdomen are valuable diagnostic signs" (Fitz).

Acute Suppurative Pancreatitis—Pancreatic Abscess.—ETIOLOGY.—The etiology in a majority of cases is doubtful. Dyspeptic disturbances and trauma have preceded the onset in some instances. Gall-stones may be present. In many of the cases it is a sequel of acute hæmorrhagic pancreatitis. In 24 cases there was a single abscess; in 14 there were numerous small abscesses. In other instances there was a diffuse purulent infiltration. Some of the sequels are peri-pancreatic abscess, perforation into the stomach, the duodenum, or the peritoneum, and thrombosis of the portal vein.

SYMPTOMS.—The symptoms of suppurative pancreatitis are not always well defined. In one case in my wards Thayer made a correct diagnosis. The patient, aged thirty-four, had had occasional attacks of severe pain and vomiting. This was followed by fever and delirium. A deep-seated mass was felt in the median line just above the umbilicus. Finney operated and found disseminated fat-necrosis and a deep-seated abscess with necrotic pancreatic tissue. The patient recovered. The course of the suppurative form is much more chronic. Icterus, fatty diarrhœa, and sugar in the urine have been met with in some cases. The presence of a tumor mass in the epigastrium is of the greatest moment.

Gangrenous Pancreatitis.—Complete necrosis of the gland, or part of it, may follow either hæmorrhage or hæmorrhagic inflammation, and in exceptional cases may occur after suppurative infiltration or after injury or the perforation of an ulcer of the stomach. In Fitz's monograph 15 cases are reported. Körte has increased its number to 40. Symptoms of hæmorrhagic pancreatitis may precede or be associated with it. Death usually follows in from ten to twenty days, with symptoms of collapse.

Anatomically the pancreas may present a dry necrotic appearance, but as a rule the organ is converted into a dark slaty-colored mass lying nearly free in the omental cavity or attached by a few shreds. In other instances the totally or partially sequestrated organ may lie in a large abscess cavity, forming a palpable tumor in the epigastric region. In two cases, reported by Chiari, the necrotic pancreas was discharged per rectum, with recovery.

V. CHRONIC PANCREATITIS

Forms.—Anatomically there are two forms:

(*a*) Interlobular pancreatitis which follows occlusion of the duct, or an infection, such as occurs in the presence of calculi, biliary or pancreatic, with which organisms of the colon group, streptococci, or occasionally the typhoid bacillus are associated. Even in advanced sclerosis of this type the islands of Langerhans are spared. It may occur as an independent affection. It is not at all uncommon in the bodies of adults to find the head of the pancreas extraordinarily hard and so dense that it feels like scirrhus; surgeons have long noted this. The condition is often present without symptoms of pancreatic disease during life. A very special form is the chronic interstitial pancreatitis which accompanies hæmochromatosis, and which is described elsewhere. Mayo Robson, Moynihan and other surgeons have called attention to the fact that sclerosis of the head of the pancreas may cause obstruction of the duct.

(*b*) Chronic interacinar pancreatitis is characterized by a diffuse fibrosis penetrating between the acini, with little or no involvement of the interlobular tissues. It may follow infection through the duct, but is more common in association with cirrhosis of the liver and arterio-sclerosis.

Symptoms.—It must be confessed that the clinical picture of chronic pancreatitis is very obscure, in spite of the good work done by our surgical colleagues. Cammidge, who has had the great advantage of seeing Mayo Robson's clinical cases, describes four types: (*a*) The dyspeptic, in which the disease is due to morbid conditions of the bowels, and the symptoms are mainly referred to the digestive organs. (*b*) The cholelithic, associated with the presence of gall-stones in the common duct; there is usually chronic jaundice and the dominant symptoms are hepatic. (*c*) A miscellaneous group in which the pancreatitis is secondary to malignant disease, etc. (*d*) The diabetic group with glycosuria, and into which the members of the preceding groups may merge in course of time.

Symptoms of pancreatic insufficiency of the internal or external secretion are generally present; there is pain after food, very often jaundice, and on deep pressure the head of the pancreas may sometimes be felt. Careful study of the urine and of the fæces gives important information. Cammidge's pancreatic reaction in the urine is, its author thinks, suggestive of active degenerative changes. Sugar may also be present. The stools may show both steatorrhœa and azotorrhœa.

Treatment.—Owing to the difficulty of diagnosis in the early stages it is impossible to speak positively in a great many cases, but in the forms which are associated with pain, jaundice, the presence of calculi, and infection of the ducts excellent results have followed free drainage of the bile passages.

So much influenced is our present picture of chronic pancreatitis by personal equation on the part of surgical and laboratory workers that we are not in a position to speak very definitely on several important points.

VI. PANCREATIC CYSTS

Of 121 cases operated upon 60 were in males and 56 in females; in 5 the sex was not given (Körte). Sixty-six of the cases occurred in the fourth decade. T. C. Railton's case (which is not in Körte's series), an infant aged six months, and Shattuck's case in a child of thirteen and a half months are the youngest in the literature. According to the origin Körte recognizes three varieties.

Varieties.—TRAUMATIC CASES.—In this list of 33 cases 30 were in men and only 3 in women. Blows on the abdomen or constantly repeated pressure are the most common forms of trauma. One case followed severe massage. Usually with the onset there are inflammatory symptoms, pain, and vomiting, sometimes suggestive of peritonitis. The contents of the cyst are usually bloody, though in 13 of the traumatic cases it was clear or yellowish.

CYSTS FOLLOWING INFLAMMATORY CONDITIONS.—In 51 cases the trouble began gradually after attacks of dyspepsia with colic, simulating somewhat that of gall-stones. Occasionally the attack set in with very severe symptoms, suggestive of obstruction of the bowel. In this group the tumor appeared in 19 cases soon after the onset of the pain; in others it was delayed for a period of from a few weeks to two or three years. McPhedran has reported a remarkable instance in which the tumor appeared in the epigastrium with signs of severe inflammation. It was opened and drained and believed to be a hydrops of the lesser peritoneal cavity. Three months later a second cyst developed, which appeared to spring directly from the pancreas.

CYSTS WITHOUT ANY INFLAMMATORY OR TRAUMATIC ETIOLOGY.—Of 33 cases in this group 26 were in women. A remarkable feature is the prolonged period of their existence—in one case for forty-seven years, in one for between sixteen and twenty years, in others for sixteen, nine, and eight years, in the majority for from two to four years.

Morbid Anatomy.—Anatomically Körte recognizes (1) *retention cysts* due to plugging of the main duct; (2) *proliferation cysts* of the pancreatic tissue —and cysto-adenoma; (3) *retention cysts* arising from the alveoli of the gland and of the smaller ducts, which become cut off and dilate in consequence of chronic interstitial pancreatitis; (4) *pseudo-cysts* following inflammatory or traumatic affections of the pancreas, usually the result of injury, causing hæmorrhage and hydrops of the lesser peritoneum.

Situation.—In its growth the cyst may (1) be in the lesser peritoneum, push the stomach upward, and reach the abdominal wall between the stomach and the transverse colon; (2) more rarely the cyst appears above the lesser curvature and pushes the stomach downward; in both of these cases the situation of the tumor is high in the abdomen; but (3) it may develop between the leaves of the transverse meso-colon and lie below both the colon and the stomach. The relation of these two organs to the tumor is variable, but in the majority of cases the stomach lies above and the transverse colon below the cyst. Occasionally, too, as in T. C. Railton's case, the cyst may arise in the tail of the pancreas and project far over in the left hypochondrium in the position of the spleen or of a renal tumor.

General Symptoms.—Apart from the features of onset already referred to, the patient may complain of no trouble unless the cyst reaches a very large size. Painful colicky attacks, with nausea and vomiting and progressive enlargement of the abdomen, have frequently been noted. Fatty diarrhœa from disturbance of the function of the pancreas is rare. Sugar in the urine has been present in a number of cases. Increased secretion of the saliva, the so-called pancreatic salivation, is also rare. Pressure of the cyst may sometimes cause jaundice, and in rare instances dyspnœa. Very marked loss of flesh has been present in a number of cases. A remarkable feature often noticed has been the transitory disappearance of the cyst. In one of Halsted's cases the girth of the abdomen decreased from 43 to 31 inches in ten days with profuse diarrhœa. Sometimes the disappearance has followed blows.

Diagnosis.—The cyst occupies the upper abdomen, usually forming a semicircular bulging in the median line, rarely to either side. In 16 cases Körte states that the chief projection was below the navel. In one case operated upon by Halsted the tumor occupied the greater part of the abdomen. The cyst is immobile, respiration having little or no influence on it. As already mentioned, the stomach, as a rule, lies above it and the colon below.

In a majority of the cases the fluid is of a reddish or dark-brown color, and contains blood or blood coloring matter, cell detritus, fat granules, and sometimes cholesterin. The consistence of the fluid is usually mucoid, rarely thin. The reaction is alkaline, the specific gravity from 1.010 to 1.020. In 22 cases Körte states that the fluid was not hæmorrhagic.

The existence of ferments is important. In 54 cases they were present in the fluid or in the material from the fistula. In 20 cases only one ferment was present, in 20 cases two, and in 14 cases all three of the pancreatic ferments were found. In view of the wide occurrence of diastatic and fat-emulsifying ferments in various exudates, the most important and only positive sign in the diagnosis of the pancreatic secretion is the digestion of fibrin and albumin.

Operation.—Of 160 cases of operation there were 150 recoveries. Incision and drainage was the operation performed in 138 cases, in 15 excision was performed.

VII. TUMORS OF THE PANCREAS

Of new growths in the organ carcinoma is the most frequent. Sarcoma, adenoma, and lymphoma are rare.

Frequency.—At the General Hospital in Vienna in 18,069 autopsies there were 22 cases of cancer of the pancreas (Biach). In 11,472 post mortems at Milan Segré found 132 tumors of the pancreas, 127 of which were carcinomata, 2 sarcomata, 2 cysts, and 1 syphiloma. In 6,000 autopsies at Guy's Hospital there were only 20 cases of primary malignant disease of the organ (Hale White). In the first 1,500 autopsies at the Johns Hopkins Hospital there were 6 cases of adeno-carcinoma, and 1 doubtful case in which the exact origin could not be stated. There were 8 cases of secondary malignant disease of the pancreas. The head of the gland is most commonly involved, but the disease may be limited to the body or to the tail. The majority of the patients are in the middle period of life.

Symptoms.—The diagnosis is not often possible. The following are the most important and suggestive features: (*a*) Epigastric pains, often occurring in paroxysms. (*b*) Jaundice, due to pressure of the tumor in the head of the pancreas on the bile-duct. The jaundice is intense and permanent, and associated with dilatation of the gall-bladder, which may reach a very large size. (*c*) The presence of a tumor in the epigastrium. This is very variable. In 137 cases Da Costa found the tumor present in only 13. Palpation under anæsthesia with the stomach empty would probably give a very much larger percentage. As the tumor rests directly upon the aorta there is usually a marked degree of pulsation, sometimes with a bruit. There may be pressure on the portal vein, causing thrombosis and its usual sequels. (*d*) Symptoms due to loss of function of the pancreas are less important. Fatty diarrhœa is not very often present. In consequence of the absence of bile the stools are usually very clay-colored and greasy. Diabetes also is not common. (*e*) A very rapid wasting and cachexia. Of other symptoms nausea and vomiting are common. In some instances the pylorus is compressed and there is great dilatation of the stomach. In a few cases there has been profuse salivation.

The points of greatest importance in the diagnosis are the intense and permanent jaundice, with dilatation of the gall-bladder, rapid emaciation, and the presence of a tumor in the epigastric region. Of less importance are features pointing to disturbance of the functions of the gland.

Of other new growths sarcoma and lymphoma have been occasionally found. Miliary tubercle is not very uncommon in the gland. Syphilis may occur as rather a chronic interstitial inflammation, or in the form of gummata.

The outlook in tumors of the pancreas is, as a rule, hopeless; but of late years a number of successful cases of operation have been reported.

VIII. PANCREATIC CALCULI

Pancreatic lithiasis is comparatively rare. In 1883 George W. Johnston collected 35 cases in the literature. In 1,500 autopsies at the Johns Hopkins Hospital there were 2 cases.

The stones are usually numerous, either round in shape or rough, spinous and coral-like. The color is opaque white. They are composed chiefly of carbonate of lime. The effects of the stones are: (1) A chronic interstitial inflammation of the gland substance with dilatation of the duct; sometimes there is cystic dilatation of the gland; (2) acute inflammation with suppuration; (3) the irritation of the stones, as in the gall-bladder, may lead to carcinoma.

Symptoms.—The cases are not often diagnosed. Pains in the epigastrium, often very severe, but not characteristic; the signs of pancreatic insufficiency already described, and the X-rays, which show the pancreatic but not the biliary concretions, are suggestive features. An analysis of the calculi passed with the stools may alone serve to distinguish a case from one of gall-stones. Operation has been performed successfully.

J. DISEASES OF THE PERITONEUM

I. ACUTE GENERAL PERITONITIS

Definition.—Acute inflammation of the peritoneum.

Etiology.—The condition may be primary or secondary.

(*a*) PRIMARY, IDIOPATHIC PERITONITIS.—Considering how frequently the pleura and pericardium are primarily inflamed, the rarity of idiopathic inflammation of the peritoneum is somewhat remarkable. It may follow cold or exposure and is then known as "rheumatic" peritonitis. In Bright's disease, gout, and arterio-sclerosis acute peritonitis may occur as a terminal event. Of 102 cases of peritonitis which came to autopsy at the Johns Hopkins Hospital, 12 were of this form.

(*b*) SECONDARY PERITONITIS is due to extension of inflammation from, or perforation of, one of the organs covered by the peritoneum. Peritonitis from extension may follow inflammation of the stomach or intestines, ulceration in these parts, cancer, acute suppurative inflammations of the spleen, liver, pancreas, retroperitoneal tissues, and the pelvic viscera.

Perforative peritonitis is the most common, following external wounds, perforation of an ulcer of the stomach or bowels, perforation of the gall-bladder, abscess of the liver, spleen, or kidneys. Two important causes are appendicitis and suppurating inflammation about the Fallopian tubes and ovaries. There are instances in which peritonitis has followed rupture of an apparently normal Graafian follicle.

Of the above 102 cases, 56 originated in an extension from some diseased abdominal viscus. The remaining 34 followed surgical operations upon the peritoneum or the contained organs.

The peritonitis of septicæmia and pyæmia is almost invariably the result of a local process. An exceedingly acute form of peritonitis may be caused by the development of tubercles on the membrane.

Morbid Anatomy.—In recent cases, on opening the abdomen the intestinal coils are distended and glued together with lymph, and the peritoneum presents a patchy, sometimes a uniform injection. The exudation may be: (*a*) Fibrinous, with little or no fluid, except a few pockets of clear serum between the coils. (*b*) Sero-fibrinous. The coils are covered with lymph, and there is in addition a large amount of a yellowish, sero-fibrinous fluid. In instances in which the stomach or intestine is perforated this may be mixed with food or fæces. (*c*) Purulent, in which the exudate is either thin and greenish yellow in color, or opaque white and creamy. (*d*) Putrid. Occasionally in puerperal and perforative peritonitis, particularly when the latter has been caused by cancer, the exudate is thin, grayish green in color, and has a gangrenous odor. (*e*) Hæmorrhagic. This is sometimes found as an admixture in cases of acute peritonitis following wounds, and occurs in the cancerous and tuberculous forms. (*f*) A rare form occurs in which the injection is present, but almost all signs of exudation are wanting. Close inspection may be necessary to detect a slight dulling of the serous surfaces.

The amount of the effusion varies from half a litre to 20 or 30 litres. There are probably essential differences between the various kinds of peritonitis.

Bacteriology.—A large number of organisms have been found in connection with the disease. In Flexner's series, in 12 primary cases the streptococcus was the prevailing organism. In the cases following operation the staphylococcus was present alone in 12 out of 33, the streptococcus in 5, and the colon bacillus in 5. Other organisms were the pneumococcus, bacillus pyocyaneus, and bacillus aerogenes. Of 56 cases of peritonitis following intestinal infections, the colon bacillus occurred in 43, usually in connection with streptococci. The bacillus lactis aerogenes has also been found as the sole organism. The gonococcus is present in the form which arises from salpingitis and may occur in the gonorrhœal infections of children.

Much attention has been paid of late to the pneumococcus as an agent in the causation of peritonitis, and many cases are of the primary form without recognizable portal of entry; but it is to be remembered that there are many latent pneumococcic lesions, particularly those of the middle ear, and of the accessory sinuses of the nose. Cameron, in a recent study, makes two groups of cases; a diffuse form setting in with abdominal pain, high fever, vomiting, diarrhœa, in which death may occur within 36 hours. In the other group the peritonitis is local, and the symptoms may suggest appendicitis. Gradually a localized abscess develops, which may rupture internally. The creamy greenish yellow odorless pus is very characteristic.

Symptoms.—In the perforative and septic cases the onset is marked by chilly feelings or an actual rigor with intense pain in the abdomen. In typhoid fever, when the sensorium is benumbed, the onset may not be noticed. The pain is general, and is usually intense and aggravated by movements and pressure. A position is taken which relieves the tension of the abdominal muscles, so that the patient lies on the back with the thighs drawn up and the shoulders elevated. The greatest pain is usually below the umbilicus, but in peritonitis from perforation of the stomach pain may be referred to the back, the chest, or the shoulder. The respiration is superficial—costal in type—as it is painful to use the diaphragm. For the same reason the action of coughing is restrained, and even the movements necessary for talking are limited. In this early stage the sensitiveness may be great and the abdominal muscles are often rigidly contracted. If the patient is at perfect rest the pain may be very slight, and there are instances in which it is not at all marked, and may, indeed, be absent.

The abdomen gradually becomes distended and tense and is tympanitic on percussion. The pulse is rapid, small, and hard, and often has a peculiar wiry quality. It ranges from 110 to 150. The temperature may rise rapidly after the chill and reach 104° or 105° F., but the subsequent elevation is moderate. In some very severe cases there may be no fever throughout. The tongue at first is white and moist, but subsequently becomes dry and often red and fissured. Vomiting is an early and prominent feature and causes great pain. The contents of the stomach are first ejected, then a yellowish and bile stained fluid, and finally a greenish and, in rare instances, a brownish black liquid with slight fæcal odor.' The bowels may be loose at the onset and then constipation may follow. Frequent micturition may be present, less often retention. The urine is usually scanty and high-colored, and contains a large quantity of indican.

The appearance of the patient when these symptoms have fully developed is very characteristic. The face is pinched, the eyes are sunken, and the expression is very anxious. The constant vomiting of fluids causes a wasted appearance, and the hands sometimes present the washer-woman's skin. Except in cholera, we see the Hippocratic facies more frequently in this than in any other disease—*"a sharp nose, hollow eyes, collapsed temples; the ears cold, contracted, and their lobes turned out; the skin about the forehead being rough, distended, and parched; the color of the whole face being brown, black, livid, or lead-colored."* There are one or two additional points about the abdomen. The tympany is usually excessive, owing to the great relaxation of the walls of the intestines by inflammation and exudation. The splenic dulness may be obliterated, the diaphragm pushed up, and the apex beat of the heart dislocated to the fourth interspace. The liver dulness may be greatly reduced, or may, in the mammary line, be obliterated. It has been claimed that this is a distinctive feature of perforative peritonitis, but the liver dulness in the middle mammary line may be obliterated by tympanites alone. In the axillary line, on the other hand, the liver dulness, though diminished, may persist. Pneumo-peritoneum following perforation more certainly obliterates the hepatic dulness. In such cases the fluid effused produces a dulness in the lateral region; but with gas in the peritoneum, if the patient is turned on the left side, a clear note is heard beneath the seventh and eighth rib. Acute peritonitis may present a flat, rigid abdomen throughout its course.

Effusion of fluid—ascites—is usually present except in some acute, rapidly fatal cases. The flanks are dull on percussion. The dulness may be movable, though this depends altogether upon the degree of adhesions. There may be considerable effusion without either movable dulness or fluctuation. A friction rub may be present, as first pointed out by Bright, but it is not nearly so common in acute as in chronic peritonitis.

Course.—The acute diffuse peritonitis usually terminates in death. The most intense forms may kill within thirty-six to forty-eight hours; more commonly death results in four or five days, or the attack may be prolonged to eight or ten days. The pulse becomes irregular, the heart-sounds weak, the breathing shallow; there are lividity with pallor, a cold skin with high rectal temperature—a group of symptoms indicating profound failure of the vital functions for which Gee has revived the old term *lipothymia*. Occasionally death occurs with great suddenness, owing, possibly, to paralysis of the heart.

Diagnosis.—In typical cases the severe pain at onset, the distention of the abdomen, the tenderness, the fever, the gradual onset of effusion, collapse, and the vomiting give a characteristic picture. Careful inquiries should at once be made concerning the previous condition, from which a clew can often be had as to the starting-point of the trouble. In young adults a considerable proportion of all cases depends upon perforating appendicitis, and there may be an account of previous attacks of pain in the iliac region, or of constipation alternating with diarrhœa. In women the most frequent causes are suppurative processes in the pelvic viscera, associated with salpingitis, abscesses in the broad ligaments, or acute puerperal infection. Perforation of gastric ulcer is a more common factor in women than in men. It is not always easy to determine the cause. Many cases come under observation for the first time with the abdomen distended and tender, and it is impossible to make a satisfactory examination. In such instances the pelvic organs should be examined with the greatest care. In typhoid fever, if the patient is conscious, the sudden onset of pain, the tenderness, rigidity, muscle spasm, and the aggravation of the general symptoms indicate what has happened. When the patient is in deep coma, on the other hand, the perforation may be overlooked. The following conditions are most apt to be mistaken for acute peritonitis:

(*a*) *Acute Entero-colitis.*—Here the pain and distention and the sensitiveness on pressure may be marked. The pain is more colicky in character, the diarrhœa is more frequent, and the collapse is more extreme.

(*b*) *The So-called Hysterical Peritonitis.*—This has deceived the very elect, as almost every feature of genuine peritonitis, even the collapse, may be simulated. The onset may be sudden, with severe pain in the abdomen, tenderness, vomiting, diarrhœa, difficulty in micturition, and the characteristic decubitus. Even the temperature may be elevated. There may be recurrence of the attack. A case has been reported by Bristowe in which four attacks occurred within a year, and it was not until special hysterical symptoms developed that the true nature of the trouble was suspected.

(*c*) *Obstruction of the bowel,* as already mentioned, may simulate peritonitis, both having pain, vomiting, tympanites, and constipation in common. It may for a couple of days really be impossible to make a diagnosis in the absence of a satisfactory history.

(*d*) *Rupture of an abdominal aneurism or embolism of the superior mesenteric artery* may cause symptoms which simulate peritonitis. In the latter, sudden onset with severe pain, the collapse symptoms, frequent vomiting, and great distention of the abdomen may be present.

(*e*) I have already referred to the fact that acute hæmorrhagic pancreatitis may be mistaken for peritonitis. Lastly, a ruptured tubal pregnancy may resemble acute peritonitis.

II. PERITONITIS IN INFANTS

Peritonitis may occur in the fetus as a consequence of syphilis, and may lead to constriction of the bowel by fibrous adhesions.

In the new-born a septic peritonitis may extend from an inflamed cord. Distention of the abdomen, slight swelling and redness about the cord, and not infrequently jaundice are present. It is an uncommon event, and existed in only 4 of 51 infants dying with inflammation of the cord and septicæmia (Runge).

During childhood peritonitis arises from causes similar to those affecting the adult. Perforative appendicitis is common. Peritonitis following blows or kicks on the abdomen occurs more frequently at this period. In boys injury while playing football may be followed by diffuse peritonitis. A rare cause in children is extension through the diaphragm from an empyema. There are on record instances of peritonitis occurring in several children at the same school, and it has been attributed to sewer-gas poisoning. It was in investigating an epidemic of this kind at the Wandsworth school, in London, that Anstie received the post mortem wound of which he died. It is to be remembered that peritonitis in children may follow the gonorrhœal vulvitis so common in infant homes and hospitals.

III. LOCALIZED PERITONITIS

Subphrenic Peritonitis.—The general peritoneum covering the right and left lobes of the liver may be involved in an extension from the pleura of suppurative, tuberculous, or cancerous processes. In various affections of the liver—cancer, abscess, hydatid disease, and in affections of the gall-bladder—the inflammation may be localized to the peritoneum covering the upper surface of the organ. These forms of localized subphrenic peritonitis in the greater sac are not so important in reality as those which occur in the lesser peritoneum. The anatomical relations of this structure are as follows: It lies behind and below the stomach, the gastro-hepatic omentum, and the anterior layer of the great omentum. Its lower limit forms the upper layer of the transverse meso-colon. On either side it reaches from the hepatic to the splenic flexure of the colon, and from the foramen of Winslow to the hilus of the spleen. Behind it covers and is tightly adherent to the front of the pancreas. Its upper limit is formed by the transverse fissure of the liver, and by that portion of the diaphragm which is covered by the lower layer of the right lateral ligament of the liver; the lobus Spigelii lies bare in the cavity. The foramen of Winslow, through which the lesser communicates with the greater peritoneum, is readily closed by inflammation.

Inflammatory processes, exudates, and hæmorrhages may be confined entirely to the lesser peritoneum. The exudate of tuberculous peritonitis may be confined to it. Perforations of certain parts of the stomach, of the duodenum, and of the colon may excite inflammation in it alone; and in various affections of the pancreas, particularly trauma and hæmorrhage, the effusion into the sac has often been confounded with cyst of this organ.

Special mention must be made of the remarkable form of subphrenic abscess containing air, which may simulate closely pneumothorax, and hence was called by Leyden *pyo-pneumothorax subphrenicus.* The affection has been thoroughly studied by Scheurlen, Mason, Meltzer, and Lee Dickinson. In 142 out of 170 recorded cases the cause was known. In a few instances, as in one reported by Meltzer, the subphrenic abscess seemed to have followed pneumonia. Pyothorax is an occasional cause. By far the most frequent condition is gastric ulcer, which occurred in 80 of the cases. Duodenal ulcer was the cause in 6 per cent. In about 10 per cent. of the cases the appendix was the starting-point of the abscess. Cancer of the stomach is an occasional cause. Other rare causes are trauma, which was present in one of my cases, perforation of an hepatic or a renal abscess, lesions of the spleen, abscess, and cysts of the pancreas.

In a majority of all the cases in which the stomach or duodenum is perforated—sometimes, indeed, in the cases following trauma, as in *Case 3* of my series—the abscess contains air.

The symptoms of subphrenic abscess vary very considerably, depending a good deal upon the primary cause. The onset, as a rule, is abrupt, particularly when due to perforation of a gastric ulcer. There are severe pain, vomiting, often of bilious or of bloody material; respiration is embarrassed, owing to the involvement of the diaphragm; then the constitutional symptoms occur associated with suppuration, chills, irregular fever, and emaciation. Subsequently perforation may take place into the pleura or into the lung, with severe cough and abundant purulent expectoration.

The perihepatic abscess beneath the arch of the diaphragm, whether to the right or left of the suspensory ligament, when it does not contain air, is almost invariably mistaken for empyema. Remarkable features are superadded when the abscess cavity contains air. On the right side, when the abscess is in the greater peritoneum, above the right lobe of the liver, the diaphragm may be pushed up to the level of the second or third rib, and the physical signs on percussion and auscultation are those of pneumothorax, particularly the tympanitic resonance and the movable dulness. The liver is usually greatly depressed and there is bulging on the right side. Still more obscure are the cases of air-containing abscesses due to perforation of the stomach or duodenum, in which the gas is contained in the lesser peritoneum. Here the diaphragm is pushed up and there are signs of pneumothorax on the left side. In a large majority of all the cases which follow perforation of a gastric ulcer the effusion lies between the diaphragm above, and the spleen, stomach, and the left lobe of the liver below.

The prognosis in subphrenic abscess is not very hopeful. Of the cases on record about 20 per cent. only have recovered.

Appendicular.—The most frequent cause of localized peritonitis in the male is inflammation of the appendix vermiformis. The situation varies with the position of this extremely variable organ. The adhesion, perforation, and intraperitoneal abscess cavity may be within the pelvis, or to the left of the median line in the iliac region, in the lower right quadrant of the umbilical region—a not uncommon situation—or, of course, most frequently in the right iliac fossa. In the most common situation the localized abscess lies upon the psoas muscle, bounded by the cæcum on the right and the terminal portion of the ileum and its mesentery in front and to the left. In many of these cases the limitation is perfect, and post mortem records show that complete healing may take place with the obliteration of the appendix in a mass of firm scar tissue.

Pelvic Peritonitis.—The most frequent cause is inflammation about the uterus and Fallopian tubes. Puerperal septicæmia, gonorrhœa, and tuberculosis are the usual causes. The tubes are the starting-point in a majority of the cases. The fimbriæ become adherent and closely matted to the ovary, and there is gradually produced a condition of thickening of the parts, in which the individual organs are scarcely recognizable. The tubes are dilated and filled with cheesy matter or pus, and there may be small abscess cavities in the broad ligaments. Rupture of one of these may cause general peritonitis, or the membrane may be involved by extension, as in tuberculosis of these parts.

IV. CHRONIC PERITONITIS

The following varieties may be recognized:

Local adhesive peritonitis, a very common condition, which occurs particularly about the spleen, forming adhesions between the capsule and the diaphragm, about the liver, less frequently about the intestines and mesentery. Points of thickening or puckering on the peritoneum occur sometimes with union of the coils or with fibrous bands. In a majority of such cases the condition is met accidentally post mortem. Two sets of symptoms may, however, be caused by these adhesions. When a fibrous band is attached in such a way as to form a loop or snare, a coil of intestine may pass through it. Thus, of the 295 cases of intestinal obstruction analyzed by Fitz, 63 were due to this cause. The second group is less serious and comprises cases with persistent abdominal pain of a colicky character, sometimes rendering life miserable.

Diffuse Adhesive Peritonitis.—This is a consequence of an acute inflammation, either simple or tuberculous. The peritoneum is obliterated. On cutting through the abdominal wall, the coils of intestines are uniformly matted together and can neither be separated from each other nor can the visceral and parietal layers be distinguished. There may be thickening of the layers, and the liver and spleen are usually involved in the adhesions.

Proliferative Peritonitis.—Apart from cancer and tubercle, which produce typical lesions of chronic peritonitis, the most characteristic form is that which may be described under this heading. The essential anatomical feature is great thickening of the peritoneal layers, usually without much adhesion. The cases are sometimes seen with sclerosis of the stomach. In one instance I found it in connection with a sclerotic condition of the cæcum and the first part of the colon. It is not uncommon with cirrhosis of the liver. In the inspection of a case of this kind there is usually moderate effusion, more rarely extensive ascites. The peritoneum is opaque white in color, and everywhere thickened, often in patches. The omentum is usually rolled and forms a thickened mass transversely placed between the stomach and the colon. The peritoneum over the stomach, intestines, and mesentery is sometimes greatly thickened. The liver and spleen may simply be adherent, or there is a condition of chronic perihepatitis or perisplenitis, so that a layer of firm, almost gristly connective tissue of from one-fourth to half an inch in thickness encircles these organs. Usually the volume of the liver is in consequence greatly reduced. The gastro-hepatic omentum may be constricted by this new growth and the calibre of the portal vein much narrowed. A serous effusion may be present. On account of the adhesions which form, the peritoneum may be divided into three or four different sacs, as is more fully described under the tuberculous peritonitis. In these cases the intestines are usually free, though the mesentery is greatly shortened. There are instances of chronic peritonitis in which the mesentery is so shortened by this proliferative change that the intestines form a ball not larger than a cocoanut situated in the middle line, and after the removal of the exudation can be felt as a solid tumor. The intestinal wall is greatly thickened and the mucous membrane of the ileum is thrown into folds like the valvulæ conniventes. This proliferative peritonitis is found frequently in the subjects of chronic alcoholism. In cases of long-continued ascites the serous surfaces generally become thickened and present an opaque, dead white color. This condition is observed especially in hepatic cirrhosis, but attends tumors, chronic passive congestion, etc.

In all forms of chronic peritonitis a friction may be felt usually in the upper zone of the abdomen. Polyorrhomenitis, polyserositis, general chronic inflammation of the serous membranes, Concato's disease (as the Italians call it) may occûr with this form as well as in the tuberculous variety. The pericardium and both pleuræ may be involved.

In some instances of chronic peritonitis the membrane presents numerous nodular thickenings, which may be mistaken for tubercles. J. F. Payne described a case of this sort associated with disseminated growths throughout the liver which were not cancerous. It has been suggested that some of the cases of tuberculous peritonitis cured by operation have been of this nature, but histological examination would, as a rule, readily determine between the conditions. Miura, in Japan, has reported a case in which these nodules contained the ova of a parasite. One case has been reported in which the exciting cause was regarded as cholesterin plates, which were contained within the granulomatous nodules.

Chronic Hæmorrhagic Peritonitis.—Blood-stained effusions in the peritoneum occur particularly in cancerous and tuberculous disease. A chronic inflammation analogous to the hæmorrhagic pachymeningitis of the brain was described first by Virchow, and is localized most commonly in the pelvis. Layers of new connective tissue form on the surface of the peritoneum with large wide vessels from which hæmorrhage occurs. This is repeated from time to time with the formation of regular layers of hæmorrhagic effusion. It is rarely diffuse, more commonly circumscribed. Probably the spontaneous peritoneal hæmorrhage with the features of an "acute abdomen" (Churchman) may represent the primary form of this rare condition.

V. NEW GROWTHS IN THE PERITONEUM

Tuberculous Peritonitis.—This has already been considered.

Cancer of the Peritoneum.—Although, as a rule, secondary to disease of the stomach, liver, or pelvic organs, cases of primary cancer have been described. It is probable that the so-called primary cancers of the serous membranes are endotheliomata and not carcinomata. Secondary malignant peritonitis occurs in connection with all forms of cancer. It is usually characterized by a number of round tumors scattered over the entire peritoneum, sometimes small and miliary, at other times large and nodular, with puckered centres. The disease most commonly starts from the stomach or the ovaries. The omentum is indurated and, as in tuberculous peritonitis, forms a mass which lies transversely across the upper portion of the abdomen. Primary malignant disease of the peritoneum is extremely rare. Colloid is said to have occurred, forming enormous masses, which in one case weighed over 100 pounds. Cancer of this membrane spreads, either by the detachment of small particles which are carried in the lymph currents and by the movements to distant parts, or by contact of opposing surfaces. It occurs more frequently in women than in men, and more commonly at the later period of life.

The *diagnosis* of cancer of the peritoneum is easy with a history of a local malignant disease; as when it occurs with ovarian tumor or with cancer of the pylorus. In cases in which there is no evidence of a primary lesion the diagnosis may be doubtful. The clinical picture is usually that of chronic ascites with progressive emaciation. There may be no fever. If there is much effusion nothing definite can be felt on examination. After tapping, irregular nodules or the curled omentum may be felt lying transversely across the upper portion of the abdomen. Multiple nodules, if large, indicate cancer, particularly in persons above middle life. Nodular tuberculous peritonitis is most frequent in children. The presence about the navel of secondary nodules and indurated masses is more common in cancer. Inflammation, suppuration, and the discharge of pus from the navel rarely occur except in tuberculous disease. Considerable enlargement of the inguinal glands may be present in cancer. The nature of the fluid in cancer and in tubercle may be much alike. It may be hæmorrhagic in both; more often in the latter. The histological examination in cancer may show large multinuclear cells or groups of cells—the sprouting cell-groups of Foulis—which are extremely suggestive. The colloid cancer may produce a totally different picture; instead of ascitic fluid, the abdomen is occupied by the semi-solid gelatinous substance, and is firm, not fluctuating.

And, lastly, there are instances of echinococci in the peritoneum which may simulate cancer very closely.

VI. ASCITES

(*Hydro-peritoneum*)

Definition.—The accumulation of serous fluid in the peritoneal cavity.

Etiology.—Local Causes.—(*a*) Chronic inflammation of the peritoneum, either simple, cancerous, or tuberculous. (*b*) Portal obstruction in the terminal branches within the liver, as in cirrhosis and chronic passive congestion, or by compression of the vein in the gastro-hepatic omentum, either by proliferative peritonitis, by new growths, or by aneurism. (*c*) Thrombosis of the portal vein. (*d*) Tumors of the abdomen. The solid growths of the ovaries may cause considerable ascites, which may completely mask the true condition. It is important to bear in mind this possibility in the obscure ascites of women. The condition is not infrequent, as I saw four cases due to this cause in 1911. The enlarged spleen in leukæmia, less commonly in malaria, may be associated with recurring ascites.

General Causes.—The ascites is part of a general dropsy, the result of mechanical effects, as in heart-disease, chronic emphysema, and sclerosis of the lung. In cardiac lesions the effusion is sometimes confined to the peritoneum, in which case it is due to secondary changes in the liver, or it has been suggested to be connected with a failure of the suction action of this organ by which the peritoneum is kept dry. Ascites occurs also in the dropsy of Bright's disease, and in hydræmic states of the blood.

Symptoms.—A gradual uniform enlargement of the abdomen is the characteristic symptom of ascites. The PHYSICAL SIGNS are usually distinctive. (*a*) *Inspection.*—According to the amount of fluid the abdomen is protuberant and flattened at the sides. With large effusions, the skin is tense and may present the lineæ albicantes. Frequently the navel itself and the parts about it are very prominent. In many cases the superficial veins are enlarged and a plexus joining the mammary vessels can be seen. Sometimes it can be determined by pressure on these veins that the current is from below upward. In some instances, as in thrombosis or obliteration of the portal vein, these superficial abdominal vessels may be extensively varicose. About the navel in cases of cirrhosis there is occasionally a large bunch of distended veins, the so-called caput Medusæ. The heart may be displaced upward.

(*b*) *Palpation.*—Fluctuation is obtained by placing the fingers of one hand upon one side of the abdomen and by giving a sharp tap on the opposite side with the other hand, when a wave is felt to strike as a definite shock against the applied fingers. Even comparatively small quantities of fluid may give this fluctuation shock. When the abdominal walls are thick or very fat, an assistant may place the edge of the hand or a piece of cardboard in front of the abdomen. A different procedure is adopted in palpating for the solid organs in case of ascites. Instead of placing the hand flat upon the abdomen, as in the ordinary method, the pads of the fingers only are placed lightly upon the skin, and then by a sudden depression of the fingers the fluid is displaced and the solid organ or tumor may be felt. By this method of "dipping" or displacement, as it is called, the liver may be felt below the costal margin, or the spleen, or sometimes solid tumors of the omentum or intestine.

(*c*) *Percussion.*—In the dorsal position with a moderate quantity of fluid in the peritoneum the flanks are dull, while the umbilical and epigastric regions, in which the intestines float, are tympanitic. This area of clear resonance may have an oval outline. Having obtained the lateral limit of the dulness on one side, if the patient turns on the opposite side, the fluid gravitates to the dependent part and the uppermost flank is now tympanitic. In moderate effusions this movable dulness changes greatly in the different postures. Small amounts of fluid, probably under a litre, would scarcely give movable dulness, as the pelvis and the renal regions hold a considerable quantity. In such cases it is best to place the patient in the knee-elbow position, when a dull note will be determined at the most dependent portion. By careful attention to these details mistakes are usually avoided.

Differential Diagnosis.—The following are among the conditions which may be mistaken for dropsy: *Ovarian tumor,* in which the sac develops, as a rule, unilaterally, though when large it is centrally placed. The dulness is anterior and the resonance is in the flanks, into which the intestines are pushed by the cyst. Examination *per vaginam* may give important indications. In those rare instances in which gas develops in the cyst the diagnosis may be very difficult. Succussion has been obtained in such cases. A *distended bladder* may reach above the umbilicus. In such instances some urine dribbles away, and suspicion of ascites or a cyst is occasionally entertained. I once saw a trocar thrust into a distended bladder, which was supposed to be an ovarian cyst, and it is stated that John Hunter tapped a bladder, supposing it to be ascites. Such a mistake should be avoided by careful catheterization prior to any operative procedures. And lastly, there are large pancreatic or hydatid cysts in the abdomen which may simulate ascites.

Nature of the Ascitic Fluid.—Usually this is a clear serum, light yellow in the ascites of anæmia and Bright's disease, often darker in color in cirrhosis of the liver. The specific gravity is low, seldom more than 1.010 or 1.015, whereas in the fluid of ovarian cysts or chronic peritonitis the specific gravity is over 1.015. It is albuminous and sometimes coagulates spontaneously. Dock has called attention to the importance of the study of the cells in the exudate. In cancer very characteristic forms, with nuclear figures, may be found. Hæmorrhagic effusion usually occurs in cancer and tuberculosis, and occasionally in cirrhosis. I have already referred to the instances of hæmorrhagic effusion in connection with ruptured tubal pregnancy.

Chylous Ascites.—Of the cases tabulated by MacKenzie, Wallis, and Scholberg, 81 were in association with tumors, 46 with the infections, chiefly tuberculosis, 37 in association with affections of the thoracic duct and lymphatic system, and 78 in connection with general diseases such as cirrhosis of the liver, cardiac disease, nephritis, amyloid disease, and thrombosis of the blood-vessels. In a certain number of cases the cause of the condition is unknown. Quincke recognized that there were two types, one in which there was a true milky or fatty fluid, the other in which the turbidity is due to fatty degeneration of cells or to chemical substances of a non-fatty nature. The fluid of the true chylous ascites is yellowish-white in color, contains fine fat globules, a creamy layer collects on standing, the specific gravity generally exceeds 1.012, and the fat content is high. As a rule, it tends to accumulate rapidly and large amounts may be removed. The fluid of pseudo-chylous ascites is milky white, the opacity often may vary at different tappings. Microscopically there are many fine refractile granules, but they do not give reactions for fat, the cellular elements may be numerous, and a creamy layer rarely forms. The specific gravity is less than 1.012, and the total solids rarely exceed 2 per cent. The fat content is low. Lecithin combined with globulin appears to be the cause of the opalescence. The authors from whom I have quoted conclude that milky ascites is characteristic of no specific morbid lesion. The prognosis is usually grave.

Treatment of the Previous Conditions.—(*a*) Acute Peritonitis.—Rest is enjoined upon the patient by the severe pain which follows the slightest movement, and he should be propped in the position which gives him greatest relief. Whether morphia should be given will depend upon the cause. In the pain of appendicitis and of perforation in typhoid fever it is best to use an ice-bag and withhold the drug. Late in the disease and in hopeless conditions it may be given freely. The opium treatment so strongly advocated by the late Alonzo Clark has gone out of vogue.

Local applications—the ice-bag, hot turpentine stupes, or cloths wrung out of ice-water—may be laid upon the abdomen.

The question of the use of purgatives in peritonitis has of late been warmly discussed. Theoretically it appears correct to give salines in concentrated form, which cause a rapid and profuse exosmosis of serum from the intestinal vessels, relieving the congestion and reducing the œdema, which is one important factor in causing the meteorism. It is also urged that the increased peristalsis prevents the formation of adhesions. In reading the reports of these successful cases, one is not always convinced, however, that peritonitis actually existed. Still, in cases of acute peritonitis due to extension or following operation or in septic conditions the judgment of many careful men is decidedly in favor of the use of salines. The majority of cases of peritonitis which come under the care of the physician follow lesions of the abdominal viscera or are due to perforation of ulcer of the stomach, the ileum, or the appendix. In such cases, particularly in the large group of appendix cases, to give saline purgatives is, to say the least, most injudicious treatment. In these instances rectal injections should be employed to relieve the large bowel. No symptom in acute peritonitis is more serious than the tympanites, and none is more difficult to meet. The use of the long tube and injections containing turpentine may be tried. Drugs by the mouth can not be retained.

For the vomiting, ice and small quantities of soda water may be employed. The patient should be fed on milk, but if the vomiting is distressing it is best not to attempt to give food by the mouth, but to use small nutrient enemata. In all cases it is best to have a surgeon in consultation early in the disease, as the question of operation may come up at any moment. In the acute forms of tuberculous peritonitis operative measures appear to be more hopeful, but they are not always successful.

(*b*) Chronic Peritonitis.—For the cases of chronic proliferative peritonitis very little can be done. The treatment is practically that of ascites. In all these forms, when the distention becomes extreme, tapping is indicated. The treatment of tuberculous peritonitis has fallen largely into the hands of the surgeons, but the results depend on the stage at which the operation is performed and the variety of the disease. With ascites the outlook is good; but when there are tuberculous tumors and many adhesions the results are not very satisfactory. Maurice Richardson, in a child aged five, with a suspected appendicitis (tumor, etc.), found the symptoms to be due to enlarged, tuberculous mesenteric glands, which were removed, and the boy remained well five years after the operation.

(*c*) Ascites.—The treatment depends somewhat on the nature of the case. In cirrhosis early and repeated tapping may give time for the establishment of the collateral circulation, and temporary cures have followed this procedure. Permanent drainage with Southey's tube, incision, and washing out the peritoneum have also been practiced. In the ascites of cardiac and renal disease the cathartics are most satisfactory, particularly the bitartrate of potash, given alone or with jalap, and the large doses of salts given an hour before breakfast with as little water as possible. These sometimes cause rapid disappearance of the effusion, but they are not so successful in ascites as in pleurisy with effusion. The stronger cathartics may sometimes be necessary. The ascites forming part of the general anasarca of Bright's disease will receive consideration under another section.

SECTION VI

DISEASES OF THE RESPIRATORY SYSTEM

A. DISEASES OF THE NOSE

I. AUTUMNAL CATARRH

(Hay Fever)

Definition.—An affection of the upper air-passages, often associated with asthmatic attacks, due to the action of the pollen of certain grasses and plants upon a hypersensitive mucous membrane.

Etiology.—This affection was first described in 1819 by Bostock, who called it *catarrhus æstivus.* Morrill Wyman, of Cambridge, Mass., wrote a monograph on the subject, and described two forms, the "June cold," or "rose cold," which comes on in the spring, and the autumnal form, which, in the United States, comes on in August and September, and never persists after a severe frost. In the Southern States cases occur all through the year. It is more common in America and in Great Britain than on the Continent. The disposition to the disease is hereditary. Women are more subject to it than men. Young and middle-aged persons are most often attacked. The tendency lessens as age advances. Dwellers in cities are chiefly attacked. The educated and highly nervous are most susceptible. The disease affects certain families, and Beard found an hereditary factor in 33 per cent. of his cases. A morbid sensitiveness of the nasal mucosa is present in many cases.

The disease must be differentiated from nervous coryza (which has been induced by suggestion) and from the attacks of irritation of the nasal, conjunctival, and bronchial mucous membranes excited by the odor of a horse, or of the "harmless necessary cat."

Dunbar's researches have placed the etiology of the disease on a scientific basis. He has shown that there is but one cause, the pollen of grasses and certain plants. The pollen of about 130 different plants has now been examined, of which that of 25 grasses and of only 7 other kinds of plants exert a definite action. The pollen of rye is the most active. Dunbar and his students have found that the severity of hay-fever attacks is in direct proportion to the quantity of pollen present in the atmosphere. In persons predisposed to the disease the pollen applied to the conjunctivæ or nasal mucosa excites characteristic attacks. He has isolated a peculiar poison of an albuminous nature from the pollen. It is so powerful that .000025 milligram excites irritation in the conjunctiva of a susceptible subject. This is the amount of toxin which corresponds to two or three pollen grains. It is entirely without influence on normal persons. In larger doses severer attacks are caused, and, injected subcutaneously, it has been followed by very unpleasant symptoms. He has succeeded in obtaining an antitoxin by injecting the poison into animals. It is capable of cutting short attacks of ordinary hay fever.

Symptoms.—These are, in a majority of the cases, very like those of ordinary coryza. There may, however, be much more headache and distress, and some patients become very low-spirited. At the outset, or even daily throughout the attack, sneezing may be frequent. Cough is a common symptom and may be very distressing. Paroxysms of asthma may occur indistinguishable from the ordinary bronchial form. The two conditions may indeed alternate, the patient having at one time an attack of common hay fever and at another, under similar circumstances, an attack of bronchial asthma.

Treatment.—This may be comprised under four heads: First, remedies may be given to improve the stability of the nervous system—such as arsenic, phosphorus, and strychnia. Secondly, climatic. Dwellers in the cities of the Atlantic seaboard and of the Central States enjoy complete immunity in the Adirondacks and White Mountains. As a rule the disease is aggravated by residence in agricultural districts. The dry mountain air is unquestionably the best; there is no general rule, and there are cases which do well at the seaside. Thirdly, the thorough local treatment of the nose, particularly the destruction of the vessels and sinuses over the sensitive areas. Fourthly, the antitoxin treatment of Dunbar in suitable cases gives excellent results when used as a prophylactic. Owing to the peculiar nature of the disease and the constant reinfection of the mucous membranes by pollen on exposure to the outside air, it is advised to sleep with the windows closed and to apply the serum in the morning before rising both to eyes and nose, and again during the day if irritation is felt in the conjunctivæ or nasal mucous membranes. Active immunization by pollen extracts is sometimes helpful.

II. EPISTAXIS

Etiology.—Bleeding from the nose may result from local or constitutional conditions. Among local causes may be mentioned traumatism, small ulcers, picking or scratching the nose, new growths, and the presence of foreign bodies. In chronic nasal catarrh bleeding is not infrequent. The blood may come from one or both nostrils. The flow may be profuse after an injury.

Among general conditions with which nose-bleeding is associated, the following are the most important: It occurs in growing children, particularly about the age of puberty; more frequently in the delicate than in the strong and vigorous. There is a family form in which many members in several generations are affected. I have described a remarkable hereditary multiple telangiectasis, a special feature of which is recurring epistaxis. The disease has nothing to do with hæmophilia, with which it has been confounded. The bleeding occurs from the telangiectasis in the nasal mucosa, and from those in the lips, tongue, and skin. A severe anæmia may be caused by the loss of blood.

Epistaxis is a very common event in persons of so-called plethoric habit. It is stated sometimes to precede, or to indicate a liability to, apoplexy. In venous engorgement epistaxis is not common and there may be a most extreme grade of cyanosis without its occurrence. It is frequent in cirrhosis hepatis. In balloon and mountain ascensions, in the very rarefied atmosphere, hæmorrhage from the nose is a common event. In hæmophilia the nose ranks first of the mucous membranes from which bleeding arises. It occurs in all forms of chronic anæmias, in chronic interstitial nephritis, and in cirrhosis of the liver. It precedes the onset of certain fevers, more particularly typhoid, with which it seems associated in a special manner. Vicarious epistaxis has been described in cases of suppression of the menses. Lastly, it is said to be brought on by certain psychical impressions, but the observations on this point are not trustworthy. The blood in epistaxis results from capillary oozing or diapedesis. The mucous membrane is deeply congested and there are often capillary angiomata situated usually in the respiratory portion of the nostril and upon the cartilaginous septum.

Symptoms.—Slight hæmorrhage is not associated with any special features. When the bleeding is protracted the patients have the more serious manifestations of loss of blood. In the slow dripping which takes place in some instances of hæmophilia, there may be formed a remarkable blood tumor projecting from one nostril and extending even below the mouth.

Death from ordinary epistaxis is very rare. The more blood is lost the greater is the tendency to clotting with spontaneous cessation of the bleeding.

Diagnosis.—The diagnosis is usually easy. One point only need be mentioned; namely, that bleeding from the posterior nares occasionally occurs during sleep and the blood trickles into the pharynx and may be swallowed. If vomited, it may be confounded with hæmatemesis; or, if coughed up, with hæmoptysis.

Treatment.—In a majority of the cases the bleeding ceases of itself. Various simple measures may be employed, such as holding the arms above the head, the application of ice to the nose, or the injection of cold or hot water into the nostrils. Astringents, such as zinc, alum, or tannin, may be used; and the tincture of the perchloride of iron, diluted with ice-water, may be introduced into the nostrils. If the bleeding comes from an ulcerated surface, an attempt should be made to apply chromic acid or the cautery. If the bleeding is at all severe and obstinate, the posterior nares should be plugged. One of the patients with epistaxis and spider angiomata of the skin and mucous membranes used a finger of a rubber glove with a small rubber tube and stopcock by which he could dilate the glove finger, inserted into the nostril, and so effectually control the bleeding. The inhalation of carbonic-acid gas may be tried or a solution of gelatine or of adrenalin injected into the nostril.

B. DISEASES OF THE LARYNX

I. ACUTE CATARRHAL LARYNGITIS

This may come on as an independent affection or in association with general catarrh of the upper respiratory passages.

Etiology.—Many cases are due to catching cold or to overuse of the voice;

others come on in consequence of the inhalation of irritating gases. It may occur in the general catarrh associated with influenza and measles. Very severe laryngitis is excited by traumatism, either injuries from without or the lodgment of foreign bodies. It may be caused by the action of very hot liquids or corrosive poisons.

Symptoms.—There is a sense of tickling referred to the larynx; the cold air irritates and, owing to the increased sensibility of the mucous membrane, the act of inspiration may be painful. There is a dry cough, and the voice is altered. At first it is simply husky, but soon phonation becomes painful, and finally the voice may be completely lost. In adults the respirations are not increased in frequency, but in children dyspnœa is not uncommon and may occur in spasmodic attacks and become urgent if there is much œdema with the inflammatory swelling.

The laryngoscope shows a swollen mucous membrane of the larynx, particularly the ary-epiglottidean folds. The vocal cords have lost their smooth and shining appearance and are reddened and swollen. Their mobility also is greatly impaired, owing to the infiltration of the adjoining mucous membrane and of the muscles. A slight mucoid exudation covers the parts. The constitutional symptoms are not severe. There is rarely much fever, and in many cases the patient is not seriously ill. Occasionally cases come on with greater intensity, the cough is very distressing, deglutition is painful, and there may be urgent dyspnœa.

Diagnosis.—There is rarely any difficulty in determining the nature of a case if a satisfactory laryngoscopic examination can be made. The severer forms may simulate œdema of the glottis. When the loss of voice is marked, the case may be mistaken for one of nervous aphonia, but the laryngoscope would decide the question at once. Much more difficult is the diagnosis of acute laryngitis in children, particularly in the very young, in whom it is so hard to make a proper examination. From ordinary laryngismus it is to be distinguished by the presence of fever, the mode of onset, and particularly the coryza and the previous symptoms of hoarseness or loss of voice. Membranous laryngitis may at first be quite impossible to differentiate, but in a majority of cases of this affection there are patches on the pharynx and early swelling of the cervical glands. The symptoms, too, are much more severe.

Treatment.—Rest of the larynx should be enjoined, so far as phonation is concerned; smoking should be forbidden. In cases of any severity the patient should be kept in bed. The room should be at an even temperature and the air saturated with moisture. Early in the disease, if there is much fever, aconite and citrate of potash may be given, and for the irritating painful cough a full dose of Dover's powder at night. An ice-bag externally often gives great relief.

II. CHRONIC LARYNGITIS

Etiology.—The cases usually follow repeated acute attacks. The most common cause is overuse of the voice, particularly in persons whose occupation necessitates shouting in the open air. The constant inhalation of irritating substances, as tobacco-smoke, may also cause it.

Symptoms.—The voice is usually hoarse and rough and in severe cases may be almost lost. There is usually very little pain; only the unpleasant sense of tickling in the larynx, which causes a frequent desire to cough. With the laryngoscope the mucous membrane looks swollen, but much less red than in the acute condition. In association with the granular pharyngitis, the mucous glands of the epiglottis and of the ventricles may be involved.

Treatment.—The nostrils should be carefully examined, since in some instances chronic laryngitis is associated with and even dependent upon obstruction to the free passage of air through the nose. Local application must be made directly to the larynx, either with a brush or by means of a spray. Among the remedies most recommended are the solutions of nitrate of silver, chlorate of potash, perchloride of zinc, and tannic acid. Insufflations of bismuth are sometimes useful.

Among directions to be given are the avoidance of heated rooms and loud speaking, and abstinence from tobacco and alcohol. The throat should not be too much muffled, and morning and evening the neck should be sponged with cold water.

III. ŒDEMATOUS LARYNGITIS

Etiology.—Œdema of the glottis, or, more correctly, of the structures which form the glottis, a very serious affection, is met with (*a*) as a rare sequence of ordinary acute laryngitis; (*b*) in chronic diseases of the larynx, as syphilis or tubercle; (*c*) in severe inflammatory diseases like diphtheria, in erysipelas of the neck, and in various forms of cellulitis; (*d*) occasionally in the acute infectious diseases—scarlet fever, typhus, or typhoid; in Bright's disease, either acute or chronic, there may be a rapidly developing œdema; (*e*) in angio-neurotic œdema.

Symptoms.—There is dyspnœa, increasing in intensity, so that within an hour or two the condition becomes very critical. There is sometimes marked stridor in respiration. The voice becomes husky and disappears. The laryngoscope shows enormous swelling of the epiglottis, which can sometimes be felt with the finger or even seen when the tongue is strongly depressed with a spatula. The ary-epiglottidean folds are the seat of the chief swelling and may almost meet in the middle line. Occasionally the œdema is below the true cords.

The diagnosis is rarely difficult, inasmuch as even without the laryngoscope the swollen epiglottis can be seen or felt with the finger. The condition is very often fatal.

Treatment.—An ice-bag should be placed on the larynx, and the patient given ice to suck. The air of the room should be moist. If the symptoms are urgent, the throat should be sprayed with a strong solution of cocaine or adrenalin and the swollen epiglottis scarified. If relief does not follow, tracheotomy should immediately be performed. The high rate of mortality is due to the fact that this operation is, as a rule, too long delayed.

IV. SPASMODIC LARYNGITIS

(*Laryngismus stridulus*)

Spasm of the glottis is met with in many affections of the larynx, but there is a special disease in children which has received the above-mentioned and other names.

Etiology.—A purely nervous affection, without any inflammatory condition of the larynx, it occurs in children between the ages of six months and three years, and is most commonly seen in connection with rickets. As Escherich has shown, the disease has close relations with tetany and may display many of the accessory phenomena of this disease. Often the attack comes on when the child has been crossed or scolded. Mothers sometimes call the attacks "passion fits" or attacks of "holding the breath." It was supposed at one time that they were associated with enlargement of the thymus, and the condition therefore received the name of *thymic asthma.*

The actual state of the larynx during a paroxysm is a spasm of the adductors, but the precise nature of the influences causing it is not yet known, whether centric or reflex from peripheral irritation. The disease is not so common in America as in England.

Symptoms.—The attacks may come on either in the night or in the day; often just as the child awakes. There is no cough, no hoarseness, but the respiration is arrested and the child struggles for breath, the face gets congested, and then, with a sudden relaxation of the spasm, the air is drawn into the lungs with a high-pitched crowing sound, which has given to the affection the name of "child-crowing." Convulsions may occur during an attack or there may be carpo-pedal spasms. Death may, but rarely does, occur during the attack. With the cyanosis the spasm relaxes and respiration begins. The attacks may recur with great frequency throughout the day.

Treatment.—The gums should be carefully examined and, if swollen and hot, freely lanced. The bowels should be carefully regulated and, as these children are usually delicate or rickety, nourishing diet and cod-liver oil should be given. By far the most satisfactory method of treatment is the cold sponging. In severe cases, two or three times a day the child should be placed in a warm bath, and the back and chest thoroughly sponged for a minute or two with cold water. Since learning this practice from Ringer, at the University Hospital, London, I have seen many cases in which it proved successful. It may be employed when the child is in a paroxysm, though if the attack is severe and the lividity is great it is much better to dash cold water into the face. Sometimes the introduction of the finger far back into the throat will relieve the spasm.

Spasmodic croup, believed to be a functional spasm of the muscles of the larynx, is an affection seen most commonly between the ages of two and five years. According to Trousseau's description, the child goes to bed well, and about midnight or in the early morning hours awakes with oppressed breathing, harsh, croupy cough, and perhaps some huskiness of voice. The oppression and distress for a time are very serious, the face is congested, and there are signs of approaching cyanosis. The attack passes off abruptly, the child falls asleep and awakes the next morning feeling perfectly well. These attacks may be repeated for several nights in succession, and usually cause great alarm to the parents. Whether this is entirely a functional spasm is, I think, doubtful. There are instances in which the child is somewhat hoarse throughout the day, and has slight catarrhal symptoms and a brazen, croupy cough. There is probably slight catarrhal laryngitis with it. These cases are not infrequently mistaken for true croup, and parents are sometimes unnecessarily disturbed by the serious view which the physician takes of the case. Too often the poor child, deluged with drugs, is longer in recovering from the treatment than he would be from the disease. To allay the spasm a whiff of chloroform may be administered, which will in a few moments give relief, or the child may be placed in a hot bath. A prompt emetic, such as wine of ipecac, will usually relieve the spasm, and is specially indicated if the child has overloaded the stomach through the day.

V. TUBERCULOUS LARYNGITIS

Etiology.—Tubercles may arise primarily in the laryngeal mucosa, but in the great majority of cases the affection is secondary to pulmonary tuberculosis, in which it is met with in a variable proportion of from 18 to 30 per cent. Laryngitis may occur very early in pulmonary tuberculosis. There may be well-marked involvement of the larynx with signs of very limited trouble at one apex. These are cases which, in my experience, run a very unfavorable course.

Morbid Anatomy.—The mucosa is at first swollen and presents scattered tubercles, which seem to begin in the neighborhood of the blood-vessels. By their fusion small tuberculous masses arise, which caseate and finally ulcerate, leaving shallow irregular losses of substance. The ulcers are usually covered with a grayish exudation, and there is a general thickening of the mucosa about them, which is particularly marked upon the arytenoids. The ulcers may erode the true cords and finally destroy them, and passing deeply may cause perichondritis with necrosis and occasionally exfoliation of the cartilages. The disease may extend laterally and involve the pharynx, and downward over the mucous membrane, covering the cricoid cartilage toward the œsophagus. Above, it may reach the posterior wall of the pharynx, and in rare cases extend to the fauces and tonsils. The epiglottis may be entirely destroyed. There are rare instances in which cicatricial changes go on to such a degree that stenosis of the larynx is induced.

Symptoms.—The first indication is slight huskiness of the voice, which finally deepens to hoarseness, and in advanced stages there may be complete loss of voice. There is something very suggestive in the early hoarseness of tuberculous laryngitis. The attention may be directed to the lungs simply by the quality of the voice.

The cough is in part due to involvement of the larynx. Early in the disease it is not very troublesome, but when the ulceration is extensive it becomes husky and ineffectual. Of the symptoms, none is more aggravating than the dysphagia, which is met with particularly when the epiglottis is involved, and when the ulceration has extended to the pharynx. There is no more distressing or painful complication in phthisis. In instances in which the epiglottis is in great part destroyed with each attempt to take food there are distressing paroxysms of cough, and even of suffocation.

With the laryngoscope there is seen early in the disease a pallor of the mucous membrane, which also looks thickened and infiltrated, particularly that covering the arytenoid cartilages. The ulcers are very characteristic. They are broad and shallow, with gray bases and ill-defined outlines. The vocal cords are infiltrated and thickened, and ulceration is very common.

The diagnosis is rarely difficult, as it is usually associated with well-marked pulmonary disease. In case of doubt the secretion from the base of an ulcer should be examined for bacilli.

Treatment.—The voice should not be used. In the early stages no method of treatment is more effectual. The ulcers should be sprayed and kept thoroughly cleansed with a solution of tannic acid, nitrate of silver, or sulphate of zinc. The insufflation, three times a day, of a powder of iodoform with morphia, after cleansing the ulcers with a spray, relieves the pain in a majority of the cases. Cocaine (4-per-cent. solution) applied with the atomizer will often enable the patient to swallow his food comfortably. There are, however, distressing cases of extensive laryngeal and pharyngeal ulceration in which even cocaine loses its good effects. When the epiglottis is lost the difficulty in swallowing becomes very great. Wolfenden states that this may be obviated if the patient hangs his head over the side of the bed and sucks milk through a rubber tube from a mug placed on the floor.

VI. SYPHILITIC LARYNGITIS

Syphilis attacks the larynx with great frequency. It may result from the inherited disease or be a secondary or tertiary manifestation of the acquired form.

Symptoms.—In secondary syphilis there is occasionally erythema of the larynx, which may go on to definite catarrh, but has nothing characteristic. The process may proceed to the formation of superficial whitish ulcers, usually symmetrically placed on the cords or ventricular bands. Mucous patches and condylomata are rarely seen. The symptoms are practically those of slight loss of voice with laryngeal irritation, as in the simple catarrhal form.

The tertiary laryngeal lesions are numerous and very serious. True gummata, varying in size from the head of a pin to a small nut, arise in the submucous tissue, most commonly at the base of the epiglottis. They go through the changes characteristic of these structures and may either break down, producing extensive and deep ulceration, or—and this is more characteristic of syphilitic laryngitis—in their healing form a fibrous tissue which shrinks and produces stenosis. The ulceration is apt to extend deeply and involve the cartilage, inducing necrosis and exfoliation, and even hæmorrhage from erosion of the arteries. Œdema may suddenly prove fatal. The cicatrices which follow the sclerosis of the gummata or the healing of the ulcers produce great deformity. The epiglottis, for instance, may be tied down to the pharyngeal wall or to the epiglottic folds, or even to the tongue; and eventually a stenosis results, which may necessitate tracheotomy.

The laryngeal symptoms of inherited syphilis have the usual course of these lesions and appear either early, within the first five or six months, or after puberty; most commonly in the former period. The gummatous infiltration leads to ulceration, most commonly of the epiglottis and in the ventricles, and the process may extend deeply and involve the cartilage. Cicatricial contraction may also occur.

The diagnosis of syphilis of the larynx is rarely difficult, since it occurs most commonly in connection with other symptoms of the disease.

Treatment.—The administration of constitutional remedies is the most important, and under mercury and iodide of potassium the local symptoms may rapidly be relieved. The tertiary laryngeal manifestations are always serious and difficult to treat. The deep ulceration is specially hard to combat, and the cicatrization may necessitate tracheotomy, or gradual dilatation, as practiced by Schroetter.

C. DISEASES OF THE BRONCHI

I. ACUTE BRONCHITIS

Acute catarrhal inflammation of the bronchial mucous membrane is a very common disease, rarely serious in healthy adults, but very fatal in the old and in the young, owing to associated pulmonary complications. It is bilateral and affects either the larger and medium sized tubes or the smaller bronchi, in which case it is known as capillary bronchitis.

We shall speak only of the former, as the latter is part and parcel of broncho-pneumonia.

Etiology.—Acute bronchitis is a common sequel of catching cold, and is often nothing more than the extension downward of an ordinary coryza. It occurs most frequently in the changeable weather of early spring and late autumn. The pneumococcus and influenza bacillus are the most common causal organisms. It may prevail as an epidemic apart from influenza, of which it is an important feature.

Acute bronchitis is associated with many other affections, notably measles. It is by no means rare at the onset of typhoid fever and malaria. It is present also in asthma and whooping-cough. The subjects of spinal curvature are specially liable to the disease. The bronchitis of Bright's disease, gout, and heart-disease is usually a chronic form. It attacks persons of all ages, but most frequently the young and the old. There are individuals who have a special disposition to bronchial catarrh, and the slightest exposure is apt to bring on an attack. Persons who live an out-of-door life are usually less subject to the disease than those who follow sedentary occupations.

Bacteriology.—The pneumococcus is responsible for many cases both in young and old. The infection may follow pneumonia, and bronchitis may recur winter after winter, with the sputum showing an almost pure culture of the pneumococcus. In one patient these germs have persisted in the sputum for seven years, with an almost daily cough, aggravated in the winter. The influenza bacillus is very common and may be found alone or with streptococci. The *Micrococcus catarrhalis* is present in a number of the ordinary cases, very often in combination with other organisms. Less frequently the staphylococci, colon bacillus, and typhoid bacilli have been found.

Morbid Anatomy.—The mucous membrane of the trachea and bronchi is reddened, congested, and covered with mucus and muco-pus, which may be seen oozing from the smaller bronchi, some of which are dilated. The finer changes in the mucosa consist in desquamation of the ciliated epithelium, swelling and œdema of the submucosa, and infiltration of the tissue with leucocytes. The mucous glands are much swollen.

Symptoms.—General.—The symptoms of an ordinary "cold" accompany the onset of an acute bronchitis. The coryza extends to the tubes, and may also affect the larynx, producing hoarseness, which in many cases is marked. A chill is rare, but there is invariably a sense of oppression, with heaviness and languor and pains in the bones and back. In mild cases there is scarcely any fever, but in severer forms the range is from 101° to 103° F. The bronchial symptoms set in with a feeling of tightness and rawness beneath the sternum and a sensation of oppression in the chest. The cough is rough at first, and often of a ringing character. It comes on in paroxysms which rack and distress the patient extremely. During the severe spells the pain may be very intense beneath the sternum and along the attachments of the diaphragm. At first the cough is dry and the expectoration scanty and viscid, but in a few days the secretion becomes muco-purulent and abundant, and finally purulent. With the loosening of the cough great relief is experienced. The sputum is made up largely of pus-cells, with a variable number of the large round alveolar cells, many of which contain carbon grains, while others have undergone the myelin degeneration.

Physical Signs.—The respiratory movements are not greatly increased in frequency unless the fever is high. There are instances, however, in which the breathing is rapid and when the smaller tubes are involved there is dyspnœa. On palpation the bronchial fremitus may often be felt. On auscultation in the early stage, piping sibilant râles are everywhere to be heard. They are very changeable, and appear and disappear with coughing. With the relaxation of the bronchial membranes and the greater abundance of the secretion, the râles change and become mucous and bubbling in quality. The bases of the lungs should be carefully examined each day, particularly in children and the aged.

Course.—The course of the disease depends on the conditions under which it arises. In healthy adults, by the end of a week the fever subsides and the cough loosens. In another week or ten days convalescence is fully established. In young children the chief risk is in the extension of the process downward. In measles and whooping-cough the ordinary bronchial catarrh is very apt to descend to the finer tubes, which become dilated and plugged with muco-pus, inducing areas of collapse, and finally broncho-pneumonia. This extension is indicated by changes in the physical signs. Usually at the base the râles are subcrepitant and numerous and there may be areas of defective resonance and of feeble or distant tubular breathing. In the aged and debilitated there are similar dangers if the process extends from the larger to the smaller tubes. In old age the bronchial mucosa is less capable of expelling the mucus, which is more apt to sag to the dependent parts and induce dilatation of the tubes with extension of the inflammation to the contiguous air-cells.

Diagnosis.—The diagnosis of acute bronchitis is rarely difficult. Although the mode of onset may be brusque and perhaps simulate pneumonia, yet the absence of dulness and blowing breathing, and the general character of the bronchial inflammation, render the diagnosis easy. The complication of broncho-pneumonia is indicated by the greater severity of the symptoms, particularly the dyspnœa, the changed color, and the physical signs.

Treatment.—In mild cases household measures suffice. The hot foot-bath, or the warm bath, a drink of hot lemonade, and a mustard plaster on the chest will often give relief. In severe cases the patient should be in bed; liquids should be taken freely. For the dry, racking cough, the symptom most complained of by the patient, Dover's powder is the best remedy. It is a popular belief that quinine, in full doses, will check an oncoming cold on the chest, but this is doubtful. It is a common custom when persons feel the approach of a cold to take a Turkish bath, and though the tightness and oppression may be relieved by it, there is in a majority of the cases great risk. Some of the severest cases of bronchitis which I have seen have followed this initial Turkish bath. No doubt, if the person could go to bed directly from the bath, its action would be beneficial, but there is great risk of catching "cold" in going home from the bath. Hydrotherapy is most useful in the form of compresses to the thorax or a wet pack. Relief is obtained from the unpleasant sense of rawness by keeping the air of the room saturated with moisture, and in this dry stage the old-fashioned mixture of the wines of antimony and ipecacuanha with liquor ammonii acetatis and nitrous ether is useful. If the pulse is very rapid, tincture of aconite may be given, particularly in the case of children. The use of inhalations, such as the compound tincture of benzoin, often gives relief. For the cough, when dry and irritating, opium should be freely used in the form of Dover's powder or paregoric. Of course, in the very young and the aged care must be exercised in the use of opium, particularly if the secretions are free; but for the distressing, irritative cough, which keeps the patient awake, opium in some form gives the only relief. Heroin is often helpful for this. As the cough loosens and the expectoration is more abundant, the patient becomes more comfortable. In this stage it is customary to ply him with expectorants of various sorts. Though useful occasionally, they should not be given as a matter of routine. A mixture of squill, ammonia, and senega is a favorite one with many practitioners at this stage. *Vaccine treatment* is not very successful, even when a single organism has been recovered.

In the acute bronchitis of children, if the amount of secretion is large and difficult to expectorate, or if there is dyspnœa and the color begins to get dusky, an emetic (a tablespoonful of ipecac wine) should be given at once and repeated if necessary.

II. CHRONIC BRONCHITIS

Etiology.—This affection may follow repeated attacks of acute bronchitis, but it is most commonly met with in chronic lung affections, heart-disease, aneurism of the aorta, gout, and renal disease. It is frequent in the aged; the young rarely are affected. Climate and season have an important influence. It is the cause of the winter cough of the aged, which recurs with regularity as the weather gets cold and changeable. Owing to the more uniform heating of the houses, it is much less common in Canada and in the United States than in England.

Morbid Anatomy.—The bronchial mucosa presents a great variety of changes, depending somewhat upon the disease with which chronic bronchitis is associated. In some cases the mucous membrane is very thin, so that the longitudinal bands of elastic tissue stand out prominently. The tubes are dilated, the muscular and glandular tissues are atrophied, and the epithelium is in great part shed.

In other instances the mucosa is thickened, granular, and infiltrated. There may be ulceration, particularly of the mucous follicles. Bronchial dilatations are not uncommon and emphysema is a constant accompaniment.

Symptoms.—In the form met with in old men, associated with emphysema, gout, or heart-disease, the chief symptoms are as follows: Shortness of breath, which may not be noticeable except on exertion. The patients "puff and blow" on going up hill or up a flight of stairs. This is due not so much to the chronic bronchitis itself as to associated emphysema or even to cardiac weakness. They complain of no pain. The cough is variable, changing with the weather and with the season. During the summer they may remain free, but each succeeding winter the cough comes on with severity and persists. There may be only a spell in the morning, or the chief distress is at night. The sputum in chronic bronchitis is very variable. In cases of the so-called dry catarrh there is no expectoration. Usually, however, it is abundant, mucopurulent, or distinctly purulent in character. There are instances in which the patient coughs up for years a thin fluid sputum. There is rarely fever. The general health may be good and the disease may present no serious features apart from the liability to induce emphysema and bronchiectasis. In many cases it is an incurable affection. Patients improve and the cough disappears in the summer time only to return during the winter months.

PHYSICAL SIGNS.—The chest is usually distended, the movements are limited, and the condition is often that which we see in emphysema. The percussion note is clear or hyperresonant. On auscultation, expiration is prolonged and wheezy and rhonchi of various sorts are heard—some high-pitched and piping, others deep-toned and snoring. Crepitant râles are common at the bases.

Clinical Varieties.—The description just given is of the ordinary chronic bronchitis which occurs in connection with emphysema and heart-disease and in many elderly men. There are certain forms which merit special description: (*a*) There is a form of CHRONIC BRONCHITIS in women, which comes on between the ages of twenty and thirty and may continue indefinitely without serious impairment of the health. In several cases the cough followed influenza, and there may be slight bronchiectasis.

(*b*) BRONCHORRHŒA.—Excessive bronchial secretion is met with under several conditions. It must not be mistaken for the profuse expectoration of bronchiectasis. The secretion may be very liquid and watery—*bronchorrhœa serosa*—and in extraordinary amount. More commonly, it is purulent though thin, and with greenish or yellow-green masses. It may be thick and uniform. This profuse bronchial secretion is usually a manifestation of chronic bronchitis, and may lead to dilatation of the tubes and ultimately to fetid bronchitis. In the young the condition may persist for years without impairment of health and without apparently damaging the lungs.

(*c*) Putrid Bronchitis.—Fetid expectoration is met with in connection with bronchiectasis, gangrene, abscess, or with decomposition of secretions within phthisical cavities and in an empyema which has perforated the lung. There are instances in which, apart from any of these states, the expectoration has a fetid character. The sputa are abundant, usually thin, grayish-white in color, and they separate into an upper fluid layer capped with frothy mucus and a thick sediment in which may sometimes be found dirty yellow masses the size of peas or beans—the so-called *Dittrich's* plugs. The affection is very rare apart from the above-mentioned conditions. In severe cases it leads to changes in the bronchial walls, pneumonia, and often to abscess or gangrene. Metastatic brain abscess has followed putrid bronchitis in a certain number of cases.

(*d*) Dry Catarrh.—The *catarrhe sec* of Laennec, a not uncommon form, is characterized by paroxysms of coughing of great intensity, with little or no expectoration. It is usually met with in elderly persons with emphysema, and is one of the most obstinate of all varieties of bronchitis.

Treatment.—Removal to a southern latitude may prevent the onset. In England the milder climate of Falmouth, Torquay, and Bournemouth is suitable for those who cannot go elsewhere. Egypt, southern France, southern California, and Florida furnish winter climates in which the subjects of chronic bronchitis live with the greatest comfort. With care chronic bronchitis may prove to be the slight ailment that, as Oliver Wendell Holmes says, promotes longevity.

The first endeavor is to ascertain, if possible, whether there are constitutional or local affections with which it is associated. In many instances the urine is found to be highly acid, perhaps slightly albuminous, and the arteries are stiff. In the form associated with this condition, sometimes called gouty bronchitis, the attacks seem related to the defective renal elimination, and to this condition the treatment should be first directed. In other instances there are heart-disease and emphysema. In the form occurring in old men much may be done in the way of prophylaxis. There is no doubt that with prudence even in the most changeable winter weather much may be done to prevent the onset of chronic bronchitis. Woollen undergarments should be used and especial care should be taken in the spring months not to change them for lighter ones before the warm weather is established.

Cure is seldom effected by medicinal remedies. There are instances in which iodide of potassium acts with remarkable benefit, and it should always be given a trial in cases of paroxysmal bronchitis of obscure origin. For the morning cough, bicarbonate of sodium (gr. xv, 1 gm.), chloride of sodium (gr. v, 0.3 gm.), spirits of chloroform (♏ v, 0.3 c. .c) in anise water and taken with an equal amount of warm water will be found useful (Fowler). When there is much sense of tightness and fullness of the chest, the portable Turkish bath may be tried. When the secretion is excessive muriate of ammonia and senega are useful. Stimulating expectorants are contraindicated. When the heart is feeble, the combination of digitalis and strychnia is very beneficial. Turpentine, the old-fashioned remedy so warmly recommended by the Dublin physicians, has in many quarters fallen undeservedly into disuse. Preparations of tar, creosote, and terebene are sometimes useful. Of other balsamic remedies, sandal-wood, the compound tincture of benzoin, copaiba, balsam of Peru or tolu may be used. Inhalations of eucalyptus and of the spray of ipecacuanha wine are often very useful. If fetor be present, carbolic acid in the form of spray (1 to 2 per cent. solution) will lessen the odor, or thymol (1 to 1,000), but the intratracheal medication is the most efficient. After the larynx is anæsthetized with a 4 per cent. cocaine solution, inject with suitable syringe about two drachms (8 c. c.) of olive oil, with gr. ½ (0.032 gm.) of iodoform, and gr. ⅛ (0.008 gm.) of morphia if there is irritating cough. For urgent dyspnœa with cyanosis, bleeding from the arm gives most relief.

III. BRONCHIECTASIS

Etiology.—The following excellent classification is given by Barty King:

- I. Bronchiolectasis
  - Acute
  - Chronic
- II. Bronchiectasis
  - A. Pure
    - 1. Chronic bronchitis
    - 2. Broncho-pneumonic
    - 3. Chronic pneumonic
    - 4. Pneumonic
    - 5. Pleuritic
  - B. Tuberculous
  - C. Traumatic
    - 1. Aneurism
    - 2. Tumor
    - 3. Foreign body
    - 4. Syphilis

In addition there is a congenital defect which Grawitz has described as *bronchiectasis universalis.*

Unquestionably the weakening of the bronchial wall is the most important, probably the essential, factor in inducing bronchiectasis, since the wall is then not able to resist the pressure of air in severe spells of coughing and in straining. In some instances the mere weight of the accumulated secretion may be sufficient to distend the terminal tubules, as is seen in compression of a bronchus by aneurism. Barty King lays great stress on pleural adherency as a factor in the initial dilatation of the tubes. The disease seems to have increased in frequency since the influenza epidemics of the past fifteen years. Of six consecutive cases in my wards in the session of 1904-05 from every one Boggs isolated the influenza bacillus.

Morbid Anatomy.—Two chief forms of bronchiectasis are recognized—the *cylindrical* and the *saccular*—which may exist together in the same lung. The condition may be general or partial. Universal bronchiectasis is always unilateral. It occurs in rare congenital cases and is occasionally seen as a sequence of interstitial pneumonia. The entire bronchial tree is represented by a series of sacculi opening one into the other. The walls are smooth and possibly without ulceration or erosion except in the dependent parts. The lining membrane of the sacculi is usually smooth and glistening. The dilatations may form large cysts immediately beneath the pleura. Intervening between the sacculi is a dense cirrhotic lung tissue. The partial dilatations—the saccular and cylindrical—are common in chronic phthisis, particularly at the apex, in chronic pleurisy at the base, and in emphysema. Here the dilatation is more commonly cylindrical, sometimes fusiform. The bronchial mucous membrane is much involved and sometimes there is a narrowing of the lumen. Occasionally one meets with a single saccular bronchiectasis in connection with chronic bronchitis or emphysema. Some of these look like simple cysts, with smooth walls, without fluid contents. Bronchiolectasis as an acute condition may follow the infectious diseases, as in the cases described by Sharkey, Carr, and others. The chronic variety is a sequel of bronchitis in old subjects.

Histologically the bronchi which are the seat of dilatation show important changes. In the large, smooth dilatations the cylindrical is replaced by a pavement epithelium. The muscular layer is stretched, atrophied, and the fibres separated; the elastic tissue is also much stretched and separated. In the large saccular bronchiectases and in some of the cylindrical forms, due to retained secretions, the lining membrane is ulcerated. The contents of some of the larger bronchiectatic cavities are horribly fetid.

Symptoms.—There are *acute* cases, usually the bronchiolectasis of children; but a case in my wards of the broncho-pneumonic form died in six weeks from the onset. The bronchi of the lower lobes were dilated; there were areas of broncho-pneumonia and one or two spots of gangrene. The patient became hemiplegic, probably from abscess of the brain. In the limited dilatations of phthisis, emphysema, and chronic bronchitis the symptoms are in great part those of the original disease, and the condition often is not suspected during life.

In extensive saccular bronchiectasis the characters of the cough and expectoration are distinctive. The patient will pass the greater part of the day without any cough and then in a severe paroxysm will bring up a large quantity of sputum. Ten of my cases showed this symptom. Of 23 of my cases the amount for twenty-four hours was in 2 less than 100 c. c., in 11 from 100-300 c. c., in 2 almost 500 c. c., in 7 over 600 c. c. In one case with over one litre per day the cavities found were very small. Sometimes change of position will bring on a violent attack, probably due to the fact that some of the secretion flows from the dilatation to a normal tube. The daily spell of coughing is usually in the morning. The expectoration is in many instances very characteristic. It is grayish or grayish brown in color, fluid, purulent, with a peculiar acid, sometimes fetid, odor. Placed in a conical glass, it separates into a thick granular layer below and a thin mucoid intervening layer above, which is capped by a brownish froth. Microscopically it consists of pus-corpuscles, often large crystals of fatty acids, which are sometimes in enormous numbers over the field and arranged in bunches. Hæmatoidin crystals are sometimes present. Elastic fibres are seldom found except when there is ulceration of the bronchial walls. Tubercle bacilli are not present. In some cases, as in 10 of my series, the expectoration is very fetid and has all the characters of that described under fetid bronchitis. Nummular expectoration, such as comes from phthisical cavities, is not common. Hæmorrhage occurred in 14 out of 35 cases analyzed by Fowler, in 17 of my 24 cases, slight in 8, and extreme in 3. Arthritis may occur, and it is one of the conditions with which the pulmonary osteo-arthropathy is commonly associated. There is a remarkable association of bronchiectasis with abscess of the brain. Among 13,700 autopsies at the London Hospital and the Brompton Hospital there were 19 instances of cerebral abscess with pulmonary disease, usually bronchiectasis (Schörstein).

Diagnosis.—In the extensive sacculated forms, unilateral and associated with interstitial pneumonia or chronic pleurisy, the diagnosis is easy. There is contraction of the side, which in some instances is not at all extreme. The cavernous signs may be chiefly at the base and may vary according to the condition of the cavity, whether full or empty. There may be the most exquisite amphoric phenomena and loud resonant râles. The condition persists for years and is not inconsistent with a tolerably active life. The patients frequently show signs of marked embarrassment of the pulmonary circulation. There is a cyanosis on exertion, the finger-tips are clubbed, and the nails incurved. A condition very difficult to distinguish from bronchiectasis is a limited pleural cavity communicating with a bronchus. The X-ray examination is an important aid in diagnosis.

Treatment.—Medical treatment is not satisfactory, since it is impossible to heal the cavities. Postural treatment is important, and the most favorable position should be studied for each patient. Sleeping with the head low favors "drainage." I have practiced the injection of antiseptic fluids in some instances with benefit. Intratracheal injections have been recommended of late. With a suitable syringe a drachm may be injected twice a day of the following solution: Menthol 10 parts, guaiacol 2 parts, olive oil 88 parts. Or better still when the odor is very offensive iodoform in olive oil. The creosote vapor bath may be given in a small room. The patient's eyes must be protected with well-fitting goggles, and the nostrils stuffed with cotton-wool. Twenty to thirty drops of creosote are poured upon water in a saucer and vaporized by placing the saucer over a spirit lamp. At first the vapor is very irritating and disagreeable, but the patient gets used to it. The bath should be taken at first every other day for fifteen minutes, then gradually increased to an hour daily. The treatment should be continued for three months. I can recommend it as a most satisfactory method. In suitable cases, as when there is a single large cavity, drainage of the cavities may be attempted, particularly if the patient is in fairly good condition. Resection of the overlying ribs has been employed. For the fetid secretion turpentine may be given, or terebene, and inhalations of carbolic acid or thymol used.

IV. BRONCHIAL ASTHMA

Asthma is a term which has been applied to various conditions associated with dyspnœa—hence the names cardiac and renal asthma—but its use should be limited to the affection known as bronchial or spasmodic asthma.

Etiology.—All writers agree that there is in a majority of cases of bronchial asthma a strong neurotic element. Many regard it as a neurosis in which, according to one view, spasm of the bronchial muscles, according to the other turgescence of the mucosa, results from disturbed innervation, pneumogastric or vaso-motor. Of the numerous theories the following are the most important:

(1) That it is due to spasm of the bronchial muscles, a theory which has perhaps the largest number of adherents. The original experiments of C. J. B. Williams, upon which it is largely based, have been confirmed by Brodie.

(2) That the attack is due to swelling of the bronchial mucous membrane —fluctionary hyperæmia (Traube), vaso-motor turgescence (Weber), diffuse hyperæmic swelling (Clark).

(3) That in many cases it is a special form of inflammation of the smaller bronchioles—*bronchiolitis exudativa* (Curschmann). Other theories which may be mentioned are that the attack depends on spasm of the diaphragm, on reflex spasm of all the inspiratory muscles, or on protein sensitization.

As already mentioned, the so-called hay fever is an affection which has many resemblances to bronchial asthma, with which the attacks may alternate. In the suddenness of onset and in many of their features these diseases have a great similarity and differ only in site, as suggested by Sir Andrew Clark and generally acknowledged by specialists. Making due allowance for anatomical differences, if the structural changes occurring in the nasal mucous membrane during an attack of hay fever were to occur also in various parts of the bronchial mucosa, their presence there would afford a complete and adequate explanation of the facts observed during a paroxysm of bronchial asthma (Clark). With this statement I fully agree, but the observations of Curschmann have directed attention to a feature in asthma which has been neglected; namely, that in a majority of the cases it is associated with an exudation, such as might be supposed to come from a turgescent mucosa and which is of a very characteristic and peculiar character. The hyperæmia and swelling of the mucosa and the extremely viscid, tenacious mucus explain well the hindrance to inspiration and expiration and also the quality of the râles. An œdema of the angio-neurotic type has been described in the hands and arms in asthma.

Some general facts with reference to etiology may be mentioned. The affection sometimes runs in families, particularly those with irritable and unstable nervous systems. The attack may be associated with neuralgia or, as Salter mentions, even alternate with epilepsy. Men are more frequently affected than women. The disease often begins in childhood and sometimes lasts until old age. For years asthmatic attacks may follow whooping-cough. One of its most striking peculiarities is the *bizarre* and extraordinary variety of circumstances which at times induce a paroxysm. Among these local conditions climate or atmosphere is most important. A person may be free in the city and invariably suffer from an attack when he goes into the country, or into one special part of the country. Such cases are by no means uncommon. Breathing the air of a particular room or a dusty atmosphere may bring on an attack. Odors, particularly of flowers and of hay, or emanations from animals, as the horse, dog, or cat, may at once cause an outbreak. Fright or violent emotion of any sort may bring on a paroxysm. Uterine and ovarian troubles were formerly thought to induce attacks and may do so in rare instances. Diet, too, has an important influence, and in persons subject to the disease severe paroxysms may be induced by overloading the stomach, or by taking certain articles of food. Chronic cases, in which the attacks recur year after year, gradually become associated with emphysema, and every fresh "cold" induces a paroxysm. And, lastly, many cases of bronchial asthma are associated with affections of the nose, particularly with hypertrophic rhinitis and nasal polypi.

Briefly stated, then, bronchial asthma is a neurotic affection, characterized by hyperæmia and turgescence of the mucosa of the smaller bronchial tubes and a peculiar exudate of mucin. The attacks may be due to direct irritation of the bronchial mucosa or may be induced, reflexly, by irritation of the nasal mucosa, and indirectly, too, by reflex influences, from stomach, intestines, or genital organs. It is important to remember that in the subjects of asthma to whom injections of diphtheria or other antitoxins are given anaphylaxis may be induced with a rapidly fatal termination.

Symptoms.—Premonitory sensations precede some attacks, such as chilly feelings, a sense of tightness in the chest, flatulence, the passage of a large quantity of urine, or great depression of spirits. Nocturnal attacks are common. After a few hours' sleep, the patient is aroused with a distressing sense of want of breath and a feeling of great oppression in the chest. Soon the respiratory efforts become violent, all the accessory muscles are brought into play, and in a few minutes the patient is in a paroxysm of the most intense dyspnœa. The face is pale, the expression anxious, speech is impossible, and in spite of the most strenuous inspiratory efforts very little air enters the lungs. Expiration is prolonged and also wheezy. The number of respirations, however, is not much increased. The asthmatic fit may last from a few minutes to several hours. When severe, the signs of defective aëration soon appear, the face becomes bedewed with sweat, the pulse is small and quick, the extremities get cold, and just as the patient seems to be at his worst the breathing begins to get easier, and often with a paroxysm of coughing relief is obtained and he sinks exhausted to sleep. The relief may be but temporary and a second attack may soon come on. In a majority of the cases even in the intervals between the asthmatic fits the respiration is somewhat embarrassed. The cough is at first very tight and dry and the expectoration is tenacious. Emphysema of the neck may occur during the violent coughing spells. Urticaria may break out over the whole body during an attack, or, as in one patient, may be confined to the skin of the interscapular regions.

The PHYSICAL SIGNS during an attack are very characteristic. On inspection the thorax looks enlarged, barrel-shaped, and is fixed, the amount of expansion being altogether disproportionate to the intensity of the inspiratory movements. The diaphragm is lowered and moves but slightly. Inspiration is short and quick, expiration prolonged. Percussion may not reveal any special difference, but there is sometimes marked hyperresonance, particularly in patients who have had repeated attacks.

On auscultation, with inspiration and expiration, there are innumerable sibilant and sonorous râles of all varieties, piping and high-pitched, low-pitched and grave. Later in the attack there are moist râles.

The *sputum* is quite distinctive, unlike that which occurs in any other affection. Early in the attack it is brought up with great difficulty and is in the form of rounded gelatinous masses, the so-called "*perles*" of Laennec.

Though ball-like, they can be unfolded and really represent moulds in mucus of the smaller tubes. The entire expectoration may be made up of these somewhat translucent-looking pellets, floating in a small quantity of thin mucus. Some of them are opaque. Often with the naked eye a twisted spiral character can be seen, particularly if the sputum is spread on a glass with a black background. Microscopically, many of these pellets have a spiral structure, which renders them among the most remarkable bodies met with in sputum. It is not a little curious that they should have been practically overlooked until described by von Curschmann. Under the microscope the spirals are of two forms. In one there is simply a twisted, spirally arranged filament of mucin, in which are entangled leucocytes, the majority of which are eosinophiles. The twist may be loose or tight. The second form is much more peculiar. In the centre of a tightly coiled skein of mucin fibrils with a few scattered cells is a filament of extraordinary clearness and translucency, probably composed of transformed mucin. These spirals are doubtless formed in the finer bronchioles and constitute the product of an acute bronchiolitis. It is difficult to explain their spiral nature. I do not know of any observations upon the course of the currents produced by the ciliated epithelium in the bronchi, but it is quite possible that their action may be rotatory, in which case, particularly when combined with spasm of the bronchial muscles, it is possible to conceive that the mucus formed in the tube might be compelled to assume a spiral form. Within two or three days the sputum changes entirely in character; it becomes muco-purulent and von Curschmann's spirals are no longer to be found. They occur in all instances of true bronchial asthma in the early period of the attack. I have never seen the true spirals either in bronchitis or pneumonia. There are, in addition, in many cases, the pointed, octahedral crystals described by Leyden and sometimes called asthma crystals. They are identical with the crystals found in the semen and in the blood in leukæmia. At one time they were supposed, by their irritating character, to induce the paroxysms. Eosinophiles in the blood are enormously increased in asthma—to 25 or 35 per cent. of the leucocytes, or even to 53.6 per cent. in one case.

Course.—This is very variable. In severe attacks the paroxysms recur for three or four nights or even more, and in the intervals and during the day there may be wheezing and cough. Early in the disease the patient may be free in the morning, without cough or much distress, and the attacks may appear at first to be of a purely nervous character. In the long-standing cases emphysema almost invariably develops and, while the pure asthmatic fits diminish in frequency the chronic bronchitis and shortness of breath become aggravated.

We have no knowledge of the morbid anatomy of true asthma. Death during the attack is unknown. In long-standing cases the lesions are those of chronic bronchitis and emphysema.

Treatment.—The asthmatic attack usually demands immediate and prompt treatment, and remedies should be administered which experience has shown are capable of relieving the condition of the bronchial mucosa. A few whiffs of chloroform will produce prompt though temporary relaxation. In a child with very severe attacks, resisting all the usual remedies, the treatment by chloroform gave immediate and finally permanent relief. Hypodermic injections of pilocarpin (gr. 1/8, 0.008 gm.) will sometimes relax the mucosa in the profuse sweating. Perles of nitrite of amyl may be broken on the handkerchief or from two to five drops of the solution may be placed upon cotton-wool and inhaled. Strong stimulants given hot or a dose of spirit of chloroform in hot whisky will sometimes induce relaxation. More permanent relief is given by the hypodermic injection of morphia or of morphia and strychnine combined. In obstinate and repeatedly recurring attacks this has proved a very satisfactory plan. The sedative antispasmodics, such as belladonna, henbane, stramonium, and lobelia, may be given in solution or used in the form of cigarettes. Nearly all the popular remedies either in this form or in pastilles contain some plant of the order *solanaceæ,* with nitrate or chlorate of potash. Excellent cigarettes are now manufactured and asthmatics try various sorts, since one form benefits one patient, another form another patient. Nitre paper made with a strong solution of nitrate of potash is very serviceable. Filling the room with the fumes of this paper prior to retiring will sometimes ward off a nocturnal attack. I have known several patients to whom tobacco smoke inhaled was quite as potent as the prepared cigarettes.

Cauterization of the mucous membrane of the nose has given great relief, particularly in cases with swelling and irritation. The use of compressed air in the pneumatic cabinet is very beneficial; oxygen inhalations may also be tried. In preventing the recurrence of the attacks there is no remedy so useful as iodide of potassium, which sometimes acts like a specific. From 10 to 20 grains (0.6 to 1.3 gm.) three times a day is usually sufficient. Persistent hydrotherapy is often of value.

Particular attention should be paid to the diet of asthmatic patients. A rule which experience generally compels them to make is to take the heavy meals in the early part of the day and not retire to bed before gastric digestion is completed. As the attacks are often induced by flatulency, the carbohydrates should be restricted. Coffee is a more suitable drink than tea. In respect to climate it is very difficult to lay down rules for asthmatics. The patients are often much better in the city than in the country. The high and dry altitudes are certainly more beneficial than the sea-shore; but in the protracted cases, with emphysema as a secondary complication, the rarefied air of high altitudes is not advantageous. In young persons I have known a residence for six months in Florida or southern California to be followed by prolonged freedom from attacks. Egypt is a peculiarly satisfactory winter climate.

V. FIBRINOUS BRONCHITIS

(*Plastic or Croupous Bronchitis*)

Definition.—An acute or chronic affection, characterized by the formation in certain of the bronchial tubes of fibrinous casts, which are expelled in paroxysms of dyspnœa and cough.

In several diseases fibrinous moulds of the bronchi are formed, as in diphtheria (with extension into the trachea and bronchi), in pneumonia, and occasionally in phthisis—conditions which, however, have nothing to do with true fibrinous bronchitis. These casts are not to be confounded with the blood-casts which occur occasionally in hæmoptysis.

Clinical Description.—Bettman, in reporting a case which occurred in Whitridge Williams's obstetrical clinic at the Johns Hopkins Hospital, analyzed all the cases from the literature since 1869, grouping them into different classes. The first and most important is *chronic idiopathic fibrinous bronchitis*. It is a rare affection. Of 27 cases, 15 were in males. It is most common at the middle period of life. The attacks may occur at definite intervals for months or years. The form and size of the casts may be identical at each attack as though each time precisely the same bronchial area was involved. The expectoration of the casts is associated with paroxysms of dyspnœa and coughing, which occur at longer or shorter intervals. Fever and hæmoptysis may be present during the attack. Physical signs usually indicate the portion of the lung affected, as there are suppressed breath sounds and numerous râles on coughing. A very dry râle, called the *"bruit de drapeau,"* has been described, caused by the vibration of a loosened portion of the cast.

In five cases there were skin lesions. Tuberculosis is sometimes present. The casts are usually rolled up and mixed with mucus and blood. When unrolled they are large white branching structures. The main stem may be as thick as the little finger. From the consistency and appearance they have been described as fibrinous, but they consist mainly of mucin. On cross-section they show a concentrically stratified structure, with leucocytes and alveolar epithelium. Leyden's crystals and von Curschmann's spirals are sometimes found, and in Bettman's case there were protozoan-like bodies. Death occurred in only one case of the series.

There is a very remarkable *acute form*, of which Bettman collected 15 cases. It comes on most frequently during some fever, as typhoid, pneumonia, or the eruptive fevers. After a preliminary bronchitis the dyspnœa increases, and then the casts are coughed up. Chills and fever have been present. Four of the 15 cases proved fatal, and the casts were found *in situ*. It is much more serious than the chronic form. There may be casts expectorated which have not the arborescent structure of the true fibrinous moulds, but which come from a single tube or its bifurcation. Sometimes they are very small and "tail off" into true spirals.

Fibrinous casts are expectorated in connection with chronic heart-disease (10 cases) and in pulmonary tuberculosis (14 cases), in the latter disease usually late in the course and of unfavorable moment. In the albuminous expectoration following tapping of a pleural exudate fibrinous casts have been coughed up.

In hæmoptysis blood-casts may be expectorated, and they are not to be confounded with the casts of true fibrinous bronchitis which may be coughed up with profuse hæmorrhage.

In pneumonia small fibrinous plugs are not uncommon in the sputum, and in a few rare instances quite large moulds of the tubes may be coughed up.

The mycelium of *Aspergillus fumigatus* may form membranous casts in the bronchi. I reported an instance of the kind in which a small partial mould of this kind was expectorated, and there is on record a case in which for long periods membranes composed of this fungus were coughed up in attacks of dyspnœa.

Pathology.—The pathology of the disease is obscure. The membrane is identical with that to which the term croupous is applied, and the obscurity relates not so much to the mechanism of the production, which is probably the same as in other mucous surfaces, as to the curious limitation of the affection to certain bronchial territories and in the chronic form to the remarkable recurrence at stated or irregular intervals throughout a period of many years.

In the fatal cases the bronchial mucous membrane may be found injected or pale. In Biermer's case the epithelial lining was intact beneath the cast, but in that of Kretschy the bronchi were denuded of their epithelium. Emphysema is almost invariably present. Evidences of recent or antecedent pleurisy are sometimes found. Model, in an article published from Bäumler's clinic, states that tuberculosis was present in 10 out of 21 autopsies.

Treatment.—In the acute cases the treatment should be that of ordinary acute bronchitis. We know of nothing which can prevent the recurrence of the attacks in the chronic form. In the uncomplicated cases there is rarely any danger during the paroxysm, even though the symptoms may be most distressing and the dyspnœa and cough very severe. Inhalations of ether, steam, or atomized lime-water aid in the separation of the membranes. Waldenberg employed the last remedy with success in one case. Ewart recommends intratracheal injections of olive oil. Pilocarpine might be useful, as in some instances it increases the bronchial secretion. The employment of emetics may be necessary, and in some cases they are effective in promoting the removal of the casts.

D. DISEASES OF THE LUNGS

I. CIRCULATORY DISTURBANCES IN THE LUNGS

Congestion.—There are two forms of congestion of the lungs—active and passive.

1. Active Congestion of the Lungs.—Much doubt and confusion still exist on this subject. French writers, following Woillez, regard it as an independent primary affection (*maladie de Woillez*), and in their dictionaries and text-books allot much space to it. English and American authors more correctly regard it as a symptomatic affection. Active fluxion to the lungs occurs with increased action of the heart, and when very hot air or irritating substances are inhaled. In diseases which interfere locally with the circulation the capillaries in the adjacent unaffected portions may be greatly distended. The importance, however, of this collateral fluxion, as it is called, is probably exaggerated. In a whole series of pulmonary affections there is this associated congestion—in pneumonia, bronchitis, pleurisy, and tuberculosis.

The symptoms of active congestion of the lungs are by no means definite. The description given by Woillez and by other French writers is of an affection which is difficult to recognize from anomalous or larval forms of pneumonia. The chief symptoms described are initial chill, pain in the side, dyspnœa, moderate cough, and temperature from 101° to 103° F. The physical signs are defective resonance, feeble breathing, sometimes bronchial in character, and fine râles. A majority of clinical physicians would undoubtedly class such cases under inflammation of the lung. In many epidemics the abnormal and larval forms are specially prevalent.

42

The occurrence of an intense and rapidly fatal congestion of the lung, following extreme heat or cold or sometimes violent exertion, is recognized by some authors. Renforth, the oarsman, is said to have died from this cause during a race at Halifax. Leuf has described cases in which, in association with drunkenness, exposure, and cold, death occurred suddenly, or within twenty-four hours, the only lesion found being an extreme, almost hæmorrhagic, congestion of the lungs. It is by no means certain that in these cases death really occurs from pulmonary congestion in the absence of specific statements with reference to the coronary arteries and the heart.

2. PASSIVE CONGESTION.—Two forms of this may be recognized, the mechanical and the hypostatic.

(*a*) *Mechanical congestion* occurs whenever there is an obstacle to the return of the blood to the heart. It is a common event in many affections of the left heart. The lungs are voluminous, russet brown in color, cutting and tearing with great resistance. On section they show at first a brownish red tinge, and then the cut surface, exposed to the air, becomes rapidly of a vivid red color from oxidation of the abundant hæmoglobin. This is the condition known as *brown induration* of the lung. Histologically it is characterized by (*i*) great distention of the alveolar capillaries; (*ii*) increase in the connective-tissue elements of the lung; (*iii*) the presence in the alveolar walls of many cells containing altered blood-pigment; (*iv*) in the alveoli numerous epithelial cells containing blood-pigment in all stages of alteration, which are also found in great numbers in the sputum.

It occasionally happens that this mechanical hyperæmia of the lung results from pressure by tumors. So long as compensation is maintained the mechanical congestion of the lung in heart disease does not produce any symptoms, but with enfeebled heart action the engorgement becomes marked and there are dyspnœa, cough, and expectoration, with the characteristic alveolar cells.

(*b*) *Hypostatic Congestion.*—In fevers and adynamic states generally it is very common to find the bases of the lungs deeply congested, a condition induced partly by the effect of gravity, the patient lying recumbent in one posture for a long time, but chiefly by weakened heart action. That it is not an effect of gravity alone is shown by the fact that a healthy person may remain in bed an indefinite time without its occurrence. The posterior parts of the lung are dark in color and engorged with blood and serum; in some instances to such a degree that the alveoli no longer contain air and portions of the lung sink in water. The terms *splenization* and hypostatic pneumonia have been given to these advanced grades. It is a common affection in protracted cases of typhoid fever and in long debilitating illness. In ascites, meteorism, and abdominal tumors the bases of the lungs may be compressed and congested. In this connection must be mentioned the form of passive congestion met with in injury to, and organic disease of, the brain. In cerebral apoplexy the bases of the lungs are deeply engorged, not quite airless, but heavy, and on section drip with blood and serum. I have twice seen this condition in an extreme grade throughout the lungs in death from morphia poisoning. In some instances the lung tissue has a blackish, gelatinous, infiltrated appearance, almost like diffuse pulmonary apoplexy. Occasionally this congestion is most marked in, and even confined to, the hemiplegic side. In prolonged coma the hypostatic congestion may be associated with patches of consolidation, due to the aspiration of portions of food into the air-passages.

The symptoms of hypostatic congestion are not at all characteristic, and the condition has to be sought for by careful examination of the bases of the lungs, when slight dulness, feeble, sometimes blowing, breathing and liquid râles can be detected.

Treatment.—The treatment of congestion of the lungs is usually that of the condition with which it is associated. In the intense pulmonary engorgement, which may possibly occur primarily, and which is met with in heart disease and emphysema, free bleeding should be practiced. From 20 to 30 ounces of blood should be taken from the arm, and if the blood does not flow freely and the condition of the patient is desperate aspiration of the right auricle may be performed.

Œdema.—In all forms of intense congestion of the lungs there is a transudation of serum from the engorged capillaries chiefly into the air-cells, but also into the alveolar walls. Not only is it very frequent in congestion, but also with inflammation, with new growths, infarcts, and tubercles. When limited to the neighborhood of an affected part, the name collateral œdema is sometimes applied to it.

Acute œdema is met with: (1) in the infections; (2) in Bright's disease; (3) in heart disease, particularly angina pectoris, myocarditis, and valve lesions; (4) in arterio-sclerosis; (5) pregnancy; (6) angio-neurotic œdema, and (7) as a complication of the epileptic fit. The theory most generally accepted is that of Welch, whose experiments seemed to indicate that pulmonary œdema is due to a disproportionate weakness of the left ventricle, so that the blood accumulates in the lung capillaries until transudation occurs. Such weakness may be brought about by paralysis or by spasm of the left ventricle. Others regard it as an effect of disturbance in the vasomotor mechanism of the lungs. In some cases there are recurring attacks of acute œdema.

Anatomically the lung is anæmic, heavy, sodden, pits on pressure, and on section a large quantity of clear or blood-tinged serum flows out. It may have in places a gelatinous aspect.

Symptoms.—The onset is sudden with a feeling of oppression and pain in the chest and rapid breathing which soon becomes dyspnœic or orthopnœic. There may be an incessant short cough and a copious frothy, sometimes blood-tinged, expectoration, which may be expelled in a gush from the mouth and nose. The face is pale and covered with a cold sweat; the pulse is feeble and the heart's action weak. Over the entire chest may be heard piping and bubbling râles. The attack may be fatal in a few hours or it may persist for twelve or twenty-four hours and then pass off. Steven, of Glasgow, has reported a case with 72 attacks in two and a half years. I have seen this recurrent form in angina pectoris, each paroxysm of which was associated with intense dyspnœa and all the features of acute œdema of the lungs.

Bleeding should be practiced at once and is often most helpful. Dry cupping may be tried. One of my patients had great relief from inhalations of chloroform. Oxygen may be used. Atropine hypodermically (gr. 1/100, 0.00065 gm.) is sometimes of value. If there is much agitation and sense of impending death, morphia may be given hypodermically.

Pulmonary Hæmorrhage.—This occurs in two forms—*broncho-pulmonary hæmorrhage,* sometimes called bronchorrhagia, in which the blood is poured out into the bronchi and is expectorated, and *pulmonary apoplexy* or pneumorrhagia, in which the hæmorrhage takes place into the air-cells and the lung tissue.

1. BRONCHO-PULMONARY HÆMORRHAGE; HÆMOPTYSIS.—Spitting of blood, to which the term hæmoptysis should be restricted, results from a variety of conditions, among which the following are the most important: (*a*) In young healthy persons hæmoptysis may occur without warning, and after continuing for a few days disappear and leave no ill traces. There may be at the time of the attack no physical signs indicating pulmonary disease. In such cases good health may be preserved for years and no further trouble occur. These cases are not very uncommon, but in spite of the good health tuberculosis may be suspected. In Ware's important contribution to this subject, of 386 cases of hæmoptysis noted in private practice 62 recovered and pulmonary disease did not subsequently develop in them. (*b*) *Hæmoptysis in pulmonary tuberculosis,* which is considered on page 194. (*c*) In connection with certain diseases of the lung, as pneumonia (in the initial stage) and cancer, occasionally in gangrene, abscess, and bronchiectasis. (*d*) In many heart affections, particularly mitral lesions. It may be profuse and recur at intervals for years. (*e*) *In ulcerative affections of the larynx, trachea, or bronchi.* Sometimes the hæmorrhage is profuse and rapidly fatal, as when the ulcer erodes a large branch of the pulmonary artery, an accident which I have known to happen in a case of chronic bronchitis with emphysema. (*f*) *Aneurism* is an occasional cause of hæmoptysis. It may be sudden and rapidly fatal when the sac bursts into the air-passages. Slight bleeding may continue for weeks or months, due to pressure on the mucous membrane or erosion of the lung; or in some cases the sac "weeps" through the exposed laminæ of fibrin. (*g*) *Vicarious hæmorrhage,* which occurs in rare instances in cases of interrupted menstruation. The instances are well authenticated. Flint mentions a case which he had had under observation for four years, and Hippocrates refers to it in the aphorism, "Hæmoptysis in a woman is removed by an eruption of the menses." Periodical hæmoptysis has also been met with after the removal of both ovaries. Even fatal hæmorrhage has occurred from the lung during menstruation when no lesion was found to account for it. (*h*) There is a form of *recurring hæmoptysis in arthritic subjects* to which Sir Andrew Clark has called special attention and which also is described by French writers. The cases occur in persons over fifty years of age who usually present signs of the arthritic diathesis. It rarely leads to fatal issue and subsides without inducing pulmonary changes. (*i*) Hæmoptysis occurs sometimes *in malignant fevers* and *in purpura hæmorrhagica.* Lastly, there is endemic hæmoptysis, due to the bronchial fluke, an affection which is confined to parts of China and Japan.

Symptoms.—Hæmoptysis sets in, as a rule, suddenly. Often without warning the patient experiences a warm, saltish taste as the mouth fills with blood. Coughing is usually induced. There may be only an ounce or so brought up before the hæmorrhage stops, or the bleeding may continue for days, the patient bringing up small quantities. In other instances, particularly when a large vessel is eroded or an aneurism bursts, the amount is large, and the patient, after a few attempts at coughing, shows signs of suffocation and death is produced by inundation of the bronchial system. Fatal hæmorrhage even may occur into a large cavity in a patient debilitated by phthisis without the production of hæmoptysis. I dissected a case of this kind at the Philadelphia Hospital. The blood from the lungs generally has characters which render it readily distinguishable from the blood which is vomited. It is alkaline in reaction, frothy, and mixed with mucus, and when coagulation occurs air-bubbles are present in the clot. Blood-moulds of the smaller bronchi are sometimes seen. Patients can usually tell whether the blood has been brought up by coughing or by vomiting, and in a majority of cases the history gives important indications. In paroxysmal hæmoptysis connected with menstrual disturbances the practitioner should see that the blood is actually coughed up, since deception may be practiced. The spurious hæmoptysis of hysteria is considered with that disease. Naturally, the patient is at first alarmed at the occurrence of bleeding, but, unless very profuse, as when due to rupture of an aortic aneurism in a pulmonary cavity, the danger is rarely immediate. The attacks, however, are apt to recur for a few days and the sputum may remain blood-tinged for a longer period. In the great majority of cases the hæmorrhage ceases spontaneously. It should be remembered that some of the blood may be swallowed and produce vomiting, and, after a day or two, the stools may be dark in color. It is not advisable to examine the chest during an attack of hæmoptysis.

2. Pulmonary Apoplexy; Hæmorrhagic Infarct.—In this condition the blood is effused into the air-cells and interstitial tissue. It is usually diffuse, the parenchyma not being broken, as is the brain tissue in cerebral apoplexy. Sometimes, in disease of the brain, in septic conditions, and in the malignant forms of fevers, the lung tissue is uniformly infiltrated with blood and has, on section, a black, gelatinous appearance.

As a rule, the hæmorrhage is limited and results from the blocking of a branch of the pulmonary artery either by a thrombus or an embolus. The condition is most common in chronic heart-disease. Although the pulmonary arteries are terminal ones, blocking is not always followed by infarction; partly because the wide capillaries furnish sufficient anastomosis, and partly because the bronchial vessels may keep up the circulation. The infarctions are chiefly at the periphery of the lung, usually wedge-shaped, with the base of the wedge toward the surface. When recent, they are dark in color, hard and firm, and look on section like an ordinary blood-clot. Gradual changes go on, and the color becomes a reddish brown. The pleura over an infarct is usually inflamed. A microscopic section shows the air-cells to be distended with red blood corpuscles, which may also be in the alveolar walls. The infarcts are usually multiple and vary in size from a walnut to an orange. Very large ones may involve the greater part of a lobe. In the artery passing to the affected territory a thrombus or an embolus is found. The globular thrombi, formed in the right auricular appendix, play an important part in the production of hæmorrhagic infarction. In many cases the source of the embolus can not be discovered, and the infarct may have resulted from thrombosis in the pulmonary artery, but, as before mentioned, it is not infrequent to find total obstruction of a large branch of a pulmonary artery without hæmorrhage into the corresponding lung area. The further history of an infarction is variable. It is possible that in some instances the circulation is re-established and the blood removed. More commonly, if the patient lives, the usual changes go on in the extravasated blood and ultimately a pigmented, puckered, fibroid patch results. Sloughing may occur with the formation of a cavity. Occasionally gangrene results. In a case at the University Hospital, Philadelphia, a gangrenous infarct ruptured and produced fatal pneumothorax.

The *symptoms* of pulmonary apoplexy are by no means definite. The condition may be suspected in chronic heart-disease when hæmoptysis occurs, particularly in mitral stenosis, but the bleeding may be due to the extreme engorgement. When the infarcts are very large, and particularly in the lower lobe, in which they most commonly occur, there may be signs of consolidation with blowing breathing and a pleuritic friction.

TREATMENT OF PULMONARY HÆMORRHAGE.—The pressure within the pulmonary artery is considerably less than that in the aortic system. The system is under vaso-motor control, but our knowledge of the mutual relations of pressure in the aorta and in the pulmonary artery, under varying conditions, is still very imperfect (Bradford). There may be an influence on the systemic blood-pressure without any on the pulmonary, and the pressure in the one may rise while it falls in the other, or it may rise and fall in both together. The researches of Brodie and Dixon indicate that drugs which raise the peripheral blood pressure by vaso-constriction increase the total blood in the lung. Thus ergot, the remedy perhaps most commonly used, causes a distinct rise in the pulmonary blood-pressure, while aconite produces a definite fall.

The question is beset with difficulties, and experimental work is by no means in accord. In a recent study Wiggers concludes that in the early stages of hæmoptysis, when the breathing is not altered, lowering of the blood pressure within the pulmonary circuit can not be accomplished by the nitrites, but this can only be done with the cardiac depressants, such as chloroform and the pituitary extracts; and in the later stages of an attack, when the heart is very rapid, pituitary extract is the only drug that raises systemic pressure while simultaneously lowering that in the pulmonary circuit.

The anatomical condition in hæmoptysis is either hyperæmia of the bronchial mucosa (or of the lung tissue) or a perforated vessel. In the latter case the patient often passes rapidly beyond treatment, though there are instances of the most profuse hæmorrhage, which must have come from a perforated artery or a ruptured aneurism, in which recovery has occurred. Practically, for treatment, we should separate these cases, as the remedies which would be applicable in the case of congested and bleeding mucosa would be as much out of place in a case of hæmorrhage from ruptured aneurism as in a cut radial artery. When the blood is brought up in large quantities, it is almost certain either that an aneurism has ruptured or a vessel has been eroded. In the instances in which the sputum is blood tinged or when the blood is in smaller quantities, bleeding comes by diapedesis from hyperæmic vessels. In such cases the hæmorrhage may be beneficial in relieving the congested blood-vessels.

The indications are to reduce the frequency of the heart-beats and to lower the blood-pressure. The truth, *Das Blut ist ein ganz besonderer Saft,* is strikingly emphasized by the frightened state of the patient. Rest of the body and peace of the mind—*"quies, securitas, silentium"* of Celsus—should be secured. If there is marked restlessness, morphia hypodermically (gr. 1/6, 0.011 gm.) is advisable. Turn the patient on the affected side, if known, as the regurgitation is less apt to occur into the bronchi of the sound lung. As Aretæus remarks, in hæmoptysis the patient despairs from the first, and needs to be strongly reassured. Death is rarely due directly to hæmoptysis; patients die after, not of it (S. West). In the majority of cases of mild hæmoptysis this is sufficient. Even when the patient insists upon going about, the bleeding may stop spontaneously. The diet should be light and unstimulating. Alcohol should not be used. The patient may, if he wishes, have ice to suck. Small doses of aromatic sulphuric acid may be given, but unless the bleeding is protracted styptic and astringent medicines are not indicated. For cough, which is always present and disturbing, opium should be freely given, and is of all medicines most serviceable in hæmoptysis. Digitalis should not be used, as it raises the blood-pressure in the pulmonary artery. Aconite, as it lowers the pressure, may be used when there is much vascular excitement. Ergot, tannic acid, and lead, which are so much employed, have little or no influence in hæmoptysis; ergot probably does harm. One of the most satisfactory means of lowering the blood-pressure is purgation, and when the bleeding is protracted salts may be freely given. In profuse hæmoptysis, such as comes from erosion of an artery or the rupture of an aneurism, a fatal result is common, and yet post mortem evidence shows that thrombosis may occur with healing in a rupture of considerable size. The fainting induced by the loss of blood is probably the most efficient means of promoting thrombosis, and it was on this principle that formerly patients were bled from the arm, or from both arms, as in the case of Laurence Sterne. Ligatures, or Esmarch's bandages, placed around the legs may serve temporarily to check the bleeding. The ice-bag on the sternum is of doubtful utility. In protracted cases pneumothorax has been induced, sometimes with success.

Briefly, then, we may say that hæmorrhage from rupture of aneurism or erosion of a blood-vessel usually proves fatal. The fainting induced by the loss of blood is beneficial, and, if the patient can be kept alive for twenty-four hours, a thrombus of sufficient strength to prevent further bleeding may form. The chief danger is the inundation of the bronchial system with the blood, so that while the hæmorrhage is profuse the cough should be encouraged. Opium should not then be used, and stimulants should be given with caution.

In the other group, in which the hæmorrhage comes from a congested area and is limited, the patient gets well if kept absolutely quiet, and fatal hæmorrhage probably never occurs from this source. Rest, reduction of the blood-pressure by minimum diet, purging, if necessary, and the administration of opium to allay the cough are the main indications.

II. CHRONIC INTERSTITIAL PNEUMONIA

(*Cirrhosis of the Lung—Fibroid Phthisis*)

A fibroid change may have its starting point in the tissue about the bronchi and blood-vessels, the interlobular septa, the alveolar walls, or in the pleura. So diverse are the forms and so varied the conditions under which this change occurs that a proper classification is extremely difficult. We may recognize, however, two chief forms—the *local*, involving only a limited area of the lung substance, and the *diffuse*, invading either both lungs or an entire organ.

Etiology.—(*a*) LOCAL fibroid change in the lungs is common. It is a constant accompaniment of tubercle, in the evolution of which interstitial changes play a very important rôle. In tumors, abscess, gummata, hydatids, and emphysema it also occurs. Fibroid processes are frequently met with at the apices of the lung and may be due either to a limited healed tuberculosis, to fibroid induration in consequence of pigment, or, in a few instances, may result from thickening of the pleura.

(*b*) DIFFUSE INTERSTITIAL PNEUMONIA is met with: (1) As a sequence of *acute fibrinous pneumonia*. Although extremely rare, this is recognized as a possible termination. From unknown causes resolution fails to take place. Organization goes on in the fibrinous plugs within the air-cells and the alveolar walls become greatly thickened by a new growth, first of nuclear and subsequently of fibrillated connective tissue. Macroscopically there is produced a smooth, grayish, homogeneous tissue which has the peculiar translucency of all new-formed connective tissue. This has been called gray induration. A majority of the cases terminate within a few months, but instances which have been followed from the outset are very rare.

(2) *Chronic Broncho-pneumonia.*—The relation of broncho-pneumonia to cirrhosis of the lung has been specially studied by Charcot, who states that it may follow the acute or subacute form of this disease, particularly in children. The fibrosis extends from the bronchi, which are usually found dilated. Bronchiectasis itself may be followed by fibrosis of the lung. The alveolar walls are thickened and the lobules converted into firm grayish masses, in which there is no trace of normal lung tissue. This process may go on and involve an entire lobe or even the whole lung. Many of these cases are tuberculous from the outset.

(3) *Pleurogenous Interstitial Pneumonia.*—Charcot applies this term to that form of cirrhosis of the lung which follows invasion from the pleura. Doubt has been expressed by some writers whether this really occurs. While Wilson Fox was probably correct in questioning whether an entire lung can become cirrhosed by the gradual invasion from the pleura, there can be no doubt that there are instances of primitive dry pleurisy, which, as Sir Andrew Clark has pointed out, gradually compresses the lung and at the same time leads to interstitial cirrhosis. This may be due in part to the fibroid change which follows prolonged compression. In some cases there seems to be a distinct connection between the greatly thickened pleura and the dense strands of fibrous tissue passing from it into the lung substance. Instances occur in which one lobe or the greater part of it presents, on section, a mottled appearance, owing to the increased thickness of the interlobar septa—a condition which may exist without a trace of involvement of the pleura. In many other cases, however, the extension seems to be so definitely associated with pleurisy that there is no doubt as to the causal connection between the two processes. In these instances the lung is removed with great difficulty, owing to the thickness and close adhesion of the pleura to the chest wall.

(4) *Chronic interstitial pneumonia,* due to inhalation of dust, which is considered in a separate section.

(5) *Syphilis* of the lung may present the features of a chronic fibrosis.

(6) Indurative changes in the lung may follow the compression by aneurism or new growth or the irritation of a foreign body in a bronchus.

Morbid Anatomy.—There are two chief forms, the massive or lobar and the insular or broncho-pneumonic form. In the massive type the disease is unilateral; the chest of the affected side is sunken, deformed, and the shoulder much depressed. On opening the thorax the heart is seen drawn far over to the affected side. The unaffected lung is emphysematous and covers the greater portion of the mediastinum. It is scarcely credible in how small a space, close to the spine, the cirrhosed lung may lie. The adhesions between the pleural membranes may be extremely dense and thick, particularly in the pleurogenous cases; but when the disease has originated in the lung there may be little thickening of the pleura. The organ is airless, firm, and hard. It strongly resists cutting, and on section shows a grayish fibroid tissue of variable amount, through which pass the blood-vessels and bronchi. The latter may be either slightly or enormously dilated. There are instances in which the entire lung is converted into a series of bronchiectatic cavities and the cirrhosis is apparent only in certain areas or at the root. The tuberculous cases can usually be differentiated by the presence of an apical cavity, not bronchiectatic, often large, and the other lung almost invariably shows tuberculous lesions. Aneurisms of the pulmonary artery are not infrequent in the cavities. The other lung is always greatly enlarged and emphysematous. The heart is hypertrophied, particularly the right ventricle, and there may be marked atheromatous changes in the vessels. An amyloid condition of the viscera is found in some cases.

In the broncho-pneumonic form the areas are smaller, often centrally placed, and most frequently in the lower lobes. They are deeply pigmented, show dilated bronchi, and when multiple are separated by emphysematous lung tissue.

A *reticular form* of fibrosis of the lung has been described by Percy Kidd and W. McCollum, in which the lungs are intersected by grayish fibroid strands following the lines of the interlobular septa.

Symptoms and Course.—The disease is essentially chronic, extending over a period of many years, and when once the condition is established the health may be fairly good. In a well marked case the patient complains only of his chronic cough, perhaps a slight shortness of breath. In other respects he is quite well, and is usually able to do light work. The cases are commonly regarded as phthisical, though there may be scarcely a symptom of that affeciton except the cough. There are instances, however, of fibroid phthisis which can not be distinguished from cirrhosis of the lung except by the presence of tubercle bacilli in the expectoration. As the bronchi are usually dilated, the symptoms and physical signs may be those of bronchiectasis. The cough is paroxysmal and the expectoration is generally copious and of a muco-purulent or sero-purulent nature. It is sometimes fetid. Hæmorrhage is by no means infrequent, and occurred in more than one-half of the cases analyzed by Bastian. Walking on the level and in the ordinary affairs of life, the patient may show no shortness of breath, but in the ascent of stairs and on exertion there may be dyspnœa.

Physical Signs.—*Inspection.*—The affected side of the chest is immobile, retracted, and shrunken, and contrasts in a striking way with the voluminous healthy one. The intercostal spaces are obliterated and the ribs may even overlap. The shoulder is drawn down and from behind it is seen that the spine is bowed. The muscles of the shoulder-girdle are wasted. The heart is greatly displaced, being drawn over by the shrinkage of the lung to the affected side. When the left lung is affected there may be a large area of visible impulse in the second, third, and fourth interspaces. Mensuration shows a great diminution in the affected side, and with the saddle-tape the expansion may be seen to be negative. The *percussion* note varies with the condition of the bronchi. It may be absolutely flat, particularly at the base or at the apex. In the axilla there may be a flat tympany or even an amphoric note over a large sacculated bronchus. On the opposite side the percussion note is usually hyperresonant. On auscultation the breath-sounds have either a cavernous or amphoric quality at the apex, and at the base are feeble, with mucous, bubbling râles. The voice-sounds are usually exaggerated. Cardiac murmurs are not uncommon, particularly late in the disease, when the right heart fails. These are, of course, the physical signs of the disease when it is well established. They naturally vary considerably, according to the stage of the process. The disease is essentially chronic, and may persist for fifteen or twenty years. Death occurs sometimes from hæmorrhage, more commonly from gradual failure of the right heart with dropsy, and occasionally from amyloid degeneration of the organs.

Diagnosis.—The diagnosis is never difficult. It may be impossible to say, without a clear history, whether the origin is pleuritic or pneumonic. Between cases of this kind and fibroid phthisis it is not always easy to discriminate, as the conditions may be almost identical. When tuberculosis is present, however, even in long-standing cases, bacilli are usually present in the sputum, and there may be signs of disease in the other lung.

Treatment.—It is only for an intercurrent affection or for an aggravation of the cough that the patient seeks relief. Nothing can be done for the condition itself. When possible the patient should live in a mild climate, and avoid exposure to cold and damp. A distressing feature in some cases is the putrefaction of the contents of the dilated tubes, for which the same measures may be used as in fetid bronchitis.

III. PNEUMONOKONIOSIS

Definition.—Under this term, introduced by Zenker, are embraced those forms of fibrosis of the lung due to the inhalation of dusts in various occupations. They have received various names, according to the nature of the inhaled particles—*anthracosis,* or coal-miner's disease; *siderosis,* due to the inhalation of metallic dusts, particularly iron; *chalicosis* and *silicosis,* due to the inhalation of mineral dusts, producing the so-called stone-cutter's phthisis, or the "grinder's rot" of the Sheffield workers.

Etiology.—The dust particles inhaled into the lungs are dealt with extensively by the ciliated epithelium and by the phagocytes, which exist normally in the respiratory organs. The ordinary mucous corpuscles take in a large number of the particles, which fall upon the trachea and main bronchi. The cilia sweep the mucus out to a point from which it can be expelled by coughing. It is doubtful if the particles ever reach the air-cells, but the swollen alveolar cells (in which they are in numbers) probably pick them up on the way. The mucous and the alveolar cells are the normal respiratory scavengers. In dwellers in the country, in which the air is pure, they are able to prevent the access of dust particles to the lung tissue, so that even in adults these organs present a rosy tint, very different from the dark, carbonized appearance of the lungs of dwellers in cities. When the impurities in the air are very abundant, a certain proportion of the dust particles escapes these cells and penetrates the mucosa, reaching the lymph spaces, where they are attacked at once by the cells of the connective-tissue stroma, which are capable of ingesting and retaining a large quantity. In coal-miners, coal-heavers, and others whose occupations necessitate the constant breathing of a very dusty atmosphere even these forces are insufficient. Vansteenberghe and Grysez have demonstrated that pulmonary anthracosis may be induced by passing an emulsion of china ink into the stomach of an animal through a catheter. From a long series of experiments they conclude that anthracosis is due to the intestinal absorption of carbon particles arrested in the nose and pharynx, and then swallowed. Their experiments further show that both the tracheal and intestinal routes are used—through the former the particles reach the bronchi and external portions of the alveoli, through the latter the parenchyma of the lung. Occasionally in anthracosis the carbon grains reach the general circulation, and the coal dust is found in the liver and spleen. As Weigert has shown, this occurs when the densely pigmented bronchial glands closely adhere to the pulmonary veins, through the walls of which the carbon particles pass to the general circulation. The lung tissue has a remarkable tolerance for these particles; but by constant exposure a limit is reached, and there is brought about a very definite pathological condition, an interstitial sclerosis. In coal-miners this may occur in patches, even before the lung tissue is uniformly infiltrated with the dust. In others it appears only after the entire organs have become so laden that they are dark in color, and an ink-like juice flows from the cut surface. The lungs of a miner may be black throughout and yet show no local lesions and be everywhere crepitant.

Morbid Anatomy.—The particles of carbon are found deposited in large numbers in the follicular cords of the tracheal and bronchial glands and of the peri-bronchial and peri-arterial lymph nodules, and in these they finally excite proliferation of the connective tissue elements. It is by no means uncommon to find in persons whose lungs are only moderately carbonized the bronchial glands sclerosed and hard. In anthracosis the fibroid changes usually begin in the peri-bronchial lymph tissue, and in the early stage of the process the sclerosis may be largely confined to these regions. A Nova Scotian miner, aged thirty-six, died under my care, at the Montreal General Hospital, of black small-pox, after an illness of a few days. In his lungs (externally coal-black) there were round and linear patches ranging in size from a pea to a hazel-nut, of an intensely black color, airless and firm, and surrounded by a crepitant tissue, slate gray in color. In the centre of each of these areas was a small bronchus. Many of them were situated just beneath the pleura, and formed typical examples of limited fibroid broncho-pneumonia. In addition there is usually thickening of the alveolar walls, particularly in certain areas. By the gradual coalescence of these fibroid patches large portions of the lung may be converted into firm areas of cirrhosis, grayish black in the case of the coal-miner, steel gray in the case of the stone-worker. In the case of a Cornish miner, aged sixty-three, who died under my care, one of these fibroid areas measured 18 by 6 cm. and 4.5 cm. in depth.

A second important factor in these cases is chronic bronchitis, which is present in a large proportion and really causes the chief symptoms. A third is the occurrence of emphysema, which is almost invariably associated with long-standing cases of pneumonokoniosis. With the changes so far described, unless the cirrhotic area is unusually extensive, the case may present the features of chronic bronchitis with emphysema, but finally another element comes into play. In the fibroid areas softening occurs, probably a process of necrosis similar to that by which softening is produced in fibro-myomata of the uterus. At first these are small and contain a dark liquid. Charcot calls them *ulcères du poumon.* They rarely attain a large size unless a communication is formed with the bronchus, in which case they may become converted into suppurating cavities.

Anthracosis and Tuberculosis.—In the Pennsylvania anthracite district tuberculosis is relatively less common among the miners, the figures for ten years at Scranton for male adults being 3.37 per cent. in mine workers, 9.97 per cent. in those of other occupations (Wainwright). Goldman in Germany, Oliver and Trotter in England, all agree upon the comparative rarity of tuberculosis among coal miners. Though this may be attributed in part to the improved ventilation of the mines, it has also probably something to do with the less favorable soil offered to the bacilli in a lung infiltrated with coal dust.

The *siderosis* induced by the oxide of iron causes an interstitial pneumonia similar to anthracosis. Workers in brass and in bronze are liable to a like affection.

Chalicosis and *silicosis,* due to the deposit of particles of silex and alumina, are found in the makers of mill-stones, particularly the French mill-stones, and also in knife and axe grinders and stone-cutters. It prevails extensively among the Rand miners of South Africa (gold-miners' phthisis), and in the workers of the Australian and Tasmanian mines. Anatomically, this form is characterized by the production of nodules of various sizes, which are cut with the greatest difficulty and sometimes present a curious grayish, even glittering, crystalloid appearance.

Workers in flax and in cotton, and grain-shovellers are also subject to these chronic interstitial changes in the lungs.

Symptoms.—The symptoms do not come on until the patient has worked for a variable number of years in the dusty atmosphere. As a rule there are cough and failing health for a prolonged period of time before complete disability. The coincident emphysema is responsible in great part for the shortness of breath and wheezy condition of these patients. The expectoration is usually muco-purulent, often profuse, and in anthracosis very dark in color—

the so-called "black spit," while in chalicosis there may be seen under the microscope the bright angular particles of silica.

Even when there are physical signs of cavity, tubercle bacilli are not necessarily, and indeed in my experience are not usually present. It is remarkable for how long a time a coal-miner may continue to bring up sputum laden with coal particles even when there are signs only of a chronic bronchitis. Many of the particles are contained in the cells of the alveolar epithelium. In these instances it appears that an attempt is made by the leucocytes to rid the lungs of some of the carbon grains.

Diagnosis.—The diagnosis of the condition is rarely difficult; the expectoration is usually characteristic. It must always be borne in mind that chronic bronchitis and emphysema form essential parts of the process and that in late stages there may be tuberculous infection.

Prophylaxis.—Much has been done to reduce the prevalence of the disease in England by proper ventilation of works and the protection of the men. The conversion of dry into wet mining prevents the distribution of the injurious dust.

Treatment.—The treatment of the condition is practically that of chronic bronchitis and emphysema.

IV. EMPHYSEMA

Definition.—The condition in which the infundibular passages and the alveoli are dilated and the alveolar walls atrophied.

Floyer of Litchfield first described the anatomical condition and spoke of the disease as "flatulent asthma" (1698), meaning a disorder in which the lungs were blown up with air.

A practical division may be made into compensatory, hypertrophic, and atrophic forms, the acute vesicular emphysema, and the interstitial forms. The last two do not in reality come under the above definition, but for convenience they may be considered here.

1. COMPENSATORY EMPHYSEMA

Whenever a region of the lung does not expand fully in inspiration, either another portion of the lung must expand or the chest wall sink in order to occupy the space. The former almost invariably occurs. We have already mentioned that in broncho-pneumonia there is a vicarious distention of the air-vesicles in the adjacent healthy lobules, and the same happens in the neighborhood of tuberculous areas and cicatrices. In general pleural adhesions there is often compensatory emphysema, particularly at the anterior margins of the lung. The most advanced example of this form is seen in cirrhosis, when the unaffected lung increases greatly in size, owing to distention of the air-vesicles. A similar though less marked condition is seen in extensive pleurisy with effusion and in pneumothorax.

At first, this distention of the air-vesicles is a simple physiological process and the alveolar walls are stretched but not atrophied. Ultimately, however, in many cases they waste and the contiguous air-cells fuse, producing true emphysema.

2. HYPERTROPHIC EMPHYSEMA

The large-lunged emphysema of Jenner, also known as substantive or idiopathic emphysema, is a well-marked clinical affection, characterized by enlargement of the lungs, due to distention of the air-cells and atrophy of their walls, and clinically by imperfect aëration of the blood and more or less marked dyspnœa.

Etiology.—Emphysema is the result of persistently high intra-alveolar tension acting upon a congenitally weak lung tissue. Strongly in favor of the view that the nutritive change in the air-cells is the primary factor are the markedly hereditary character of the disease and the frequency with which it starts early in life. To James Jackson, Jr., of Boston, we owe the first observations on the hereditary character of emphysema. Working under Louis' direction, he found that in 18 out of 28 cases one or both parents were affected.

In childhood it may follow recurring asthmatic attacks due to adenoid vegetations. It may occur, too, in several members of the same family. We are still ignorant as to the nature of this congenital pulmonary weakness. Cohnheim thinks it probably due to a defect in the development of the elastic-tissue fibres—a statement which is borne out by Eppinger's observations.

Heightened pressure within the air-cells may be due to forcible inspiration or expiration. Much discussion has taken place as to the part played by these two acts in the production of the disease. The inspiratory theory was advanced by Laennec and subsequently modified by Gairdner, who held that in chronic bronchitis areas of collapse were induced, and compensatory distention took place in the adjacent lobules. This unquestionably does occur in the vicarious or compensatory emphysema, but it probably is not a factor of much moment in the form now under consideration. The expiratory theory, which was supported by Mendelssohn and Jenner, accounts for the condition in a much more satisfactory way. In all straining efforts and violent attacks of coughing the glottis is closed and the chest walls are strongly compressed by muscular efforts, so that the strain is thrown upon those parts of the lung least protected, as the apices and the anterior margins, in which we always find the emphysema most advanced. The sternum and costal cartilages gradually yield to the heightened intrathoracic pressure and are, in advanced cases, pushed forward, giving the characteristic rotundity to the thorax.

FREUND'S THEORY.—A primary disease of the costal cartilages—a chronic hyperplasia with premature ossification is believed to bring about gradually a state of rigid dilatation of the chest, to which the emphysema is secondary. Recent observations make it probable that there is a group of cases in which such changes occur in young persons, particularly in the cartilages of the first three ribs. Niemeyer says that he had met with a few such cases, and there have been reported recently instances in which the cartilages increased in size and stood out prominently. For such a condition what is now called Freund's operation (of resection) would be indicated.

Of other etiological factors occupation is the most important. The disease is met with in players on wind instruments, in glass-blowers, and in occupations necessitating heavy lifting or straining. Whooping-cough and bronchitis play an important rôle, not so much in the changes which they induce in the bronchi as in consequence of the prolonged attacks of coughing.

Morbid Anatomy.—The thorax is capacious, usually barrel-shaped, and the cartilages are calcified. On removal of the sternum, the anterior mediastinum is found completely occupied by the margins of the lungs, and the pericardial sac may not be visible. The organs are very large and have lost their elasticity, so that they do not collapse either in the thorax or when placed on the table. The pleura is pale and there is often an absence of pigment, sometimes in patches, termed by Virchow *albinism* of the lung. To the touch they have a peculiar, downy, feathery feel, and pit readily on pressure. This is one of the most marked features. Beneath the pleura greatly enlarged air-vesicles may be readily seen. They vary in size from .5 to 3 mm., and irregular bullæ, the size of a walnut or larger, may project from the free margins. The best idea of the extreme rarefaction of the tissue is obtained from sections of a lung distended and dried. At the anterior margins the structure may form an irregular series of air-chambers, resembling the frog's lung. On careful inspection with the hand-lens, remnants of the interlobular septa or even of the alveoli may be seen on these large emphysematous vesicles. Though general, the distention is more marked, as a rule, at the anterior margins, and is often specially marked at the inner surface of the lobe near the root, where in extreme cases air-spaces as large as a hen's egg may sometimes be found. Microscopically there is seen atrophy of the alveolar walls, by which is produced a coalescence of neighboring air-cells. In this process the capillary network disappears before the walls are completely atrophied. The loss of the elastic tissue is a special feature. It is stated, indeed, that in certain cases there is a congenital defect in the development of this tissue. The epithelium of the air-cells undergoes a fatty change, but the large distended air-spaces retain a pavement layer.

The bronchi show important changes. In the larger tubes the mucous membrane may be rough and thickened from chronic bronchitis; often the longitudinal lines of submucous elastic tissue stand out prominently. In the advanced cases many of the smaller tubes are dilated, particularly when, in addition to emphysema, there are peri-bronchial fibroid changes. Bronchiectasis is not, however, an invariable accompaniment of emphysema, but, as Laennec remarks, it is difficult to understand why it is not more common. Of associated morbid changes the most important are found in the heart. The right chambers are dilated and hypertrophied, the tricuspid orifice is large, and the valve segments are often thickened at the edges. In advanced cases the cardiac hypertrophy is general. The pulmonary artery and its branches may be wide and show marked atheromatous changes.

The changes in the other organs are those commonly associated with prolonged venous congestion. Pneumothorax may follow the rupture of an emphysematous bleb.

Symptoms.—The disease may be tolerably advanced before any special symptoms occur. A child, for instance, may be somewhat short of breath on going up-stairs or may be unable to run and play as other children without great discomfort; or, perhaps, has attacks of slight lividity. Doubtless much depends upon the completeness of cardiac compensation. When this is perfect, there may be no special interruption of the pulmonary circulation and, except with violent exertion, there is no interference with the aëration of the blood. In well-marked cases the following are the most important symptoms: *Dyspnœa,* which may be felt only on slight exertion, or may be persistent, and aggravated by intercurrent attacks of bronchitis. The respirations are often harsh and wheezy, and expiration is distinctly prolonged.

Cyanosis of an extreme grade is more common in emphysema than in other affections with the exception of congenital heart-disease. So far as I know it is the only disease in which a patient may be able to go about and even to walk into the hospital or consulting-room with a lividity of startling intensity. The contrast between the extreme cyanosis and the comparative comfort of the patient is very striking. In other affections of the heart and lungs associated with a similar degree of cyanosis the patient is invariably in bed and usually in a state of orthopnœa. One condition must be here referred to, viz., the extraordinary cyanosis in cases of poisoning by aniline products, which is in most part due to the conversion of the hæmoglobin into methæmoglobin.

Bronchitis with associated cough is a frequent symptom and often the direct cause of the pulmonary distress. The contrast between emphysematous patients in the winter and summer is marked in this respect. In the latter they may be comfortable and able to attend to their work, but with the cold and changeable weather they are laid up with attacks of bronchitis. Finally, in fact, the two conditions become inseparable and the patient has persistently more or less cough. The acute bronchitis may produce attacks not unlike asthma. In some instances this is true spasmodic asthma, with which emphysema is frequently associated.

As age advances, and with successive attacks of bronchitis, the condition grows slowly worse. In hospital practice it is common to admit patients over sixty with well marked signs of advanced emphysema. The affection can generally be told at a glance—the rounded shoulders, barrel chest, the thin yet oftentimes muscular form, and sometimes, I think, a very characteristic facial expression.

There is another group of younger patients from twenty-five to forty years of age who, winter after winter, have attacks of intense cyanosis in consequence of an aggravated bronchial catarrh. On inquiry we find that these patients have been short-breathed from infancy, and they belong to a category in which there has been a primary defect of structure in the lung tissue.

Physical Signs.—*Inspection.*—The thorax is markedly altered in shape; the antero-posterior diameter is increased and may be even greater than the lateral, so that the chest is barrel-shaped. The appearance is somewhat as if the chest was in a permanent inspiratory position. The sternum and costal cartilages are prominent. The lower zone of the thorax looks large and the intercostal spaces are much widened, particularly in the hypochondriac regions. The sternal fossa is deep, the clavicles stand out with great prominence, and the neck looks shortened from the elevation of the thorax and the sternum. A zone of dilated venules may be seen along the line of attachment of the diaphragm. Though this is common in emphysema, it is by no means peculiar to it or indeed to any special affection.

The curve of the spine is increased and the back is remarkably rounded, so that the scapulæ seem to be almost horizontal. Mensuration shows the rounded form of the chest and the very slight expansion on deep inspiration. The respiratory movements, which may look energetic and forcible, exercise little or no influence. The chest does not expand, but there is a general elevation. The inspiratory effort is short and quick; the expiratory movement is prolonged. There may be retraction instead of distention in the upper abdominal region during inspiration, and there is sometimes seen a transverse curve crossing the abdomen at the level of the twelfth rib. The apex beat of the heart is not visible, and there is usually marked pulsation in the epigastric region. The cervical veins stand out prominently and may pulsate.

Palpation.—The vocal fremitus is somewhat enfeebled but not lost. The apex beat can rarely be felt. There is a marked shock in the lower sternal region and very distinct pulsation in the epigastrium. *Percussion* gives greatly increased resonance, full and drum-like—what is sometimes called hyperresonance. The note is not often distinctly tympanitic in quality. The percussion note is greatly extended, the heart dulness may be obliterated, the upper limit of liver dulness is greatly lowered, and the resonance may extend to the costal margin. Behind, a clear percussion note extends to a much lower level than normal. The level of splenic dulness, too, may be lowered.

On *auscultation* the breath-sounds are usually enfeebled and may be masked by bronchitic râles. The most characteristic feature is the prolongation of the expiration, and the normal ratio may be reversed—4 to 1 instead of 1 to 4. It is often wheezy and harsh and associated with coarse râles and sibilant rhonchi. It is said that in interstitial emphysema there may be a friction sound heard, not unlike that of pleurisy. The heart-sounds are usually feeble but clear; in advanced cases, when there is marked cyanosis, a tricuspid regurgitant murmur may be heard. Accentuation of the pulmonary second sound may be present.

Course.—The course of the disease is slow but progressive, the recurring attacks of bronchitis aggravating the condition. Death may occur from intercurrent pneumonia, either lobar or lobular, and dropsy may supervene from cardiac failure. Occasionally death results from overdistention of the heart, with extreme cyanosis. Duckworth has called attention to the occasional occurrence of fatal hæmorrhage in emphysema. In an old emphysematous patient at the Montreal General Hospital death followed the erosion of a main branch of the pulmonary artery by an ulcer near the bifurcation of the trachea.

Treatment.—Practically, the measures mentioned in connection with bronchitis should be employed. In children with asthma and emphysema the nose should be carefully examined. No remedy is known which has any influence over the progress of the condition itself. Bronchitis is the great danger of these patients, and therefore when possible they should live in an equable climate. They do well in southern California and in Egypt. In consequence of the venous engorgement they are liable to gastric and intestinal disturbance, and it is particularly important to keep the bowels regulated and to avoid flatulency, which often seriously aggravates the dyspnœa. Patients who come into the hospital in a state of urgent dyspnœa and lividity, with great engorgement of the veins, particularly if they are young and vigorous, should be bled freely. Inhalation of oxygen may be used. Strychnine will be found specially useful, and breathing exercises are sometimes helpful. Breathing of compressed air in a pneumatic cabinet gives temporary relief. Resection of the first costal cartilage or of the first three cartilages on either side has been practiced (Freund's operation). It is not likely to be of any benefit in the aged in whom the condition is established, but in a special group in the young in which the primary trouble appears to be in the cartilages—what has been called *Freund's Disease*—the operation may be practiced and good results have followed.

3. ATROPHIC EMPHYSEMA

A senile change, called by Sir William Jenner small-lunged emphysema, is really a primary atrophy of the lung, coming on in advanced life, and scarcely constitutes a special affection. It occurs in "withered-looking old persons" who may perhaps have had a winter cough and shortness of breath for years. In striking contrast to the essential hypertrophic emphysema, the chest is small and the ribs obliquely placed. The thoracic muscles are usually atrophied. The lung presents a remarkable appearance, being converted into a series of large vesicles, on the walls of which the remnants of air-cells may be seen.

4. ACUTE VESICULAR EMPHYSEMA

When death occurs from bronchitis of the smaller tubes, when strong inspiratory efforts have been made, the lungs are large in volume and the air-cells are much distended. Clinically, this condition may occur rapidly in cases of cardiac asthma and angina pectoris. The area of pulmonary resonance is much increased, and on auscultation there are heard everywhere piping râles and prolonged expiration. A similar condition may follow pressure on the vagi.

5. INTERSTITIAL EMPHYSEMA

Beads of air are seen in the interlobular and subpleural tissue, sometimes forming large bullæ beneath the pleura. A rare event is rupture close to the root of the lung, and the passage of air along the trachea into the subcutaneous tissues of the neck. After tracheotomy just the reverse may occur and the air may pass from the tracheotomy wound along the windpipe and bronchi and appear beneath the surface of the pleura. From this interstitial emphysema spontaneous pneumothorax may arise in healthy persons.

V. GANGRENE OF THE LUNG

Etiology.—Gangrene of the lung is not an affection *per se*, but occurs in a variety of conditions when necrotic areas undergo putrefaction. It is not easy to say why sphacelus should occur in one case and not in another, as the germs of putrefaction are always in the air-passages, and yet necrotic territories rarely become gangrenous. Total obstruction of a pulmonary artery, as a rule, causes infarction, and the area shut off does not often, though it may, sphacelate. Another factor would seem to be necessary—probably a lowered tissue resistance, the result of general or local causes. It is met with (1) as a sequence of lobar pneumonia. This rarely occurs in a previously healthy person—more commonly in the debilitated or in the diabetic subject. (2) Gangrene is very prone to follow the aspiration pneumonia, since the foreign particles rapidly undergo putrefactive changes. Of a similar nature are the cases of gangrene due to perforation of cancer of the œsophagus into the lung or into the bronchus. (3) The putrid contents of a bronchiectatic, more commonly of a tuberculous, cavity may excite gangrene in the neighboring tissues. The pressure bronchiectasis following aneurism or tumor may lead to extensive sloughing. (4) Gangrene may follow simple embolism of the pulmonary artery. More commonly, however, the embolus is derived from a part which is mortified or comes from a focus of bone disease. In typhus and in typhoid fever gangrene of the lung may follow thrombosis of one of the larger branches of the pulmonary artery. A case occurred in my wards in October, 1897, in connection with a typhoid septicæmia. Typhoid bacilli were isolated from the lung. Lastly, gangrene of the lung may occur in conditions of debility during convalescence from protracted fever—occasionally, indeed, without our being able to assign any reasonable cause.

Morbid Anatomy.—Laennec, who first accurately described pulmonary gangrene, recognized a diffuse and a circumscribed form. The former, though rare, is sometimes seen in connection with pneumonia, more rarely after obliteration of a large branch of the pulmonary artery. It may involve the greater part of a lobe, and the lung tissue is converted into a horribly offensive greenish-black mass, torn and ragged in the centre. In the circumscribed form there is well-marked limitation between the gangrenous area and the surrounding tissue. The focus may be single or there may be two or more. The lower lobe is more commonly affected than the upper, and the peripheral more than the central portion of the lung. A gangrenous area is at first uniformly greenish brown in color; but softening rapidly takes place with the formation of a cavity with shreddy, irregular walls and a greenish, offensive fluid. The lung tissue in the immediate neighborhood shows a zone of deep congestion, often consolidation, and outside this an intense œdema. In the embolic cases the plugged artery can sometimes be found. When rapidly extending, vessels may be opened and a copious hæmorrhage ensue. Perforation of the pleura is not uncommon. The irritating decomposing material usually excites the most intense bronchitis. Embolic processes are not infrequent. There is a remarkable association in some cases between circumscribed gangrene of the lung and abscess of the brain. It has been referred to under the section on bronchiectasis.

Symptoms and Course.—Usually definite symptoms of local pulmonary disease precede the characteristic features of gangrene. These, of course, are very varied, depending on the nature of the trouble. The sputum is very characteristic. It is intensely fetid—usually profuse—and, if expectorated into a conical glass, separates into three layers—a greenish brown, heavy sediment; an intervening thin liquid, which sometimes has a greenish or a brownish tint; and, on top, a thick, frothy layer. Spread on a glass plate, the shreddy *débris* of lung tissue can readily be picked out. Even large fragments of lung may be coughed up. Robertson, of Onancock, Va., sent me one several centimetres in length, which had been expectorated by a lad of eighteen, who had severe gangrene and recovered. Microscopically, elastic fibres are found in abundance, with granular matter, pigment grains, fatty crystals, bacteria, and leptothrix. It is stated that elastic tissue is sometimes absent, but I have never met with such an instance. The peculiar plugs of sputum which occur in bronchiectasis are not found. Blood is often present, and, as a rule, is much altered. The sputum has, in a majority of the cases, an intensely fetid odor, which is communicated to the breath and may permeate the entire room. It is much more offensive than in fetid bronchitis or in abscess of the lung. The fetor is particularly marked when there is free communication between the gangrenous cavities and the bronchi. On several occasions I have found, post mortem, localized gangrene, which had been unsuspected during life, and in which there had been no fetor of the breath.

The physical signs, when extensive destruction has occurred, are those of cavity, but the limited circumscribed areas may be difficult to detect. Bronchitis is always present. The X-ray examination may aid in diagnosis.

Among the general symptoms may be mentioned fever, usually of moderate grade; the pulse is rapid, and very often the constitutional depression is severe. But the only special features indicative of gangrene are the sputum and the fetor of the breath. The patient generally sinks from exhaustion. Fatal hæmorrhage may ensue.

Treatment.—The treatment of gangrene is very unsatisfactory. The indications, of course, are to disinfect the gangrenous area, but this is often impossible. An antiseptic spray of carbolic acid may be employed. A good plan is for the patient to use over the mouth and nose an inhaler, which may be charged with a solution of carbolic acid or with guaiacol; the latter drug has also been used hypodermically, with, it is said, happy results in removing the odor. If the signs of cavity are distinct an attempt should be made to cleanse it by direct injections of an antiseptic solution. If the patient's condition is good and the gangrenous region can be localized, surgical interference may be indicated. Successful cases have been reported. The general condition of the patient is always such as to demand the greatest care in the matter of diet and nursing.

VI. ABSCESS OF THE LUNG

Etiology.—Suppuration occurs in the lung under the following conditions: (1) As a sequence of inflammation, either lobar or lobular. Apart from the purulent infiltration this is unquestionably rare, and even in lobar pneumonia the abscesses are of small size and usually involve, as Addison remarked, several points at the same time. On the other hand, abscess formation is extremely frequent in the deglutition and aspiration forms of lobular pneumonia. After wounds of the neck or operations upon the throat, in suppurative disease of the nose or larynx, occasionally even of the ear (Volkmann), infective particles reach the bronchial tubes by aspiration and excite an intense inflammation which often ends in abscess. Cancer of the œsophagus, perforating the root of the lung or into the bronchi, may produce extensive suppuration. The abscesses vary in size from a walnut to an orange, and have ragged and irregular walls, and purulent, sometimes necrotic, contents.

(2) Embolic, so-called metastatic, abscesses, the result of infective emboli, are extremely common in pyæmia. They may be numerous and present very

definite characters. As a rule they are superficial, beneath the pleura, and often wedge-shaped. At first firm, grayish red in color, and surrounded by a zone of intense hyperæmia, suppuration soon follows with the formation of a definite abscess. The pleura is usually covered with greenish lymph, and perforation sometimes takes place with the production of pneumothorax.

(3) Perforation of the lung from without, lodgment of foreign bodies, and, in the right lung, perforation from abscess of the liver or a suppurating echinococcus cyst are occasionally causes of pulmonary abscess.

(4) Suppurative processes play an important part in chronic pulmonary tuberculosis, many of the symptoms of which are due to them.

Symptoms.—Abscess following pneumonia is easily recognized by an aggravation of the general symptoms and by the physical signs of cavity and the characters of the expectoration. Embolic abscesses can not often be recognized, and the local symptoms are generally masked in the general pyæmic manifestations. The character of the sputum is of great importance in determining the presence of abscess. The odor is offensive, yet it rarely has the horrible fetor of gangrene or of putrid bronchitis. In the pus fragments of lung tissue can be seen, and the elastic tissue may be very abundant. The presence of this with the physical signs rarely leaves any question as to the nature of the trouble. Embolic cases usually run a fatal course. Recovery occasionally occurs after pneumonia. In a case following typhoid fever which I saw at the Garfield Hospital Kerr removed two ribs and found free in the pus of a localized empyema a sequestered piece of lung, the size of the palm of the hand, which had sloughed off from the lower lobe. The patient made a good recovery.

Medicinal treatment is of little avail in abscess of the lung. When well defined and superficial, an attempt should always be made to open and drain it. A number of successful cases have already been treated in this way.

VII. NEW GROWTHS IN THE LUNGS

Etiology and Morbid Anatomy.—While primary tumors are rare, secondary growths are not uncommon. Carcinoma is the most common primary form. Endothelium and sarcoma are less frequently met with.

Varieties.—The following groups may be recognized:

(*a*) Acute galloping pleuro-pneumonic form, with a very rapid course —dyspnœa, cough, asphyxia, rapid emaciation and death in from six to twelve weeks. Most of these cases are secondary, sometimes to unrecognized disease elsewhere, but there are instances of the primary disease of this type. It is a remarkable fact that cobalt miners of Schneeberg are very liable to a primary carcinoma of the lung which may run this acute course.

(*b*) Chronic pleuro-pulmonary carcinoma, of which there are several types:

(1) *Broncho-pulmonary Form.*—This, the most typical variety, begins with bronchial symptoms, bloody sputum, loss of weight and strength, and anæmia. The physical signs may be suggestive of tuberculosis, but the earliest indications are usually at the root of the lung. Later there may be cavity formation, with a bronchiectatic type of sputum. Tubercle bacilli are absent

and there may be very large round cells with many fatty granules, representing degenerate cancer cells. The X-ray picture is not distinctive and the cases are usually taken for tuberculosis.

(2) *Mediastinal Type.*—Quite early in this form the glands become involved, increase rapidly, compress the adjoining structures and the type of the disease is that of a mediastinal tumor with its dominant pressure symptoms.

(3) *Pleuritic Type.*—The earliest and dominant symptoms are at the back with pleuritic pain, cough, friction, progressive effusion, and shortness of breath. On tapping, the effusion is usually bloody, though I have known it at first to be clear. In other instances the pleura is early involved with rapid extension, but no effusion. There may be little or no cough, and very slight dyspnœa, with progressive weakness, emaciation, and anæmia as the chief features. Subcutaneous nodules may occur along the ribs, with involvement of both cervical and axillary glands.

From the standpoint of treatment not much is to be expected. The new surgical technique has made the thoracic cavity accessible, and it is quite possible that early explorations may become common in doubtful cases. In a few instances carcinoma of the lung has been operated upon; in Lenhartz' case the patient remained well for a year, and died two and a half years after operation.

E. DISEASES OF THE PLEURA

I. ACUTE PLEURISY

Anatomically, the cases may be divided into dry or adhesive pleurisy and pleurisy with effusion. Another classification is into primary or secondary forms. According to the course of the disease, a division may be made into *acute* and *chronic pleurisy,* and as it is impossible, at present, to group the various forms etiologically, this is perhaps the most satisfactory division. The following forms of acute pleurisy may be considered:

1. FIBRINOUS OR PLASTIC PLEURISY

In this the pleural membrane is covered by a sheeting of lymph of variable thickness, which gives it a turbid, granular appearance, or the fibrin may exist in distinct layers. It occurs (1) as an independent affection, following cold or exposure. This form of acute plastic pleurisy without fluid exudate is not common in perfectly healthy individuals. Cases are met with, however, in which the disease sets in with the usual symptoms of pain in the side and slight fever, and there are the physical signs of pleurisy as indicated by the friction. After persisting for a few days, the friction murmur disappears and no exudation occurs. Union takes place between the membranes, and possibly the pleuritic adhesions which are found in such a large percentage of all bodies examined after death originate in these slight fibrinous pleurisies.

Fibrinous pleurisy occurs (2) as a secondary process in acute diseases of the lung, such as pneumonia, which is always accompanied by a certain amount of pleurisy, usually of this form. Cancer, abscess, and gangrene also cause plastic pleurisy when the surface of the lung becomes involved. This condition is specially associated in a large number of cases with tuberculosis. Pleural pain, stitch in the side, and a dry cough, with marked friction sounds on auscultation, are the initial phenomena in many instances of phthisis. The signs are usually basic.

2. SERO-FIBRINOUS PLEURISY

In a majority of cases of inflammation of the pleura there is, with the fibrin, a variable amount of fluid exudate, which produces the condition known as pleurisy with effusion.

Etiology.—Of 194 cases in fifteen years in my wards, there were 161 males and 33 females. Under twenty years of age there were 20 patients; 18 were over sixty years of age. The greatest number was in the fifth decade, 59. Cold acts as a predisposing agent, which permits the action of various micro-organisms. We have not yet, however, brought all the acute pleurisies into the category of microbic affections, and the fact remains that pleurisy does follow with great rapidity a sudden wetting or a chill. A majority of the cases are tuberculous. This view is based upon: (1) Post mortem evidence. Tubercles have been found in acute cases, thought to have been rheumatic or due to cold. (2) The not infrequent presence of tuberculous lesions, often latent, in the lung or elsewhere. (3) The character of the exudate. If coagulated and the coagulum digested and centrifugalized (Inoscopy), tubercle bacilli are frequently found. Injected into a guinea pig, in amounts of 15 c. c. or more, tuberculosis followed in 62 per cent. (Eichhorst). The cyto-diagnosis shows that as in other tuberculous exudates the mono-nuclear leucocytes predominate. (4) The tuberculin reaction is given in a considerable percentage of the cases. (5) The subsequent history. Of 90 cases of acute pleurisy which had been under the observation of H. I. Bowditch between 1849 and 1879, 32 died of or had phthisis. Among 130 patients with primary pleurisy with effusion, followed for a period of seven years by Hedges, 40 per cent. became tuberculous.

Of 300 uncomplicated cases of pleural effusion in the Massachusetts General Hospital, followed by R. C. Cabot, the subsequent history was ascertained in 221; followed five years until death or phthisis, 117; well after five years, 96.

In 172 of the cases of pleurisy with effusion in the Johns Hopkins Hospital Hamman got reports from 88; of these 48 were living and well, 30 later became tuberculous, in 2 the result was questionable, and 8 died of other diseases. Twelve of the 88 had tubercle bacilli in the sputum while in the hospital without discoverable pulmonary lesion; 3 of the 12 were living and well; in 8 the signs became well marked; one died of unknown cause. Hamman has collected 562 cases (including the above) in which the subsequent history was sought; of these 167, 29.7 per cent. became tuberculous.

Bacteriology of Acute Pleurisy.—From a bacteriological standpoint we may recognize three groups of cases, caused by the tubercle bacillus, the pneumococcus, and the streptococcus, respectively.

Bacillus tuberculosis is present in a very large proportion of all cases of primary or so-called idiopathic pleurisy. The exudate is usually sterile on cover slips or in the culture and inoculation tests made in the ordinary way, as the bacilli are very scanty. It has been demonstrated clearly that a large amount of the exudate must be taken to make the test complete, either in cultures or in the inoculation of animals. Eichhorst found that more than 62 per cent. were demonstrated as tuberculous when as much as 15 c. c. of the exudate was inoculated into test animals, while less than 10 per cent. of the cases showed tuberculosis when only 1 c. c. of the exudate was used. This is a point to which observers should pay very special attention. Le Damany has demonstrated the tuberculous character of all but 4 in 55 primary pleurisies. He used large quantities of the fluid for his inoculation experiments.

The pneumococcus pleurisy is almost always secondary to a focus of inflammation in the lung. It may, however, be primary. The exudate is usually purulent and the outlook is very favorable.

The streptococcus pleurisy is the typical septic form which may occur either from direct infection of the pleura through the lung in broncho-pneumonia, or in cases of streptococcus pneumonia; in other instances it follows infection of more distant parts. The acute streptococcus pleurisy is the most serious and fatal of all forms.

Among other bacteria which have been found are the staphylococcus, Friedländer's bacillus, the typhoid bacillus, and the diphtheria bacillus.

Morbid Anatomy.—In sero-fibrinous pleurisy the serous exudate is abundant and the fibrin is found on the pleural surfaces and scattered through the fluid in the form of flocculi. The proportions of these constituents vary a great deal. In some instances there is very little membranous fibrin; in others it forms thick, creamy layers and exists in the dependent part of the fluid as whitish, curd-like masses. The fluid of sero-fibrinous pleurisy is of a lemon color, either clear or slightly turbid, depending on the number of formed elements. In some instances it has a dark brown color. The microscopic examination of the fluid shows leucocytes, occasional swollen cells, which may possibly be derived from the pleural endothelium, shreds of fibrillated fibrin, and a variable number of red blood-corpuscles. A large number of cells undergoing mitotic division is diagnostic of malignant disease. On boiling, the fluid is found to be rich in albumin. Sometimes it coagulates spontaneously. Its composition closely resembles that of blood serum. Cholesterin, uric acid, and sugar are occasionally found. The amount of the effusion varies from ½ to 4 litres. Enormous amounts are sometimes removed, 188 ounces in one case (E. C. Carter). The lung in acute sero-fibrinous pleurisy is more or less compressed. If the exudation is limited the lower lobe alone is atelectatic; but in an extensive effusion which reaches to the clavicle the entire lung will be found lying close to the spine, dark and airless, or even bloodless—*i. e.,* carnified.

In large exudations the adjacent organs are displaced; the liver is depressed and the heart dislocated. With reference to the position of the heart, the following statements may be made: (1) Even in the most extensive left sided exudation there is no rotation of the apex of the heart, which in no case was to the right of the mid-sternal line; (2) the relative position of the apex and base is usually maintained; in some instances the apex is lifted, in others the whole heart lies more transversely; (3) the right chambers of the heart occupy the greater portion of the front, so that the displacement is rather a definite dislocation of the mediastinum, with the pericardium, to the right, than any special twisting of the heart itself; (4) the kink or twist in the inferior vena cava described by Bartels was not present in any of my cases.

Symptoms.—Prodromes are not uncommon, but the disease may set in abruptly with a chill, followed by fever and a severe pain in the side. In very many cases, however, the onset is insidious, particularly in children and in elderly persons. A little dyspnœa on exertion and an increasing pallor may be the only features. Washbourn has called attention to the frequency with which the pneumococcus pleurisy sets in with the features of pneumonia. The pain in the side is the most distressing symptom, and is usually referred to the nipple or axillary regions. It must be remembered, however, that pleuritic pain may be felt in the abdomen or low down in the back, particularly when the diaphragmatic surface of the pleura is involved. It is lancinating, sharp, and severe, and is aggravated by cough. At this early stage, on auscultation, sometimes indeed on palpation, a dry friction rub can be detected. The fever rarely rises so rapidly as in pneumonia, and does not reach the same grade. A temperature of from 102° to 103° F. is an average pyrexia. It may drop to normal at the end of a week or ten days without the appearance of any definite change in the physical signs, or it may persist for several weeks. The temperature of the affected is higher than that of the sound side. Cough is an early symptom in acute pleurisy, but is rarely so distressing or so frequent as in pneumonia. There are instances in which it is absent. The expectoration is usually slight in amount, mucoid in character, and occasionally streaked with blood.

At the outset there may be dyspnœa, due partly to the fever and partly to the pain in the side. Later it results from the compression of the lung, particularly if the exudation has taken place rapidly. In the cases with very rapid effusion the dyspnœa may be very marked. When, however, the fluid is effused slowly, one lung may be entirely compressed without inducing shortness of breath, except on exertion, and the patient will lie quietly in bed without evincing the slightest respiratory distress. When the effusion is large the patient usually prefers to lie upon the affected side.

Physical Signs.—Inspection shows some degree of immobility on the affected side, depending upon the amount of exudation; and in large effusions an increase in volume, which may appear to be much more than it really is as determined by mensuration. The intercostal depressions are obliterated. In the right sided effusions the apex beat may be lifted to the fourth interspace or be pushed beyond the left nipple, or may even be seen in the axilla. When the exudation is on the left side, the heart's impulse may not be visible; but if the effusion is large it is seen in the third and fourth spaces on the right side, and sometimes as far out as the nipple, or even beyond it.

Palpation enables us more successfully to determine the deficient movements on the affected side, and the obliteration of the intercostal spaces, and more accurately to define the position of the heart's impulse. In simple serofibrinous effusion there is rarely any œdema of the chest walls. It is scarcely ever possible to obtain fluctuation. Tactile fremitus is greatly diminished or abolished. If the effusion is slight there may be only enfeeblement. The absence of the voice vibrations in effusions of any size constitutes one of the most valuable of physical signs. In children there may be much effusion with retention of fremitus. In rare cases the vibrations may be communicated to the chest walls through localized pleural adhesions.

Mensuration.—With the cyrtometer, if the effusion is excessive, a difference of from half an inch to an inch, or even, in large effusions, an inch and a half, may be found between the two sides. Allowance must be made for the fact that the right side is naturally larger than the left. With the saddle tape the difference in expansion between the two sides can be conveniently measured.

Percussion.—Early in the disease there may be no alteration in the note, but with the gradual accumulation of the fluid the resonance becomes defective, and finally gives place to absolute flatness. From day to day the gradual increase in height of the fluid may be studied. In a pleuritic effusion rising to the fourth rib in front the percussion signs are usually very suggestive. In the subclavicular region the attention is often aroused at once by a tympanitic note, the so-called Skoda's resonance, which is heard perhaps more commonly in this situation with pleural effusion than in any other condition. It shades insensibly into a flat note in the lower mammary and axillary regions. Skoda's resonance may be obtained also behind, just above the limit of effusion. The dulness has a peculiarly resistant, wooden quality, differing from that of pneumonia and readily recognized by skilled fingers. It has long been known that when the patient is in the erect posture the upper line of dulness is not horizontal, but is higher behind than it is in front, forming a parabola. The curve marking the intersection of the plane of contact of lung and fluid with the chest wall is known as "Ellis's line of flatness," which Garland has verified clinically and by animal experiments. With medium-sized effusions this line begins lowest behind, advances upward and forward in a letter-S curve to the axillary region, whence it proceeds in a straight decline to the sternum. This curve is demonstrable only when the patient is in the erect position. Grocco, in 1902, called attention to the existence in pleural effusion of a triangular area of relative dulness, along the spine, on the side opposite to the pleurisy, in width from 2 to 5 cm., and with the apex upward. It can be demonstrated in a large majority of all cases, particularly in the young and in thin persons. It is possibly due to the bulging of the mediastinum, by the fluid, across the middle line, the anatomical possibility of which has been pointed out by Calvert.

On the right side the dulness passes without change into that of the liver. On the left side in the nipple line it extends to and may obliterate Traube's semilunar space. If the effusion is moderate, the phenomenon of movable dulness may be obtained by marking carefully, in the sitting posture, the upper limit in the mammary region, and then in the recumbent posture, noting the change in the height of dulness. This infallible sign of fluid can not always be obtained. In very copious exudation the dulness may reach the clavicle and even extend beyond the sternal margin of the opposite side.

Auscultation.—Early in the disease a friction rub can usually be heard, which disappears as the fluid accumulates. It is a to-and-fro dry rub, close to the ear, and has a leathery, creaking character. There is another pleural friction sound which closely resembles, and is scarcely to be distinguished from, the fine crackling crêpitus of pneumonia. This may be heard at the commencement of the disease, and also, as pointed out in 1844 by MacDonnell,

Sr., of Montreal, when the effusion has receded and the pleural layers come together again.

With even a slight exudation there is weakened or distant breathing. Often inspiration and expiration are distinctly audible, though distant, and have a tubular quality. Sometimes only a puffing tubular expiration is heard, which may have a metallic or amphoric quality. Loud resonant râles accompanying this may forcibly suggest a cavity. These pseudo-cavernous signs are met with more frequently in children, and often lead to error in diagnosis. Above the line of dulness the breath sounds are usually harsh and exaggerated, and may have a tubular quality.

The vocal resonance is usually diminished or absent. The whispered voice is said to be transmitted through a serous and not through a purulent exudate (Baccelli's sign), but this is not always true. This author advises direct auscultation in the antero-lateral region of the chest. There may, however, be intensification—bronchophony. The voice sometimes has a curious nasal, squeaking character, which was termed by Laennec *ægophony,* from its supposed resemblance to the bleating of a goat. In typical form this is not common, but it is by no means rare to hear a curious twang-like quality in the voice, particularly at the outer angle of the scapula.

In the examination of the heart in cases of pleuritic effusion it is well to bear in mind that when the apex of the heart lies beneath the sternum there may be no impulse. The determination of the situation of the organ may rest with the position of maximum loudness of the sounds. Over the displaced organ a systolic murmur may be heard. When the lappet of lung over the pericardium is involved on either side there may be a pleuro-pericardial friction.

Blood Count in Pleural Effusion.—Emerson has looked over for me the histories of 89 cases of acute pleurisy with effusion in which the blood counts were made before the temperature reached normal. Only 26 had a leucocytosis between 10,000 and 15,000; one only above 15,000. In 12 of the cases the count was below 5,000.

The X-ray pictures are of great interest and of much value in diagnosis. They have shown that the effusion is not always in the lower portion of the chest with the patient in the upright position, but that it may represent a vertical column in the lateral aspect of the chest, compressing the lung toward the spine. The effusion is not always mobile, but may be fixed by adhesions in one position.

Course.—The course of acute sero-fibrinous pleurisy is very variable. After persisting for a week or ten days the fever subsides, the cough and pain disappear, and a slight effusion may be quickly absorbed. In cases in which the effusion reaches as high as the fourth rib recovery is usually slower. Many instances come under observation for the first time, after two or three weeks' indisposition, with the fluid at a level with the clavicle. The fever may last from ten to twenty days without exciting anxiety, though, as a rule, in ordinary pleurisy from cold, as we say, the temperature in cases of moderate severity is normal within eight or ten days. Left to itself, the natural tendency is to resorption; but this may take place very slowly. With the absorption of the fluid there is a redux-friction crepitus, either leathery and creaking or crackling and râle-like, and for months, or even longer, the defective resonance and feeble breathing are heard at the base. Rare modes of termination are perforation and discharge through the lung, and externally through the chest wall, examples of which have been recorded by Sahli.

The immediate prognosis in pleurisy with effusion is good. Of 320 cases at St. Bartholomew's Hospital, only 6.1 per cent. died before leaving the hospital (Hedges).

A sero-fibrinous exudate may persist for months without change, particularly in tuberculous cases, and will sometimes reaccumulate after aspiration and resist all treatment. After persistence for more than twelve months, in spite of repeated tapping, a serous effusion was cured by incision without deformity of the chest (S. West). When one pleura is full and the heart is greatly dislocated, the condition, although in a majority of cases producing remarkably little disturbance, is not without risk.

3. PURULENT PLEURISY

(*Empyema*)

Etiology.—Pus in the pleura is due to (*a*) infection from within, as a rule directly from a patch of pneumonia or a septic focus due to the pneumococcus or the pus organisms, in some cases a tuberculous broncho-pneumonia; (*b*) involvement from without, as in fracture of a rib, penetrating wound, disease of œsophagus, etc.

It frequently follows the infectious diseases, particularly scarlet fever. It is very often latent, and due to undiscovered foci of lobar or lobular pneumonia. It is common in children, more in boys than in girls, and between the ages of one and five and eight and nine.

The pneumococcus is the most common organism, then the ordinary pus organisms and the tubercle bacilli. The pneumococcus has been found and in rare cases the influenza bacillus, and even psorosperms.

Morbid Anatomy.—On opening an empyema post mortem we usually find that the effusion has separated into a clear, greenish yellow serum above and the thick, cream-like pus below. The fluid may be scarcely more than turbid, with flocculi of fibrin through it. In the pneumococcus empyema the pus is usually thick and creamy. It usually has a heavy, sweetish odor, but in some instances—particularly those following wounds—it is fetid. In cases of gangrene of the lung or pleura the pus has a horribly stinking odor. Microscopically it has the characters of ordinary pus. The pleural membranes are greatly thickened, and present a grayish white layer from 1 to 2 mm. in thickness. On the costal pleura there may be erosions, and in old cases fistulous communications are common. The lung may be compressed to a very small limit, and the visceral pleura also may show perforations.

Symptoms.—Purulent pleurisy may begin abruptly, with the symptoms already described. More frequently it comes on insidiously in the course of other diseases or follows an ordinary sero-fibrinous pleurisy. There may be no pain in the chest, very little cough, and no dyspnœa, unless the side is very full. Symptoms of septic infection are rarely wanting. If in a child, there is a gradually developing pallor and weakness; sweats occur, and there is irregular fever. A cough is by no means constant. The leucocytes are usually much increased; in one fatal case they numbered 115,000 per cubic millimetre.

Physical Signs.—Practically they are those already considered in pleurisy with effusion. There are, however, one or two additional points to be mentioned. In empyema, particularly in children, the disproportion between the sides may be extreme. The intercostal spaces may not only be obliterated, but may bulge. Not infrequently there is œdema of the chest walls. The network of subcutaneous veins may be very distinct. It must not be forgotten that in children the breath-sounds may be *loud and tubular* over a purulent effusion of considerable size. The dislocation of the heart and the displacement of the liver are more marked in empyema than in sero-fibrinous effusion—probably, as Senator suggests, owing to the greater weight of the fluid.

A curious phenomenon associated generally with empyema, but sometimes occurring in the sero-fibrinous exudate, is *pulsating pleurisy,* first described by MacDonnell, Sr., of Montreal. In 95 cases collected by Sailer it was much more frequent in males than in females. In 38 there was a tumor; that is, empyema necessitatis. In all but one case the fluid was purulent. Pneumothorax may be present. There are two groups of cases, the intrapleural pulsating pleurisy and the pulsating *empyema necessitatis,* in which there is an external pulsating tumor. No satisfactory explanation has been offered how the heart impulse is thus forcibly communicated through the effusion.

Empyema is a chronic affection, which in a few instances terminates naturally in recovery, but a majority of cases, if left alone, ends in death. The following are some modes of natural cure: (*a*) By absorption of the fluid. In small effusions this may take place gradually. The chest wall sinks. The pleural layers become greatly thickened and enclose between them the inspissated pus, in which lime salts are gradually deposited. Such a condition may be seen once or twice a year in the post mortem room of any large hospital. (*b*) By perforation of the lung. Although in this event death may take place rapidly, by suffocation, as Aretæus says, yet in cases in which it occurs gradually recovery may follow. Since 1873, when I saw a case of this kind in Traube's clinic, and heard his remarks on the subject, I have seen a number of instances of the kind and can corroborate his statement as to the favorable termination of many of them. Empyema may discharge either by opening into the bronchus and forming a fistula, or, as Traube pointed out, by producing necrosis of the pulmonary pleura, sufficient to allow the soaking of the pus through the spongy lung tissue into the bronchi. In the first way pneumothorax usually, though not always, develops. In the second way the pus is discharged, without formation of pneumothorax. Even with a bronchial fistula recovery is possible. (*c*) By perforation of the chest wall—*empyema necessitatis.* This is by no means an unfavorable method, as many cases recover. The perforation may occur anywhere in the chest wall, but is, as Cruveilhier remarked, more common in front. It may be anywhere from the third to the sixth interspace, usually, according to Marshall, in the fifth. It may perforate in more than one place, and there may be a fistulous communication which opens into the pleura at some distance from the external orifice. The tumor, when near the heart, may pulsate. The discharge may persist for years. In Copeland's Dictionary is mentioned an instance of a

Bavarian physician who had a pleural fistula for thirteen years and enjoyed fairly good health.

An empyema may perforate the neighboring organs, the œsophagus, peritoneum, pericardium, or the stomach. A remarkable sequel is a pleuro-œsophageal fistula, of which cases have been reported by Voelcker, Thursfield, and myself. In my case there was a fistulous communication through the chest wall. Very remarkable cases are those which pass down the spine and along the psoas into the iliac fossa, and simulate a psoas or lumbar abscess.

4. TUBERCULOUS PLEURISY

This has already been considered (p. 178), and the symptoms and physical signs do not require any description other than that already given in connection with the sero-fibrinous and purulent forms.

5. OTHER VARIETIES OF PLEURISY

Hæmorrhagic Pleurisy.—A bloody effusion is met with under the following conditions: (*a*) In the pleurisy of asthenic states, such as cancer, Bright's disease, and occasionally in the malignant fevers. It is interesting to note the frequency with which hæmorrhagic pleurisy is found in cirrhosis of the liver. It occurred in the very patient in whom Laennec first accurately described this disease. While this may be a simple hæmorrhagic pleurisy, in a majority of the cases which I have seen it has been tuberculous. (*b*) Tuberculous pleurisy, in which the bloody effusion may result from the rupture of newly formed vessels in the soft exudate accompanying the eruption of miliary tubercles, or it may come from more slowly formed tubercles in a pleurisy secondary to extensive pulmonary disease. (*c*) Cancerous pleurisy, whether primary or secondary, is frequently hæmorrhagic. (*d*) Occasionally hæmorrhagic exudation is met with in perfectly healthy individuals, in whom there is not the slightest suspicion of tuberculosis or cancer. In one such case, a large, able-bodied man, the patient was to my knowledge healthy and strong eight years afterward. And, lastly, it must be remembered that during aspiration the lung may be wounded and blood in this way get mixed with the sero-fibrinous exudate. The condition of hæmorrhagic pleurisy is to be distinguished from hæmothorax, due to the rupture of aneurism or the pressure of a tumor on the thoracic veins.

Diaphragmatic Pleurisy.—The inflammation may be limited partly or chiefly to the diaphragmatic surface. This is often a dry pleurisy, but there may be effusion, either sero-fibrinous or purulent, which is circumscribed on the diaphragmatic surface. In these cases the pain is low in the zone of the diaphragm and may simulate that of acute abdominal disease. It may be intensified by pressure at the point of insertion of the diaphragm at the tenth rib. The diaphragm is fixed and the respiration is thoracic and short. Andral noted in certain cases severe dyspnœa and attacks simulating angina. As mentioned, the effusion is usually plastic, not serous. Serous or purulent effusions of any size limited to the diaphragmatic surface are extremely rare. Intense subjective with trifling objective features are always suggestive of diaphragmatic pleurisy.

Encysted Pleurisy.—The effusion may be circumscribed by adhesions or separated into two or more pockets or loculi, which communicate with each other. This is most common in empyema. In these cases there have usually been, at different parts of the pleura, multiple adhesions by which the fluid is limited. In other instances the recent false membranes may encapsulate the exudation on the diaphragmatic surface, for example, or the part of the pleura posterior to the mid-axillary line. The condition may be very puzzling during life, and present special difficulties in diagnosis. In some cases the tactile fremitus is retained along certain lines of adhesion. The exploratory needle should be freely used.

Interlobar pleurisy forms an interesting and not uncommon variety. In nearly every instance of acute pleurisy the interlobar serous surfaces are also involved and closely agglutinated together, and sometimes the fluid is encysted between them. In this position tubercles are to be carefully looked for. In a case of this kind following pneumonia there was between the lower and upper and middle lobes of the right side an enormous purulent collection, which looked at first like a large abscess of the lung. These collections may perforate the bronchi, and the cases present special difficulties in diagnosis.

Diagnosis of Pleurisy

Acute plastic pleurisy is readily recognized. In the diagnosis of pleuritic effusion the first question is, Does a fluid exudate exist? the second, What is its nature? In large effusions the increase in the size of the affected side, the immobility, the absence of tactile fremitus, together with the displacement of organs, give infallible indications of the presence of fluid. The chief difficulty arises in effusions of moderate extent, when the dulness, the presence of bronchophony, and, perhaps, tubular breathing may simulate *pneumonia.* The chief points to be borne in mind are: (*a*) Differences in the onset and in the general characters of the two affections, more particularly the initial chill, the higher fever, more urgent dyspnœa, and the rusty expectoration, which characterize pneumonia. As already mentioned, some of the cases of pneumococcus pleurisy set in like pneumonia. (*b*) Certain physical signs—the more wooden character of the dulness, the greater resistance, and the marked diminution or the absence of tactile fremitus in pleurisy. The auscultatory signs may be deceptive. It is usually, indeed, the persistence of tubular breathing, particularly the high-pitched, even amphoric expiration, heard in some cases of pleurisy, which has raised the doubt. The intercostal spaces are more commonly obliterated in pleuritic effusion than in pneumonia. As already mentioned, the displacement of organs is a very valuable sign. Nowadays with the hypodermic needle the question is easily settled. A separate small syringe with a capacity of two drachms should be reserved for exploratory purposes, and the needle should be longer and firmer than in the ordinary hypodermic instrument. With careful preliminary disinfection the instrument can be used with impunity, and in cases of doubt the exploratory puncture should be made without hesitation. Pneumothorax is an occasional sequence. The hypodermic needle is especially useful in those cases in which there are pseudo-cavernous signs at the base. In cases, too, of massive pneumonia, in which the bronchi are plugged with fibrin, if the patient has not been seen from the outset, the diagnosis may be impossible without it.

On the left side it may be difficult to differentiate a very large pericardial from a pleural effusion. The retention of resonance at the base, the presence of Skoda's resonance toward the axilla, the absence of dislocation of the heart-beat to the right of the sternum, the feebleness of the pulse and of the heart-sounds, and the urgency of the dyspnœa, out of all proportion to the extent of the effusion, are the chief points to be considered. Unilateral hydrothorax, which is not at all uncommon in heart-disease, presents signs identical with those of sero-fibrinous effusion. Certain tumors within the chest may simulate pleural effusion. It should be remembered that many intrathoracic growths are accompanied by exudation. Malignant disease of the lung and of the pleura and hydatids of the pleura produce extensive dulness, with suppression of the breath-sounds, simulating closely effusion.

On the right side, abscess of the liver, subdiaphragmatic abscess, and hydatid cysts may rise high into the pleura and produce dulness and enfeebled breathing. Often in these cases there is a friction sound, which should excite suspicion, and the upper outline of the dulness is sometimes plainly convex. In a case of cancer of the kidney the growth involved the diaphragm very early, and for months there were signs of pleurisy before our attention was directed to the kidney. In all cases of doubt the X-ray examination is a great aid; exploratory puncture should be done without hesitation.

The second question, as to the nature of the fluid, is quickly decided by the use of the needle. The persistent fever, the occurrence of sweats, a leucocytosis, and the increase in the pallor suggest the presence of pus. In children the complexion is often sallow and earthy. In protracted cases, even in children, when the general symptoms and the appearance of the patient have been most strongly suggestive of pus, the syringe has withdrawn clear fluid. On the other hand, effusions of short duration may be purulent, even when the general symptoms do not suggest it. In pneumonia the practitioner should be on the alert if the crisis is delayed or the temperature rises after the crisis, if chills and sweats follow, or if the cough changes to one of paroxysmal type of great intensity. There are three groups: (*a*) The presence of the empyema is readily detected. (*b*) It is suspected, but it is not possible to locate the pus by the ordinary physical means. The exploratory needle should be freely used with the aid of a local anæsthetic; many punctures may be made without discomfort. (*c*) In a few instances small interlobar collections, small mural abscesses, and the diaphragmatic form may escape detection until an operation is performed. The prognostic import of the bacteriological examination of the aspirated fluid is as follows: The pneumococcus is of favorable significance, as such cases usually get well rapidly, even with a single aspiration. The streptococcus empyema is the most serious form, and even after a free drainage the patient may succumb to a general septicæmia. A sterile fluid indicates in a majority of instances a tuberculous origin.

Treatment

At the onset the severe pain may be relieved by hot or cold applications, but a hypodermic of morphia is more effective. The Paquelin cautery may be lightly but freely applied. It is well to administer a mercurial or saline purge. Fixing the side by careful strapping with long strips of adhesive plaster, which should pass well over the middle line, drawn tightly and evenly, gives great relief, and I can corroborate the statement of F. T. Roberts as to its efficacy. Cupping, wet or dry, is now seldom employed. Blisters are of no special service in the acute stages, although they relieve the pain. The ice-bag may be used as in pneumonia. The open-air treatment should be begun early, as a majority of the cases are tuberculous. Medicines are rarely required and mercurials are not indicated. A Dover's powder may be given at night.

When effusion has taken place, mustard plasters or iodine, producing slight counter-irritation, appear useful, particularly in the later stages. Iodide of potassium is of doubtful benefit. By some the salicylates are believed to be of special efficacy; but the drug treatment of the disease is most unsatisfactory. The dry diet and frequent saline purges (given in concentrated form before breakfast in Hay's method) may be tried. Recently it has been advised to use a salt-free diet.

Early and if necessary repeated aspiration of the fluid is the most satisfactory method of treatment. The results obtained by Delafield in 200 cases treated by early aspiration have never been equalled by any other method. The credit of introducing aspiration in pleuritic effusions is due to Morrill Wyman, of Cambridge, Mass., and Henry I. Bowditch, of Boston. Years prior to Dieulafoy's work, aspiration was in constant use at the Massachusetts General Hospital and was advocated repeatedly by Bowditch. As the question is one of some historical interest, I give Bowditch's conclusions concerning aspiration, expressed more than sixty years ago, and which practically represent the opinion of to-day: "(1) The operation is perfectly simple, but slightly painful, and can be done with ease upon any patient in however advanced a stage of the disease. (2) It should be performed forthwith in *all* cases in which there is complete filling up of one side of the chest. (3) He had determined to use it in *any* case of even *moderate* effusion lasting more than a few weeks and in which there should seem to be a disposition to resist ordinary modes of treatment. (4) He urged this practice upon the profession as a very important measure in practical medicine; believing that by this method death may frequently be prevented from ensuing either by sudden attack of dyspnœa or subsequent phthisis, and, finally, from the gradual wearing out of the powers of life or inability to absorb the fluid." When the fluid reaches to the clavicle the indication for aspiration is imperative. Fever is not a contra-indication; indeed, sometimes with serous exudates the temperature falls after aspiration.

The operation is extremely simple and is practically without risk. The spot selected for puncture should be either in the sixth intercostal space in the mid-axilla or at the outer angle of the scapula in the eighth space. The arm of the patient should be brought forward with the hand on the opposite shoulder, so as to widen the spaces. The needle should be thrust in close to the upper margin of the rib, so as to avoid the intercostal artery, the wounding of which, however, is an exceedingly rare accident. The fluid should be withdrawn slowly. The amount will depend on the size of the exudate. If the fluid reaches to the clavicle a litre or more may be withdrawn with safety. In chronic cases of serous pleurisy after the failure of repeated tappings S. West has shown the great value of free incision and drainage. He has reported cases of recovery after effusions of fifteen and eighteen months' standing.

Repeated tapping may be required in some cases. In the chronic cases the injection of adrenalin solution (20 to 30 drops of a 1 to 1,000 solution) into the pleural cavity after aspiration has proved of value.

SYMPTOMS AND ACCIDENTS DURING PARACENTESIS.—Pain is usually complained of after a certain amount of fluid has been withdrawn; it is sharp and cutting in character. *Coughing* occurs toward the close, and may be severe and paroxysmal. *Pneumothorax* may follow an exploratory puncture with a hypodermic needle; it is rare during aspiration. *Subcutaneous emphysema* may develop from the point of puncture, without the production of pneumothorax. *Cerebral symptoms.*—Faintness is not uncommon. Epileptic convulsions may occur either during the withdrawal or while irrigating the pleura. These symptoms are very difficult to explain and are regarded by most authors as of reflex origin. Hemiplegia may follow. And lastly *sudden death* may occur either from syncope or during the convulsions.

As A. E. Russell has pointed out, these serious and even fatal events may follow exploratory puncture of the lung. Such accidents of paracentesis and of washing out the pleura are explained by the studies of Capp and Lewis, who have shown that a sudden and sometimes fatal fall in blood pressure may follow the experimental irrigation of the pleura in dogs. Occasionally toxic symptoms arise resembling those of the "serum illness"—pains in the joints, albumin in the urine, and œdema—suggestive of the absorption of toxins that act like a heterogenous serum. Expectoration of a large quantity of *albuminous fluid* may occur suddenly after the tapping, associated with dyspnœa. Some cases have proved rapidly fatal, with the features of an acute œdema of the lungs. It has occurred only once in my practice.

The after-treatment of pleurisy is important and the patients should be handled exactly as if they had an early tuberculous lung lesion.

Empyema.—A majority of the cases get well, provided that free drainage is obtained, and it makes no difference practically what measures are followed so long as this indication is met. The good results in any method depend upon the thoroughness with which the cavity is drained. Irrigation of the cavity is rarely necessary unless the contents are fetid. In the subsequent treatment a point of great importance in facilitating the closure of the cavity is the distention of the lung on the affected side. This may be accomplished by the method advised by Ralston James, which has been practiced with great success in the surgical wards of the Johns Hopkins Hospital. The patient daily, for a certain length of time, increasing gradually with the increase of his strength, transfers by air-pressure water from one bottle to another. The bottles should be large, holding at least a gallon each, and by the arrangement of tubes, as in the Wolff's bottle, an expiratory effort of the patient forces the water from one bottle into the other. Equally efficacious is the plan advised by Naunyn. The patient sits in an arm-chair grasping strongly one of the rungs with the hand and forcibly compressing the sound side against the arm of the chair; then forcible inspiratory efforts are made which act chiefly on the compressed lung, as the sound side is fixed. The abscess cavity is gradually closed, partly by the falling in of the chest wall and partly by the expansion of the lung. In some instances it is necessary to resect portions of one or more ribs.

Until recently efficient drainage has been regarded as the most important consideration, and both operative and drainage proceedings have been directed toward making the chest wall conform to the lung. While thoracotomy and free drainage have done a great deal, it must be confessed that in a not inconsiderable number of cases the obliteration of the pus cavity has been a long and sometimes hopeless matter. In its place continuous drainage and intermittent siphonage have been used. It looks as if surgeons have made an important departure in the method of negative tension drainage as devised by von Eberts.

The physician is often asked, in cases of empyema with emaciation, hectic and feeble, rapid pulse, whether the patient could stand the operation. Even in the most desperate cases the surgeon should never hesitate to make a free incision.

II. CHRONIC PLEURISY

This affection occurs in two forms:

Chronic pleurisy with effusion in which the disease may set in insidiously or may follow an acute sero-fibrinous pleurisy. There are cases in which the liquid persists for months or even years without undergoing any special alteration and without becoming purulent. Such cases have the characters which we have described under pleurisy with effusion.

Chronic Dry Pleurisy.—The cases are met with (*a*) *as a sequence of ordinary pleural effusion.* When the exudate is absorbed and the layers of the pleura come together there is left between them a variable amount of fibrinous material which gradually undergoes organization, and is converted into a layer of firm connective tissue. This process goes on at the base, and is represented clinically by a slight grade of flattening, deficient expansion, defective resonance on percussion, and enfeebled breathing. After recovery from empyema the flattening and retraction may be still more marked. In both cases it is a condition which can be greatly benefited by pulmonary gymnastics. In these firm, fibrous membranes calcification may occur, particularly after empyema. It is not very uncommon to find between the false membranes a small pocket of fluid forming a sort of pleural cyst. In the great majority of these cases the condition is one which need not cause anxiety. There may be an occasional dragging pain at the base of the lung or a stitch in the side, but patients may remain in perfectly good health for years. The most advanced grade of this secondary dry pleurisy is seen in those cases of empyema which have been left to themselves and have perforated and ultimately healed by a gradual absorption or discharge of the pus, with retraction of the side of the chest and permanent carnification of the lung. Traumatic lesions, such as gunshot wounds, may be followed by an identical condition. Post mortem, it is quite impossible to separate the layers of the pleura, which are greatly thickened, particularly at the base, and surround a compressed, airless, fibroid lung. Bronchiectasis may gradually ensue, and in one remarkable case which I saw on several occasions with Blackader, of Montreal, not only on the affected side, but also in the lower lobe of the other lung.

(*b*) *Primitive dry pleurisy.*—This condition may directly follow the acute plastic pleurisy already described; but it may set in without any acute symptoms whatever, and the patient's attention may be called to it by feeling the pleural friction. A constant effect of this primitive dry pleurisy is the adhesion of the layers. This is probably an invariable result, whether the pleurisy is primary or secondary. The organization of the thin layer of exudation in a pneumonia will unite the two surfaces by delicate bands. Pleural adhesions are extremely common, and it is rare to examine a body entirely free from them. They may be limited in extent or universal. Thin fibrous adhesions do not produce any alteration in the percussion characters, and, if limited, there is no special change heard on auscultation. When, however, there is general synechia on both sides the expansile movement of the lung is considerably impaired. We should naturally think that universal adhesions would interfere materially with the function of the lungs, but practically we see many instances in which there has not been the slightest disturbance. The physical signs of total adhesion are by no means constant. It has been stated that there is a marked disproportion between the degree of expansion of the chest walls and the intensity of the vesicular murmur, but the latter is a very variable factor, and under perfectly normal conditions the breath-sounds, with very full chest expansion, may be extremely feeble. The diaphragm phenomenon—Litten's sign—is absent.

As already stated, it is possible, as the late Sir Andrew Clark held, that a primitive dry pleurisy may gradually lead to great thickening of the membranes, and ultimate invasion of the lung, causing a cirrhosis.

Lastly, there is a primitive dry pleurisy of tuberculous origin. In it both parietal and costal layers are greatly thickened—perhaps from 2 to 3 mm. each—and present firm fibroid, caseous masses and small tubercles, while uniting these two greatly thickened layers is a reddish-gray fibroid tissue, sometimes infiltrated with serum. This may be a local process confined to one pleura, or it may be in both. These cases are sometimes associated with a similar condition in the pericardium and peritoneum.

Occasionally remarkable vaso-motor phenomena occur in chronic pleurisy, whether simple or in connection with tuberculosis of an apex. Flushing or sweating of one cheek or dilatation of the pupil are the common manifestations. They appear to be due to involvement of the first thoracic ganglion at the top of the pleural cavity.

III. HYDROTHORAX

Hydrothorax is a transudation of simple non-inflammatory fluid into the pleural cavities, and occurs as a secondary process in many affections. The fluid is clear, without any flocculi of fibrin, and the membranes are smooth. It is met with more particularly in connection with general dropsy, either renal, cardiac, or hæmic. It may, however, occur alone, or with only slight œdema of the feet. A child was admitted to the Montreal General Hospital with urgent dyspnœa and cyanosis, and died the night after admission. She had extensive bilateral hydrothorax, which had come on early in the nephritis of scarlet fever. In renal disease hydrothorax is almost always bilateral, but in heart affections one pleura is more commonly involved. The physical signs are those of pleural effusion, but the exudation is rarely excessive. In kidney and heart-disease, even when there is no general dropsy, the occurrence of dyspnœa should at once direct attention to the pleura, since many patients are carried off by a rapid effusion. In chronic valvular disease the effusion is usually on the right side, and may recur for months. Stengel attributes the greater frequency of the dextral effusion to compression of the azygos veins. Post mortem records show the frequency with which this condition is overlooked. The saline purges will in many cases rapidly reduce the effusion, but, if necessary, aspiration should be practiced repeatedly.

IV. PNEUMOTHORAX

(*Hydro-Pneumothorax and Pyo-Pneumothorax*)

Air alone in the pleural cavity, to which the term pneumothorax is strictly applicable, is an extremely rare condition. It is almost invariably associated with a serous fluid—hydro-pneumothorax, or with pus—pyo-pneumothorax.

Etiology.—There exists normally within the pleural cavity of an adult a negative pressure of several (3 to 5) millimetres of mercury, due to the recoil of the distended, perfectly elastic lung. Hence, through any opening connecting the pleural cavity with the external air we should expect air to rush in until this negative pressure is relieved. To explain the absence of pneumothorax in a few cases of external injury laying the pleura bare, in which it would be expected, S. West has assumed the existence of a cohesion between the pleuræ, but this force has not as yet been satisfactorily demonstrated.

In a case of pneumothorax, if the opening causing it remain patent, which occurs only in some external wounds, or especially perforations through consolidated areas of the lungs, the intrathoracic pressure will be that of the atmosphere, the lung will be found to have collapsed as much as possible by virtue of its own elastic tension, the intercostal grooves obliterated, the heart displaced to the other side, and the diaphragm lower than normal, because the negative pressure by reason of which these organs are partly retained in their ordinary position has been relieved. If the opening becomes closed the intrathoracic pressure may rise above the atmospheric and the above-mentioned displacements be much increased. But most perforations through the lung are valvular, a property of lung tissue, and the intrapleural pressure is soon about 7 mm. of mercury. If there be a fluid exudate the pressure may be higher, but the high pressures supposed are more apparent than real, and that measured at the autopsy table is quite surely not that during life. It is more a question of the amount of distention than the actual pressure which determines the discomfort of the patient.

Pneumothorax arises: (1) In perforating wounds of the chest, in which case it is sometimes associated with extensive cutaneous emphysema. It may follow exploratory puncture either with a small needle or an aspirator. There were ten cases in my series. Pneumothorax rarely follows fracture of the rib, even though the lung may be torn. (2) In perforation of the pleura through the diaphragm, usually by malignant disease of the stomach or colon, or abscess of the liver perforating lung and pleura. The pleura may also be perforated in cases of cancer of the œsophagus. (3) When the lung is perforated. This is by far the most common cause, and may occur: (*a*) In the normal lung from rupture of the air-vesicles during straining or even when at rest. Special attention has been called to this accident by S. West and De H. Hall. The air may be absorbed and no ill effect follow. It does not necessarily excite pleurisy, as pointed out many years ago by Gairdner, but inflammation and effusion are the usual result. In one of my cases the condition developed as the patient was going down-stairs; no effusion followed; he did not react to tuberculin. (*b*) From perforation due to local disease of the lung, either the softening of a caseous focus or the breaking of a tuberculous cavity. According to S. West, 90 per cent. of all the cases are due to this cause. Less common are the cases due to septic broncho-pneumonia and to gangrene. A rare cause is the breaking of a hæmorrhagic infarct in chronic heart-disease, of which I met an instance a few years ago. (*c*) Perforation of the lung from the pleura, which arises in certain cases of empyema and produces a pleuro-bronchial fistula. (4) Spontaneously, by the development in pleural exudates of the gas bacillus (*B. aërogenes capsulatus* Welch). Of 48 cases, the basis of Emerson's exhaustive monograph (J. H. H. Reports, vol. xi), 22 were tuberculous, 6 were the result of trauma, 10 of aspiration, 2 were spontaneous, 2 followed bronchiectasis, 2 abscess of the lung, 1 gangrene, 2 an empyema, and 1 abscess of the liver perforating through the lung.

Pneumothorax occurs chiefly in adults, though cases are met with in very young children. It is more frequent in males than in females.

A remarkable recurrent variety has been described by S. West, Goodhart, and Furney. In Goodhart's case the pneumothorax developed first in one side and then in the other.

Morbid Anatomy.—If the trocar or blow-pipe is inserted between the ribs, there may be a jet of air of sufficient strength to blow out a lighted match. On opening the thorax the mediastinum and pericardium are seen to be pushed, or rather, as Douglas Powell pointed out, "drawn over" to the opposite side; but, as before mentioned, the heart is not rotated, and the relation of its parts is maintained much as in the normal condition. A serous or purulent fluid is usually present, and the membranes are inflamed. The cause of the pneumothorax can usually be found without difficulty. In the great majority of instances it is the perforation of a tuberculous cavity or a breaking of a superficial caseous focus. The orifice of rupture may be extremely small. In chronic cases there may be a fistula of considerable size communicating with the bronchi. The lung is usually compressed and carnified.

Symptoms.—The onset is usually sudden and characterized by severe pain in the side, urgent dyspnœa, and signs of general distress, as indicated by slight lividity and a very rapid and feeble pulse—the pneumothorax acutissimus of Unverricht. There may, however, be no urgent symptoms, particularly in cases of long-standing phthisis.

Physical Signs.—The physical signs are very distinctive. *Inspection* shows marked enlargement of the affected side with immobility. The heart impulse is usually much displaced. On *palpation* the fremitus is greatly diminished or more commonly abolished. On *percussion* the resonance may be tympanitic or even have an amphoric quality. This, however, is not always the case. It may be a flat tympany, resembling Skoda's resonance. In some instances it may be a full, hyperresonant note, like emphysema; while in others—and this is very deceptive—there is dulness. These extreme variations depend doubtless upon the degree of intrapleural tension. On several occasions I have known an error in diagnosis to result from ignorance of the fact that, in certain instances, the percussion note may be "muffled, toneless, almost dull" (Walshe). There is usually dulness at the base from effused fluid, which can readily be made to change the level by altering the position of the patient. Movable dulness can be obtained much more readily in pneumothorax than in a simple pleurisy. On *auscultation* the breath-sounds are suppressed. Sometimes there is only a distant feeble inspiratory murmur of marked amphoric quality. The contrast between the loud exaggerated breath-sounds on the normal side and the absence of the breath-sounds on the other is very suggestive. The râles have a peculiar metallic quality, and on coughing or deep inspiration there may be what Laennec termed the metallic tinkling. The voice, too, has a curious metallic echo. What is sometimes called the coin-sound, termed by Trousseau the *bruit d'airain*, is very characteristic. To obtain it the auscultator should place one ear on the back of the chest wall while the assistant taps one coin on another on the front of the chest. The metallic echoing sound which is produced in this way is one of the most constant and characteristic signs of pneumothorax. And, lastly, the Hippocratic succussion splash may be obtained when the auscultator's head is placed upon the chest while the patient's body is shaken. A splashing sound is produced, which may be audible at a distance. A patient may himself notice it in making abrupt changes in posture. The signs, distention, immobility, lack of vocal fremitus, hyperresonance, absence of breath-sounds and coin-sound, are those of the pure pneumothorax of Laennec. The metallic phenomena may be present, *e. g.*, the metallic tinkling and amphoric respiration, but these are best heard in cases with a consolidated lung and thickened pleura, such as occur in tuberculosis. The movable dulness and splash on succussion depend on fluid. Of other physical signs displacement of organs is most constant. As already mentioned, the heart may be much "drawn over" to the opposite side, and the liver greatly displaced, so that its upper surface is below the level of the costal margin, a degree of dislocation never seen in simple effusion.

Diagnosis.—The diagnosis of pneumothorax rarely offers any difficulty, as the signs are very characteristic. In cases in which the percussion note is dull the condition may be mistaken for effusion. Diaphragmatic or congenital hernia following a crush or other accident may closely simulate pneumothorax.

In cases of very large phthisical cavities with tympanitic percussion resonance and râles of an amphoric, metallic quality, the question of pneumothorax is sometimes raised. In those rare instances of total excavation of one lung the amphoric and metallic phenomena may be most intense, but the absence of dislocation of the organs, of the succussion splash, and of the coin-sound suffices to differentiate this condition. While this is true in the great majority of cases, I have heard the *bruit d'airain* over a large cavity in the right upper lobe. The condition of pyo-pneumothorax subphrenicus may simulate closely true pneumothorax.

The X-ray examination is of great help, and the picture in ordinary pneumothorax is very characteristic. There is a remarkable condition, described by Newton Pitt, associated with aneurism of the aorta, in which the sac pressing on the bronchus causes inflation of one lung with a picture simulating pneumothorax very closely.

Prognosis.—The prognosis in cases of pneumothorax depends largely upon the cause. S. West gives a mortality of 70 per cent. The tuberculous cases usually die within a few weeks. Of 39 cases, 29 died within a fortnight (West) ; 10 patients died on the first day, 2 within twenty and thirty minutes respectively of the attack. Of our 22 tuberculous cases 20 died, and 5 of the 10 cases following aspiration. Pneumothorax in a healthy individual often ends in recovery. There are tuberculous cases in which the pneumothorax, if occurring early, seems to arrest the progress of the tuberculosis. There is a chronic pneumothorax which may last for between three and four years. It may be a chronic condition, as in the case just mentioned, and a fair measure of health may be enjoyed.

Treatment.—There are three groups of cases: First, in the pneumothorax acutissimus, with urgent dyspnœa, great displacement of the heart, cyanosis, and low blood pressure, an opening should be made in the pleura and kept open, converting a valvular into an open variety. Immediate aspiration with a trocar has saved life. Secondly, the spontaneous cases which usually do well, as the air is quickly absorbed; so also with the traumatic variety. Very many of the tuberculous cases are best let alone, if the patient is doing well, or if the disease in the other lung is advanced. Thirdly, when there is pus, and the patient is not doing well, or in the tuberculous variety if the other lung is not involved, pleurotomy, or resection of one or two ribs, may be done. Of nine cases in my series two recovered.

V. AFFECTIONS OF THE MEDIASTINUM

Lymphadenitis.—The greater number of glands are on the right side, and the right bronchus passes off at a higher level (fifth dorsal vertebra) than the left. The glands are constantly enlarged in all inflammatory affections of the lungs. In all the acute affections of childhood they are found swollen. They are almost constantly involved in tuberculosis of the lungs and they are not infrequently the only organs of the body found tuberculous. Often in children the glands on the lung root become enlarged and caseous and penetrate deeply into the hilus and into the lung itself.

The symptoms of enlarged mediastinal glands are very uncertain in the simple and tuberculous forms. On the other hand in Hodgkin's disease and in sarcoma pressure symptoms are the rule.

Much attention has been paid recently to the diagnosis of this condition and authors speak quite lightly of the possibility of recognizing by percussion the various grades of enlargement. Indeed, it is claimed by Kronig and others that the pressure of the glands on the right bronchus may cause a dulness in the right lung apex due to slight collapse. The shadows on the X-ray picture cast by enlarged glands are believed to be distinctive, and examined in this way the percentage of cases in children is very high, 50 to 60 in some series.

D'Espine says there is a change in the whispered voice which has a bronchial ring at the level of the seventh cervical and last dorsal, and the respiratory murmur may be rougher and harsher.

Suppurative Lymphadenitis.—Occasionally abscess in the bronchial or tracheal lymph-glands is found. It may follow the simple adenitis, but is most frequently associated with the presence of tubercle. The liquid portion may gradually become absorbed and the inspissated contents undergo calcification. Serious accidents occasionally occur, as perforation into the œsophagus or into a bronchus, or in rare instances, as in the case reported by Sidney Phillips, perforation of the aorta, as well as a bronchus, which, it is remarkable to say, did not prove fatal rapidly, but caused repeated attacks of hæmoptysis during a period of sixteen months.

Tumors: Cancer and Sarcoma.—In Hare's elaborate study of 520 cases of disease of the mediastinum there were 134 cases of cancer, 98 cases of sarcoma, 21 cases of lymphoma, 7 cases of fibroma, 11 cases of dermoid cysts, 8 cases of hydatid cysts and instances of lipoma, gumma and enchondroma. From this we see that cancer is the most common form of growth. The tumor occurred in the anterior mediastinum alone in 48 of the cases of cancer and in 33 of the cases of sarcoma. There are three chief points of origin, the thymus, the lymph-glands, and the pleura and lung. Sarcoma is more frequently primary than cancer. Males are more frequently affected than females. The age of onset is most commonly between thirty and forty.

SYMPTOMS.—The signs of mediastinal tumor are those of intrathoracic pressure. In some cases almost the entire chest is filled with the masses. The heart and lungs are pushed back and it is marvelous how life can be maintained with such dislocation and compression of the organs. *Dyspnœa* is one of the earliest and most constant symptoms, and may be due either to pressure on the trachea or on the recurrent laryngeal nerves. It may, indeed, be cardiac, due to pressure upon the heart or its vessels. In a few cases it results from the pleural effusion which so frequently accompanies intrathoracic growths. Associated with the dyspnœa is a cough, often severe and paroxysmal in character, with the brazen quality of the so-called aneurismal cough when a recurrent nerve is involved. The voice may also be affected from a similar cause. Pressure on the vessels is common. The superior vena cava may be compressed and obliterated, and when the process goes on slowly the collateral circulation may be completely established. Less commonly the inferior vena cava or one or other of the subclavian veins is compressed. The arteries are much more rarely obstructed. There may be dysphagia, due to compression of the œsophagus. In rare instances there are pupillary changes, either dilatation or contraction, due to involvement of the sympathetic. Expectoration of blood, pus, and hair is characteristic of the dermoid cyst, of which Christian has collected 40 cases.

Physical Signs.—On inspection there may be orthopnœa and marked cyanosis of the upper part of the body. In such instances, if of long duration, there are signs of collateral circulation and the superficial mammary and epigastric veins are enlarged. In these cases of chronic obstruction the finger-tips may be clubbed. There may be bulging of the sternum or the tumor may erode the bone and form a prominent subcutaneous growth. The rapidly growing lymphoid tumors more commonly than others perforate the chest wall. In 4 of 13 cases of Hodgkin's disease there was mediastinal growth, and in 3 instances the sternum was eroded and perforated. The perforation may be on one side of the breast-bone. The projecting tumor may pulsate; the heart may be dislocated and its impulse much out of place. Contraction of one side of the thorax has been noted in a few instances. On palpation the fremitus is absent wherever the tumor reaches the chest wall. If pulsating, it rarely has the forcible, heaving impulse of an aneurismal sac. On auscultation there is usually silence over the dull region. The heart-sounds are not transmitted and the respiratory murmur is feeble or inaudible, rarely bronchial. Vocal resonance is, as a rule, absent. Signs of pleural effusion occur in a great many instances of mediastinal growth, and in doubtful cases the aspirator needle should be used.

Tumors of the anterior mediastinum originate usually in the thymus, or its remnants, or in the connective tissue; the sternum is pushed forward and often eroded. The growth may be felt in the suprasternal fossa; the cervical glands are usually involved. The pressure symptoms are chiefly upon the venous trunks. Dyspnœa is a prominent feature.

Intrathoracic tumors in the middle and posterior mediastinum originate most commonly in the lymph-glands. The symptoms are out of all proportion to the physical signs; there is urgent dyspnœa and cough, which is sometimes loud and ringing. The pressure symptoms are chiefly upon the gullet, the recurrent laryngeal, and sometimes upon the azygos vein.

In a third group, tumors originating in the pleura and the lung, the pressure symptoms are not so marked. Pleural exudate is very much more common; the patient becomes anæmic and emaciation is rapid. There may be secondary involvement of the lymph-glands in the neck.

Diagnosis.—The diagnosis of mediastinal tumor from aneurism is sometimes extremely difficult. An interesting case reported and figured by Sokolosski, in Bd. 19 of the Deutsches Archiv für klinische Medicin, in which Oppolzer diagnosed aneurism and Skoda mediastinal tumor, illustrates how in some instances the most skillful of observers may be unable to agree. Scarcely a sign is found in aneurism which may not be duplicated in mediastinal tumor. This is not strange, since the symptoms in both are largely due to pressure. The cyanosis, the venous engorgement, the signs of collateral circulation are, as a rule, much more marked in tumor. The time element is important. If a case has persisted for more than eighteen months the disease is probably aneurism. There are, however, exceptions to this. By far the most valuable sign of aneurism is the diastolic shock so often to be felt, and in a majority of cases to be heard, over the sac. This is rarely, if ever, present in mediastinal growths, even when they perforate the sternum and have communicated pulsation. Tracheal tugging is rarely present in tumor. Another point of importance is that a tumor, advancing from the mediastinum, eroding the sternum, and appearing externally, if aneurismal, has forcible, heaving, and distinctly expansile pulsations. The radiating pain in the back and arms and neck is rather in favor of aneurism, as is also a beneficial influence on it of iodide of potassium. The remarkable traumatic cyanosis of the upper half of the body which follows compression injuries of the thorax could scarcely be mistaken for the effect of tumor. In skillful hands the X-ray picture gives us now a means of differentiating aneurism and tumor which is rarely at fault.

The frequency of pleural effusion in connection with mediastinal tumor is to be constantly borne in mind. It may give curiously complex characters to the physical signs—characters which are profoundly modified after aspiration of the liquid. Occasionally a tumor of the mediastinum is operable.

Abscess of the Mediastinum.—Hare collected 115 cases of mediastinal abscess, in 77 of which there were details sufficient to permit the analysis. Of these cases the great majority occurred in males. Forty-four were instances of acute abscess. The anterior mediastinum is most commonly the seat of the suppuration. The cases are most frequently associated with trauma. Some have followed erysipelas or occurred in association with eruptive fevers. Many cases, particularly the chronic abscesses, are of tuberculous origin. Of *symptoms,* pain behind the sternum is the most common. It may be of a throbbing character, and in the acute cases is associated with fever, sometimes with chills and sweats. If the abscess is large there may be dyspnœa. The pus may burrow into the abdomen, perforate through an intercostal space, or it may erode the sternum. Instances are on record in which the abscess has discharged into the trachea or œsophagus. In many cases, particularly of chronic abscess, the pus becomes inspissated and produces no ill effect. The *physical signs* may be very indefinite. A pulsating and fluctuating tumor may appear at the border of the sternum or at the sternal notch. The absence of *bruit,* of the diastolic shock, and of the expansile pulsation usually enables a correct diagnosis to be made. When in doubt a fine hypodermic needle may be inserted.

Indurative Mediastino-Pericarditis.—Harris has reviewed the subject. In one form there are adherent pericardium and great increase in the fibrous tissues of the mediastinum; in another there is adherent pericardium with union to surrounding parts, but very little mediastinitis; in a third the pericardium may be uninvolved. The disease is rare; of 22 cases 17 were in males; only 2 were above thirty years of age. The symptoms are essentially those of that form of adhesive pericardium which is associated with great hypertrophy and dilatation of the heart, and in which the patients present a picture of cyanosis, dyspnœa, anasarca, etc. The pulsus paradoxus, described by Kussmaul, is not distinctive. Occasionally there is also a proliferative peritonitis. Mediastinal friction is sometimes heard in patients with adhesive mediastino-pericarditis—dry, coarse, crackling râles heard along the sternum, particularly when the arms are raised.

Miscellaneous Affections.—In Hare's monograph there were 7 instances of fibroma, 11 cases of dermoid cyst, 8 cases of hydatid cyst, and cases of lipoma and gumma.

Emphysema of the Mediastinum.—Air in the cellular tissues of the mediastinum is met with in cases of trauma, and occasionally in fatal cases of diphtheria and in whooping-cough. It may extend to the subcutaneous tissues. Champneys has called attention to its frequency after tracheotomy, in which, he says, the conditions favoring the production are division of the deep fascia, obstruction in the air-passages, and inspiratory efforts. The deep fascia, he says, should not be raised from the trachea. It is often associated with pneumothorax, and more often in rupture of the lung without pneumothorax, the pleura remaining intact and the air dissecting its way along the bronchi into the mediastinum and into the neck. The condition seems by no means uncommon. Angel Money found it in 16 of 28 cases of tracheotomy, and in 2 of these pneumothorax also was present.

SECTION VII

DISEASES OF THE KIDNEYS

I. MALFORMATIONS

Newman classifies the malformations of the kidney as follows: A. Displacements without mobility—(1) congenital displacement without deformity; (2) congenital displacement with deformity; (3) acquired displacements. B. Malformations of the kidney. I. Variations in number—(*a*) supernumerary kidney; (*b*) single kidney, congenital absence of one kidney, atrophy of one kidney; (*c*) absence of both kidneys. II. Variations in form and size—(*a*) general variations in form, lobulation, etc.; (*b*) hypertrophy of one kidney; (*c*) fusion of two kidneys—horseshoe kidney, sigmoid kidney, disk-shaped kidney. C. Variations in pelvis, ureters, and blood-vessels.

The fused kidneys may form a large mass, which is often displaced, being either in an iliac fossa or in the middle line of the abdomen, or even in the pelvis. Under these circumstances it may be mistaken for a new growth. In Polk's case the organ was removed under the belief that it was a floating kidney. The patient lived eleven days, had complete anuria, and it was found post mortem that a single fused kidney had been removed. A second case of the same kind has been reported.

II. MOVABLE KIDNEY

(*Floating Kidney; Palpable Kidney; Ren mobilis; Nephroptosis*)

Known to Riolan in the 17th century and to Matthew Baillie and to Rayer in the first half of the 19th century, it is only during the past quarter of a century that the condition has attracted widespread attention.

The kidney is held in position by its fatty capsule, by the peritoneum which passes in front of it, and by the blood-vessels. Normally the kidney is firmly fixed, but under certain circumstances one or the other organ, more rarely both, becomes movable. In very rare cases the kidney is surrounded, to a greater or less extent, by the peritoneum, and is anchored at the hilus by a mesonephron. Some would limit the term floating kidney to this condition.

Movable kidney is almost always acquired. It is more common in women. Of the 667 cases collected in the literature by Kuttner, 584 were in women and only 83 in men. It is more common on the right than on the left side. Of 727 cases analyzed by this author, it occurred on the right in 553 cases, on the left in 81, and on both sides in 93. The greater frequency of the condition in women may be attributed to compression of the lower thoracic zone by tight lacing, and, more important still, to the relaxation of the abdominal walls which follows repeated pregnancies. This does not account for all the cases, as movable kidney is by no means uncommon in nulliparæ. In many cases there is a congenitally relaxed condition of the peritoneal attachments. The condition has been met with in infants and in children. Wasting of the fat about the kidney may be a cause. Trauma and the lifting of heavy weights are occasionally factors. The kidney is sometimes dragged down by tumors. The greater frequency on the right side is probably associated with the position of the kidney just beneath the liver, and the depression to which the organ is subjected with each descent of the diaphragm in inspiration.

And, lastly, movable kidney is met with in many cases which present that combination of neurasthenia with gastro-intestinal disturbance which has been described by Glénard as *enteroptosis* (see p. 548).

To determine the presence of a movable kidney the patient should be placed in the dorsal position, with the head moderately low and the abdominal walls relaxed. The left hand is placed in the lumbar region behind the eleventh and twelfth ribs; the right hand in the hypochondriac region, in the nipple line, just under the edge of the liver. Bimanual palpation may detect the presence of a firm, rounded body just below the edge of the ribs. If nothing can be felt, the patient should be asked to draw a deep breath, when, if the organ is palpable, it is touched by the fingers of the right hand. Various grades of mobility may be recognized. It may be possible barely to feel the lower edge on deep palpation—*palpable kidney*—or the organ may be so far displaced that on drawing the deepest breath the fingers of the right hand may be, in a thin person, slipped above the upper end of the organ, which can be readily held down, but can not be pushed below the level of the navel—*movable kidney*. In a third group of cases the organ is freely movable, and may even be felt just above Poupart's ligament, or may be in the middle line of the abdomen, or can even be pushed over beyond this point. To this the term *floating kidney* is appropriate.

The movable kidney is not painful on pressure, except when it is grasped very firmly, when there is a dull pain, or sometimes a sickening sensation. Examination of the patient from behind may show a distinct flattening in the lumbar region on the side in which the kidney is mobile.

Symptoms.—In a large majority of cases there are no symptoms, and if detected accidentally it is well not to let the patient know of its presence. Far too much stress has been laid upon the condition of late years. In other instances there is pain in the lumbar region or a sense of dragging and discomfort, or there may be intercostal neuralgia. In a large group the symptoms are those of neurasthenia with dyspeptic disturbance. In women the hysterical symptoms may be marked, and in men various grades of hypochondriasis; and various forms of insanity have been attributed to it! The gastric disturbance is usually a form of nervous dyspepsia. Dilatation of the stomach has been observed, owing, as suggested by Bartels, to pressure of the dislocated kidney upon the duodenum. The association with a *depressed* stomach is common in women. Constipation is not infrequent. Some writers have described pressure upon the gall-ducts, with jaundice, but this is very rare. Fæcal accumulation and even obstruction may be associated with the displaced organ.

DIETL'S CRISES.—In connection with movable kidney, nearly always in women, and on the right side, there are remarkable attacks characterized by pain, chill, nausea, vomiting, fever, and collapse. They were described first by Dietl, in 1864, and attributed to twist or kink of the renal vessels or of the ureter. In the subject of movable kidney they may recur at intervals for months or years. A sudden exertion, an error in diet, or standing for a long time may bring on an attack. The pain is in the renal region, of great intensity, simulating colic, and radiates down to the ureter and through to the back. The patient feels nauseated and cold, or there may be a severe chill; vomiting is common. The urine is scanty and contains an excess of urate and oxalates; sometimes it is bloody. Locally there are two conditions, the affected side is tender, the muscular tension increases, and the kidney may be felt enlarged, sensitive to pressure and less movable; but there is no positive tumor. In other cases a tumor rapidly forms from dilatation of the pelvis of the kidney. Appearing, first anteriorly, at the edge of the epigastric region, it may gradually reach the size of a large orange or a cocoanut and fills the entire renal region. This may happen within thirty-six or forty-eight hours. The nausea persists, there is fever, the patient looks ill, and the urine may be scanty or bloody. The general symptoms abate, the local tenderness lessens, the amount of urine may increase rapidly, and in ten or twelve hours the tumor may disappear. In a month or two with a return of the symptoms the tumor re-appears, and again subsides. This is the well-known condition of *intermittent hydronephrosis*, which is one of the most serious and distressing of the sequels of movable kidney.

Diagnosis.—The diagnosis of movable kidney is rarely doubtful, as the shape of the organ is usually distinctive and the mobility marked. Tumors of the gall-bladder, ovarian growths, and tumors of the bowels may in rare instances be confounded with it.

Treatment.—In many instances the greatest relief is experienced from a bandage and pad. It should be applied in the morning, with the patient in the dorsal or knee-breast position, and she should be taught how to push up the kidney. An air pad may be used if the organ is sensitive. In other cases a broad bandage well padded in the lower abdominal zone pushes up the intestines and makes them act as a support. In the attacks of severe colic morphia is required. When dependent, as seems sometimes the case, upon an excess of uric acid or the oxalates, the diet must be carefully regulated. The intermittent hydronephrosis may be relieved by the pad and bandage. It rarely demands immediate operation. The kidney may have to be stitched in position.

Stitching of the kidney—nephrorrhaphy—is the most suitable procedure for severe cases, and relief is afforded in many instances by the operation, though not in all. Treatment designed to increase fat-formation often helps to hold the kidney in place. In the neurasthenic cases a prolonged rest treatment is indicated.

III. CIRCULATORY DISTURBANCES

Normally the secretion of urine is accomplished by the maintenance of a certain blood pressure within the glomeruli and by the activity of the renal epithelium. The watery elements are filtered from the glomeruli, the amount depending on the rapidity and the pressure of the blood current; the quality, whether normal or abnormal, depending upon the condition of the capillary and glomerular epithelium; while the greater portion of the solid ingredients are excreted by the epithelium of the convoluted tubules. The integrity of the epithelium covering the capillary tufts within Bowman's capsule is essential to the production of a normal urine. If under any circumstances their nutrition fails, as when, for example, the rapidity of the blood current is lowered, so that they are deprived of the necessary amount of oxygen, the material which filters through is no longer normal (i. e., water), but contains serum albumin. Cohnheim has shown that the renal epithelium is extremely sensitive to circulatory changes, and that compression of the renal artery for only a few minutes causes serious disturbance.

The circulation of the kidney is remarkably influenced by reflex stimuli coming from the skin. Exposure to cold causes heightened blood pressure within the kidneys and increased secretion of urine. Bradford has shown that after excision of portions of the kidney, to as much as one-third of the total weight, there is a remarkable increase in the flow of urine.

Congestion of the Kidneys.—(1) ACTIVE CONGESTION; HYPERÆMIA.—Acute congestion of the kidney is met with in the early stage of nephritis, whether due to cold or to the action of poisons and severe irritants. Turpentine, cubebs, cantharides, and copaiba cause extreme hyperæmia of the organ. The most typical congestion of the kidney which we see post mortem is that in the early stage of acute Bright's disease, when the organ may be large, soft, of a dark color, and on section blood drips from it freely.

It has been held that in all the acute fevers the kidneys are congested, and that this explained the scanty, high colored, and often albuminous urine. On the other hand, by Roy's oncometer, Walter Mendelson has shown that the kidney in acute fever is in a state of extreme anæmia, small, pale, and bloodless; and that this anæmia, increasing with the pyrexia and interfering with the nutrition of the glomerular epithelium, accounts for the scanty, dark-colored urine of fever and for the presence of albumin. In the prolonged fevers, however, it is probable that relaxation of the arteries again takes place. Certainly it is rare to find post-mortem such a condition of the kidney as is described by Mendelson. On the contrary, the kidney of fever is commonly swollen, the blood-vessels are congested, and the cortex frequently shows traces of cloudy swelling. However, the circulatory disturbances in acute fevers are probably less important than the irritative effects of either the specific agents of the disease or the products produced in their growth or in the altered metabolism of the tissues. The urine is diminished in amount, and may contain albumin and tube-casts, sometimes much of the former and few of the latter.

(2) PASSIVE CONGESTION; MECHANICAL HYPERÆMIA.—This is found in cases of chronic disease of the heart or lung, with impeded circulation, and as

a result of pressure upon the renal veins by tumors, the pregnant uterus, or ascitic fluid. In the cardiac kidney, as it is called, the cyanotic induration associated with chronic heart disease, the organs are enlarged and firm, the capsule strips off, as a rule, readily, the cortex is of a deep red color, and the pyramids of a purple red. The section is coarse looking, the substance is very firm, and resists cutting and tearing. The interstitial tissue is increased, and there is a small-celled infiltration between the tubules. Here and there the Malpighian tufts have become sclerosed. The blood-vessels are usually thickened, and there may be more or less granular, fatty, or hyaline changes in the epithelium of the tubules. The condition is indeed a diffuse nephritis. The urine is usually reduced, is of high specific gravity, and contains more or less albumin. Hyaline tube casts and blood corpuscles are not uncommon. In some cases (over half) with macroscopically no signs of chronic or acute nephritis the urinary features lead to the diagnosis of acute nephritis (Emerson). In uncomplicated cases of the cyanotic induration uræmia is rare. On the other hand, in the cardiac cases with extensive arterio-sclerosis, the kidneys are more involved and the renal function is likely to be disturbed.

IV. ANOMALIES OF THE URINARY SECRETION

1. ANURIA

Total suppression of urine occurs under the following conditions:

(*a*) As an event in the intense congestion of acute nephritis. For a time no urine may be formed; more often the amount is greatly reduced.

(*b*) More commonly complete anuria is seen in subjects of renal stone, fragments of which block both ureters; or as in a case reported by Monod the calculus blocked the only kidney, the other being represented by a shell of tissue. In this "obstructive suppression," as it is called, there is a condition which has been called latent uræmia. There may be very little discomfort, and the symptoms are very unlike those of ordinary uræmia. Convulsions occurred in only 5 of 41 cases (Herter); headache in only 6; vomiting in only 12. Consciousness is retained; the pupils are usually contracted; the temperature may be low; there are twitchings and perhaps occasional vomiting. Of 41 cases in the literature, 35 occurred in males. Of 36 cases in which there was absolute anuria, in 11 the condition lasted more than four days, in 18 cases from seven to fourteen days, and in 7 cases longer than fourteen days (Herter). Obstructive suppression is met with also when cancer compresses both ureters and involves their orifices in the bladder.

(*c*) Cases occur occasionally in which the suppression is prerenal. The following are among the more important conditions with which this form of anuria may be associated: Fevers and inflammations; acute poisoning by phosphorus, lead, and turpentine; in the collapse after severe injuries or after operations, or, indeed, after the passing of a catheter; in the collapse stage of cholera and yellow fever; and, lastly, there is an hysterical anuria, of which Charcot reports a case in which the suppression lasted for eleven days. Bailey reports the case of a young girl, aged eleven, inmate of an orphan asylum, who passed no urine from October 10th to December 12th (when 8 ounces were withdrawn), and again from this date to March 1st! The question of hysterical deception was considered in the case.

A patient may live for from ten days to two weeks with complete suppression. In Polk's case, in which the only kidney was removed, the patient lived eleven days. It is remarkable that in many instances there are no toxic features. Adams reports a case of recovery after nineteen days of suppression.

In the obstructive cases surgical interference should be resorted to. In the non-obstructive cases, particularly when due to extreme congestion of the kidney, cupping over the loins, hot applications, free purging, and sweating with pilocarpine and hot air are indicated. When the secretion is once started diuretin often acts well. Large hot irrigations, with normal salt solution, with Kemp's double-current rectal tubes, should be tried, as they are stated to stimulate the activity of the kidneys in a remarkable way.

2. HÆMATURIA

Etiology.—The following division may be made of the condition in which hæmaturia occurs:

(1) Essential Hæmaturia.—To this condition much attention has been paid of late, as the surgeons have taught us to recognize its frequency. The not very happy name of renal hæmophilia has been given to it. In this condition bleeding takes place from one or both of the kidneys without any evidence of disease to the naked eye or to the microscope. Angioma and capillary nævi of the renal papillæ and of the pelves of the kidney are excluded. The subjects are usually under the age of thirty. The bleeding is spontaneous, often associated with pain, though in many cases the attacks are painless. The X-ray picture is negative, the hæmorrhage ceases of itself, and only in a few cases do the attacks recur with such frequency that the patient becomes anæmic. The condition has been referred to under Gull's name of renal epistaxis in several previous editions. It is rarely serious, and many cases recover spontaneously, in others the nephrotomy stops the tendency to bleeding, though why it should do so is difficult to say. The outlook for patients is good (see Hale White, *Q. J. M.*, 1911).

(2) General Diseases.—In the malignant specific fevers, in purpura, and occasionally in leukæmia.

(3) Renal Causes.—Acute congestion and inflammation, as in Bright's disease, or the effect of toxic agents, such as turpentine, carbolic acid, and cantharides. When the carbolic spray was in use many surgeons suffered from hæmaturia in consequence of this poison. Renal infarction, as in ulcerative endocarditis. New growths, in which the bleeding is usually profuse. In tuberculosis at the onset, when the papillæ are involved, there may be bleeding. Stone in the kidney is a frequent cause. Parasites: The *Filaria sanguinis hominis* and the *Bilharzia* cause a form of hæmaturia met with in the tropics. The echinococcus is rarely associated with hæmorrhage. It is sometimes met with in floating kidney.

(4) Affections of the Urinary Passages.—Stone in the ureter, tumor or ulceration of the bladder, the presence of a calculus, parasites, and, very rarely, ruptured veins in the bladder. Bleeding from the urethra occasionally occurs in gonorrhœa and as a result of the lodgment of a calculus. Re-

curring hæmaturia may be an early symptom in enlarged prostate. An unusual cause is the painful, villous tumor of the renal pelvis, of which Savory and Nash report a remarkable case and have collected 49 others from the literature. It would be difficult to recognize the condition from stone. Angioma and capillary nævi of the papillæ may cause bleeding.

(5) TRAUMATISM.—Injuries may produce bleeding from any part of the urinary passages. By a fall or blow on the back the kidney may be ruptured, and this may be followed by very free bleeding; less commonly the blood comes from injury of the bladder or of the prostate. Blood from the urethra is frequently due to injury by the passage of a catheter, or sometimes to falls. Transient hæmaturia follows all operations on the kidney.

The malarial hæmaturia has already been considered.

Diagnosis.—The diagnosis of hæmaturia is usually easy. The color of the urine varies from a light smoky to a bright red, or it may have a dark porter color. Examined with the microscope, the blood-corpuscles are readily recognized, either plainly visible and retaining their color, in which case they are usually crenated, or simply as shadows. In ammoniacal urine or urines of low specific gravity the hæmoglobin is rapidly dissolved from the corpuscles, but in normal urine they remain for many hours unchanged.

It is important to distinguish between blood coming from the bladder and from the kidneys, though this is not always easy. From the bladder the blood may be found only with the last portions of urine, or only at the termination of micturition. In hæmorrhage from the kidneys the blood and urine are intimately mixed. Clots are more commonly found in the blood from the kidneys, and may form moulds of the pelvis or of the ureter. When the seat of the bleeding is in the bladder, on washing out this organ, the water is more or less blood-tinged; but if the source of the bleeding is higher, the water comes away clear. In many instances it is difficult to settle the question by the examination of the urine alone, and the symptoms and the physical signs must also be taken into account. Cystoscopic examination of the bladder, paying especial attention to the urine flowing from each ureteral orifice, and catheterization of the ureters are aids in the diagnosis of doubtful cases.

3. HÆMOGLOBINURIA

This condition is characterized by the presence of blood-pigment in the urine. The blood-cells are either absent or in insignificant numbers. The coloring matter is not hæmatin, as indicated by the old name, *hæmatinuria,* nor in reality always hæmoglobin, but it is most frequently methæmoglobin. The urine has a red or brownish-red, sometimes quite black, color, and usually deposits a very heavy brownish sediment. When the hæmoglobin occurs only in small quantities, it may give a lake or smoky color to the urine. Microscopic examination shows the presence of granular pigment, sometimes fragments of blood disks, epithelium, and very often darkly pigmented urates. The urine is also albuminous. The number of red blood corpuscles bears no proportion whatever to the intensity of the color of the urine. Examined spectroscopically, there are either the two absorption bands of oxyhæmoglobin, which is rare, or, more commonly, there are the three absorption bands of methæmoglobin, of which the one in the red near *C* is characteristic. Two clinical groups may be distinguished.

Toxic Hæmoglobinuria.—This is caused by poisons which produce rapid dissolution of the blood corpuscles, such as potassium chlorate in large doses, pyrogallic acid, carbolic acid, arseniuretted hydrogen, carbon monoxide, naphthol, and muscarine; also the poisons of scarlet fever, yellow fever, typhoid fever, malaria, and syphilis. It has also followed severe burns. Exposure to excessive cold and violent muscular exertion are stated to produce hæmoglobinuria. A most remarkable toxic form occurs in horses, coming on with great suddenness and associated with paresis of the hind legs. Death may occur in a few hours or a few days. The animals are attacked only after being stalled for some days and then taken out and driven, particularly in cold weather. The form of hæmoglobinuria from cold and exertion is extremely rare. No instance of it, even in association with frost-bites, came under my observation in Canada. Blood transfused from one mammal into another causes dissolution of the corpuscles with the production of hæmoglobinuria; and, lastly, there is the *epidemic hæmoglobinuria* of the newborn, associated with jaundice, cyanosis, and nervous symptoms.

Paroxysmal Hæmoglobinuria.—This rare disease is characterized by the occasional passage of bloody urine, in which the coloring matter only is present. It is more frequent in males than in females, and occurs chiefly in adults. It seems specially associated with cold and exertion, and has often been brought on, in a susceptible person, by the use of a cold foot-bath. It occurs, too, in persons subject to the various forms of Raynaud's disease, and the relation between these two affections is extremely close; some hold that they are manifestations of one and the same disorder. Druitt, the author of the well-known Surgical Vade-mecum, has given a graphic description of his sufferings, which lasted for many years, and were accompanied with local asphyxia and local syncope. The connection, however, is not very common. In only one of the cases of Raynaud's disease which I have seen was paroxysmal hæmoglobinuria present, and in it epileptic attacks occurred at the same time. The relation of hæmoglobinuria to malaria has been considered.

The attacks may come on suddenly after exposure to cold or as a result of mental or bodily exhaustion. They may be preceded by chills and pyrexia. In other instances the temperature is subnormal. There may be vomiting and diarrhœa. Pain in the lumbar region is not uncommon. The hæmoglobinuria rarely persists for more than a day or two—sometimes, indeed, not for a day. There are instances in which, even in the course of a single day, there have been two or three paroxysms, and in the intervals clear urine has been passed. Jaundice has been present in a number of cases. The disease is rarely if ever fatal.

Much has been done latterly to clear up the nature of this remarkable disease by the studies of Eason, Donath, Landsteiner, Hoover and Stone, and Moss. Briefly, the blood serum of these patients contains a complex hæmolysin, a potential toxin, capable of dissolving the patient's own corpuscles and those of other individuals. It is an amboceptor component of the hæmolysin, not the complement, that is peculiar, and this amboceptor differs "from other known hæmolytic amboceptors in that it will unite with the red blood-corpuscles only at a low temperature in the presence of complement, and furthermore in that it is capable of bringing about the solution of the patient's own cells (auto-hæmolytic action), and those of other members of the group to which the patient belongs, as well as the cells of members of other groups" (Moss). Atmospheric cold and congestion of the peripheral vessels, as in Raynaud's disease, will reduce the temperature of the blood sufficiently to permit of the union of the amboceptor and corpuscles, and hæmolysis occurs when the blood passes to the internal organs.

In a certain number of cases syphilis is present, usually congenital.

Treatment.—In all forms of hæmaturia rest is essential. In that produced by renal calculi the recumbent posture may suffice to check the bleeding. Full doses of acetate of lead and opium should be tried, then calcium lactate, adrenalin, ergot, gallic acid and tannic acid, and the dilute sulphuric acid. The oil of turpentine, sometimes recommended, is a risky remedy in hæmaturia. Extr. hamamelis virgin. and extr. hydrastis canad. are also recommended. Cold may be applied to the loins or dry cups in the lumbar region. Incision of the kidney has cured the so-called "renal epistaxis."

The treatment of paroxysmal hæmoglobinuria is unsatisfactory. Amyl nitrite will sometimes cut short or prevent an attack (Chvostek). During the paroxysm the patient should be kept warm and given hot drinks. If there is a syphilitic history, iodide of potassium in full doses may be tried. In a warm climate the attacks are much less frequent. It is possible that an antitoxin may be obtained to neutralize the hæmolytic amboceptor of the disease.

4. ALBUMINURIA

"Reasons drawn from the urine are as brittle as the urinal" is a dictum of Thomas Fuller peculiarly appropriate in connection with this subject.

The presence of albumin in the urine, formerly regarded as indicative of Bright's disease, is now recognized as occurring under many circumstances without the existence of serious organic change in the kidney. Two groups of cases may be recognized—those in which the kidneys show no coarse lesions, and those in which there are evident anatomical changes.

Albuminuria without Coarse Renal Lesions.—(*a*) FUNCTIONAL, SO-CALLED PHYSIOLOGICAL ALBUMINURIA.—In a normal condition of the kidney only the water and the salts are allowed to pass from the blood. When albuminous substances transude there is probably disturbance in the nutrition of the epithelium of the capillaries of the tuft, or of the cells surrounding the glomerulus. This statement is still, however, in dispute, and many hold that there is a physiological albuminuria which may follow muscular work, the ingestion of food rich in albumin, violent emotions, cold bathing, and dyspepsia. On one point all agree, that the cause must be something unusual and excessive, as a very hard tramp, a football match, a race, etc. The presence of albumin in the urine, in any form and under any circumstance, may be regarded as indicative of change in the renal or glomerular epithelium, a change, however, which may be transient, slight, and unimportant, depending upon variations in the circulation or upon the irritating effects of substances taken with the food or temporarily present, as in febrile states.

Albuminuria of adolescence and cyclic albuminuria, in which the albumin is present only at certain times during the day—orthostatic albuminuria—

are interesting forms. A majority of the cases occur in young persons—boys more commonly than girls—and the condition is often discovered accidentally. These are often the children of neurotic parents, and have well-marked vasomotor instability. Some cases last only during puberty, some throughout life. The condition is very common, particularly in young men in training—the athletic albuminuria to which Collier has called attention. Of 156 men in training 130 had albumin in the urine. Erlanger and Hooker have shown that the albumin is excreted only during periods with low pulse pressure. The urine, as a rule, contains only a very small amount of albumin, but in some instances large quantities are present. The most striking feature is the variability. It may be absent in the morning and present only after exertion; or it may be greatly increased after taking food, particularly proteins. Even the change to the upright position (orthostatic) may suffice to cause it, and in such cases there may be tension on the renal veins by increase of the lumbar curve, since it has been shown that a spinal jacket will prevent the appearance of the albumin. The quantity of urine may be but little, if at all, increased, the specific gravity is usually normal, and the color may be high. Occasionally hyaline casts may be found, and in some instances there has been transient glycosuria. As a rule, the pulse is not of high tension and the second aortic sound is not accentuated.

Various forms of this affection have been recognized by writers, such as neurotic, dietetic, cyclic, intermittent, and paroxysmal—names which indicate the characters of the different varieties.

Goodhart, from a study of the after history of more than 250 cases, holds that albuminuria of the adolescent has no sinister effect on health or upon duration of life, and that with due circumspection such cases ought not to be excluded from the advantages of life insurance, or from clerkships in banks and private offices. This is a very important and gratifying statement from a man who has made a special study of the subject.

In a few cases the albumin is persistent, the amount is larger, though it may vary from day to day, and the pulse tension is increased, and there are probably indications of organic changes in the kidney.

(*b*) Febrile Albuminuria.—Pyrexia, by whatever cause produced, may cause slight albuminuria. The presence of the albumin is due to slight changes in the glomeruli induced by the fever, such as cloudy swelling, which can not be regarded as an organic lesion. It is extremely common, occurring in pneumonia (in about 70 per cent. of our cases), diphtheria, typhoid fever (about 60 per cent. of our cases), malaria, especially the æstivo-autumnal type, and even in the fever of acute tonsillitis. The amount of albumin is slight, and it usually disappears from the urine with the cessation of the fever. Hyaline and even epithelial casts accompany the condition.

(*c*) Hæmic Changes.—Purpura, scurvy, chronic poisoning by lead or mercury, syphilis, leukæmia, and profound anæmia may be associated with slight albuminuria. Abnormal ingredients in the blood, such as bile pigment and sugar, may cause the passage of small amounts of albumin.

The transient albuminuria of pregnancy may belong to this hæmic group, although in a majority of such cases there are changes in the renal tissue. Albumin may be found sometimes after the inhalation of ether or chloroform.

(*d*) Nervous System.—Under many morbid conditions of the nervous system, albumin may be present in the urine, and there are instances in young nervous persons which are not easy to separate from the so-called orthostatic forms. In brain tumors, following epileptic attacks, in various types of meningitis, albumin has been present. In meningeal hæmorrhage, as pointed out by Guillain, the albumin may be very abundant, 5 to 20 grams in the litre.

Albuminuria with Definite Lesions of the Urinary Organs.—(*a*) Congestion of the kidney, either active, such as follows exposure to cold and is associated with the early stages of nephritis, or passive, due to obstructed outflow in disease of the heart or lungs, or to pressure on the renal veins by the pregnant uterus or tumors.

(*b*) Organic disease of the kidneys—acute and chronic Bright's disease, amyloid and fatty degeneration, suppurative nephritis, and tumors.

(*c*) Affections of the pelvis, ureters, bladder, and prostate, when associated with the formation of pus.

Albumosuria.—Albumose, peptone, and globulin are occasionally found in the urine, but are of very slight clinical significance. They are found in many febrile diseases, in chronic suppuration, and whenever protein materials are undergoing autolysis, as in pneumonia, acute yellow atrophy, and during the involution of the uterus.

Myelopathic albumosuria, *"Kahler's disease,"* is characterized by multiple myelomata with persistent excretion of what is known as the Bence-Jones body, a proteid discovered by him in 1848. There are now many cases on record. Males above forty years of age are usually affected. The Bence-Jones body appears rarely with other tumors of the bones. The myeloma is a true tumor, the cells of which resemble the plasma rather than the myelocytes of the bone marrow (Christian). In a case which I saw with Hamburger the persistent albumosuria led to the diagnosis of multiple myelomata before any bone tumors could be felt. The disease runs a fatal course. The simplest reaction is the white precipitate formed on adding nitric acid to the urine; when boiled it disappears, to reappear on cooling. As in one of Bradshaw's cases, the urine may be of a milky white color when passed.

Prognosis.—Febrile albuminuria is transient, and in a majority of the cases depending upon hæmic causes the condition disappears and leaves the kidneys intact. A trace of albumin in a man over forty, with or without a few hyaline casts, is not of much significance, except as an indication that his kidneys, like his hair, are beginning to turn "gray" with age. In many instances the discovery is a positive advantage, as the man is made to realize, perhaps for the first time, that he has been living carelessly. I have discussed the question from this standpoint in a paper with the paradoxical title "On the Advantages of a Trace of Albumin and a Few Tube-casts in the Urine of Men over Fifty Years of Age" (*N. Y. Med. Jour.*, vol. lxxiv).

The persistence of a slight amount of albumin in young men without increased arterial tension is less serious, as even after continuing for years it may disappear. The outlook in the so-called cyclic albuminuria has been discussed.

Practically in all cases the presence of albumin indicates a change of some sort in the glomeruli, the nature, extent, and gravity of which it is difficult to estimate; so that other considerations, such as the presence of tube-casts, the existence of increased tension, the general condition of the patient, and the influence of digestion upon the albumin, must be carefully considered.

The physician is daily consulted as to the relation of albuminuria and life assurance. As his function is to protect the interests of the company, he should reject all cases in which albumin occurs in the urine, except in young persons with transient albuminuria. Naturally, companies lay great stress upon the presence or absence of albumin, but in the most serious and fatal malady with which they have to deal—chronic interstitial nephritis—the albumin is often absent or transient, even when the disease is well developed. After the fortieth year, from a standpoint of life insurance, the state of the arteries and the blood pressure are far more important than the condition of the urine.

5. BACTERIURIA

Described first by Roberts in 1881, much attention has been paid to it of late years, and its importance recognized both as a secondary and a primary affection. The secondary form is best illustrated by the common bacilluria of typhoid fever already described. In the cases in which there is no recognizable cause or primary focus of the disease, the colon bacillus, streptococci, and the gonococcus are the commonest organisms. The bacilli may come directly from the blood, as in typhoid fever, and probably multiply in the urinary passages, or they may come from a focus of infection anywhere from Bowman's capsule to the prostate.

Clinically there are two groups of cases, the bacilluria pure and simple and the bacilluric cystitis or pyelitis. In the former there may be no symptoms; the urine may have a slight haziness due to the enormous number of organisms, but there is no pus. In the other there are signs of inflammatory reaction in the urinary passages and there is pus. Usually with the *Bacillus coli* infection the urine is acid, with the staphylococcus alkaline and often with marked phosphaturia. The cases are often very intractable. Without cystitis or pyelitis there may be no symptoms, but in too many instances there are all the aggravated phenomena of these two affections. Many cases clear up rapidly with hexamethylenamine. Vaccine therapy has been extensively used but not with very good results.

6. PYURIA

(Pus in the Urine)

Causes.—(*a*) Pyelitis and Pyelonephritis.—In large abscesses of the kidney, pyonephrosis, the pus may be intermittent, while in calculus and tuberculous pyelitis the pyuria is usually continuous, though varying in intensity. In cases due to the colon or tubercle bacillus the urine is acid, in those due to the proteus bacillus alkaline, while in the staphylococcus cases the urine is either less acid than normal, or alkaline. In the pyelitis and pyelonephritis following cystitis the urine is alkaline or acid, depending upon the infecting micro-organism; more mucus, frequent micturition, and a previous bladder history are aids in diagnosis.

(*b*) CYSTITIS.—The urine is usually acid, especially in women, since the colon bacillus is a very common cause of these infections. The pus and mucus are more ropy, and triple phosphate crystals are found in the freshly passed urine in the alkaline infections.

(*c*) URETHRITIS, particularly gonorrhœa. The pus appears first, is in small quantities, and there are signs of local inflammation.

(*d*) In LEUCORRHŒA the quantity of pus is usually small, and large flakes of vaginal epithelium are numerous. In doubtful cases, when leucorrhœa is present, the urine should be withdrawn through a catheter.

(*e*) RUPTURE OF ABSCESSES INTO THE URINARY PASSAGES.—In such cases as pelvic or perityphlitic abscess there have been previous symptoms of pus formation. A large amount is passed within a short time, then the discharge stops abruptly or rapidly diminishes within a few days.

Pus gives to the urine a white or yellowish-white appearance. On settling, the sediment is sometimes ropy, the supernatant fluid usually turbid. In cases due to urea-decomposing microbes (proteus bacillus, various staphylococci) the odor may be ammoniacal even in fresh urine. Examination with the microscope reveals the presence of a large number of pus-corpuscles, which are usually, when the pus comes from the bladder, well formed; the protoplasm is granular, and often shows many translucent processes.

The only sediment likely to be confounded with pus is that of the phosphates; but it is whiter and less dense, and is distinguished immediately by microscopic examination or by the addition of acid.

With the pus there is always more or less epithelium from the bladder and pelves of the kidneys, but since in these situations the forms of cells are practically identical, they afford no information as to the locality from which the pus has come.

The treatment of pus in the urine is considered under the conditions in which it occurs.

7. CHYLURIA—NON-PARASITIC

This is a rare affection, occurring in temperate regions and unassociated with the *Filaria bancrofti*. The urine is of an opaque white color; it resembles milk closely, is occasionally mixed with blood (hæmatochyluria), and sometimes coagulates into a firm, jelly-like mass. In other instances there is at the bottom of the vessel a loose clot which may be distinctly blood tinged. Under the microscope the turbidity seems to be caused by numerous minute granules—more rarely oil droplets similar to those of milk. In Montreal I made the dissection in a case of thirteen years' duration and could find no trace of parasites. The urine may be much more milky shortly after taking food, and the recumbent posture increases the milkiness. It has been shown in one case that the urine only became chylous in the bladder, and Hertz found obstruction of the thoracic duct and a communicating ruptured lymphatic vessel in the bladder.

8. LITHURIA

The general relations of uric acid have already been considered in speaking of gout.

Occurrence in the Urine.—The uric acid occurs in combination chiefly with ammonium and sodium, forming the acid urates. In smaller quantities are the potassium, calcium, and lithium salts. The uric acid may be separated from its bases and crystallizes in rhombs or prisms, which are usually of a deep red color, owing to the staining of the urinary pigments. The sediment formed is granular and the groups of crystals look like grains of Cayenne pepper. It is very important not to mistake a deposit of uric acid for an excess. The deposition of numerous grains in the urine within a few hours after passing is more likely to be due to conditions which diminish the solvent power than to increase in the quantity. Of the conditions which cause precipitation of the uric acid Roberts gives the following: "(1) High acidity; (2) poverty in mineral salts; (3) low pigmentation; and (4) high percentage of uric acid." The grade of acidity is probably the most important element.

In health the weight of uric acid excreted bears a fairly constant ratio to the weight of urea eliminated. According to von Noorden, the average ratio is 1 to 50, while the average ratio of the nitrogen of uric acid to the total nitrogen eliminated in the urine is 1 to 70. In several of the cases of gout in my wards Futcher found that in the intervals between the acute arthritic attacks the uric acid was reduced to a much greater extent than the urea, so that the ratio of the former to the latter often varied between 1 to 300 up to (in one case) 1 to 1,500, a return to about the normal proportions occurring during the acute attacks.

More common is the precipitation of amorphous urates, forming the so-called brick-dust or lateritious deposit, which has a pinkish color, due to the presence of urinary pigment. It is composed chiefly of the acid sodium urates. It occurs particularly in very acid urine of a high specific gravity. As the urates are more soluble in warm solutions, they frequently deposit as the urine cools. Here, too, the deposition does not necessarily, indeed usually does not, mean an excessive excretion, but the existence of conditions favoring the deposit.

9. OXALURIA

The discovery of calcium oxalate crystals in the urine by Donné in 1838 led to the description of the so-called oxalic-acid diathesis. It is claimed that all the oxalic acid found in the urine is taken into the body with the food (Dunlop). In health none, or only a trace, is formed in the body. The amount fluctuates with the quantity of food taken, and is usually below 10 milligrams daily (H. Baldwin). It seems to be formed in the body when there is an absence of free hydrochloric acid in the gastric juice, and in connection with excessive fermentation in the intestines. It never forms a heavy deposit, but the crystals—usually octahedral, rarely dumb-bell-shaped—collect in the mucous cloud and on the sides of the vessel.

When in excess and present for any considerable time, the condition is known as oxaluria, the chief interest of which is in the fact that the crystals may be deposited before the urine is voided, and form a calculus. It is held by many that there is a special diathesis associated with its presence in excess and manifested clinically by dyspepsia, particularly the nervous form, irritability, depression of spirits, lassitude, and sometimes marked hypochondriasis. There may be in addition neuralgic pains and the general symptoms of neurasthenia. The local and general symptoms are probably dependent upon some disturbance of metabolism of which the oxaluria is one of the manifestations. It is a feature also in many gouty persons, and in the condition called lithæmia.

10. CYSTINURIA

This rare condition, a sort of chemical malformation (Garrod), is of clinical importance because cystin is very sparingly soluble and calculi may be formed, renal or vesical. It is strongly hereditary and has been traced through three generations. The quantity excreted is about 0.5 gram per diem, and the excretion persists for years, or even for life, without causing disturbance of health. Cystin is one of the primary fractions of protein, and its excretion is one of the as yet unexplained errors of protein metabolism. In the urinary sediment the colorless hexagonal crystals of cystin are readily detected.

11. PHOSPHATURIA

The phosphoric acid is excreted from the body in combination with potassium, sodium, calcium, and magnesium, forming two classes, the alkaline phosphates of sodium and potassium and the earthy phosphates of lime and magnesia. The amount of phosphoric acid (P_2O_5) excreted in the twenty-four hours varies, according to Hammarsten, between 1 and 5 grams, with an average of 2.5 grams. It is derived mainly from the phosphoric acid taken in the food, but also in part as a decomposition product from nuclein, protagon, and lecithin. Of the alkaline phosphates, those in combination with sodium are the most abundant. The alkaline phosphates of the urine are more abundant than the earthy phosphates.

Of the *earthy phosphates,* those of lime are abundant, of magnesium scanty. In urine which has undergone the ammoniacal fermentation, either inside or outside the body, there is in addition the ammonio-magnesium or triple phosphate, which occurs in triangular prisms or in feathery or stellate crystals; hence the term of stellar phosphates given to this form. The earthy phosphates occur as a sediment in the urine when the alkalinity is due to a fixed alkali, or under certain circumstances the deposit may take place within the bladder, and then the phosphates are passed at the end of micturition as a whitish fluid, which is popularly confounded with spermatorrhœa. Recent study of these cases with symptoms of neurasthenia and a phosphate sediment in the fresh urine would indicate an abnormality in the calcium metabolism, an absolute increase of this with a decrease of the phosphoric acid. The calcium phosphate may be precipitated by heat and produce a cloudiness which may be mistaken for albumin, but is at once dissolved upon making the urine acid. This condition is very frequent in persons suffering from dyspepsia or from debility of any kind. The phosphates may be in great excess, rising in the twenty-four hours to from 7 to 9 grams (Teissier), whereas the normal amount is not more than 2.5 grams. And, lastly, the phosphates may be deposited in urine which has undergone decomposition, in which the carbonate of ammonia from the urea combines with the magnesium phosphates, forming the triple salt. This is seen in *cystitis,* due to a urea decomposing microbe.

The clinical significance of an excess of phosphates, to which the term phosphaturia is applied, has been much discussed. It must be remembered that a deposit does not necessarily mean an excess, to determine which a careful analysis of the twenty four hours' secretion should be made. It has long been thought that there is a relation between the activity of the nerve tissues and the output of phosphoric acid; but the question can not yet be considered settled. The amount is increased in wasting diseases, such as phthisis, acute yellow atrophy of the liver, leukæmia, and severe anæmia, whereas it is diminished in acute diseases and during pregnancy.

Teissier, of Lyons, in 1876, described a condition to which he gave the name of "essential phosphaturia," and it has been called "phosphatic diabetes," the symptoms of which are polyuria, thirst, emaciation, and a great increase in the excretion of phosphates, which would rise to as much as 7 to 9 grams a day. The condition sometimes simulates true diabetes very closely, even to the pruritis and dry skin. In a remarkable case of this kind, under my observation for several years, Barker studied the metabolism very thoroughly, and found it normal for carbohydrates, but the organic phosphorus percentage was high; the chief abnormality, however, was an abnormally large amount of organic acids, so that chemically the condition was suggestive of an acidosis.

12. INDICANURIA

The substance in the urine which has received this name is the indoxylsulphate of potassium, in which form it appears in the urine and is colorless. When concentrated acids or strong oxidizing agents are added to the urine, this substance is decomposed and the indigo set free. It is present only in small quantities in healthy urine. It is derived from the indol, a product formed in the intestine by the decomposition of the albumin under the influence of bacteria. When absorbed, this is oxidized in the tissues to indoxyl, which combines with the potassium sulphate, forming the above named substance.

It is a common condition met with accidentally in persons of good health or with slight digestive complaints. It is not specially associated with constipation (Allen Jones). In gall-stone attacks, in hyperchlorhydria, in recurring appendicitis, in wasting diseases, in peritonitis, and in empyema it is usually present. In a few cases it is constantly present and in excess. In a recent study Barr found only 32 such cases among 2,092 patients, and in these the clinical symptoms did not suggest an intestinal auto-intoxication, nor did the lacto-bacillary treatment of Metschnikoff have the slightest influence on the condition.

Indican has occasionally been found in calculi. Though, as a rule, the urine is colorless when passed, there are instances in which the decomposition has taken place within the body, and a blue color has been noticed immediately after the urine was voided. Sometimes, too, in alkaline urine on exposure there is a bluish film on the surface. Methylene blue, a coloring matter for candy, etc., must be excluded.

13. MELANURIA

Black urine may be dark when passed or may become so later. In the following conditions melanuria may occur: (1) Jaundice. Only in very chronic cases of deeply bronzed icterus do we see the urine quite dark, due to the presence of large quantities of biliverdin. (2) Hæmaturia and hæmoglobinuria. Here it is a matter of the exaggeration of the smoky tint due to the presence of blood in various quantities. (3) Hæmatoporphyrinuria, to be considered later. (4) Melanuria, in which the urine has, as a rule, the normal color when passed, and on standing becomes black as ink. In some instances it is black when passed. Melanuria of this type only occurs with the presence of melanotic tumors. (5) Alkaptonuria. (6) Indicanuria. When rich in indoxyl sulphate the urine is brown in color, or becomes so after standing, due to the oxidation products of indol. This is by far the most common cause of black urine, and in any disease leading to an abundant secretion of indican, as in intestinal obstruction, etc., black urine may be passed. As Garrod suggests, it is probable that the black urine in cases of tuberculosis is of an allied nature. (7) After certain articles of diet and drugs. Some dark colored vegetable pigments, as black cherries and plums and bilberries, cause darkening of the urine. Resorcin may do the same. Carboluria is by no means uncommon, and was frequently seen in the days of the antiseptic spray. It has been ascribed to hydrochinone formed from phenol. Naphthalene, creosote, and the salicylates may cause darkening of the urine, or even blackness.

14. ALKAPTONURIA

"Alkaptonuria is not the manifestation of a disease, but is rather of the nature of an alternative course of metabolism, harmless and usually congenital and lifelong" (Garrod). Of 40 known examples, 19 occurred in seven families, and several were the offspring of first cousins (Garrod). There are two points of clinical interest. The alkapton urine reduces Fehling's solution, and diabetes may be suggested, but it does not ferment, and it is optically inactive. The linen may be stained by the urine, which in some cases is dark when passed. In 1866 Virchow recorded a case of blackening of the cartilages and ligaments—ochronosis, which is considered elsewhere.

15. PNEUMATURIA

Gas may be passed with the urine—

1. After mechanical introduction of air in vesical irrigation or cystoscopic examination in the knee elbow position.

2. As a result of the introduction of gas forming organisms in catheterization or other operation. Glycosuria has been present in a majority of the cases. The yeast fungus, the colon bacillus, and the *Bacillus aërogenes capsulatus* have been found.

3. In cases of vesico-enteric fistula.

In gas production within the bladder the symptoms are those of a mild cystitis, with the passage of gas at the end of micturition, sometimes with a loud sound. The diagnosis is readily made by causing the patient to urinate in a bath or by plunging the end of the catheter under water.

16. OTHER SUBSTANCES

Lipuria.—Fat in the urine, or lipuria, occurs, first, without disease of the kidneys, as in excess of fat in the food, after the administration of cod liver oil, in fat embolism occurring after fractures, in the fatty degeneration in phosphorus poisoning, in prolonged suppuration, as in phthisis and pyæmia, in the lipæmia of diabetes mellitus; secondly, with disease of the kidneys, as in the fatty stage of chronic Bright's disease, in which fat casts are sometimes present, and, according to Ebstein, in pyonephrosis; and, thirdly, in the affection known as chyluria. The urine is usually turbid, but there may be fat drops as well, and fatty crystals have been found. In a few rare instances calculi composed of fat and coated with phosphates have been found.

Lipaciduria is a term applied by von Jaksch to the condition in which there are volatile fatty acids in the urine, such as acetic, butyric, formic, and propionic acid.

The occurrence of *acetone, diacetic acid,* and *β-oxybutyric acid* has been sufficiently considered under Diabetes.

Choluria and **glycosuria** have already been considered under jaundice and diabetes.

Hæmatoporphyrin occasionally occurs in the urine. It was first recognized by Hoppe-Seyler. Nencki and Sieler determined its exact formula, and the former demonstrated that the only chemical difference between hæmatin and hæmatoporphyrin is that the latter is simply hæmatin free from iron. It has been found in the urine in pulmonary tuberculosis, pleurisy with effusion, acute rheumatism, lead poisoning, and intestinal hæmorrhages. This pigment has been found very frequently after the administration of sulphonal, and sometimes imparts a very dark color to the urine.

V. URÆMIA

Definition.—A toxæmia developing in the course of nephritis or in conditions associated with anuria. The nature of the poison or poisons is as yet unknown, whether they are the retained normal products or the products of an abnormal metabolism.

Theories of Uræmia.—There are four chief views: (*a*) That it is due to the accumulation in the blood of body poisons which should be excreted by the kidney. What these substances are is not known, but neither the urea, nor the salts, nor the various extractives appear to be capable of producing the symptoms. (*b*) That it is a disturbance of the normal kidney metabolism. Brown-Séquard suggested that the kidney had an internal secretion, to the disturbance of which it is thought that the symptoms of uræmia may be due. Rose Bradford's experiments show how profoundly the kidneys influence the body metabolism, particularly that of the muscles. If more than two-thirds of the total kidney weight is removed, there is an extraordinary increase in the production of urea and of the nitrogenous bodies of the creatin class. From a study of the question Hughes and Carter conclude that the poison is of an albuminous nature, and quite different from anything in normal urine. (*c*) Uræmia has been attributed to nephrolysins. Broken up renal substance contains a material which, when injected into an animal, exerts a specific destructive action upon the renal cells. This substance may be found in the serum, and such a blood serum injected into another animal sets up nephritis and albuminuria. It is suggested that the phenomena of uræmia may result from the action of these nephrolysins upon the nerve centres. F. Müller has pointed out that uræmia is most apt to occur in those forms of renal disease in which the destruction of tissue is most extensive. (*d*) Lastly, there is the old view of Traube that the symptoms of uræmia, particularly the coma and convulsions, are due to localized œdema of the brain.

Symptoms.—Clinically, we may recognize latent, acute, and chronic forms. The latent form has been considered under the section on anuria. Acute uræmia may arise in any form of nephritis. It is more common in the post-febrile varieties. Bradford thinks that it is specially associated with a form of contracted white kidney in young subjects. Chronic forms of uræmia are more frequent in the arterio-sclerotic and granular kidney. For convenience the symptoms of uræmia may be described under cerebral, dyspnœic, and gastro-intestinal manifestations.

Among the CEREBRAL symptoms of uræmia may be described:

(*a*) *Mania.*—This may come on abruptly in an individual who has shown no previous indications of mental trouble, and who may not be known to have Bright's disease. In one case of this kind the patient became suddenly maniacal and died in six days. More commonly the delirium is less violent, but the patient is noisy, talkative, restless, and sleepless.

(*b*) *Delusional Insanity* (*Folie Brightique*).—Cases are by no means uncommon, and excellent clinical reports have been issued on the subject from several of the asylums, particularly by Bremer, Christian, and Alice Bennett. Delusions of persecution are common. One of my patients committed suicide by jumping out of a window. The condition is of interest medico-legally because of its bearing on testamentary capacity. Profound melancholia may also supervene.

(*c*) *Convulsions.*—These may come on unexpectedly or be preceded by pain in the head and restlessness. The attacks may be general and identical with those of ordinary epilepsy, though the initial cry may not be present. The fits may recur rapidly, and in the interval the patient is usually unconscious. Sometimes the temperature is elevated, but more frequently it is depressed, and may sink rapidly after the attack. Local or Jacksonian epilepsy may occur in most characteristic form in uræmia. A remarkable sequence of the convulsions is blindness—*uræmic amaurosis*—which may persist for several days. This, however, may occur apart from the convulsions. It usually passes off in a day or two. There are, as a rule, no ophthalmoscopic changes. Sometimes uræmic deafness supervenes, and is probably also a cerebral manifestation. It may also occur in connection with persistent headache, nausea, and other gastric symptoms.

(*d*) *Coma.*—Unconsciousness invariably accompanies the general convulsions, but a coma may develop gradually without any convulsive seizures. Frequently it is preceded by headache, and the patient gradually becomes dull and apathetic. In these cases there may have been no previous indications of renal disease, and unless the urine is examined the nature of the case may be overlooked. Twitchings of the muscles occur, particularly in the face and hands, but there are many cases of coma in which the muscles are not involved. In some of these cases a condition of torpor persists for weeks or even months. The tongue is usually furred and the breath very foul and heavy.

(*e*) *Local Palsies.*—In the course of chronic Bright's disease hemiplegia or monoplegia may come on spontaneously or follow a convulsion, and post mortem no gross lesions of the brain be found, but only a localized or diffused œdema. These cases, which are not very uncommon, may simulate almost every form of organic paralysis of cerebral origin.

(*f*) Of other cerebral symptoms, HEADACHE is important. It is most often occipital and extends to the neck. It may be an early feature and associated with giddiness. Other nervous symptoms of uræmia are intense itching of the skin, numbness and tingling in the fingers, and cramps in the muscles of the calves, particularly at night. An erythema may be present.

URÆMIC DYSPNŒA is classified by Palmer Howard as follows: (*a*) Continuous dyspnœa; (*b*) paroxysmal dyspnœa; (*c*) both types alternating; and (*d*) Cheyne-Stokes breathing. The attacks of dyspnœa are most commonly nocturnal; the patient may sit up, gasp for breath, and evince as much distress as in true asthma. Occasionally the breathing is noisy and stridulous. The Cheyne-Stokes type may persist for weeks or months. One patient, up and about, could feed himself only in the apnœa period. Though usually of serious omen and occurring with coma and other symptoms, recovery may follow even after persistence for a long period.

The GASTRO-INTESTINAL manifestations of uræmia often set in with abruptness. Uncontrollable vomiting may come on and its cause be quite unrecognizable. The attacks may be preceded by nausea and may be associated with diarrhœa. In some instances the diarrhœa may come on without the vomiting; sometimes it is profuse and associated with an intense catarrhal or even diphtheritic inflammation of the colon.

A special URÆMIC STOMATITIS has been described in which the mucosa of the lips, gums, and tongue is swollen and erythematous. The saliva may be increased, and there is difficulty in swallowing and in mastication. The tongue is usually very foul and the breath heavy and fetid. A cutaneous erythema may occur and a remarkable urea "frost" on the skin.

FEVER is not uncommon in uræmic states, and may occur with the acute nephritis, with the complications, and as a manifestation of the uræmia itself.

Very many patients with chronic uræmia succumb to what I have called terminal infections—acute peritonitis, pericarditis, pleurisy, meningitis, or endocarditis.

Diagnosis.—Herter called attention to the value of the clinical determination of the urea in the blood (for which purpose only a few cubic centimetres are required) as an index of the degree of renal inadequacy. In but 2 of 96 cases could the urea determination in the urine have been of any value in predicting uræmia, and equal drops in the urea occurred without this symptom (Emerson). The test of the functional capacity of the kidney by the use of phenol-sulphonephthalein (Rowntree and Geraghty) is of great value both in differential diagnosis and in giving warning of impending uræmia. In uræmia the elimination of phthalein is nil or only a faint trace in two hours. In patients with chronic nephritis in whom the elimination in two hours is below 10 per cent. there is grave danger of uræmia.

Uræmia may be confounded with:

(*a*) Cerebral lesions, such as hæmorrhage, meningitis, or even tumor. In apoplexy, which is so commonly associated with kidney disease and stiff arteries, the sudden loss of consciousness, particularly if with convulsions, may simulate a uræmic attack; but the mode of onset, the existence of complete hemiplegia, with conjugate deviation of the eyes, suggest hæmorrhage. As already noted, there are cases of uræmic hemiplegia or monoplegia which can not be separated from those of organic lesion and which post mortem show no trace of coarse disease of the brain. Indeed, in some of these cases it is quite impossible to distinguish between the two conditions. So, too, cases of meningitis, in a condition of deep coma, with perhaps slight fever, furred tongue, but without localizing symptoms, may readily be confounded with uræmia.

(*b*) With certain infectious diseases. Uræmia may persist for weeks or months and the patient lies in a condition of torpor or even unconsciousness, with a heavily coated, perhaps dry, tongue, muscular twitchings, a rapid feeble pulse, with slight fever. This state not unnaturally suggests the existence of one of the infectious diseases. Cases of the kind are not uncommon, and I have known them to be mistaken for typhoid fever and for miliary tuberculosis.

(*c*) Uræmic coma may be confounded with poisoning by alcohol or opium. In opium poisoning the pupils are contracted; in alcoholism they are more commonly dilated. In uræmia they are not constant; they may be either widely dilated or of medium size. The examination of the eye grounds should be made to determine the presence or absence of albuminuric retinitis. The urine should be drawn off and examined. The odor of the breath sometimes gives an important hint.

The condition of the heart and arteries should also be taken into account. Sudden uræmic coma is more common in the chronic interstitial nephritis. The character of the delirium in alcoholism is sometimes important, and the coma is not so deep as in uræmia or opium poisoning. It may for a time be impossible to determine whether the condition is due to uræmia, profound alcoholism, or hæmorrhage into the pons Varolii.

And, lastly, in connection with sudden coma, it is to be remembered that insensibility may occur after prolonged muscular exertion, as after running a ten-mile race. In some instances unconsciousness has come on rapidly with stertorous breathing and dilated pupils. Cases have occurred under conditions in which sun-stroke could be excluded; and Poore considers that the condition is due to the too rapid accumulation of waste products in the blood, and to hyperpyrexia from suspension of sweating.

The treatment will be considered under Chronic Bright's Disease.

VI. ACUTE BRIGHT'S DISEASE

Definition.—Acute diffuse nephritis, due to the action of cold or of toxic agents upon the kidneys.

In all instances changes exist in the epithelial, vascular, and intertubular tissues, which vary in intensity in different forms; hence writers have described a tubular, a glomerular, and an acute interstitial nephritis. Delafield recognizes *acute exudative* and *acute productive* forms, the latter characterized by proliferation of the connective-tissue stroma and of the cells of the Malpighian tufts.

Etiology.—The following are the principal causes of acute nephritis:

(1) Cold. Exposure to cold and wet is one of the most common causes. It is particularly prone to follow exposure after a drinking-bout.

(2) The poisons of the specific fevers, particularly scarlet fever, less commonly typhoid fever, measles, diphtheria, small-pox, chicken-pox, malaria, cholera, yellow fever, meningitis, and, very rarely, dysentery. Acute nephritis may be associated with syphilis and with acute tuberculosis, particularly the former. Bradford suggests that many of the idiopathic cases and those ascribed to cold may be of syphilitic origin. It may also occur in septicæmia and in acute tonsillitis. In exudative erythema and the allied purpuric affections acute nephritis is not uncommon. Among 1,832 cases of malaria at the Johns Hopkins Hospital there were 26 of nephritis (Thayer). A primary infective epidemic nephritis has been met with in Italy.

(3) Toxic agents, such as turpentine, cantharides, potassium chlorate, and carbolic acid, may cause an acute congestion which sometimes terminates in nephritis. Alcohol probably never excites an acute nephritis.

(4) Pregnancy, in which the condition is probably due to toxic products as yet undetermined.

(5) Acute nephritis occurs occasionally in connection with extensive lesions of the skin, as in burns or in chronic skin-diseases, and also after trauma. It may follow operations on the kidney.

Morbid Anatomy.—The kidneys may present to the naked eye in mild cases no evident alterations. When seen early in more severe forms the organs are congested, swollen, dark, and on section may drip blood. Bright's original description is as follows:

"The kidneys, . . . stripped easily out of their investing membrane, were large and less firm than they often are, of the darkest chocolate color, interspersed with a few white points, and a great number nearly black; and this, with a little tinge of red in parts, gave the appearance of a polished fine-grained porphyry or greenstone. . . . On (section) these colors were found to pervade the whole cortical part; but the natural striated appearance was not lost, and the external part of each mass of tubuli was particularly dark . . . a very considerable quantity of blood oozed from the kidney, showing a most unusual accumulation in the organ."

In other instances the surface is pale and mottled, the capsule strips off readily, and the cortex is swollen, turbid, and of a grayish red color, while the pyramids have an intense beefy red tint. The glomeruli in some instances stand out plainly, being deeply swollen and congested; in other instances they are pale.

The histology may be thus summarized: (*a*) *Glomerular changes.* The tufts suffer first, and there is either an acute intracapillary glomerulitis, in which the capillaries become filled with cells and thrombi, or involvement of the epithelium of the tuft and of Bowman's capsule, the cavity of which contains leucocytes and red blood-corpuscles.

(*b*) The *alterations in the tubular epithelium* consist in cloudy swelling, fatty change, and hyaline degeneration. In the convoluted tubules, the accumulation of altered cells with leucocytes and blood-corpuscles causes the enlargement and swelling of the organ.

(*c*) *Interstitial changes.* In the milder forms a simple inflammatory exudate—serum mixed with leucocytes and red blood-corpuscles—exists between the tubules. In severer cases areas of small celled infiltration occur about the capsules and between the convoluted tubes.

Symptoms.—The onset is usually sudden, and, when the nephritis follows cold, dropsy may be noticed within twenty-four hours. After fevers the onset is less abrupt, but the patient gradually becomes pale and a puffiness of the face or swelling of the ankles is first noticed. In children there may be convulsions at the outset. Chilliness or rigors initiate the attack in a limited number of cases. Pain in the back, nausea, and vomiting may be present. The fever is variable. Many cases in adults have no rise in temperature. In young children with nephritis from cold or scarlet fever the temperature may, for a few days, range from 101° to 103°.

The most characteristic symptoms are the *urinary changes.* There may at first be suppression; more commonly the urine is scanty, highly colored, and contains blood, albumin, and tube casts. The quantity is reduced and only 4 or 5 ounces may be passed in the twenty-four hours; the specific gravity is high—1.025, or even more; the color varies from a smoky to a deep porter color, but is seldom bright red. On standing there is a heavy deposit; microscopically there are blood corpuscles, epithelium from the urinary passages, and hyaline, blood, and epithelial tube casts. The albumin is abundant, forming a curdy, thick precipitate. The largest amounts of albumin are seen in the early acute nephritis of syphilis, in which it may reach 8.5 per cent. The total excretion of urea is reduced, though the percentage is high.

Œdema is an early and marked symptom. In cases of extensive dropsy effusion may take place into the pleuræ and peritoneum. There are cases of scarlatinal nephritis in which the dropsy of the extremities is trivial and effusion into the pleuræ extensive. The lungs may become œdematous. In rare cases there is œdema of the glottis. Epistaxis may occur or cutaneous ecchymoses may develop in the course of the disease.

The pulse may be hard, the tension increased, and the second sound in the aortic area accentuated. Occasionally dilatation of the heart comes on rapidly and may cause sudden death. The skin is dry and it may be difficult to induce sweating.

Uræmic symptoms occur in a limited number of cases, either at the onset with suppression, more commonly later in the disease. Ocular changes are not so common in acute as in chronic Bright's disease, but hæmorrhagic retinitis may occur and occasionally papillitis.

The course of acute Bright's disease varies considerably. The description just given is of the form which most commonly follows cold or scarlet fever. In many of the febrile cases dropsy is not a prominent symptom, and the diagnosis rests rather with the examination of the urine. Moreover, the condition may be transient and less serious. In other cases, as in the acute nephritis of typhoid fever, there may be hæmaturia and pronounced signs of interference with the renal function. The most intense acute nephritis may exist without anasarca.

In scarlatinal nephritis, in which the glomeruli are most seriously affected, suppression of the urine may be an early symptom, the dropsy is apt to be extreme, and uræmic manifestations are common. Acute Bright's disease in children, however, may set in very insidiously and be associated with transient or slight œdema, and the symptoms may point rather to affection of the digestive system or to brain disease.

Diagnosis.—It is very important to bear in mind that the most serious involvement of the kidneys may be manifested only by slight œdema of the feet or puffiness of the eyelids, without impairment of the general health. On the other hand, from the urine alone a diagnosis can not be made with certainty, since simple cloudy swelling, and circulatory changes may cause a similar condition of urine. The first indication of trouble may be a uræmic convulsion. This is particularly the case in the acute nephritis of pregnancy, and it is a good rule for the practitioner, when engaged to attend a case, invariably to ask that during the seventh and eighth months the urine should occasionally be sent for examination.

In nephritis from cold and in scarlet fever the symptoms are usually marked and the diagnosis is rarely in doubt. As already mentioned, every case in which albumin is present should not be called acute Bright's disease, not even if tube casts be present. Thus the common febrile albuminuria, although it represents the first link in the chain of events leading to acute Bright's disease, should not be placed in the same category.

There are occasional cases of acute Bright's disease with anasarca, in which albumin is either absent or present only as a trace. This is a rare condition. Tube casts are usually found, and the absence of albumin is rarely permanent. The urine may be reduced in amount.

The character of the casts is of use in the diagnosis of the form of Bright's disease, but scarcely of such extreme value as has been stated. Thus, the hyaline and granular casts are common to all varieties. The blood and epithelial casts, particularly those made up of leucocytes, are most common in the acute cases.

Prognosis.—The outlook varies somewhat with the cause of the disease. Recoveries in the form following exposure to cold are much more frequent than after scarlatinal nephritis. In younger children the mortality is high, amounting to at least one-third of the cases. Serious symptoms are low arterial tension, the occurrence of uræmia, and effusion into the serous sacs. The persistence of the dropsy after the first month, intense pallor, and a large amount of albumin indicate the possibility of the disease becoming chronic. For some months after the disappearance of the dropsy there may be traces of albumin and a few tube casts.

In a case of scarlatinal nephritis, if the progress is favorable, the dropsy diminishes in a week or ten days, the urine increases, the albumin lessens, and by the end of a month the dropsy has disappeared and the urine is nearly free. In very young children the course may be rapid, and I have known the urine to be free from albumin in the fourth week. Other cases are more insidious, and though the dropsy may disappear, the albumin persists in the urine, the anæmia is marked, and the condition becomes chronic, or, after several recurrences of the dropsy, improves and complete recovery takes place.

Treatment.—The patient should be in bed and there remain until all traces of the disease have disappeared. As sweating plays such an important part in the treatment, it is well, if possible, to accustom the patient to blankets. He should also be clad in thin Canton flannel.

The diet should consist of milk or butter-milk, gruels made of arrow-root or oat-meal, barley water, and, if necessary, beef tea and chicken broth. It is better, if possible, to confine the patient to a strictly milk diet. As convalescence is established, bread and butter, lettuce, water cress, grapes, oranges, and other fruits may be given. Meats should be used very sparingly. As there is marked retention of the chlorides, which seem to bear a relation to the dropsy, salt should be withheld.

The patient should drink freely of alkaline mineral waters, ordinary water, or lemonade. The fluids keep the kidneys flushed and wash out the *débris* from the tubes. A useful drink is a drachm of cream of tartar in a pint of boiling water, to which may be added the juice of half a lemon and a little sugar. Taken when cold, this is a pleasant and satisfactory diluent drink. Fluid may be given by the bowel or by saline infusion if it is not well taken by mouth.

No remedies, so far as known, control directly the changes which are going on in the kidneys. The indications are: (1) To give the excretory function of the kidney rest by utilizing the skin and the bowels, in the hope that the natural processes may be sufficient to effect a cure; (2) to meet the symptoms as they arise.

In a case of scarlet fever it may occasionally be possible to avert an attack, the premonitory symptoms of which are marked increase in the arterial tension and the presence of blood coloring matter in the urine (Mahomed). An active saline cathartic may completely relieve this condition.

At the onset, when there is pain in the back or hæmaturia, the Paquelin cautery or the dry or wet cups give relief. The last should not be used in children. Warm poultices are often grateful. In cases which set in with suppression of urine these measures should be adopted, and in addition the hot bath with subsequent pack, copious diluents, and a free purge. The dropsy is best treated by hydrotherapy—either the hot bath, the wet pack, or the hot-air bath. In children the wet pack is usually satisfactory. It is applied by wringing a blanket out of hot water, wrapping the child in it, covering this with a dry blanket, and then with a rubber cloth. In this the child may remain for an hour. It may be repeated daily. In the case of adults, the hot air bath or the vapor bath may be conveniently given by allowing the vapor or air to pass from a funnel beneath the bed clothes, which are raised on a low cradle. More efficient, as a rule, is a hot bath of from fifteen or twenty minutes, after which the patient is wrapped in blankets. The sweating produced by these measures is usually profuse, rarely exhausting, and in a majority of cases the dropsy can in this way be relieved. There are some cases, however, in which the skin does not respond to the baths, and if the symptoms are serious, particularly if uræmia supervenes, jaborandi or its active principle, pilocarpine, may be used. The latter may be given hypodermically, in doses of from a sixth to an eighth of a grain (0.01 to 0.008

gm.) in adults, and from a twentieth to a twelfth of a grain (0.003 to 0.005 gm.) in children of from two to ten years.

The bowels should be kept open by a morning saline purge; in children the fluid magnesia is readily taken; in adults the sulphate of magnesia may be given by Hay's method, in concentrated form, in the morning, before anything is taken into the stomach. In Bright's disease it not infrequently causes vomiting. The compound powder of jalap (gr. xx, 1.3 gm.) or, if necessary, elaterium may be used. If the dropsy is not extreme, the urine not very concentrated, and uræmic symptoms are not present, the bowels should be kept loose without active purgation. If these measures fail to reduce the dropsy and it has become extreme, the skin may be punctured with a lancet or drained by a small silver cannula (Southey's tube), which is inserted beneath it. A fine aspirator needle may be used, and the fluid allowed to drain through a piece of long, narrow rubber tubing into a vessel beneath the bed. If the dyspnœa is marked, owing to pressure of fluid in the pleuræ, aspiration should be performed. In rare instances the ascites is extreme and may require paracentesis, or a Southey's tube may be inserted and the fluid gradually withdrawn. If uræmic convulsions occur, the intensity of the paroxysms may be limited by the use of chloroform; to an adult a pilocarpine injection should be at once given, and from a robust, strong man 20 ounces of blood may be withdrawn. In children the loins may be dry cupped, the wet pack used, and a brisk purgative given. Bromide of potassium and chloral sometimes prove useful.

Vomiting may be relieved by ice and by restricting the amount of food. Drop doses of creosote, iodine, and carbolic acid may be given. The dilute hydrocyanic acid with bismuth is often effectual.

The question of the use of diuretics in acute Bright's disease is not yet settled. The best diuretic, after all, is water, which may be taken freely with the citrate of potash or the benzoate of soda, salts which are held to favor the conversion of the urates into less irritating and more easily excreted compounds. Digitalis and strophanthus are useful diuretics, and may be employed without risk when the arterial tension is low and the cardiac impulse is not forcible. I have never seen any injurious effects from their employment after the early symptoms had lessened in intensity.

For the persistent albuminuria, I agree with Roberts and Rosenstein that we have no remedy of the slightest value. Nothing indicates more clearly our helplessness in controlling kidney metabolism than inability to meet this common symptom. Astringents, alkalies, nitroglycerin, and mercury have been recommended.

For the anæmia associated with acute Bright's disease iron should be employed. It should not be given until the acute symptoms have subsided. In the adult it may be used in the form of the perchloride in increasing doses, as convalescence proceeds. In children, the syrup of the iodide of iron or the syrup of the phosphate of iron are better preparations. Tyson has recently urged caution in the too free use of iron in kidney disease. The dilatation of the heart is best treated with digitalis, strophanthus, and strychnia.

In the convalescence from acute Bright's disease, care should be taken to guard the patient against cold. The diet should still consist chiefly of milk and a return to mixed food should be gradual. A change of air is often beneficial, particularly a residence in a warm, equable climate.

VII. CHRONIC BRIGHT'S DISEASE

Here, too, in all forms we deal with a diffuse process, involving epithelial, interstitial, and glomerular tissues. Clinically two groups are recognized—(*a*) the chronic parenchymatous nephritis, which follows the acute attack or comes on insidiously, is characterized by marked dropsy, and post mortem by the *large white kidney.* In the later stages of this process the kidney may be smaller—a condition known as the *small white kidney;* (*b*) chronic interstitial nephritis, in which dropsy is not common and the cardio-vascular changes are pronounced. Delafield recognizes a chronic diffuse nephritis with exudation and a chronic productive diffuse nephritis without exudation, the latter corresponding to the contracted kidney of authors.

The amyloid kidney is usually spoken of as a variety of Bright's disease, but in reality it is a degeneration which may accompany any form of nephritis.

1. CHRONIC PARENCHYMATOUS NEPHRITIS

(*Chronic Desquamative and Chronic Tubal Nephritis; Chronic Diffuse Nephritis with Exudation*)

Etiology.—In many cases the disease follows the acute nephritis of cold, scarlet fever, or pregnancy. More frequently than is usually stated the disease has an insidious onset and occurs independently of any acute attack. The fevers may play an important rôle in certain of these cases. Rosenstein, Bartels, I. E. Atkinson, and Thayer have laid special stress upon malaria as a cause. The use of alcohol is believed to lead to this form of nephritis. In chronic suppuration, syphilis, and tuberculosis the diffuse parenchymatous nephritis is not uncommon, and is usually associated with amyloid disease. Males are rather more subject to the affection than females. It is met with most commonly in young adults, and is by no means infrequent in children as a sequence of scarlatinal nephritis.

Morbid Anatomy.—Several varieties of this form have been recognized. The *large white kidney* of Wilks, in which the organ is enlarged, the capsule is thin, and the surface white with the stellate veins injected, is not very common in America. On section the cortex is swollen and yellowish white in color, and often presents opaque areas. The pyramids may be deeply congested. On microscopic examination it is seen that the epithelium is granular and fatty, and the tubules of the cortex are distended, and contain tube casts. Hyaline changes are also present in the epithelial cells. The glomeruli are large, the capsules thickened, the capillaries show hyaline changes, and the epithelium of the tuft and of the capsule is extensively altered. The interstitial tissue is everywhere increased, though not to an extreme degree.

The second variety of this form results from the gradual increase in the connective tissue and the subsequent shrinkage, forming what is called the *small white kidney* or the pale granular kidney. It is doubtful whether this is always preceded by the large white kidney. Some observers hold that it may be a primary independent form. The capsule is thickened and the surface is rough and granular. On section the resistance is greatly increased, the cortex is reduced and presents numerous opaque white or whitish yellow foci, consisting of accumulations of fatty epithelium in the convoluted tubules. This combination of contracted kidney with the areas of marked fatty degeneration has given the name of small granular fatty kidney to this form. The interstitial changes are marked, many of the glomeruli are destroyed, the degeneration of epithelium in the convoluted tubules is widespread, and the arteries are greatly thickened.

Belonging to this chronic tubal nephritis is a variety known as the *chronic hæmorrhagic nephritis,* in which the organs are enlarged, yellowish white in color, and in the cortex are many brownish red areas, due to hæmorrhage into and about the tubes. In other respects the changes are identical with those in the large white kidney.

Of changes in the other organs the most marked are thickening of the blood vessels and hypertrophy of the left heart.

Symptoms.—Following an acute nephritis, the disease may present, in a modified way, the symptoms of that affection. In many cases it sets in insidiously, and after an attack of dyspepsia or a period of failing health and loss of strength the patient becomes pale, and puffiness of the eyelids or swollen feet are noticed in the morning.

The symptoms are as follows: The urine is, as a rule, diminished in quantity, averaging 500 c. c., often scanty. It has a dirty yellow, sometimes smoky, color, and is turbid from the presence of urates. On standing, a heavy sediment falls, in which are found numerous tube casts of various forms and sizes, hyaline, both large and small, epithelial, granular, and fatty casts. Leucocytes are abundant; red blood-corpuscles are frequently met with, and epithelium from the kidneys and pelves. The albumin is abundant and may be from 4 to 6 per cent. It is more abundant in the urine passed during the day. The specific gravity may be high in the early stages—from 1.020 to 1.025, even 1.040—though in the later stages it is lower. The urea is always reduced in quantity. As the case improves from 5 to 6 litres of urine a day may be voided.

Dropsy is a marked and obstinate symptom of this form of Bright's disease. The face is pale and puffy, and in the morning the eyelids are œdematous. The anasarca is general, and there may be involvement of the serous sacs. In these chronic cases associated with large white kidney there is often a distinctive appearance in the face; the complexion is pasty, the pallor marked, and the eyelids are œdematous. The dropsy is peculiarly obstinate. Uræmic symptoms are common, though convulsions are perhaps less frequent than in the interstitial nephritis.

The tension of the pulse is usually increased; the vessels ultimately become stiff and the heart hypertrophied, though there are instances of this form of nephritis in which the heart is not enlarged. The aortic second sound is accentuated. Retinal changes, though less frequent than in the chronic interstitial nephritis, occur in a considerable number of cases.

Gastro-intestinal symptoms are common. Vomiting is frequently a distressing and serious symptom, and diarrhœa may be profuse. Ulceration of the colon may occur and prove fatal.

It is sometimes impossible to determine, even by the most careful examination of the urine or by analysis of the symptoms, whether the condition of the kidney is that of the large white or of the small white form. In cases, however, which have lasted for several years, with the progressive increase in the renal connective tissue and the cardio-vascular changes, the clinical picture may approach, in certain respects, that of the contracted kidney. The urine is increased, with low specific gravity. It is often turbid, may contain traces of blood, the tube casts are numerous and of every variety of form and size, and the albumin is abundant. Dropsy is usually present, though not so extensive as in the early stages.

Prognosis.—The prognosis is extremely grave. In a case which has persisted for more than a year recovery rarely takes place. Death is caused either by great effusion with œdema of the lungs, by uræmia, or by secondary inflammation of the serous membranes. Occasionally in children, even when the disease has persisted for two years, the symptoms disappear and recovery takes place.

Treatment.—Essentially the same treatment should be carried out as in acute Bright's disease. Milk or buttermilk should constitute for a time the chief article of food. Later more food may be allowed, oysters, fresh vegetables, and fruit. The dropsy should be treated by the hot baths, and a salt-free diet. Iron preparations should be given when there is marked anæmia. It is to be remembered that the pallor of the face may not be a good index of the blood condition. The acetate of potash, digitalis, and diuretin are useful in increasing the flow of urine. Basham's mixture given in plenty of water will be found beneficial.

2. CHRONIC INTERSTITIAL NEPHRITIS

(*Secondary Contracted Kidney; Red Granular Kidney; Gouty Kidney; Arterio-sclerotic Kidney; Senile Kidney*)

Etiology and Morbid Anatomy.—Sclerosis of the kidney is met with (*a*) as a sequence of the large white kidney, forming the so-called pale granular or secondary contracted kidney; (*b*) as a primary independent affection, the red granular kidney; (*c*) as a sequence of arterio-sclerosis; and (*d*) as a senile change.

(*a*) Secondary Form.—The small white kidney, as it is called, has already been described as a sequel to chronic parenchymatous nephritis.

(*b*) In the primary form, known also as the red granular kidney, the organ is smaller than in the secondary interstitial nephritis, the capsule is very adherent, the granulations small, the organ of a reddish brown color, the cysts numerous, the arteries very sclerotic, and the cortex greatly reduced in volume. The chief reason for calling this primary is that one can find no history of previous renal disease. It is met with in the members of gouty families, and there are doubtless hereditary influences at work, for Dickinson reported a remarkable family in which this interstitial nephritis occurred in four generations. Syphilis, alcohol, and overeating are mentioned as contributary causes. Lead is a rare cause in America, but a more common cause in parts of England. It is by no means always easy to differentiate between the secondary and the primary forms. As a rule, the former is paler and not so small. Of 174 cases of chronic interstitial nephritis from my wards which came to autopsy, in 79 the combined weight of the kidneys was about 300 grams, in 57 cases 200 to 300 grams, in 30 cases 150 to 200 grams, and below 150 grams in 8 cases (Emerson). Unilateral nephritis in my experience is extremely rare, not occurring once in the series.

(*c*) ARTERIO-SCLEROTIC KIDNEY.—This is not necessarily a contracted kidney. The organ is very hard, red, and often heavier than normal. Of the cases from my wards, studied by Emerson, in 61 per cent. the combined weight was above 300 grams, and in only 6 per cent. was it below 200 grams. The surface may be smooth or the capsule only slightly thickened and adherent, tearing the substance very little as it is stripped off. In other cases the atrophy is in spots, affecting certain vascular districts, so that there is a large, sunken, deep red patch on the surface, or one pole of the kidney is shrunken, or the process is general in both kidneys, but the resulting contraction gives a warty rather than a granular surface.

(*d*) In the SENILE FORM, met with in the aged, the organs are reduced in size, the capsules thickened and adherent, the pelvic fat much increased, both cortical and pyramidal portions uniformly wasted, and the arteries of the kidney substance very prominent.

Almost invariably associated with chronic interstitial nephritis are general arterio-sclerosis and hypertrophy of the heart. The changes in the arteries will be described elsewhere. In the red granular kidney the left ventricle is specially hypertrophied, but in all forms the heart is greatly enlarged, constituting one of the largest forms met with. In many cases the disease is latent, and the patients die of apoplexy or of acute uræmia. In the arterio-sclerotic form death is more commonly cardiac, and the condition of the kidneys may be entirely overlooked.

Much discussion has taken place as to the association of hypertrophy of the heart and sclerosis of the blood-vessels with the renal changes. A complete solution of the many problems has scarcely yet been offered. Briefly, there are two views—the mechanical and the chemical. Dating from the time of Bright it was thought that the heart had greater difficulty in driving the impure blood through the capillary system. Traube held that the obliteration of a large number of capillary territories in the kidney raised the arterial pressure and in this way led to hypertrophy of the heart. In explanation of the muscular hypertrophy of the walls of the smaller arteries George Johnson introduced the view of a stop-cock action of these vessels under the influence of irritating ingredients in the blood. The mechanical view was thus put by Cohnheim. The activity of the circulation through the kidneys at any moment does not depend upon the need of these organs for blood, but solely upon the amount of material for the urinary secretion existing in the blood. When parts of both kidneys have undergone atrophy, the blood flow in the parts remaining must be as great as it would have been to the whole of the organs, had they been intact; but in order that such a quantity of blood should pass through the restricted capillary area now open to it an excessive pressure is necessary. This can be brought to bear only by the exertion of an increased force on the part of the left ventricle with the maintenance of a corresponding resistance in all other arterial territories. In this way both the high arterial pressure and the cardio-vascular changes are explained.

The chemical view, which has been much discussed of late, supposes the production (*a*) by the kidneys, (*b*) by the supra-renal glands, of certain pressor substances. So far as the kidney is concerned, the observations are by no means in accord. Practically we know only that the kidney does contain substances capable of raising the blood-pressure. According to Bingel those so-called rennin preparations act in a manner very different from adrenalin. In chronic interstitial nephritis there is often hyperplasia of the cortical substance of the supra-renals, and many recent writers have claimed to have discovered in the blood of chronic nephritics an increase in the pressor substances, an adrenalinæmia. Through their influence, from one or both of these sources, the blood-pressure is raised, with the inevitable sequence of hypertrophy of the heart and sclerosis of the arteries. As already mentioned, the question is still under discussion.

Symptoms.—Many cases are latent, and are not recognized until the occurrence of one of the serious or fatal complications. Even an advanced grade of contracted kidney may be compatible with great mental and bodily activity. There may have been no symptoms whatever to suggest to the patient the existence of a serious malady. In other cases the general health is disturbed. The patient complains of lassitude, is sleepless, has to get up at night to micturate; the digestion is disordered, the tongue is furred; there are complaints of headache, failing vision, and breathlessness on exertion.

So complex and varied is the clinical picture of chronic Bright's disease that it will be best to consider the symptoms under the various systems.

Urinary System.—In the *small contracted kidney* polyuria is common. Frequently the patient has to get up two or three times during the night to empty the bladder, and there is increased thirst. It is for these symptoms occasionally that relief is sought. And yet in many cases with very small kidneys this feature has not been present. A careful study of the cases from my wards, of the urine and the anatomical condition, showed that almost no parallelism could be made between the weight of the kidney, its appearance, and the urine it secreted before death. Of the 174 cases with autopsy, in almost a third the renal changes were so slight that the nephritis was not mentioned as a part of the clinical diagnosis (Emerson). The color of the urine is a light yellow, and the specific gravity ranges from 1.005 to 1.012. Persistent low specific gravity is one of the most constant and important features of the disease. Traces of albumin are found, but may be absent at times, particularly in the early morning urine. It is often simply a slight cloudiness, and may be apparent only with the more delicate tests. The sediment is scanty, and in it a few hyaline or granular casts are found. The quantity of the solid constituents of the urine is, as a rule, diminished, though in some instances the urea may be excreted in full amount. In attacks of dyspepsia or bronchitis, or in the later stages when the heart fails, the quantity of albumin may be greatly increased and the urine diminished. Occasionally blood occurs in the urine, and there may even be hæmaturia (S. West). Slight leakage, represented by the constant presence of a few red cells, may be present early in the disease and persist for years. In the *arterio-sclerotic form* the quantity of urine is normal, or reduced rather than increased; the specific gravity is normal or high, the color of the urine is good, and there are hyaline and finely granular casts. The amount of albumin varies greatly with the food and exercise, and is usually much in excess of that seen with the contracted kidneys, and does not show so often the albumin free intervals of that form, also it is more common to find albumin without casts, while in the contracted kidney casts may occur without albumin.

Circulatory System.—The pulse is hard, the tension increased, and the vessel wall, as a rule, thickened. As already mentioned, a distinction must be made between increased tension and thickening of the arterial wall. The tension may be plus in a normal vessel, but in chronic Bright's disease it is more common to have increased tension in a stiff artery.

A pulse of increased tension has the following characters: It is hard and incompressible, requiring a good deal of force to overcome it; it is persistent, and in the intervals between the beats the vessel feels full and can be rolled beneath the finger. These characters may be present in a vessel the walls of which are little, if at all, increased in thickness. To estimate the latter the pulse wave should be obliterated in the radial, and the vessel wall felt beyond it. In a perfectly normal vessel the arterial coats, under these circumstances, can not be differentiated from the surrounding tissue; whereas, if thickened, the vessel can be rolled beneath the finger. Persistent high blood pressure is one of the earliest and most important symptoms of interstitial nephritis. During the disease the pressure may rise to 250 mm. or even 300 mm. With dropsy and cardiac dilatation the pressure may fall, but not necessarily. The cardiac features are equally important, though often less obvious. Hypertrophy of the left ventricle occurs to overcome the resistance offered in the arteries. The enlargement of the heart ultimately becomes more general. The apex is displaced downward and to the left; the impulse is forcible and may be heaving. In elderly persons with emphysema the displacement of the apex may not be evident. The first sound at the apex may be duplicated; more commonly the second sound at the aortic cartilage is accentuated, a very characteristic sign of increased tension. The sound in extreme cases may have a bell-like quality. In many cases a systolic murmur develops at the apex, probably as a result of relative insufficiency. It may be loud and transmitted to the axilla. Finally the hypertrophy fails, the heart becomes dilated, gallop rhythm is present, and the general condition is that of a chronic heart-lesion. In the arterio-sclerotic form the picture may be cardiac from beginning to close—dyspnœa and signs of dilated heart.

Respiratory System.—Sudden œdema of the glottis may occur. Effusion into the pleuræ or sudden œdema of the lungs may prove fatal. Acute pleurisy and pneumonia are not uncommon. Bronchitis is a frequent accompaniment, particularly in the winter. Sudden attacks of oppressed breathing, particularly at night, are not infrequent. This is often a uræmic symptom, but is sometimes cardiac. The patient may sit up in bed and gasp for breath, as in true asthma. Cheyne-Stokes breathing may be present, most commonly toward the close, but the patient may be walking about and even attending to his occupation.

Digestive System.—Dyspepsia and loss of appetite are common. Severe and uncontrollable vomiting may be the first symptom. This is usually regarded as a manifestation of uræmia, but it may occur without any other indications, and I have known it to prove fatal without any suspicion that chronic Bright's disease was present. Severe and even fatal diarrhœa may develop. The tongue may be coated and the breath heavy and urinous.

NERVOUS SYSTEM.—Various cerebral manifestations have already been mentioned under uræmia. Headache, sometimes of the migraine type, may be an early and persistent feature of chronic Bright's disease. Cerebral apoplexy is closely related to interstitial nephritis. The hæmorrhage may take place into the meninges or the cerebrum. It is usually associated with marked changes in the vessels. Neuralgias, in various regions, are not uncommon.

SPECIAL SENSES.—Troubles in vision may be the first symptom of the disease. It is remarkable in how many cases of interstitial nephritis the condition is diagnosed first by the ophthalmic surgeon. The flame shaped retinal hæmorrhages are the most common. Less frequent is diffuse retinitis or papillitis. Sudden blindness may supervene without retinal changes—uræmic amaurosis. Diplopia is a rare event. Recurring conjunctival and palpebral hæmorrhages are fairly common, particularly in the arterio-sclerotic form. Auditory troubles are by no means infrequent in chronic Bright's disease. Ringing in the ears, with dizziness, is not uncommon. Various forms of deafness may occur. Epistaxis is not infrequent, either alone, or of a severe type in association with purpura.

SKIN.—Œdema is not common in interstitial nephritis. Slight puffiness of the ankles may be present, but in a majority of the cases dropsy does not supervene. When extensive, it is almost always the result of gradual failure of the hypertrophied heart. The skin is often dry and pale, and sweats are not common. In some instances the sweat may deposit a white frost of urea on the surface of the skin. Eczema is a common accompaniment of chronic interstitial nephritis. Tingling of the fingers or numbness and pallor—the dead fingers—are not, as some suppose, in any way peculiar to Bright's disease. Intolerable itching of the skin may be present, and cramps in the muscles are by no means rare.

Hæmorrhages are not infrequent; epistaxis may prove serious and extensive; purpura may occur. Broncho-pulmonary hæmorrhages are said, by some French writers, to be common, but no instance of it has come under my observation. Ascites is rare except in association with cirrhosis of the liver.

Diagnosis.—The autopsy often discloses the true nature of the disease, one of the many intercurrent affections of which may have proved fatal. The early stages of interstitial nephritis are not recognizable. In a patient with increased pulse tension (particularly if the vessel wall is sclerotic), with the apex beat of the heart dislocated to the left, the second aortic sound ringing and accentuated, the urine abundant and of low specific gravity, with a trace of albumin and an occasional hyaline or granular cast, the diagnosis of interstitial nephritis may be safely made. Of all the indications, that offered by the pulse is the most important. Persistent high tension with thickening of the arterial wall in a man under fifty means that serious mischief has already taken place, that cardio-vascular changes are certainly, and renal most probably, present. In the arterio-sclerotic cases the history is of the "strenuous life"—work, alcohol, tobacco, Venus—and not of an infection or of lead or gout. The urine is not of persistently low specific gravity, there may be little or no albumin except in intercurrent attacks; the symptoms are cardiac rather than renal or cerebral; the ocular changes are hæmorrhagic, not the true albuminuric retinitis

Prognosis.—Chronic Bright's disease is an incurable affection, and the anatomical conditions on which it depends are quite as much beyond the reach of medicines as wrinkled skin or gray hair. Interstitial nephritis, however, is compatible with the enjoyment of life for many years, and it is now universally recognized that increased tension, thickening of the arterial walls, and polyuria with a small quantity of albumin, neither doom a man to death within a short time nor necessarily interfere with the pursuits of an active life so long as proper care be taken. I know patients who have had high tension and a little albumin in the urine with hyaline casts for ten, twelve, or even fifteen years. Serious indications are the occurrence of uræmic symptoms, dilatation of the heart, the onset of serous effusions, the onset of Cheyne-Stokes breathing, persistent vomiting, and diarrhœa. The phenolsulphonephthalein test gives valuable information as to the functional capacity of the kidneys and is a material aid in prognosis.

Treatment.—Patients without local indications or in whom the condition has been accidentally discovered should so regulate their lives as to throw the least possible strain upon heart, arteries, and kidneys. A quiet life without mental worry, with gentle but not excessive exercise, and residence in an equable climate, should be recommended. In addition they should be told to keep the bowels regular, the skin active by a daily tepid bath with friction, and the urinary secretion free by drinking daily a definite amount of either distilled water or some pleasant mineral water. Alcohol should be strictly prohibited. Tea and coffee are allowable.

The diet should be light and nourishing, and the patient should be warned not to eat excessively, and not to take meat more than once a day. Care in food and drink is probably the most important element in the treatment of these early cases.

A patient in good circumstances may be urged to go away during the winter months, or, if necessary, to move altogether to a warm equable climate, like that of Southern California. There is no doubt of the value in these cases of removal from the changeable, irregular weather which prevails in the temperate regions from November until April.

At this period medicines are not required unless for certain special symptoms. Patients derive much benefit from an annual visit to certain mineral springs, such as Poland, Bedford, Saratoga, in America, and Vichy and others in Europe. Mineral waters have no curative influence upon chronic Bright's disease; they simply help the interstitial circulation and keep the drains flushed. In this early stage, when the patient's condition is good, the tension not high, and the quantity of albumin small, medicines are not indicated, since no remedies are known to have the slightest influence upon the progress of the disease. Sooner or later SYMPTOMS arise which demand treatment. Of these the following are the most important:

(*a*) *Greatly Increased Arterial Tension.*—It is to be remembered that a certain increase of tension is not only necessary but unavoidable in chronic Bright's disease, and probably the most serious danger is too great lowering of the blood tension. The happy medium must be sought between such heightened tension as throws a serious strain upon the heart and risks rupture of the vessels and the low tension which, under these circumstances, is specially liable to be associated with serous effusions. In cases with persistent high tension the diet should be light, an occasional saline purge should be given, and sweating promoted by means of hot air or the hot bath. If these measures do not suffice, nitroglycerin may be tried, beginning with 1 minim of the 1-per-cent. solution three times a day, and gradually increasing the dose if necessary. Patients vary so much in susceptibility to this drug that in each case it must be tested, the limit of dosage being that at which the patient experiences the physiological effect. As much as 10 minims of the 1-per-cent. solution may be given three times a day. In many cases I have given it in much larger doses for weeks at a time. I have never seen any ill effects from it. If the dose is excessive the patients complain at once of flushing or headache. Its use may be kept up for six or seven weeks, then stopped for a week and resumed. Its value is seen not only in the reduction of the tension, but also in the striking manner in which it relieves the headache, dizziness, and dyspnœa. The sodium nitrite may be given in doses of grs. ii-v (0.13 to 0.3 gm.) three times a day.

(*b*) More or less *anæmia* is present in advanced cases, and is best met by the use of iron. Weir Mitchell, who had a unique experience in certain forms of chronic Bright's disease, gave the tincture of the perchloride of iron in large doses—from half a drachm to a drachm three times a day. He thought that it not only benefits the anæmia, but that it also is an important means of reducing the arterial tension.

(*c*) Many patients with Bright's disease present themselves for treatment with signs of cardiac dilatation; there is a gallop rhythm or the heart-sounds have a fetal character, the breath is short, the urine scanty and highly albuminous, and there are signs of local dropsy. In these cases the treatment must be directed to the heart. A morning dose of salts or calomel may be given, and digitalis in 10-minim doses, three or four times a day. Strychnia may be used with benefit in this condition. In some instances other cardiac tonics may be necessary, but as a rule the digitalis acts promptly and well.

(*d*) *Uræmic Symptoms.*—Even before marked manifestations are present there may be extreme restlessness, mental wandering, a heavy, foul breath, and a coated tongue. Headache is not often complained of, though intense frontal headache may be an early symptom of uræmia. In this condition, too, the patient may complain of palpitation, feelings of numbness, and sometimes nocturnal cramps. For these symptoms the saline purgatives should be ordered, and hot baths, so as to induce copious sweating. Grandin states that irrigation of the bowel with water at a temperature from 120° to 150° is most useful. Nitroglycerin also may be used to reduce the tension. For the uræmic convulsions, if severe, inhalations of chloroform may be used. If the patient is robust and full-blooded, from 12 to 20 ounces of blood should be removed. The patient should be freely sweated, and if the convulsions tend to recur chloral may be given, either by the mouth or per rectum, or, better still, morphia. Uræmic coma must be treated by active purgation, and sweating should be promoted by the use of pilocarpine or the hot bath. For the restlessness and delirium morphia is indispensable. Since its recommendation in uræmic states some years ago, by Stephen MacKenzie, I have used this remedy extensively and can speak of its great value in these cases. I have never seen ill effects or any tendency to coma follow. It is of special value in the dyspnœa and Cheyne-Stokes breathing of advanced arterio-sclerosis with chronic uræmia.

SURGICAL TREATMENT.—Edebohls introduced the operation of decapsultation of the kidneys in Bright's disease in order to establish new vascular connections, and so influence the nutrition and work of the organs. In his work records are given of 72 cases; 7 died within two weeks, 22 died at periods more or less remote, 3 disappeared from observation, and 40 were known to be living—one eleven years and eight months after the operation. As Edebohls said the difficult thing to determine is the existence of chronic Bright's disease before operation. No case should be regarded as such on the urine examination alone. The cardio-vascular condition and the retinæ should be studied. There is probably a small group of suitable cases—the subacute and chronic forms which follow the acute infections—in which the outlook is hopeless from medical treatment.

VIII. AMYLOID DISEASE

Amyloid (lardaceous or waxy) degeneration of the kidneys is simply an event in the process of chronic Bright's disease, most commonly in the chronic parenchymatous nephritis following fevers, or of cachectic states. It has no claim to be regarded as one of the varieties of Bright's disease. The affection of the kidneys is generally a part of a widespread amyloid degeneration occurring in prolonged suppuration, as in disease of the bone, in syphilis, tuberculosis, and occasionally leukæmia, lead poisoning, and gout. It varies curiously in frequency in different localities.

Anatomically the amyloid kidney is large and pale, the surface smooth, and the venæ stellatæ well marked. On section the cortex is large and may show a peculiar glistening, infiltrated appearance, and the glomeruli are very distinct. The pyramids, in striking contrast to the cortex, are of a deep red color. A section soaked in dilute tincture of iodine shows spots of a walnut or mahogany brown color. The Malpighian tufts and the straight vessels may be most affected. In lardaceous disease of the kidneys the organs are not always enlarged. They may be normal in size or small, pale, and granular. The amyloid change is first seen in the Malpighian tufts, and then involves the afferent and efferent vessels and the straight vessels. It may be confined entirely to them. In later stages of the disease the tubules are affected, chiefly the membrane, rarely, if ever, the cells themselves.

Symptoms.—The renal features alone may not indicate the presence of this degeneration. Usually the associated condition gives a hint of the nature of the process. The urine, as a rule, shows important changes; the quantity is increased, and it is pale, clear, and of low specific gravity. The albumin is usually abundant, but it may be scanty, and in rare instances absent. Possibly the variations in the situation of the amyloid changes may account for this, since albumin is less likely to be present when the change is confined to the vasa recta. In addition to ordinary albumin globulin may be present. The tube casts are variable, usually hyaline, often fatty or finely granular. Occasionally the amyloid reaction can be detected in the hyaline casts. Dropsy is present in many instances, particularly when there is much anæmia or profound cachexia. It is not, however, an invariable symptom, and there are cases in which it does not develop. Diarrhœa is a common accompaniment.

Increased arterial tension and cardiac hypertrophy are not usually present, except in those cases in which amyloid degeneration occurs in the secondary contracted kidney; under which circumstances there may be uræmia and retinal changes, which, as a rule, are not met with in other forms.

Diagnosis.—By the condition of the urine alone it is not possible to recognize amyloid changes in the kidney. Usually, however, there is no difficulty, since the Bright's disease comes on in association with syphilis, prolonged suppuration, disease of the bone, or tuberculosis, and there is evidence of enlargement of the liver and spleen. A suspicious circumstance is the existence of polyuria with a large amount of albumin in the urine and few casts, or when, in these constitutional affections, a large quantity of clear, pale urine is passed, even without the presence of albumin.

The prognosis depends rather on the condition with which the nephritis is associated. As a rule it is grave.

IX. PYELITIS

(*Consecutive Nephritis; Pyelonephritis; Pyonephrosis*)

Definition.—Inflammation of the pelvis of the kidney and the conditions which result from it.

Etiology.—Pyelitis in almost all cases is induced by bacterial invasion and multiplication, rarely by the irritation of various substances such as turpentine, cubebs, or sugar (diabetes). Normally the kidney can eliminate without harm to itself, apparently, various bacteria carried to it by the blood-current from the intestinal tract or some focus of infection; and it probably becomes infected only when its resistance is lowered, as a result of some general cause, as anæmia, malnutrition, or intercurrent disease, or of some local cause, as nephritis, displacement, congestion due to pressure of neoplasms upon the ureter, twisted ureter (Dietl's crisis), or of operation, or when the number or virulence of the micro-organisms is increased. These same factors probably play an important rôle also in the other common causes of pyelitis, ascending infection from an infected bladder (cystitis), and tuberculous infection. Other causes described are various fevers, cancer, hydatids, the ova of certain parasites, cold, and overexertion. Calculus seems not to be a common cause. It is a not uncommon complication of pregnancy (French). In T. R. Brown's series of 20 cases the colon bacillus was obtained 7 times, the tubercle bacillus 6, the proteus bacillus 4, a white staphylococcus twice, while in 1 case cultures were negative.

Morbid Anatomy.—In the early stages of pyelitis the mucous membrane is turbid, somewhat swollen, and may show ecchymoses or a grayish pseudomembrane. The urine in the pelvis is cloudy, and, on examination, numbers of epithelial cells are seen.

In the calculous pyelitis there may be only slight turbidity of the membrane, which has been called by some catarrhal pyelitis. More commonly the mucosa is roughened, grayish in color, and thick. Under these circumstances there is almost always more or less dilatation of the calyces and flattening of the papillæ. Following this condition there may be (*a*) extension of the suppurative process to the kidney itself, forming a pyelonephritis; (*b*) a gradual dilatation of the calyces with atrophy of the kidney substance, and finally the production of the condition of pyonephrosis, in which the entire organ is represented by a sac of pus with or without a thin shell of renal tissue. (*c*) After the kidney structure has been destroyed by suppuration, if the obstruction at the orifice of the pelvis persists, the fluid portions may be absorbed and the pus become inspissated, so that the organ is represented by a series of sacculi containing grayish, putty like masses, which may become impregnated with lime salts.

Tuberculous pyelitis, as already described, usually starts upon the apices of the pyramids, and may at first be limited in extent. Ultimately the condition produced may be similar to that of calculous pyelitis. Pyonephrosis is quite as frequent a sequence, while the final transformation of the pus into a putty-like material impregnated with salts, forming the so-called scrofulous kidney, is even commoner.

The pyelitis consecutive to cystitis is generally bilateral, and the kidneys are sometimes involved, forming the so-called *surgical kidneys*—acute suppurative nephritis. There are lines of suppuration extending along the pyramids, or small abscesses in the cortex, often just beneath the capsule; or there may be wedge shaped abscesses. The pus organisms either pass up the tubules or, as Steven has shown, through the lymphatics.

Symptoms.—The forms associated with the fevers rarely cause any symptoms, even when the process is extensive. In mild grades there is pain in the back or there may be tenderness on deep pressure on the affected side. The urine, turbid and containing pus cells, some mucus, and occasional red blood-cells, is acid or alkaline, depending on the infecting microbe; usually the albuminuria is of higher grade comparatively than the pyuria.

Before the condition of pyuria is established there may be attacks of pain on the affected side (not reaching the severe agony of renal colic), rigors, high fever, and sweats. Under these circumstances the urine, which may have been clear, becomes turbid or smoky from the presence of blood, and may contain large numbers of mucus cells and transitional epithelium.

The statement is not infrequently made that the epithelium in the urine in pyelitis is distinctive and characteristic. This is erroneous, as may be readily demonstrated by comparing scrapings of the mucosa of the renal pelvis and of the bladder. In both the epithelium belongs to what is called the transitional variety, and in both regions the same conical, fusiform, and irregular cells with long tails are found, and yet in pyelitis more of these tailed cells occur, for in cystitis one must often search long for them.

When the pyelitis, whether calculous or tuberculous, has become chronic and discharges, the symptoms are:

(*a*) *Pyuria.*—The pus is in variable amount, and may be intermittent. Thus, as is often the case when only one kidney is involved, the ureter may be temporarily blocked, and normal urine is passed for a time; then there is a sudden outflow of the pent up pus and the urine becomes purulent. Coincident with this retention, a tumor mass may be felt on the side affected. The pus has the ordinary characters, but the transitional epithelium is not so abundant at this stage and comes from the bladder or from the pelvis of the healthy side. Occasionally, in rapidly advancing pyelonephritis, portions of the kidney tissue, particularly of the apices of the pyramids, may slough away and appear in the urine; or, as in a remarkable specimen shown to me by Tyson, solid cheesy moulds of the calyces are passed. Casts from the kidney tubules are sometimes present. The reaction of the urine depends entirely upon the infecting microbe, whether the condition is unilateral or bilateral, and whether the bladder is also infected, when vesical irritability and frequent micturition may be present. Polyuria is usually present in the chronic cases.

(*b*) Intermittent fever associated with rigors is usually present in cases of suppurative pyelitis. The chills may recur at regular intervals, and the cases are often mistaken for malaria. Owen-Rees called attention to the frequent occurrence of these rigors, which form a characteristic feature of both calculous and tuberculous pyelitis. Ultimately the fever assumes a hectic type and the rigors may cease.

(*c*) The general condition of the patient often indicates prolonged suppuration. There is more or less wasting with anæmia and a progressive failure of health. Secondary abscesses may develop and the clinical picture becomes that of pyæmia. In some instances, particularly of tuberculous pyelitis, the clinical course may resemble that of typhoid fever. There are instances of pyuria recurring, at intervals, for many years without impairment of the bodily vigor. Some of the chronic cases have practically no discomfort.

(*d*) Physical examination in chronic pyelitis usually reveals tenderness on the affected side or a definite swelling, which may vary much in size and ultimately attain large dimensions if the kidney becomes enormously distended, as in pyonephrosis.

(*e*) Occasionally nervous symptoms, which may be associated with dyspnœa, supervene, or the termination may be by coma, not unlike that of diabetes. These have been attributed to the absorption of the decomposing materials in the urine, whence the so-called ammoniæmia. A form of paraplegia has been described in connection with some cases of abscess of the kidney, but whether due to a myelitis or to a peripheral neuritis has not yet been determined.

In suppurative nephritis or surgical kidney following cystitis, the patient complains of pain in the back, the fever becomes high, irregular, and associated with chills, and in acute cases a typhoid state may precede the fatal event.

Diagnosis.—Between the tuberculous and the calculous forms of pyelitis it may be difficult or impossible to distinguish, except by the detection of tubercle bacilli in the pus. The examination for bacilli should be made systematically, and in suspicious cases intraperitoneal injections of guinea-pigs should also be made. From perinephric abscess pyonephrosis is distinguished by the more definite character of the tumor, the absence of œdematous swelling in the lumbar region, and, most important of all, the history of the case. The urine, too, in perinephric abscess may be free from pus. There are cases, however, in which it is difficult indeed to make a satisfactory diagnosis.

Suppurative pyelitis and cystitis are apt to be confounded, and perineal section is not infrequently performed on the supposition of the existence of the latter. The two conditions may, of course, coexist and prove puzzling, but the history, the higher relative grade of albuminuria in pyelitis, the polyuria, the mode of development, the local signs in one lumbar region, and the absence of pain in the bladder should be sufficient to differentiate the affections. By catheterization of the ureters, it may be definitely determined whether the pus comes from the kidneys or from the bladder. The cystoscope may be used for this purpose.

Much may be done with X-ray examinations to determine the condition of the pelves of the kidneys. When a 2-per-cent. solution of collargol is injected by means of the ureteral catheter a shadow is cast giving a very accurate outline of the pelvis of the organ.

Prognosis.—Cases coming on during the fevers usually recover. Tuberculous pyelitis may terminate favorably by inspissation of the pus and conversion into a putty-like substance with deposition of lime salts. With pyonephrosis the dangers are increased. Perforation may occur into the peritoneum, the patient may be worn out by the hectic fever, or amyloid disease may develop.

Treatment.—Fluids should be taken freely, particularly the alkaline mineral waters, to which potassium citrate may be added.

The treatment of the calculous form will be considered later. Practically there are no remedies which have much influence upon the pyuria. Some of the urinary antiseptics seem to be of value, especially in the acute cases. Urotropin should be given in full doses (gr. xv, 1 gm., three or four times a day); watch should be kept for signs of irritation and the dose reduced if they appear. Vaccine therapy is sometimes of value. Tonics should be given, a nourishing diet, and milk and butter-milk may be taken freely. When the tumor has formed or even before it is perceptible, if the symptoms are serious and severe, the kidney should be explored, and, if necessary, nephrotomy or nephrectomy should be performed.

X. HYDRONEPHROSIS

Definition.—Dilatation of the pelvis and calyx of the kidney with atrophy of its substance, caused by the accumulation of non-purulent fluids, the result of obstruction.

Etiology.—The condition may be congenital, owing to some abnormality in the ureter or urethra. The tumor produced may be large enough to retard labor. Sometimes it is associated with other malformations. There is a condition of moderate dilatation, apparently congenital, which is not connected with any obstruction in the ducts.

In some instances there has been contraction or twisting of the ureter, or it has been inserted into the kidney at an acute angle or at a high level. In adult life the condition may be due to lodgment of a calculus, or to a cicatricial stricture following ulcer.

There is a remarkable condition of hypertrophy and dilatation of the bladder and ureters associated with congenital defect of the abdominal muscles. The bladder may form a large abdominal tumor and the ureters may be as large and visible as coils of the small intestine.

New growths, such as tubercle or cancer, occasionally induce hydronephrosis; more commonly, pressure upon the ureter from without, particularly tumors of the ovaries and uterus. Occasionally cicatricial bands compress the ureter. Obstruction within the bladder may result from cancer, from hypertrophy of the prostate with cystitis, and in the urethra from stricture. It is stated that slight grades of hydronephrosis have been found in patients with excessive polyuria.

In whatever way produced, when the ureter is blocked the secretion accumulates in the pelvis and infundibula. Sometimes acute inflammation follows, but more commonly the slow, gradual pressure causes atrophy of the papillæ with gradual distention and wasting of the organ. In acquired cases from pressure, even when dilatation is extreme, there may usually be seen a thin layer of renal structure. In the most extreme stages the kidney is represented by a large cyst, which may perhaps show on its inner surface imperfect septa. The fluid is thin and yellowish in color, and contains traces of urinary salts, urea, uric acid, and sometimes albumin. The secretion may be turbid from admixture with small quantities of pus.

Total occlusion does not always lead to a hydronephrosis, but may be followed by atrophy of the kidney. It appears that when the obstruction is intermittent or not complete the greatest dilatation is apt to follow. The sac may be enormous, and cause an abdominal tumor of the largest size. The condition has even been mistaken for ascites. Enlargement of the other kidney may compensate for the defect. Hypertrophy of the left side of the heart usually follows.

Symptoms.—When small, it may not be noticed. The congenital cases when bilateral usually prove fatal within a few days; when unilateral, the tumor may not be noticed for some time. It increases progressively and has all the characters of a tumor in the renal region. In adult life many of the cases, due to pressure by tumors, as in cancer of the uterus and enlargement of the prostate, etc., give rise to no symptoms.

In *intermittent* hydronephrosis the tumor suddenly disappears with the discharge of a large quantity of clear fluid; the sac gradually refills, and the process may be repeated for years. In these cases the obstruction is unilateral; a cicatricial stricture exists, or a valve is present in the ureter, or the ureter enters the upper part of the pelvis. Many of the cases are in women and associated with movable kidney.

The examination of the abdomen shows, in unilateral hydronephrosis, a tumor occupying the renal region. When of moderate size it is readily recognized, but when large it may be confounded with ovarian or other tumors. In young children it may be mistaken for sarcoma of the kidney or of the retroperitoneal glands, the common cause of abdominal tumor in early life. Aspiration alone would enable us to differentiate between hydronephrosis and tumor. The large hydronephrotic sac is frequently mistaken for ovarian tumor. The latter is, as a rule, more mobile, and rarely fills the deeper portion of the lumbar region so thoroughly. The ascending colon can often be detected passing over the renal tumor, and examination per vaginam, particularly under ether, will give important indications as to the condition of the ovaries. In doubtful cases the sac should be aspirated. The fluid of the renal cyst is clear, or turbid from the presence of cell elements, rarely colloid in character; the specific gravity is low; albumin and traces of urea and uric acid are usually present; and the epithelial elements in it may be similar to those found in the pelvis of the kidney. In old sacs, however, the fluid may not be characteristic, since the urinary salts disappear, but in one case of several years' duration oxalates of lime and urea were found.

Perhaps the greatest difficulty is offered by the condition of hydronephrosis in a movable kidney. Here, the history of sudden disappearance of the tumor with the passage of a large quantity of clear fluid would be a point of great importance in the diagnosis. In those rare instances of an enormous sac filling the entire abdomen, and sometimes mistaken for ascites, the character of the fluid might be the only point of difference. The tumor of pyonephrosis may be practically the same in physical characteristics. Fever is usually present, and pus is often found in the urine. In these cases, when in doubt, exploratory puncture should be made.

The outlook in hydronephrosis depends much upon the cause. When single, the condition may never produce serious trouble, and the intermittent cases may persist for years, and finally disappear. Occasionally the cyst ruptures into the peritoneum, more rarely through the diaphragm into the lung. A remarkable case of this kind was under the care of my colleague, Halsted. A man, aged twenty-one, had, from his second year, attacks of abdominal pain in which a swelling would appear between the hip and costal margin and subside with the passage of a large amount of urine. In January, 1888, the sac discharged through the right lung. Reaccumulations occurred on several occasions, and on June 9, 1891, the sac was opened and drained. He remains well, though there is still a sinus through which a clear, probably urinous, fluid is discharged.

The sac may discharge spontaneously through the ureter and the fluid never reaccumulate. In bilateral hydronephrosis there is a danger that uræmia may supervene. There are instances, too, in which blocking of the ureter on the sound side by calculus has been followed by uræmia. And, lastly, the sac may suppurate, and the condition change to one of pyonephrosis.

Treatment.—Cases of intermittent hydronephrosis which do not cause serious symptoms should be let alone. It is stated that, in sacs of moderate size, the obstruction has been overcome by massage, but, if practiced, it should be done with great care. When the sac reaches a large size aspiration may be performed and repeated if necessary. Puncture should be made in the flank, midway between the ilium and the last rib. If the fluid reaccumulates and the sac becomes large, it may be incised and drained, or, as a last resort, the kidney may be removed. In women a carefully adapted pad and bandage will sometimes prevent the recurrence of an intermittent hydronephrosis.

XI. NEPHROLITHIASIS

(*Renal Calculus*)

Definition.—The formation in the kidney or in its pelvis of concretions, by the deposition of certain of the solid constituents of the urine.

Etiology and Pathology.—In the kidney substance itself the separation of the urinary salts produces a condition to which, unfortunately, the term infarct has been applied. Three varieties may be recognized: (1) The uric acid infarct, usually met with at the apices of the pyramids in new born children and during the first weeks of life. The priapism and attacks of crying in the new-born have been attributed to the passage of these infarcts; (2) the sodium urate infarct, sometimes associated with ammonium urate, which forms whitish lines at the apices of the pyramids and is met with chiefly, but not always, in gouty persons; and (3) the lime infarcts, forming very opaque white lines in the pyramids, usually in old people.

In the pelvis and calyces concretions of the following forms occur: (*a*) Small gritty particles, *renal sand,* ranging in size from the individual grains of the uric acid sediment to bodies 1 or 2 mm. in diameter. These may be passed in the urine for long periods without producing any symptoms, since they are too fine to be arrested in their downward passage.

(*b*) Larger concretions, ranging in size from a small pea to a bean, and either solitary or multiple in the calyces and pelvis. It is the smaller of these calculi which, in their passage, produce the attacks of renal colic. They may be rounded and smooth, or present numerous irregular projections.

(*c*) The dendritic form of calculus. The orifice of the ureter may be blocked by a Y-shaped stone. The pelvis itself may be occupied by the concretion, which forms a more or less distinct mould. These are the remarkable *coral calculi,* which form in the pelvis complete moulds of infundibula and calyces, the latter even presenting cup-like depressions corresponding to the apices of the papillæ. Some of these casts in stone of the renal pelvis are as beautifully moulded as Hyrtl's corrosion preparations.

Chemically the varieties of calculi are: (1) Uric acid and urates, most important, and forming the renal sand, the small solitary, or the large dendritic stones. They are very hard, the surface is smooth, and the color reddish. The larger stones are usually stratified and very dense. Usually the uric acid and the urates are mixed, but in children stones composed of urates alone may occur.

(2) Oxalate of lime, which forms mulberry-shaped calculi, studded with points and spines. They are often very dark in color, intensely hard, and are a mixture of oxalate of lime and uric acid.

(3) Phosphatic calculi are composed of the calcium phosphate and the ammonio-magnesium phosphate, sometimes mixed with a small amount of calcium carbonate. They are quite common, although the phosphatic salts are often deposited about the uric acid or the calcium oxalate stones.

(4) Rare forms of calculi are made up of cystine, xanthine, carbonate of lime, indigo, and urostealith.

The mode of formation of calculi has been much discussed. They may be produced by an excess of a sparingly soluble abnormal ingredient, such as cystine or xanthine; more frequently by the presence of uric acid in a very acid urine which favors its deposition. Sir William Roberts thus briefly states the conditions which lead to the formation of the uric acid concretions: high acidity, poverty in salines, low pigmentation, and high percentage of uric acid. Ord suggests that albumin, mucus, blood, and epithelial threads may be the starting point of stone. The demonstration of organisms in the centre of renal calculi renders it probable that in many cases the nucleus of the stone is an agglutinated mass of bacteria.

Renal calculi are most common in the early and later periods of life. They are moderately frequent in the United States, but there do not appear to be special districts, corresponding to the "stone counties" in England. Men are more often affected than women. Sedentary occupations seem to predispose to stone.

The effects of the calculi are varied. It is by no means uncommon to find a dozen or more stones of various sizes in the calyces without any destruction of the mucous membrane or dilatation of the pelvis. A turbid urine fills the pelvis, in which there are numerous cells from the epithelial lining. There are cases of this sort in which, apparently, the stones may go on forming and are passed for years without seriously impairing the health and without inconvenience, except the attacks of renal colic. Still more remarkable are the cases of coral like calculi, which may occupy the entire pelvis and calyces without causing pyelitis, but which gradually lead to more or less induration of the kidney. The most serious effects are when the stone excites a suppurative pyelitis and pyonephrosis.

Symptoms.—Patients may pass gravel for years without having an attack of renal colic, and a stone may never lodge in the ureter. In other instances, the formation of calculi goes on year by year and the patient has recurring attacks such as have been so graphically described by Montaigne in his own case. A patient may pass enormous numbers of calculi. A patient may pass a single calculus, and never be troubled again. The large coral calculi may excite no symptoms. In a remarkable specimen of the kind, presented to the McGill Medical Museum by J. A. Macdonald, the patient, a middle-aged woman, died suddenly with uræmic symptoms. There was no pyelitis, but the kidneys were sclerotic.

Renal colic ensues when a stone enters the ureter, or follows an acute pyelitis. An attack may set in abruptly without apparent cause, or may follow a strain in lifting. It is characterized by agonizing pain, which starts in the flank of the affected side, passes down the ureter, and is felt in the testicle and along the inner side of the thigh. The pain may also radiate through the abdomen and chest, and be very intense in the back. In severe attacks there are nausea and vomiting and the patient is collapsed. The perspiration breaks out upon the face and the pulse is feeble and quick. A chill may precede the outbreak, and the temperature may rise as high as 103°. No one has more graphically described an attack of "the stone" than Montaigne,* who was a sufferer for many years: "Thou art seen to sweat with pain, to look pale and red, to tremble, to vomit well-nigh to blood, to suffer strange contortions and convulsions, by starts to let tears drop from thine eyes, to urine thick, black, and frightful water, or to have it suppressed by some sharp and craggy stone, that cruelly pricks and tears thee." From personal experience I can describe three sorts of pain in an attack of renal colic: (*a*) A constant localized, dull pain, the area of which could be covered on the skin of the back in the renal region by a penny piece, and which could be imitated exactly by deep firm pressure on a superficial bone. (*b*) Paroxysms of pain radiating in the course of the ureter or into the flank, and as they increase accompanied by sweating, fainting, and nausea. (*c*) Flushes or

*Essays, Book 111, 13.

rushes of hot pain at intervals, often momentary, usually passing to the back, less often toward the groin. Dozens of these flushes relieved the monotony of (*b*). The symptoms persist for a variable period. In short attacks they do not last longer than an hour; in other instances they continue for a day or more, with temporary relief. Micturition is frequent, occasionally painful, and the urine, as a rule, is bloody. There are instances in which a large amount of clear urine is passed, probably from the other kidney. In rare cases the secretion of urine is completely suppressed, even when the kidney on the opposite side is normal, and death may occur from uræmia. This most frequently happens when the second kidney is extensively diseased, or when only a single kidney exists.

After the attack of colic has passed there is more or less aching on the affected side, and the patient can usually tell from which kidney the stone has come. Examination during the attack is usually negative. Very rarely the kidney becomes palpable. Tenderness on the affected side is common. In very thin persons it may be possible, on examination of the abdomen, to feel the stone in the ureter; or the patient may complain of a grating sensation.

When the calculi remain in the kidney they may produce very definite and characteristic symptoms, of which the following are the most important:

(*a*) *Pain*, usually in the back, which is often no more than a dull soreness, but which may be severe and come on in paroxysms. It is usually on the side affected, but may be referred to the opposite kidney, and there are instances in which the pain has been confined to the sound side. It radiates in the direction of the ureter, and may be felt in the scrotum or even in the penis. Pains of a similar nature may occur in movable kidneys, and there are several instances on record in which surgeons have incised the kidney for stone and found none. In an instance in which pain was present for a couple of years the exploration revealed only a contracted kidney.

(*b*) *Hæmaturia.*—Although this occurs most frequently when the stone becomes engaged in the ureter, it may also come on when the stones are in the pelvis. The bleeding is seldom profuse, as in cancer, but in some instances may persist for a long time. It is aggravated by exertion and lessened by rest. Frequently it only gives to the urine a smoky hue. The urine may be free for days, and then a sudden exertion or a prolonged ride may cause smokiness, or blood may be passed in considerable quantities.

(*c*) *Pyelitis.*—(1) There may be attacks of severe pain in the back, not amounting to actual colic, which are initiated by a heavy chill followed by fever, in which the temperature may reach 104° or 105°, followed by profuse sweating. The urine, which has been clear, may become turbid and smoky and contain blood and abundant epithelium from the pelvis. Attacks of this description may recur at intervals for months or even years, and are generally mistaken for malaria, unless special attention is paid to the urine and to the existence of the pain in the back. This renal intermittent fever, due to the presence of calculi, is analogous to the hepatic intermittent fever, due to gall-stones, and in both it is important to remember that the most intense paroxysms may occur without any evidence of suppuration.

(2) More frequently the symptoms of purulent pyelitis, which have already been described, are present; pain in the renal region, recurring chills, and pus in the urine, with or without indications of pyonephrosis.

(*d*) *Pyuria.*—There are instances of stone in the kidney in which pus occurs continuously or intermittently in the urine for many years.

Patients with stone in the kidney are often robust, high livers, and gouty. Attacks of dyspepsia are not uncommon, or they may have severe headaches.

Diagnosis.—The X-ray picture is rarely at fault, and specialists in this department are becoming more and more skillful, so that mistakes are now rare. Renal may be mistaken for intestinal colic, particularly if the distention of the bowels is marked, or for biliary colic. The situation and direction of the pain, the retraction and tenderness of the testicle, the occurrence of hæmaturia, and the altered character of the urine are distinctive features. Attention may again be called to the fact that attacks simulating renal colic are associated with movable kidney, or even, it has been supposed, without mobility of the kidney, with the accumulation of the oxalates or uric acid in the pelvis of the kidney. The diagnosis between a stone in the kidney and stone in the bladder is not always easy, though in the latter the pain is particularly about the neck of the bladder, and not limited to one side. In the uric acid or uratic renal stone, the urine is acid, thus aiding us in differentiating it from a bladder stone, when alkaline urine is the rule. It is stated that certain differences occur in the symptoms produced by different sorts of calculi. The large uric acid calculi less frequently produce severe symptoms. On the other hand, as the oxalate of lime is a rougher calculus, it is apt to produce more pain (often of a radiating character) than the lithic acid form, and to cause hæmorrhage. In both these forms the urine is acid. The phosphatic calculi are stated to produce the most intense pain, and the urine is commonly alkaline.

Treatment.—In the attacks of renal colic great relief is experienced by the hot bath, which is sometimes sufficient to relax the spasm. When the pain is very intense morphia should be given hypodermically and inhalations of chloroform may be necessary until the effects of the anodyne are manifest. Local applications are sometimes grateful—hot poultices, or cloths wrung out of hot water. The patient may drink freely of hot lemonade, soda water, or barley water. Occasionally change in posture or inversion will give great relief. Surgical interference should be considered in all cases, especially when the stone is large or the associated pyelitis severe.

In the intervals the patient should, as far as possible, live a quiet life, avoiding sudden exertion of all sorts. The essential feature in the treatment is to keep the urine abundant and, in the uric acid or uratic cases, alkaline. The patient should drink daily a large but definite quantity of mineral waters* or distilled water, which is just as satisfactory. The citrate or bicarbonate of potash may be added. The aching pains in the back are often greatly relieved by this treatment. Many patients find benefit from a stay at Saratoga, Bedford, Poland, or other mineral springs in the United States, or at Vichy or Ems in Europe.

The diet should be carefully regulated, and similar to that indicated in the early stages of gout. Sir William Roberts recommends what is known as the solvent treatment for uric acid calculi. The citrate of potash is given in large doses, half a drachm to a drachm, every three hours in a tumblerful of

*Some of these, if we judge by the laudatory reports, are as potent as the waters of Corsena, declared by Montaigne to be "powerful enough to break stones."

water. This should be kept up for several months. I have had no success with this treatment, nor, when one considers the character of the uric acid stones usually met with in the kidney, does it seem likely that any solvent action could be exercised upon them by changes in the urine. This treatment should be abandoned if the urine becomes ammoniacal.

The value of piperazine as a solvent of uric acid gravel or of uric acid stones has been much discussed. While outside the body a watery solution of the drug has this power in a marked degree, the amount excreted in the urine as given in the ordinary doses of 15 grains daily seems to have very little influence. Several observers have shown that the percentage of piperazine excreted in the urine, when taken in doses of from 1 to 2 grams, has, when tested outside of the body, little or no influence as a solvent (Fawcett, Gordon).

XII. TUMORS OF THE KIDNEY

These are benign and malignant. Of the benign tumors, the most common are the small nodular *fibromata* which occur frequently in the pyramids, and occasionally *lipoma, angioma,* or *lymphadenoma.* The *adenomata* may be congenital. In one of my cases the kidneys were greatly enlarged, contained small cysts, and numerous adenomatous structures throughout both organs.

Malignant growths—*cancer* or *sarcoma*—may be either primary or secondary. The sarcomata are the most common, either alveolar sarcoma or the remarkable form containing striped muscular fibres—rhabdomyoma. One of the most common and important renal tumors is the *hypernephroma,* growing in or upon the organ from the adrenal tissue—the aberrant "rests" of Grawitz. Of 163 cases only 6 were extra-renal (Ellis). They may be small and in the renal cortex or form large tumors with extensive metastases, particularly in the lungs. Most of the primary carcinomas and alveolar sarcomas of the kidney are really hypernephromata. Adami holds that they may arise from either renal or adrenal tissues.

The tumors attain a very large size, and almost fill the abdomen. In children they may be enormous. They grow rapidly, are often soft, and hæmorrhage frequently takes place into them. In the sarcomata, invasion of the pelvis or of the renal vein is common. The rhabdomyomata rarely form very large tumors, and death occurs shortly after birth. In one of my cases the child at the age of three years and a half died suddenly of embolism of the pulmonary artery and tricuspid orifice by a fragment of the tumor, which had grown into the renal vein.

Symptoms.—The following are the most important: (*a*) Hæmaturia in one-half the cases, which may be the first indication. The blood is fluid or clotted, and there may be very characteristic moulds of the pelvis of the kidney and of the ureter. It would no doubt be possible for such to form in the hæmaturia from calculus, but I have never met with a case of blood casts of the pelvis and of the ureter, either alone or together, except in cancer. It is rare, indeed, that cancer elements can be recognized in the urine, and yet the diagnosis has been made in this way.

(*b*) Pain is an uncertain symptom. In several of the largest tumors which have come under my observation there has been no discomfort from beginning to close. When present, it is of a dragging, dull character, situated in the flank and radiating down the thigh. The passage of the clots may cause great pain. In one case the growth was at first upward, and the symptoms for some months were those of pleurisy.

(*c*) Progressive emaciation. The loss of flesh is usually marked and advances rapidly. There may, however, be a very large tumor without emaciation.

Physical Signs.—In almost all instances tumor is present. When small and on the right side, it may be very movable; in some instances, occupying a position in the iliac fossa, it has been mistaken for ovarian tumor. The large growths fill the flank and gradually extend toward the middle line, occupying the right or left half of the abdomen. Inspection may show two or three hemispherical projections corresponding to distended sections of the organ. In children the abdomen may reach an enormous size and the veins are prominent and distended. On bimanual palpation the tumor is felt to occupy the lumbar region and can usually be lifted slightly from its bed; in some cases it is very movable, even when large; in others it is fixed, firm, and solid. The respiratory movements have but slight influence upon it. Rapidly growing renal tumors are soft, and on palpation may give a sense of fluctuation. A point of considerable importance is the fact that the colon crosses the tumor, and can usually be detected without difficulty.

Diagnosis.—In children very large abdominal tumors are either renal or retroperitoneal. The retroperitoneal sarcoma (Lobstein's cancer) is more central, but may attain as large a size. If the case is seen only toward the end, a differential diagnosis may be impossible; but, as a rule, the sarcoma is less movable. It is to be remembered that these tumors may invade the kidney. On the left side an enlarged spleen is readily distinguished, as the edge is very distinct and the notch or notches well marked; it descends during respiration, and the colon lies behind, not in front of it. On the right side growths of the liver are occasionally confounded with renal tumors; but such instances are rare, and there can usually be detected a zone of resonance between the upper margin of the renal tumor and the ribs. Late in the disease, however, this is not possible, for the renal tumor is in close union with the liver.

A malignant growth in a movable kidney may be very deceptive and may simulate cancer of the ovary or myoma of the uterus. The great mobility upward of the renal growth and the negative result of examination of the pelvic viscera are the reliable points.

When the growth is small and the patient in good condition removal of the organ may be undertaken, but the percentage of cases of recovery is very small, only 5.4 per cent. (G. Walker).

XIII. CYSTIC DISEASE OF THE KIDNEY

The following varieties of cysts are met with:

Small Cysts.—The small cysts, already described in connection with the chronic nephritis, which result from dilatation of obstructed tubules or of Bowman's capsules. There are cases very difficult to classify, in which the kidneys are greatly enlarged, and very cystic in middle-aged or elderly persons, and yet not so large as in the congenital form.

Solitary Cysts.—Solitary cysts, ranging in size from a marble to an orange, or even larger, are occasionally found in kidneys which present no other changes. In exceptional cases they may form tumors of considerable size. Newman operated on one which contained 25 ounces of blood. They, too, in all probability, result from obstruction.

Polycystic Kidneys.—The polycystic kidneys, in which the greatly enlarged organs, weighing even as much as six pounds, are represented by a conglomeration of cysts, varying in size from a pea to a marble. Little or no renal tissue may be noticeable, although in microscopic sections it is seen that a considerable amount remains in the interspaces. The cysts contain a clear or turbid fluid, sometimes reddish brown or even blackish in color, and may be of a colloidal consistence. Albumin, blood crystals, cholesterin, with triple phosphates and fat drops, are found in the contents. Urea and uric acid are rarely present. The cysts are lined by a flattened epithelium. They occur in the fetus, and sometimes are of such a size as to obstruct labor. In the adult they are usually bilateral, and there is every reason to believe that they begin in early life and increase gradually. Indeed, a progressive growth has been noticed in some cases (Alfred King). They may be found in connection with cystic disease of the liver and other organs. It is difficult to account for the origin of this remarkable condition, which some regard as a defect of development rather than a pathological change, and point to the association in the fetal cases of other anomalies, as imperforate anus. Others believe the condition to be a new growth—a sort of mucoid endothelioma.

It is interesting to note that several members of a family may be affected. I have reported an instance in which mother and son were the subjects of the disease.

Symptoms.—Of five cases which I have seen in adults the condition was recognized during life in four. The features are characteristic.

(*a*) Bilateral tumors in the renal regions, which may increase in size under observation. They may cause great enlargement of the upper zone of the abdomen. The colon and stomach are in front of the tumors, on the surface of which in very thin subjects the cysts may be palpable.

(*b*) Hæmaturia, which may recur at intervals for years.

(*c*) The signs of a chronic interstitial nephritis—(1) pallor or muddy complexion; in rare instances a bronzing of the skin; (2) sclerosis of the arteries; (3) hypertrophy of the heart with accentuated second sound; (4) urine abundant, of low specific gravity, with albumin, and hyaline and granular tube casts, and in one of my cases there were cholesterin crystals. Death occurs from uræmia or the cardio-vascular complications of chronic Bright's disease. A rare event is rupture of a cyst with the formation of a perinephric abscess and peritonitis. In two of my cases the skin became much pigmented.

While both kidneys are, as a rule, involved, one may be much smaller than the other.

Operation, by exposing the kidney and draining the cysts, has been successful. When the condition is unilateral the kidney has been removed and the patients have remained well for years.

Other Varieties.—Occasionally the kidneys and liver present numerous small cysts scattered through the substance. The spleen and the thyroid also may be involved, and there may be congenital malformation of the heart. The cysts in the kidney are small, and neither so numerous nor so thickly set as in the conglomerate form, though in these cases the condition is probably the result of some congenital defect. There are cases, however, in which the kidneys are very large. It is more common in the lower animals than in man. I have seen several instances of it in the hog; in one case the liver weighed 40 pounds, and was converted into a mass of simple cysts. The kidneys were less involved. Charles Kennedy found references to 12 cases of combined cystic disease of the liver and kidneys.

The echinococcus cysts have been described under the section on parasites. Paranephric cysts (external to the capsule) are rare; they may reach a large size.

XIV. PERINEPHRIC ABSCESS

Suppuration in the connective tissue about the kidney may follow (1) blows and injuries; (2) the extension of inflammation from the pelvis of the kidney, the kidney itself, or the ureters; (3) perforation of the bowel, most commonly the appendix, in some instances the colon; (4) extension of suppuration from the spine, as in caries, or from the pleura, as in empyema; (5) as a sequel of the fevers, particularly in children.

Post mortem the kidney is surrounded by pus, particularly at the posterior part, though the pus may lie altogether in front, between the kidney and the peritoneum. Usually the abscess cavity is extensive. The pus is often offensive and may have a distinctly fæcal odor from contact with the large bowel. It may burrow in various directions and burst into the pleura and be discharged through the lungs. A more frequent direction is down the psoas muscle, when it appears in the groin, or it may pass along the iliacus fascia and appear at Poupart's ligament. It may perforate the bowel or rupture into the peritoneum; sometimes it penetrates the bladder or vagina.

Post mortem we occasionally find a condition of *chronic perinephritis* in which the fatty capsule of the kidney is extremely firm, with numerous bands of fibrous tissue, and is stripped off from the proper capsule with the greatest difficulty. Such a condition probably produces no symptoms.

Symptoms.—There may be intense pain, aggravated by pressure, in the lumbar region. In other instances the onset is insidious, without pain in the renal region; on examination signs of deep seated suppuration may be detected. On the affected side there is usually pain, which may be referred to the neighborhood of the hip joint or to the joint itself, or radiate down the thigh and be associated with the retraction of the testis. The patient lies with the thigh flexed, so as to relax the psoas muscle, and in walking throws, as far as possible, the weight on the opposite leg. He also keeps the spine immobile, assumes a stooping posture in walking, and has great difficulty in voluntarily adducting the thigh (Gibney).

There may be pus in the urine if the disease has extended from the pelvis or the kidney, but in other forms the urine is clear. When pus has formed there are usually chills with irregular fever and sweats. On examination, deep seated induration is felt between the last rib and the crest of the ilium. Bimanual palpation may reveal a distinct tumor mass. Œdema or puffiness of the skin is frequently present.

Diagnosis.—The diagnosis is usually easy; when doubt exists the aspirator needle should be used. We can not always differentiate the primary forms from those due to perforation of the kidney or of the bowel. This, however, makes but little difference, for the treatment is identical. It is usually possible by the history and examination to exclude diseases of the vertebra. In children hip-joint disease may be suspected, but the pain is higher, and there is no fullness or tenderness over the hip-joint itself.

Treatment.—The treatment is clear—early, free, and permanent drainage.

SECTION VIII

DISEASES OF THE BLOOD

I. ANÆMIA

Anæmia, a reduction of the amount of blood as a whole or of its corpuscles, or of certain of its constituents, may be due to failure in the manufacture, to increase in the consumption, or to a sudden loss, as in hæmorrhage. Defective formation, hæmatogenesis, is responsible for a large group of what are known as the primary anæmias. Increased destruction, or hæmolysis, is the basis of the majority of all cases in which anæmia is secondary to some existing disease.

Anæmia may be local, confined to certain parts, or general, involving the entire body.

LOCAL ANÆMIA

Tissue irrigation with blood is primarily from the heart, but in all extensive systems of this sort provision is made at the local territories for variations in the supply, according to the needs of a part. The sluices are arranged by means of the stop-cock action of the arteries, which contract or expand under the influence of the vaso-motor ganglia, central and peripheral. If the sluices of one large district are too widely open, so much blood may enter that other important regions have not enough to keep them at work. Local anæmia of the brain, causing swooning, ensues when the mesenteric channels, capable of holding all the blood of the body, are wide open. Emotional stimuli, reflex from pain, etc., removal of pressure, as after tapping in ascites, may cause this. It is probable that many of the nervous and other symptoms in enteroptosis are due to the relative anæmia of the cerebral and spinal systems, owing to the persistent overfilling of the mesenteric reservoir. We know very little of local anæmia of the various organs, but possibly functional disturbance in the liver, kidneys, pancreas, heart, etc., may result from a permanently low pressure in the local blood "mains." Anæmia from spasm of the arterial walls is seen in Raynaud's disease, which usually affects the peripheral vessels, causing local syncope of the fingers, but it may occur in the visceral vessels, particularly of the brain, and cause temporary hemiplegia, aphasia, etc.

In local anæmia we are sometimes deceived by the appearance of the skin and mucous membranes. A marked pallor may exist with normal corpuscles and hæmoglobin; for example, the pallor after a drinking bout, or of nausea; in certain cases of heart disease, in lead-workers, and in the morphia habitué the skin is often permanently pale. There are a few healthy people who are always pale, and yet have a practically normal blood count and color index.

GENERAL ANÆMIA

The general anæmias may be divided into the secondary or symptomatic, and the primary or essential.

Acute Secondary Anæmia

Etiology.—Hæmorrhage, certain acute infections, and intoxications are the important causes. A typical form is that which follows hæmorrhage, either traumatic or spontaneous. In rupture of a large vessel, or of an aneurism, in the peptic ulcer, or in injury to blood vessels the loss of three or four pounds of blood may prove fatal. Seven and a half pounds is the largest quantity I have known shed into one cavity (rupture of an aneurism into the pleura). A patient with hæmatemesis lost ten pounds of blood in one week, and yet recovered from the immediate effects. Even after the severest traumatic hæmorrhage the blood count is rarely so low as in certain forms of primary anæmia. Thus in the case of hæmatemesis just mentioned the red blood-corpuscles were 1,390,000 per c. mm.

Acute secondary anæmia may follow hæmolysis in certain infections, as malaria, acute endocarditis, sepsis, and a profound anæmia may be induced in the course of a week. Less often do we see an acute secondary anæmia follow toxic substances, such as mercury or nitro-benzol.

Symptoms.—Dyspnœa, rapid action of the heart, and faintness are the prominent symptoms of an acutely produced anæmia. There is marked pallor of the skin and mucous membranes, the pulse becomes small, the temperature is low, the patient feels giddy and faint and has noises in the ears. If the bleeding continues there may be nausea, vomiting, and, with the rapid loss of large quantities of blood, convulsions. Examination of the blood shows a great diminution of the red blood-corpuscles, often in severe hæmorrhage to two millions per c. mm. The hæmoglobin is proportionately lower, giving a color index of about 0.8. Irregularity in the red blood-corpuscles is seen; nucleated red corpuscles, usually normoblasts, appear early; the leucocytes are increased, usually the multi-nuclear neutrophiles. The process of regeneration goes on with great rapidity; the watery and saline constituents are readily restored by absorption; the albuminous elements are quickly renewed, but it may take weeks or months for the red blood-corpuscles to reach the normal standard. Thus in a case of purpura the red blood-corpuscles fell between the 20th and 30th April to below two millions, and the leucocytes rose to 12,000. It was not until July that the red blood-corpuscles reached four million, and the blood was not normal until September. The hæmoglobin is always restored more slowly than the corpuscles. This is very well illustrated in the accompanying chart (page 729).

In repeated hæmorrhages the picture depends upon the interval between the losses of blood. If long enough to allow of complete regeneration each time the total amount of blood lost may be very great. Ehrlich mentions the case of a patient with hæmoptysis who lost 20 kilograms of blood in 6½ months. If, however, the intervals are short, so that complete recovery from each loss of blood is not possible, a chronic anæmia is soon induced with a very watery plasma, a low color index, and lymphocytosis.

Chronic Secondary Anæmia

Etiology.—There are very many causes, of which the following are the most important:

(*a*) *Inanition.*—This may be brought about by defective food supply, or by conditions which interfere with the proper reception and preparation of

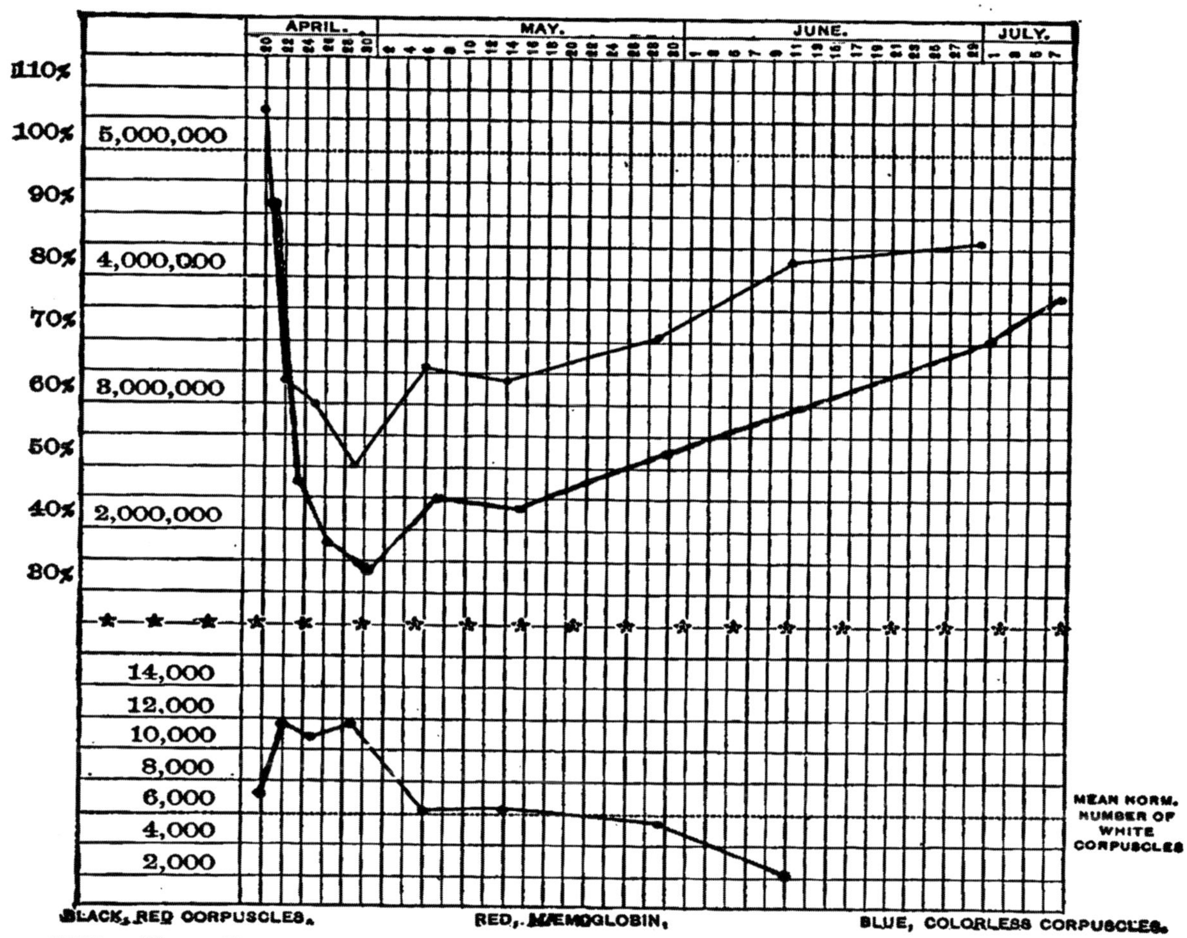

CHART XV.—THE RAPIDITY WITH WHICH ANÆMIA IS PRODUCED IN PURPURA HÆMORRHAGICA, AND THE GRADUAL RECOVERY.

the food, as in cancer of the œsophagus and chronic dyspepsia. The reduction of the blood mass may be extreme, but the plasma suffers proportionately more than the corpuscles, which, even in the wasting of cancer of the œsophagus, may not be reduced more than one-half to three-fourths. The reduction in the plasma may be so great that the corpuscles show a relative increase.

(*b*) *Infections.*—In nearly all acute fevers anæmia is produced, which may persist after the infection has subsided. We see this particularly in typhoid fever, rheumatic fever, sepsis, syphilis, and malaria. Certain forms of animal parasites, as the anchylostoma and bothriocephalus, cause a profound anæmia.

(*c*) *Intoxications.*—Inorganic poisons, such as lead, mercury, arsenic; organic poisons, as the toxins of various fevers; and certain autogenous poisons occurring in chronic affections, such as nephritis and jaundice.

(*d*) *Hæmorrhage.*—This, if repeated, may cause severe anæmia. This is particularly shown in cases of persistent bleeding from hæmorrhoids.

(*e*) Long continued drains upon the system, as in chronic suppuration, prolonged lactation, and in rapidly growing tumors of all sorts.

Symptoms.—Loss of bodily and mental vigor with loss of weight and obvious anæmia are the important features. The patient tires easily, the appetite is poor, digestion often faulty, palpitation is complained of, and there may be feelings of faintness, and, as the anæmia progresses, swelling of the feet. There is not infrequently slight fever. Petechiæ on the skin are not uncommon, and retinal hæmorrhages may occur. The blood picture is distinctive. The red blood-corpuscles are reduced, but rarely below two millions per c. mm. In 59 cases of cancer of the stomach the average count was 3,712,186 per c. mm. In only 8 cases was the count below two millions, in none below one million per c. mm. The hæmoglobin is proportionately low in the cases just mentioned; the average was 44.9 per cent.; in only 9 cases was it below 30 per cent. The red blood-corpuscles are irregular in shape, nucleated forms are present, and the leucocytes are usually increased in number.

PRIMARY OR ESSENTIAL ANÆMIA

1. *Chlorosis*

Definition.—An anæmia of unknown cause, occurring in young girls, characterized by a marked relative diminution of the hæmoglobin.

Etiology.—It is a disease of girls, more often of blondes than of brunettes. It is doubtful if males are ever affected. The age of onset is between the fourteenth and seventeenth years; under the age of twelve cases are rare. Recurrences, which are common, may extend into the third decade. Of the essential cause of the disease we know nothing. There exists a lowered energy in the blood-making organs, associated in some obscure way with the evolution of the sexual apparatus in women. Hereditary influences, particularly chlorosis and tuberculosis, play a part in some cases. Sometimes, as Virchow pointed out, the condition exists with a defective development (hypoplasia) of the circulatory and generative organs.

The disease is most common among the ill-fed, overworked girls of large towns, who are confined all day in close, badly lighted rooms, or have to do much stair-climbing. Cases occur, however, under the most favorable conditions of life, but not often in country-bred girls, as Maudlin sings in the *Compleat Angler.* Lack of proper exercise and of fresh air and the use of improper food are important factors. Emotional and nervous disturbances may be prominent—so prominent that certain writers have regarded the disease as a neurosis. De Sauvages speaks of a *chlorose par amour.* Newly arrived Irish girls were very prone to the disease in Montreal. The "corset and chlorosis" expresses O. Rosenbach's opinion. Menstrual disturbances are not uncommon, but are probably a sequence, not a cause, of chlorosis. Sir Andrew Clark believed that constipation played an important rôle and that the condition is in reality a *copræmia* due to the absorption of poisons from the large bowel.

Symptoms.—(*a*) GENERAL.—The symptoms of chlorosis are those of anæmia. The subcutaneous fat is well retained or even increased in amount. The complexion is peculiar; neither the blanched aspect of hæmorrhage nor the muddy pallor of grave anæmia, but a curious yellow green tinge, which has given to the disease its name, and its popular designation, the green sickness. Occasionally the skin shows areas of pigmentation, particularly about the joints. In cases of moderate grade the color may be deceptive, as the

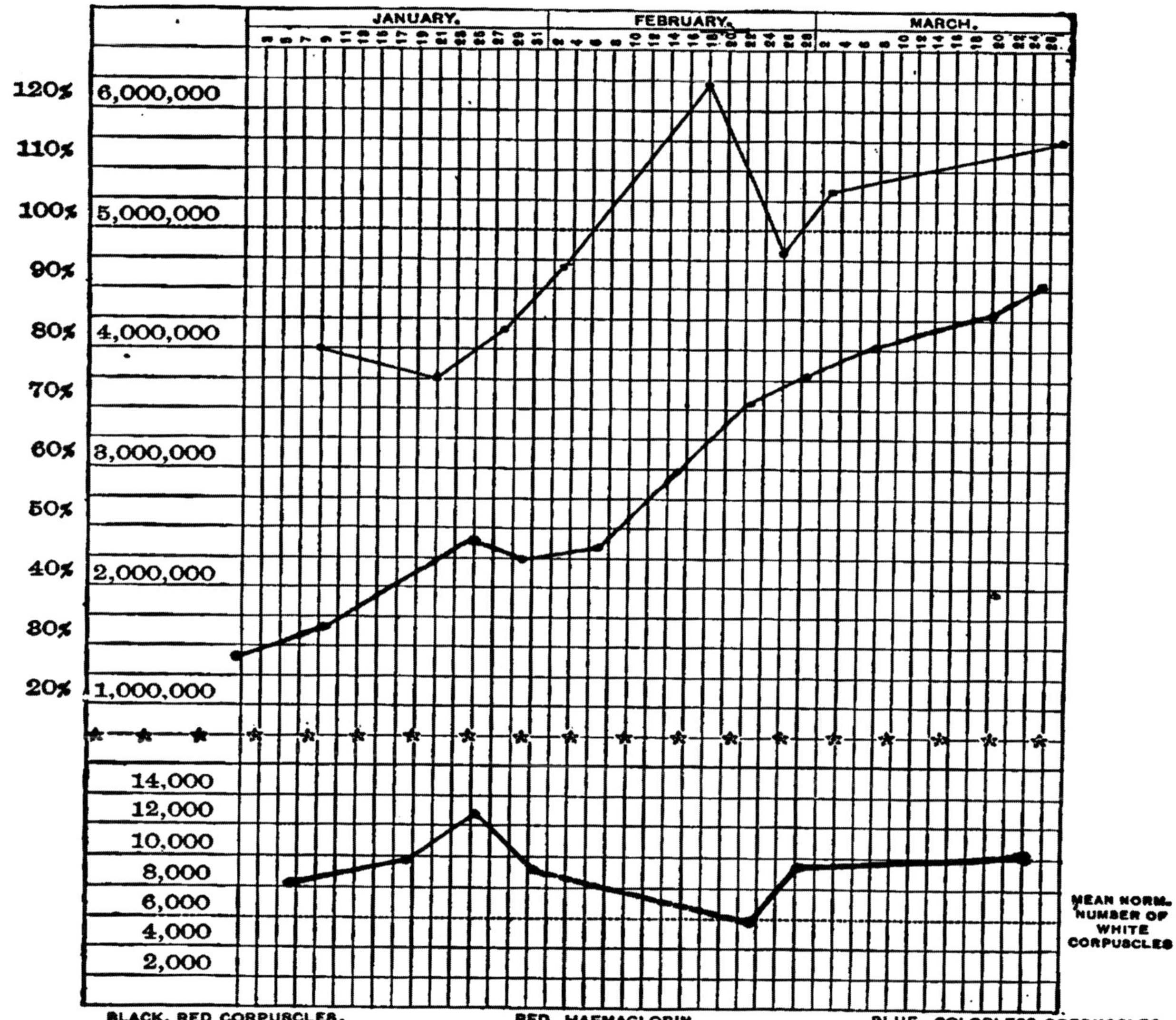

CHART XVI.—CHLOROSIS.

cheeks have a reddish tint, particularly on exertion (chlorosis rubra). The subjects complain of breathlessness and palpitation, and there may be a tendency to fainting—symptoms which often lead to the suspicion of heart or lung disease. Puffiness of the face and swelling of the ankles may suggest nephritis. The disposition often changes, and the girl becomes low-spirited and irritable. The eyes have a peculiar brilliancy and the sclerotics are of a bluish color.

(*b*) SPECIAL FEATURES.—*Blood.*—The drop as expressed looks pale. Johann Duncan, in 1867, first called attention to the fact that the essential feature was not a great reduction in the number of the corpuscles, but a quantitative change in the hæmoglobin. The corpuscles themselves look pale. In 63 consecutive cases examined at my clinic by Thayer the average number per cubic millimetre of the red blood-corpuscles was 4,096,544, or over 80 per cent., whereas the percentage of hæmoglobin for the total number was 42.3 per cent. The accompanying chart illustrates well these striking differences. There may, however, be well-marked actual anæmia. The lowest blood-count in the series of cases referred to above was 1,932,000. There may be all the physical characteristics and symptoms of a profound anæmia with the number of the blood-corpuscles nearly at the normal standard. Thus in one instance the globular richness was over 85 per cent., with the hæmoglobin about 35. No other form of anæmia presents this feature, at least with the same constancy and in the same degree. The importance of the reduction in the hæmoglobin depends upon the fact that it is the iron-containing elements of the blood with which in respiration the oxygen enters into combination. This marked diminution in the iron has also been determined by chemical analysis of the blood. The microscopic characteristics of the blood are as follows: In severe cases the corpuscles may be extremely irregular in size and shape—poikilocytosis, which may occasionally be as marked as in some cases of pernicious anæmia. The large forms of red blood cells are not as common, and the average size is stated to be below normal. The color of the corpuscles is noticeably pale and the deficiency may be seen either in individual corpuscles or in the blood mixture prepared for counting. Nucleated red corpuscles (normoblasts) are not very uncommon, and may vary greatly in numbers in the same case at different periods. The leucocytes may show a slight increase; the average in the 63 cases above referred to was 8,467 per cubic millimetre.

(*c*) Gastro-intestinal Symptoms.—The appetite is capricious, and patients often have a longing for unusual articles, particularly acids. In some instances they eat all sorts of indigestible things, such as chalk or even earth. Superacidity of the gastric juice is common. Distress after eating and even cardialgic attacks may be present. Constipation is a common symptom, and, as already mentioned, has been regarded as an important element in causing the disease. A majority of chlorotic girls who wear corsets have gastroptosis, and on inflation the stomach will be found vertically placed; sometimes the organ is very much dilated. The motor power is usually well retained. Enteroptosis with palpable right kidney is not uncommon.

(*d*) Circulatory Symptoms.—Palpitation of the heart occurs on exertion, and may be the most distressing symptom of which the patient complains. Percussion may show slight increase in the transverse dulness. A systolic murmur is heard at the apex or at the base; more commonly at the latter, but in extreme cases at both. A diastolic murmur is rarely heard. The systolic murmur is usually loudest in the second left intercostal space, where there is sometimes a distinct pulsation. The exact mode of production is still in dispute. Balfour holds that it is produced at the mitral orifice by relative insufficiency of the valves in the dilated condition of the ventricle. On the right side of the neck over the jugular vein a continuous murmur may be heard, the *bruit de diable*, or humming-top murmur.

The pulse is usually full and soft. Visible impulse is present in the veins of the neck, as noted by Lancisi. Pulsation in the peripheral veins is sometimes seen. Thrombosis in the veins may occur, most commonly in the femoral, but occasionally in the cerebral sinuses. In 86 cases the veins of the legs were affected in 48, the cerebral sinuses in 29 (Lichtenstern). The chief danger in thrombosis of the extremities is pulmonary embolism, which occurred in 13 of 52 cases collected by Welch.

As in all forms of essential anæmia, fever is not uncommon. Chlorotic patients suffer frequently from headache and neuralgia, which may be paroxysmal. The hands and feet are often cold. Dermatographia is common. Hysterical manifestations are not infrequent. Menstrual disturbances are very common—amenorrhœa or dysmenorrhœa. With the improvement in the blood condition this function is usually restored.

Diagnosis.—The green sickness, as it is sometimes called, is in many instances recognized at a glance. The well-nourished condition of the girl, the peculiar complexion, which is most marked in brunettes, and the white or bluish sclerotics are very characteristic. A special danger exists in mistaking the apparent anæmia of the early stage of pulmonary tuberculosis for chlorosis. Mistakes of this sort may often be avoided by the very simple test furnished by allowing a drop of blood to fall on a white towel or a piece of blotting paper—a deficiency in hæmoglobin is readily appreciated. The palpitation of the heart and shortness of breath frequently suggest heart-disease, and the œdema of the feet and general pallor cause the cases to be mistaken for Bright's disease. In the great majority of cases the characters of the blood readily separate chlorosis from other forms of anæmia.

2. *Idiopathic or Pernicious Anæmia*

Definition.—A recurring and usually fatal anæmia of unknown origin, characterized by hæmolysis and imperfect action of the blood-making organs.

History.—Addison (1855) gave the first accurate account, and it is sometimes known as Addison's anæmia. Channing described cases of severe anæmia in the puerperal state. The writings of Gusserow and Biermer in the early seventies did much to awaken interest in the disease. The studies of Pepper (Secundus), H. C. Wood, and Palmer Howard made the disease very familiar to American and Canadian physicians. The special methods introduced by Ehrlich have greatly increased our knowledge of the state of the blood and the bone marrow in the disease.

Distribution.—It is a common and widespread disease. It was of frequent occurrence in Montreal; I saw many cases in Philadelphia and also at the Johns Hopkins Hospital, and it seems quite as common, or even more so, in England. As Cabot remarks, the incidence of the disease is a good deal a matter of keenness on the part of the practitioners of any district.

Etiology.—The figures here quoted are from Cabot's analysis of some 1,200 cases given in his article in my "System of Medicine." It is a disease of middle life; a great majority—922—occurred over the age of 36. The youngest patient I have seen was a boy of ten years. Two or three cases may occur in one family, as a father and two girls.

Of special etiological factors much stress has been laid upon pregnancy and the puerperal state. Doubtless many of the patients reported by Channing and Gusserow do not belong in this group. Of the true disease it forms a very small fraction, according to Cabot only 18 among the 1,200 cases of his series.

Sex.—It is twice as common in males as in females, but it is slightly commoner in women under the age of 36.

Buccal and Gastro-intestinal Infection.—William Hunter, who has done so much good work on the subject, claims that a large number of cases grouped as pernicious anæmia are really of an infective nature, and not related to the true Addisonian anæmia, which he regards as a chronic infection due to a specific glossitis with oral, gastric, and intestinal sepsis. In a few cases there is a history of long standing diarrhœa.

Intestinal Parasites.—Anæmia of a very severe, and even of a pernicious, type may be induced by the bothriocephalus and by the hookworm.

Atrophy of the Stomach.—In a certain number of cases—61 in Cabot's series—there was atrophy of the gastro-intestinal mucosa, but it seems not improbable, as he suggests, that when these two diseases are associated the atrophy is a result rather than a cause of the anæmia.

Hæmorrhage.—As a rule the anæmia which follows repeated hæmorrhages is of the secondary type with a very different blood picture, but in every long series of cases of Addison's anæmia there will be found a few with a history of bleeding piles, of recurring nose bleeding, or of repeated hæmorrhages from other sources.

Nervous shock and emotional strain have been present in a few instances.

We have not got much beyond the position of Addison, who characterized the disease which he was describing as "a general anæmia occurring without any discoverable cause whatever; cases in which there had been no previous loss of blood, no existing diarrhœa, no chlorosis, no purpura, no renal, splenic, myasmatic, glandular, strumous, or malignant disease."

Pathology and Morbid Anatomy.—The body is rarely emaciated. A lemon tint of the skin is present in a majority of the cases. The muscles often are intensely red in color, like horse flesh, while the fat is light yellow. Hæmorrhages are common on the skin and serous surfaces. The heart is usually large, flabby, and empty. In one instance I obtained only 2 drachms of blood from the right heart, and between 3 and 4 from the left. The muscle substance of the heart is intensely fatty, and of a pale, light yellow color. In no affection do we see more extreme fatty degeneration. The lungs show no special changes. The stomach in many instances is normal, but in some cases of fatal anæmia the mucosa has been extensively atrophied. In the case described by Henry and myself the mucous membrane had a smooth, cuticular appearance, and there was complete atrophy of the secreting tubules. The liver may be enlarged and fatty. In most of my autopsies it was normal in size, but usually fatty. The iron is in excess, a striking contrast to the condition in cases of secondary anæmia. It is deposited in the outer and middle zones of the lobules.

The spleen shows no important changes. In one of Palmer Howard's cases the organ weighed only 1 ounce and 5 drachms. The iron pigment is usually in excess. The lymph glands may be of a deep red color (hæmo-lymph gland). The amount of iron pigment is increased in the kidneys, chiefly in the convoluted tubules. The bone-marrow is usually red, lymphoid in character, showing great numbers of nucleated red corpuscles, especially the larger forms called by Ehrlich gigantoblasts. There are cases in which the bone-marrow shows no signs of activity—*aplastic anœmia.*

Spinal cord lesions were present in 84 per cent. of the post mortems collected by Cabot. They affect chiefly the posterior columns of the cervical region.

The exact nature of the disease is unknown. Two views prevail: one that it is a hæmolysis produced by poisons intestinal or metabolic. Bunting has shown that a picture very similar to that of pernicious anæmia may be produced experimentally in animals by the injection of small doses of ricin. The investigations of Schaumann and others have shown the bothriocephalus anæmia to be a hæmolysis caused by a lipoid substance that may be extracted from the segments of the worm. From the intestinal mucosa of persons dead of pernicious anæmia lipoid substances have been extracted with hæmolytic action of remarkable potency, causing anæmia of a severe and fatal type in animals. These are interesting and suggestive facts, the only ones I know in favor of a special hæmolytic body. The majority of patients with pernicious anæmia have good appetites and good digestion, and usually get well from the first and second attacks without any special change in the condition of the bowels.

The view has been put forward by Moffitt and others that pernicious anæmia is an infection, possibly protozoal in character, in favor of which are the facts that anæmia is a very striking feature in many protozoal diseases, the occurrence of fever, the remarkable remissions, the nervous lesions, and the value of arsenic in treatment.

Symptoms.—The first thing that often attracts attention in a case of pernicious anæmia is the combination of pallor with good nutrition. As a rule there is very slight loss in weight and the fat layer is well preserved, so that the condition offers a striking contrast to most of the secondary anæmias, with which wasting is associated. The description given by Addison presents the chief features of the disease in a masterly way: "It makes its approach in so slow and insidious a manner that the patient can hardly fix a date to the earliest feeling of that languor which is shortly to become so extreme. The countenance gets pale, the whites of the eyes become pearly, the general frame flabby rather than wasted, the pulse perhaps large, but remarkably soft and compressible, and occasionally with a slight jerk, especially under the slightest excitement. There is an increasing indisposition to exertion, with an uncomfortable feeling of faintness or breathlessness in attempting it; the heart is readily made to palpitate; the whole surface of the body presents a blanched, smooth, and waxy appearance; the lips, gums, and tongue seem bloodless, the flabbiness of the solids increases, the appetite fails, extreme languor and faintness supervene, breathlessness and palpitations are produced by the most trifling exertion or emotion; some slight œdema is probably perceived about the ankles; the debility becomes extreme—the patient can no longer rise from bed; the mind occasionally wanders; he falls into a prostrate and half-torpid state, and at length expires; nevertheless, to the very last, and after a sickness of several months' duration, the bulkiness of the general frame and the amount of obesity often present a most striking contrast to the failure and exhaustion observable in every other respect."

A surprising fact is that there are patients with extreme anæmia who are remarkably vigorous. I recently saw a powerfully built man with 2,300,000 red blood-corpuscles per c. mm., who insisted that he was able to do everything as usual except that he was a little short of breath.

The appearance of the patient is usually very characteristic. The combination of a lemon-yellow tint of the skin with retention of the fat gives a very suggestive picture. Sometimes the tint is icteroid. In rare cases there is a white, anæmic pallor, and in a third group a brownish tinge of the skin (which is sometimes associated with leucoderma) deep enough to suggest Addison's disease. Muscular weakness, palpitation, headache, dyspnœa, vertigo, and œdema of the feet are common in this as in other types of anæmia.

Gastro-intestinal symptoms are not uncommon. Paroxysms of pain in the stomach with or without diarrhœa may occur in crises. In fully one-half of the cases diarrhœa occurs at some time during the course. The hydrochloric acid is usually greatly diminished or absent, and there may be complete achylia. A sore mouth and tongue, a feature to which attention was called especially by William Hunter, has not been common in my experience. There may be marked glossitis and ulcers. Pyorrhœa alveolaris may be said to be present in all cases, and the teeth are often very bad. Not infrequently the patients come for palpitation and disturbance of the heart. Slight dilatation is common; murmurs are rarely missed, generally hæmic and basic.

Apex diastolic murmurs may occur without valve lesions. Extraordinary throbbing of the arteries may occur, so that aneurism may be suspected; the pulse may be collapsing. Œdema is common, usually in the feet, sometimes in the hands.

The urine is usually of low specific gravity, pale, and with diminished pigments. Sometimes, as pointed out by Hunter and Mott, it is of a deep sherry color, due to great excess of urobilin.

Nervous Symptoms.—Numbness and tingling are common. Sometimes there are marked neuritic pains. Anatomically it has been shown that lesions of the spinal cord are not at all uncommon. There are three groups of cases:

(*a*) The patient may have had no special symptoms pointing to involvement of the nervous system, but post mortem well marked lesions of the cord are found.

(*b*) With the anæmia there are signs of spinal cord lesions, either of a lateral sclerosis with spastic features and increased reflexes, or the picture may be rather of the tabetic type—lightning pains, girdle sensation, areas of anæsthesia, loss of the reflexes.

(*c*) There is a remarkable group carefully described by Risien Russell, Batten, and Collier, in which the nervous symptoms, usually those of a posterolateral sclerosis, precede the anæmia.

As the disease progresses there may be great depression, sometimes delusions, but mental symptoms, as a rule, are not marked.

Hæmorrhages are not very uncommon, chiefly in the form of small petechiæ in the skin. Retinal hæmorrhages are frequent. Optic neuritis is very rare.

Blood.—The total quantity in the body is much diminished. The drop may look of good color, but it is abnormally fluid. The red blood-corpuscles are greatly diminished; the average count in 81 cases, when they came under observation, was 1,575,000 per c. mm. As Cabot says, there is no other disease which so often reduces the number of red blood-corpuscles below two millions per c. mm. In 12 per cent. of my cases the count was under one million. The lowest count on record is in a patient of Quincke's, 143,000 per c. mm.

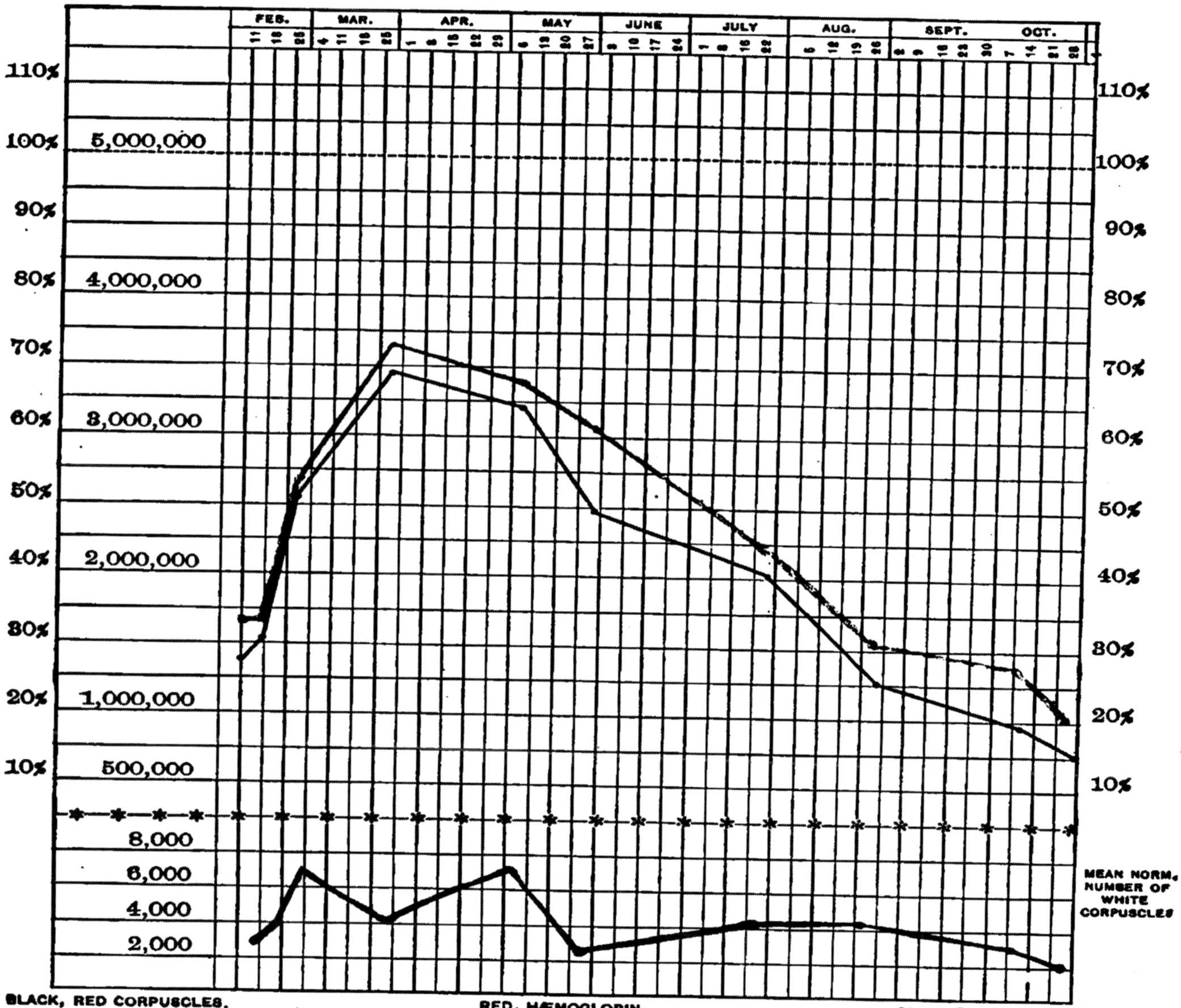

CHART XVII.—PERNICIOUS ANÆMIA.

The hæmoglobin, though quantitatively reduced, is relatively high. This is one of the most constant and distinctive features of the disease, connected probably with an average increase in the size of the red blood-corpuscles. Stained films of the blood show great variation in the shape of the red blood-corpuscles—poikilocytosis. There are large giant forms, megalocytes, ovoid, measuring 8, 11, or even 15 μ. As Laache showed, this is one of the most pathognomonic features of the disease. On the other hand, there are a great many very small red corpuscles—microcytes, from 2 to 6 μ in diameter, and of a deep red color. The irregularity in the shape of the red corpuscles is remarkable. Some are elongated, rod-like, others pyriform; one end of the corpuscle may be of normal shape, while the other is extended like the neck of a bottle. Stippling of the red blood-corpuscles is common with dark blue or blackish discoloration—the so-called polychromatophilia.

Nucleated red blood-corpuscles are constantly present, varying very much in numbers from day to day. There are two types—normoblasts of the average size, and the megaloblasts, which are much larger. There are frequently intermediate forms between these two groups. These nucleated red cells vary extraordinarily in different cases, and there may be what have been called blood crises, in which a large number of the nucleated reds appear. In one such crisis there were 14,388 normoblasts, 460 intermediates, and 138 megaloblasts per c. mm. These crises are sometimes followed by gains in the blood count, but they may be terminal events, and not specially indicative of active blood regeneration.

The leucocytes are generally normal or diminished in number. Polynuclear cells are rarely reduced. Occasionally there is a marked increase in the small mononuclear forms. Myelocytes are frequently present, even up to 8 and 10 per cent. Blood-platelets are usually low; counts of 100,000 and less are not uncommon (Pratt).

Chart XVIII gives a very good idea of the blood condition in a case during nine months.

Aplastic Anæmia.—A certain number of cases of primary anæmia run a rapid and progressive course, without remissions; and death occurs within a few months from the beginning of the attack. Post mortem, instead of an active hyperplasia of the bone marrow, there is atrophy or aplasia. To these cases the term "aplastic anæmia" has been given. It is a sub-type of pernicious anæmia with identical clinical features, except that it runs a more rapid course, is met with in younger persons, the color index may be low, hæmorrhages are more common, there may be leucopenia, and erythroblasts are usually absent. The hæmorrhages may be very severe, and some of the cases are of a pronounced purpuric type.

The diagnosis is only certain after an examination of the bones, when it is found that the marrow of the long bones is fatty, and even the red marrow may have disappeared from the short bones.

Forms of splenic anæmia, suggesting the primary pernicious form, and leukanæmia will be discussed elsewhere.

Prognosis and Course.—The disease sometimes runs a very acute course. In a patient seen with Finley in Montreal the fatal termination occurred within ten days of the onset of the symptoms. In other cases the course is from six to twelve weeks, but, as a rule, it is a chronic malady with remarkable remissions. It is rare to meet with a case in which recovery does not take place from the first attack. The number of remissions varies from two or three to five or six. In 524 cases analyzed by Cabot for this special point, 296 had one remission, 118 two, 65 three, 21 four, and 24 five. The duration of the remission may be from three months to four years. In 81 cases treated in my wards death occurred in 27 while under observation. The average duration in these cases was about a year.

The ultimate prognosis in a great majority of cases is bad; only one case in our series appears to have recovered completely, another was alive and in good health six years after the last attack, and a third four years after. In Cabot's series there were ten cases which had lasted seven years or more, but there were only 6 out of the 1,200 cases analyzed which he regarded as having completely recovered.

Diagnosis.—Few diseases are more readily recognized at sight. There is something very characteristic about the general appearance of a patient with Addisonian anæmia, and nowadays practitioners are much more alert, and the disease is better known. The lemon colored tint of the skin may suggest jaundice; the anæmia, puffy face, swollen ankles, and albumin in the urine, Bright's disease; the pigmentation, Addison's disease; the shortness of breath and palpitation, heart disease; the pallor and gastric symptoms, cancer of the stomach. The retention of fat, the insidious onset, the absence of signs of local disease, and the blood features already discussed are the important diagnostic points. From cancer of the stomach pernicious anæmia is distinguished by the absence of wasting, the high color index of the blood, the lower corpuscular count, and by the marked improvement in the first attacks under proper treatment.

TREATMENT OF ANÆMIA

Secondary Anæmia.—The traumatic cases do best, and with plenty of good food and fresh air the blood is readily restored. The extraordinary rapidity with which the normal percentage of red blood-corpuscles is reached without any medication whatever is an important lesson. The cause of the hæmorrhage should be sought and the necessary indications met. The large group depending on the drain on the albuminous materials of the blood, as in Bright's disease, suppuration, and fever, is difficult to treat successfully, and so long as the cause keeps up it is impossible to restore the normal blood condition. The anæmia of inanition requires plenty of nourishing food. When dependent on organic changes in the gastro-intestinal mucosa not much can be expected from either food or medicine. In the toxic cases due to mercury and lead the poison must be eliminated and a nutritious diet given with full doses of iron. In a great majority of these cases there is deficient blood formation, and the indications are briefly three: plenty of food, an open-air life, and iron. As a rule, it makes but little difference what form of the drug is administered. In severe forms the patient should be at rest in bed and in the open air, if possible.

Chlorosis.—The treatment of chlorosis affords one of the most brilliant instances—of which we have but three or four—of the specific action of a remedy. Apart from the action of quinine in malarial fever, and of mercury and iodide of potassium in syphilis, there is no other drug the beneficial effects of which we can trace with the accuracy of a scientific experiment. It is a minor matter *how* the iron cures chlorosis. In a week we give to a case as much iron as is contained in the entire blood, as even in the worst case of chlorosis there is rarely a deficit of more than 2 grams of this metal. Iron is present in the fæces of chlorotic patients before they are placed upon any treatment, so that the disease does not result from any deficiency of available iron in the food. Bunge believes that it is the sulphur which interreres with the digestion and assimilation of this natural iron. The sulphides are produced in the process of fermentation and decomposition in the fæces, and interfere with the assimilation of the normal iron contained in the food. By the administration of an inorganic preparation of iron, with which these sulphides unite, the natural organic combinations in the food are spared.

In studying charts of chlorosis, it is seen that there is an increase in the red blood-corpuscles under the influence of the iron, and in some instances the globular richness rises above normal. The increase in the hæmoglobin is slower and the maximum percentage may not be reached for a long time. I have for years in the treatment of chlorosis used with the greatest success Blaud's pills, made and given according to the formula in Niemeyer's text-book, in which each pill contains 2 grains of the sulphate of iron. During the first week one pill is given three times a day; in the second week, two pills; in the third week, three pills, three times a day. This dose should be continued for four or five weeks at least before reduction. An important feature in the treatment is to persist in the use of the iron for at least three months, and, if necessary, subsequently to resume it in smaller doses, as recurrences are so common. The diet should consist of good, easily digested food. Special care should be directed to the bowels, and if constipation is present a saline purge should be given each morning. The dyspeptic symptoms may be relieved by alkalies. Dilute hydrochloric acid, manganese, phosphorus, and oxygen have been recommended. Rest in bed is important in severe cases.

Pernicious Anæmia.—There are five essentials: first, a diagnosis; secondly, rest in bed for weeks or even months, if possible (thirdly) in the open air; fourthly, all the good food the patient can take; the outlook depends largely on the stomach; fifthly, arsenic; Fowler's solution in increasing doses, beginning with ♏ iii or v (0.2 to 0.3 c. c.) three times a day, and increasing ♏ i each week until the patient takes ♏ xv (1 c. c.) three times a day. Other forms of arsenic may be tried, as the sodium cacodylate or the atoxyl hypodermically. Atoxyl can be given in doses of gr. ss (0.032 gm.) every five days, and the amount gradually increased. Accessories are oil inunctions; bone-marrow, which has the merit of a recommendation by Galen; in some cases iron seems to do good. Care should be taken of the mouth and teeth. Gastric lavage and irrigations of the colon are useful in some cases.

Splenectomy has been done in a number of cases, but it is well to be cautious in judging of its value. Some patients have been helped for a time, but it is not yet proved that permanent benefit results.

Injections of blood serum and defibrinated blood have been given. The serum is given in small amounts, 10 to 20 c. c., usually into a vein; rabbit serum is perhaps the best. Defibrinated human blood should be given intravenously in large amounts, up to 500 c. c. This is better than to attempt direct transfusion. It is important to test the blood so that there is certainty of using a homologous serum (see Moss, *Johns Hopkins Hosp. Bull.*, 1911, xxii, p. 238). This treatment should only be carried out by those who are familiar with the problems involved and is not advisable for general use.

After recovery the patient should be told to watch the earliest indications of return of the trouble and at once resume the arsenic.

II. LEUKÆMIA

Definition.—A disease characterized by a permanent increase in the leucocytes of the blood, associated with hyperplasia of the leucoblastic tissues.

History.—In October, 1845, Hughes Bennett recorded a case of "suppuration of the blood with enlargement of the spleen and liver," and he afterward gave the disease the name of "leukocythæmia." A month later Virchow described a similar condition of "white blood" to which he gave the name of "leukæmia." In 1870 Neumann determined the importance of the changes in the bone marrow in connection with the disease.

Varieties.—The whole hæmatopoietic system—marrow, spleen, and lymph glands—is involved in the disease. Formerly we spoke of three different groups—the splenic, lymphatic, and medullary, but we now recognize that the leucoblastic hyperplasia may begin in any part of the blood-glandular system, marrow, lymph glands, and probably in the spleen. The differences in the types of the disease depend upon the dominance of the lymphoid or the myeloid process, so that we now divide the cases roughly into two great groups: (1) the myelocytic or myeloid, corresponding to the spleno-medullary type, and (2) the lymphoid, which represents the lymphatic variety. Some cases not fitting accurately into either are spoken of as "atypical" or "transitional" forms.

The nature of the disease is unknown. The acutely fatal cases resemble an infection, but no organisms have been determined. Banti, Warthin, and others regard the disease as related to myeloma and sarcoma.

I. Myeloid Leukæmia.—*Etiology.*—The disease is not very rare. There were 24 cases in my wards at the Johns Hopkins Hospital in fifteen years. It certainly is not more frequent in malarial regions.

It is rather more common in males than in females, and between the 30th and 50th years. The youngest of my patients was a child of eight months.

In some instances it has followed a blow. Some of the patients have had a tendency to hæmorrhage, but, as a rule, the disease appears in fairly healthy persons without any recognizable cause. It may occur during pregnancy, and a leukæmic patient of Cameron's of Montreal passed through three pregnancies, bearing on each occasion a non-leukæmic child. One of this patient's children had leukæmia before the mother showed signs of the disease, and another died of it. This patient's grandmother, mother, and brother suffered from symptoms strongly suggestive of leukæmia.

Morbid Anatomy.—Dropsy is sometimes present. There is in many cases a condition of polyæmia; the heart and veins are distended with large blood-clots. In Case XI of my series the weight of blood in the heart chambers alone was 620 grams. There may be remarkable distention of the portal, cerebral, pulmonary, and subcutaneous veins. The blood is usually clotted, and the enormous increase in the leucocytes gives a pus like appearance to the coagula, so that it has happened more than once, as in Virchow's memorable case, that on opening the right auricle the observer at first thought he had cut into an abscess. The coagula have a peculiar greenish color, somewhat like the fat of a turtle. Sometimes this is so intense as to suggest the color of chloroma, described later. The alkalinity of the blood is diminished.

The fibrin is increased. Charcot's octahedral crystals may separate from the blood after death.

In the myelitic form the spleen is greatly enlarged, the capsule may be thickened, and the vessels at the hilus enlarged. The weight may range from 2 to 18 pounds. The organ is in a condition of chronic hyperplasia. It cuts with resistance, has a uniformly reddish brown color, and the Malpighian bodies are invisible. Grayish white, circumscribed, lymphoid tumors may occur throughout the organ, contrasting strongly with the reddish brown matrix. Instead of a fatty tissue, the medulla of the long bones may resemble the consistent matter which forms the core of an abscess, or it may be dark brown in color. There may be hæmorrhagic infarctions. There may be much expansion of the shell of bone, and localized swellings which are tender and may even yield to firm pressure.

In some instances there are leukæmic enlargements in the solitary and agminated glands of Peyer. In a case of Willcocks' there were growths on the surface of the stomach and gastro-splenic omentum. The thymus is rarely involved, though it has been enlarged in some of the acute cases. The liver may be greatly enlarged, due to a diffuse leukæmic infiltration. There may be definite leukæmic growths. There are rarely changes of importance in the lungs. The kidneys are often enlarged and pale, the capillaries may be distended with leucocytes, and leukæmic tumors may occur. The skin may present leukæmic tumors.

Leukæmic tumors in the organs are not common. In 159 cases collected by Gowers there were only 13 instances of leukæmic nodules in the liver and 10 in the kidneys.

Symptoms.—The onset is insidious, and, as a rule, the patient seeks advice for progressive enlargement of the abdomen and shortness of breath, or the pallor, palpitation, and other symptoms of anæmia. Bleeding at the nose is common. Gastro-intestinal symptoms may precede the onset. Occasionally the first symptoms are of a very serious nature. In one of the cases of my series the boy played lacrosse two days before the onset of the final hæmatemesis; and in another case a girl, who had, it was supposed, only a slight chlorosis, died of fatal hæmorrhage from the stomach before any suspicion had been aroused as to the true condition.

Anæmia is not a necessary accompaniment of all stages of the disease; the subjects may look very healthy and well.

The gradual increase in the volume of the spleen is the most prominent feature in a majority of the cases. Pain and tenderness are common, though the progressive enlargement may be painless. A creaking fremitus may be felt on palpation. The enlarged organ extends downward to the right, and may be felt just at the costal edge, or when large it may extend as far over as the navel. In many cases it occupies fully one half of the abdomen, reaching to the pubes below and extending beyond the middle line. As a rule, the edge, in some the notch or notches, can be felt distinctly. Its size varies greatly from time to time. It may be perceptibly larger after meals. A hæmorrhage or free diarrhœa may reduce the size. The pressure of the enlarged organ may cause distress after eating; in one case it caused fatal obstruction of the bowels. On auscultation a murmur may sometimes be heard over the spleen, and Gerhardt has described a pulsation in it.

The pulse is usually rapid, soft, compressible, but often full in volume. There are rarely any cardiac symptoms. The apex beat may be lifted an interspace by the enlarged spleen. Toward the close œdema may occur in the feet or general anasarca. Hæmorrhage is common. There may be most extensive purpura, or hæmorrhagic exudate into pleura or peritoneum. Epistaxis is the most frequent form. Hæmoptysis and hæmaturia are rare. Bleeding from the gums may be present. Hæmatemesis proved fatal in two of my cases, and in a third a large cerebral hæmorrhage rapidly killed. The leukæmic retinitis is a part of the hæmorrhagic manifestations. J. Hughes Bennet's first leukæmic patient died suddenly, without obvious cause.

Local gangrene may develop, with signs of intense infection and high fever. There are very few pulmonary symptoms. The shortness of breath is due, as a rule, to the anæmia. Toward the end there may be œdema of the lungs, or pneumonia may carry off the patient. The gastro-intestinal symptoms are rarely absent. Nausea and vomiting are early features in some cases, and diarrhœa may be very troublesome, even fatal. Intestinal hæmorrhage is not common. There may be a dysenteric process in the colon. Jaundice rarely occurs, though in one case of my series there were recurrent attacks. Ascites may be a prominent symptom, probably due to the presence of the splenic tumor. A leukæmic peritonitis also may be present, due to new growths in the membranes.

The nervous system is not often involved. Facial paralysis has been noted. Headache, dizziness, and fainting spells are due to anæmia. The patients are usually tranquil. Coma may follow cerebral hæmorrhage.

The special senses are often affected. There is a peculiar retinitis, due chiefly to the extravasation of blood, but there may be aggregations of leucocytes, forming small leukæmic growths. Optic neuritis is rare. Deafness has frequently been observed; it may appear early and possibly is due to hæmorrhage. Features suggestive of Ménière's disease may come on quite suddenly, due to leukæmic infiltration or hæmorrhage into the semi-circular canal.

The urine presents no constant changes. The uric acid excreted is always in excess.

Priapism is a curious symptom which has been present in a large number of cases. It may, as in one of our patients, be the first symptom. In one of my patients it persisted for seven weeks. The cause is not known.

Fever was present in two-thirds of my series. Periods of pyrexia may alternate with prolonged intervals of freedom. The temperature may range from 102° to 103° F.

Blood.—In all forms of the disease the diagnosis must be made by the examination of the blood, as it alone offers distinctive features.

The striking change is an increase in the colorless corpuscles. The average in my series was 298,700 per c. mm., and the average ratio to the red cells was 1 to 10. Counts above 500,000 per c. mm. are common, and they may rise above 1,000,000 per c. mm. The proportion of white to red cells may be 1 to 5, or may even reach 1 to 1. There are instances on record in which the number of leucocytes has exceeded that of the red corpuscles.

The increase is in all the forms. The polynuclear neutrophiles make up from 30 to 50 per cent.; both the small and the large lymphocytes are increased; the eosinophiles and the mast cells show both a percentage and absolute increase. The abnormal cells, the myelocytes, range from 30 to 50 per cent. Normoblasts and megaloblasts are common. There is no anæmia at first. The red cell count may be normal, but sooner or later anæmia comes on, and the count may fall to 2,000,000 per c. mm. The color index is usu-

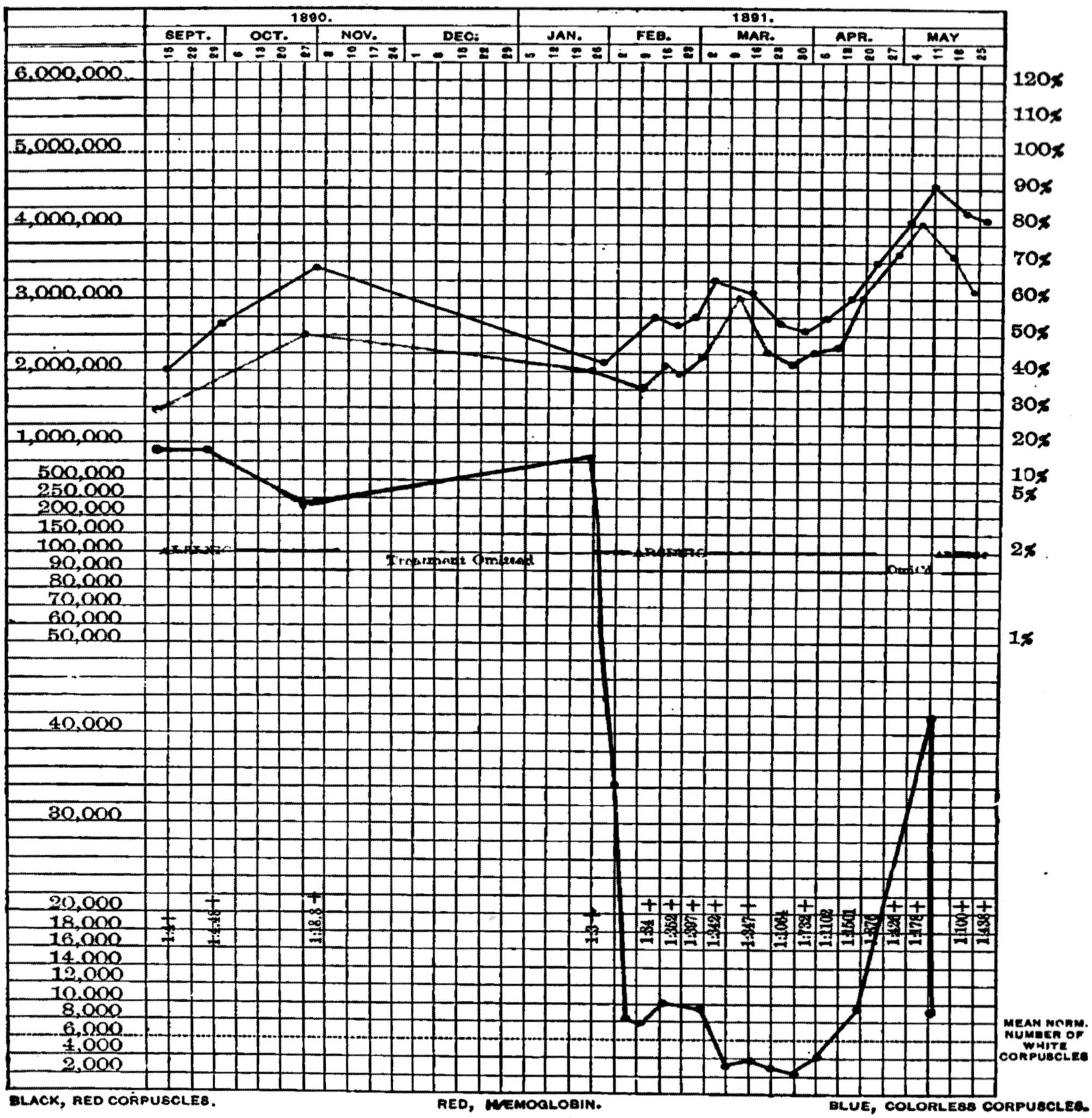

CHART XVIII.—LEUKÆMIA.

ally low. The blood platelets are increased. Charcot-Leyden crystals may separate from the clots and the hæmoglobin shows a remarkable tendency to crystalize.

II. LYMPHOID LEUKÆMIA.—*Symptoms.*—This less common form occurs more frequently in males. There are two varieties, the acute and the chronic.

Acute lymphatic leukæmia, one of the most terrible of all the blood diseases, may run a malignant course unparalleled by any of them. Among the early symptoms are angina, often of an ulcerative character, involving the tonsils and the pharynx. Hæmorrhages occur early, usually into the skin, or there is profuse nose-bleeding. The swelling of the glands, most commonly of the neck, is then noticed; the patient rapidly becomes anæmic, and death has occurred as early as the seventh day. There may be marked fever, to 103° or 105° F., and the case may be mistaken for malignant typhoid or typhus fever. The real nature of the disease may not be evident until the lymph glands begin to swell; in some cases there is no evident glandular enlargement.

The chronic form is a very different disease, occurring later in life, and beginning with a general enlargement of the lymph glands, first the cervical, then the axillary. The spleen may be slightly enlarged, and anæmia eventually comes on, but the disease may last for years without any special anæmia. Hæmorrhages are rare. Fever is not common. A pruritus of great intensity may be present, sometimes with ecthymatous patches. The skin may become deeply pigmented. Localized leukæmic tumors of the skin have been described.

Blood.—The drop may be sticky and viscous, spreading with difficulty. The most remarkable feature is the increase of lymphocytes, which are very often above 90 per cent., and may reach even 99 per cent. There are two chief forms, the large and the small mononuclear. The majority of the chronic cases have the small lymphocytes, and the total percentage is rarely so high. The number of leucocytes is less than in the myeloid form, the average in 34 cases being 180,000 (Cabot). In 20 cases the first count was below 60,000.

ATYPICAL LEUKÆMIAS.—(1) *Mixed leukæmias,* in part myeloid and in part lymphoid; but in nearly all cases of the ordinary spleno-medullary leukæmia a certain percentage of lymphocytes are present, which toward the end may be materially increased.

(2) *Cases with atypical blood changes,* such as a very high percentage of eosinophiles, or a condition with a very high proportion of plasma cells.

(3) *Chloroma* is an atypical lymphoid leukæmia in which the lymphatic tumors have a greenish color. The tumor growths occur chiefly in the skull, the orbit, the long bones, and throughout the viscera. The blood picture is like that of leukæmia and the condition is generally fatal within six or eight months.

(4) In a few rare instances a condition of leukæmia has been found without changes in the blood-making organs.

(5) *Leukanæmia.*—This term was invented by Leube to describe a condition showing features both of leukæmia and severe anæmia. The cases are now regarded as a myeloid leukæmia with severe anæmia. Glandular enlargement is usually present; the onset may be like the acute types of leukæmia, and the blood picture may be either of the lymphoid or of the myeloid type.

Diagnosis.—The recognition of the acute forms may be difficult, particularly those which begin with marked angina and cutaneous hæmorrhages. It may not be until a blood examination is made or the glands enlarge that suspicion is aroused. The chronic forms are easily recognized. The enlarged spleen at once suggests a blood count, upon which alone the diagnosis rests. Twice I have had cases of leukæmia sent from the ophthalmic surgeon, one case with the diagnosis. In the lymphatic form, too, the diagnosis rests with the blood examination. One has to recognize that there are certain cases of sepsis with marked lymphocytosis, in which the white blood-corpuscles may reach 30,000 or 40,000 per c. mm. When the regional lymph glands are involved this may raise a doubt. Cabot gives an instance of a child in whom after pneumonia and whooping-cough there was a leucocytosis of 94,000 per c. mm. It is important to remember that in the ordinary myelitic forms under treatment with arsenic or with X-rays the increase of leucocytes may disappear, but the differential count may still be characteristic.

Prognosis.—Recovery in leukæmia is practically unknown. The acute cases die within three months; the chronic forms last from six months to four or five years. The chronic lymphatic form seems to be the most protracted. One case in my hospital series lasted three years. A private patient with accurate blood counts, in whom the diagnosis was made by W. H. Draper, was seen by me ten years subsequently; the cervical, axillary, and inguinal glands were greatly enlarged; the leucocytes were 242,000 per c. mm., above 90 per cent. being lymphocytes.

Association with Other Diseases.—Tuberculosis is not uncommon. Dock has collected 27 cases, in none of which did the tuberculosis show any special influence. Intercurrent infections are not rare, such as influenza, erysipelas, or sepsis—often with a remarkable effect upon the disease. In a case reported by Dock, after an attack of influenza the leucocytes fell from 367,000 to 7,500 per c. mm. Various other conditions influence the disease, and the leucocytes have disappeared under the use of arsenic, quinine, tuberculin, and the X-rays.

Treatment.—Fresh air, good diet, and abstention from mental worry and care are the important general indications. The *indicatio morbi* can not be met. There are certain remedies which have an influence upon the disease. Of these, arsenic, given in large doses, is the best. I have repeatedly seen improvement under its use. On the other hand, there are curious remissions in the disease, as mentioned above, which render therapeutic deductions very fallacious.

Quinine may be given in cases with a malarial history. Iron may be of value in some cases, as may also inhalations of oxygen. Treatment with the X-rays should be tried. Some observers have reported very good results. Personally, I have not seen any very striking permanent improvement.

Excision of the leukæmic spleen has been performed 43 times, with 5 recoveries (J. C. Warren).

III. HODGKIN'S DISEASE

Definition.—A disease characterized by enlargement of the lymph-glands with progressive anæmia and a fatal termination.

Anatomically there is an increase in the adenoid tissue of the glands, proliferation of the endothelial cells, formation of mononuclear and multinuclear giant cells, the presence of eosinophiles, and thickening of the fibrous reticulum.

History.—In 1832 Hodgkin recorded a series of cases of enlargement of the lymphatic glands and spleen. From the motley group that Hodgkin described, Wilks picked out the disease and called it *anæmia lymphatica*. Other names that have been given to it are *adénie* by Trousseau, *pseudo-leukæmia* by Cohnheim, and *generalized lymphadenoma*.

Etiology.—A widely spread disease in Europe and America, a majority of the cases occur in young adults, and more frequently in males than in females. Twins and sisters have been known to be attacked. The cause is unknown. Certain features suggest an acute infection: the rapid course of some cases, the association with local irritation in the mouth and tonsils, the frequency with which the disease starts in the cervical glands, the gradual extension from one gland group to another, and the recurring exacerbations of fever. Various organisms have been described, but nothing definite has been determined. Possibly the disease is a spirillosis—in favor of which are the presence of eosinophilia, so characteristic of infection with animal parasites, the presence of eosinophilic cells in the glands, and the influence of arsenic on the disease. Sternberg suggested that the disease was a special form of tuberculosis; but the histological changes in the glands are quite characteristic, tubercle bacilli are not present in uncomplicated cases, the tuberculin test may be negative, and when present the tuberculosis appears to be a terminal infection.

Morbid Anatomy.—The superficial lymph glands are found most extensively involved, and from the cervical groups they form continuous chains uniting the mediastinal and axillary glands. The masses may pass beneath the pectoral muscles and even beneath the scapulæ. Of the internal glands, those of the thorax are most often affected, and the tracheal and bronchial groups may form large masses. The trachea and the aorta with its branches may be completely surrounded; the veins may be compressed, rarely the aorta itself. The masses perforate the sternum and invade the lung deeply. The retroperitoneal glands may form a continuous chain from the diaphragm to the inguinal canals. They may compress the ureters, the lumbar and sacral nerves, and the iliac veins. They may adhere to the broad ligament and the uterus and simulate fibroids. At an early stage the glands are soft and elastic; later they may become firm and hard. Fusion of contiguous glands does not often occur, and they tend to remain discrete, even after attaining a large size. The capsule may be infiltrated, and adjacent tissues invaded. On section the gland presents a grayish white semi-translucent appearance, broken by intersecting strands of fibrous tissue; there is no caseation or necrosis unless a secondary infection has occurred.

The spleen is enlarged in 75 per cent. of the cases; in young children the enlargement may be great, but the organ rarely reaches the size of the spleen in ordinary leukæmia. In more than half of the cases lymphoid growths are present.

The marrow of the long bones may be converted into a rich lymphoid tissue. The lymphatic structures of the tonsillar ring and of the intestines may show marked hyperplasia. The liver is often enlarged, and may present scattered nodular tumors, which may also occur in the kidneys.

Histology.—The studies of Andrewes and of Dorothy Reed show a very characteristic microscopic picture—proliferation of the endothelial and reticular cells, with the formation of lymphoid cells of uniform size and shape, and characteristic giant cells, the so-called lymphadenoma cells, containing four or more nuclei. Eosinophiles are always present, and proliferation of the stroma leads to fibrosis of the gland. The difference between the soft and hard forms depends largely upon the stage of the disease. When tuberculosis occurs as a secondary infection the two processes may be readily distinguished in sections of the gland.

Symptoms.—A tonsillitis may precede the onset. Enlargement of the cervical glands is usually an initial symptom; it is rare to find other superficial groups or the deeper glands attacked first. Months or even several years may elapse before the glands in the axillæ and groin become involved. During what may be called the first stage the patient's general condition is good; then anæmia comes on, not marked at first, but usually progressive. In the majority of cases the spleen is enlarged, but it never reaches the dimension of the leukæmic organ. There may be very little pain until the internal glands become involved. With swelling of the mediastinal glands there are cough, dyspnœa, and often intense cyanosis, with all the signs of intrathoracic tumor. There may be moderate fever. Bronzing of the skin may occur, apart altogether from the use of arsenic. Pruritis may be a very depressing symptom, and boils and ecthymatous blebs may occur. The leucocytes show no characteristic changes. There may be a moderate eosinophilia and, as the anæmia progresses, nucleated red corpuscles appear, and toward the end there are instances of a great increase in the lymphocytes. As the disease progresses there is marked emaciation with great asthenia, and sometimes anasarca. This represents the common clinical course, but there are many variations, among which the following are the most common:

(*a*) An ACUTE FORM has been described. I saw a remarkable case beginning, like so many cases of lymphatic leukæmia, with angina, in which the whole course was less than ten weeks. Ziegler mentions two cases of death within a month.

(*b*) LOCALIZED FORM.—The enlargement may be localized to certain groups, those in the neck, the groin, the retroperitoneum, or the thorax. Some of these cases present great difficulty in diagnosis, particularly when there are febrile paroxysms with very slight involvement of the external groups. The disease may be confined to one region for a year or more before there is any extension. The localized mediastinal group often presents a very remarkable picture—pressure signs, pain, orthopnœa—and, unless there are other groups involved, or enlargement of the spleen, it may be impossible to make the diagnosis during life.

(*c*) WITH RELAPSING PYREXIA.—To this remarkable type Pel and afterward Ebstein called attention. MacNalty has recently made a very careful study of this syndrome, which is one of the most remarkable met with in the practice of medicine. The relapsing pyrexia may occur in cases with involvement of the internal glands alone, or, more frequently, with a general involvement of all the groups. "Following on a period of low pyrexia, or of normal or subnormal temperature, there is a steady rise occupying two or four days to a maximum, which may reach 105°. For about three days the temperature remains at a high level, and then there is a gradual fall by lysis occupying about three days, and the temperature then becomes sub-normal" (MacNalty). An afebrile period of ten days or two weeks then occurs, to be followed by another bout of fever. This may be repeated for many months. In one of my cases the pyrexia lasted for accurately fourteen days for many successive paroxysms. During the fever the glands swell and may become hot and tender. This febrile type may occur in connection with involvement of the internal glands alone. In one patient whose cervical glands had been thoroughly removed there were typical Pel-Ebstein paroxysms, and we could find no enlarged glands, internal or external.

(*d*) Latent Type.—In his recent monograph Ziegler has called attention to the importance of this form, in which anæmia, fever, and constitutional symptoms may be present with enlargement of the internal glands. One of my early cases was of this type—a very stout man, in whom the retroperitoneal glands alone were involved. Symmers has reported an instance in which the glands and the hilus of the liver were attacked.

(*e*) Splenomegalic Form.—Enlargement of the spleen is present in a large proportion of cases of Hodgkin's disease. Whether or not there is a type involving the spleen alone without the lymph glands is still a question. Formerly, under the name pseudo-leukæmia of Cohnheim, many cases of simple enlargement of the spleen with or without anæmia were spoken of as *pseudo-leukœmia splenica*. It is not improbable that the disease may originate in the lymphoid tissue of the spleen, and several cases have been reported of late years by Ziegler, Symmers, Warrington, and others. It must be very difficult to distinguish such cases clinically from the early stages of Banti's disease.

(*f*) Lastly, a lymphadenia ossium has been described—cases in which there have been multiple bone tumors of the bone marrow and of the periosteum with enlargement of the glands and spleen. How far these should be grouped with Hodgkin's disease seems to me very doubtful.

Diagnosis.—(*a*) Tuberculosis.—There are both acute and chronic forms of general tuberculous adenitis (already described), but they do not often present difficulty in diagnosis. In the case of enlargement of the glands on one side of the neck beginning in a young person, it is often not at all easy to determine whether the disease is tuberculosis or beginning Hodgkin's disease. Two points should be decided. First, under cocaine one of the small glands of the affected side should be excised and the structure carefully studied. The histological changes differ markedly in Hodgkin's disease from those in tuberculosis. Secondly, tuberculin should be used if the patient is afebrile. In early tuberculosis of the glands of the neck the reaction is prompt and decisive. In the later stages, when many groups of glands are involved and the cachexia is well advanced, the tuberculin reaction may be present in Hodgkin's disease, but even then the histological changes are distinctive. Other points to be noted are the tendency in the tuberculous adenitis to coalescence of the glands, adhesion to the skin, with suppuration, etc., and the liability to tuberculosis of the lung or pleura.

(*b*) Leukæmia.—As a rule, the blood examination gives the diagnosis at a glance, as Hodgkin's disease presents only a slight leucocytosis. A difficulty arises only in those rare instances of leukæmia, usually the acute lymphatic form, in which the leucocytes gradually decrease or in which the number for a time may become normal. Histologically there are striking differences between the structure of the glands in the two conditions.

(*c*) LYMPHO-SARCOMA.—Clinically the cases may resemble Hodgkin's disease very closely, and in the literature the two diseases have been confounded. The glands, as a rule, form larger masses, the capsules are involved, and adjacent structures are attacked, but this may be the case in Hodgkin's disease. Pressure signs in the chest and abdomen are much more common in lympho-sarcoma. But the easiest and most satisfactory mode of diagnosis is examination of sections of a gland, as the structure is very different from that seen in Hodgkin's disease. The blood condition, the type of fever, etc., need a more careful study in this group of cases.

Course.—There are acute cases in which the enlargements spread rapidly and death follows in a few months. As a rule, the disease lasts for two or three years. Remarkable periods of quiescence may occur, in which the glands diminish in size, the fever disappears, and the general condition improves. Even a large group of glands may almost completely disappear, or a tumor mass on one side of the neck may subside while the inguinal glands are enlarging. Usually a cachexia with anæmia and swelling of the feet precedes death. A fatal event may occur early from great enlargement of the mediastinal glands.

Treatment.—When the glands are small and limited to one side of the neck, operation should be advised; even when both sides of the neck are involved, if there are no signs of mediastinal growth, operation is justifiable. The course of the disease may be delayed, even if cure does not follow.

There is a possibility that the X-rays may do good in selected cases. Certainly the glands have been reduced in size, but I know of no case in which complete cure has been reported. Local treatment of the glands seems to do but little good.

Arsenic is the only drug which has a positive value in the disease. In some cases the effects on the glands are striking. It may be given in the form of Fowler's solution in increasing doses. Recoveries have been reported (?). Ill effects from the larger doses are rare. Peripheral neuritis followed the use of ℥ iv, ʒj, ♏ xviij during a period of less than three months. Phosphorus is recommended by Gowers and Broadbent, and may be tried if arsenic is not well borne. Quinine, iron, and cod-liver oil are useful as tonics. For the pressure pains morphia should be given.

IV. PURPURA

Strictly speaking, purpura is a symptom, not a disease; but under this term are conveniently arranged a number of affections characterized by extravasations of the blood into the skin. In the present state of our knowledge a satisfactory classification can not be made. W. Koch groups all forms, including hæmophilia, under the designation *hæmorrhagic diathesis,* believing that intermediate forms link the mild purpura simplex and the most intense purpura hæmorrhagica. For a full discussion of the subject and an analysis of my cases, see Pratt's article in my "System of Medicine," Vol. IV.

The purpuric spots vary from 1 to 3 or 4 mm. in diameter. When small and pin-point-like they are called petechiæ; when large, they are known as ecchymoses. At first bright red in color, they become darker, and gradually fade to brownish stains. They do not disappear on pressure.

In some forms of purpura the coagulation time of the blood is retarded to ten or fifteen minutes, and in hæmophilia it has been delayed to fifty minutes.

The following is a provisional grouping of the cases:

Symptomatic Purpura.—(*a*) Infectious.—In pyæmia, septicæmia, and malignant endocarditis (particularly in the last affection) ecchymoses may be very abundant. In typhus fever the rash is always purpuric. Measles, scarlet fever, and more particularly small-pox and cerebro-spinal fever, have each a variety characterized by an extensive purpuric rash.

(*b*) Toxic.—The virus of snakes produces extravasation of blood with great rapidity—a condition which has been very carefully studied by Weir Mitchell. Certain medicines, particularly copaiba, quinine, belladonna, mercury, ergot, and the iodides occasionally, are followed by a petechial rash. Purpura may follow the use of comparatively small doses of iodide of potassium. A fatal event may be caused by a small amount, as in a case reported by Stephen Mackenzie of a child which died after a dose of 2½ grains. An erythema may precede the hæmorrhage. It is not always a simple purpura, but may be an acute febrile eruption of great intensity. Workers with benzol, which is used as a solvent for rubber, may be attacked with severe purpura. Cases such as those reported by Selling have been in connection with the coating of tin cans, while the Swedish cases occurred in connection with the manufacture of bicycle tires. Under this division, too, comes the purpura so often associated with jaundice.

(*c*) Cachectic.—Under this heading are best described the instances of purpura which occur in the constitutional disturbance of cancer, tuberculosis, Hodgkin's disease, Bright's disease, scurvy, and in the debility of old age. In these cases the spots are usually confined to the extremities. They may be very abundant on the lower limbs and about the wrists and hands. This constitutes, probably, the commonest variety of the disease, and many examples of it can be seen in the wards of any large hospital.

(*d*) Neurotic.—One variety is met with in cases of organic disease. It is the so-called myelopathic purpura, which is seen occasionally in locomotor ataxia, particularly following attacks of the lightning pains, and, as a rule, involving the area of the skin in which the pains have been most intense. Cases have been met with also in acute myelitis and in transverse myelitis, and occasionally in severe neuralgia. Another form is the remarkable hysterical condition in which stigmata, or bleeding points, appear upon the skin.

(*e*) Mechanical.—This variety is most frequently seen in venous stasis of any form, as in the paroxysms of whooping cough and in epilepsy and about tight bandages.

Arthritic Purpura.—This form is characterized by involvement of the joints. It is usually known, therefore, as rheumatic, though in reality the evidence upon which this view is based is not conclusive. Of 200 cases of purpura analyzed by Stephen Mackenzie, 61 had a history of rheumatism. For the present it seems more satisfactory to use the designation arthritic. Three groups of cases may be recognized:

(*a*) Purpura Simplex.—A mild form, often known as *purpura simplex*, seen most commonly in children, in whom, with or without articular pain, a crop of purpuric spots appears upon the legs, less commonly upon the trunk and arms. As pointed out by Graves, this form is not infrequently associated with diarrhœa. The disease is seldom severe. There may be loss of appetite, and slight anæmia. Fever is not, as a rule, present, and the patients get well in a week or ten days. Usually regarded as rheumatic, and certainly associated, in some instances, with undoubted rheumatic manifestations, yet in a majority of the patients the arthritis is slighter than in the ordinary rheumatism of children, and no other manifestations are present.

(*b*) Purpura (Peliosis) Rheumatica (*Schönlein's Disease*).—This remarkable affection is characterized by multiple arthritis and an eruption which varies greatly in character, sometimes *purpuric*, more commonly associated with *urticaria* or with *erythema exudativum*. The disease is most common in males between the ages of twenty and thirty. It not infrequently sets in with sore throat, a fever from 101° to 103°, and articular pains. The rash, which makes its appearance first on the legs or about the affected joints, may be a simple purpura or may show ordinary urticarial wheals. In other instances there are nodular infiltrations, not to be distinguished from erythema nodosum. The combination of wheals and purpura, the *purpura urticans*, is very distinctive. Much more rarely vesication is met with, the so-called *pemphigoid purpura*. The amount of œdema is variable; occasionally it is excessive. These are the cases which have been described as *febrile purpuric œdema*. The temperature range, in mild cases, is not high, but may reach 102° or 103° F.

The urine is sometimes reduced in amount and may be albuminous. The joint affections are usually slight, though associated with much pain, particularly as the rash comes out. Relapses may occur and the disease may return at the same time for several years in succession.

The diagnosis of Schönlein's disease offers no difficulty. The association of multiple arthritis with purpura and urticaria is very characteristic.

Schönlein's peliosis is thought by most writers to be of rheumatic origin, and certainly many of the cases have the characters of ordinary rheumatic fever, *plus* purpura. By many, however, it is regarded as a special affection, of which the arthritis is a manifestation analogous to that which occurs in hæmophilia and in scurvy. The frequency with which sore throat precedes the attack, and the occasional occurrence of endocarditis or pericarditis, are certainly very suggestive of true rheumatism.

The cases usually do well, and a fatal event is extremely rare. The throat symptoms may persist and give trouble. In two instances I have seen necrosis and sloughing of a portion of the uvula.

Visceral Lesions in Purpura.—In any form of purpura, in the erythemas, and in urticaria visceral lesions may occur. (*a*) Gastro-intestinal crises, pain, vomiting, melæna, and diarrhœa. The attacks have often been mistaken for appendicitis or for intussusception, and at operation the condition has been found to be an acute sero-hæmorrhagic infiltration of a limited area of the stomach or bowel. Identical attacks occur in angio-neurotic œdema. These crises may occur for years in children before an outbreak of purpura or urticaria gives a clue to their nature. (*b*) Enlargement of the spleen is usually present in these cases. (*c*) Albuminuria and acute nephritis may occur and form the most serious complication, of which seven cases in my series died (*Am. J. Med. Sciences,* Jan., 1904). The combination of purpura with colic is usually spoken of as Henoch's purpura.

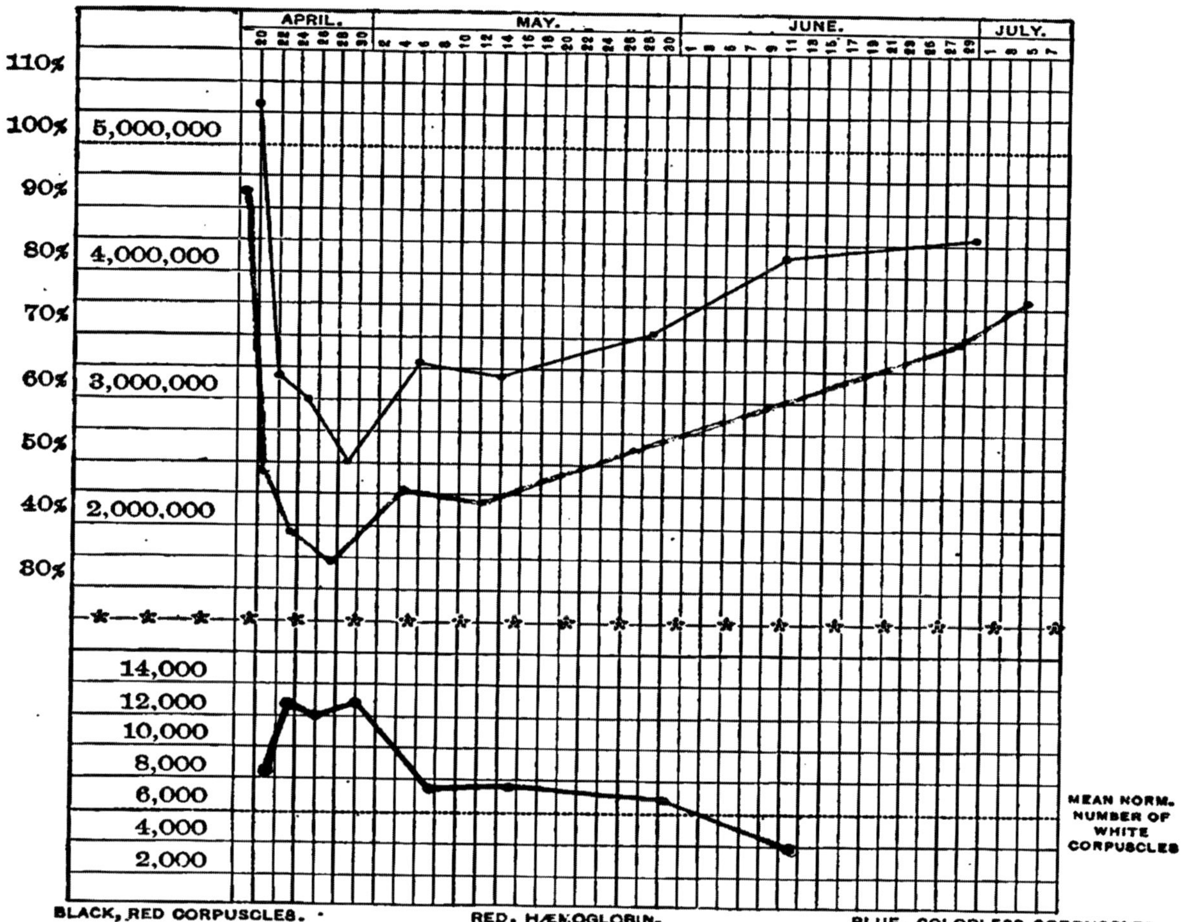

CHART XIX.—THE RAPIDITY WITH WHICH ANÆMIA IS PRODUCED IN PURPURA HÆMORRHAGICA, AND THE GRADUAL RECOVERY.

Purpura Hæmorrhagica.—Under this heading may be considered cases of very severe purpura with hæmorrhages from the mucous membranes. The affection, known as the *morbus maculosus* of Werlhof, is most commonly met with in young and delicate individuals, particularly in girls; but the disease may attack adults in full vigor. After a few days of weakness and debility, purpuric spots appear on the skin and rapidly increase in number and size. Bleeding from the mucous surfaces sets in, and the epistaxis, hæmaturia, and hæmoptysis may cause profound anæmia. Death may take place from loss of blood, or from hæmorrhage into the brain. Slight fever usually accompanies the disease. In favorable cases the affection terminates in from ten days to two weeks. There are instances of purpura hæmorrhagica of great malignancy, which may prove fatal within twenty-four hours—*purpura fulminans.* This form is most commonly met with in children, and is characterized chiefly by cutaneous hæmorrhages, and death may occur before any bleeding takes place from the mucous membranes.

In the *diagnosis* of purpura hæmorrhagica it is important to exclude scurvy, which may be done by the consideration of the previous health, the circumstances under which the disease occurs, and by the absence of swelling of the gums. The malignant forms of the fevers, particularly small-pox and measles, are distinguished by the prodromes and the higher temperature.

Treatment.—In symptomatic purpura attention should be paid to the conditions under which it occurs, and measures should be employed to increase the strength and to restore a normal blood condition. Tonics, good food, and fresh air meet these indications. In the simple purpura of children, or that associated with slight articular trouble, arsenic in full doses should be given. No good is obtained from the small doses, but the Fowler's solution should be pushed freely until physiological effects are obtained. In peliosis rheumatica the sodium salicylate may be given, but with discretion. I confess not to have seen any special control of the hæmorrhages by this remedy.

Aromatic sulphuric acid, ergot, turpentine, acetate of lead, or tannic and gallic acids may be given, and in some instances they seem to check the bleeding. Oil of turpentine is perhaps the best remedy, in 10 or 15-minim (1 c. c.) doses three or four times a day. The calcium salts, preferably the lactate, may be given in doses of 15 grains (1 gm.) three or four times a day for a few days, to increase the coagulability of the blood. In bleeding from the mouth, gums, and nose the inhalation of carbon dioxide, irrigations with 2-per-cent. gelatin solution, and adrenalin should be tried. The last remedy has often acted promptly. The treatment of the severe forms is the same as that given in hæmophilia.

HÆMORRHAGIC DISEASES OF THE NEW-BORN

Syphilis Hæmorrhagica Neonatorum.—The child may be born healthy, or there may be signs of hæmorrhage at birth. Then in a few days there are extensive cutaneous extravasations and bleeding from the mucous surfaces and from the navel. The child may become deeply jaundiced. The post mortem shows numerous extravasations in the internal organs and extensive syphilitic changes in the liver and other organs.

Epidemic Hæmoglobinuria (*Winckel's Disease*).—Hæmoglobinuria in the new-born, which occasionally occurs in epidemic form in lying-in institutions, is a very fatal affection, which sets in usually about the fourth day after birth. The child becomes jaundiced, and there are marked gastro-intestinal symptoms, with fever, jaundice, rapid respiration, and sometimes cyanosis. The urine contains albumin and blood coloring matter—methæmoglobin. The disease has to be distinguished from the simple icterus neonatorum, with which there may sometimes be blood or blood coloring matter in the urine. The post mortem shows an absence of any septic condition of the umbilical vessels, but the spleen is swollen, and there are punctiform hæmorrhages in different parts. Some cases have shown in a marked degree acute fatty degeneration of the internal organs—the so-called Buhl's disease.

Morbus Maculosus Neonatorum.—Apart from the common visceral hæmorrhages, the result of injuries at birth, bleeding from one or more of the surfaces is a not uncommon event in the new-born, particularly in hospital practice. Forty-five cases occurred in 6,700 deliveries (C. W. Townsend).

The bleeding may be from the navel alone, but more commonly it is general. Of Townsend's 50 cases, in 20 the blood came from the bowels (*melæna neonatorum*), in 14 from the stomach, in 14 from the mouth, in 12 from the nose, in 18 from the navel, in 3 from the navel alone. The bleeding begins within the first week, but in rare instances is delayed to the second or third. Thirty-one of the cases died and 19 recovered. The disease is usually of brief duration, death occurring in from one to seven days. The temperature is often elevated. The nature of the disease is unknown. As a rule, nothing abnormal is found post mortem. The general and not local nature of the affection, its self limited character, the presence of fever, and the greater prevalence of the disease in hospitals suggest an infectious origin (Townsend). The bleeding may be associated with intense hæmatogenous jaundice. Not every case of bleeding from the stomach or bowels belongs in this category. Ulcers of the œsophagus, stomach, and duodenum have been found in the new-born dead of *melæna neonatorum*. The child may draw the blood from the breast and subsequently vomit it.

V. HÆMOPHILIA

Definition.—A disease characterized by excessive and chronic liability to immoderate hæmorrhage. The liability is hereditary, and is confined to the male sex (Bulloch and Fildes).

History.—The origin of our knowledge of this remarkable condition dates from 1803, when John C. Otto, a Philadelphia physician, published "an account of an hæmorrhagic disposition occurring in certain families"; and he first used the word "bleeder." The works of Grandidier and of Wickham Legg give full clinical details, and the monograph of Bulloch and Fildes (Dulan & Co., London, 1911) presents in extraordinary detail every aspect of the disease.

Distribution.—A majority of the cases have been reported from Germany, Switzerland, and the United States. Jews are supposed to be more prone than others to the disease, but this Bulloch doubts, and he discredits the negro cases.

SEX.—Bulloch and Fildes claim to have established by their researches the fact of immunity in females, denying the authenticity of all the published cases (19). "In none of the families of bleeders . . . do we find any unequivocal evidence of abnormality in the women, that is to say, any abnormality beyond what might be expected in any collection of females taken at random."

INHERITANCE.—Otto pointed out in his original paper that while the females do not themselves bleed they alone transmit the tendency. Of 171 recorded instances of transmission, 160 conform to the "law of Nasse" that the disease is transmitted by the unaffected female—"the conductor" (Bulloch and Fildes). They explain the 11 exceptions, and conclude that the disease is not capable of being propagated through a male. Instances of hæmophilia without demonstrable inheritance are very rare.

Pathology.—Recent studies point to disturbance in the fibrin forming factors as the essential feature of the disease. Almroth Wright showed that the coagulation time in hæmophilics was much delayed, and the recent observations of Addis in 12 cases have shown that the delay may be as much as 40 to 60 minutes. According to the development of Buchanan and Schmidt's views the factors in coagulation are fibrinogen, prothrombin, thrombokinase, and calcium, and by the interaction of the last three thrombin is produced, which, acting on the fibrinogen, precipitates fibrin. Set free when a wound takes place, the thrombokinase present in the tissues in the presence of calcium rapidly forms a new body—thrombin. Sahli, whose studies on hæmophilia have been most important and interesting, believes that there is an anomaly of the cellular elements of the blood, and of certain other cells, especially in the walls of the vessels, so that the thrombokinase is not produced. Morowitz believes that thrombokinase is derived from the leucocytes or from the platelets. One of the difficulties in explaining the bleeding in hæmophilia is the fact that the hæmorrhage continues in spite of the presence of clots in and about the wound. Addis believes that a higher amount of thrombokinase is required to produce rapid clotting in hæmophilic than in normal blood. In a wound, coagulation may occur only in those parts, as at the side, where the concentration of this material is highest; but the clot itself prevents the addition of further quantities of the thrombokinase from the tissues, and when the quantity of thrombin set free from the primary clot is insufficient completely to coagulate the blood in the centre of the wound, the bleeding may continue indefinitely.

Symptoms.—"The cardinal symptoms are three in number . . . an *inherited* tendency in *males* to *bleed*" (Bulloch and Fildes). A trifling injury, of no moment in a normal person, determines a hæmorrhage, which has no tendency to stop, but the blood trickles or oozes until death follows or there is spontaneous arrest. The bleeding may be external, internal, or into joints. A majority of the attacks may be traced to trauma but spontaneous bleeding may occur. The liability is first noticed in children and persists to adult life, gradually diminishing and eventually disappearing. Tooth extraction is a very common cause. Epistaxis is a frequent occurrence, heading the list in Grandidier's series of 334 cases. Other localities were: mouth 43, stomach 15, bowels 36, urethra 16, lungs 17, and a few instances of bleeding from the tongue, finger-tips, tear papilla, eyelids, external ear, vulva, navel, and scrotum. Trivial operations, as circumcision, have been followed by fatal hæmorrhage.

Hæmarthrosis and periarticular bleedings are common. The knee is most commonly attacked, and the affection has been mistaken for tuberculosis. König distinguishes three stages—hæmarthrosis, panarthritis, and deformity.

Diagnosis.—Karl Pearson's new iatro-mathematical school of medicine has done good work in making the profession more careful about its facts, as well as its figures. Bulloch's monograph should be read by all who value accuracy of observation and of investigation. Forms of bleeding are so common that it is a simple matter to construct a pedigree showing an inherited "hæmorrhagic diathesis." It is essential for the diagnosis that the individual should have been more or less subject to bleeding from various parts throughout his life. "No solitary hæmorrhage, however inexplicable, should, in our opinion, be regarded as hæmophilia; it is necessary to show that the individual has been repeatedly attacked, if not from birth, from infancy" (Bulloch and Fildes).

Treatment.—Recent work of a most encouraging character indicates that injections of serum or of defibrinated blood, or direct transfusion have remarkable effects in these severe hæmorrhagic cases, particularly in hæmophilia. The method has been introduced by Weil, who recommends the subcutaneous injection of 30 c. c. of fresh human or animal serum or the intravenous injection of 15 c. c. The method has been successful in the hæmorrhagic diseases of the new-born, injecting subcutaneously 10 c. c., and giving as much as 100 or even 200 c. c. in four or five days (Moss). The serum may be applied locally to the bleeding spot in hæmophilia. Cure has followed the use of the anti-diphtheritic serum. Injection of defibrinated blood has been successful in several cases, and melæna neonatorum has been cured by direct transfusion. Lambert's case is remarkable, as the hæmorrhage had been going on for three days and the child was dying. In the severer cases the direct transfusion should be tried and the technique is not now a matter of difficulty.

VI. ERYTHRÆMIA

(*Vaquez' Disease, Polycythæmia Vera*)

Definition.—A disease characterized by a persistent increase of the red blood-corpuscles, a condition of plethora, splenomegaly, and at times cyanosis. Cases were reported by Rendu and Widal, Vaquez, Cabot, McKeen, Saundby and Russell, and since 1903, when I tried to put the disease on a firm clinical basis, great interest has been aroused in the condition.

Pathology.—We see polycythæmia as a secondary condition in high altitudes, and in stasis of the blood in congenital heart disease, and in emphysema of the lungs. The high altitude hyperglobulism is compensatory to lack of oxygen in the air, and there is an increased activity of the bone marrow. In erythræmia proper this same increased activity of the bone marrow is present, and the disease is regarded as a primary lesion of the erythroblastic tissues of the bone marrow, just as leukæmia is an affection of the leucoblastic elements. There is also an increased viscosity of the blood which favors the stasis and capillary engorgement.

Symptoms.—The three cardinal features are a change in the appearance of the patient, enlargement of the spleen, and hyperglobulism. The superficial blood vessels, capillaries, and veins look full, so that the skin is always congested, in warm weather of a brick red color, in cold weather cyanosed. The engorgement of the face may be extreme, extending to the conjunctivæ, and in the cold the cyanosis of the face and hands may be as marked as any that is ever seen. There is often, too, a remarkable vasomotor instability, e. g., the hand becoming deeply engorged when held down, and rapidly anæmic when held up.

The spleen is usually enlarged, but not to the great extent of leukæmia. It may vary in size from time to time. It is hard, firm, and painless.

The total bulk of blood is enormously increased, and the ratio of corpuscles to plasma is high. The polycythæmia ranges from 7 to 12 or even 13 millions of red corpuscles per c. mm. As a rule, they are normal in appearance and shape; nucleated red blood-corpuscles may be present, the hæmoglobin ranging from 130 to 160 per cent., but the color index is relatively low. Moderate leucocytosis is the rule without any characteristic differential change; a few myelocytes may be present. The specific gravity is high.

Of other symptoms the most common are headache, flushing, and giddiness. Constipation is common, and albuminuria is usually present. The blood pressure is high; occasionally there may be hæmorrhages into the skin and from the mucous membranes. Recurring ascites, probably in association with splenic tumor, was present in two of my cases.

Morris has reported a couple of cases with the general appearance of the disease and with slight enlargement of the spleen, but without polycythæmia. Geisböck has described a variety, *polycythæmia hypertonica*, with increased tension, arterio-sclerosis, and nephritis.

Diagnosis.—The triad of features above referred to are sufficient in the absence of congenital heart disease, emphysema, and forms of cyanosis associated with poisoning by coal tar products. In a few rare cases the polycythæmia has been associated with tuberculosis of the spleen.

Prognosis.—The prognosis is bad for cure, but the condition may persist for years with reasonably good health. Cardiac failure, hæmorrhage, and recurring ascites have been the usual modes of death.

Treatment.—When there is much fullness of the head and vertigo, repeated bleedings have given relief. Inhalations of oxygen may be tried when the cyanosis is extreme. Saline purges and low diet are also helpful. The X-rays have done no good in my cases. Splenectomy should not be performed.

VII. ENTEROGENOUS CYANOSIS

(*Methæmoglobinæmia and Sulphæmoglobinæmia*)

Definition.—A form of permanent cyanosis due to changes in the composition of the hæmoglobin of the blood.

Etiology.—It has long been known that with the use of certain drugs changes were induced in the hæmoglobin. In poisoning by potassium chlorate methæmoglobinæmia occurs often with an active hæmolysis. Carbon monoxide, sulphuretted hydrogen, the coal-tar products, acetanilide, phenacetin, sulphonal, and trional may cause a chronic cyanosis. Stokvis brought forward evidence to show that certain cases of chronic cyanosis are associated with intestinal disturbances, and he gives this form the name "enterogenous." Some of the forms are associated with methæmoglobinæmia, others with sulphæmoglobinæmia. In a doubtful case, with absence of lesions of the heart or lungs, a spectroscopic examination of the blood will determine if the cyanosis is of this nature, and which of the two derivatives of hæmoglobin is causing it.

There have been some 15 or 20 cases now on record of both forms (see Garrod, Allbutt and Rolleston's System).

Methæmoglobinæmia.—Several of the patients have had chronic diarrhœa, in two associated with parasites. In Stokvis' case there was clubbing of the fingers without any recognizable cause. Gibson and Douglas obtained from the blood of their patient a pure culture of a colon organism and suggested the name "Microbic cyanosis." In connection with this observation it may be mentioned that methæmoglobinæmia has been met with in Winckel's disease, in one case of which the staphylococcus has been isolated from the blood. But a still more striking confirmation is Boycott's discovery of an infective methæmoglobinæmia in rats, caused by Gaertner's bacillus, which gives a remarkable bluish tint to the skin of white rats.

Sulphæmoglobinæmia.—The appearance of the patients is very much the same. They look very badly, even death-like, but feel comfortable, and there is no shortness of breath. The absence of symptoms at once suggests a drug habit as a cause, but the history is negative. In the case reported by Wood Clarke, the first in this country, the cultures were negative. Intestinal disturbances have been present in a number of cases, and Garrod suggests that it is a chronic poisoning by hydrogen sulphide, possibly absorbed from the intestines.

SECTION IX

DISEASES OF THE CIRCULATORY SYSTEM

A. DISEASES OF THE PERICARDIUM

I. PERICARDITIS

Pericarditis is the result of infective processes, primary or secondary, or arises by extension of inflammation from contiguous organs.

Etiology.—PRIMARY, so-called idiopathic, inflammation is rare; but it has been met with in children without any evidence of rheumatism or of any local or general disease. Certain of the cases are tuberculous.

Pericarditis from injury usually comes under the care of the surgeon in connection with the primary wound. The trauma may be from within, due to the passage of a foreign body—a needle, a pin, or a bone—through the œsophagus—a variety exceedingly common in cows and horses.

SECONDARY: (*a*) Occurs most frequently in connection with rheumatic fever. The percentage given by different authors ranges from thirty to seventy. In our 330 cases of rheumatic fever (Johns Hopkins Hospital) pericarditis occurred in twenty—practically 6 per cent. The articular trouble may be slight or, indeed, the disease may be associated with acute tonsillitis in rheumatic subjects. Certain of the so-called idiopathic cases have their origin in an acute tonsillitis. The pericarditis may precede the arthritis. (*b*) In septic processes; in the acute necrosis of bone and in puerperal fever it is not uncommon. (*c*) In tuberculosis, in which the disease may be primary or part of a general involvement of the serous sacs or associated with extensive pulmonary disease. (*d*) In the fevers. Not infrequent after scarlatina, it is rare in measles, small-pox, typhoid fever, and diphtheria. In pneumonia it is not uncommon, occurring in 31 among 665 in my clinic (J. A. Chatard). In 184 post mortems there were 29 instances of pericarditis. It is most frequent in double pneumonia, and in our series with disease of the right side, if only one lung was involved. Pericarditis sometimes complicates chorea; it was present in 19 of 73 autopsies which I collected; in only 8 of these was arthritis present. (*e*) Terminal pericarditis. In gout, in chronic Bright's disease —*pericardite brightique* of the French—in arterio-sclerosis, in scurvy, in diabetes, and in chronic illness of all sorts a latent pericarditis is common and is usually overlooked.

(*f*) *By Extension.*—In pleuro-pneumonia it forms a serious complication, and was present in 5 cases of 100 post mortems. It is most often met with in the pleuro-pneumonia of children and of alcoholics. With simple pleurisy it is rare. In ulcerative endocarditis, purulent myocarditis, and in aneurism of the aorta pericarditis is occasionally found. It may also follow extension of the disease from the mediastinal glands, the ribs, sternum, vertebræ, and even from the abdominal viscera.

The ordinary pus cocci, the pneumococcus, and the tubercle bacillus are the chief organisms met with in acute pericarditis.

Pericarditis occurs at all ages. Cases have been reported in the fetus. In the new-born it may result from septic infection through the navel. Throughout childhood the incidence of rheumatic fever and scarlet fever makes it a frequent affection, whereas late in life it is most often associated with tuberculosis, Bright's disease, and gout. Males are somewhat more frequently attacked than females. The so-called epidemics of pericarditis have been outbreaks of pneumonia with this as a frequent complication.

ACUTE FIBRINOUS PERICARDITIS

This, the most common and benign form, is distinguished by the small amount of exudate which coats the surface in a thin layer.

It may be partial or general. In the mildest grades the membrane looks lustreless and roughened, due to the presence of a thin fibrinous sheeting, which can be lifted with the knife, showing beneath an injected or ecchymotic serosa. As the fibrinous sheeting increases in thickness the constant movement of the adjacent surfaces gives to it sometimes a ridge-like, at others a honeycombed appearance. With more abundant fibrinous exudation the membranes present an appearance resembling buttered surfaces which have been drawn apart. The fibrin is in long shreds, and the heart presents a curiously shaggy appearance—the hairy heart of old writers, *cor villosum.*

In mild grades the subjacent muscle looks normal, but in the more prolonged and severe cases there is myocarditis, and for 2 or 3 mm. beneath the visceral layer the muscle presents a pale, turbid appearance. Many of these acute cases are tuberculous and the granulations are easily overlooked in a superficial examination.

There is usually a slight amount of fluid entangled in the meshes of fibrin, but there may be very thick exudate without much serous effusion.

Symptoms.—Unless sought for there may be no objective signs, and for this reason it is often overlooked, and in hospitals the disease is relatively more common in the post mortem room than in the wards.

Pain is a variable symptom, not usually intense, and in this form rarely excited by pressure. It is more marked in the early stage, and may be referred either to the præcordia or to the region of the xiphoid cartilage. Instances are recorded of pain of an aggravated and most distressing character resembling angina. Fever is usually present, but it is not always easy to say how much depends upon the primary disease, and how much upon the pericarditis. It is as a rule not high, rarely exceeding 102.5° F. In rheumatic cases hyperpyrexia has been observed.

PHYSICAL SIGNS.—*Inspection* is negative; *palpation* may reveal the presence of a distinct fremitus caused by the rubbing of the roughened pericardial surfaces. This is usually best marked over the right ventricle. It is not always to be felt, even when the friction sound on auscultation is loud and clear. *Auscultation:* The friction sound, due to the movement of the pericardial surfaces upon each other, is one of the most distinctive of physical signs. It is double, corresponding to the systole and diastole; but the synchronism with the heart sounds is not accurate, and the to and fro murmur usually outlasts the time occupied by the first and second sound. In rare instances the friction is single; more frequently it appears to be triple in character—a sort of canter rhythm. The sounds have a peculiar rubbing, grating quality, characteristic when once recognized, and rarely simulated by endocardial murmurs. Sometimes instead of grating there is a creaking quality—the *bruit de cuir neuf*—the new leather murmur of the French. The pericardial friction appears superficial, very close to the ear, and is usually intensified by pressure with the stethoscope. It is best heard over the right ventricle, the part of the heart which is most closely in contact with the front of the chest—that is, in the fourth and fifth interspaces and adjacent portions of the sternum. There are instances in which the friction is most marked at the base, over the aorta, and at the superior reflection of the pericardium. Occasionally it is best heard at the apex. It may be limited to a very narrow area, or it may be transmitted up and down the sternum. There are, however, no definite lines of transmission as in endocardial murmurs. An important point is the variability of the sounds, both in position and quality; they may be heard at one visit and not at another. The maximum of intensity will be found to vary with position. Friction may be present with a thin, almost imperceptible, layer of exudate; on the other hand it may not be present with a thick, buttery layer. The rub may be entirely obscured by the loud bronchial râles in pneumonia, in which disease pericarditis is not recognized clinically in more than half the cases, only 13 in 31 cases in my series.

Diagnosis.—There is rarely any difficulty in determining the presence of a dry pericarditis, for the friction sounds are distinctive. The double murmur of aortic incompetency may simulate closely the to and fro pericardial rub. I recall several instances in which this mistake was made. The constant character of the aortic murmur, the direction of transmission, the phenomena in the arteries, and the associated conditions of the disease should be sufficient to prevent this error.

Pleuro-pericardial friction is very common, and may be associated with endo-pericarditis, particularly in cases of pleuro-pneumonia. It is frequent, too, in tuberculosis. It is best heard over the left border of the heart, and is much affected by the respiratory movement. Holding the breath or taking a deep inspiration may annihilate it. The rhythm is not the simple to and fro diastolic and systolic, but the respiratory rhythm is superadded, usually intensifying the murmur during expiration and lessening it on inspiration. In tuberculosis of the lungs there are instances in which, with the friction, a loud systolic click is heard, due to the compression of a thin layer of lung and the expulsion of a bubble of air from a small softening focus or from a bronchus.

And, lastly, it is not very uncommon, in the region of the apex beat, to hear a series of fine crepitant sounds, systolic in time, often very distinct, suggestive of pericardial adhesions, but heard too frequently for this cause.

Course and Termination.—Simple fibrinous pericarditis never kills, but it occurs so often in connection with serious affections that we have frequent opportunities to see all stages of its progress. In the majority of cases the inflammation subsides and the thin fibrinous laminæ gradually become converted into connective tissue, which unites the pericardial leaves firmly together. A very thin layer may "clear" without leaving adhesions. In other instances the inflammation progresses, with increase of the exudation, and the condition is changed from a "dry" to a "moist" pericarditis, or the pericarditis with effusion.

In a few instances—probably always tuberculous—the simple plastic pericarditis becomes chronic, and great thickening of both visceral and parietal layers is gradually induced.

PERICARDITIS WITH EFFUSION

Etiology.—Commonly a direct sequence of the dry or plastic pericarditis, of which it is sometimes called the second stage, this form is found most frequently in association with rheumatic fever, tuberculosis, and septicæmia, and sets in usually with the symptoms above described, namely, præcordial pain, with slight fever or a distinct chill.

In children the disease may, like pleurisy, come on without local symptoms, and, after a week or two of failing health, slight fever, shortness of breath, and increasing pallor, the physician may find, to his astonishment, signs of most extensive pericardial effusion. These latent cases are often tuberculous. W. Ewart has called special attention to latent and ephemeral pericardial effusions, which he thinks are often of short duration and of moderate size, with an absence of the painful features of pericarditis.

Morbid Anatomy.—The effusion may be sero-fibrinous, hæmorrhagic, or purulent. The amount varies from 200 to 300 c. c. to 2 litres. In the cases of sero-fibrinous exudation the pericardial membranes are covered with thick, creamy fibrin, which may be in ridges or honeycombed, or may present long, villous extensions. The parietal layer may be several millimetres in thickness and may form a firm, leathery membrane. The hæmorrhagic exudation is usually associated with tuberculous, or with cancerous pericarditis, or with the disease in the aged. The lymph is less abundant, but both surfaces are injected and often show numerous hæmorrhages. Thick, curdy masses of lymph are usually found in the dependent part of the sac. In many cases the effusion is really sero-purulent, a thin, turbid exudation containing flocculi of fibrin.

The pericardial layers are greatly thickened and covered with fibrin. When the fluid is pus, they present a grayish, rough, granular surface. Sometimes there are distinct erosions on the visceral membrane. The heart muscle in these cases becomes involved to a greater or less extent and, on section, the tissue, for a depth of from 2 to 3 mm., is pale and turbid, and shows evidence of fatty and granular change. Endocarditis coexists frequently, but rarely results from the extension of the inflammation through the wall of the heart.

Symptoms.—Even with copious effusion the onset and course may be so insidious that no suspicion of the true nature of the disease is aroused.

As in the simple pericarditis, pain may be present, either sharp and stabbing or as a sense of distress and discomfort in the cardiac region. It is more frequent with effusion than in the plastic form. Pressure at the lower end of the sternum usually aggravates it. Dyspnœa is a common and important symptom, one which, perhaps, more than any other, excites suspicion of grave disorder and leads to careful examination of heart and lungs. The patient is restless, lies upon the left side or, as the effusion increases, sits up in bed. Associated with the dyspnœa is in many cases a peculiarly dusky, anxious countenance. The pulse is rapid, small, sometimes irregular, and may present the characters known as *pulsus paradoxus,* in which during each inspiration the pulse beat becomes very weak or is lost. These symptoms are due, in great part, to the direct mechanical effect of the fluid within the pericardium which embarrasses the heart's action. Other pressure effects are distention of the veins of the neck, dysphagia, which may be a marked symptom, and irritative cough from compression of the trachea. Aphonia is not uncommon, owing to compression or irritation of the recurrent laryngeal as it winds round the aorta. In massive effusion the pericardial sac occupies a large portion of the antero-lateral region of the left side and the condition has frequently been mistaken for pleurisy. Even in moderate grades the left lung is somewhat compressed, an additional element in the production of the dyspnœa.

Great restlessness, insomnia, and in the later stages low delirium and coma are symptoms in the more severe cases. Delirium and marked cerebral symptoms are associated with the hyperpyrexia of rheumatic cases, but apart from the ordinary delirium there may be peculiar mental symptoms. The patient may become melancholic and show suicidal tendencies. In other cases the condition resembles closely delirium tremens. Sibson, who has specially described this condition, states that the majority of such cases recover. Chorea may also occur, as was pointed out by Bright. Epilepsy is a rare complication which has occurred during paracentesis.

PHYSICAL SIGNS.—*Inspection.*—In children the præcordia bulges and with copious exudation the antero-lateral region of the left chest becomes enlarged. A wavy impulse may be seen in the third and fourth interspaces, or there may be no impulse visible. The intercostal spaces bulge somewhat and there may be marked œdema of the wall. The epigastrium may be more prominent. Perforation externally through a space is very rare. Owing to the compression of the lung, the expansion of the left side is greatly diminished. The diaphragm and left lobe of the liver may be pushed down and may produce a distinct prominence in the epigastric region.

Palpation.—A gradual diminution and final obliteration of the cardiac impulse is a striking feature in progressive effusion. The position of the apex beat is not constant. In large effusions it is usually not felt. In children as the fluid collects the pulsation may be best seen in the fourth space, but this may not be the apex itself. The pericardial friction may lessen with the effusion, though it often persists at the base when no longer palpable over the right ventricle, or may be felt in the erect and not in the recumbent posture. Fluctuation can rarely, if ever, be detected.

Percussion gives most important indications. The gradual distention of the pericardial sac pushes aside the margins of the lungs so that a large area comes in contact with the chest wall and gives a greatly increased percussion dulness. The form of this dulness is irregularly pear-shaped; the base or broad surface directed downward and the stem or apex directed upward toward the manubrium. There is a disproportionate extension of dulness upward and to the right, with dulness in the right fifth interspace extending one or two inches to the right of the sternum (Rotch's sign). The dulness may extend to the left beyond the apex beat. There may be marked differences in the area of flatness in the erect and recumbent postures. In large effusions there may be impaired resonance in the left axilla, and Bamberger called attention to an area of dulness near the angle of the scapula with bronchial breathing, which may alter when the patient leans forward.

Auscultation.—The friction sound heard in the early stages may disappear when the effusion is copious, but often persists at the base or at the limited area of the apex. It may be audible in the erect and not in the recumbent posture. With the absorption of the fluid the friction returns. One of the most important signs is the gradual weakening of the heart sounds, which with the increase in the effusion may become so muffled and indistinct as to be scarcely audible. The heart's action is usually increased and the rhythm disturbed. Occasionally a systolic endocardial murmur is heard. Early and persistent accentuation of the pulmonary second sound may be present.

Important accessory signs in large effusion are due to pressure on the left lung. The antero-lateral margin of the lower lobe is pushed aside and in some instances compressed, so that percussion in the axillary region, in and just below the transverse nipple line, gives a modified percussion note, usually a flat tympany. Variations in the position of the patient may change materially this modified percussion area, over which on auscultation there is either feeble or tubular breathing.

Course.—Cases vary extremely in the rapidity with which the effusion takes place. In every instance, when a pericardial friction murmur has been detected, the practitioner should first outline with care—using the aniline pencil—the upper and lateral limits of cardiac dulness, secondly mark the position of the apex beat, and thirdly note the intensity of the heart sounds. In many instances the exudation is slight in amount, reaches a maximum within forty-eight hours, and then gradually subsides. In other instances the accumulation is more gradual and progressive, increasing for several weeks. To such cases the term *chronic* has been applied. The rapidity with which a sero-fibrinous effusion may be absorbed is surprising. The possibility of the absorption of a purulent exudate is shown by the cases in which the pericardium contains semi-solid grayish masses in all stages of calcification. With sero-fibrinous effusion, if moderate in amount, recovery is the rule, with inevitable union, however, of the pericardial layers. In some of the septic cases there is a rapid formation of pus and a fatal result may follow in three or four days. More commonly, when death occurs with large effusion, it is not until the second or third week and takes place by gradual asthenia.

Prognosis.—In the sero-fibrinous effusions the outlook is good, and a large majority of all the rheumatic cases recover. The purulent effusions are, of course, more dangerous; the septic cases are usually fatal, and recovery is rare in the slow, insidious tuberculous forms.

Diagnosis.—Probably no serious disease is so frequently overlooked by the practitioner. Post mortem experience shows how often pericarditis is not recognized, or goes on to resolution and adhesion without attracting notice. In a case of rheumatic fever, watched from the outset, with the attention directed daily to the heart, it is one of the simplest of diseases to diagnose;

but when one is called to a case for the first time and finds perhaps an increased area of præcordial dulness, it is often very hard to determine with certainty whether or not effusion is present.

The difficulty usually lies in distinguishing between dilatation of the heart and pericardial effusion. Although the differential signs are simple enough on paper, it is notoriously difficult in certain cases, particularly in stout persons, to say which of the conditions exists. The points which deserve attention are:

(*a*) The character of the impulse, which in dilatation, particularly in thin-chested people, is commonly visible and wavy.

(*b*) The shock of the cardiac sounds is more distinctly palpable in dilatation.

(*c*) The area of dulness in dilatation rarely has a triangular form; nor does it, except in cases of mitral stenosis, reach so high along the left sternal margin or so low in the fifth and sixth interspaces *without visible or palpable impulse.* An upper limit of dulness shifting with change of position speaks strongly for effusion.

(*d*) In dilatation the heart sounds are clearer, often sharp, valvular, or fetal in character; gallop rhythm is common, whereas in effusion the sounds are distant and muffled.

(*e*) Rarely in dilatation is the distention sufficient to compress the lung and produce the tympanitic note in the axillary region, or flatness behind.

(*f*) The X-ray picture may be very definite, and unlike any form of dilatation or hypertrophy of the heart.

The number of excellent observers who have acknowledged that they have failed sometimes to discriminate between these two conditions, and who have indeed performed paracentesis *cordis* instead of paracentesis *pericardii,* is perhaps the best comment on the difficulties.

Massive (1½ to 2-litre) exudations have been confounded with a pleural effusion. On more than one occasion the pericardium has been tapped under the impression that the exudate was pleuritic. The flat tympany in the infrascapular region, the absence of well defined movable dulness, and the feeble, muffled sounds are indicative points. Followed from day to day there is rarely much difficulty, but it is different when a patient seen for the first time presents a large area of dulness in the antero-lateral region of the left chest, and there is no to and fro pericardial friction murmur. Many of the cases have been regarded as encapsulated pleural effusions.

A special difficulty exists in recognizing the large exudate in pneumonia. The effusion may be very much larger than the signs indicate, and the involvement of the adjacent lung and pleura is confusing. In at least three cases in our series we should have tapped the sac; post mortem the effusion was more than a litre.

The nature of the fluid can not positively be determined without aspiration; but a fairly accurate opinion can be formed from the nature of the primary disease and the general condition of the patient. In rheumatic cases the exudation is usually sero-fibrinous; in septic and tuberculous cases it is often purulent from the outset; in senile, nephritic, and tuberculous cases the exudate may be hæmorrhagic.

Treatment.—The patient should have absolute quiet, mentally and bodily, so as to reduce to a minimum the heart's action. Drugs given for this purpose, such as aconite or digitalis, are of doubtful utility. Local bloodletting by cupping or leeches is certainly advantageous in robust subjects, particularly in the cases of extension in pleuro-pneumonia. The ice bag is of great value. It may be applied to the præcordia at first for an hour or more at a time, and then continuously. It reduces the frequency of the heart's action and seems to retard the progress of an effusion. Blisters are not indicated in the early stage.

When effusion is present, the following measures to promote absorption may be adopted: Blisters to the præcordia, a practice not so much in vogue now as formerly. It is surprising, however, in some instances, how quickly an effusion will subside on their application. Purges and iodide of potassium are of doubtful utility. The diet should be light, dry, and nutritious. The action of the kidneys may be promoted by the infusion of digitalis and potassium acetate.

With an effusion, so soon as signs of serious impairment of the heart occur, as indicated by dyspnœa, small, rapid pulse, dusky, anxious countenance, paracentesis, or incision of the pericardium, should be performed. With the sero-fibrinous exudate, such as commonly occurs after rheumatism, aspiration is sufficient; but when the exudate is purulent, the pericardium should be freely incised and freely drained. The puncture may be made in the fourth or fifth interspace, in or outside the nipple line. In large effusions the pericardium can be readily reached without danger by thrusting the needle upward and backward close to the costal margin in the left costo-xiphoid angle; or the needle may be introduced outside the left nipple line. The results of paracentesis of the pericardium have so far not been satisfactory. With an earlier operation in many instances and a more radical one in others —incision and free drainage, not aspiration, when the fluid is purulent— the percentage of recoveries will be greatly increased. Repeated tapping may be needed. One case of tuberculous effusion, tapped three times, recovered completely and was alive three years afterward.

CHRONIC ADHESIVE PERICARDITIS

(*Adherent Pericardium, Indurative Mediastinopericarditis*)

The remote prognosis in pericarditis is very variable. A large majority of these cases get well and have no further trouble, but in young persons serious results sometimes follow adhesions and thickening of the layers. As Sequira has pointed out, the danger is here directly in proportion to the amount of dilatation and weakening of the pericardium in consequence of the inflammation. The loss of the firm support afforded to the heart by the rigid fibrous bag in which it is inclosed is the important factor. There are two groups of cases of adherent pericardium.

(*a*) Simple adhesion of the peri- and epicardial layers, a common sequence of pericarditis, met with post mortem as an accidental lesion. It is not necessarily associated with disturbance in the function of the heart, which in a large proportion of the cases is neither dilated nor hypertrophied.

(*b*) Adherent pericardium with chronic mediastinitis and union of the outer layer of the pericardium to the pleura and to the chest walls. This constitutes one of the most serious forms of cardiac disease, particularly in early life, and may lead to an extreme grade of hypertrophy and dilatation of the heart. The peritoneum may be involved with perihepatitis, cirrhosis, and ascites (Pick's disease).

Symptoms.—The symptoms of adherent pericardium are those of hypertrophy and dilatation of the heart, and later of cardiac insufficiency. G. D. Head in a careful study of 59 cases divides them into (1) a small silent group with no symptoms, (2) a larger group with all the features of cardiac disease, and (3) a group comprising 11 cases in his series in which the features were hepatic. To this last group much attention has been paid since Pick's description. The hepatic features dominate the picture and the diagnosis of cirrhosis of the liver is usually made. Recurring ascites is the special feature. One of my patients was tapped one hundred and twenty-one times. There is chronic peritonitis, with great thickening of the capsule of the liver and consequent contraction of the organ.

Diagnosis.—The following are important points in the diagnosis: *Inspection.*—A majority of the signs of value come under this heading. (*a*) The præcordia is prominent and there may be marked asymmetry, owing to the enormous enlargement of the heart. (*b*) The extent of the cardiac impulse is greatly increased, and may sometimes be seen from the third to the sixth interspaces, and in extreme cases from the right parasternal line to outside the left nipple. (*c*) The character of the cardiac impulse. It is undulatory, wavy, and in the apex region there is marked systolic retraction. (*d*) Diaphragm phenomena. Walter Broadbent has called attention to a very valuable sign in adherent pericardium. When the heart is adherent over a large area of the diaphragm there is with each pulsation a systolic tug, which may be communicated through the diaphragm to the points of its attachment on the wall, causing a visible retraction. This has long been recognized in the region of the seventh or eighth rib in the left parasternal line, but Broadbent called attention to the fact that it was frequently best seen on the left side behind, between the eleventh and twelfth ribs. This is a very valuable and quite common sign, and may sometimes be very localized. One difficulty is that, as A. W. Tallant has pointed out, it may occur in thin chested persons with great hypertrophy of the heart. Sir William Broadbent called attention to the fact that owing to the attachment of the heart to the central tendon of the diaphragm this part does not descend with inspiration, during which act there is not the visible movement in the epigastrium. (*e*) Diastolic collapse of the cervical veins, the so-called Friedreich's sign. This is not of much moment.

Palpation.—The apex beat is fixed, and turning the patient on the left side does not alter its position. On placing the hand over the heart there is felt a diastolic shock or rebound, which some have regarded as the most reliable of all signs of adherent pericardium.

Percussion.—The area of cardiac dulness is usually much increased. In a majority of instances there are adhesions between the pleura and the pericardium, and the limit of cardiac dulness above and to the left may be fixed and is uninfluenced by deep inspiration. This, too, is an uncertain sign, inasmuch as there may be close adhesions between the pleura and the pericardium and between the pleura and the chest wall, which at the same time allow a very considerable degree of mobility to the edge of the lung.

Auscultation.—The phenomena are variable and uncertain. In the cases in children with a history of rheumatism endocarditis has usually been present. Even in the absence of chronic endocarditis, when the dilatation reaches a certain grade, there are murmurs of relative insufficiency, which, as in one case I have recorded, may be present not only at the mitral but also at the tricuspid and pulmonary orifices. Theodore Fisher has called attention to the fact that there may be a well-marked presystolic murmur in connection with adherent pericardium. Occasionally the layers of the pericardium are united in places by strong fibrous bands, 5-7 mm. long by 3-5 mm. wide. In one such case Drasche heard a remarkable whirring, systolic murmur with a twanging quality.

The pulsus paradoxus, in which during inspiration the pulse-wave is small and feeble, is sometimes present, but it is not a diagnostic sign of either simple pericardial adhesion or of the cicatricial mediastino-pericarditis.

Cardiolysis, Brauer's operation, has been proposed for this condition and has been helpful in a few cases. Four or five centimetres of the fourth, fifth, and sixth left ribs with a couple of centimetres of the corresponding cartilages are resected, by which means the heart's action is less embarrassed. It is a justifiable procedure in selected cases—in, for example, a child with a very large, tumultuously acting heart, with much bulging of the chest.

II. OTHER AFFECTIONS OF THE PERICARDIUM

Hydropericardium.—The pericardial sac contains post mortem a few cubic centimetres of clear, citron colored fluid. In connection with general dropsy, due to kidney or heart disease, more commonly the former, the effusion may be excessive, adding to the embarrassment of the heart and the lungs, particularly when the pleural cavities are the seat of similar transudation. There are rare instances in which effusion into the pericardium occurs after scarlet fever with few, if any, other dropsical symptoms. Hydropericardium is frequently overlooked.

In rare cases the serum has a milky character—chylopericardium.

Hæmopericardium.—This condition is met with in aneurism of the first part of the aorta, of the cardiac wall, or of the coronary arteries, and in rupture and wounds of the heart. Death usually follows before there is time for the production of symptoms other than those of rapid heart failure due to compression. In rupture of the heart the patient may live for many hours or even days with symptoms of progressive heart failure, dyspnœa, and the physical signs of effusion.

In the pericarditis of tuberculosis, of cancer, of Bright's disease, and of old people the inflammatory exudate is often blood stained.

Pneumopericardium.—This is an excessively rare condition, of which Walter James was able to collect only 38 cases in 1903. I have met with but one instance, from rupture of a cancer of the stomach. Perforation of the sac occurred in all but 5, in which the gas bacillus was the possible cause, as in Nicholl's case at the Royal Victoria Hospital, Montreal, this organism was isolated. Seven cases were due to perforation of the œsophagus and eight to penetrating wounds from without. The physical signs are most characteristic. A tympany replaces the normal pericardial flatness. On auscultation there is a splashing, gurgling, churning sound, called by the French *bruit de moulin*. This was described in 19 of the cases collected by James. Of the 38 cases, 26 died.

Calcified Pericardium.—This remarkable condition may follow pericarditis, particularly the suppurative and tuberculous forms; occasionally it extends from the calcified valves. It may be partial or complete. Of 59 cases collected by A. E. Jones, in 38 there were no cardiac symptoms. Adherent pericardium was diagnosed in one case. Jones's careful study shows that the condition is usually latent and unrecognized.

B. DISEASES OF THE HEART

I. FUNCTIONAL AFFECTIONS OF THE HEART

1. PALPITATION

In health we are unconscious of the action of the heart. One of the first indications of debility or overwork is the consciousness of the cardiac pulsations, which may, however, be perfectly regular and orderly. This is not palpitation. The term is properly limited to irregular or forcible action of the heart perceptible to the individual. The condition of extra-systole described in the next section is present in many cases.

Etiology.—The expression "perceptible to the individual" covers the essential element in palpitation of the heart. The most extreme disturbance of rhythm, a condition even of what is termed *delirium cordis,* may be unattended with subjective sensations of distress, and there may be no consciousness of disturbed action. On the other hand, there are cases in which complaint is made of the most distressing palpitation and sensations of throbbing, in which the physical examination reveals a regularly acting heart, the sensations being entirely subjective. We meet with this symptom in a large group of cases in which there is increased excitability of the nervous system. Palpitation may be a marked feature at the time of puberty, at the climacteric, and occasionally during menstruation. It is a very common symptom in hysteria and neurasthenia, particularly in the form of the latter which is associated with dyspepsia. Emotions, such as fright, are common causes of palpitation. It may occur as a sequence of the acute fevers. Females are more liable to the affection than males.

In a second group the palpitation results from the action upon the heart of certain substances, such as tobacco, coffee, tea, and alcohol. And, lastly, palpitation may be associated with organic disease of the heart, either of the myocardium or of the valves. As a rule, however, it is a purely nervous phenomenon—seldom associated with organic disease—in which the most violent action and the most extreme irregularity may exist without that subjective element of consciousness of the disturbance which constitutes the essential feature of palpitation.

The irritable heart described by Da Costa, which was so common among the young soldiers during the civil war, is a neurosis of this kind. The chief symptoms were palpitation with great frequency of the pulse on exertion, a variable amount of cardiac pain, and dyspnœa. The factors at work in producing this condition appeared to be the mental excitement, the unwonted muscular exertion associated with the drill, and diarrhœa. The condition is not infrequent in civil life among young men, and when persistent it may lead to hypertrophy of the heart.

Symptoms.—In the mildest form, such as occurs during a dyspeptic attack, there are slight fluttering of the heart and a sense of what patients sometimes call "goneness." In more severe attacks the heart beats violently, its pulsations against the chest wall are visible, the rapidity of the action is much increased, the arteries throb forcibly, and there is a sense of great distress. In some instances the heart's action is not at all quickened. The most striking cases are in neurasthenic women, in whom the mere entrance of a person into the room may cause the most violent action of the heart and throbbing of the peripheral arteries. The pulse may be rapidly increased until it reaches 150 or 160. A diffuse flushing of the skin may appear at the same time. After such attacks there may be the passage of a large quantity of pale urine. In many cases of palpitation, particularly in young men, the condition is at once relieved by exertion. A patient with extreme irregularity of the heart may, after walking quickly 100 yards or running upstairs, return with the pulse perfectly regular. This is not infrequently seen, too, in the irregular action of the heart in mitral valve disease.

The physical examination of the heart is usually negative. The sounds, the shock of which may be very palpable, are on auscultation clear, ringing, and metallic, but not associated with murmurs. The second sound at the base may be greatly accentuated. A murmur may sometimes be heard over the pulmonary artery or even at the apex in cases of rapid action in neurasthenia or in severe anæmia. The attacks may be transient, lasting only for a few minutes, or may persist for an hour or more. In some instances any attempt at exertion renews the attack. Sometimes in vigorous young adults who are upset nervously, especially after exertion or during excitement, the signs of mitral stenosis are simulated. There is a systolic shock preceded by a suggestion of a thrill. On auscultation it may be difficult to decide whether or not there is a short presystolic murmur. A short period of observation usually removes the uncertainty.

The *prognosis* is usually good, though it may be extremely difficult to remove the conditions underlying the palpitation.

2. ARRHYTHMIA

The work of Gaskell and of Engelmann on the functions of the heart muscle, and the clinical studies of James Mackenzie, Wenckebach, and others, have modified the older views of the neurogenic cardiac mechanism with its musculo-motor nerve centres upon which the higher centres played through the vagi and the sympathetic nerves. The source of the action of the heart is now placed in the muscle itself—myogenic—and Gaskell describes as its functions rhythmicity, excitability, contractility, conductivity, and tonicity; "that is to say, the muscular fibres of the heart possess the power of rhythmically creating a stimulus, of being able to receive a stimulus, of responding to a stimulus by contracting, of conveying the stimulus from muscle fibre to muscle fibre, and of maintaining a certain ill-defined condition called tone." Wenckebach and James Mackenzie have studied the disturbances of these functions of the heart clinically, and have endeavored to classify them in harmony with the myogenic theory. I am indebted to Erlanger for the following classification based on that of Wenckebach:

I. *Arrhythmia resulting from decreased conductivity in the auriculo-ventricular junction—heart-block.* Characteristics: Auricular rhythm perfect, rate normal or accelerated; ventricular rhythm may or may not be perfect; if perfect its rate will be one half of that of the auricles, or less; if not perfect the irregularities will bear some direct relation to the contractions of the auricles.

A. Partial heart-block: (1) Occasional ventricular silence; (2) regularly recurring ventricular silence, either one ventricular beat missed in 7, 6, 5, 4, etc., auricular beats, or a 2 :1, 3 :1, 4 :1 rhythm, or either of these alternating.

B. Complete heart-block: Auricular and ventricular rhythms perfect but independent.

C. Paroxysmal bradycardia (Stokes-Adams disease) affecting the ventricular rate alone.

II. *Arrhythmia resulting from increased irritability of the heart.*

A. Ventricular extra-systoles, characterized by an early systole, which is associated with the phenomena of a retrograde impulse. There may be one or more extra-systoles following a normal systole; when regularly recurring, one or more extra-systoles after 5, 4, 3, 2, or 1 normal systoles, the last giving the bigeminal or trigeminal pulse, or there may be irregularly recurring extra-systoles causing delirium cordis.

B. Auricular extra-systoles.

C. Nodal extra-systoles, causing the auricle and ventricle to contract at nearly the same time.

III. *Arrhythmia resulting from a deficiency of contractility in the cardiac muscle.*

A. Alternating pulse.

B. Omissions of ventricular systole, e. g., in the halved rate seen after large doses of digitalis.

IV. *Arrhythmia resulting from the influence of extrinsic nerves upon the heart-rate.* (1) Vagus effect, and (2) accelerator effects. These are seen in the irregularities synchronous with respiration in the youthful type of irregularity, in "sinus" irregularity, and in certain forms of paroxysmal tachycardia (vagal). Extra-systoles seen in nervous persons are probably due to a slight excess of accelerator action.

V. *Arrhythmia resulting from disturbed diastolic filling of the heart.*

A. Disturbed filling resulting from violent respiratory movements: may give the paradoxical pulse.

B. Disturbed filling from adherent pericardium or mediastinal tumor: may give the paradoxical pulse.

Intermittency; Extra-systoles.—The commonest type of arrhythmia is that now known as the extra-systole, to explain which it must be remembered that to a stimulus strong enough to set up a contraction the heart answers with all the contractility of which it is capable at the moment (Bowditch's law of maximal contraction). A second property of the heart muscle is that it possesses a "refractory phase" in which normally it is not excitable, or answers only to very strong stimuli. During this refractory stage, beginning shortly before the systole and continuing a short time after it, the heart is inexcitable. When not refractory it may again contract during this phase and produce an

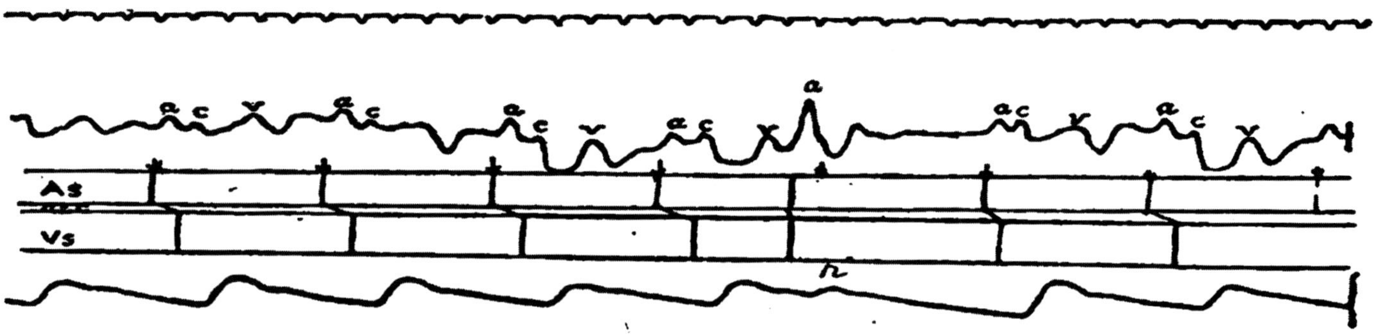

FIG. 1.—A "NODAL" EXTRA-SYSTOLE. The auricular and ventricular systoles are premature and simultaneous (Mackenzie).

extra-systole, which is followed by a long pause. Engelmann explains this long pause as follows: "In consequence of the extra-systole the ventricle is still in the refractory stage when the next physiological stimulus reaches it. This stimulus, therefore, has no effect, no contraction takes place, and it is not till the next stimulus after it that a contraction can again be produced. Thus the normal systole that would follow the extra-systole is missed; then the first systole that comes after the compensatory pause occurs exactly at the moment at which it would have occurred had no extra-systole preceded it" (Wenckebach). The irregularity, inequality, and intermission of the pulse as

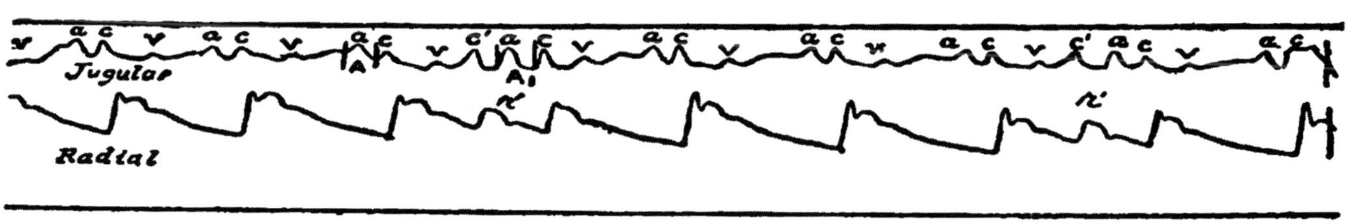

FIG. 2.—EXTRA-SYSTOLES OF VENTRICULAR TYPE AT c′ and r′ (Mackenzie).

met with in every day clinical experience are largely due to the occurrence of these extra-systoles, which may present all sorts of combinations and groupings, bigeminal, trigeminal, etc., depending upon whether the extra pulse beats are perceptible or not. And yet in spite of this most extreme irregularity there may be no actual pathological change, and so far as the maintenance of the circulation is concerned the heart may be acting in a most satisfactory manner. Patients may feel the extra-systole as a definite thud, and the compensatory pause is perceptible, but very often there are no subjective sensations.

Extra-systoles occur at all ages and under the most varied conditions in health and disease. Mackenzie recognizes a youthful and an adult type of arrhythmia, which in the latter is due chiefly to the presence of extra-systoles, There are several classes of cases. The arrhythmia may be a life-long condition. Without any recognizable disease, without any impairment of the action of the heart, there is permanent irregularity. This may be a peculiarity of the heart-muscle of the individual, who has extra-systole for the same reason—physiological but not well understood—as the dog and horse, in which animals this phenomenon is common. The late Chancellor Ferrier, of McGill University, who died at the age of eighty seven, had an extremely irregular heart action for the last fifty years of his life. I know several men who have

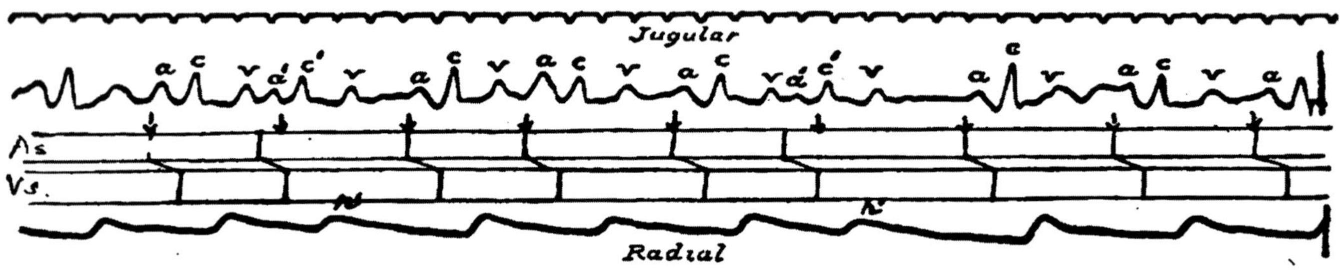

Fig. 3.—Extra-systoles (*a'*) Followed by Ventricular Contractions (*c'*, *v'*). The arrows in the diagram represent the sinus stimulation, and the long pauses after the extra-systoles are seen to be due to the fact that the auricle did not respond to the sinus stimulation after the extra-systole (as, auricular systole vs. ventricular systole) (Mackenzie).

had for many years irregularity without the slightest discomfort. In debilitated and neurasthenic persons there may be an irritable weakness of the heart associated with extra-systole, and palpitation of a most distressing character. In a second group toxic agents, as tobacco, tea, coffee, or the poisons of the infectious diseases or those originating in the intestines or metabolic poisons cause arrhythmia. Even reflexly, as in flatulent dyspepsia, extra-systoles may arise. Thirdly, a high blood pressure can set up extra-systoles; also change in posture. And, lastly, organic disease of the heart itself, "dilatation, inflammation, poor blood supply to the muscle, overexertion, can all supply stimuli to set up extra-systoles either directly or reflexly" (Wenckebach). Too much stress should not be laid upon arrhythmia *per se* in the absence of organic disease.

3. FIBRILLATION OF THE HEART

(*Cardiac Flutter, Nodal Rhythm, Pulsus Irregularis Perpetuus*)

This common manifestation of cardiac irregularity is exceedingly important to recognize clinically. In the most pronounced form it is seen in the last stages of mitral stenosis, in which the pulse shows extreme irregularity, which, when once established, seldom returns to normal. A study of its features in this condition gave Mackenzie the clue to its explanation. He found that in certain cases the transition from regular to irregular pulse of this type occurred with suddenness, and that, whereas before the irregularity supervened the jugular pulse showed the normal features in the presence of auricular carotid and ventricular waves, with a marked presystólic murmur and thrill at the apex, after the irregularity was established, the auricular wave disappeared from the jugular pulse and the presystolic murmur from the apex. The inference drawn from these facts was that the right auricle of the heart was so dilated as to prevent the formation of a normal auricular contraction. The stimulus normally produced at or near the superior vena cava was prevented from passing down the junctional tissues to the ventricle; hence the stimulus arose in another and slightly less excitable part of the heart, which Mackenzie supposed to be the auriculo-ventricular node of Tawara on the right side of the auricular septum. Complete proof of the cause of this condition has been supplied by Lewis, who found that patients with this irregularity showed in galvanometric tracings from the auricle numerous small and continuous waves, exactly similar to those obtained in the dog after fibrillation of the auricle has been induced by faradic stimulation of the appendix, of the right auricle, or by ligation of the right coronary artery. Very small auricular beats are occasionally to be seen in the jugular tracings from such patients. As no co-ordinated contraction of the auricle is present, the arrival of the stimuli at the junctional tissues has no orderly sequence, the ventricle is stimulated without regularity, and in consequence the pulse is irregular.

True nodal rhythm is a comparatively rare condition, in which the stimulus production arises in the junctional tissues; the diagnostic feature is the simultaneous contraction of auricle and ventricle as shown by the superposition of the *a* and *c* waves of the jugular pulse. The radial pulse in this condition is regular.

Auricular fibrillation forms a large proportion of the cases showing cardiac irregularity. Of 114 cases of all forms of irregularity studied by Lewis 57 were of this type. Of etiological factors the most important are mitral stenosis, whether in the rheumatic form or that seen in women with no history of rheumatism and cardio-stenosis. The average age of onset in those with a previous history of rheumatism is 30 to 40; in the non-rheumatic group it is between 50 and 60. In the older patients it may show a paroxysmal form or at least prolonged intermissions.

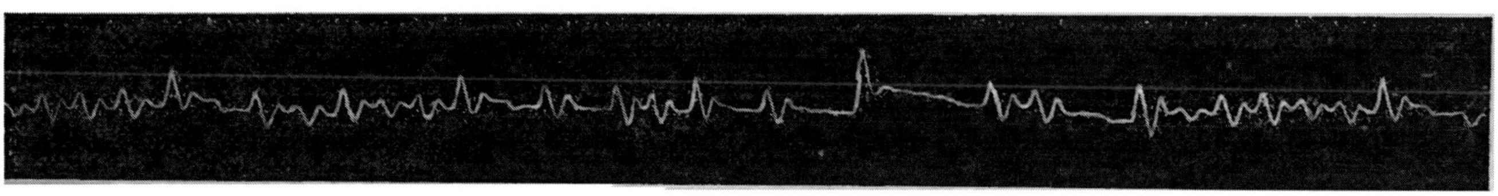

FIG. 4.—PULSE TRACING FROM A CASE OF AURICULAR FIBRILLATION.

The symptoms due to the fibrillation itself cannot be appreciated in the cases of mitral stenosis, but may be seen in those not so accompanied. Here the symptoms may be absent, or consist in some limitation in the field of cardiac response: the patient more easily becomes breathless on exertion, and there may be a tendency to much greater fatigue. The inception of fibrillation may be associated with great dyspnœa, orthopnœa, and the features of right heart failure. The condition may last for many years when once established, and the patient may be able to follow an arduous occupation. An unduly grave view must not, therefore, be taken, unless there be marked evidence of cardiac failure. The patient should be cautioned against undue exertion.

4. RAPID HEART—TACHYCARDIA

The rapid action may be perfectly natural. There are individuals whose normal heart action is at 100 or even more per minute. Emotional causes, violent exercise, and fevers all produce great increase in the rapidity of the heart's action. The extremely rapid action which follows fright may persist for days or even weeks. Traube reports an instance in which, after violent exercise, the rapidity of the heart continued. Cases are not uncommon at the menopause.

There are cases again in which the condition can hardly be termed a neurosis, since it depends upon definite changes in the pneumogastrics or in the medulla. Cases have been reported in which tumor or clot in or about the medulla or pressure upon the vagi has been associated with heart hurry. Some of the cases of frequent action of the heart in women have been thought to be due to reflex irritation from ovarian or uterine disease. Other cases are almost certainly due to lesions of the heart itself and are now and then seen subsequent to an influenzal attack; young and old persons are affected. The tachycardia may persist for months or indefinitely, and there is serious interference with the amount of muscular exertion such persons can take; in addition there is a sense of weakness and sometimes fainting attacks.

Paroxysmal Tachycardia.—Modern methods enable us to subdivide the cases of paroxysmal tachycardia into three groups, corresponding to the types of extra-systole—the auricular, the nodal, and the ventricular. In the auricular type there is a well marked auricular wave in the venous pulse in its normal relation to the carotid wave; in the nodal type the auricular and carotid wave occur at the same time, giving a large double wave in the venous tracing; the third type has not been seen in man, but from experimental work on the dog (Lewis) it may be predicted that it will be found. These three types are due to an irritable focus in the cardiac musculature, the auricular in the auricular muscle, the nodal in the functional (auriculo-ventricular) tissues which form the muscular bridge between the auricle and the ventricle, and the ventricular in the ventricular muscle. In many cases it may be due to slight or transitory ischæmia from a sclerosed artery or one whose muscle is liable to spasm, for Lewis has shown that on tying the right coronary artery in the dog attacks of ventricular tachycardia are almost invariably seen. "A hyper-excitability of some focus in the cardiac musculature as the direct exciting cause of paroxysmal tachycardia is a probable explanation of its production. The degree of response to stimulation depends not only on the intensity of the stimulus, but also on the excitability of the tissue itself. In the known increased excitability of the auricle as compared to the ventricle may possibly be found an explanation of the increased frequency of auricular over other forms of tachycardia" (Lea).

The pulse rate may reach 200 and over. The cases are not common. The attack may be quite short and persist only for an hour or so. A patient at the Philadelphia Infirmary for Nervous Diseases was attacked every week or two; the pulse would rise to 220 or 230, and there were such feelings of distress and uneasiness that the patient always had to lie down. There may be, however, no subjective disturbance, and in another case the patient was able to walk about during the paroxysm and had no dyspnœa. One of the most remarkable cases is reported by H. C. Wood. A physician in his eighty-seventh year had had attacks at intervals from his thirty-seventh year. The onset was abrupt and the pulse would rapidly rise to 200 a minute. For more than twenty years the taking of ice-water or strong coffee would arrest the attacks. Bouveret, who has analyzed a number of cases of this essential or idiopathic form, finds that a permanent cure is rare, and that the patients suffer for ten or more years. Four instances terminated fatally from heart-failure. One of the most remarkable features is the abruptness of onset and the abruptness with which an attack may end. One of my patients had recurring attacks lasting ten to thirty days, and the heart would suddenly "flop," as she expressed it, the rate falling from 180 to 80 or 90 per minute.

5. SLOW HEART—BRADYCARDIA

Slow action of the heart is sometimes normal and may be a family peculiarity. Napoleon is stated to have had a pulse of only 40 per minute.

In any case of slow pulse it is important first to make sure that the number of heart and arterial beats correspond. In many instances this is not the case, and with a radial pulse at 40 the cardiac pulsations may be 80, half the beats not reaching the wrist. The heart contractions, not the pulse wave, should be taken into account.

Physiological Bradycardia.—As age advances the pulse rate becomes slow. In the puerperal state the pulse may beat from 44 to 60 per minute, or may even be as low as 34. It is seen in premature labor as well as at term. The explanation of its occurrence at this period is not clear. Slowness of the pulse is associated with hunger. Bradycardia depending on individual peculiarity is extremely rare.

Pathological bradycardia, which is met with under the following conditions: (*a*) In convalescence from acute fevers. This is extremely common, particularly after pneumonia, typhoid fever, rheumatic fever, and diphtheria. It is most frequently seen in young persons and in cases which have run a normal course. (*b*) In diseases of the digestive system, such as chronic dyspepsia, ulcer or cancer of the stomach, and jaundice. (*c*) In diseases of the respiratory system. Here it is by no means so common, but it is seen not infrequently in emphysema. (*d*) In diseases of the circulatory system. Excluding all cases of irregularity of the heart, bradycardia is not common in diseases of the valves. It is most frequently seen in fatty and fibroid changes in the heart, but is not constant in them. (*e*) In diseases of the urinary organs. It occurs occasionally in nephritis and may be a feature of uræmia. (*f*) From the action of toxic agents. It occurs in uræmia, poisoning by lead, alcohol, and follows the use of tobacco, coffee, and digitalis. (*g*) In constitutional disorders, such as anæmia, chlorosis, and diabetes. (*h*) In diseases of the nervous system. Apoplexy, epilepsy, the cerebral tumors, affections of the medulla, and diseases and injuries of the cervical cord may be associated with very slow pulse. In general paresis, mania, and melancholia it is not infrequent. (*i*) It occurs occasionally in affections of the skin and sexual organs, and in sunstroke, or in prolonged exhaustion from any cause.

6. HEART-BLOCK. STOKES-ADAMS DISEASE

The impulse causing the heart to beat originates at the venous end of the heart and is transmitted in such a way that the auricles contract first, the ventricles a moment later, the impulse being propagated like a peristaltic wave through the heart walls. In passing from the auricle to the ventricle the stimulus traverses a narrow band of muscle, the only demonstrable muscular connection between the venous and arterial chambers. In the adult heart this auriculo-ventricular bundle of His is 18 mm. long, 2.5 mm. broad, and 1.5 mm. thick; it arises in the septum of the auricles below the foramen ovale and passes downward and forward through the trigonum fibrosum of the auriculo-ventricular junction, where it comes into close relation with the mesial leaflet of the tricuspid valve. Passing along the upper edge of the

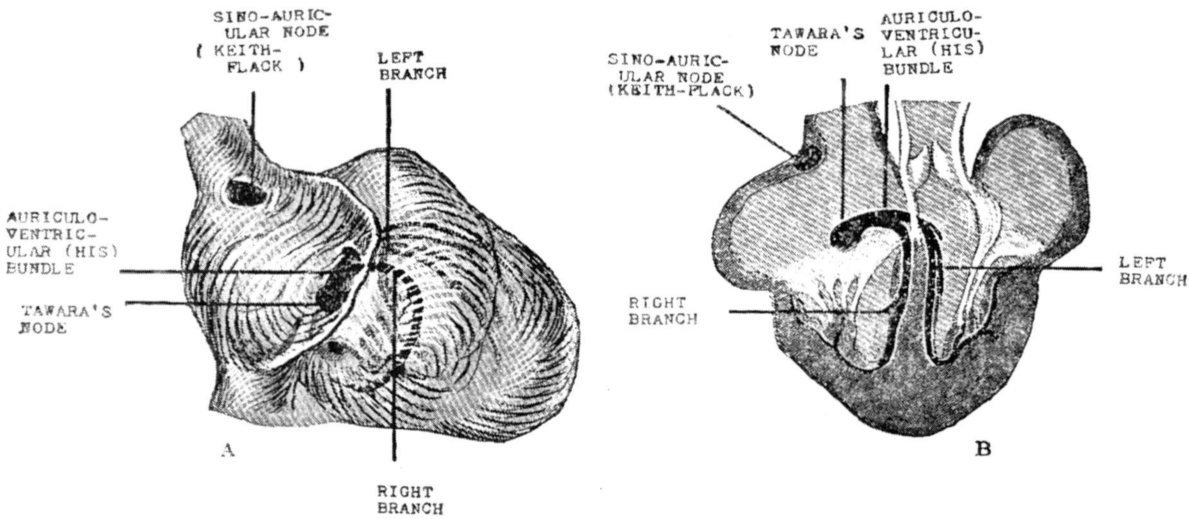

Fig. 5.—Diagram Showing the Sino-auricular Node and the Auricular Bundle. A, viewed from the right; B, cross section of the heart, viewed from the front. (Kindness of A. D. Hirschfelder.)

muscular septum, just where it joins with the posterior edge of the membranous septum, it radiates from this point throughout the heart as the junctional system of Tawara. In the dog destruction of the bundle prevents the passage from the auricle to the ventricle of the impulse which normally causes the ventricles to contract. They immediately assume a rate of beating which is very much slower than that of the auricles and is totally independent, as they possess their own automatic rhythmicity. Under ordinary circumstances this inherent rhythmicity can not manifest itself because the much more rapidly beating venous end of the heart sets the pace for the sluggish arterial end. But if the auricular impulse is blocked, the ventricles, released from the control of their normal pace maker, assume their own rate. This condition has been called complete heart-block. By an ingenious contrivance Erlanger has been able in the dog gradually to compress the auriculo-ventricular bundle and produce various stages of this condition, namely, one ventricular silence with every other auricular beat, giving a 2:1 rhythm, and proceeding to a 3:1 and a 4:1 rhythm. Finally, complete block may result, in which no impulses pass from the auricles, but the ventricles beat with their own inherent rate, which Erlanger estimates from a study of cases of heart-block in my wards, to be about 23 to 28 beats to the minute in man. The explanation of the phenomenon is based upon one suggested by Gaskell. The bundle of His, like all muscle tissue, becomes fatigued when it is made to contract repeatedly. Under normal circumstances sufficient time elapses between successive beats to permit the bundle to return to its normal state, but when from injury or any cause the irritability of the bundle is greatly reduced, it may not react to the auricular stimulus, which thus fails to reach the ventricles. Occasionally while compressing the auriculo-ventricular bundle in the dog, the ventricle alone may suddenly stop beating for as long as twenty seconds. The explanation is here to be sought for the syncopal attacks in Stokes-Adams disease. In this condition the relaxed ventricles are distended rhythmically by the beats of the auricles until the distention may be extreme. The veins become engorged and pulsate synchronously with the auricles. Each of the infrequent contractions of the ventricles relieves the condition temporarily. When the heart-block is complete the vagi still exert their normal control over the rate of the auricles, but they have lost almost completely their influence over the ventricles, and in Stokes-Adams disease we find the pulse rate is little influenced by conditions which normally alter it, as exercise, posture, etc.

Clinically Stokes-Adams disease presents three features: (*a*) slow pulse, usually permanent, but sometimes paroxysmal, falling to 40, 20, or even 6 per minute; (*b*) cerebral attacks—vertigo of a transient character, syncope, pseudo-apoplectiform attacks or epileptiform seizures; (*c*) visible auricular impulses in the veins of the neck, as noted by Stokes—the beats varying greatly; a 2:1 or 3:1 rhythm is the most common. There are several groups of cases. It is usually a senile manifestation associated with arterio-sclerosis. The cases in young adults and middle aged men are often myocardial and of syphilitic origin. There is a neurotic group in which all the features may be present, and in which post mortem no lesions have been found (Edes and Councilman). In the attacks of slow pulse in this group the auricular as well as the ventricular rate may be slow and equal, the normal sequence of events being preserved; the origin of the condition is probably vagal. The outlook in this class of cases is good; in the others it is a serious disease and usually fatal, though it may last for many years. The cerebral attacks are due to anæmia of the brain or of the medulla in consequence of the imperfect ventricular action. In one of my cases Baetjer could see with the fluoroscope the more frequent contraction of the auricles.

TREATMENT OF PALPITATION AND ARRHYTHMIA

An important element in many cases is to get the patient's mind quieted, and he can be assured that there is no actual danger. The mental element is often very strong. In palpitation, before using medicines, it is well to try the effect of hygienic measures. As a rule, moderate exercise may be taken with advantage. Regular hours should be kept, and at least ten hours out of the twenty four should be spent in the recumbent posture. A tepid bath may be taken in the morning, or, if the patient is weakly and nervous, in the evening, followed by a thorough rubbing. Hot baths and the Turkish bath should be avoided. The dietetic management is most important. It is best to prohibit alcohol, tea, and coffee absolutely. The diet should be light and the patient should avoid taking large meals. Articles of food known to cause flatulency should not be used. If a smoker, the patient should give up tobacco. Sexual excitement is particularly pernicious, and the patient should be warned specially on this point. For the distressing attacks of palpitation which occur with neurasthenia, particularly in women, a rigid Weir Mitchell course is the most satisfactory. It is in these cases that we find the most distressing throbbing in the abdomen, which is apt to come on after meals, and is very much aggravated by flatulency. The cases of palpitation due to excesses or to errors in diet and dyspepsia are readily remedied by hygienic measures.

A course of iron is often useful. Strychnia is particularly valuable, and is perhaps best administered as the tincture of nux vomica in large doses. Very little good is obtained from the smaller quantities. It should be given freely, 20 minims (1.3 c. c.) three times a day.

If there is great rapidity of action, aconite may be tried. There are cases associated with sleeplessness and restlessness which are greatly benefited by bromide of potassium. Digitalis is very rarely indicated, but in obstinate cases it may be tried with the nux vomica. Ammonium bromide is very efficacious in the tachycardias and arrythmias of nervous people.

Cases of heart hurry are often extremely obstinate, as may be judged from the case of the physician reported by H. C. Wood, in whom the condition persisted in spite of all measures for fifty years. The bromides are sometimes useful; the general condition of neurasthenia should be treated, and during the paroxysm an ice bag may be placed upon the heart, or Leiter's coil, through which ice water is passed. Electricity, in the form of galvanism, is sometimes serviceable, and for its mental effect the Franklinic current. For the condition of slow pulse but little can be done. A great majority of the cases are not dangerous.

II. AFFECTIONS OF THE MYOCARDIUM

1. HYPERTROPHY

Varieties.—The heart enlarges to meet a demand for extra work, either general, as in the continuous strain of athletics (the hypertrophy of work), or special to combat a deficiency of cardiac structure, such as a damaged valve. There are two forms, one in which the cavity or cavities are of normal size, and the other in which the cavities are enlarged and the walls increased in thickness (eccentric hypertrophy). The so-called concentric hypertrophy in which there is diminution of the size of the cavity with thickening of the walls is, as a rule, a post mortem change.

The enlargement may affect the entire organ, or one side, or only one chamber. Naturally, as the left ventricle does the chief work the change is most frequently found here. Though its production is assisted by adequate nutrition, hypertrophy may appear even under conditions of starvation, given otherwise healthy organs. In the debilitated the limits to which hypertrophy may progress are small, though very marked hypertrophy is sometimes seen in the aged.

HYPERTROPHY OF THE LEFT VENTRICLE ALONE, or with general enlargement of the heart, is brought about by—

Conditions affecting the heart itself: (*a*) Disease of the aortic valve; (*b*) mitral insufficiency; (*c*) pericardial adhesions; (*d*) sclerotic myocarditis; (*e*) disturbed innervation with overaction, as in exophthalmic goitre, in long-continued nervous palpitation, and as a result of the action of certain articles, such as tea, coffee, tobacco, and probably alcohol, as in the Munich beer heart. In all of these the work of the heart is increased. In the case of the valve lesions the increase is due to the increased intraventricular pressure; in the case of the adherent pericardium and myocarditis, to direct interference with the symmetrical and orderly contraction of the chambers.

Conditions acting upon the blood-vessels: (*a*) General arterio-sclerosis, with or without renal disease, especially sclerosis of the aorta, the renal arteries, and the vessels of the splanchnic area; (*b*) all states of increased arterial tension induced by the contraction of the smaller arteries under the influence of certain toxic substances, which, as Bright suggested, "by affecting the minute capillary circulation, render great action necessary to send the blood through the distant subdivisions of the vascular system"; (*c*) prolonged muscular exertion, which enormously increases the blood pressure in the arteries; (*d*) narrowing of the aorta, as in the congenital stenosis.

HYPERTROPHY OF THE RIGHT VENTRICLE is met with under the following conditions—

(*a*) *Lesions of the mitral valve,* either incompetence or stenosis, which act by increasing the resistance in the pulmonary vessels. (*b*) *Pulmonary lesions,* obliteration of any number of blood vessels within the lungs, such as occurs in emphysema or cirrhosis, is followed by hypertrophy of the right ventricle. (*c*) *Valvular lesions* on the right side occasionally cause hypertrophy in the adult, not infrequently in the fetus. (*d*) *Chronic valvular disease of the left heart and pericardial adhesions* are sooner or later associated with hypertrophy of the right ventricle.

In the auricles simple hypertrophy is never seen; there is always dilatation with hypertrophy. In the left auricle the condition develops in lesions at the mitral orifice, particularly stenosis. The right auricle hypertrophies when there is greatly increased blood pressure in the lesser circulation, whether due to mitral stenosis or pulmonary lesions. Narrowing of the tricuspid orifice is a less frequent cause.

Symptoms.—There may be no complaint attributable to the hypertrophy, and if associated with renal disease or arterio-sclerosis there may be a marked sense of well-being. If, however, the cardiac defect be not fully compensated, the patient may complain of slight giddiness, headache, a sense of palpitation in the thorax, and some dyspnœa on exertion.

In hypertrophy of the right auricle the venous pulsation in the neck may be more evident, and a tracing may show a marked increase in the size of the auricular wave. An increase in dulness to the right of the sternum in the third and fourth interspaces may be detected, and on very rare occasions a sound preceding that of the ventricle over that area. Hypertrophy of the right ventricle causes a slight bulging of the costal angle with a positive instead of a negative pulsation at this spot. The apex beat may be diffuse, as the enlarged right ventricle prevents the left ventricle from coming into contact with the chest wall. The venous pulsation in the neck is usually marked, and the first sound over the tricuspid area louder than normal. Hypertrophy of the left auricle, which is seldom marked and never unassociated with dilatation, may be detected occasionally by dulness toward the base of the left lung behind; it is easily diagnosed by the extension backward of the cardiac shadow in oblique illumination of the chest by the X-rays. Hypertrophy of the left ventricle is usually easy to diagnose. There is a forcible impulse at the apex beat, both visible and palpable. This impulse may cause a movement of a large area of the chest wall. The apex beat, if there be only slight dilatation, is usually displaced downward, and is found in the 6th and 7th spaces; but if the dilatation be marked, the apex beat becomes more diffuse and is found well outside the nipple line in the 4th, 5th, and 6th spaces. The first sound is usually marked and has been discribed by Michell as "L-lumb"; sometimes it has a distinct booming sound. The second sound at the base is accentuated. The pulse is full and of high tension at the height of the ventricular impulse. The blood pressure is raised.

2. DILATATION

As with other hollow muscular organs, the size of the chambers of the heart varies greatly within normal limits. Dilatation may be an acute process and quite transitory, as after severe muscular effort, or it may be chronic, in which case it is associated with hypertrophy. Not always, however; there is an extraordinary heart in the McGill College Museum showing a parchment like thinning of the walls with uniform dilatation of all the chambers; in places in the right auricle and ventricle only the epicardium remains. Dilatation is pathological only when permanent. Increase in capacity means increased work for the walls and in consequence hypertrophy to meet the demand.

Etiology.—Two important causes combine to produce dilatation—increased pressure within the cavities and impaired resistance, due to weakening of the muscular wall—which may act singly, but are often combined. A normal wall may yield under a heightened blood pressure, or a weakened wall may yield to a normal distending force, the weakened wall being due either to structural change in the cardiac muscle, or to a diminution of its natural tonus.

(*a*) Heightened endocardiac pressure results either from an increased quantity of blood to be moved, or an obstacle to be overcome, and is the more frequent cause of weakening. It does not necessarily bring about dilatation; simple hypertrophy may follow, as in the early period of aortic stenosis, and in the hypertrophy of the left ventricle in Bright's disease.

The size of the cardiac chambers varies in health. With slow action of the heart the dilatation is complete and fuller than it is with rapid action. Moderate exertion in a normal heart, or even prolonged exertion in a well-trained heart, lessens the heart size, but in conditions of ill health dilatation occurs. Physiologically, the limits of dilatation are reached when the chamber does not empty itself during the systole. This may occur as an acute, transient condition in severe exertion in an untrained or feeble condition—during, for example, the ascent of a mountain.

There may be great dilatation of the right heart, as shown by the increased epigastric pulsation, and even increase in the cardiac dulness. The safety valve action of the tricuspid valves may here come into play, relieving the lungs by permitting regurgitation into the auricle. With rest the condition is removed, but, if it has been extreme, the heart may suffer a strain from which it may recover slowly, or, indeed, the individual may never be able again to undertake severe exertion. In the process of training the getting wind, as it is called, is largely a gradual increase in the capability of the heart, particularly of the right chambers. A degree of exertion can be safely maintained in full training which would be quite impossible under other circumstances, because, by a gradual process of what we may call physical education, the heart has strengthened its reserve force—widened enormously its limit of physiological work. Endurance in prolonged contests is measured by the capabilities of the heart, which by increasing its tonus has increased its resistance to dilatation. We have no positive knowledge of the nature of the changes in the heart which occur in this process, but it must be in the direction of increased muscular and nervous energy. The large heart of athletes may be due to the prolonged use of their muscles, but no man becomes a great runner or oarsman who has not naturally a capable if not a large heart. Master McGrath, the celebrated greyhound, and Eclipse, the race horse, both famous for endurance rather than speed, had very large hearts.

Excessive dilatation during severe muscular effort results in *heart-strain.* A man, perhaps in poor condition, calls upon his heart for extra work during the ascent of a high mountain, and is at once seized with pain about the heart and a sense of distress in the epigastrium. He breathes rapidly for some time, is "puffed," as we say, but the symptoms pass off after a night's quiet. An attempt to repeat the exercise is followed by another attack, or, indeed, an attack of cardiac dyspnœa may come on while he is at rest. For months such a man may be unfitted for severe exertion, or he may be permanently incapacitated. In some way he has overstrained his heart and become "broken-winded." Exactly what has taken place in these hearts we can not say, but their reserve force is lost, and with it the power of meeting the demands exacted in maintaining the circulation during severe exertion. The "heart-shock" of Latham includes cases of this nature—sudden cardiac breakdown during exertion, not due to rupture of a valve. It seems probable that sudden death in men during long continued efforts, as in a race, is sometimes due to overdistention and paralysis of the heart.

Acute dilatative heart weakness is seen in many conditions, as in Graves' disease, in paroxysmal tachycardia, in old myocardial cases following exertion, and in angina pectoris. There is usually a striking contrast between the wide and forcible cardiac impulse and the small, feeble, irregular pulse.

Dilatation occurs in all forms of *valve lesions.* In aortic incompetency blood enters the left ventricle during diastole from the unguarded aorta and from the left auricle, and the quantity of blood at the termination of diastole subjects the walls to an extreme degree of pressure, under which they inevitably yield. In time they augment in thickness, and present the typical eccentric hypertrophy of this condition.

In mitral insufficiency blood which should have been driven into the aorta is forced into and dilates the auricle from which it came, and then in the diastole of the ventricle a large amount is returned from the auricle, and with increased force. In mitral stenosis the left auricle is the seat of greatly increased tension during diastole, and dilates as well as hypertrophies; the distention, too, may be enormous. Dilatation of the right ventricle is produced by a number of conditions, which were considered under hypertrophy. All circumstances, such as mitral stenosis, emphysema, etc., which permanently increase the tension of the blood in the pulmonary vessels cause its dilatation.

The idiopathic dilatation and hypertrophy of beer drinkers also comes in this group, as it is brought about gradually by increased endocardial pressure.

(*b*) Impaired nutrition of the heart walls may lead to a diminution of the resisting power so that dilatation readily occurs.

The loss of tone due to parenchymatous degeneration or myocarditis in fevers may lead to a fatal condition of acute dilatation. It is a recognized cause of death in scarlatinal dropsy (Goodhart), and may occur in rheumatic fever, typhus, typhoid, erysipelas, etc. The changes in the heart muscle which accompany acute endocarditis or pericarditis may lead to dilatation, especially in the latter disease. In anæmia, leukæmia, and chlorosis the dilatation may be considerable. In sclerosis of the walls the yielding is always where this process is most advanced, as at the left apex. Under any of these circumstances the walls may yield with normal blood pressure.

Pericardial adhesions are a cause of dilatation, and we generally find in cases with extensive and firm union considerable hypertrophy and dilatation. There is usually here some impairment as well of the superficial layers of muscle.

3. CARDIAC INSUFFICIENCY

Etiology.—With lessening of the muscular power of the heart the rapidity with which the blood circulates is diminished, and the tissues fail to receive their proper supply of oxygen and food, and to be adequately relieved of their waste products—this is cardiac failure. The same effect may be produced in another way. The amount of blood in the body is much less than the total capacity of the vascular bed, and an adequate blood supply is only kept up by a general constriction of arterioles which dam the blood in the arterial system, but if by any chance there is a general vaso-dilatation of the arterioles, especially those in the splanchnic area, the heart does not receive an amount of blood sufficient to supply the bodily needs, with the same effect on the organs as in certain forms of cardiac failure. This condition, which is probably the essence of shock, does not concern us here, but it must be mentioned to avoid the impression that all failure of the circulation means failure of the heart.

The failure in muscular power may affect any cavity singly or the whole heart. Weakness of the left ventricle fails to give proper filling of the arterial system and general anæmia of the tissues results. Failure of the left auricle means stasis in the lung vessels with deficient aeration of the blood, and a tendency to œdema of the lung or to effusion into the pleural cavity.

Failure of the right auricle and ventricle gives cyanosis of the organs, dyspnœa at rest and on slight exertion, with stasis in the abdominal organs and œdema.

The reserve power with which the cardiac muscle is endowed disappears in heart failure. This reserve, greatest in youth, is increased by adequate nutrition, certain congenital endowments, and, apart from other defects, by hypertrophy. It is lessened by defects in the cardiac structure, gross or minute, by defective nutrition, by certain bacterial and other poisons, and with advancing years. We have at present no means of gauging this reserve power of the organ as a whole or in its different parts.

The failure may be sudden or slow, according to the kind and rapidity of the lesion which causes it. When the left ventricle fails the effect may vary from immediate death, through all forms of fainting, giddiness, sense of dissolution, to a mild sense of bodily or mental fatigue; when the right ventricle fails the effect varies from a sudden dyspnœa to a dyspnœa which comes on with slight exertion.

As to the actual condition in cardiac failure generally, it is by no means easy in all cases to say what has been the cause. The lesions to which the cardiac musculature is liable are described further on, yet there is a proportion of cases in which neither by post mortem examination nor careful microscopic search can the source of the failure be even suggested. It is well to bear in mind a suggestion which has been made by Aschoff, namely, that in certain cases the failure is due not so much to the implication of the general musculature as to an affection of the conducting muscular system of Tawara's node in the inter-auricular septum, and of the bundle of His with its ramifications which stretch to all parts of the right and left ventricles, and whose function is to distribute the muscular impulses which at each contraction spread from the venous to the arterial end of the heart.

The blood pressure in cardiac insufficiency shows no uniform figures. The maximum pressure, which is that usually estimated, may be high even in a failing heart. In serious degrees of myocardial affection, such as fatty degeneration or chloroform poisoning, it is low. In cases in which there has been a raised blood pressure, the maximum may be lower or higher than the normal for the patient. We must recognize that probably in early stages of failure the heart is stimulated to put forth increased energy at each beat, and that the maximum pressure at the height of the beat slightly over-compensates the circulatory defect.

Acute Cardiac Insufficiency.—Causes: (*a*) Wounds of the heart, (*b*) spontaneous rupture or rupture of valves, (*c*) rapid effusion into the pericardium of blood or serous fluid, (*d*) access of air to the chambers of the heart, as from operations at the root of the neck or decomposition after exposure to a high atmospheric pressure, (*e*) large thrombi quickly formed in a heart cavity, (*f*) sudden interference with the coronary circulation, especially the left coronary artery, (*g*) mechanical interference with the heart from obliteration of the trachea or larynx, as in strangulation, (*h*) acute infections, such as diphtheria or pericarditis, (*i*) certain poisons, such as pilocarpin, cocaine, phosphorus, etc., (*j*) stimulation of the vagus nerve, its centre in the medulla, or its termination in the heart.

Chronic Cardiac Insufficiency.—Causes: (*a*) Lesions of the heart muscle, which will be described in more detail in a subsequent paragraph.

Essentially all cardiac failure is muscular. The myocardium may be insufficiently nourished, as in the starvation atrophy of new growths or in diabetes, or there may be recognizable gross or microscopic lesions. One or more of the functions of the cardiac muscle may be interfered with without producing any changes that can be detected by the microscope, such as the failure associated with aortic disease. (*b*) Lesions of the valves. (*c*) Lesions affecting the vascular fields of the efferent arteries. Emphysema, chronic bronchitis, asthma, sclerosis of the lungs, chest deformities, and mitral disease produce an embarrassment of the right heart; atheroma of the aorta and arterio-sclerosis, especially of the splanchnic and renal area, produce failûre of the left heart. (*d*) Over-exertion. (*e*) Certain poisons, such as alcohol (especially beer) and phosphorus. (*f*) Other causes, such as adherent pericardium and exophthalmic goitre.

Anatomical Basis of Cardiac Insufficiency.—I. Lesions Due to Disease of the Coronary Arteries.—A knowledge of the changes produced in the myocardium by disease of the coronary vessels gives a key to the understanding of many problems in cardiac pathology. The terminal branches of the coronary vessels are end arteries; that is, the communication between neighboring branches is through capillaries only. J. H. Pratt has shown that the vessels of Thebesius, which open from the ventricles and auricles into a system of fine branches and thus communicate with the cardiac capillaries and coronary veins, may be capable of feeding the myocardium sufficiently to keep it alive even when the coronary arteries are occluded. The blocking of one of these vessels by a thrombus or an embolus leads usually to a condition which is known as—

(*a*) *Anæmic necrosis,* or white infarct. When this does not occur the reason may be sought in (1) the existence of abnormal anastomoses, which by their presence take the coronary system out of the group of end arteries; or (2) the vicarious flow through the vessels of Thebesius and the coronary veins. The condition is most commonly seen in the left ventricle and in the septum, in the territory of distribution of the anterior coronary artery. The affected area has a yellowish white color, sometimes a turbid, parboiled aspect, at other times a grayish red tint. It may be somewhat wedge-shaped, more often it is irregular in contour and projects above the surface. Microscopically the changes are very characteristic. The nuclei either disappear from the muscle fibres or they undergo fragmentation. Leucocytes wander in from the surrounding tissue, and these may suffer disintegration. At a later stage a new growth of fibrous tissue is found in the periphery of the infarct which ultimately may entirely replace the dead fibres. The fibres present a homogeneous, hyaline appearance. In some instances there is complete transformation, and even to the naked eye a firm white patch of hyaline degeneration may appear in the centre of the area. Rupture of the heart may be associated with anæmic necrosis.

(*b*) The second important effect of coronary-artery disease upon the myocardium is seen in the production of *fibrous myocarditis.* This may result from the gradual transformation of areas of anæmic necrosis. More commonly it is caused by the narrowing of a coronary branch in a process of obliterative endarteritis. Where the process is gradual evidences of granulation tissue are often wanting, and any distinction between the necrotic muscle fibres and the new scar tissue is difficult to establish. J. B. MacCallum showed that the muscle fibres undergo a change the reverse of that of their normal development and lose their fibril bundles preliminary to their complete replacement by connective tissue. The sclerosis is most frequently seen at the apex of the left ventricle and in the septum, but it may occur in any portion. In the septum and walls there are often streaks and patches which are only seen in carefully made serial sections. Hypertrophy of the heart is commonly associated with this degeneration. It is the invariable precursor of aneurism of the heart.

(*c*) *Sudden Death in Coronary Artery Disease.*—Complete obliteration of one coronary artery, if produced suddenly, is usually fatal. When induced slowly, either by arterio-sclerosis at the orifice of the artery at the root of the aorta or by an obliterating endarteritis in the course of the vessel, the circulation may be carried on through the other vessel. Sudden death is not uncommon, owing to thrombosis of a vessel which has become narrowed by sclerosis. *In medico-legal cases it is a point of primary importance to remember that this is one of the common causes of sudden death.* This condition should be carefully sought for, inasmuch as it may be the sole lesion, except a general, sometimes slight, arterio-sclerosis. In the most extreme grade one coronary artery may be entirely blocked, with the production of extensive fibroid disease, and a main branch of the other also may be occluded. A large, powerfully built imbecile, aged thirty five, at the Elwyn Institution, Pennsylvania, who had for years enjoyed doing the heavy work about the place, died suddenly, without any preliminary symptoms. The heart weighed over 600 grams; the anterior coronary artery was practically occluded by obliterating endarteritis, and of the posterior artery one main branch was blocked.

(*d*) *Septic Infarcts.*—In pyæmia the smaller branches of the coronary arteries may be blocked with emboli which give rise to infectious or septic infarcts in the myocardium in the form of abscesses, varying in size from a pea to a pin's head. These may not cause any disturbance, but when large they may perforate into the ventricle or into the pericardium, forming what has been called acute ulcer of the heart.

II. Acute Interstitial Myocarditis.—In some infectious diseases and in acute pericarditis the intermuscular connective tissue may be swollen and infiltrated with small round cells and leucocytes, the blood vessels dilated, and the muscle fibres the seat of granular, fatty, and hyaline degeneration. Occasionally, in pyæmia the infiltration with pus cells has been diffuse and confined chiefly to the interstitial tissue. Councilman has described this condition of the heart wall in gonorrhœa, and succeeded in demonstrating the gonococcus in the diseased areas. The commonest examples are found in diphtheria, typhoid fever, and acute endocarditis, as shown by the studies of Romberg. The foci may be the starting points of patches of fibrous myocarditis.

III. Fragmentation and Segmentation.—This condition was described by Renaut and Landouzy in 1877, and has been carefully studied by different pathologists. Two forms are met with: 1. Segmentation. The muscle fibres have separated at the cement line. 2. Fragmentation. The fracture has been across the fibre itself, and perhaps at the level of the nucleus. Longitudinal division is unusual. Although the condition doubtless arises in some instances during the death agony, as in cases of sudden death by violence, in others it would seem to have clinical and pathological significance. It is found associated with other lesions, fibrous myocarditis, infarction, and fatty degeneration. J. B. MacCallum distinguished a simple from a degenerative fragmentation. The first takes place in the normal fibre, which, however, shows irregular extensions and contractions. The second succeeds degeneration in the fibre. Hearts the seat of marked fragmentation are lax, easily torn, the muscle fibres widely separated, and often pale and cloudy.

IV. Parenchymatous Degeneration.—This is usually met with in fevers, or in connection with endocarditis or pericarditis, and in infections and intoxications generally. It is characterized by a pale, turbid state of the cardiac muscle, which is general, not localized. Turbidity and softness are the special features. It is the softened heart of Laennec and Louis. Stokes speaks of an instance in which "so great was the softening of the organ that when the heart was grasped by the great vessels and held with the apex pointing upward, it fell down over the hand, covering it like a cap of a large mushroom."

Histologically, there is a degeneration of the muscle fibres, which are infiltrated to a various extent with granules which resist the action of ether, but are dissolved in acetic acid. Sometimes this granular change in the fibres is extreme, and no trace of the striæ can be detected. It is probably the effect of a toxic agent, and is seen in its most exquisite form in the lumbar muscles in cases of toxic hæmoglobinuria in the horse. It is met with in cases of typhoid, typhus, small-pox, and other infectious diseases, particularly when the course is protracted. There is no definite relation between it and the high temperature.

V. Fatty Heart.—Under this term are embraced fatty degeneration and fatty overgrowth.

(*a*) *Fatty degeneration* is a very common condition, and mild grades are met with in many diseases. It is found in the failing nutrition of old age, of wasting diseases, and of cachectic states; in prolonged infectious fevers, in which it may follow or accompany the parenchymatous change. In pernicious anæmia and in phosphorus poisoning the most extreme degrees are seen. Pericarditis is usually associated with fatty or parenchymatous changes in the superficial layers of the myocardium. Disease of the coronary arteries is a much more common cause of fibroid degeneration than of fatty heart. Lastly, in the hypertrophied ventricular wall in chronic heart-disease fatty change is by no means infrequent. This degeneration may be limited to the heart or it may be more or less general in the solid viscera. The diaphragm may also be involved, even when the other muscles show no special changes. There appears to be a special proneness to fatty degeneration in the heart muscle, which may perhaps be connected with its incessant activity. So great is its need of an abundant oxygen supply that it feels at once any deficiency, and is in consequence the first muscle to show nutritional changes.

Anatomically the condition may be local or general. The left ventricle is most frequently affected. If the process is advanced and general, the heart looks large and is flabby and relaxed. It has a light yellowish brown tint, or, as it is called, a faded leaf color. Its consistence is reduced and the substance tears easily. In the left ventricle the papillary columns and the muscle beneath the endocardium show a streaked or patchy appearance. Microscopically, the fibres are seen to be occupied by minute globules distributed in rows along the line of the primitive fibres (Welch). In advanced grades the fibres seem completely occupied by the minute globules.

(*b*) *Fatty Overgrowth.*—This is usually a simple excess of the normal subpericardial fat, to which the term *cor adiposum* was given by the older writers. In pronounced instances the fat infiltrates between the muscular substance and, separating the strands, may reach even to the endocardium. In corpulent persons there is always much pericardial fat. It forms part of the general obesity, and occasionally leads to dangerous or even fatal impairment of the contractile power of the heart. Of 122 cases analyzed by Forchheimer there were 88 males and 34 females. Over 80 per cent. occurred between the fortieth and seventieth years.

The entire heart may be enveloped in a thick sheeting of fat through which not a trace of muscle substance can be seen. On section the fat infiltrates the muscle, separating the fibres, and in extreme cases—particularly in the right ventricle—reaches the endocardium. In some places there may be even complete substitution of fat for the muscle substance. In rare instances the fat may be in the papillary muscles. The heart is usually much relaxed and the chambers are dilated. Microscopically the muscle fibres may show, in addition to the atrophy, marked fatty degeneration.

VI. Other Degenerations of the Myocardium.—(*a*) *Brown Atrophy.*—This is a common change in the heart muscle, particularly in chronic valvular lesions and in the senile heart. When advanced the color of the muscles is a dark red brown, and the consistence is usually increased. The fibres present an accumulation of yellow brown pigment chiefly about the nuclei. The cement substance is often unusually distinct, but seems more fragile than in healthy muscle.

(*b*) *Amyloid degeneration of the heart* is occasionally seen. It occurs in the intermuscular connective tissue and in the blood vessels, not in the fibres.

(*c*) The *hyaline transformation of Zenker* is sometimes met with in prolonged fevers. The affected fibres are swollen, homogeneous, translucent, and the striæ are very faint.

(*d*) *Calcareous degeneration* occasionally occurs in the myocardium, and the muscle fibres may be infiltrated with lime salts and yet retain their appearance.

Symptoms of Cardiac Insufficiency.—As indicated above, the symptoms of left sided cardiac failure differ from those of the right side, and in each we may distinguish a number of types, which, however, merge gradually the one into the other. Failure of the left ventricle is seen in its severest forms in the abrupt death stroke of angina pectoris, in the sudden faints with sweats and heart pain of fatty or fibroid hearts, or in the fainting and convulsive attacks of Stokes-Adams disease. Less severe failure may be seen in athletes after a hard race, when vomiting and a feeling of dissolution are present—a type which is sometimes seen in angina, when it is liable to be mistaken for a gastro-intestinal upset. The milder degrees show themselves in an inability to take much exercise or to suffer much mental work without the sense of great fatigue. Sudden and slow types are also seen in failure of the right side. Subjected to a slight strain, great hyperpnœa and distress may come on, and one form of cardiac dyspnœa which attacks the patient at night is of this nature. The severer forms show an increasing inability to undergo slight extra exertion, such as mounting stairs, or hyperpnœa even when at rest in bed, in both of which there is usually some œdema of the feet, especially at night, if the patient is on his feet most of the day.

Grouped under their special systems the symptoms complained of by patients with cardiac failure are as follows: (*a*) Cardio-vascular system: Pain in the cardiac area or extending to the shoulders and down the arms, a sense of weight in the præcordium; palpitation is seldom complained of. (*b*) Respiratory system: Dyspnœa at rest or on exertion, or orthopnœa, Cheyne-Stokes respiration, cough, loss of voice from pressure of a dilated left auricle on the left recurrent laryngeal nerve, hæmoptysis (as resulting from lung infarcts). (*c*) Central nervous system; in addition to those given above are sleeplessness, mental symptoms, delusions, melancholia, and especially toward the end stupor and drowsiness. (*d*) Cyanosis, pallor, œdema, and occasionally purpura in the lower limbs. (*e*) Alimentary system: The stasis in the abdominal organs in right heart failure produces loss of appetite, indigestion, flatulence, vomiting, constipation, diarrhœa, abdominal pain, hæmorrhoids, etc. (*f*) Renal system: The urine is scanty, high colored, and contains a slight amount of albumin.

Physical examination of the heart may reveal an apex-beat which is feeble, outside the nipple line, diffuse, and whose maximum intensity is not easily localized. The pulsation may be marked on inspection and cover a very wide area; arterial pulsation in the neck in the left heart failure may be great; in right heart failure the jugular veins may be very dilated and their pulsations may be normal, indicating three waves, or regurgitant. On percussion the cardiac area may be much increased to the right or to the left, or both. On auscultation the sounds may be difficult to hear, or feebler than normal; murmurs, usually soft, may be present at both apex and base. Gallop rhythm may be present. The pulse may show great variations; marked failure may exist with a full bounding pulse; more usually it is feeble with diminished tension; it may be irregular, intermittent, slow, or rapid. No one sign or combination of signs is significant of cardiac failure. A heart may be insufficient and yet perhaps nothing can be detected by physical examination except feeble sounds and a low tension pulse.

The myocardial lesion is not always proportionate to the intensity of the symptoms. A patient may present enfeebled, irregular action and signs of dilatation—shortness of breath, œdema, and the general symptoms believed to be characteristic of cases of fibroid and fatty heart—and the post mortem show little or no change in the myocardium.

Cardio-sclerosis or fibroid heart is in some cases characterized by a feeble, irregular, slow pulse, with dyspnœa on exertion and occasional attacks of angina. Irregularity is present in many, but not in all cases. The pulse may be very slow, even 30 or 40 per minute, and the features those of Stokes-Adams disease. A man with advanced fibroid myocarditis may die suddenly while at work, without having ever complained of heart trouble. Ultimately the cases come under observation with the symptoms of cardiac insufficiency. The arrhythmia, which may have been present, becomes aggravated and, according to Riegel, may not only precede, but also persist after the cardiac insufficiency has passed away.

Fatty degeneration of the heart presents the same difficulties. Extreme fatty changes, as in pernicious anæmia, may be present with a full pulse and regularly acting heart. The fat does not appear to interfere seriously with the function of the organ. The truth is, it may be present in an extreme grade without producing symptoms, so long as great dilatation of the chambers does not occur. The cardiac irregularity, the dyspnœa, palpitation and small pulse are in reality not symptoms of the fatty degeneration, but of dilatation which has supervened. The fatty *arcus senilis* is of no moment in the diagnosis of fatty heart. The heart sounds may be weak and the action irregular.

When dilatation occurs there is gallop rhythm, shortening of the long pause, and a systolic murmur at the apex. Shortness of breath on exertion is an early feature in many cases, and anginal attacks may occur. There is sometimes a tendency to syncope, and in both fibroid and fatty heart there are attacks in which the patient feels cold and depressed and the pulse sinks to 40 or 30, or even, as in one case which I saw, to 26. The patient may wake from sleep in the early morning with an attack of severe "cardiac asthma." These "spells" may be associated with nausea and may alternate with others in which there are anginal symptoms. These are the cases, too, in which for weeks there may be mental symptoms. The patient has delusions and may even become maniacal. Toward the close the type of breathing known as Cheyne-Stokes may occur. It was described in the following terms by John Cheyne, speaking of a case of fatty heart (Dublin Hospital Reports, vol. ii, p. 221, 1818): "For several days his breathing was irregular; it would entirely cease for a quarter of a minute, then it would become perceptible, though very low, then by degrees it became heaving and quick, and then it would gradually cease again: this revolution in the state of his breathing lasted about a minute, during which there were about thirty acts of respiration." It is seen much more frequently in arterio-sclerosis and uræmic states than in fatty heart.

Fatty overgrowth of the heart is a condition certain to exist in very obese persons. It produces no symptoms until the muscular fibre is so weakened that dilatation occurs. These patients may for years present a feeble but regular pulse; the heart sounds are weak and muffled, and a murmur may be heard at the apex. Attacks of "cardiac asthma" are not uncommon, and the patient may suffer from bronchitis. Dizziness and pseudo-apoplectic seizures may occur. Sudden death may result from syncope or from rupture of the heart. The physical examination is often difficult because of the great increase in the fat, and it may be impossible to define the area of dulness.

For clinical purposes we may group the cases of failure from myocardial disease as follows:

(1) Those in which sudden death occurs with or without previous indications of heart-trouble. Sclerosis of the coronary arteries exists—in some instances with recent thrombus and white infarcts; in others, extensive fibroid disease; in others again, fatty degeneration. Many patients never complain of cardiac distress, but, as in the case of Chalmers, the celebrated Scottish divine, enjoy unusual vigor of mind and body.

(2) Cases in which there are cardiac arrhythmia, shortness of breath on exertion, attacks of dyspnœa, sometimes anginal attacks, collapse symptoms

with sweats and extremely slow pulse, and occasionally marked mental symptoms.

(3) Cases with general arterio-sclerosis and hypertrophy and dilatation of the heart. They are robust men of middle age who have worked hard and lived carelessly Dyspnœa, cough, and swelling of the feet are the early symptoms, and the patient comes under observation either with a gallop rhythm, embryocardia, or an irregular heart with an apex systolic murmur of mitral insufficiency. Recovery from the first or second attack is the rule. It is one of the most common forms of heart-disease.

Prognosis.—Each case must be judged on its own merits, special notice being taken of the age, probable origin, and anatomical basis of the insufficiency. The outlook in affections of the myocardium occurring late in life is extremely grave. Patients recover, however, in a surprising way from the most serious attacks, particularly those of the third group.

Treatment.—Many cases never come under treatment; the first are the final symptoms. Other cases with well marked failure, if treated on general lines according to the routine measures, recover quickly.

Much more difficult is the management of those cases in which there is marked cardiac arrhythmia, with a feeble, irregular, very slow pulse, and syncope or angina. Dropsy is not, as a rule, present; the heart sounds may be clear and there are no signs of dilatation.

The following are the general methods to be observed in the treatment of cardiac failure:

(*a*) Rest.—Disturbed compensation may be completely restored by rest of the body. In many cases with œdema of the ankles, moderate dilatation of the heart, and irregularity of the pulse, rest in bed, a few doses of the compound tincture of cardamon, and a saline purge suffice, within a week or ten days, to restore the compensation.

(*b*) Diet.—In acute conditions it is usually well to limit this in amount, especially the fluids. With marked passive congestion liquid diet may be advisable; otherwise small amounts of simple food may be given at short intervals. In any case with dilatation it is well to limit the total daily intake of fluids to 1,500 c. c. A "dry diet" for a few days is sometimes useful.

(*c*) The relief of the embarrassed circulation.

(1) *By Venesection.*—In cases of dilatation, from whatever cause, in mitral or aortic lesions or distention of the right ventricle in emphysema, when signs of venous engorgement are marked and when there is orthopnœa with cyanosis, the abstraction of from 20 to 30 ounces of blood is indicated. This is the occasion in which timely venesection may save the patient's life. It is particularly helpful in the dilated heart of arterio-sclerosis.

(2) *By Depletion through the Bowels.*—This is particularly valuable when dropsy is present. Of the various purges the salines are to be preferred, and may be given by Matthew Hay's method. Half an hour to an hour before breakfast from half an ounce to an ounce and a half of Epsom salts may be given in a concentrated form. This usually produces from three to five liquid evacuations. The compound jalap powder in half drachm doses, or elaterium, may be employed for the same purpose. Even when the pulse is very feeble these hydragogue cathartics are well borne, and they deplete the portal system rapidly and efficiently.

(3) *The Use of Remedies Which Stimulate the Heart's Action.*—Of these by far the most important is digitalis, which was introduced into practice by Withering. The indication for its use is weakness of the heart muscle; the contra-indication is a perfectly balanced compensatory hypertrophy, such as we see in all forms of valvular disease. Broken compensation in valvular disease, no matter what the lesion may be, is the signal for its use. It acts upon the heart, slowing and at the same time increasing the force of the contractions. It acts on the peripheral arteries, raising their tension, so that a steady and equable flow of blood is maintained in the capillaries, which, after all, is the prime aim and object of the circulation. High blood pressure is not a contra-indication to its use. The beneficial effects are best seen in cases of mitral disease with small, irregular pulse and cardiac dropsy. Its effects are not less striking in the dilatation of the left ventricle, in the failing compensation of aortic insufficiency or of arterio-sclerosis. On theoretical grounds it has been urged that its use is not so advantageous in aortic insufficiency, since it prolongs the diastole and leads to greater distention. This need not be considered, and digitalis is just as serviceable in this as in any other condition associated with progressive dilatation; larger doses are often required. It may be given as the tincture or the infusion. In cases of cardiac dropsy, from whatever cause, 15 minims (1 c. c.) of the tincture or half an ounce (15 c. c.) of the infusion may be given every three hours for two days, after which the dose may be reduced. Some prefer the tincture, others the infusion; it is a matter of indifference if the drug is good. The urine of a patient taking digitalis should be carefully estimated each day. As a rule, when its action is beneficial, there is within twenty-four hours an increase in the amount; often the flow is very great. Under its use the dyspnœa is relieved, the dropsy gradually disappears, the pulse becomes firmer, fuller in volume, and sometimes, if it has been very intermittent, regular.

Ill effects sometimes follow digitalis. There is no such thing as a cumulative action of the drug manifested by sudden symptoms. Toxic effects are seen in the production of nausea and vomiting. Digipuratum is less disturbing to the stomach and may be given when there is gastric irritability. The pulse becomes irregular and small, and there may be two beats of the heart to one of the pulse, which, as pointed out by Broadbent, is found particularly in cases of mitral stenosis when they are under the influence of this drug. The urine is reduced in amount. These symptoms subside on the withdrawal of the digitalis, and are rarely serious. There are patients who take digitalis uninterruptedly for years, and feel palpitation and distress if the drug is omitted. In mitral disease, even when it does good, it does not always steady the pulse. There are many cases in which the irregularity is not affected by the digitalis. When the compensation has been re-established the drug may be omitted. When there is dyspnœa on exertion and cardiac distress, from 5 to 10 minims (0.3 to 0.6 c. c.) three times a day may be advantageously given for prolonged periods, but the effects should be carefully watched. In cardiac dropsy digitalis should be used at the outset with a free hand. Small doses should not be given, but from the first half-ounce doses of the infusion every three hours, or from 15 to 20 minims of the tincture. Digitalin, hypodermically (gr. 1/30, 0.002 gm.), every three or four hours, may be substituted.

Of other remedies strophanthus alone is of service, but as its effect is uncertain when given by mouth it should be administered by intramuscular injection. Doses of 10 to 15 minims (0.6 to 1 c. c.) of the tincture or strophanthin gr. 1/100 (0.00065 gm.) are given and repeated once or twice after intervals of twenty-four hours. The intramuscular is safer than the intravenous administration. It certainly will sometimes steady the intermittent heart of mitral valve disease when digitalis fails to do so. Convallaria, citrate of caffeine, and adonis vernalis and sparteine are warmly recommended as substitutes for digitalis, but their inferiority is so manifest that their use is rarely indicated.

There are two valuable adjuncts in the treatment of valvular disease—iron and strychnia. When anæmia is a marked feature iron should be given in full doses. In some instances of failing compensation this is the only medicine needed to restore the balance. Arsenic is occasionally an excellent substitute, and one or other of them should be administered in all instances of heart trouble when pallor is present. Strychnia is a heart tonic of very great value. It may be given alone or in combination with the digitalis in 1 or 2 drop doses of the 1 per cent. solution, or hypodermically in doses of 1/40-1/10 gr. (0.0016 to 0.006 gm.). Alcoholic stimulants in moderation are occasionally useful, especially in tiding over a period of acute cardiac weakness.

Treatment of Special Symptoms.—(*a*) DROPSY.—The increased arterial tension and activity of the capillary circulation under the influence of digitalis hasten the interstitial lymph flow and favor resorption of the fluid. The hydragogue cathartics, by rapidly depleting the blood, promote, too, the absorption of the fluid from the lymph spaces and the lymph sacs. These two measures usually suffice to rid the patient of the dropsy. In some cases, however, it can not be relieved, and then Southey's tubes may be used or the legs punctured by ordinary aspirating needles with rubber tubing attached, which may be inserted and left for hours; they often drain away large amounts. If done with care, after a thorough washing of the parts, and if antiseptic precautions are taken, scarification is a very serviceable measure, and should be resorted to more frequently than it is. Canton flannel bandages may be applied on the œdematous legs. In case of marked hydrothorax or ascites tapping is advisable before digitalis is given.

(*b*) DYSPNŒA.—The patients are usually unable to lie down. A comfortable bed-rest should therefore be provided—if possible, one with lateral projections, so that in sleeping the head can be supported as it falls over. The shortness of breath is associated with dilatation, chronic bronchitis, or hydrothorax. The chest should be carefully examined in all these cases, as hydrothorax of one side or of both is a common cause of shortness of breath. There are cases of mitral regurgitation with recurring hydrothorax usually on the right side, which is relieved, week by week or month by month, by tapping. For the nocturnal dyspnœa, particularly when combined with restlessness, morphia is invaluable and may be given without hesitation. The value of the calming influence of opium in all conditions of cardiac insufficiency is not sufficiently recognized. There are instances of cardiac dyspnœa unassociated with dropsy, particularly in mitral valve disease, in which nitroglycerin is of great service, if given in the 1 per cent. solution in increasing doses. It is especially serviceable in the cases in which the pulse tension is high.

(*c*) Palpitation and Cardiac Distress.—In instances of great hypertrophy and in the throbbing which is so distressing in some cases of aortic insufficiency, aconite is of service in doses of from 1 to 3 drops every two or three hours. An ice bag over the heart or Leiter's coil is also of service in allaying the rapid action and the throbbing. For the pains, which are often so marked in aortic lesions, iodide of potassium in 10-grain (0.6 gm.) doses, three times a day, or nitroglycerin may be tried. Small blisters are sometimes advantageous. It must be remembered that an important cause of palpitation and cardiac distress is flatulent distention of the stomach or colon, against which suitable measures must be directed.

(*d*) Gastric Symptoms.—The cases of cardiac insufficiency which do badly and fail to respond to digitalis are most often those in which nausea and vomiting are prominent features. The liver is often greatly enlarged in these cases; there is more or less stasis in the hepatic vessels, and but little can be expected of drugs until the venous engorgement is relieved. If the vomiting persists, it is best to stop the food and give small bits of ice, small quantities of milk and lime water, and effervescing drinks, such as Apollinaris water and champagne. The bowels should be freely moved and drugs given hypodermically, if possible.

(*e*) Cough and Hæmoptysis.—The former is almost a necessary concomitant of cardiac insufficiency, owing to engorgement of the pulmonary vessels and more or less bronchitis. It is allayed by measures directed rather to the heart than to the lungs. Hæmoptysis in chronic valvular disease is sometimes a salutary symptom. An army surgeon, who was invalided during the American civil war on account of hæmoptysis, supposed to be due to tuberculosis, had for many years, in association with mitral insufficiency and enlarged heart, many attacks of hæmoptysis. He assured me that his condition was invariably better after the attack. It is rarely fatal, except in some cases of acute dilatation, and seldom calls for special treatment.

(*f*) Sleeplessness.—One of the most distressing features of valvular lesions, even in the stage of compensation, is disturbed sleep. Patients may wake suddenly with throbbing of the heart, often in an attack of nightmare. Subsequently, when the compensation has failed, it is also a worrying symptom. The sleep is broken, restless, and frequently disturbed by frightful dreams. Sometimes a dose of the spirit of chloroform or of ether, with half a drachm of spirit of camphor, given in a little hot whisky, will give a quiet night. The compound spirit of ether, Hoffmann's anodyne, though very unpleasant to take, is frequently a great boon in the intermediate period when compensation has partially failed and the patients suffer from restless and sleepless nights. Paraldehyde and amylene hydrate are sometimes serviceable, but it is best, after a few trials, particularly if the paraldehyde does not answer, to resort to morphia. It may be given in combination with atropine.

(*g*) Renal Symptoms.—With broken compensation and lowering of the tension in the aorta, the urinary secretion is greatly diminished, and the amount may sink to 5 or 6 ounces in the day. Digitalis and strophanthus usually increase the flow. A brisk purge may be followed by augmented secretion. The combination in pill form of digitalis, squill, and calomel will sometimes prove effective when the infusion or tincture of digitalis alone has failed. Calomel acts well in some cases, given in 3 grain (0.2 gm.) doses every six hours for three or four days.

The DIET in chronic valve diseases is often very difficult to regulate. Widal and others have shown that retention of the chlorides is an important factor in cardiac dropsy and heart failure. A milk diet, 2 litres a day, favors their elimination, and in the intervals between attacks a salt free diet as far as possible should be used. Starchy foods and all articles likely to cause flatulency should be forbidden. Stimulants are often necessary, either whisky or brandy.

In certain cases of weak heart, particularly when it is due to fatty overgrowth, the plans recommended by Oertel and by Schott are advantageous. They are invaluable methods in those forms of heart weakness due to intemperance in eating and drinking and defective bodily exercise. The Oertel plan consists of three parts: First, the reduction in the amount of liquid. This is an important factor in reducing the fat in these patients. It also slightly increases the density of the blood. Oertel allows daily about 36 ounces of liquid, which includes the amount taken with the solid food. Free perspiration is promoted by bathing (if advisable, the Turkish bath), or even by the use of pilocarpine.

The second important point in his treatment is the diet, which should consist largely of proteids.

Morning.—Cup of coffee or tea, with a little milk, about 6 ounces altogether. Bread, 3 ounces.

Noon.—Three to 4 ounces of soup, 7 to 8 ounces of roast beef, veal, game, or poultry, salad or a light vegetable, a little fish; 1 ounce of bread or farinaceous pudding; 3 to 6 ounces of fruit for dessert. No liquids at this meal, as a rule, but in hot weather 6 ounces of light wine may be taken.

Afternoon.—Six ounces of coffee or tea, with as much water. As an indulgence an ounce of bread.

Evening.—One or 2 soft-boiled eggs, an ounce of bread, perhaps a small slice of cheese, salad, and fruit; 6 to 8 ounces of wine with 4 or 5 ounces of water (Yeo).

The most important element of all is graduated exercise, not on the level, but up hills of various grades. The distance walked each day is marked off and is gradually lengthened. In this way the heart is systematically exercised and strengthened.

The Schott Treatment.—This consists in a combination of baths with exercises at Nauheim. The water has a temperature of from 82°-95° F., and is very richly charged with CO_2. The good effects of the bath are claimed by Schott to come from a cutaneous excitation, induced by the mineral and gaseous constituents of the bath, and a stimulation of the sensory nerves. There is no question that the bath, in suitable cases, will alter the position of the apex beat, and that it lessens the area of cardiac dulness; this means that it diminishes the dilatation of the heart. Artificial baths are used, consisting of forty gallons of water, with various strengths of sodium chloride and calcium chloride. The exercises, resistance gymnastics, consist in slow movements executed by the patient and resisted by the operator. The best cases for the Nauheim treatment are those with myocardial weakness from whatever cause. For valvular heart diseases in the stage of broken compensation with dropsy, etc., it is not so suitable. The neurotic heart is often much benefited.

III. ENDOCARDITIS

Inflammation of the lining membrane of the heart is usually confined to the valves, so that the term is practically synonymous with valvular endocarditis. It occurs in two forms—*acute*, characterized by the presence of vegetations with loss of continuity or of substance in the valve tissues; *chronic*, a slow sclerotic change, resulting in thickening, puckering, and deformity.

ACUTE ENDOCARDITIS

This occurs in rare instances as a primary, independent affection; but in the great majority of cases it is an accident in various infective processes, so that in reality the disease does not constitute an etiological entity.

For convenience of description we speak of a simple or benign, and a malignant, ulcerative, or infective endocarditis, between which, however, there is no essential anatomical difference, as all gradations can be traced, and they represent but different degrees of intensity of the same process.

Etiology.—SIMPLE ENDOCARDITIS does not constitute a disease of itself, but is invariably found with some other affection. In 330 cases of rheumatic fever at the Johns Hopkins Hospital there were 110 cases of endocarditis. Bouillaud first emphasized the frequency of the association of simple endocarditis with rheumatic fever. Before him, however, the association had been noticed. Possibly it is nothing in the disease itself, but simply an altered state of the fluid media—a reduction perhaps of the lethal influences which they normally exert—permitting the invasion of the blood by certain microorganisms. Tonsillitis, which in some forms is regarded as a rheumatic affection, may be complicated with endocarditis. Of the specific diseases of childhood it is not uncommon in scarlet fever, while it is rare in measles and chicken-pox. In diphtheria simple endocarditis is rare. In small-pox it is not common. In typhoid fever it occurred six times among 1,500 cases.

In pneumonia both simple and malignant endocarditis are common. In 100 autopsies in this disease made at the Montreal General Hospital there were 5 instances of the former. Among 61 cases of endocarditis studied bacteriologically in Welch's laboratory, pneumococci were found in 21 (Marshall). Of 517 fatal cases of acute endocarditis, 115 were in connection with pneumonia—22.3 per cent. (E. F. Wells). Acute endocarditis is by no means rare in phthisis. I found it in 12 cases in 216 post mortems.

In chorea simple warty vegetations are found on the valves in a large majority of all fatal cases, in 62 of 73 cases collected by me. There is no disease in which, post mortem, acute endocarditis has been so frequently found. And, lastly, simple endocarditis is met with in diseases associated with loss of flesh and progressive debility, as cancer, and such disorders as gout, diabetes, and Bright's disease.

A very common form is that which occurs on the sclerotic valves in old heart-disease—the so-called recurring endocarditis.

MALIGNANT OR INFECTIVE ENDOCARDITIS is met with: (*a*) As a primary disease of the lining membrane of the heart or of its valves.

(*b*) As a secondary affection in rheumatic fever, pneumonia, in various specific fevers, in septic processes of all sorts, and most frequently of all as an infection on old sclerotic valves. In a majority of all cases it is a local process in an acute infection. Congenital lesions are very prone to the severer types of endocarditis, particularly affections of the orifice of the pulmonary artery and the margins of the imperfect ventricular septum (C. Robinson).

The existence of a primary endocarditis has been doubted; but there are instances in which persons previously in good health, without any history of affections with which endocarditis is usually associated, have been attacked with symptoms resembling severe typhus or typhoid. In one case which I saw death occurred on the sixth day and no lesions were found other than those of malignant endocarditis.

The simple endocarditis of rheumatic fever or of chorea rarely progresses into the malignant form. In only 24 of 209 cases the symptoms of severe endocarditis arose in the progress of acute rheumatism. Of all acute diseases complicated with severe endocarditis pneumonia probably heads the list. Gonorrhœa is a much more common cause than has been supposed. There have been at least ten instances in my wards.

The affection may complicate erysipelas, septicæmia (from whatever cause), and puerperal fever. Malignant endocarditis is very rare in tuberculosis, typhoid fever, and diphtheria. In dysentery, in small-pox, and in scarlet fever, with which simple endocarditis is not infrequently complicated, the malignant form is extremely rare.

Morbid Anatomy of Simple and Malignant Endocarditis.—SIMPLE ENDOCARDITIS is characterized by the presence on the valves or on the lining membrane of the chambers of minute vegetations, ranging from 1 to 4 mm. in diameter, with an irregular and fissured surface, giving to them a warty or verrucose appearance. Often these little cauliflower-like excrescences are attached by very narrow pedicles. They are more common on the left side of the heart than the right, and occur on the mitral more often than on the aortic valves. The vegetations are upon the line of closure of the valves—i. e., on the auricular face of the auriculo-ventricular valves, a little distance from the margin, and on the ventricular side of the sigmoid valves, festooned on either half of the valve from the corpora Arantii. It is rare to see any swelling or macroscopic evidence of infiltration of the endocardium in the neighborhood of even the smallest of the granulations, or of redness, indicative of distention of the vessels, even when they occur upon valves already the seat of sclerotic changes, in which capillary vessels extend to the edges. With time the vegetations may increase greatly in size, but in what may be called simple endocarditis the size rarely exceeds that mentioned above. Hirschfelder has shown experimentally that they may form with great rapidity, even in a few hours.

The earliest vegetations consist of elements derived from the blood, and are composed of blood platelets, leucocytes, and fibrin in varying proportions. At a later stage they appear as small outgrowths of connective tissue. The transition of one form into the other can often be followed. The process consists of a proliferation of the endothelial cells and the cells of the subendothelial layer which gradually invade the fresh vegetation, and ultimately entirely replace it. The blood cells and fibrin undergo disintegration and gradually they are removed. The whole process has received the name of "organization." Even when the vegetation has been entirely converted into connective tissue it is often found at autopsy to be capped with a thin layer of fibrin and leucocytes.

Micro-organisms are generally, even if not invariably, found associated with the vegetations. They tend to be entangled in the granular and fibrillated fibrin or in the older ones to cap the apices.

SUBSEQUENT CHANGES.—(*a*) The vegetations may become organized and the valve restored to a normal state (?). (*b*) The process may extend, and a simple may become an ulcerative endocarditis. (*c*) The vegetations may be broken off and carried in the circulation to distant parts. (*d*) The vegetations become organized and disappear, but they initiate a nutritive change in the valve tissue which ultimately leads to sclerosis, thickening, and deformity. The danger in any case of simple endocarditis is not immediate, but remote, and consists in this perversion of the normal processes of nutrition which results in sclerosis of the valves.

A gradual transition from the simple to a more severe affection, to which the name MALIGNANT OR ULCERATIVE ENDOCARDITIS has been given, may be traced. Practically in every case of ulcerative endocarditis vegetations are present. In this form the loss of substance in the valve is more pronounced, the deposition—thrombus formation—from the blood is more extensive, and the micro-organisms are present in greater number and often show increased virulence. Ulcerative endocarditis is often found in connection with heart valves already the seat of chronic proliferative and sclerotic changes.

In this form there is much loss of substance, which may be superficial and limited to the endocardium, or, what is more common, it involves deeper structures, and not very infrequently leads to perforation of a valve, the septum, or even of the heart itself.

Upon microscopic examination the affected valve shows necrosis, with more or less loss of substance; the tissue is devoid of preserved nuclei and presents a coagulated appearance. Upon it a mixture of blood platelets, fibrin—granular or fibrillated—and leucocytes enclosing masses of micro-organisms are met with. The subjacent tissue often shows sclerotic thickening and always infiltration with exuded cells.

PARTS AFFECTED.—The following figures, taken from my Goulstonian lectures, give an approximate estimate of the frequency with which in 209 cases different parts of the heart were affected in malignant endocarditis: Aortic and mitral valves together, in 41; aortic valves alone, in 53; mitral valves alone, in 77; tricuspid in 19; the pulmonary valves in 15; and the heart walls in 33. In 9 instances the right heart alone was involved, in most cases the auriculo-ventricular valves.

Mural endocarditis is seen most often at the upper part of the septum of the left ventricle. Next in order is the endocarditis of the left auricle on the postero-external wall. The vegetations may extend, as in a case in my wards, along the intima of the pulmonary artery into the hilum of the lung. A common result of the ulceration is the production of valvular aneurism. In three fourths of the cases the affected valves present old sclerotic changes. The process may extend to the aorta, producing, as in one of my cases, extensive endarteritis with multiple acute aneurisms.

ASSOCIATED LESIONS.—The associated changes are those of the primary disease, those due to embolism, and the changes in the myocardium. In the endocarditis of septic processes there is the local lesion—an acute necrosis, a suppurative wound, or puerperal disease. In many cases the lesions are those of pneumonia, rheumatism, or other febrile processes.

The changes due to embolism constitute the most striking features, but it is remarkable that in some instances, even with endocarditis of a markedly ulcerative character, there may be no trace of embolic processes. The infarcts may be few in number—only one or two, perhaps, in the spleen or kidney—or they may exist in hundreds throughout the various parts of the body. They may present the ordinary appearance of red or white infarcts of a suppurative character. They are most common in the spleen and kidneys, though they may be numerous in the brain, and in many cases are very abundant in the intestines. In right sided endocarditis there may be infarcts in the lungs. In many of the cases there are innumerable miliary abscesses. Acute suppurative meningitis was met with in 5 of 23 of the Montreal cases, and in over 10 per cent. of the 209 cases analyzed in the literature. Acute suppurative parotitis also may occur. And, lastly, as Romberg has pointed out, the oft accompanying myocarditis plays an important rôle. The valvular insufficiency in an acute endocarditis is probably not due to the row of little vegetations, but to the associated myocarditis, which interferes with the proper closure of the orifice.

Bacteriology.—No distinction in the micro-organisms found in the two forms of endocarditis can be made. In both the pyogenic cocci—streptococci, staphylococci, pneumococci, and gonococci—are the most frequent bacteria met with. More rarely, especially in the simple vegetative endocarditis, the bacilli of tuberculosis, typhoid fever, and anthrax have been encountered. The colon bacillus has also been found, and Howard has described a case of malignant endocarditis due to an attenuated form of the diphtheria bacillus. Marshall in 61 cases found the pneumococci in 21, streptococci alone or with other bacteria in 26, staphylococcus pyogenes aureus in 12. The meningococcus may cause endocarditis, of which there are at least 5 cases in the literature (Cecil and Soper); only 3 of these were associated with meningitis. Combined infections are not uncommon. In the chronic infective form the *Streptococcus mitior* is the common organism (Libman).

As a rule no organisms are found in the simple endocarditis in many chronic diseases, as carcinoma, tuberculosis, nephritis, etc. They may have been present and died out, or the lesions may be caused by the toxins.

Symptoms.—Neither the clinical course nor the physical signs of SIMPLE ENDOCARDITIS are in any respect characteristic. The great majority of the cases are latent and there is no indication whatever of cardiac mischief. Experience has taught us that endocarditis is frequently found post mortem in persons in whom it was not suspected during life. There are certain features, however, by which its presence is indicated with a degree of probability. The patient, as a rule, does not complain of any pain or cardiac distress. In a case of rheumatic fever, for example, the symptoms to excite suspicion would be increased rapidity of the heart's action, perhaps slight irregularity, and an increase in the fever, without aggravation of the joint trouble. Rows of tiny vegetations on the mitral or on the aortic segments seem a trifling matter to excite fever, and it is difficult in the endocarditis of febrile processes to say definitely in every instance that an increase in the fever depends upon this complication; but a study of the recurring endocarditis—which is of the warty variety, consisting of minute beads on old sclerotic valves—shows that the process may be associated, for days or weeks at a time, with slight fever ranging from 100° to 102½°. Palpitation may be a marked feature and is a symptom upon which certain authors lay great stress.

The *diagnosis* of the condition rests upon physical signs, which are notoriously uncertain. The presence of a murmur at one or other of the cardiac areas in a case of fever is often taken as proof of the existence of endocarditis—a common mistake which has arisen from the fact that the *bruit de souffle* or bellows murmur is common to it and to a number of other conditions. At first there may be only a slight roughening of the first sound, which may gradually increase to a distinct murmur. The apex systolic bruit is probably more often the result of a myocarditis. It may not be present in the endocarditis of such chronic maladies as tuberculosis and carcinoma, since in them the muscle involvement is less common (Krehl). Reduplication and accentuation of the pulmonic second sound are frequently present.

It is difficult to give a satisfactory clinical picture of MALIGNANT ENDOCARDITIS because the modes of onset are so varied and the symptoms so diverse. Arising in the course of some other disease, there may be simply an intensification of the fever or a change in its character. In a majority of the cases there are present certain general features, such as irregular pyrexia, sweating, delirium, and gradual failure of strength.

Embolic processes may give special characters, such as delirium, coma, or paralysis from involvement of the brain or its membranes, pain in the side and local peritonitis from infarction of the spleen, bloody urine from implication of the kidneys, impaired vision from retinal hæmorrhage and suppuration, and even gangrene in various parts from the distribution of the emboli.

Two special types of the disease have been recognized—the septic or pyæmic and the typhoid. In some the cardiac symptoms are most prominent, while in others again the main symptoms may be those of an acute affection of the cerebro-spinal system.

The *septic type* is met with usually in connection with an external wound, the puerperal process, or an acute necrosis or gonorrhœa. There are rigors, sweats, irregular fever, and all of the signs of septic infection. The heart symptoms may be completely masked by the general condition, and attention called to them only on the occurrence of embolism. In many cases the features are those of a severe septicæmia, and the organisms may be isolated from the blood. Optic neuritis is not uncommon, and was present in 15 cases of chronic septic endocarditis examined by Faulkner, and in four of these recurrent retinal hæmorrhages were present.

The *typhoid type* is by far the most common and is characterized by a less irregular temperature, early prostration, delirium, somnolence, and coma, relaxed bowels, sweating, which may be of a most drenching character, petechial and other rashes, and occasionally parotitis. The heart symptoms may be completely overlooked, and in some instances the most careful examination has failed to discover a murmur.

Under the *cardiac group*, as suggested by Bramwell, may be considered those cases in which patients with chronic valve disease are attacked with marked fever and evidence of recent endocarditis. Many such cases present symptoms of the pyæmic and typhoid character and run a most acute course. In others there may be only slight fever or even after a period of high fever recovery takes place.

In what may be termed the *cerebral group* of cases the clinical picture may simulate a meningitis, either basilar or cerebro-spinal. There may be acute delirium or, as in three of the Montreal cases, the patient may be brought into the hospital unconscious. Heineman reports an instance, with autopsy, in which the clinical picture was that of an acute cerebro-spinal meningitis.

Certain special symptoms may be mentioned. The fever is not always of a remittent type, but may be high and continuous. Petechial rashes are very common and render the similarity very strong to certain cases of typhoid and cerebro-spinal fever. In one case the disease was thought to be hæmorrhagic small-pox. Erythematous rashes are not uncommon. The sweating may be most profuse, even exceeding that which occurs in phthisis and ague. Diarrhœa is not necessarily associated with embolic lesions in the intestines. Jaundice has been observed, and cases are on record which were mistaken for acute yellow atrophy.

The heart symptoms may be entirely latent and are not found unless a careful search be made. Even on examination there may be no murmur present. Instances are recorded by careful observers in which the examination of the heart has been negative. Cases with chronic valve disease usually present no difficulty in diagnosis.

The course of the disease is varied, depending largely upon the nature of the primary trouble. Except in the disease grafted upon chronic valvulitis the course is rarely extended beyond five or six weeks. The most rapidly fatal case on record is described by Eberth, the duration of which was scarcely two days.

Chronic Infective Endocarditis.—This is almost always engrafted on an old, sometimes an unrecognized, valve lesion. At first fever is the only symptom; in a few cases there have been chills at onset or recurring chills may arouse the suspicion of malaria. The patient may keep at work for months with a daily rise of temperature, or perhaps an occasional sweat. The heart features may be overlooked. The murmur of the old valve lesion may show no change, and even with the most extensive disease of the mitral cusps the heart's action may be very little disturbed. For months—six, eight, ten, even thirteen!—fever and progressive weakness may be the only symptoms. These are the cases in which, with recurring chills, the diagnosis of malaria is made. With involvement of the aortic segments the signs of a progressive lesion are more common. Embolic features are not common, occurring only toward the close. Ephemeral cutaneous nodes, red raised painful spots on the skin of hands or feet and lasting a few days, rarely occur except in this form. Post mortem there has been found in my cases a remarkable vegetative endocarditis, involving usually the mitral valves, sometimes with much encrusting of the chordæ tendineæ, and large irregular firm vegetations quite different to those of the ordinary ulcerative form of the disease. In some cases the aortic and tricuspid segments are also involved, and the vegetations may extend on to the walls of the heart.

Diagnosis.—In many cases the detection of the disease is very difficult; in others, with marked embolic symptoms, it is easy. From simple endocarditis it is readily distinguished, though confusion occasionally occurs in the transitional stage, when a simple is developing into a malignant form. The constitutional symptoms are of a graver type, the fever is higher, rigors are common, and septic and typhoid symptoms occur. Perhaps a majority of the cases not associated with puerperal processes or bone disease are confounded with typhoid fever. A differential diagnosis may even be impossible, particularly when we consider that in typhoid fever infarctions and parotitis may occur. The diarrhœa and abdominal tenderness may also be present, which with the stupor and progressive asthenia make a picture not to be distinguished from this disease. Points which may guide us are: The more abrupt onset in endocarditis, the absence of any regularity of the pyrexia in the early stage of the disease, and the cardiac pain. Oppression and shortness of breath may be early symptoms in malignant endocarditis. Rigors, too, are not uncommon. There is a marked leucocytosis in infective endocarditis. Between pyæmia and malignant endocarditis there are practically no differential features, for the disease really constitutes an *arterial pyæmia* (Wilks). In the acute cases resembling malignant fevers the diagnosis is usually made of typhus, typhoid, cerebro-spinal fever, or even of hæmorrhagic small-pox. The intermittent pyrexia, occurring for weeks or months, has led in some cases to the diagnosis of malaria, but this disease can be positively excluded by the blood examination. Blood cultures may aid greatly in the diagnosis.

The cases usually terminate fatally. The instances of recovery are those more subacute forms, the so-called recurring endocarditis developing on old sclerotic valves in cases of chronic heart disease.

Treatment.—We know no measures by which in rheumatic fever, chorea, or the eruptive fevers the onset of endocarditis can be prevented. As it is probable that many cases arise, particularly in children, in mild forms of these diseases, it is well to guard the patients against taking cold and insist upon rest and quiet, and to bear in mind that of all complications an acute endocarditis, though in its immediate effects harmless, is perhaps the most serious. This statement is enforced by the observations of Sibson that on a system of absolute rest the proportion of cases of rheumatic fever attacked by endocarditis was less than of those who were not so treated. It is doubtful whether in rheumatic fever the salicylates have an influence in reducing the liability to endocarditis. Considering the extremely grave after results of simple endocarditis in children, the question arises whether it is possible to do anything to avert the onset of progressive sclerosis of the affected valve. Caton recommends a systematic plan of treatment: (1) Prolonged rest in bed, three months, to keep the heart quiet; (2) a series of small blisters over the heart; and (3) the iodide of potassium in moderate doses for many months. If there is much vascular excitement aconite may be given and an ice bag placed over the heart. The salicylates are strongly advised by some writers. The treatment of malignant endocarditis is practically that of septicæmia—useless and hopeless in a majority of the cases. Blood cultures should be taken as soon as possible and a vaccine prepared. Horder and others have reported good results. Personally I have not seen a successful case.

CHRONIC ENDOCARDITIS

Definition.—A sclerosis of the valves leading to shrinking, thickening, and adhesion of the cusps, often with the deposition of lime salts, with shortening and thickening of the chordæ tendineæ, leading to insufficiency and to narrowing of the orifice. It may be primary, but is oftener secondary to acute endocarditis, particularly the rheumatic form.

Etiology.—It is a mistake to regard every case of sclerotic valve as a sequel to an acute endocarditis. It is long ago since Roy and Adami called attention to the possibility that sclerosis of the valve segments might be a sequel of high pressure. The preliminary endocarditis may be a factor in weakening the valve, the progressive thickening of which may be a direct consequence of the strain. As age advances the valves begin to lose their pliancy, show slight sclerotic changes and foci of atheroma and calcification. Certain poisons appear capable of initiating the change, such as alcohol, lead, syphilis, and gout, though we are at present ignorant of the way in which they act. The poisons of the specific fevers may initiate the change. A very important factor, particularly in the case of the aortic valves, is the strain of prolonged and heavy muscular exertion. In no other way can be explained the occurrence of sclerosis of these valves in young and middle aged men whose occupations necessitate the overuse of the muscles. In the aortic segments it may be only the valvular part of a general arterio-sclerosis.

The *frequency* with which chronic endocarditis is met with may be gathered from the following figures: In the statistics, amounting to from 12,000 to 14,000 autopsies, reported from Dresden, Würzburg, and Prague, the percentage ranged from four to nine. The relative frequency of involvement of the various valves is thus given in the collected statistics of Parrot: The mitral orifice was involved in 621, the aortic in 380, the tricuspid in 46, and the pulmonary in 11. This gives 57 instances in the right to 1,001 in the left heart.

Morbid Anatomy.—Vegetations in the form in which they occur in acute endocarditis are not present. In the early stage, which we have frequent opportunities of seeing, the edge of the valve is a little thickened and perhaps presents a few small nodular prominences, which in some cases may represent the healed vegetations of the acute process. In the aortic valves the tissue about the corpora Arantii is first affected, producing a slight thickening with an increase in the size of the nodules. The substance of the valve may lose its translucency, and the only change noticeable be a grayish opacity and a slight loss of its delicate tenuity. In the auriculo-ventricular valves these early changes are seen just within the margin and here it is not uncommon to find swellings of a grayish red, somewhat infiltrated appearance, almost identical with the similar structures on the intima of the aorta in arterio-sclerosis. Even early there may be seen yellow or opaque white subintimal fatty degenerated areas. As the sclerotic changes increase, the fibrous tissue contracts and produces thickening and deformity of the segment, the edges of which become round, curled, and incapable of that delicate apposition necessary for perfect closure. A sigmoid valve, for instance, may be narrowed one fourth or even one third across its face, the most extreme grade of insufficiency being induced without any special deformity and without any narrowing of the arterial orifice. In the auriculo-ventricular segments a simple process of thickening and curling of the edges of the valves, inducing a failure to close without forming any obstruction to the normal course of the blood-flow, is less common. Still, we meet with instances at the mitral orifice, particularly in children, in which the edges of the valves are curled and thickened, so that there is extreme insufficiency without any material narrowing of the orifice. More frequently, as the disease advances, the chordæ tendineæ become thickened, first at the valvular ends and then along their course. The edges of the valves at their angles are gradually drawn together and there is a narrowing of the orifice, leading in the aorta to more or less stenosis and in the left auriculo-ventricular orifice—the two sites most frequently involved—to constriction. Finally, in the sclerotic and necrotic tissues lime salts are deposited and may even reach the deeper structures of the fibrous rings, so that the entire valve becomes a dense calcareous mass with scarcely a remnant of normal tissue. The chordæ tendineæ may gradually become shortened, greatly thickened, and in extreme cases the papillary muscles are implanted directly upon the sclerotic and deformed valve. The apices of the papillary muscles usually show marked fibroid change.

In all stages of the process the vegetations of simple endocarditis may be present, and the severer, ulcerative forms are very apt to attack these sclerotic valves.

Chronic *mural* endocarditis produces cicatrical like patches of a grayish white appearance which are sometimes seen on the muscular trabeculæ of the ventricle or in the auricles. It often occurs in association with myocarditis.

The endocarditis of the fetus is usually of the sclerotic form and involves the valves of the right more frequently than those of the left side.

IV. CHRONIC VALVULAR DISEASE

GENERAL INTRODUCTION

Effects of Valve Lesions.—The general influence on the work of the heart may be briefly stated as follows: The sclerosis induces insufficiency or stenosis, which may exist separately or in combination. The narrowing retards in a measure the normal outflow and the insufficiency permits the blood current to take an abnormal course. The result in the former case is difficulty in the expulsion of the normal contents of the chamber through the narrow orifice; in the other, the overfilling of a chamber by blood flowing into it from an improper source as, for instance, in mitral insufficiency, when the left auricle receives blood both from the pulmonary veins and from the left ventricle. In both instances the effect is dilatation of a chamber, and to expel the normal amount of blood from a dilated chamber a relatively greater amount of mechanical energy is required, which by various adjustments the muscle is stimulated to do.

The cardiac mechanism is fully prepared to meet ordinary grades of dilatation which constantly occur during sudden exertion. A man, for instance, at the end of a hundred yard race has his right chambers greatly dilated and his reserve cardiac power worked to its full capacity. The slow progress of the sclerotic changes brings about a gradual, not an abrupt, insufficiency, and the moderate dilatation which follows is at first overcome by the exercise of the ordinary reserve strength of the heart muscle. Gradually a new factor is introduced. The constant increase in the energy put forth by the heart is a stimulus to the muscle fibres to increase in bulk and probably also in number; the heart hypertrophies, and the effect of the valve lesion becomes, as we say, *compensated*. The equilibrium of the circulation is in this way maintained.

The nature of the process with which we have to deal is graphically illustrated in the accompanying diagram, from Martius. The perpendicular lines in the figures represent the power of work of the heart. While the muscle

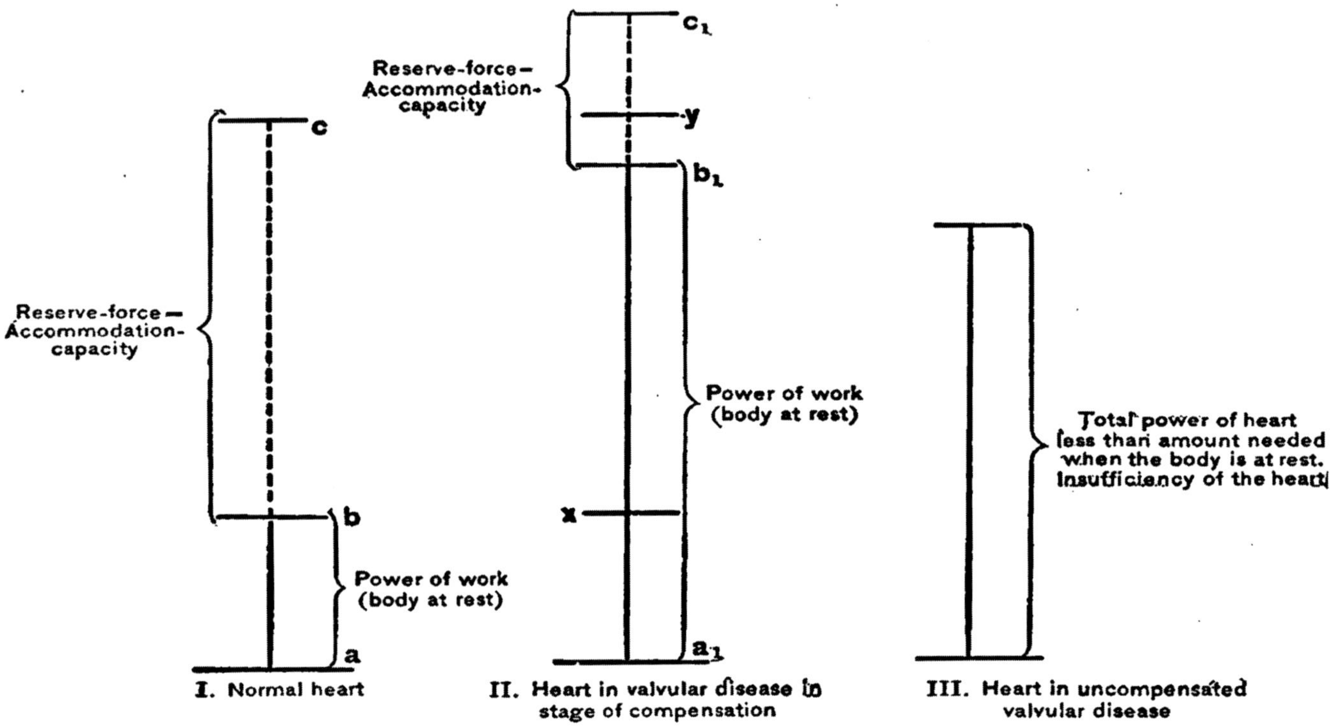

FIG. 6.—DIAGRAMMATIC PRESENTATION SHOWING THE FORCE OF THE HEART FOR WORK UNDER NORMAL CONDITIONS AND IN VALVULAR LESIONS.

in the healthy heart (Diagram I) has at its disposal the maximal force, *a c*, it carries on its work under ordinary circumstances (when the body is at rest) with the force *a b* and *c* is the reserve force by means of which the heart accommodates itself to greater exertion.

If now there be a gross valvular lesion, the force required to do the ordinary work of the heart (at rest) becomes very much increased (Diagram II). But in spite of this enormous call for force, insufficiency of the heart muscle does not necessarily result, for the working force required is still within the limits of the maximal power of the heart, $a_1\ b_1$ being less than $a_1\ c_1$. The muscle accommodates itself to the new conditions by making its reserve force mobile. If nothing further occurred, however, this condition could not be permanently maintained, for there would be left over for emergencies only the small reserve force, $b_1\ y$. Even when at rest the heart would be using continuously almost its entire maximal force. Any slight exertion requiring more extra force than that represented by the small value $b_1\ y$ (say the effort required on walking or on going upstairs) would bring the heart to the limit of its working power, and palpitation and dyspnœa would appear. Such a condition does not last long. The working power of the heart gradually increases. More and more exertion can be borne without causing dyspnœa, for *the heart hypertrophies.* Finally, a new, more or less permanent condition is attained, in that the hypertrophied heart possesses the maximal force, $a_1\ c_1$. Owing to the increase in volume of the heart muscle, the total force of the heart is greater *absolutely* than that of the normal heart by the amount $y\ c_1$. It is, however, *relatively* less efficient, for its reserve force is much less than that of the healthy heart. Its capacity for accommodating itself to unusual calls upon it is accordingly permanently diminished.

Turning now to the disturbances of compensation, it is to be distinctly borne in mind that any heart, normal or diseased, can become insufficient whenever a call upon it exceeds its maximal working capacity. The liability to such disturbance will depend, above all, upon the accommodation limits of the heart—the less the width of the latter, the easier will it be to go beyond the heart's efficiency. A comparison of Diagrams I and II will immediately make it clear that the heart in valvular disease will much earlier become insufficient than the heart of a healthy individual. If the heart muscle is compelled to do maximal or nearly maximal work for a long time, it becomes exhausted. It is obvious that the heart in valvular disease, on account of its small amount of reserve force, has to do maximal or nearly maximal work far more frequently than does the normal heart. The power of the heart may become decreased to the amount necessary simply to carry on the work of the heart when the body is at rest, or it may cease to be sufficient even for this. The reserve force gained through the compensatory process may be entirely lost (Diagram III). If the loss be only temporary, the exhausted heart muscle quickly recovering, the condition is spoken of as a "disturbance of compensation." The term "loss of compensation" is reserved for the condition in which the disturbance is continuous.

The schema of Martius (Fig. 7) will enable the student to understand the relation of the pathological phenomena to the normal cardiac cycle. The contraction of the ventricle takes an appreciable period of time, seven-hundredths of a second (*a-b*) to overcome the strong arterial pressure which keeps the aortic (and pulmonary) doors tightly shut. This closure-time is the only brief period in the cycle in which both the auriculo-ventricular valves and the semilunar valves are shut, the former as a result of the beginning of the systole, the latter until the intra-ventricular has overcome the aortic pressure. With this closure-time correspond the first sound and the heart beat. In the second period of the ventricular systole the blood is driven into the arteries—the expulsion-time (*b-c*)—and this corresponds with the beginning of the aortic pulse. During this there may be seen at the apex in a forcibly beating heart the "back stroke," as Hope called it. Following the expulsion-time there is a brief period—waiting-time (*c-d*)—before the diastole begins. Clinically the murmur of mitral insufficiency (*A*) coincides, at any rate in its beginning, with the closure-time, the murmur of aortic stenosis with the expulsion-time. The semilunar valves close at the moment when the ventricles begin to relax (*d*) and with this coincides the second sound. At the same moment the auriculo-ventricular valves open. The murmur of aortic insufficiency (*C*) is heard through the first part of the diastole, sometimes more, while the murmur of mitral stenosis (*D*) corresponds with the latter part of the diastole of the ventricles and with the systole of the auricles (*D*).

The *incidence* of valvular lesions may be gathered from the following figures compiled by Gillespie from the records of the Royal Infirmary, Edinburgh: Of 2,368 cases with cardiac lesions, valvular disease occurred in 80.8 per cent.; endocarditis and pericarditis in 5.3; myocardial lesions in 11.9 per cent.; 66.2 per cent. of the cases were in males.

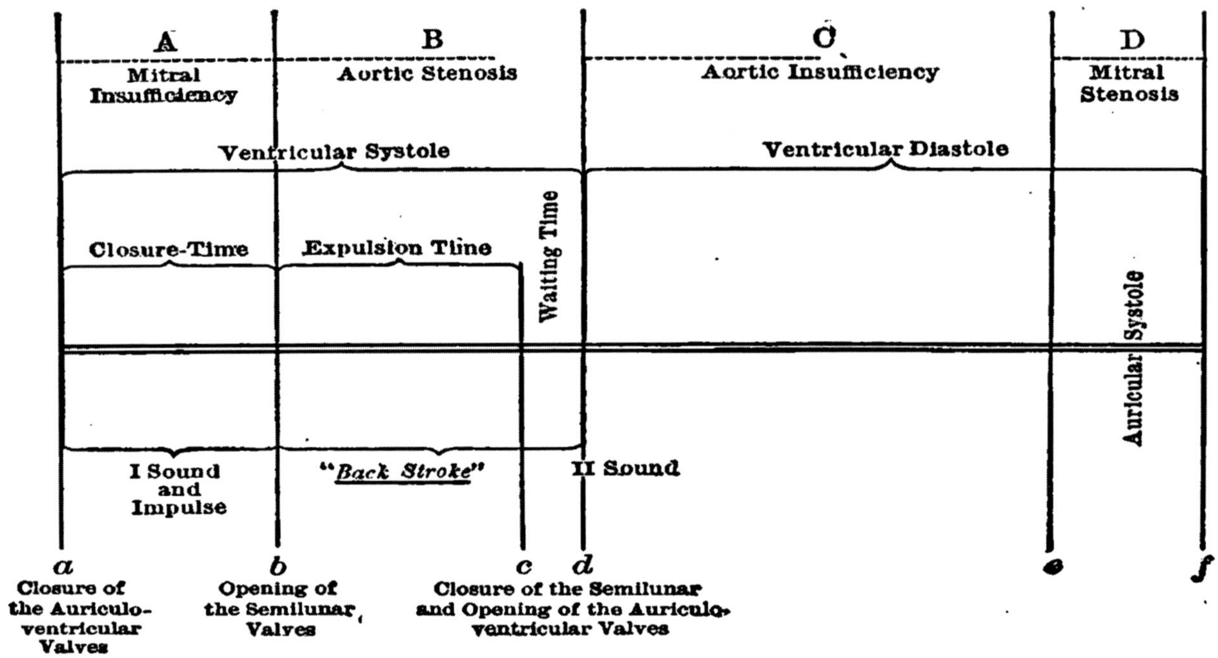

FIG. 7.—SCHEMATIC DIVISION OF THE PHASES OF THE HEART'S ACTION (Martius).

AORTIC INCOMPETENCY

Incompetency of the aortic valves arises either from inability of the valve segments to close an abnormally large orifice or more commonly from disease of the segments themselves. This best-defined and most easily recognized of valvular lesions was first carefully studied by Corrigan, whose name it sometimes bears.

Etiology and Morbid Anatomy.—It is more frequent in males than in females, affecting chiefly able bodied, vigorous men at the middle period of life. The ratio which it bears to other valve diseases has been variously given as from 30 to 50 per cent.

There are five groups of cases: I. Those due to *congenital malformation,* particularly fusion of two of the cusps—most commonly those behind which the coronary arteries are given off. It is probable that an aortic orifice may be competent with this bicuspid state of the valves, but a great danger is the liability of these malformed segments to sclerotic endocarditis. Of 17 cases which I have reported all presented sclerotic changes, and the majority of them had, during life, the clinical features of chronic heart-disease.

II. The *endocarditic group.* Endocarditis may produce an acute insufficiency by ulceration and destruction of the valves; in one case the aortic valves were completely eroded away. The valvulitis of rheumatism and of the fevers, while more rarely aortic, is common enough in children, and the insufficiency is caused by nodular excrescences at the margins or in the valves, which may ultimately become calcified; more often it induces a slow sclerosis of the valves with adhesions, causing also some degree of narrowing.

III. The *arterio-sclerotic group.* By far the most frequent cause of insufficiency is a slow, progressive sclerosis of the segments, resulting in a curling of the edges, which lessens the working surface of the valve. Most frequent in strong, able bodied men, there are three main factors in its production: First, *strain*—not a sudden, forcible strain, but a persistent increase of the normal tension to which the segments are subject during the diastole of the ventricle. Of circumstances increasing this tension, repeated and excessive use of the muscles is perhaps the most important. So often is this form of heart disease found in persons devoted to athletics that it is sometimes called the "athlete's heart." Secondly, *alcohol,* the action of which is probably direct as a poison to the vessel wall and not, as we have supposed heretofore, in keeping up a high blood pressure. Thirdly, *syphilis,* which is of importance equal to alcohol and strain combined. The Wassermann reaction is present in a very large proportion of all cases of aortic insufficiency in young and middle aged men.

In a small group, usually in young men, syphilis causes a localized arteriosclerosis at the root of the aorta, involving the valves secondarily or causing dilatation of the aortic ring with relative insufficiency. The endarteritis may be singularly localized, even annular, sometimes patchy. The spirochætes have been found in the lesions.

The condition of the valves is such as has already been described in chronic endocarditis. It may be noted, however, how slight a grade of curling may produce serious incompetency. Associated with the valve disease is, in a majority of cases, a more or less advanced arterio-sclerosis of the arch of the aorta, one serious effect of which may be a narrowing of the orifices of the coronary arteries. The sclerotic changes are often combined with atheroma, either in a fatty or calcareous stage. This may exist at the attached margin of the valves without inducing insufficiency. In other instances insufficiency may result from a calcified spike projecting from the aortic attachment into the body of the valve, and so preventing its proper closure. Some writers (Peter) have laid great stress upon the extension of the endarteritis to the valve, and would separate the instances of this kind from those of simple valvular endocarditis. Anatomically one can usually recognize the arterio-sclerotic variety by the smooth surface, the rounded edges, and the absence of excrescences.

IV. Insufficiency may be induced by *rupture of a segment*—a very rare event in healthy valves, but not uncommon in disease, either from excessive effort during heavy lifting or from the ordinary endarterial strain on a valve eroded and weakened by ulcerative endocarditis.

V. *Relative insufficiency,* due to dilatation of the aortic ring and adjacent arch, is not very frequent. It occurs in extensive arterial sclerosis of the ascending portion of the arch with great dilatation just above the valves. The valve segments are usually involved with the arterial coats, but the changes in them may be very slight. In aneurism just above the aortic ring relative insufficiency of the valve may be present.

It would appear from the careful measurements of Beneke that the aortic orifice, which at birth is 20 mm., increases gradually with the growth of the heart until at one and twenty it is about 60 mm. At this it remains until the age of forty, beyond which date there is a gradual increase in the size up to the age of eighty, when it may reach from 68 to 70 mm. There is thus at the very period of life in which sclerosis of the valve is most common a physiological tendency toward the production of a state of relative insufficiency.

The insufficiency may be combined with various grades of narrowing, particularly in the endocarditic group. In a majority of the cases of the arteriosclerotic form there is no stenosis. On the other hand, aortic stenosis almost without exception is associated with some grade, however slight, of regurgitation.

Non-valvular incompetency is met with in two groups of cases, in one of which there is a stretching of the aortic ring in connection with dilatation of the ascending portion of the arch. Whether insufficiency occurs apart from this in cases of dilatation of the left ventricle has been much discussed—a relative incompetency similar to that which occurs at the pulmonary orifice. Cases are reported in which transient diastolic murmurs have occurred in connection with dilatation of the heart, of which Anders has reported and collected corroborative cases. Some years ago J. B. MacCallum, whose untimely death was a great loss to science, described a sphincter-like band of muscle encircling the opening of the left ventricle into the aorta, and in these cases the relaxation of this ring muscle may be associated with insufficiency of the valve.

Effects.—The direct effect of aortic insufficiency is the regurgitation of blood from the artery into the ventricle, causing an overdistention of the cavity and a reduction of the blood column; that is, a relative anæmia in the arterial tree. The amount returning varies with the size of the opening. The double blood flow into the left ventricle causes dilatation of the chamber, and finally hypertrophy, the grade depending upon the lesion. In this way the valve defect is compensated, and, as with each ventricular systole a larger amount of blood is propelled into the arterial system, the regurgitation of a certain amount during diastole does not, for a time at least, seriously impair the nutrition of the peripheral parts. For a time at least there is little or no resistance offered to the blood flow from the auricle—the ventricle accommodates itself readily to the extra amount, and there is no disturbance in the lesser circulation. In acute cases, on the other hand, with rapid destruction of the segments, there may be the most intense dyspnœa and even profuse hæmoptysis. In this lesion dilatation and hypertrophy reach their most extreme limit. The heaviest hearts on record are described in connection with this affection. The so-called bovine heart, *cor bovinum,* may weigh 35 or 40 ounces, or even, as in a case of Dulles's, 48 ounces. The dilatation is usually extreme and is in marked contrast to the condition of the chamber in cases of pure aortic stenosis. The papillary muscles may be greatly flattened. The mitral valves are usually not seriously affected, though the edges may present slight sclerosis, and there is often relative incompetency, owing to distention of the mitral ring. Dilatation and hypertrophy of the left auricle are common, and secondary enlargement of the right heart occurs in all cases of long standing. In the arterio-sclerotic group there is an ever present possibility of narrowing of the orifices of the coronary arteries or an extension of the sclerosis to their branches, leading to fibroid myocarditis. In the endocarditis cases, particularly those following rheumatism, the intima is perfectly smooth, and the arch with its main branches not dilated. A normal aorta may be found post mortem when during life there have been the most characteristic signs of enlargement of the arch and of dilatation of the innominate and right carotid. The so-called dynamic dilatation of the arch is best seen in these cases. A young girl, whose case had been reported as one of aneurism, had forcible pulsation and a tumor which could be grasped above the sternum —post mortem the innominate artery did not admit the little finger and the arch was not dilated!

Although the coronary arteries, as shown by Martin and Sedgwick, are filled during the ventricular systole, the circulation in them must be embarrassed in aortic incompetency. They must miss the effect of the blood pressure in the sinuses of Valsalva during the elastic recoil of the arteries, which surely aids in keeping the coronary vessels full. The arteries of the body usually present more or less sclerosis consequent upon the strain which they undergo during the forcible ventricular systole.

Symptoms.—The condition is often discovered accidentally in persons who have not presented any features of cardiac disease.

Headache, dizziness, flashes of light, and a feeling of faintness on rising quickly are among the earliest symptoms. Palpitation and cardiac distress on slight exertion are common. Long before any signs of failing compensation pain may become a marked and troublesome feature. It is extremely variable in its manifestations. It may be of a dull, aching character confined to the præcordia. More frequently, however, it is sharp and radiating, and is transmitted up the neck and down the arms, particularly the left. Attacks of true angina pectoris are more frequent in this than in any other valvular disease. Anæmia is also common, much more so than in aortic stenosis or in mitral affections.

As compensation fails more serious symptoms are shortness of breath and œdema of the feet. The attacks of dyspnœa are liable to come on at night, and the patient has to sleep with his head high or even in a chair. Cyanosis is rare. It is most commonly due to complicating valve disease, or it is stated that it may result from bulging of the septum ventriculorum and encroachment upon the right ventricle. Of respiratory symptoms cough is common, due to the congestion of the lungs or œdema. Hæmoptysis is less frequent than in mitral disease. I have reported a case in which it was profuse and believed to be due to tuberculosis of the lungs, inasmuch as the patient was admitted in a state of emaciation and profound exhaustion. General dropsy is not common, but œdema of the feet may occur early and is sometimes due to the anæmia, sometimes to the venous stasis, at times to both. Unless there is coexisting disease of the mitral valve, it is rare in aortic incompetency for the patient to die with general anasarca. Sudden death is frequent; more so in this than in other valvular diseases. As compensation fails the patient takes to bed and slight irregular fever, associated usually with a recurring endocarditis, is not uncommon toward the close. Embolic symptoms are not infrequent—pain in the splenic region with enlargement of the organ, hæmaturia, and in some cases paralysis. Distressing dreams and disturbed sleep are more common in this than in other forms of valvular disease.

Mental symptoms are often seen with this lesion; toward the close there may be delirium, hallucinations, and morbid impulses. It is important to bear this in mind, for patients occasionally display suicidal tendencies. I have twice had patients throw themselves from a window of the ward.

Physical Signs.—*Inspection* shows a wide and forcible area of cardiac impulse with the apex beat in the sixth or seventh interspace, and perhaps as far out as the anterior axillary line. In young subjects the præcordia may bulge. There may be slight visible pulsation in the second right interspace, or, in some acute cases of insufficiency or ulcerative endocarditis, a couple of inches from the sternal margin. In very slight insufficiency there may be little or no enlargement to be determined clinically. On *palpation* a thrill, diastolic in time, is occasionally felt, but is not common. The impulse is usually strong and heaving, unless in conditions of extreme dilatation, when it is wavy and indefinite. Occasionally two or three interspaces between the nipple line and sternum will be depressed with the systole as the result of atmospheric pressure. *Percussion* shows a greater increase in the area of heart dulness than is found in any other valvular lesion. It extends chiefly downward and to the left.

Auscultation.—A murmur is heard during the diastole of the ventricles at the base of the heart and propagated down the sternum. It may be feeble or inaudible at the aortic cartilage, and is usually heard best at midsternum opposite the third costal cartilage or along the left border of the sternum as low as the ensiform cartilage. It is usually soft, blowing in quality, and is prolonged, or "long drawn," as the phrase is. It is produced by the reflux of blood into the ventricle. In some cases it is loudly transmitted to the axilla at the level of the fourth interspace, not by way of the apex. The second sound may be well heard or it may be replaced by the murmur, or with a dilated and calcified arch the second sound may have a ringing metallic or booming quality, and the diastolic murmur is well heard, or even loudest, over the manubrium.

The first sound may be clear at the base; more commonly there is a soft, short, systolic murmur. In the arterio-sclerotic group the systolic bruit is, as a rule, short and soft, while in the endocarditic group, in which the valve segments are united and often covered with calcified vegetations and excrescences, the systolic murmur is rough and may be accompanied by a thrill.

At the apex, or toward it, the diastolic murmur may be faintly heard propagated from the base. With full compensation the first sound is usually clear at the apex; with dilatation there is a loud systolic murmur of relative mitral insufficiency, which may disappear under observation as the dilatation lessens.

A second murmur at the apex, probably produced at the mitral orifice, is not uncommon. Attention was called to this by the late Austin Flint, and the murmur usually goes by his name. It is of a rumbling, echoing character, occurring in the middle or latter part of diastole, usually presystolic in time, and limited to the apex region. It is similar to, though less intense than, the louder presystolic murmurs of mitral stenosis, and is often associated with a palpable thrill. It is probably caused by the impinging of the regurgitant current from the aortic orifice on the large, anterior flap of the mitral valve, so as to cause interference with the entrance of blood at the time of auricular contraction. The condition is thus essentially the same as in a moderate mitral stenosis. This late diastolic echoing or rumbling murmur is present in about half of the cases of uncomplicated aortic insufficiency (Thayer). It is very variable, disappearing and reappearing again without apparent cause. The sharp, valvular first sound and abrupt systolic shock, so common in true mitral stenosis, are rarely present, while the pulse is characteristic of uncomplicated aortic insufficiency.

Arteries.—The examination of the arteries in aortic insufficiency is of great value. Visible pulsation is more commonly seen in the peripheral vessels in this than in any other condition. The carotids may be seen to throb forcibly, the temporals to dilate, and the brachials and radials to expand with each heart-beat. With the ophthalmoscope the retinal arteries are seen to pulsate. Not only is the pulsation evident, but the characteristic jerking quality is apparent. In the throat the throbbing carotids may lead to the diagnosis of aneurism. In many cases the pulsation can be seen in the suprasternal notch, and prominent, forcibly throbbing vessels beneath the right sterno-mastoid muscle. The abdominal aorta may lift the epigastrium with each systole. In severe cases with great hypertrophy, particularly if anæmia is present, the vascular throbbing may be of an extraordinary character,

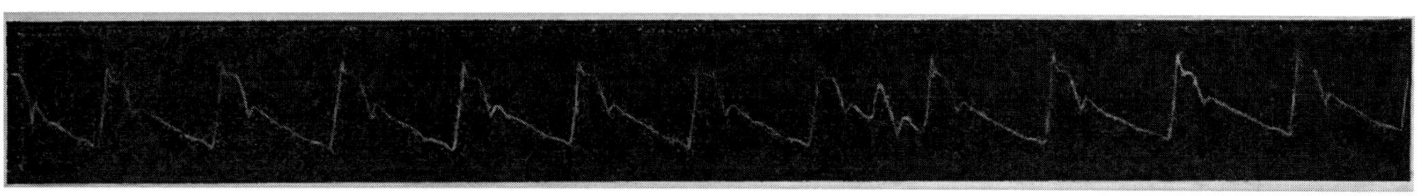

FIG. 8.—PULSE TRACING IN AORTIC INSUFFICIENCY; AN EXTRA-SYSTOLE IS SHOWN.

jarring the whole front of the chest, causing the head to nod, the pulsation may lift the foot when the knees are crossed, and even the tongue may throb rhythmically. To be mentioned with this is the capillary pulse, met very often in the aortic insufficiency, and best seen in the finger nails or by drawing a line upon the forehead, when the margin of hyperæmia on either side alternately blushes and pales. In extreme grades the face or the hand may blush visibly at each systole. It is met with also in profound anæmia, occasionally in neurasthenia, and in health in conditions of great relaxation of the peripheral arteries. Pulsation may also be present in the peripheral veins. On palpation the characteristic water-hammer or Corrigan pulse is felt. In the majority of instances the pulse wave strikes the finger forcibly with a quick jerking impulse, and immediately recedes or collapses. The characters of this are sometimes best appreciated by grasping the arm above the wrist and holding it up. Moreover, the pulse of aortic regurgitation is usually retarded or delayed—i. e., there is an appreciable interval between the beat of the heart and the pulsation in the radial artery, which varies according to the extent of the incompetence. Occasionally in the carotid artery the second sound is distinctly audible when absent at the aortic cartilage. Indeed, according to Broadbent, it is at the carotid that we must listen for the second aortic sound, for when heard it indicates that the regurgitation is small in amount, and is consequently a very favorable prognostic element. In the larger arteries a systolic thud or shock may be heard and sometimes a double murmur, as pointed out by Duroziez. The systolic pressure is high and the diastolic much decreased. The sphygmographic tracing is very characteristic. The high ascent, the sharp top, the quick drop in which the dicrotic notch and wave are very slightly marked.

The recent studies of Stewart and of W. G. MacCallum have shown that in aortic insufficiency the low position of the dicrotic notch in the descending arm of the pulse wave and the characteristic collapsing character of the pulse are not due, as was formerly supposed, to the regurgitation in the left ventricle, but to the dilatation of the peripheral arteries, which is a sort of protective adaptation under the vaso-motor influences.

Aortic insufficiency may for years be fully *compensated*. Persons do not necessarily suffer any inconvenience, and the condition is often found accidentally. So long as the hypertrophy just equalizes the valvular defect there may be no symptoms and the individual may even take moderately heavy exercise without experiencing sensations of distress about the heart. The cases which last the longest are those in which the insufficiency follows endocarditis and is not a part of a general arterio-sclerosis. The age of the patient, too, at the time of onset, is a most important consideration, as in youth the lesion is not often from sclerosis, and the coronary arteries are unaffected. Coexistent lesions of the mitral valves tend early to disturb the compensation. Pure aortic insufficiency is consistent with years of average health and with a tolerably active life.

With the onset of myocardial changes, with increasing degeneration of the arteries, particularly with a progressive sclerosis of the arch and involvement of the orifices of the coronary arteries, the compensation becomes disturbed. The insufficiency of the circulation is seen first on the arterial side in occasional faintings, giddiness, or mental irritability and enfeeblement; later there may be mitral regurgitation and embarrassment of the right side of the heart with its usual features. In advanced cases the changes about the aortic ring may be associated with alterations in the cardiac nerves and ganglia, and so introduce an important factor.

AORTIC STENOSIS

Narrowing or stricture of the aortic orifice is not nearly so common as insufficiency. The two conditions, as already stated, may occur together, however, and probably in almost every case of stenosis there is some leakage.

Etiology and Morbid Anatomy.—In the milder grades there is adhesion between the segments, which are so stiffened that during systole they can not be pressed back against the aortic wall. The process of cohesion between the segments may go on without great thickening, and produce a condition in which the orifice is guarded by a comparatively thin membrane, on the aortic face of which may be seen the primitive raphes separating the sinuses of Valsalva. In some instances this membrane is so thin and presents so few traces of atheromatous or sclerotic changes that the condition looks as if it had originated during fetal life. More commonly the valve segments are thickened and rigid, and have a cartilaginous hardness. In advanced cases they may be represented by stiff, calcified masses obstructing the orifice, through which a circular or slit like passage can be seen. The older the patient the more likely it is that the valves will be rigid and calcified.

We may speak of a relative stenosis of the aortic orifice when with normal valves and ring the aorta immediately beyond is greatly dilated. A stenosis due to involvement of the aortic ring in sclerotic and calcareous changes without lesion of the valves is referred to by some authors. I have never met with an instance of this kind. A subvalvular stenosis, the result of endocarditis in the mitro-sigmoidean sinus, usually occurs as the result of fetal endocarditis. In comparison with aortic insufficiency, stenosis is a rare disease. It is usually met with at a more advanced period of life than insufficiency, and the most typical cases of it are found associated with extensive calcareous changes in the arterial system in old men.

Owing to the impeded blood flow the ventricle has to work against an increased resistance and its walls become hypertrophied, usually at first with little or no dilatation. We see in this condition the most typical instances of what is called concentric hypertrophy, in which, without much, if any, enlargement of the cavity, the walls are greatly thickened, in contradistinction to the so-called eccentric hypertrophy, in which, with the increase in the thickness of the walls, the chamber itself is greatly dilated. The systole is prolonged, even as much as twenty-five per cent. There may be no changes in the other cardiac cavities if compensation is well maintained; but with its failure come dilatation, impeded auricular discharge, pulmonary congestion, and increased work for the right heart. The arterial changes are, as a rule, not so marked as in aortic insufficiency, for the walls have not to withstand the impulse of greatly increased blood-wave with each systole. On the contrary, the amount of blood propelled through the narrow orifice may be smaller than normal, though when compensation is fully established the pulse wave may be of medium volume.

Symptoms.—PHYSICAL SIGNS.—*Inspection* may fail to reveal any area of cardiac impulse. Particularly is this the case in old men with rigid chest walls and large emphysematous lungs. Under these circumstances there may be a high grade of hypertrophy without any visible impulse. Even when the apex beat is visible, it may be, as Traube pointed out, feeble and indefinite. In many cases the apex is seen displaced downward and outward, and the impulse looks strong and forcible.

Palpation reveals in many cases a thrill at the base of the heart of maximum force in the aortic region. With no other condition do we meet with thrills of greater intensity. The apex beat may not be palpable under the conditions above mentioned, or there may be a slow, heaving, forcible impulse.

Percussion never gives the same wide area of dulness as in aortic insufficiency. The extent of it depends largely on the state of the lungs, whether emphysematous or not.

Auscultation.—A rough systolic murmur, of maximum intensity at the aortic cartilage, and propagated into the great vessels, is the most constant physical sign in aortic stenosis. One of the last lessons learned by the student of physical diagnosis is to recognize that the systolic murmur at the aortic area does not necessarily mean obstruction at the orifice. Roughening of the valves, or of the intima of the aorta, and hæmic states are much more frequent causes. In aortic stenosis the murmur often has a much harsher quality, is louder, and is more frequently musical than in the conditions just mentioned. When compensation fails and the ventricle is dilated and feeble, the murmur may be soft and distant. The second sound is rarely heard at the aortic cartilage, owing to the thickening and stiffness of the valve. A diastolic murmur is not uncommon, but in many cases it can not be heard. Occasionally, as noted by W. H. Dickinson, there is a musical murmur of greatest intensity in the region of the apex, due probably to a slight regurgitation at high pressure through the mitral valves. The pulse in pure aortic stenosis is small, usually of good tension, well sustained, regular, and perhaps slower than normal.

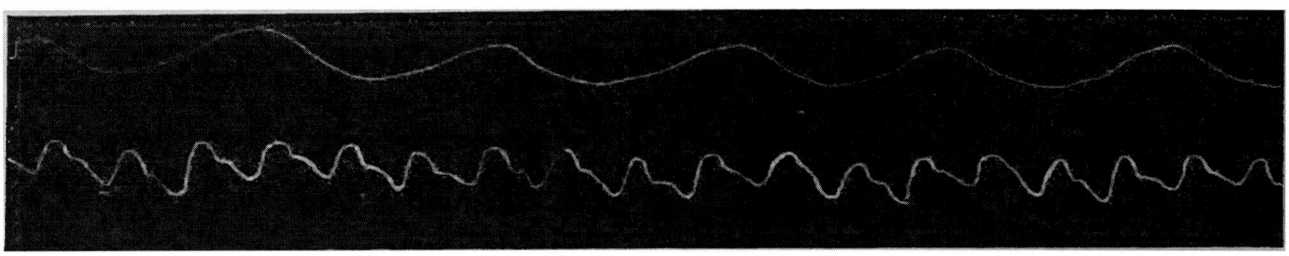

FIG. 9.—PULSE TRACING IN AORTIC STENOSIS.

The condition may be latent for an indefinite period, as long as the hypertrophy is maintained. Early symptoms are those due to defective blood supply to the brain, dizziness, and fainting. Palpitation, pain about the heart, and anginal symptoms are not so marked as in insufficiency. With degeneration of the heart-muscle and dilatation relative insufficiency of the mitral valve is established, and the patient may present all the features of engorgement in the lesser and systemic circulations, with dyspnœa, cough, rusty expectoration, and the signs of anasarca in the lower part of the body. Many of the cases in old people, without presenting any dropsy, have symptoms pointing rather to general arterial disease. Cheyne-Stokes breathing is not uncommon with or without signs of uræmia.

Diagnosis.—With an extremely rough or musical murmur of maximum intensity at the aortic region and signs of hypertrophy of the left ventricle, a thrill, and especially a hard, slow pulse of moderate volume and fairly good tension, which in a sphygmographic tracing gives a curve of slow rise, a broad, well sustained summit and slow decline, a diagnosis of aortic stenosis can be made with some degree of certainty, particularly if the subject is an old man. Mistakes are common, however, and a roughened or calcified valve segment, or, in some instances, a very roughened and prominent calcified plate in the aorta, and hypertrophy associated with renal disease, may produce similar symptoms. Seldom is there difficulty in distinguishing the murmur due to anæmia, since it is rarely so intense and is not associated with thrill or with marked hypertrophy of the left ventricle. In aortic insufficiency a systolic murmur is usually present, but has neither the intensity nor the musical quality, nor is it accompanied with a thrill. With roughening and dilatation of the ascending aorta the murmur may be very harsh or musical; but the existence of a second sound, accentuated and ringing in quality, is usually sufficient to differentiate this condition.

MITRAL INCOMPETENCY

Etiology.—Insufficiency of the mitral valve ensues: (*a*) From changes in the segments whereby they are contracted and shortened, usually combined with changes in the chordæ tendineæ, or with more or less narrowing of the orifice. (*b*) As a result of changes in the muscular walls of the ventricle, either dilatation, so that the valve segments fail to close an enlarged orifice, or changes in the muscular substance, so that the segments are imperfectly coapted during the systole—muscular incompetency. The common lesions producing insufficiency result from endocarditis, which causes a gradual thickening at the edges of the valves, contraction of the chordæ tendineæ, and union of the edges of the segments, so that in a majority of the instances there is not only insufficiency, but some grade of narrowing as well. Except in children, we rarely see the mitral leaflets curled and puckered without narrowing of the orifice. Calcareous plates at the base of the valve may prevent perfect closure of one of the segments. In long-standing cases the entire mitral structures are converted into a firm calcareous ring. From this valvular insufficiency the other condition of muscular incompetency must be carefully distinguished. It is met with in all conditions of extreme dilatation of the left ventricle, and also in weakening of the muscles in prolonged fevers and in anæmia.

Morbid Anatomy.—The effects of incompetency of the mitral segment upon the heart and circulation are as follows: (*a*) The imperfect closure allows a certain amount of blood to regurgitate from the ventricle into the auricle, so that at the end of auricular diastole this chamber contains not only the blood which it has received from the lungs, but also that which has regurgitated from the left ventricle. This necessitates dilatation, and, as increased work is thrown upon it in expelling the augmented contents, hypertrophy as well.

(*b*) With each systole of the left auricle a larger volume of blood is forced into the left ventricle, which also dilates and subsequently becomes hypertrophied.

(*c*) During the diastole of the left auricle, as blood is regurgitated into it from the left ventricle, the pulmonary veins are less readily emptied. In consequence the right ventricle expels its contents less freely, and in turn becomes dilated and hypertrophied.

(*d*) Finally, the right auricle also is involved, its chamber is enlarged, and its walls are increased in thickness.

(*e*) The effect upon the pulmonary vessels is to produce dilatation both of the arteries and veins—often in long-standing cases, atheromatous changes; the capillaries are distended, and ultimately the condition of brown induration is produced. Perfect compensation may be effected, chiefly through the hypertrophy of both ventricles, and the effect upon the peripheral circulation may not be manifested for years, as a normal volume of blood is discharged from the left heart at each systole. The time comes, however, when, owing either to increase in the grade of the incompetency or to failure of the compensation, the left ventricle is unable to send out its normal volume into the aorta. Then there are overfilling of the left auricle, engorgement in the lesser circulation, embarrassed action of the right heart, and congestion in the systemic veins. For years this somewhat congested condition may be limited to the lesser circulation, but finally the right auricle becomes dilated, the tricuspid valves incompetent, and the systemic veins are engorged. This gradually leads to the condition of cyanotic induration in the viscera and, when extreme, to dropsical effusion.

Muscular incompetency, due to impaired nutrition of the mitral and papillary muscles, is rarely followed by such perfect compensation. There may be in acute destruction of the aortic segments an acute dilatation of the left ventricle with relative incompetency of the mitral segments, great dilatation of the left auricle, and intense engorgement of the lungs, under which circumstances profuse hæmorrhage may result. In these cases there is little chance for the establishment of compensation. In cases of hypertrophy and dilatation of the heart, without valvular lesions, but associated with heavy work and alcohol, the insufficiency of the mitral valve may be extreme and lead to great pulmonary congestion, engorgement of the systemic veins, and a condition of cardiac dropsy, which can not be distinguished by any feature from that of mitral incompetency due to lesion of the valve itself. In chronic Bright's disease the hypertrophy of the left ventricle may gradually fail, leading, in the later stages, to relative insufficiency of the mitral valve, and the production of a condition of pulmonary and systemic congestion, similar to that induced by the most extreme grade of lesion of the valve itself. Adherent pericardium, especially in children, may lead to like results.

Symptoms.—During the development of the lesion, unless the incompetency comes on acutely in consequence of rupture of the valve segment or of ulceration, the compensatory changes go hand in hand with the defect, and there are no subjective symptoms. So, also, in the stage of perfect compensation, there may be the most extreme grade of mitral insufficiency with enormous hypertrophy of the heart, yet the patient may not be aware of the existence of heart trouble, and may suffer no inconvenience except perhaps a little shortness of breath on exertion or on going upstairs. It is only when from any cause the compensation has not been perfectly effected, or, having been so, is broken abruptly or gradually, that the patients begin to be troubled. The symptoms may be divided into two groups:

(*a*) The minor manifestations while compensation is still good. Patients with extreme incompetency often have a congested appearance of the face, the lips and ears have a bluish tint, and the venules on the cheeks may be enlarged—signs in many cases very suggestive. In long standing cases, particularly in children, the fingers may be clubbed, and there is shortness of breath on exertion. This is one of the most constant features in mitral insufficiency and may exist for years, even when the compensation is perfect. Owing to the somewhat congested condition of the lungs these patients have a tendency to attacks of bronchitis or hæmoptysis. There may also be palpitation of the heart. As a rule, however, in well balanced lesions in adults, this period of full compensation or latent stage is not associated with symptoms which call the attention to an affection of the heart, and with care the patient may reach old age in comparative comfort without being compelled to curtail seriously his pleasures or his work.

(*b*) Sooner or later comes a period of disturbed or broken compensation, in which the most intense symptoms are those of venous engorgement. There are palpitation, weak, irregular action of the heart, and signs of dilatation. Dyspnœa is an especial feature, and there may be cough. A distressing symptom is the cardiac "sleep-start," in which, just as the patient falls asleep, he wakes gasping and feeling as if the heart were stopping. There is usually a slight cyanosis, and even a jaundiced tint to the skin. The most marked symptoms, however, are those of venous stasis. The overfilling of the pulmonary vessels accounts in part for the dyspnœa. There is cough, often with bloody or watery expectoration, and the alveolar epithelium containing brown pigment-grains is abundant. Dropsical effusion usually sets in, beginning in the feet and extending to the body and the serous sacs. Right sided hydrothorax may recur and require repeated tapping. The urine is usually scanty and albuminous, and contains tube casts and sometimes blood corpuscles. With judicious treatment the compensation may be restored and all the serious symptoms may pass away. Patients usually have recurring attacks of this kind, and die of a general dropsy; or there is progressive dilatation of the heart, and death from asystole. Sudden death in these cases is rare. Some cases of mitral disease—stenosis and insufficiency—reach what may be called the hepatic stage, when all the symptoms are due to the secondary changes in the liver.

Physical Signs.—*Inspection.*—In children the præcordia may bulge and there may be a large area of visible pulsation. The apex beat is to the left of the nipple, in some cases in the sixth interspace, in the anterior axillary line. A localized right ventricle impulse may sometimes be seen below the right costal border in the parasternal line. There may be a wavy impulse in the cervical veins, which are often full, particularly when the patient is recumbent.

Palpation.—A thrill is rare; when present it is felt at the apex, often in a limited area. The force of the impulse may depend largely upon the stage in which the case is examined. In full compensation it is forcible and heaving; when the compensation is disturbed, usually wavy and feeble.

Percussion.—The dulness is increased, particularly in a lateral direction. There is no disease of the valves which produces, in long standing cases, a more extensive transverse area of heart dulness. It does not extend so much upward along the left margin of the sternum as beyond the right margin and to the left of the nipple line.

Auscultation.—At the apex there is a systolic murmur which wholly or partly obliterates the first sound. It is loudest here, and has a blowing, sometimes musical character, particularly toward the latter part. The murmur is transmitted to the axilla and may be heard at the back, in some instances over the entire chest. There are cases in which, as pointed out by Naunyn, the murmur is heard best along the left border of the sternum. Usually in diastole at the apex the loudly transmitted second sound may be heard. Occasionally there is also a soft, sometimes a rough or rumbling presystolic murmur. As a rule, in cases of extreme mitral insufficiency from valvular lesion with great hypertrophy of both ventricles, there is heard only a loud blowing murmur during systole. A murmur of mitral insufficiency may vary a great deal according to the position of the patient. It may be present in the recumbent and absent in the erect posture. In cases of dilatation, particularly when dropsy is present, there may be heard at the ensiform cartilage and in the lower sternal region a soft systolic murmur due to tricuspid regurgitation. An important sign on auscultation is the accentuated pulmonary second sound. This is heard to the left of the sternum in the second interspace, or over the third left costal cartilage.

The pulse in mitral insufficiency, during the period of full compensation, may be full and regular, often of low tension. Usually with the first onset of the symptoms the pulse becomes irregular, a feature which then dominates the case throughout. There may be no two beats of equal force or volume. Often after the disappearance of the symptoms of failure of compensation the irregularity of the pulse persists.

The three important physical signs then of mitral regurgitation are: (*a*) Systolic murmur of maximum intensity at the apex, which is propagated to the axilla and heard at the angle of the scapula; (*b*) accentuation of the pulmonary second sound; (*c*) evidence of enlargement of the heart, particularly the increase in the transverse diameter, due to hypertrophy of both right and left ventricles.

Diagnosis.—There is rarely any difficulty in the diagnosis of mitral insufficiency. The physical signs just referred to are quite characteristic and distinctive. Two points are to be borne in mind. First, a murmur, systolic in character, and of maximum intensity at the apex, and propagated even to the axilla, does not necessarily indicate incompetency of the mitral valve. There is heard in this region a large group of what are termed accidental murmurs, the precise nature of which is still doubtful. They are probably formed, however, in the ventricle, and are not associated with hypertrophy, or accentuation of the pulmonary second sound.

Second, it is not always possible to say whether the insufficiency is due to lesion of the valve segment or to dilatation of the mitral ring and relative incompetency. Here neither the character of the murmur, the propagation, the accentuation of the pulmonary second sound, nor the hypertrophy assists in the differentiation. The history is sometimes of greater value in this matter than the physical examination. The cases most likely to lead to error are those of the so-called idiopathic dilatation and hypertrophy of the heart (in which the systolic murmur may be of the greatest intensity), and the instances of arterio-sclerosis with dilated heart. Balfour and others, however, maintain that organic disease of the mitral leaflets sufficient to produce incompetency is always accompanied with a certain degree of narrowing of the orifice, so that the only unequivocal proof of the actual disease of the mitral valve is the presence of a presystolic murmur.

MITRAL STENOSIS

Etiology.—There are two groups of cases, one following an acute endocarditis, the other the result of a slow sclerosis of the valves without any history of rheumatic fever or other infection. It is very much more common in women than in men—in 63 of 80 cases noted by Duckworth, while in 4,791 autopsies at Guy's Hospital during ten years there were 196 cases, of which 107 were females and 89 males (Samways). This is not easy to explain, but there are at least two factors to be considered. Rheumatism prevails more in girls than in boys, and, as is well known, endocarditis of the mitral valve is more common in rheumatism. Chorea, also, as suggested by Barlow, has an important influence, occurring more frequently in girls and being often associated with endocarditis. Anæmia and chlorosis, which are prevalent in girls, have been regarded as possible factors. In a surprising number of cases of what the French call *pure* mitral stenosis no recognizable etiological factor can be discovered. This has been regarded by some writers as favoring the view that they may be of congenital origin, but congenital affections of the mitral valve are notoriously rare. Whooping-cough, with its terrible strain on the heart-valves, may be accountable for certain cases. While met with at all ages, stenosis is certainly most frequent in young adult women.

Morbid Anatomy.—The valve segments and chordæ may be fused together, the result of repeated attacks of endocarditis. The condition varies a good deal, according to the amount of atheromatous change. In many cases the curtains are so welded together and the whole valvular region so thickened that the orifice is reduced to a mere chink—Corrigan's button-hole contraction. In non-endocarditic cases the curtains are not much thickened, but narrowing has resulted from gradual adhesion at the edges, and thickening of the chordæ tendineæ, so that from the auricle it looks cone like—the so-called funnel shaped variety of stenosis. The instances in which the valve segments are very slightly deformed, but in which the orifice is considerably narrowed, are regarded by some as possibly of congenital origin. Occasionally the curtains are in great part free from disease, but the narrowing results from large calcareous masses, which project into them from the ring. The involvement of the chordæ tendineæ is usually extreme, and the papillary muscles may be inserted directly upon the valve. In moderate grades of constriction the orifice will admit the tip of the index finger; in more extreme forms the tip of the little finger; and occasionally one meets with a specimen in which the orifice seems almost obliterated, admitting only a medium sized probe. The heart is not greatly enlarged, rarely weighing more than 14 or 15 ounces. Occasionally, in an elderly person, it may seem only slightly, if at all, enlarged, and again there are instances in which the weight may reach as much as 20 ounces. The left ventricle is usually small, and may look very small in comparison with the right ventricle, which forms the greater portion of the apex. In cases in which with the narrowing there is very considerable incompetency the left ventricle may be moderately dilated and hypertrophied.

It is not uncommon at the examination to find white thrombi in the appendix of the left auricle. Occasionally a large part of the auricle is occupied by an ante-mortem thrombus. Still more rarely the remarkable ball thrombus is found, in which a globular concretion, varying in size from a walnut to a small egg, lies free in the auricle, two examples of which have come under my observation.

The left auricle discharges its blood with greater difficulty and in consequence dilates, and its walls reach three or four times their normal thickness.

Although the auricle is by structure unfitted to compensate an extreme lesion, the probability is that for some time during the gradual production of stenosis the increasing muscular power of the walls is sufficient to counterbalance the defect. In 36 cases of well-marked stenosis Samways found the auricle hypertrophied in 26, dilatation coexisting in 14. Eventually the tension is increased in the pulmonary circulation, owing to impeded outflow from the veins and this to heightened pressure in the pulmonary artery. Extra work is thus thrown on the right ventricle, which gradually hypertrophies. Relative incompetency of the tricuspid and congestion of the systemic veins at last supervene.

Symptoms.—PHYSICAL SIGNS.—*Inspection.*—In children the lower sternum and the fifth and sixth left costal cartilages are often prominent, owing to hypertrophy of the right ventricle. The apex beat may be ill defined. Usually it is not dislocated far beyond the nipple line, and the chief impulse is over the lower sternum and adjacent costal cartilages. Often in thin chested persons there is pulsation in the third and fourth left interspaces close to the sternum. When compensation fails, the præcordial impulse is much feebler, and in the veins of the neck there may be marked systolic regurgitation or the right jugular near the clavicle may stand out as a prominent tumor. In the later stage there is great enlargement with pulsation of the liver or pulmonary pulsation seen in the intercostal spaces.

Palpation reveals in a majority of the cases a characteristic, well defined fremitus or thrill, which is best felt, as a rule, in the fourth or fifth interspace within the nipple line. It is of a rough, grating quality, often peculiarly limited in area, most marked during expiration, and can be felt to terminate in a sharp, sudden shock, synchronous with the impulse. This most characteristic of physical signs is pathognomonic of narrowing of the mitral orifice, and is perhaps the only instance in which the diagnosis of a valvular lesion can be made by palpation alone. The cardiac impulse is felt most forcibly in the lower sternum and in the fourth and fifth left interspaces. The impulse is felt very high in the third and fourth interspaces, or in rare cases even in the second, and it has been thought that in the latter interspace the impulse is due to pulsation of the auricle. It is always the impulse of the conus arteriosus of the right ventricle; even in the most extreme grades of mitral stenosis there is never such tilting forward of the auricle or its appendix as would enable it to produce an impression on the chest wall.

Percussion gives an increase in the cardiac dulness to the right of the sternum and along the left margin; not usually a great increase beyond the nipple line, except in extreme cases, when the transverse dulness may reach from 5 cm. beyond the right margin of the sternum to 10 cm. beyond the nipple line.

Auscultation.—To the inner side of the apex beat, often in a very limited region, there is heard a rough, vibratory or purring murmur, cumulative or crescendo in character, which terminates abruptly in the first sound. By combining palpation and auscultation the purring murmur is found to be synchronous with the thrill and the loud shock with the first sound. The murmur is auricular systolic, due to the blood passing through the narrow orifice. Some have thought it to be early systolic in time, but the majority of observers hold to the former view with Gairdner. The presystolic murmur may occupy the entire period of the diastole, or the middle or only the latter half, corresponding to the auricular systole. The difference may sometimes be noted between the first and second portions of the murmur, when it occupies the entire time. Often there is a peculiar rumbling or echoing quality, which in some instances is very limited and may be heard only over a single bell-space of the stethoscope. A rumbling, echoing presystolic murmur at the apex is heard in some cases of aortic insufficiency (Flint murmur), occasionally in adherent pericardium with great dilatation of the heart, and in upward dislocation of the organ.

A systolic murmur may be heard at the apex or along the left sternal border, often of extreme softness and audible only when the breath is held. Sometimes the systolic murmur is loud and distinct and is transmitted to the axilla. The second sound in the second left interspace is loudly accentuated, and often reduplicated. It may be transmitted far to the left and be heard with great clearness beyond the apex. In uncomplicated cases of mitral stenosis there are usually no murmurs audible at the aortic region, at which spot the second sound is less intense than at the pulmonary area. In advanced cases at the lower sternum and to the right a systolic tricuspid murmur is sometimes heard. Other points to be noted are the following: The unusually sharp, clear first sound which follows the presystolic murmur, the cause of which is by no means easy to explain. It can scarcely be a valvular sound produced chiefly at the mitral orifice, since it may be heard with great intensity in cases in which the valves are rigid and calcified. It has been suggested by A. E. Sansom and others that it is a loud "snap" of the tricuspid valves caused by the powerful contraction of the greatly hypertrophied right ventricle. Broadbent thinks it may be due to the abrupt contraction of a partially filled left ventricle. The valvular sound may be audible at a distance, as one sits at the bedside of the patient (Graves). In a patient I saw with C. J. Blake the first sound was audible six feet, by measurement, from the chest wall.

These physical signs, it is to be borne in mind, are characteristic only of the stage in which compensation is maintained. The murmur may be soft, almost inaudible, and only brought out after exertion. Finally there comes a period in which, with the establishment of auricular fibrillation, the presystolic murmur disappears and there is heard in the apex region a sharp first sound, or sometimes a gallop rhythm. The marked systolic shock may be present after the disappearance of the thrill and the characteristic murmur. Under treatment, with gradual recovery of compensation, probably with increasing vigor of contraction of the right ventricle and left auricle, the presystolic murmur reappears. In cases seen at this stage of the disease the nature of the valve lesion may be entirely overlooked. As Mackenzie and Lewis have shown, auricular fibrillation is the rule in the arrhythmia of mitral stenosis.

Stenosis of the mitral valve may for years be efficiently compensated by the hypertrophy of the right ventricle. Many persons with the characteristic physical signs of this lesion present no symptoms. They may for years perhaps be short of breath on going upstairs, but are able to pass through the ordinary duties of life without discomfort. The pulse is smaller in volume than normal, and very often irregular. A special danger of this stage is the recurring endocarditis. Vegetations may be whipped off into the circulation and, blocking a cerebral vessel, may cause hemiplegia or aphasia, or both. This, unfortunately, is not an uncommon sequence in women. Patients with mitral stenosis may survive this accident for an indefinite period. A woman, above seventy years of age, died in one of my wards at the Philadelphia Hospital, who had been in the almshouse, hemiplegic, for more than thirty years. The heart presented an extreme grade of mitral stenosis which had probably existed at the time of the hemiplegic attack.

Pressure of the enlarged auricle on the left recurrent laryngeal nerve, causing paralysis of the vocal cord on the corresponding side, has been described by Ortner and by Herrick. It is a point to be borne in mind, as the diagnosis of aneurism of the arch of the aorta may be made. On the other hand, Fetterolf and Norris conclude that it is not the pressure of the left auricle directly, but the squeezing of the nerve between the pulmonary artery and the aortic arch, and that the paralysis is due to the neuritis so excited.

Failure of compensation brings in its train the group of symptoms which have been discussed under cardiac insufficiency. Briefly enumerated, they are: Rapid and irregular action of the heart, shortness of breath, cough, signs of pulmonary engorgement, and very frequently hæmoptysis. Attacks of this kind may recur for years. Bronchitis or a febrile attack may cause shortness of breath or slight blueness. Inflammatory affections of the lungs or pleura seriously disturb the right heart, and these patients stand pneumonia very badly. Many, perhaps a majority of, cases of mitral stenosis do not have dropsy. The liver may be greatly enlarged, and in the late stages ascites is not uncommon, particularly in children. General anasarca is most frequently met with in those cases in which there is secondary narrowing of the tricuspid orifice (Broadbent).

TRICUSPID VALVE DISEASE

Tricuspid Regurgitation.—Occasionally this results from acute or chronic endocarditis with puckering; more commonly the condition is one of relative insufficiency, and is secondary to lesions of the valves on the left side, particularly of the mitral. It is met with also in all conditions of the lungs which cause obstruction to the circulation, such as cirrhosis and emphysema, particularly in combination with chronc bronchitis. The symptoms are those of obstruction in the lesser circulation with venous congestion in the systemic veins, such as has already been described in connection with mitral insufficiency. The signs of this condition are:

(*a*) Systolic regurgitation of the blood into the right auricle and the transmission of the pulse wave into the veins of the neck. If the regurgitation is slight or the contraction of the ventricle is feeble there may be no venous throbbing, but in other cases there is marked systolic pulsation in the cervical veins. That in the right jugular is more forcible than that in the left. It may be seen both in the internal and the external vein, particularly in the latter. Marked pulsation in these veins occurs only when the valves guarding them become incompetent. Slight oscillations are by no means uncommon, even when the valves are intact. The distention is sometimes enormous, particularly in the act of coughing, when the right jugular at the root of the neck may stand out, forming an extraordinarily prominent ovoid mass. Occasionally the regurgitant pulse wave may be widely transmitted and be seen in the subclavian and axillary veins, and even in the subcutaneous veins over the shoulder, or in the superficial mammary veins.

Regurgitant pulsation through the tricuspid orifice may be transmitted to the inferior cava, and so to the hepatic veins, causing a systolic distention of the liver. This is best appreciated by bimanual palpation, placing one hand over the fifth and sixth costal cartilages and the other in the lateral region of the liver in the mid-axillary line. The rhythmical expansile pulsation may be readily distinguished, as a rule, from the systolic depression of the liver due to communicated pulsation from the left ventricle.

(*b*) The second important sign of tricuspid regurgitation is the occurrence of a systolic murmur of maximum intensity in the lower sternum. It is usually a soft, low murmur, often to be distinguished from a coexisting mitral murmur by differences in quality and pitch, and may be heard to the right as far as the axilla. Sometimes it is very limited in its distribution.

Together these two signs positively indicate tricuspid regurgitation. In addition, the percussion usually shows increase in the area of dulness to the right of the sternum, and the impulse in the lower sternal region is forcible. In the great majority of cases the symptoms are those of the associated lesions. In cirrhosis of the lung and in chronic emphysema the failure of compensation of the right ventricle with insufficiency of the tricuspid not infrequently leads either to acute asystole or to gradual failure with cardiac dropsy.

Tricuspid Stenosis.—The condition is rare both clinically and anatomically, and it is not often recognized during life. Of 26,000 medical admissions in the Johns Hopkins Hospital there were only 8 with either clinical or post mortem diagnosis of this condition; and in a total of 3,500 autopsies, only 5 cases were found, all in females. Of a total of 195 collected cases, there were 141 females, 38 males, 16 sex unknown. In a majority of the cases—104—the mitral and tricuspid were affected together, in 14 the tricuspid alone, in 64 the tricuspid and aortic. A definite history of rheumatism was present in only 66 cases (Futcher).

The diagnosis is not often made; extreme cyanosis and dyspnœa are common, and toward the end the ordinary signs of cardiac failure. Among the important physical signs are presystolic pulsation in the jugular veins and in the enlarged liver. A presystolic thrill may be felt at the tricuspid area with a marked systolic shock. The cardiac dulness is greatly increased to the right, a rumbling presystolic murmur may be present over the lower sternum with an extension to the right border. This, with a very snappy first sound, great increase of dulness to the right, and chronic breathlessness with cyanosis, are the important features.

PULMONARY VALVE DISEASE

Murmurs in the region of the pulmonary valves are extremely common; lesions of the valves are exceedingly rare. Balfour has well called the pulmonic area the region of auscultatory romance. A systolic murmur is heard here under many conditions—(1) very often in health, in thin chested persons, particularly in children, during expiration and in the recumbent posture; (2) when the heart is acting rapidly, as in fever and after exertion; (3) it is a favorite situation of the cardio-respiratory murmur; (4) in anæmic states; and (5), as mentioned previously, the systolic murmur of mitral insufficiency may be transmitted along the left sternal margin. Actual lesions of the valves of the pulmonary artery are rare.

Stenosis is almost invariably a congenital anomaly. It constitutes one of the most important of the congenital cardiac affections. The valve segments are usually united, leaving a small, narrow orifice. In adults cases occasionally occur. The congenital lesion is commonly associated with patency of the ductus Botalli and imperfection of the ventricular septum. There may also be tricuspid stenosis. Acute endocarditis not infrequently attacks the sclerotic valves.

The physical signs are extremely uncertain. There may be a systolic murmur with a thrill heard best to the left of the sternum in the second intercostal space. This murmur may be very like a murmur of aortic stenosis, but is not transmitted into the vessels. Naturally the pulmonary second sound is weak or obliterated, or may be replaced by a diastolic murmur. Usually there is hypertrophy of the right heart.

Pulmonary Insufficiency.—This rare affection is occasionally due to congenital malformation, particularly fusion of two of the segments. It is sometimes present, as Bramwell has shown, in cases of malignant endocarditis. Barie has collected 58 cases.

The physical signs are those of regurgitation into the right ventricle, but, as a rule, it is difficult to differentiate the murmur from that of aortic insufficiency, though the maximum intensity may be in the pulmonary area. The absence of the vascular features of aortic insufficiency is the most suggestive feature. Both Gibson and Graham Steell have called attention to the possibility of leakage through these valves in cases of great increase of pressure in the pulmonary artery, and to a soft diastolic murmur heard under these circumstances, which Steell calls "the murmur of high pressure in the pulmonary artery."

COMBINED VALVULAR LESIONS

Valvular lesions are seldom single or pure; combined lesions are more common. This is particularly the case in congenital disease. In young children mitral and aortic lesions, the result of rheumatic fever, are common. Pure mitral insufficiency and pure mitral stenosis may exist for years, but in time the tricuspid becomes involved, at first in sclerosis and later narrowing of the orifice. Aortic valve lesions are more commonly uncombined than mitral lesions. The added lesion may be hurtful or helpful. The stenosis which so often accompanies the endocarditic variety may lessen the regurgitation in aortic insufficiency; and a progressive narrowing of the mitral orifice may be beneficial in mitral regurgitation.

Prognosis in Valvular Disease.—The question is entirely one of efficient compensation. So long as this is maintained the patient may suffer no inconvenience, and even with the most serious forms of valve lesion the function of the heart may be little, if at all, disturbed.

Practitioners who are not adepts in auscultation and feel unable to estimate the value of the various heart murmurs should remember that the best judgment of the conditions may be gathered from inspection and palpation.

With an apex beat in the normal situation and regular in rhythm the auscultatory phenomena may be practically disregarded.

A murmur *per se* is of little or no moment in determining the prognosis in any given case. There is a large group of patients who present no other symptoms than a systolic murmur heard over the body of the heart, or over the apex, in whom the left ventricle is not hypertrophied, the heart rhythm is normal, and who may not have had rheumatism. Indeed, the condition is accidentally discovered, often during examination for life insurance. Among the conditions influencing prognosis are:

(*a*) AGE.—Children under ten are bad subjects. Compensation is well effected, and they are free from many of the influences which disturb compensation in adults. The coronary arteries are healthy, and nutrition of the heart muscle can be readily maintained. Yet, in spite of this, the outlook in cardiac lesions developing in very young children is usually bad. One reason is that the valve lesion itself is apt to be rapidly progressive, and the limit of cardiac reserve force is in such cases early reached. There seems to be proportionately a greater degree of hypertrophy and dilatation. Among other causes of the risks of this period are to be mentioned insufficient food in the poorer classes, the recurrence of rheumatic attacks, and the existence of pericardial adhesions. The outlook in a child who can be carefully supervised and prevented from damaging himself by overexertion is naturally better than in one who is constantly overtasking his muscles. The valvular lesions which occur at, or subsequent to, the period of puberty are more likely to be permanently and efficiently compensated. Sudden death from heart disease is very rare in children.

(*b*) SEX.—Women bear valve lesions, as a rule, better than men, owing partly to the fact that they live quieter lives, partly to the less common involvement of the coronary arteries, and to the greater frequency of mitral lesions. Pregnancy and parturition are disturbing factors, but are, I think, less serious than some writers would have us believe.

(*c*) VALVE AFFECTED.—The relative prognosis of the different valve lesions is very difficult to estimate. Each case must, therefore, be judged on its own merits. Aortic insufficiency is unquestionably the most serious; yet for years it may be perfectly compensated. Favorable circumstances in any case are the moderate grade of hypertrophy and dilatation, the absence of all symptoms of cardiac distress, and the absence of extensive arterio-sclerosis and of angina. The prognosis rests in reality with the condition of the coronary arteries. Rheumatic lesions of the valves, inducing insufficiency, are less apt to be associated with endarteritis at the root of the aorta; and in such cases the coronary arteries may escape for years. On the other hand, when the aortic insufficiency is only a part of an extensive arterio-sclerosis at the root of the aorta, the coronary arteries are almost invariably involved, and the outlook in such cases is much more serious. Sudden death is not uncommon, either from acute dilatation during some exertion, or, more frequently, from blocking of one of the branches of the coronary arteries. The liability of this form to be associated with angina pectoris also adds to its severity. Aortic stenosis is a comparatively rare lesion, most commonly met with in middle aged or elderly men, and is, as a rule, well compensated. In Broadbent's series of cases, in which autopsy showed definite aortic narrowing, forty years was the average age at death, and the oldest was but fifty-three.

In mitral lesions the outlook on the whole is much more favorable than in aortic insufficiency. Mitral insufficiency, when well compensated, carries with it a better prognosis than mitral stenosis. Except aortic stenosis, it is the only lesion commonly met with in patients over three-score years. It must be borne in mind that the cases which last the longest are those in which the valve orifice is more or less narrowed, as well as incompetent. There is, in reality, no valve lesion so poorly compensated and so rapidly fatal as that in which the mitral segments are gradually curled and puckered until they form a narrow strip around a wide mitral ring—a condition specially seen in children. There are many cases of mitral insufficiency in which the defect is thoroughly balanced for thirty or even forty years, without distress or inconvenience. Even with great hypertrophy and the apex beat almost in the mid-axillary line, there may be little or no distress, and the compensation may be most effective. Women may pass safely through repeated pregnancies, though here they are liable to accidents associated with the severe strain. I have had under observation for many years a patient who had her first attack of rheumatism at the age of fifteen, when she already had a well marked mitral murmur. She first came under my observation over thirty years ago, with signs of hypertrophy of the left ventricle and a loud systolic murmur. She has lived a very active life, has been unusually vigorous, has borne eleven children, and has passed through three subsequent attacks of rheumatism. The loud mitral systolic murmur persists, but she is very well, only a little short of breath on exertion.

In mitral stenosis the prognosis is usually regarded as less favorable. My own experience has led me, however, to place this lesion almost on a level, particularly in women, with the mitral insufficiency. It is found very often in persons in perfect health, who have had neither palpitation nor signs of heart-failure, and who have lived laborious lives. The figures given, too, by Broadbent indicate that the date of death in mitral stenosis is comparatively advanced. Of 53 cases abstracted from the post mortem records of St. Mary's Hospital, thirty three was the age for males, and thirty seven or thirty eight for females. These women, too, pass through repeated pregnancies with safety. There are, of course, those too common accidents, the result of cerebral embolism, which are more likely to occur in this than in other forms.

Hard and fast lines can not be drawn in the question of prognosis in valvular disease. Every case must be judged separately, and all the circumstances carefully balanced. There is no question which requires greater experience and more mature judgment, and even the most experienced are sometimes at fault.

The following conditions justify a favorable prognosis: Good general health and good habits; no exceptional liability to rheumatic or catarrhal affections; origin of the valvular lesion independently of degeneration; existence of the valvular lesion without change for over three years; sound ventricles, of moderate frequency, and general regularity of action; sound arteries, with a normal amount of blood and tension in the smaller vessels; and, lastly, freedom from pulmonary, hepatic, and renal congestion.

Treatment of Valvular Lesions.—(*a*) Stage of Compensation.—Medicinal treatment at this period is not necessary and is often hurtful. A very common error is to administer cardiac drugs, such as digitalis, on the discovery of a murmur or of hypertrophy. If the lesion has been found accidentally, it may be best not to tell the patient, but rather an intimate friend. Often it is necessary, however, to be perfectly frank in order that the patient may take certain preventive measures. He should lead a quiet, regulated, orderly life, free from excitement and worry, and the risk of sudden death makes it imperative that the patient suffering from aortic disease should be specially warned against overexertion and hurry. An ordinary wholesome diet in moderate quantities should be taken; tobacco may be allowed in moderation, but stimulants should be interdicted or used in very small amount. Exercise should be regulated entirely by the feelings of the patient. So long as no cardiac distress or palpitation follows, moderate exercise will prove very beneficial. The skin should be kept active by a daily bath. Hot baths should be avoided and the Turkish bath should be interdicted. In the case of full-blooded, somewhat corpulent individuals, an occasional saline purge should be taken. Patients with valvular lesions should not go into very high altitudes. The act of coition has serious risks, particularly in aortic insufficiency. Knowing that the causes which most surely and powerfully disturb the compensation are overexertion, mental worry, and malnutrition, the physician should give suitable instructions in each case. As it is always better to have the coöperation of an intelligent patient, he should, as a rule, be told of the condition, but in this matter the physician must be guided by circumstances, and there are cases in which reticence is the wiser policy.

(*b*) Stage of Broken Compensation.—The break may be immediate and final, as when sudden death results from acute dilatation or from blocking of a branch of the coronary artery, or it may be gradual. Among the first indications are shortness of breath on exertion or attacks of nocturnal dyspnœa. These are often associated with impaired nutrition, particularly with anæmia, and a course of iron or change of air may suffice to relieve the symptoms.

Irregularity of the action of the heart can not always be termed an indication of failing compensation, particularly in instances of mitral disease. It has greater significance in aortic lesions. Serious failure of compensation is indicated by signs of dilatation of the heart, marked cyanosis, the gallop rhythm, or various forms of arrhythmia, with or without the existence of dropsy. Under these circumstances the same measures are to be carried out as are indicated under treatment in cardiac insufficiency.

V. SPECIAL PATHOLOGICAL CONDITIONS

1. ANEURISM OF THE HEART

Aneurism of a valve results from acute endocarditis, which produces softening or erosion and may lead either to perforation of the segment or to gradual dilatation of a limited area under the influence of the blood pressure. The aneurisms are usually spheroidal and project from the ventricular face of a sigmoid valve. They are much less common on the mitral segments. They frequently rupture and produce extensive destruction and incompetency of the valves.

Aneurism of the walls results from the weakening induced by chronic myocarditis, or occasionally it follows acute mural endocarditis, which more commonly, however, leads to perforation. It has followed a stab wound, a gumma of the ventricle, and, according to some authors, pericardial adhesions. The left ventricle near the apex is usually the seat, this being the situation in which fibrous degeneration is most common. Fifty nine of the 60 cases collected by Legg were situated here. In the early stages the anterior wall of the ventricle, near the septum, sometimes even the septum itself, is slightly dilated, the endocardium opaque, and the muscular tissue sclerotic. In a more advanced stage the dilatation is pronounced and layers of thrombi occupy the sac. Ultimately a large rounded tumor may project from the ventricle and may attain a size equal to that of the heart. Occasionally the aneurism is sacculated and communicates with the ventricle through a very small orifice. The sac may be double, as in the cases of Janeway and Sailer. In the museum of Guy's Hospital there is a specimen showing the wall of the ventricle covered with aneurismal bulgings. Rupture occurred in 7 of the 90 cases collected by Legg.

The **symptoms** produced by aneurism of the heart are indefinite. Occasionally there is marked bulging in the apex region and the tumor may perforate the chest wall. In mitral stenosis the right ventricle may bulge and produce a visible pulsating tumor below the left costal border, which I have known to be mistaken for cardiac aneurism. When the sac is large and produces pressure upon the heart itself, there may be a marked disproportion between the strong cardiac impulse and the feeble pulsation in the peripheral arteries.

2. RUPTURE OF THE HEART

This rare event is usually associated with fatty infiltration or degeneration of the heart-muscle. In some instances acute softening in consequence of embolism of a branch of the coronary artery, suppurative myocarditis, or a gummatous growth has been the cause. Of 100 cases collected by Quain, fatty degeneration was noted in 77. Two thirds of the patients were over sixty years of age. It may occur in infants. Schaps reports a case in an infant of four months associated with an embolic infarct of the left ventricle. Harvey, in his second letter to Riolan (1649), described the case of Sir Robert Darcy, who had distressing pain in the chest and syncopal attacks with suffocation, and finally cachexia and dropsy. Death occurred in one of the paroxysms. The wall of the left ventricle of the heart was ruptured, "having a rent in it of size sufficient to admit any of my fingers, although the wall itself appeared sufficiently thick and strong."

The rent may occur in any of the chambers, but is found most frequently in the left ventricle on the anterior wall, not far from the septum. The accident usually takes place during exertion. There may be no preliminary symptoms, but without any warning the patient may fall and die in a few moments. Sudden death occurred in 71 per cent. of Quain's cases. In other instances there may be in the cardiac region a sense of anguish and suffocation, and life may be prolonged for several hours. In a Montreal case, which I examined, the patient walked up a steep hill after the onset of the symptoms, and lived for thirteen hours. A case is on record in which the patient lived for eleven days.

3. NEW GROWTHS AND PARASITES

Tubercle and syphilis have already been considered. Primary cancer or sarcoma is extremely rare. Secondary tumors may be single or multiple, and are usually unattended with symptoms, even when the disease is most extensive. In one case I found in the wall of the right ventricle a mass which involved the anterior segment of the tricuspid valve and partly blocked the orifice. The surface was eroded and there were numerous cancerous emboli in the pulmonary artery. In another instance the heart was greatly enlarged, owing to the presence of innumerable masses of colloid cancer the size of cherries. The mediastinal sarcoma may penetrate the heart, though it is remarkable how extensive the disease of the mediastinal glands may be without involvement of the heart or vessels.

Cysts in the heart are rare. They are found in different parts, and are filled either with a brownish or a clear fluid. Blood cysts occasionally occur.

The parasites have been discussed under the appropriate section, but it may be mentioned here that both the *cysticercus cellulosæ* and the echinococcus cysts occur occasionally.

4. WOUNDS AND FOREIGN BODIES

Wounds of the heart may be caused by external injuries, as stabs and bullet wounds, by foreign bodies passing from the gullet or œsophagus, or by puncture for therapeutic purposes.

(*a*) Bullet wounds of the heart are common. Recovery may take place, and bullets have been found encysted in the organ. Stab wounds are still more common. A medical student, while on a spree, passed a pin into his heart. The pericardium was opened, and the head of the pin was found outside of the right ventricle. It was grasped and an attempt made to remove it, but it was withdrawn into the heart and, it is said, caused the patient no further trouble (Moxon). In recent stab wounds the practice now is to expose the heart and attempt to suture the wound. The results have been progressively improving. In a case of stab wound Pagenstecher tied the left coronary artery, which had been divided.

(*b*) Hysterical girls sometimes swallow pins and needles, which, passing through the œsophagus and stomach, are found in various parts of the body. A remarkable case is reported by Allen J. Smith of a girl from whom several dozen needles and pins were removed, chiefly from subcutaneous abscesses. Several years later she developed symptoms of chronic heart disease. At the post mortem needles were found in the tissues of the adherent pericardium, and between thirty and forty were embedded in the thickened pleural membranes of the left side.

(*c*) Puncture of the heart (cardiocentesis) has been recommended as a therapeutic procedure, as in chloroform narcosis, and experimental evidence has been brought forward by B. A. Watson in favor of the operation. He advises abstraction of blood in combination with the puncture—cardiocentesis. The proceeding is not without risk. Hæmorrhage may take place from the puncture, though it is not often extensive. Sloane has recently urged its use in all cases of asphyxia and in suffocation by drowning and from coal gas. The successful case which he reports illustrates forcibly its stimulating action.

VI. CONGENITAL AFFECTIONS OF THE HEART

These have only a limited clinical interest, as in a large proportion of the cases the anomaly is not compatible with life, and in others nothing can be done to remedy the defect or even to relieve the symptoms.

The congenital affections result from interruption of the normal course of development or from inflammatory processes—endocarditis; sometimes from a combination of both.

General Anomalies.—Of general anomalies of development the following conditions may be mentioned: *Acardia,* absence of the heart, which has been met with in the monstrosity known by the same name; *double heart,* which has occasionally been found in extreme grades of fetal deformity; *dextrocardia,* in which the heart is on the right side, either alone or as part of a general transportation of the viscera; *ectopia cordis,* a condition associated with fission of the chest wall and of the abdomen. The heart may be situated in the cervical, pectoral, or abdominal regions. Except in the abdominal variety, the condition is very rarely compatible with extra-uterine life. Occasionally, as in a case reported by Holt, the child lives for some months, and the heart may be seen and felt beating beneath the skin in the epigastric region. This infant was five months old at the date of examination.

Anomalies of the Cardiac Septa.—The septa of both auricles and ventricles may be defective, in which case the heart consists of but two chambers, the *cor biloculare* or reptilian heart. In the septum of the auricles there is a very common defect, owing to the fact that the membrane closing the foramen ovale has failed at one point to become attached to the ring, and leaves a valvular slit which may be large enough to admit the handle of a scalpel. Neither this nor the small cribriform perforations of the membrane are of any significance.

The foramen ovale may be patent without a trace of membrane closing it. In some instances this exists with other serious defects, such as stenosis of the pulmonary artery, or imperfection of the ventricular septum. In others the patent foramen ovale is the only anomaly, and in many instances it does not appear to have caused any embarrassment, as the condition has been found in persons who have died of various affections. The ventricular septum may be absent, the condition known as trilocular heart. Much more frequently there is a small defect in the upper portion of the septum, either in the situation of the membranous portion known as the "undefended space" or in the region situated just anterior to this. The anomaly is very frequently associated with narrowing of the pulmonary orifice or of the conus arteriosus of the right ventricle.

Apart from the instances in association with narrowing of the orifice of the pulmonary artery, or of the conus, there are cases in which defect of the membranous septum is the only lesion, a condition not incompatible with long and fairly active life. The late Professor Brooks of the Johns Hopkins University knew from early manhood that he had heart trouble, but he accomplished an extraordinary amount of work, and lived to be about 60. Imperfect septum was the only lesion. The physical signs are fairly distinctive, with usually some enlargement of the heart, and a murmur first described by Roger in the following terms: "It is a loud murmur, audible over a large area, and, commencing with systole, is prolonged so as to cover the normal tic-tac. It has its maximum, not at the base to the right, as in aortic stenosis, or to the left, as in pulmonary stenosis, but at the upper third of the præcordial region. It is central, like the septum, and from this central point gradually diminishes in intensity in every direction. The murmur does not vary at any time, and it is not conducted into the vessels." In several of my cases there has been a distinct systolic intensification of this loud continuous murmur.

Anomalies and Lesions of the Valves.—Numerical anomalies of the valves are not uncommon. The semilunar segments at the arterial orifices are not infrequently increased or diminished in number. Supernumerary segments are more frequent in the pulmonary artery than in the aorta. Four, or sometimes five, valves have been found. The segments may be of equal size, but, as a rule, the supernumerary valve is small.

Instead of three there may be only two semilunar valves, or, as it is termed, the *bicuspid condition*. In my experience this is more frequent in the aortic valve. Of 21 instances only 2 occurred at the pulmonary orifice. Two of the valves have united, and from the ventricular face show either no trace of division or else a slight depression indicating where the union has occurred. From the aortic side there is usually to be seen some trace of division into two sinuses of Valsalva. There has been a discussion as to the origin of this condition, whether it is really an anomaly or whether it is not due to endocarditis, fetal or post-natal. The combined segment is usually thickened, but the fact that this anomaly is met with in the fetus without a trace of sclerosis or endocarditis shows that it may, in some cases at least, result from a developmental error.

Clinically this is a very important congenital defect, owing to the liability of the combined valve to sclerotic changes. Except two fetal specimens, all of my cases showed thickening and deformity, and in 15 of those which I have reported death resulted directly or indirectly from the lesion.

The little fenestrations at the margins of the sigmoid valves have no significance; they occur in a considerable proportion of all bodies.

Anomalies of the auriculo-ventricular valves are not often met with.

Fetal endocarditis may occur either at the arterial or auriculo-ventricular orifices. It is nearly always of the chronic or sclerotic variety. Very rarely, indeed, is it of the warty or verrucose form. There are little nodular bodies, sometimes six or eight in number, on the mitral and tricuspid segments—the nodules of Albini—which represent the remains of fetal structures, and must not be mistaken for endocardial outgrowths. The little rounded, bead like hæmorrhages of a deep purple color, which are very common on the heart valves of children, are also not to be mistaken for the products of endocarditis. In fetal endocarditis the segments are usually thickened at the edges, shrunken, and smooth. In the mitral and tricuspid valves the cusps are found united and the chordæ tendineæ are thickened and shortened. In the semilunar valves all trace of the segments has disappeared, leaving a stiff membranous diaphragm perforated by an oval or rounded orifice. It is sometimes very difficult to say whether this condition has resulted from fetal endocarditis or whether it is an error in development. In very many instances the processes are combined; an anomalous valve becomes the seat of chronic sclerotic changes, and, according to Rauchfuss, endocarditis is more common on the right side of the heart only because the valves are here more often the seat of developmental errors.

Lesions at the Pulmonary Orifice.—*Stenosis* of this orifice is one of the commonest and most important of congenital heart affections. A slow endocarditis causes gradual union of the segments and narrowing of the orifice to such a degree that it admits only the smallest sized probe. In some of the cases the smooth membranous condition of the combined segments is such that it would appear to be the result of faulty development. In some instances vegetations occur. The condition is compatible with life for many years, and in a considerable proportion of the cases of congenital heart disease above the tenth year this lesion is present. With it there may be defect of the ventricular septum. Pulmonary tuberculosis is a very common cause of death. Obliteration or *atresia* of the pulmonary orifice is a less frequent but more serious condition than stenosis. It is associated with persistence of the ductus arteriosus, together with patency of the foramen ovale or defect of the ventricular septum with hypertrophy of the right heart. *Stenosis of the conus arteriosus* of the right ventricle exists in a considerable proportion of the cases of obstruction at the pulmonary orifice. At the outset a developmental error, it may be combined with sclerotic changes. The ventricular septum is imperfect, the foramen ovale is usually open, and the ductus arteriosus patent. These three lesions at the pulmonary orifice constitute the most important group of all congenital cardiac affections. Of 181 instances of various congenital anomalies collected by Peacock, 119 cases came under this category, and, according to this author, in 86 per cent. of the patients living beyond the twelfth year the lesion is at this orifice.

Congenital lesions of the aortic orifice are not very frequent. Rauchfuss has collected 24 cases of stenosis and atresia; stenosis of the left conus arteriosus may also occur, a condition which is not incompatible with prolonged life. Ten of the 16 cases tabulated by Dilg were over thirty years of age.

Transposition of the large arterial trunks is a not uncommon anomaly. There may be neither hypertrophy, cyanosis, nor heart murmur.

Symptoms of Congenital Heart Disease.—Cyanosis occurs in over 90 per cent. of the cases, and forms so distinctive a feature that the terms "blue disease" and "morbus cæruleus" are practically synonyms for congenital heart-disease. The lividity in a majority of cases appears only within the first week of life, and may be general or confined to the lips, nose, and ears, and to the fingers and toes. In some instances there is in addition a general dusky suffusion, and in the most extreme grades the skin is almost purple. It may vary a good deal and may be intense only on exertion. The external temperature is low. Dyspnœa on exertion and cough are common symptoms. A great increase in the number of the red corpuscles has been noted by Gibson and by Vaquez. In a case of Gibson's there were above eight millions of red blood corpuscles to the cubic millimetre. The children rarely thrive, and often display a lethargy of both mind and body. The fingers and toes are clubbed to a degree rarely met with in any other affection. The cause of the cyanosis has been much discussed. Morgagni referred it to the general congestion of the venous system due to obstruction, and this view was supported in a paper, one of the ablest that has been written on the subject, by Moreton Stillé. Morrison's analysis of 75 cases of congenital heart disease shows that closure of the pulmonary orifice with patency of the foramen ovale and the ventricular septum is the condition most frequently associated with cyanosis, and he concludes that the deficient aeration of the blood owing to diminished lung function is the most important factor. Another view, often attributed erroneously to William Hunter, was that the discoloration was due to the admixture in the heart of venous and arterial blood; but lesions may exist which permit of very free mixture without producing cyanosis. The question of the cause of cyanosis really can not be considered as settled. Variot has recently made the suggestion that the cause is not entirely cardiac, but is associated with disturbance throughout the whole circulatory system, and particularly a vaso-motor paresis and malaeration of the red blood corpuscles.

Diagnosis.—In the case of children, cyanosis, with or without enlargement of the heart, and the existence of a murmur, are sufficient, as a rule, to determine the presence of a congenital heart lesion. The cyanosis gives us no clew to the precise nature of the trouble, as it is a symptom common to many lesions and it may be absent in certain conditions. The murmur is usually systolic in character. It is, however, not always present, and there are instances on record of complicated congenital lesions in which the examination showed normal heart sounds. In two or three instances fetal endocarditis has been diagnosed *in gravida* by the presence of a rough systolic murmur, and the condition has been corroborated subsequent to the birth of the child. Hypertrophy is present in a majority of the cases of congenital defect. The fatal event may be caused by abscess of the brain. For a full discussion of the subject the senior student is referred to the exhaustive monograph of Dr. Maude Abbott in Vol. IV of my "System of Medicine." I here abstract the conclusions of Hochsinger:

"(1) In childhood, loud, rough, musical heart murmurs, with normal or only slight increase in the heart dulness, occur only in congenital heart disease. The acquired endocardial defects with loud heart murmurs in young children are almost always associated with great increase in the heart dulness. In the transposition of the large arterial trunks there may be no cyanosis, no heart murmur, and an absence of hypertrophy.

"(2) In young children heart murmurs with great increase in the cardiac dulness and feeble apex beat suggest congenital changes. The increased dulness is chiefly of the right heart, whereas the left is only slightly altered. On the other hand, in the acquired endocarditis in children, the left heart is chiefly affected and the apex beat is visible; the dilatation of the right heart comes late and does not materially change the increased strength of the apex beat.

"(3) The entire absence of murmurs at the apex, with their evident presence in the region of the auricles and over the pulmonary orifice, is always an important element in differential diagnosis, and points rather to septum defect or pulmonary stenosis than to endocarditis.

"(4) An abnormally weak second pulmonic sound associated with a distinct systolic murmur is a symptom which in early childhood is only to be explained by the assumption of a congenital pulmonary stenosis, and possesses therefore an importance from a point of differential diagnosis which is not to be underestimated.

"(5) Absence of a palpable thrill, despite loud murmurs which are heard over the whole præcordial region, is rare except with congenital defects in the septum, and it speaks, therefore, against an acquired cardiac affection.

"(6) Loud, especially vibratory, systolic murmurs, with the point of maximum intensity over the upper third of the sternum, associated with a lack of marked symptoms of hypertrophy of the left ventricle, are very important for the diagnosis of a persistence of the ductus Botalli, and can not be explained by the assumption of an endocarditis of the aortic valve."

Escherich suggests that the systolic basic murmur heard sometimes in the newborn, particularly if premature, may originate in the ductus Botalli before its closure.

Treatment.—The child should be warmly clad and guarded from all circumstances liable to excite bronchitis. In the attacks of urgent dyspnœa with lividity blood should be freely let. Saline cathartics are also useful. Digitalis must be used with care; it is sometimes beneficial in the later stages. When the compensation fails, the indications for treatment are those of valvular disease in adults.

VII. ANGINA PECTORIS

(*Stenocardia, Breast Pang*)

Definition.—A disease characterized by paroxysmal attacks of pain, usually pectoral, associated with changes in the vascular walls, organic or functional.

History.—In 1768 Heberden described a "disorder of the breast," to which he gave the name of "Angina Pectoris." Before this date Morgagni and Rougnon had described cases. The association with coronary artery disease was early shown by Jenner. John Hunter died in an attack. The connection with aortitis as demonstrated by Corrigan and Allbutt, the recognition of extra-pectoral forms, and the introduction of nitrites in treatment by Lauder Brunton are the important contributions of the nineteenth century.

Etiology.—The disease is not uncommon, about 700 dying yearly of it in England and Wales. In the United States it is more common, the average number of deaths per million of the population being more than double that of England.

It is a rare disease in hospitals; a case a year is about the average, even in the large metropolitan hospitals. It is a disease of the better classes, and a consultant in active work may see a dozen or more cases a year.

Age.—In my series of 268 cases there were, under 30, 9 cases; between 30 and 40, 41; between 40 and 50, 59; between 50 and 60, 81; between 60 and 70, 62; between 70 and 80, 13; above 80, 3. The fifth and sixth decades are the fatal periods, as shown by the Registrar General's statistics.

Sex.—Women are rarely attacked. Of my cases 231 were men and 37 women.

RACE.—As mentioned, the disease seems to be relatively more frequent in the United States. Jews are particularly prone, 37 of my 268 cases.

OCCUPATION.—It is not an affection of the working classes. The life of stress and strain, particularly of worry, seems to predispose to it, and this is perhaps why it is so common in our profession. In my series of 268 cases there were 33 physicians, a very large proportion. From John Hunter onward a long list of distinguished physicians have been its victims, among whom may be mentioned in recent years Charcot, Nothnagel, and William Pepper.

CARDIO-VASCULAR DISEASE.—In persons under forty syphilis is an important feature, causing an aortitis, often limited to the root of the vessel. Whatever the cause, arterio-sclerosis predisposes to angina. A majority of the patients have sclerosis, many high blood pressure. Business men leading lives of great strain, and eating, drinking, and smoking to excess, form the large contingent of angina cases. Slight attacks may occur with high blood pressure alone.

HEREDITY.—The disease may occur in members of three generations, as in the Arnold family.

Imitative Features.—Outbreaks of angina-like attacks have been described. After the death of one member of a family from the disease, another may have somewhat similar attacks. Two of his physicians had angina after Senator Sumner's fatal attack. One of them died within two weeks; the other, a young man, recovered completely.

Symptoms.—Gaged by the severity of the attacks, cases may be grouped in three categories:

(*a*) MILDEST FORM (*"Les Formes Frustes"* of the French).—There is a feeling of substernal tension, uneasiness, or distress, rising at times to positive pain, usually associated with emotion, sometimes with exertion, but soon passing off. There may be slight pallor, or a feeling of faintness. When rising to speak in public there may be a feeling of substernal tension—it is a common experience—which passes off. Muscular effort, as in climbing a hill or a stair, may bring on the sensation. In the high pressure life a man may experience for weeks or months this sense of substernal tension, not pain, and without accurate localization or radiation, and not increased by exercise or emotion. It is, as one patient expressed it, a "hot-box" indicating too great pressure and too high speed. It is away after the night's rest, and may disappear entirely when the "harness" is taken off.

(*b*) MILD FORM (*Angina Minor*).—Pain in the heart of moderate severity with radiation to the arm is met with in many nervous and hysterical persons, in tobacco smokers, sometimes following the acute infections, particularly influenza. The attacks are rarely prolonged, are brought on by emotion, are more frequent in women, and are never fatal. Often called pseudo, false, functional, or toxic angina, the difference in the character of the attacks may be one of degree only. The conditions under which the attacks come on are of greater importance than the nature of the attack itself. There may be marked vaso-motor disturbance, with cold, numb, and blue extremities, followed by præcordial pain and a feeling of faintness. In persons addicted to tea, coffee, and tobacco heart pain is not infrequent, sharp and shooting, associated with palpitation, or severe and truly anginal.

(*c*) Severe Angina (*Angina Major*).—The two special features in this group are the existence in a large proportion of all the cases of organic disease of heart or vessels and the liability to sudden death. An exciting cause of the attack can usually be traced; muscular effort is the most common. Mental emotion is a second potent cause. John Hunter used to say that "his life was in the hands of any rascal who chose to worry him," and his fatal attack occurred in a fit of anger. A third very common excitant is flatulent distention of the stomach. Many patients are very sensitive to cold, and the chill of getting out of bed or of the bath may bring on a paroxysm.

Phenomena of the Attack.—During exertion or intense mental emotion the patient is seized with an agonizing pain in the region of the heart and a sense of constriction, as if the heart had been seized in a vice. The pains radiate to the neck and down the arm, and there may be numbness of the fingers or in the cardiac region. The face is usually pallid and may assume an ashy gray tint, and not infrequently a profuse sweat breaks out over the surface. The paroxysm lasts from several seconds to a minute or two, during which, in severe attacks, the patient feels as if death were imminent. As pointed out by Latham, there are two elements in it, the pain—*dolor pectoris*—and the indescribable feeling of anguish and sense of imminent dissolution—*angor animi.* There are great restlessness and anxiety, and the patient may drop dead at the height of the attack or faint and pass away in syncope. The condition of the heart during the attack is variable; the pulsations may be uniform and regular. The pulse tension, however, is usually increased, but it is surprising, even in the cases of extreme severity, how slightly the character of the pulse may be altered. After the attack there may be eructations, or the passage of a large quantity of clear urine. The patient usually feels exhausted, and for a day or two may be badly shaken; in other instances in an hour or two the patient feels himself again. While dyspnœa is not a constant feature, the paroxysm is not infrequently associated with a form of asthma; there is wheezing in the bronchial tubes, which may come on very rapidly, and the patient gets short of breath.

Death may occur in the first attack, as in the well known case of Thomas Arnold; or at the end of a series of attacks, the so-called *status angiosus.* Paroxysms may occur at intervals of a few weeks for a year or more before the fatal attack.

There is a chronic form represented by ten cases in my series, in which attacks occur irregularly. John Hunter's first seizure was in 1773, and he had many in the 20 years before his death. Sometimes life is a terrible burden, as any emotion or effort may bring on an attack. And, lastly, after paroxysms of great severity recurring for months, or even for so long as two years, as in one of my cases, complete recovery takes place.

Extra-pectoral Features of Angina.—In the attack the pain usually radiates up the neck and down the left arm. As the studies of Mackenzie and Head have shown in disease of the heart and of the aorta, the pain is referred to the 1st, 2d, 3d, and 4th dorsal areas; and in angina it may be also in areas of the distribution of the 5th to the 9th dorsal nerves. The pain may begin in the left arm, or in the jaw, even in the front teeth, or in one testis. Sometimes the pain remains in these distant parts, and yet the attack presents, as noted by Heberden, all the features of angina. I have known the attack to begin with agonizing pain in the left leg; in another case in the left pectoral muscle. The entire features of the attack may be sub-diaphragmatic—the so-called *angina abdominis.* In at least ten of my series the pains were abdominal, and, as first pointed out by Leared, gastralgia may be diagnosed.

The *pulmonary features* of angina are remarkable. A condition like acute emphysema may come on, with wheezing and an inflated state of the lungs. Acute œdema may follow with the expectoration of large quantities of a thin, bloody fluid. The blood pressure may be extraordinarily high—340 mm. Hg. in one case. *Cerebral features* are not common, but unconsciousness may occur. Transient monoplegia, or hemiplegia and aphasia, occurred in three of my cases.

Morbid Anatomy and Pathology.—The 17 post mortems in my series illustrate the usual lesions:

(*a*) *Coronary artery disease* was present in 13 cases. The orifices only may be involved in a sclerotic aortitis. In one case they were narrowed to admit only a bristle, while the vessels beyond were normal. Blocking of a branch with a fresh thrombus, or with an embolus, is not uncommon. During an attack an infarct may soften, with perforation of the ventricular wall. Obliterative endarteritis, *the* lesion of the disease, was present in 9 of my cases. In elderly subjects the coronary vessels may be calcified—the condition found by Jenner in John Hunter.

(*b*) *Aortitis* was present in four of my cases, in syphilitic subjects, all under 40 years of age. Corrigan first called attention to this lesion in angina, the great importance of which has been emphasized by Clifford Allbutt. It is usually limited to the supra-sigmoidal area, and has the characteristic features of the syphilitic aortitis.

(*c*) In a few instances no lesions have been found. In one case of my list a man aged 26 had attacks, which were regarded as functional, on and off for two years. Death occurred after a series of paroxysms. The aorta was small, otherwise there were no changes.

No completely satisfactory explanation of the phenomena of the angina attack has yet been offered. It has been regarded as a neuralgia of the cardiac nerves, a cramp of the heart muscle, or of certain parts of it, or an expression of tension of the ventricular walls in extreme dilatation. In some ways the intermittent claudication theory of Allan Burns meets the case. This may be defined as a state in which an artery admits enough blood to a muscular structure for quiet work, but not enough for increased work, so that the contractile function of the muscle is disturbed and pain results. Burns remarked that " . . . If we can call into vigorous action a limb around which we have with moderate tightness applied a ligature, we find that then the member can only support its action for a very short time, for now the supply of energy and its expenditure do not balance each other. . . A heart, the coronary arteries of which are cartilaginous or ossified, is nearly in a similar condition; it can, like the limb begirt with a moderately tight ligature, discharge its functions so long as its action is moderate and equal. Increase. however, the action of the whole body, and along with the rest that of the heart, and you will soon see exemplified the truth of what has been said."

Angina results from an alteration in the working of the muscle fibres of any part of the cardio-vascular system, whereby painful afferent stimuli are excited. Cold, emotion, or toxic agents interfering with the orderly action of the peripheral circulation increase the tension in the heart walls or in the larger central mains, causing strain and a type of contraction capable of exciting in the involuntary muscles painful afferent stimuli. In disturbance of this all-important Gaskellian function, in the stretching, in the alteration of the wall tension at any point, sufficient to excite a pain-producing resistance to this by the muscle elements, are to be sought an explanation of the phenomenon of the attack. Spasm, or narrowing of a coronary artery, or of one branch, may so modify the action of a section of the heart that it works with disturbed tension, and with stretching and strain sufficient to rouse painful sensations. Or the heart may be in the same state as the leg muscles of a man with intermittent claudication, working smoothly when quiet, but the instant an effort is made, or if a wave of emotion touches the peripheral vessels, the normal contraction is disturbed and a crisis of pain excited.

There are three modes of dying in angina—one, as Walshe says, "is sudden, instantaneous, coeval with a single pang." The functions of life stop abruptly, and with a gasp all is over. In a second mode, following a series of attacks, the heart grows weaker and the patient dies in a progressive asthenia; while in a third there is a gradually induced cardiac insufficiency with dyspnœa.

Prognosis.—In men under 40 syphilis must be suspected, and with appropriate treatment recovery may be complete (see my Lumleian Lectures, Lancet, 1910, I). In men in the 5th and 6th decades who have lived the high pressure life a change of habits may bring relief; but, as Walshe remarked, "the cardinal fact in real angina is its uncertainty." Even after attacks of the greatest severity recovery is possible. The circumstances that bring on an attack are important. Emotion is of the least importance. The angina of effort that follows any slight exertion is, as a rule, more serious than that which comes on spontaneously, or is excited by emotion; yet one of my patients who could never dress without having what he called "angor de toilette" lived for 11 years. The cardio-vascular condition is of the first importance in prognosis. Very high blood pressure, advanced arterio-sclerosis, valvular disease, signs of myocardial weakness are of serious import. It is to be remembered that a large proportion of all cases have no obvious signs of cardiac disease; and the coronary arteries may be extensively diseased with clear heart sounds and a good pulse. In women the forms of angina with marked vaso-motor disturbance as a rule do well, and when neurotic or hysterical manifestations are prominent the outlook is good.

Treatment.—Syphilitic cases require active treatment—salvarsan in the subjects under 40, mercury and iodide of potassium in older persons. In the neurotic cases with a recognition of the basic disturbance in the vaso-motor system a Weir Mitchell cure and hydrotherapy are indicated. A persistent course of wet packs I have often seen helpful. When high tension is present, as is not infrequently the case in neurasthenia, the nitrites may be given; and ergotin grs. ii (0.13 gm.) three times a day has a definite value in vaso-motor instability. In the severer types of the disease the treatment is concerned with the attack and with the general condition afterward. In the attack inhalation of nitrite of amyl, introduced by Lauder Brunton, may give instant relief. We see its benefit particularly in cases with widespread arterial constriction. In the recurring terrible paroxysms it may lose its effect, but many milder forms are relieved promptly, and it gives great comfort and confidence to the patient to carry the *perles*. Morphia should be used freely when amyl nitrite fails and when the attacks recur with great frequency. As Burney Yeo pointed out, angina patients are very resistant to this drug, and between 10 p. m. and 1 p. m. the next day I have known five grains administered with relief to the pain, but without causing sleep. Chloroform may have to be used, and my experience coincides with that of the late George Balfour of Edinburgh, that it is always helpful, never harmful. With a dusky cyanosis and asthma like breathing oxygen inhalations may be given.

For the general condition, if high tension is present, iodide of potassium and the nitrites in all forms are useful. The use of theobromine has been warmly advocated by Marchiafava, grs. xv (1 gm.) three times a day, and I have tried it in a few cases with benefit, particularly in two cases of the angina of effort.

C. DISEASES OF THE ARTERIES

I. ARTERIO-SCLEROSIS

(*Arterio-capillary Fibrosis*)

The conception of arterio-sclerosis as an independent affection—a general disease of the vascular system—is due to Gull and Sutton.

Definition.—A condition of thickening of the arterial coats, with degeneration, diffuse or circumscribed. The process leads, in the larger arteries, to what is known as atheroma and to endarteritis deformans, and seriously interferes with the normal functions of various organs.

Etiology.—Among the important factors in causing arterio-sclerosis the following may be considered:

(*a*) Hypertension.—The blood pressure, the tension or force with which the blood circulates, depends upon five factors: The heart pump supplies the force; the elastic coats of the large arteries store and convert an intermittent into a continuous stream; the small arteries act as sluices or taps regulating the control to different parts; the capillary bed is the irrigation field over which the nutritive fluid is distributed; and the drainage system is represented by the veins and lymph channels.

Galen first grasped the fact that life depends upon the maintenance of a due pressure in these irrigation fields: "Many canals dispersed throughout all the parts of the body convey to them blood as those of a garden convey moisture, and the intervals separating those canals are wonderfully disposed by nature in such a way that they should neither lack a sufficient quantity of blood for absorption, nor be overloaded at any time with an excessive supply."

The blood pressure varies greatly in different individuals, and in the same individual under varying conditions. The normal blood pressure is from 120 to 130 mm. of mercury, but in persons over 50 it is very often from 140 to 160 mm. A permanent pressure above the latter figure may be called high, but there are great regional variations. Permanently low blood pressure may be met with in asthenia from any cause, in the various toxæmias of the infectious diseases, and there are persons in apparently good health with chronic hypotension.

High tension is met with in many chronic diseases, in various forms of cardiac and renal disease, in lead poisoning, and, above all, in connection with general arterio-sclerosis. The relation to arterio-sclerosis has been much discussed. Briefly, there are three groups of cases: (1) First, the simple high tension without signs of arterial or renal disease—what Clifford Allbutt calls hyperpyesis. In this well recognized condition, met with in individuals otherwise healthy, the blood pressure is permanently high—above 180—but, so far as can be ascertained, there are no arterial, cardiac, or renal changes. It is difficult, of course, to exclude internal, not discernible alterations in the splanchnic and other vessels, since, as is well known, vascular disease may be very localized. But clinically the group is well defined and very important. The condition is met with most frequently in keen business men, who work hard, drink hard, and smoke hard.

The exact cause of this high tension we do not know. Some have attributed it to over-activity of the adrenals, but it is much more likely that the primary difficulty is somewhere in the capillary bed—in that short space in which the real business of life is transacted. However produced, the important point here is that this hypertension itself leads to arterio-sclerosis, which can be produced experimentally by the injection of adrenalin and other hypertensive substances.

(2) In the second group of cases the high tension is associated with an arterio-sclerosis with consecutive cardiac and renal disease.

(3) In the third group the high tension is secondary to forms of chronic nephritis in association with cardio-vascular disease.

(*b*) As an INVOLUTION PROCESS arterio-sclerosis is an accompaniment of old age, and is the expression of the natural wear and tear to which the tubes are subjected. Longevity is a vascular question, which has been well expressed in the axiom that "a man is only as old as his arteries." To a majority of men death comes primarily or secondarily through this portal. The onset of what may be called physiological arterio-sclerosis depends, in the first place, upon the quality of arterial tissue (vital rubber) which the individual has inherited, and secondly upon the amount of wear and tear to which he has subjected it. That the former plays a most important rôle is shown in the cases in which arterio-sclerosis sets in early in life in individuals in whom none of the recognized etiological factors can be found. Thus, for instance, a man of twenty eight or twenty nine may have the arteries of a man of sixty, and a man of forty may present vessels as much degenerated as they should be at eighty. Entire families sometimes show this tendency to early arterio-sclerosis—a tendency which can not be explained in any other way than that in the makeup of the machine bad material was used for the tubing. More commonly the arterio-sclerosis results from the bad use of good vessels.

(*c*) Chronic Intoxications.—Alcohol, lead, and gout play an important rôle in the causation of arterio-sclerosis, although the precise mode of their action is not yet very clear. They may act, as Traube suggests, by increasing the peripheral resistance in the smaller vessels and in this way raising the blood tension, or possibly, as Bright taught, they alter the quality of the blood and render more difficult its passage through the capillaries. The observations of Cabot have thrown doubt on the importance of alcohol as a factor.

The poisons of the acute infections may produce degenerative changes in the media and adventitia. Thayer has recently called attention to the frequency of arterial changes as a sequence of typhoid fever.

(*d*) Syphilis, one of the most important single causes, will be spoken of under morbid anatomy.

(*e*) Overeating.—I am more and more impressed with the part played by overeating in inducing arterio-sclerosis. There are many cases in which there is no other factor. George Cheyne's advice, quoted at page 451, was never more needed than by the present generation.

(*f*) The Stress and Strain of Modern Life.—There are men in the fifth decade who have not had syphilis or gout, who have eaten and drunk with discretion, and in whom none of the ordinary factors are present—men in whom the arterio-sclerosis seems to come on as a direct result of a high pressure life.

(*g*) Overwork of the muscles, which acts by increasing the peripheral resistance and by raising the blood pressure.

(*h*) Renal Disease.—The relation between the arterial and kidney lesions has been much discussed, some regarding the arterial degeneration as secondary, others as primary. There are two groups of cases, one in which the arterio-sclerosis is the first change, and the other in which it is secondary to a primary affection of the kidneys.

Morbid Anatomy.—The affection is met with most frequently in the aorta and its main branches. It is comparatively less frequent in the mesenteric and rare in the pulmonary arteries. Several different forms may be recognized:

(*a*) Nodular.—The aorta presents in the early stages, from the ring to the bifurcation, numerous flat projections, yellowish or yellowish white in color, and situated particularly about the orifices of the branches. In the early stage these patches are scattered and do not involve the entire intima. In more advanced stages the patches undergo atheromatous changes. The material constituting the button undergoes softening and breaks up into granular material, consisting of molecular débris—the so-called atheromatous abscess.

(*b*) Diffuse Arterio-sclerosis.—In this form, met with usually in middle-aged men, or younger persons, the affection is widespread throughout the arteries. In the aorta the media shows necrotic and hyaline changes, while the intima may be smooth or show very slight thickenings—scattered elevated areas of an opaque white color, some of which undergo atheromatous changes. The smaller arteries show thickening of the walls, due particularly to increase in the sub-endothelial connective tissue. The muscular coat may be at first hypertrophied, but later undergoes hyaline and calcareous changes. In this group of cases the heart hypertrophies and later fibrous myocarditis is often present. The semilunar valves are opaque and sclerotic. The kidneys are sclerotic and may be increased in size, and are usually very firm. In places the surface may be rough, or present atrophied depressed areas of a deep red color.

(*c*) SENILE ARTERIO-SCLEROSIS.—In this the larger arteries are dilated and tortuous, the walls thin and stiff, and the smaller vessels, as the radials, converted into rigid tubes like pipe-stems. The intima of the aorta may be occupied by rough, calcareous plaques, with here and there fissures and loss of substance. There may be sub-endothelial softening with the formation of atheromatous ulcers on which thrombi may deposit; though, as a rule, there may be the most extreme calcification and roughness with erosions of the aorta without thrombus formation. In the smaller vessels, as the radicals, there are degeneration and calcification of the media—the so-called Monckeberg type.

The SYPHILITIC ARTERIO-SCLEROSIS is usually a mesaortitis with definite characteristics. Macroscopically it may be limited in extent, localized at the root of the aorta, or about the orifice of an aneurism, or there is a band of an inch in width on some portion of the tube, while other parts of the aorta and its branches are normal. In other instances the intima is involved, not with the usual plaque-like areas of atheroma, but there are shallow depressions of a bluish tint, and short transverse or longitudinal puckerings, sometimes with a stellate arrangement; or the intima is pitted and scarred with small depressions and linear sulci. Microscopically the most important changes are found in the media and adventitia: (*a*) perivascular infiltration of the vasa vasorum; (*b*) small-celled infiltration in areas of the media, with (*c*) splitting, separation, and destruction of elastic fibres and the muscle cells. The intima over these areas may be perfectly normal, but it often shows signs of thickening with fatty degeneration and the production of hyaline. Similar changes have been described by Klotz in the larger blood vessels in cases of congenital syphilis. And, lastly, the specific nature of this mesaortitis has been determined by the detection of the spirochætes. Other forms affecting the smaller vessels have been referred to under syphilis.

SCLEROSIS OF THE PULMONARY ARTERY is met with in all conditions which for a long time increase the tension in the lesser circulation, particularly in mitral valve disease and in emphysema. Sometimes the sclerosis reaches a high grade and is accompanied with aneurismal dilatation of the primary and secondary branches, more rarely with insufficiency of the pulmonary valve. Leonard Rogers has shown that in India it is not uncommon as a primary affection. In a remarkable case of a young man of twenty four, reported by Romberg from Curschmann's clinic, the pulmonary arteries were involved in most extensive arterio-sclerosis; the main branches were dilated, and the smaller branches were the seat of the most extreme sclerotic changes. On the other hand, the aorta and its branches were normal.

In many cases of arterio-sclerosis the condition is not confined to the arteries, but extends not only to the capillaries but also to the veins, and may properly be termed an *angio-sclerosis.*

Sclerosis of the veins—*phlebo-sclerosis*—is not at all an uncommon accompaniment of arterio-sclerosis. It is seen in conditions of heightened blood pressure, as in the portal system in cirrhosis of the liver and in the pulmonary veins in mitral stenosis. The affected vessels are usually dilated, and the intima shows, as in the arteries, a compensatory thickening, which is particularly marked in those regions in which the media is thinned. The new-formed tissue in the endophlebitis may undergo hyaline degeneration, and is sometimes extensively calcified. Without existing arterio-sclerosis the peripheral veins may be sclerotic, usually in conditions of debility, but not infrequently in young persons.

Symptoms.—Increased Tension.—The pressure with which the blood flows in the arteries depends upon the degree of peripheral resistance and the force of the ventricular contraction. A high-tension pulse may exist with very little arterio-sclerosis; but, as a rule, when the condition has been persistent, the sclerosis and high tension are found together. On the other hand, a very low or normal tension may be present in extremely sclerotic vessels.

General Symptoms.—The early symptoms are interesting. Stengel has called attention to the pallor, and there may be dyspeptic symptoms. It is remarkable with what rapidity the disease may progress. I have known the peripheral arteries to stiffen and grow old in a couple of years.

The combination of heightened blood pressure, a palpable thickening of the arteries, hypertrophy of the left ventricle, and accentuation of the aortic second sound are signs pathognomonic of arterio-sclerosis. From this period of establishment the course of the disease may be very varied. For years the patient may have good health, and be in a condition analogous to that of a person with a well compensated valvular lesion. There may be no renal symptoms, or there may be the passage of a larger amount of urine than normal, with transient albuminuria, and now and then hyaline tube casts. The subsequent history is extraordinarily diverse, depending upon the vascular territory in which the sclerosis is most advanced, or upon the accidents which are so liable to happen, and the symptoms may be cardiac, cerebral, renal, etc.

(*a*) *Cardiac.*—The involvement of the coronary arteries may lead to the various symptoms already referred to under that section—thrombosis with sudden death, fibroid degeneration of the heart, aneurism of the heart, rupture, and angina pectoris. Angina pectoris is not uncommon, and the organic variety is almost always associated with arterio-sclerosis. A second important group of cardiac symptoms results from the dilatation which finally gets the better of the hypertrophy. The patient then presents all the symptoms of cardiac insufficiency—dyspnœa, scanty urine, and very often serous effusions. If the case has come under observation for the first time the clinical picture is that of chronic valvular disease, and the existence of a loud blowing murmur at the apex may throw the practitioner off his guard. Many cases terminate in this way.

(*b*) The *cerebral* symptoms of arterio-sclerosis are varied and important, and embrace those of many degenerative diseases, acute and chronic (which follow sclerosis of the smaller branches), and cerebral hæmorrhage.

Transient hemiplegia, monoplegia, or aphasia may occur in advanced arterio-sclerosis. The attacks are very characteristic, often brief, lasting twenty four hours or less. Recovery may be perfect. Recurrence is the rule, and a patient may have a score or more attacks of aphasia, or in the course of a couple of years there may be half a dozen transient hemiplegic attacks or one or two monoplegias, or paraplegia for a day or two. Much attention has of late been given to these cases, which seem best explained on the view of transient spasm as originally suggested by Peabody. Vertigo occurs frequently, and may be either simple, or is associated with slow pulse and syncopal or epileptiform attacks—the Stokes-Adams syndrome.

(*c*) *Renal* symptoms supervene in a large number of the cases. A sclerosis, patchy or diffuse, is present in a majority of the cases at the time of autopsy, and the condition is practically that of contracted kidney. It is seen in a typical manner in the senile form, and not infrequently develops early in life as a direct sequence of the diffuse variety. It is often difficult to decide clinically (and the question is one upon which good observers might not agree in a given case) whether the arterial or the renal disease has been primary.

(*d*) *Abdominal Arterio-sclerosis.*—It is believed to be associated particularly with overeating and chronic overtaxing of the stomach and intestines with work. The condition is by no means uncommon, and the sclerosis of the splanchnic vessels may be advanced out of all proportion to that elsewhere. The symptoms are indefinite, sometimes resembling those of the ordinary neurosis with marked constipation, features that are by no means certainly associated with sclerosis; on the other hand, there is much more reason to connect the attacks of severe abdominal pain, the gastric crises of lead and of tabes with spasm of the vessels in this condition. There are cases of angina pectoris with abdominal pain which may be due to angiospasm of the sclerotic vessels.

(*e*) Among other events in arterio-sclerosis may be mentioned gangrene of the extremities, due either directly to endarteritis or to the dislodgment of thrombi. Sudden transient paralysis may occur.

(*f*) *Intermittent lameness or claudication,* the dysbasia angio-sclerotica of Erb, the crural angina of Walton, is seen most frequently in connection with arterio-sclerosis. In the horse, in which the intermittent lameness was first described by Bouley, verminous aneurisms are present in the iliac arteries. In man Charcot described the condition in 1856 in an old soldier who was not able to walk for more than a quarter of an hour without severe cramps in the legs. The post mortem showed a traumatic aneurism of one iliac artery. The loss of function and the pain in the muscles were due to the relative ischemia. Erb has shown that intermittent lameness is not at all infrequent, particularly among private patients, only 2 of his 45 cases not coming in this class. Of 127 cases there were only 7 in women. Hebrews seem more frequently affected. Syphilis, alcohol, and tobacco are common factors. Muscular weakness after exertion or complete disability, numbness, tingling, and paræsthesia of various forms are the common symptoms. Pulsation may be absent in the dorsal arteries of the feet and the vessels are sclerotic. Vaso-motor changes may be present, and in the dependent position the feet and legs become deeply congested.

Treatment.—In the late stages the conditions must be treated as they arise in connection with the various viscera. In the early stages, before any local symptoms are manifest, the patient should be enjoined to live a quiet, well regulated life, avoiding excesses in food and drink. It is usually best to explain frankly the condition of affairs, and so gain his intelligent coöperation. Special attention should be paid to the state of the bowels and urine, and the secretion of the skin should be kept active by daily baths. Alcohol in all forms should be prohibited, and the food should be restricted to plain, wholesome articles. The use of mineral waters or a residence every year at one of the mineral springs is usually serviceable. If there has been a syphilitic history the persistent use of iodide of potassium is indicated; indeed, even in the non-syphilitic cases it seems to do good. It is best given in small doses, grains v to x (0.3 to 0.6 gm.). Whenever the blood pressure is high nitroglycerin or the sodium nitrite may be given to relieve symptoms rather than with any hope of essentially influencing the disease.

In cases which come under observation for the first time with dyspnœa, slight lividity, and signs of cardiac insufficiency, venesection is indicated. In some instances, with very high tension, striking relief is afforded by the abstraction of 10 to 20 ounces of blood. Cardiac failure, renal symptoms, etc., require the usual treatment.

II. ANEURISM

Definition.—A tumor containing fluid or solid blood in direct communication with the cavity of the heart, the surface of a valve, or the lumen of an artery.

History.—Galen knew external aneurism well, and in the second century A. D., Antyllos devised his operation of incising and emptying the sac inclosed between ligatures. Internal aneurism was recognized by Fernelius in the 16th century, and Vesalius was very familiar with the disease. Ambroise Paré suggested the relation of aneurism to syphilis, which was insisted upon in the great monograph of Lancisi in 1728. Morgagni in 1761 described very fully the symptoms and morbid anatomy. The modern views date from the studies of Helmstedter and Köster, who showed that the primary change was in the media. The researches of Eppinger, Thoma, and Welch emphasized the importance of these changes in the media, particularly as brought about by syphilis.

Classification.—For practical purposes the following classification may be adopted:

I. TRUE ANEURISM (aneurisma verum or aneurisma spontaneum), in which one or more of the coats of the vessel form the wall of the tumor: (*a*) *Dilatation-aneurism*—(1) Limited to a certain portion of the vessel, fusiform, cylindroid; (2) extending over a whole artery and its branches—cirsoid aneurism. (*b*) *Circumscribed saccular aneurism*, which is the common form of aneurism of the aorta. (*c*) *Dissecting aneurism*, with splitting of the media, and occasionally with the formation of a new tube lined with intimal endothelium.

II. FALSE ANEURISM, following a wound or the rupture of an artery, or of a true aneurism, causing a diffuse, or circumscribed, hæmatoma.

III. ARTERIO-VENOUS ANEURISM, either with direct communication between an artery and vein, or with the intervention of a sac, varicose aneurism.

IV. Special forms, such as the parasitic, the erosion, the traction, the mycotic.

Etiology.—Predisposing Causes.—*Age.*—Nearly one half of the deaths in England and Wales from aneurism in males occur between the ages of 30 and 45. In the young and in the very old the disease is rare, but it may occur at any age. Congenital aneurism has been described.

Sex.—Males are attacked much more frequently than females—in a ratio of 5 to 1.

Race and Locality.—The disease is more common in Great Britain than on the Continent. Among about 19,000 post mortems at Vienna there were 230 cases of aneurism, while among 18,678 at Guy's Hospital there were 325 cases. It is more common in the negroes of the Southern States of America than among the whites. Of 345 admissions for aneurism to my wards at the Johns Hopkins Hospital 132 were in colored and 213 in white patients—a ratio of 1 to 1.6, while the ratio of white to colored in the hospital at large was 5 to 1. In India aneurism is rare, though syphilis and arterial disease are common. Possibly, as Rogers suggests, the low blood pressure in the natives may have something to do with this comparative immunity.

Occupation.—Soldiers, sailors, draymen, iron and steel workers, and dock workers are particularly prone. In soldiers and sailors, who are peculiarly liable, the disease appears to be in direct proportion to the prevalence of syphilis.

Determining Causes.—These are three in number:

I. *The Acute Infections.*—In the specific fevers areas of degeneration are common in the aorta. Fortunately in most instances they are confined to the intima, but occasionally, as Thayer has pointed out in typhoid fever, the changes may be in the media. *The* infection with which aneurism is especially connected is syphilis—a fact recognized in the eighteenth century by Lancisi and by Morgagni, and dwelt upon specially in 1876 by Francis H. Welch, of the British Army. All recent figures show a very high percentage of syphilis in the subjects of aneurism—as high as 80 or 85 per cent.; and nowadays it is rare not to find a positive Wassermann reaction in an aneurismal patient under fifty. The lesion, a mesaortitis, has been described under arterio-sclerosis.

Other infections play a very minor rôle in the disease. With rheumatic fever, pneumonia, and septicæmia, the mycotic aneurism may be associated.

The various toxic factors which favor arterial degeneration, such as alcohol, lead, tobacco, and the chronic endogenous toxæmias, as gout and Bright's disease, are rare determining causes.

II. The second determining factor is *strain,* particularly the internal strain associated with sudden and violent muscular effort. The media is the protecting coat of the artery, and during a violent effort, as in lifting or jumping, laceration or splitting of the intima may occur over a weak spot. If small this leads to a local bulging of the media and the gradual production of a sac, or the tear of the intima may heal completely, or a dissecting aneurism may form. In other instances a widespread mesaortitis leads to a gradual, diffuse distention of the artery. This type of aneurism, frequently seen in the aged, may follow ordinary chronic atheroma.

III. *Occasional Causes.*—(*a*) Embolism: The emboli may consist of vegetations or calcified fragments from the valves. This form of aneurism, often multiple, is met with in infective endocarditis, as in the remarkable case which was described by me in 1888. In infective endocarditis the emboli probably pass to the vasa vasorum, causing mesaortitis with weakening of the wall; but in the smaller vessels the aneurisms are caused by the direct lodgment of the emboli which infect and weaken the wall. (*b*) External Injury: A blow on the chest, a sudden fall, or the jar of an accident may cause a rupture of the intima over a weak spot in the aorta, with the production of a dissecting or sacculated aneurism. (*c*) External Erosion: A tuberculous focus may involve the wall of the aorta; or a bullet lodged near the wall of an artery may weaken it and be followed by aneurism. (*d*) In the horse there is a *parasitic aneurism* common in the mesenteric vessels, due to growth in them of the *Strongylus armatus*. (*e*) Thoma has described a "traction" aneurism at the concavity of the arch at the point of insertion of the ductus Botalli.

Morbid Anatomy and Pathology.—Number.—Usually there is one aneurism, but three or four or even a dozen may be present. Multiple cup-shaped tumors in the aorta are always syphilitic. The mycotic are usually multiple, and in the peripheral vessels there may be a dozen or more.

Form.—There are two great types—one in which the lumen of the vessel is dilated, and the other in which a limited section of the wall gives way with the formation of a sac. Typical cylindrical and spindle shaped aneurisms are seen in the aorta and in the vessels of the second and third dimensions. The sacculated form is the more common. They are either flat, saucer-shaped, or cup-shaped, or sometimes beyond a very narrow orifice is a cylindrical tumor of variable size, from a pin's head in the smaller vessels, as in the brain, to a huge sac which may fill one half of the chest.

Vessels Affected.—Of a series of 551 cases studied by Crisp, the thoracic aorta was involved in 175, the abdominal aorta in 59, the femoral-iliac in 66, the popliteal in 137, the innominate in 20, the carotids in 25, subclavians in 23, axillary in 18. The other smaller vessels are rarely attacked. Of late years aneurism of the external vessels appears to have become much less frequent.

ANEURISM OF THE THORACIC AORTA

I. Dilatation Aneurism.—New interest has been attached to this form since the introduction of the X-rays in diagnosis. Formerly it was very often overlooked. The shape may be a single fusiform, or tent-shaped, or there may be multiple spindles. The condition was accurately noted by Hodgson, who called it "a preternatural permanent enlargement of the cavity of an artery," and distinguished it clearly from ordinary aneurism. It is very often associated with insufficiency of the aortic valves—a combination to which the French gave the name "Maladie de Hodgson." It is more common in elderly people, and may follow diffuse arterio-sclerosis from any cause. In syphilitic subjects it may be limited to the ascending portion of the arch, or may involve the entire arch.

Symptoms.—The cases are often latent, met with accidentally in medicolegal work, and the dilatation may reach an extreme grade without any symptoms. In other cases, particularly in the syphilitic aortitis in men, angina pectoris is an early symptom, and dilatation may be present in the senile form. In a third group the features are those of organic disease of the heart, usually of aortic insufficiency. Of 60 cases analyzed by T. McCrae there were 18 patients under 40; the majority of the cases were in elderly persons. Pressure effects are not uncommon; the trachea may be flattened and the œsophagus compressed. Erosion of the bones is rare.

The PHYSICAL SIGNS are often characteristic. Visible pulsation in the episternal notch is usually present, and it may even extend to the right sterno-clavicular articulation. Pulsation may sometimes be seen in the first and second right interspaces. In about one half of the cases a diffuse pulsation over the manubrium is present, but in old persons with rigid chest walls there may be extreme dilatation without any visible impulse. A rough thrill is not infrequently present, or a diastolic thrill when the valves are insufficient. A sharp diastolic shock may be felt.

Dulness over the manubrium is the most constant single sign. The second sound may be of a clanging, metallic, or even amphoric quality. When a diastolic murmur is present it may be heard loudly over the manubrium and perhaps transmitted into the vessels of the neck. The blood pressure is often low—below 140 mm. in 35 of 40 cases studied by McCrae. Examination with the X-rays in skilled hands is the most satisfactory means of diagnosis, as the dilated aorta casts a very definite shadow much larger than the normal aorta, and showing very little difference in extent during systole and diastole.

II. Dissecting Aneurism.—The majority of aneurisms of the aorta begin with a split or crack of the intima over a spot of syphilitic mesaortitis. Once this split has started the aorta may rupture in all its coats, or an aneurism may form at the site, or the fracture of the intima, though large and often circumferential, may heal; or the blood may extend between the coats, separating them for many inches, or in the entire extent, forming a dissecting aneurism; and, lastly, such a dissecting aneurism may heal perfectly.

RUPTURE OF THE AORTA is not very infrequent, as medico-legal work indicates. Usually there is agonizing pain with features of shock, and death may take place instantly; but in fully half of the cases there are two very characteristic stages, the first corresponding to the rupture of the inner coats, the second eight to ten hours, or as long as fifteen or sixteen days later, to fatal rupture of the external layer.

Dissecting aneurism is not very common. There were only two cases in 16 years at the Johns Hopkins Hospital, where aneurism may be said to be exceptionally frequent. The primary split is most frequently in the arch, not far above the valves, and is in the form of a transverse, or vertical, clean cut incision, as if made with a razor. The extent of the separation of the coats is variable. If the adventitia is reached, rupture is certain to take place, as only the structures of the middle coat can resist for any time the pressure of the blood. The blood may pass for three or four or more inches, separating the media, and then burst internally or externally. In other cases the dissection reaches from the ascending arch to the bifurcation of the aorta, even passing down the iliac and femorals into the smaller vessels of the leg. The splitting of the coats may, indeed, as in a case described by Rokitansky, reach to all the subdivisions of the aorta. The symptoms are those spoken of under rupture; but a very remarkable condition may follow, leading to:

Healed Dissecting Aneurism.—The earlier observers of this remarkable condition regarded it as an anatomical anomaly of a double aorta. Adami has collected 39 cases, in a majority of which there was no advanced disease of the aorta itself. The outer tube formed by the dissecting aneurism may extend the entire length of the aorta, occupying the full extent of the circumference. The most extraordinary feature is that the outer tube may present a perfectly smooth and natural appearance, and be lined with a new intima. The condition may last for many years.

III. Sacculated Aneurism of the Aorta: Aneurism of the Arch.—For purposes of discussion this part of the vessel may be divided into the sinuses of Valsalva, ascending, transverse, and descending portions.

(*a*) Aneurism of the sinuses of Valsalva, a common and important variety, is met with most frequently in young syphilitic subjects. There may be pouching of one or of all three sinuses; the aortic ring is apt to be involved and one or more of the valves rendered incompetent. The special features may be thus summarized: (1) It is often latent, causing sudden death by perforation into the pericardium. (2) It is a medico-legal aneurism met with most frequently in coroner's cases. (3) Angina pectoris is not uncommon and may be the only symptom. (4) Aortic insufficiency is often associated with it. (5) In a majority of all cases syphilitic mesaortitis is present.

(*b*) Aneurism of the Ascending Arch.—Along the convex border aneurism frequently arises and may grow to a large size, either passing out into the right pleura or forward, pointing at the second or third interspace, eroding the ribs and sternum, and producing large external tumors. In this situation the sac may compress the superior vena cava, causing engorgement of the vessels of the head and arm; sometimes it compresses only the subclavian vein, and causes enlargement and œdema of the right arm. Perforation may take place into the superior vena cava, of which accident Pepper and Griffith have collected 29 cases. In rare instances, when the aneurism springs from the concave side of the vessels, the tumor may appear to the left of the sternum. Large aneurisms in this situation may cause much dislocation of the heart, pushing it down and to the left, and sometimes compressing the inferior vena cava, and causing swelling of the feet and ascites. The right recurrent laryngeal nerve is often compressed. The innominate artery is rarely involved. Death commonly follows from rupture into the pericardium, the pleura, or into the superior cava; less commonly from rupture externally, sometimes from syncope.

(*c*) Aneurism of the Transverse Arch.—The direction of growth is most commonly backward, but the sac may grow forward, erode the sternum, and form a large tumor. The sac presents in the middle line and to the right of the sternum much more often than to the left, which occurred in only 4 of 35 aneurisms in this situation (O. A. Browne). Even when small and producing no external tumor it may cause marked pressure signs in its growth backward toward the spine, involving the trachea and the œsophagus, and giving rise to cough, which is often of a paroxysmal character, and dysphagia. The left recurrent laryngeal is often involved in its course round the arch. A small aneurism from the lower or posterior wall of the arch may compress a bronchus, inducing bronchorrhœa, gradual bronchiectasis, and suppuration in the lung—a process which by no means infrequently causes death in aneurism, and a condition which at the Montreal General Hospital we were in the habit of terming aneurismal phthisis. Occasionally enormous aneurisms arise in this situation, and grow into both pleuræ, extending between the manubrium and the vertebræ; they may persist for years. The sac may be evident at the sternal notch. The innominate artery, less commonly the left carotid and subclavian, may be involved in the sac, and the radial or carotid pulse may be absent or retarded. Pressure on the sympathetic may at first cause dilatation and subsequently contraction of the pupil. Sometimes the thoracic duct is compressed.

The ascending and transverse portions of the arch are not infrequently involved together, usually without the branches; the tumor grows upward, or upward and to the right.

(*d*) Aneurism of the Descending Portion of the Arch.—It is not infrequently the traction aneurism of Thoma. The sac projects to the left and backward, and often erodes the vertebræ from the third to the sixth dorsal, causing great pain and sometimes compression of the spinal cord. Dysphagia is common. Pressure on a bronchus may induce bronchiectasis, with retention of secretions, and fever. A tumor may appear externally in the region of the scapula, and here attain an enormous size. Death not infrequently occurs from rupture into the pleura, or the sac may grow into the lung and cause hæmoptysis.

(*e*) Aneurism of the Descending Thoracic Aorta.—This is the least common situation of aortic aneurism. The larger number occur close to the diaphragm, the sac lying upon or to the left of the bodies of the lower dorsal vertebræ, which are often eroded. It is frequently latent, in 3 of 14 cases reported by me, and is often overlooked; pulmonary and pleural symptoms are common. Pain in the back is severe; dysphagia is not infrequent. The sac may reach an enormous size and form a subcutaneous tumor in the left back.

Physical Signs.—Inspection.—A good light is essential; cases are often overlooked owing to a hasty inspection. The face is often suffused, the conjunctivæ injected, and veins of the chest and of one arm engorged. One pupil may be enlarged. In many instances inspection is negative. On either side of the sternum there may be abnormal pulsation, due to dislocation of the heart, to deformity of the thorax, or to retraction of the lung. Three sorts of pulsation may be seen in the chest: (1) A general shock, such as is seen in the violent throbbing of the heart or of an aneurism. In anæmia, in neurasthenia, and in great hypertrophy this widespread shock may suggest aneurism. (2) A diffuse impulse localized in a certain part of the chest, which may be caused by a deep-seated aneurism but which is met with also in tumors, in pulsating pleurisy, and in a few cases without evident cause (see "Modern Medicine," Vol. IV, p. 474). (3) The punctate, heaving true aneurismal impulse which when of any extent is visibly expansile. It is seen most frequently above the level of the third rib to the right of the sternum, in the second left interspace, over the manubrium, and behind in the left interscapular region. When the innominate is involved the throbbing may be seen at the right sterno-clavicular joint and above it. An external tumor is present in many cases, projecting either through the upper part of the sternum or to the right, sometimes involving the sternum and costal cartilages on both sides, forming a swelling the size of a cocoanut or even larger. The skin is thin, often blood stained, or it may have ruptured, exposing the laminæ of the sac. The apex beat may be much dislocated, particularly when the sac is large. It is more commonly a dislocation from pressure than from enlargement of the heart itself.

Palpation.—The area and degree of pulsation are best determined by palpation. When the aneurism is deep seated and not apparent externally, the bimanual method should be used, one hand upon the spine and the other on the sternum. There may be only a diffuse impulse. When the sac has perforated the chest wall the impulse is, as a rule, forcible, slow, heaving, and expansile, and has the same qualities as a forcible apex beat. The resistance may be very great if there are thick laminæ beneath the skin; more rarely the sac is soft and fluctuating. The hand upon the sac, or on the region in which it is in contact with the chest wall, may feel a diastolic shock, often of great intensity, which forms one of the valuable physical signs of aneurism. A systolic thrill is sometimes present, not so often in saccular aneurisms as in the dilatation of the arch. The pulsation may sometimes be felt in the suprasternal notch.

Percussion.—The small and deep seated aneurisms are in this respect negative. In the larger tumors, as soon as the sac reaches the chest wall, there is produced an area of abnormal dulness, the position of which depends upon the part of the aorta affected. Aneurisms of the ascending arch grow forward and to the right, producing dulness on one side of the manubrium; those from the transverse arch produce dulness in the middle line, extending toward the left of the sternum, while aneurisms of the descending portion most commonly produce dulness in the left interscapular and scapular regions. The percussion note is flat and gives a feeling of increased resistance.

Auscultation.—Adventitious sounds are not always to be heard. Even in a large sac there may be no murmur. Much depends upon the thickness of the laminæ of fibrin. An important sign, particularly if heard over a dull region, is a ringing, accentuated second sound, a phenomenon rarely missed in large aneurisms of the aortic arch. A systolic murmur may be present; sometimes a double murmur, in which case the diastolic *bruit* is usually due to associated aortic insufficiency. The systolic murmur alone is of little moment in the diagnosis of an aneurismal sac. A continuous humming top murmur with systolic intensification is heard when the aneurism communicates with the vena cava or the pulmonary artery. With the single stethoscope the shock of the impulse with the first sound is sometimes very marked.

Among other physical signs of importance are retardation of the pulse in the arteries beyond the aneurism, or in those involved in the sac. There may, for instance, be a marked difference between the right and left radial, both in volume and time. The blood pressure on the two sides may be unequal. A physical sign of large thoracic aneurism, which I have not seen referred to, is obliteration of the pulse in the abdominal aorta and its branches. My attention was called to this in a patient who was stated to have aortic insufficiency. There was a well-marked diastolic murmur, but in the femorals and in the aorta I was surprised to find no trace of pulsation, and not the slightest throbbing in the abdominal aorta or in the peripheral arteries of the leg. The circulation was, however, unimpaired in them and there was no dilatation of the veins. Attracted by this, I then made a careful examination of the patient's back, when the circumstance was discovered, which neither the patient himself nor any of his physicians had noticed, that he had a very large area of pulsation in the left scapular region. The sac probably was large enough to act as a reservoir annihilating the ventricular systole, and converting the intermittent into a continuous stream.

A remarkable condition suggestive of pneumothorax may be caused by compression of one bronchus by the sac (Newton Pitt). The air is inspired beyond the obstruction, but has difficulty in getting out, so that the lung is gradually distended, causing enlargement of the side with a hyperresonant note on percussion, and on auscultation absence of breath sounds. The X-ray picture may alone decide the diagnosis.

The *tracheal tugging,* a valuable sign in deep-seated aneurisms, was described by Surgeon-Major Oliver, and was specially studied by my colleagues Ross and MacDonnell at the Montreal General Hospital. Oliver gives the following directions: "Place the patient in the erect position, and direct him to close his mouth and elevate his chin to almost the full extent; then grasp the cricoid cartilage between the finger and thumb, and use steady and gentle upward pressure on it, when, if dilatation or aneurism exists, the pulsation of the aorta will be distinctly felt transmitted through the trachea to the hand." The tug is sometimes felt more easily if the chin is held down. This is a sign of great value in the diagnosis of deep-seated aneurisms, though it may occasionally be felt in tumors and in the extreme dynamic dilatation of aortic insufficiency. It may be visible in the thyroid cartilage. The trachea may be pushed to one side.

Occasionally a systolic murmur may be heard in the trachea, as pointed out by David Drummond, or even at the patient's mouth, when opened. This is either the sound conveyed from the sac, or is produced by the air as it is driven out of the wind pipe during the systole. Feeble respiration in one lung is a common effect of pressure.

Symptoms.—Broadbent made the useful division of aneurisms of symptoms and aneurisms of physical signs; the former is more commonly seen when the transverse arch is involved, the latter when the ascending portion. There may be no symptoms. A man may present a tumor which has eroded the chest wall without pain or any discomfort. On the other hand, every physical sign may be present without a single symptom.

An important but variable feature in thoracic aneurism is *pain,* which is particularly marked in deep seated tumors. It is usually paroxysmal, sharp, and lancinating, often very severe when the tumor is eroding the vertebræ, or perforating the chest wall. In the latter case after perforation the pain may cease. Anginal attacks are not uncommon, particularly in aneurisms at the root of the aorta. Frequently the pain radiates down the left arm or up the neck, sometimes along the upper intercostal nerves. Superficial tenderness may be felt in the skin over the heart or over the left sternomastoid muscle. *Cough* results either from the direct pressure on the trachea, or is associated with bronchitis. The expectoration in these instances is abundant, thin, and watery; subsequently it becomes thick and turbid. Paroxysmal cough of a peculiar brazen, ringing character is a characteristic symptom in some cases, particularly when there is pressure on the recurrent laryngeal nerves, or the cough may have a peculiar wheezy quality—the "goose cough."

Dyspnœa, which is common in cases of aneurism of the transverse portion, is not necessarily associated with pressure on the recurrent laryngeal nerves, but may be due directly to compression of the trachea or the left bronchus. It may occur with marked stridor. Loss of voice and hoarseness are consequences of pressure on the recurrent laryngeal, usually the left, inducing either a spasm in the muscles of the left vocal cord or paralysis.

Paralysis of an abductor on one side may be present without any symptoms. It is more particularly, as Semon states, when the paralytic contractures supervene that the attention is called to laryngeal symptoms.

Hæmorrhage in thoracic aneurism may come from (*a*) the soft granulations in the trachea at the point of compression, in which case the sputum is blood tinged, but large quantities of blood are not lost; (*b*) from rupture of the sac into the trachea or a bronchus; (*c*) from perforation into the lung or erosion of the lung tissue. The bleeding may be profuse, rapidly proving fatal, and is a common cause of death. It may persist for weeks or months, in which case it is simply hæmorrhagic weeping through the sac, which is exposed in the trachea. In some instances, even after a very profuse hæmorrhage, the patient recovers and may live for years. A man with well-marked thoracic aneurism, whom I showed to my class at the University of Pennsylvania and who had had several brisk hæmorrhages, died four years after, having in the meantime enjoyed average health. Death from hæmorrhage is relatively more common in aneurism of the third portion of the arch and of the descending aorta.

Difficulty of swallowing is a comparatively rare symptom, and may be due either to spasm or to direct compression. The sound should never be passed in these cases, as the œsophagus may be almost eroded and perforation of the sac has taken place.

Heart Symptoms.—Pain has been referred to; it is often anginal in character, and is most common when the root of the aorta is involved. The heart is hypertrophied in less than one half the cases. The aortic valves are sometimes incompetent, either from disease of the segments or from stretching of the aortic ring.

Among other signs and symptoms, venous compression, which has already been mentioned, may involve one subclavian or the superior vena cava. A curious phenomenon in intrathoracic aneurism is the clubbing of the fingers and incurving of the nails of one hand, of which two examples have been under my care, both without any special distention or signs of venous engorgement. Tumors of the arch may involve the pulmonary artery, producing compression, or in some instances adhesion of the pulmonary segments and insufficiency of the valve; or the sac may rupture into the artery, an accident which happened in two of my cases, producing instantaneous death.

Pupil Symptoms.—These may be due to, first, pressure on the sympathetic, which may cause dilatation of one pupil when the cord is irritated, contraction when the nerve is paralyzed. Flushing of the side of the face and ear, increased temperature, and sweating may be present. Secondly, as Ainley Walker and Wall have shown, the anisocoria is most frequently due to vascular conditions—with low blood pressure in one carotid the pupil on that side is dilated, with high pressure contracted, and in 26 cases of aneurism they found a relation between the state of the pupil and the arteries on the same side. Thirdly, in a few cases the anisocoria is a parasyphilitic manifestation associated with the Argyll-Robertson phenomenon and absent knee-jerks—the Babinski syndrome.

An X-ray examination should be made in all doubtful cases. The fluoroscope gives an accurate picture of the situation, the size, and the relation to the heart. Even a small sac may be seen. In several cases I have known the diagnosis to rest upon it alone in cases in which scarcely a physical sign was present. Sailer and Pfahler have shown that a condition of tortuosity of the aorta, due to arterio-sclerosis, may exist, suggesting very strongly the presence of aneurism, particularly on examination with the fluoroscope.

The clinical picture of aneurism of the aorta is extremely varied. Many cases present characteristic symptoms and no physical signs, while others have well-marked physical signs and no symptoms.

Diagnosis.—Aneurism of the aorta may be confounded with: (*a*) The violent throbbing impulse of the arch in aortic insufficiency. I have already referred to a case of this kind in which the diagnosis of aneurism was made by several good observers.

(*b*) *Simple Dynamic Pulsation.*—This is common in the abdominal aorta, but is rare in the arch. A case which came under the care of William Murray and Bramwell presented, without any pain or pressure symptoms, pulsation and dulness over the aorta. The condition gradually disappeared and was thought to be neurotic.

(*c*) Dislocation of the heart in curvature of the spine may cause great displacement of the aorta, so that it has been known to pulsate forcibly to the right of the sternum.

(*d*) *Solid Tumors.*—When the tumor projects externally and pulsates the difficulty may be considerable. In tumor the heaving, *expansile* pulsation is absent, and there is not that sense of force and power which is so striking in the throbbing of a perforating aneurism. There is not to be felt, as in aortic aneurism, the shock of the heart sounds, particularly the diastolic shock. Auscultatory sounds are less definite, as large aneurisms may occur without murmurs; and, on the other hand, murmurs may be heard over tumors. The greatest difficulty is in the deep seated thoracic tumors, and here the diagnosis may be impossible. The physical signs may be indefinite. The ringing aortic second sound is of great importance and is rarely, if ever, heard over tumor. Tracheal tugging is here a valuable sign. Pressure phenomena are less common in tumor, whereas pain is more frequent. The general appearance of the patient in aneurism is much better than in tumor, in which there may be cachexia and enlargement of the glands in the axilla or in the neck. Healthy, strong males who have worked hard and have had syphilis are the most common subjects of aneurism. Occasionally cancer of the œsophagus may simulate aneurism, producing pressure on the left bronchus.

(*e*) *Pulsating Pleurisy.*—In cases of *empyema necessitatis,* if the projecting tumor is in the neighborhood of the heart and pulsates, the condition may readily be mistaken for aneurism. The absence of the heaving, firm distention and of the diastolic shock would, together with the history and the existence of pleural effusion, determine the nature of the case. If necessary, puncture may be made with a fine hypodermic needle. In a majority of the cases of pulsating pleurisy the throbbing is diffuse and widespread, moving the whole side.

Prognosis.—The outlook in thoracic aneurism is always grave. Life may be prolonged for some years, but the patients are in constant jeopardy. Spontaneous cure is not very infrequent in the small sacculated tumors of the ascending and thoracic portions. The cavity becomes filled with laminæ of firm fibrin, which become more and more dense and hard, the sac shrinks considerably, and finally lime salts are deposited in the old fibrin. The laminæ of fibrin may be on a level with the lumen of the vessel, causing complete obliteration of the sac. The cases which rupture externally, as a rule, run a rapid course, although to this there are exceptions; the sac may contract, become firm and hard, and the patient may live for five, or even for ten or twenty years. The cases which have lasted longest in my experience have been those in which a saccular aneurism has projected from the ascending arch. One patient in Montreal had been known to have aneurism for eleven years. The aneurism may be enormous, occupying a large area of the chest, and yet life be prolonged for many years. One of the most remarkable instances is the case of dissecting aneurism reported by Graham. The patient was invalided after the Crimean War with aneurism of the aorta, and for years was under the observation of J. H. Richardson, of Toronto, under whose care he died in 1885. The autopsy showed a healed aneurism of the arch, with a dissecting aneurism extending the whole length of the aorta, which formed a double tube.

Treatment.—In a large proportion of the cases this can only be PALLIATIVE. Still in every instance measures should be taken which are known to promote clotting and consolidation within the sac. In any large series of cured aneurisms a considerable majority of the patients have not been known to be subjects of the disease, but the obliterated sac has been found accidentally at the post mortem.

The most satisfactory plan in early cases, when it can be carried out thoroughly, is the modified Valsalva method advised by the late Mr. Tufnell, of Dublin, the essentials of which are rest and a restricted diet. The rest should, as far as possible, be absolute. The reduction of the daily number of heart beats, when a patient is recumbent and without exertion, amounts to many thousands, and is one of the principal advantages of this plan. Mental quiet should also be enjoined. The diet advised by Tufnell is extremely rigid—for breakfast, 2 ounces of bread and butter and 2 ounces of milk or tea; dinner, 3 ounces of mutton and 3 of potatoes or bread and 4 ounces of claret; supper, 2 ounces of bread and butter and 2 ounces of tea. This low diet diminishes the blood volume and is thought also to render the blood more fibrinous. "Total per diem, 10 ounces of solid food and 8 ounces of fluid, and *no more.*" This treatment should be pursued for several months, but, except in persons of a good deal of mental stamina, it is impossible to carry it out for more than a few weeks at a time. It is a form of treatment adapted only to the saccular form of aneurism, and in cases of large sacs communicating with the aorta by a comparatively small orifice the chances of consolidation are fairly good. Unquestionably rest and the restriction of the liquids are the important parts of the treatment, and a greater variety and quantity of food may be allowed with advantage. If this plan can not be thoroughly carried out, the patient should at any rate be advised to live a very quiet life, moving about with deliberation and avoiding all sudden mental or bodily excitement. The bowels should be kept regular, and constipation and straining should be carefully avoided. Of medicines, iodide of potassium, as advised by Balfour, is of great value. It may be given in doses of from 10 to 20 grains (0.6 to 1.3 gm.) three times a day. Larger doses are not necessary. The mode of action is not well understood. It may act by increasing the secretions and so inspissating the blood, by lowering the blood pressure, or, as Balfour thinks, by causing thickening and contraction of the sac. The most striking effect of the iodide in my experience has been the relief of the pain. The evidence is conclusive that the syphilitic cases are more benefited by it than the non-syphilitic. All these measures have little value unless the sac is of a suitable form and size. The large tumors with wide mouths communicating with the ascending portion of the aorta may be treated on the most approved plans for months without the slightest influence other than reduction in the intensity of the throbbing. A patient with a tumor projecting into the right pleura remained on the most rigid Tufnell treatment for more than one hundred days, during which time he also took iodide of potassium faithfully. The pulsations were greatly reduced and the area of dulness diminished, and we congratulated ourselves that the sac was probably consolidating. Sudden death followed rupture into the pleura, and the sac contained only fluid blood, not a shred of fibrin. In cases in which the tumor is large, or in which there seems to be very little prospect of consolidation, it is perhaps better to advise a man to go on quietly with his occupation, avoiding excitement and worry. Our profession has offered many examples of good work, thoroughly and conscientiously carried out, by men with aneurism of the aorta, who wisely, I think, preferred, as did the late Hilton Fagge, to die in harness.

Surgical Measures.—In a few cases consolidation may be promoted in the sac by the introduction of a foreign body, such as wire, horse-hair, or by the combination of wiring and electrolysis. Moore, in 1864, first wired a sac, putting in 78 feet of fine wire. Death occurred on the fifth day. Corradi proposed the combined method of wiring with electrolysis, which was first used by Burresi in 1879. His patient lived for three and a half months. Horse-hair, watch-spring wire, catgut, and Florence silk have been used. Hunner reports the statistical results of both methods up to October, 1900. With Moore's method (wiring) 14 cases were treated, 8 of thoracic aneurism, all fatal; 6 aneurisms of the abdominal aorta, 3 of which were successful. Of 23 cases treated by wiring and electrolysis (Moore-Corradi method) 17 were thoracic and 6 abdominal. The thoracic cases of Rosenstirn, Stewart, and Kerr, and the abdominal cases of Noble and Finney (Case V), were successful. In 3 of the 23 cases there were amelioration of symptoms and probable prolongation of life. The most favorable cases are those in which the aneurism is sacculated, but this is a point not easily determined, and often from a sac particularly favorable for wiring there may be secondary projections of great thinness. The sudden filling by clot of an aneurism of the cœliac axis of the superior mesenteric artery may result fatally from infarct of the intestine.

Other Conditions Requiring Treatment.—Pressure on veins causing engorgement, particularly of the head and arms, is sometimes promptly relieved by free venesection, and, at any time during the course of a thoracic aneurism, if attacks of dyspnœa with lividity supervene, bleeding may be resorted to with great benefit. It has the advantage also of promptly checking the pain, for which symptom, as already mentioned, the iodide of potassium often gives relief. In the final stages morphia is, as a rule, necessary. Dyspnœa, if associated with cyanosis, is best relieved by bleeding. Chloroform inhalations may be necessary. The question sometimes comes up with reference to tracheotomy in these cases of urgent dyspnœa. If it can be shown by laryngoscopic examination that it is due to bilateral abductor paralysis the trachea may be opened, but this is extremely rare, and in nearly every instance the urgent dyspnœa is caused by pressure about the bifurcation. When the sac appears externally and grows large, an ice bag or a belladonna plaster may be applied to allay the pain. In some instances an elastic support may be used with advantage, and I saw a physician with an enormous external aneurism in the right mammary region who for many months had obtained great relief by an elastic support, passing over the shoulder and under the arm of the opposite side.

The calcium salts may be given to influence coagulation, and the nitrites if the blood pressure is high, but rest and diet, restriction of the fluids, and free purgation are usually more effectual than drugs in reducing blood pressure.

ANEURISM OF THE ABDOMINAL AORTA

Of 233 cases collected by Nixon, 207 were in males, 26 in females; 121 were between the ages of twenty-five and forty-five. Nixon reports a case in a syphilitic girl of twenty. Sixteen cases occurred among 16,000 admissions at the Johns Hopkins Hospital.

Pathology.—The sac is most common just below the diaphragm in the neighborhood of the cœliac axis. The tumor may be fusiform or sacculated, and it is sometimes multiple. Projecting backward, it erodes the vertebræ and may cause numbness and tingling in the legs and finally paraplegia, or it may pass into the thorax and burst into the pleura. More commonly the sac is on the anterior wall and projects forward as a definite tumor, which may be either in the middle line or a little to the left. The tumor may project in the epigastric region (which is most common), in the left hypochondrium, in the left flank, or in the lumbar region. When high up beneath the pillar of the diaphragm it may attain considerable size without being very apparent on palpation. When it ruptures into the retro-peritoneal tissues a tumor in the flank may be formed gradually, which enlarges with very little pulsation. It may be mistaken for a rapidly growing sarcoma or for appendicitis, and an operation may be performed.

The **symptoms** are chiefly pain, very often of a neuralgic nature, passing round to the sides or localized in the back, and more persistent and intense than in any other variety of aneurism. Gastric symptoms, particularly vomiting, may be early and deceptive features. Retardation of the pulse in the femoral artery is a very common symptom.

Diagnosis and Physical Signs.—Inspection may show marked pulsation in the epigastric region, sometimes a definite tumor. A thrill is not uncommon. The pulsation is forcible, expansile, and sometimes double when the sac is large and in contact with the pericardium. On palpation a *definite tumor can be felt.* If large, there is some degree of dulness on percussion, which usually merges with that of the left lobe of the liver. On auscultation, a systolic murmur is, as a rule, audible, and is sometimes best heard at the back. A diastolic murmur is occasionally present, usually very soft in quality. One of the commonest of clinical errors is to mistake a throbbing aorta for an aneurism. It is to be remembered that no pulsation, however forcible, or the presence of a thrill or a systolic murmur, justifies the diagnosis of abdominal aneurism unless there is a *definite tumor which can be grasped and which has an expansile pulsation.* Attention to this rule will save many errors. The throbbing aorta—the "preternatural pulsation in the epigastrium," as Allan Burns calls it—is met with in all neurasthenic conditions, particularly in women. In anæmia, particularly in some instances of traumatic anæmia, the throbbing may be very great. Very frequently a tumor of the pylorus, of the pancreas, or of the left lobe of the liver is lifted with each impulse of the aorta and may be confounded with aneurism. The absence of the forcible expansile impulse and the examination in the knee elbow position, in which the tumor, as a rule, falls forward, and the pulsation is not then communicated, suffice for differentiation. The tumor of abdominal aneurism, though usually fixed, may be very freely movable.

Prognosis.—The outlook in abdominal aneurism is bad. A few cases heal spontaneously. Death may result from (*a*) complete obliteration of the lumen by clots; (*b*) compression paraplegia; (*c*) rupture (which occurred in 152 of the 233 cases in Nixon's series) either into the pleura, retroperitoneal tissues, peritoneum, or the intestines, most commonly into the duodenum; (*d*) embolism of the superior mesenteric artery, producing infarction of the intestines.

The **treatment** is such as already advised in thoracic aneurism. When the aneurism is low down pressure has been successfully applied in a case by Murray, of Newcastle. It must be kept up for many hours under chloroform. The plan is not without risk, as patients have died from bruising and injury of the sac. Nine cases in my series were treated surgically. In two the wiring and electrolysis were followed by great improvement; one man lived for three years.

ANEURISM OF THE BRANCHES OF THE ABDOMINAL AORTA

The **cœliac axis** is itself not infrequently involved in aneurism of the first portion of the abdominal aorta. Of its branches, the **splenic artery** is occasionally the seat of aneurism. This rarely causes a tumor large enough to be felt; sometimes, however, the tumor is of large size. I have reported a case in a man, aged thirty, who had an illness of several months' duration, severe epigastric pain and vomiting, which led his physicians in New York to diagnose gastric ulcer. There was a deep seated tumor in the left hypochondriac region, the dulness of which merged with that of the spleen. There was no pulsation, but it was thought on one occasion that a *bruit* was heard. The chief symptoms while under observation were vomiting, severe epigastric pain, occasional hæmatemesis, and finally severe hæmorrhage from the bowels. An aneurism of the splenic artery the size of a cocoanut was situated between the stomach above and the transverse colon below, and extended to the right as far as the level of the navel. The sac contained densely laminated fibrin. It had perforated the colon. I have twice seen small aneurisms on the splenic artery. Of 39 instances of aneurism on the branches of the abdominal aorta collected by Lebert, 10 were of the splenic artery.

Of aneurism of the **hepatic artery** Rolland has collected 40 cases (1908), of which 24 were extra-hepatic. In Rolland's case there were three sacs—all intra-hepatic. Rupture took place in 32 cases—in 16 into the peritoneal cavity, in 13 into the bile passages. The sac is rarely large, but in the case of Wollmann's it was as large as a child's head. No case has been diagnosed. Cholelithiasis and duodenal ulcer are the conditions for which it is most likely to be mistaken. In Ross and Osler's case the liver was enlarged, with symptoms of pyæmia.

Aneurism of the **superior mesenteric artery** is not very uncommon. The diagnosis is scarcely possible from aneurism of the arch. Plugging of the branches or of the main stem may cause infarction of the bowel.

Renal Artery.—Henry Morris has collected 21 instances of aneurism, 12 of which arose from injury. Many of them were false. Pulsation and a *bruit* are not always present. Four cases were operated upon; three recovered. In a case of Keen's the tumor and the kidney were removed together.

Pulmonary Artery.—Primary aneurism of the trunk is very rare. Of the branches there are two varieties: (*a*) The acute embolic, which may be multiple, arising in connection with thrombi in the veins or a septic endocarditis in the right heart. (*b*) The small aneurisms in the walls of pulmonary cavities, already considered.

ARTERIO-VENOUS ANEURISM

In this form, known to Galen, but first accurately described by the great William Hunter, there is abnormal communication between an artery and a vein. When a tumor lies between the two it is known as *varicose aneurism;* when there is a direct communication without tumor the vein is chiefly distended and the condition is known as *aneurismal varix.*

While it may occur in the aorta, it is much more common in the peripheral arteries as a result of stab or gunshot wounds.

An aneurism of the ascending portion of the arch may open directly into the vena cava. Twenty-nine cases of this lesion have been analyzed by Pepper and Griffith. Cyanosis, œdema, and great distention of the veins of the upper part of the body are the most frequent symptoms, and develop, as a rule, with suddenness. Of the physical signs a thrill is present in some cases. A continuous murmur with systolic intensification is of great diagnostic value. Thurnam (Medico-Chirurgical Transactions, 1840) gave the first accurate account of this murmur and of this characteristic type of cyanosis. There is only one condition with which it could be confounded, viz., the remarkable cyanosis of the upper part of the body which follows crushing accidents to the thorax. Perforation between the aorta and pulmonary artery causes very much the same symptoms. In a few cases an aneurism of the abdominal aorta perforates the inferior vena cava—œdema and cyanosis of the legs and lower half of the body, and the distinctive thrill and murmur are present.

In the arterio-venous aneurisms which follow stab and bullet wounds of the subclavian, axillary, carotid, femoral, and popliteal arteries the clinical features are most characteristic. First, the veins enlarge as the arterial blood flows under high pressure into them. The affected limb may be greatly swollen and in a young person may lengthen, and the growth of hair is increased. Secondly, a strong thrill is felt, of maximum intensity at the site of the aneurism, but sometimes to be felt at the most distant parts of a limb. Thirdly, the characteristic continuous murmur with systolic intensification is heard. In the external arteries the condition may persist for years before disability is caused by enlargement of the veins and swelling of the limb.

POLYARTERITIS ACUTA NODOSA

(*Periarteritis Nodosa*)

A series of cases has been described in which small aneurisms occur on the arteries of the muscles and viscera. The first case was reported by Kussmaul and Maier, and about 19 cases in all have been described (Dickson). A case, agreeing clinically with the others, has occurred in my wards. No autopsy was permitted, but the nodules were felt in the abdominal wall before death. The case is reported by Sabin (J. H. H. Bulletin, 1901). There are marked thickening of the intima and infiltration of the other coats, with a nuclear growth almost sarcomatous. There are two theories: one, that the nodules are aneurisms due to syphilis or to congenital weakening of the arteries; the other, that they are aneurisms secondary to an inflammatory process like the infectious granulomata.

The cases have occurred chiefly in men between the ages of twenty seven and fifty two; the course is from eight to twelve weeks. The patients complain of weakness. The symptoms correspond with the situation of the lesions; thus their presence in the muscles is associated with pain, weakness, and sometimes paralysis and atrophy. The nodules are abundant in the alimentary tract. The severest symptom is epigastric pain; there is loss of appetite, thirst, vomiting, constipation, or diarrhœa. The disease is febrile at first, but the temperature sinks to subnormal, while the pulse remains rapid. When the cerebral vessels are involved there are headache, excitement, convulsions, and optic neuritis, and the diagnosis of meningitis is made. The anæmia is extreme. In our case the hæmoglobin was 21 per cent., the red blood-cells 1,704,000. The leucocytes reached 116,000, of which 91 per cent. were polymorphonuclear forms. The urine is scanty, of low specific gravity, with albumin and casts. Urea is excreted in small quantities, but the mind is clear.

SECTION X

DISEASES OF THE DUCTLESS GLANDS

I. DISEASES OF THE SUPRARENAL BODIES

1. ADDISON'S DISEASE

Definition.—A disease characterized by muscular and vascular asthenia, irritation of the stomach, and pigmentation of the skin; due either to tuberculosis or atrophy of the adrenals, or to degenerative changes in the chromaffin system generally.

The recognition of the disease is due to Addison of Guy's Hospital, whose monograph on "The Constitutional and Local Effects of Disease of the Suprarenal Capsules" was published in 1855.

Etiology.—The disease is rare. Only 17 cases came under my observation in the United States. In large clinics a year or more may pass without a case. Males are more frequently attacked than females. In Greenhow's analysis of 183 cases, 119 were males and 64 females. The majority of cases occur between the twentieth and fortieth years. A congenital case has been described, in which the child lived for eight weeks, and post mortem the adrenals were found to be large and cystic. In a few cases a blow on the abdomen or back has preceded the onset. A certain number of cases have been associated with Pott's disease.

Pathology.—To understand the remarkable character of Addison's disease it is necessary to have an idea of the structure and function of the suprarenal bodies. The cortex of the gland is an epithelial structure, the medulla consists of an irregular meshwork of consecutive tissue, including large multinucleated cells, non-medullated nerve fibres and nerve cells, and in addition large polymorphous cells, which in chromic acid solution take on a brownish pigmentation, and are spoken of as chromaffin cells. Extra-adrenal chromaffin cells are found in the ganglia of the abdominal sympathetic system and in certain structures situated along the course of the aorta and are known as paraganglia or Zuckerkandl's bodies. These chromaffin cells have also been found in the carotid glands and, according to some authors, in the coccygeal gland, the parovarium and the epidydimis. Collectively these structures are spoken of as the "chromaffin system."

Removal of the suprarenal causes death in animals by progressive weakness and toxæmia.

The specific function of the medullary portion of the gland and of the chromaffin system is to furnish an internal secretion known as epinephrin, which controls blood pressure, acting on peripheral neuro-muscular elements in the arterioles, promotes the activity of the skeletal muscles, and in some way controls the metabolism of the pigment of the skin. The remarkable discovery of Schäfer and Oliver of the blood pressure raising property of these glands is almost the only positive fact we know in connection with their functions.

Glycosuria is also caused by the injection of epinephrin, and in animals a form of arterio-sclerosis, probably due to the high blood pressure. Following this discovery many theoretical conceptions have been entertained of the relation between a defect of the adrenal secretion and asthenic affections, and it is suggested that adrenal insufficiency itself plays an important rôle in acute infections, in tuberculosis, and many wasting diseases, with which it is interesting to note that increased pigmentation may be associated.

Epinephrin has been shown to be present in the chromaffin bodies, so that we may take it that the chromaffin system has everywhere the special function of providing a material which keeps up the vascular tone.

In some way, too, it controls the pigment metabolism. Abolition of the function of the suprarenals, or marked irritation in the chromaffin tissues in the abdomen, as in tuberculous peritonitis or in aneurism, is associated with a great increase in the pigmentation of the skin.

We have no positive knowledge as to the function of the cortex of the glands. Apparently it has some influence upon sexual activity and pregnancy. This portion of the capsules becomes twice its normal thickness in pregnant rabbits. Hyperplasia of the cortex or tumor formations may be associated with precocious sexual development, and hypoplasia of this part with infantilism. It is also suggested that the cortex produces bodies which neutralize the poisonous products of nitrogenous metabolism and in this way prevent auto-intoxication.

Morbid Anatomy.—There is rarely emaciation or anæmia. Rolleston thus summarizes the condition of the suprarenal bodies in Addison's disease:

"1. The fibro-caseous lesion due to tuberculosis—far the commonest condition found. 2. Simple atrophy. 3. Chronic interstitial inflammation leading to atrophy. 4. Malignant disease invading the capsules, including Addison's case of malignant nodule compressing the suprarenal vein. 5. Blood extravasated into the suprarenal bodies. 6. No lesion of the suprarenal bodies themselves, but pressure or inflammation involving the semilunar ganglia.

"The first is the only common cause of Addison's disease. The others, with the exception of simple atrophy, may be considered as very rare."

The nerve-cells of the semilunar ganglia have been found degenerated and deeply pigmented, and the nerves sclerotic. The ganglia are not uncommonly entangled in the cicatricial tissue about the adrenals. The chromaffin cells in the sympathetic ganglia and in the abdominal plexuses generally disappear. The cases of extensive destruction of the glands without Addison's disease are explained by a persistence of the chromaffin structures elsewhere, while extensive involvement of the extra-capsular chromaffin system may itself be sufficient to cause the symptoms, the adrenals themselves being intact.

Few changes of importance are found in other organs. The spleen is occasionally enlarged; the thymus may be persistent. The other organs show only the alterations associated with a protracted illness.

Symptoms.—In the words of Addison, the characteristic symptoms are "anæmia, general languor or debility, remarkable feebleness of the heart's action, irritability of the stomach, and a peculiar change of color in the skin."

The onset is, as a rule, insidious. The feelings of weakness, as a rule, precede the pigmentation. In other instances the gastro-intestinal symptoms, the weakness, and the pigmentation come on together. There are a few cases in the literature in which the whole process has been acute, following a shock or some special depression. There are three important symptoms:

(*a*) Pigmentation of the Skin.—This, as a rule, first attracts the attention of the patient's friends. The grade of coloration ranges from a light yellow to a deep brown, or even black. In typical cases it is diffuse, but always deeper on the exposed parts and in the regions where the normal pigmentation is more intense, as the areolæ of the nipples and about the genitals; also wherever the skin is compressed or irritated, as by the waistband. At first it may be confined to the face and hands. Occasionally it is absent. Patches showing atrophy of pigment, leucoderma, may occur. The pigmentation is found on the mucous membranes of the mouth, conjunctivæ, and vagina. Pigmentation of the mucous membrane is not distinctive. It has been found in chronic stomach troubles, etc. (Fr. Schultze), and is common in the negro. A patchy pigmentation of the serous membranes has often been found. Over the diffusely pigmented skin there may be little mole like spots of deeper pigmentation, and upon the trunk, particularly on the lower abdomen, it may be "ribbed" like the sand on the seashore.

(*b*) Gastro-intestinal Symptoms.—The disease may set in with attacks of nausea and vomiting, spontaneous in character. Toward the close there may be pain with retraction of the abdomen, and even features suggestive of peritonitis. A marked anorexia may be present. The gastric symptoms are variable throughout the course; occasionally they are absent. Attacks of diarrhœa are frequent and come on without obvious cause.

(*c*) Asthenia, the most characteristic feature of the disease, may be manifested early as a feeling of inability to carry on the ordinary occupation, or the patient may complain constantly of feeling tired. The weakness is specially marked in the muscular and cardio-vascular systems. There may be an extreme degree of muscular prostration in an individual apparently well nourished, whose muscles feel firm and hard. The cardio-vascular asthenia is manifest in a feeble, irregular action of the heart, which may come on in paroxysms, in attacks of vertigo, or of syncope, in one of which the disease may prove fatal. The blood pressure is low, falling to 70 or 80 mm. of Hg. Headache is a frequent symptom; convulsions occasionally occur. Pain in the back may be an early and important symptom.

Anæmia, a symptom specially referred to by Addison, is not common. In a majority of the patients the blood count is normal. McMunn has described an increase in the urinary pigments, and a pigment has been isolated of very much the same character as the melanin of the skin.

The mode of termination is either by syncope, which may occur even early in the disease, by gradual progressive asthenia, or by the development of tuberculous lesions. In two cases I have known a noisy delirium with urgent dyspnœa to precede the fatal event.

Diagnosis.—Pigmentation of the skin is not confined to Addison's disease. The following conditions may give rise to an increase in the pigment; some of which, *e. g.*, *a* and *b*, are due, as in Addison's disease, to disturbance in the chromaffin system.

(*a*) Abdominal growths—tubercle, cancer, or lymphoma. In tuberculosis of the peritoneum pigmentation is not uncommon.

(*b*) Pregnancy, in which the discoloration is usually limited to the face, the so-called *masque des femmes enceintes.* Uterine disease is a common cause of a patchy melasma.

(*c*) *Hæmochromatosis,* associated with hypertrophic cirrhosis, pigmentation of the skin, and diabetes.

(*d*) In overworked persons of constipated habit and with sluggish livers there may be a patchy staining of the face and forehead.

(*e*) The vagabond's discoloration, caused by the irritation of lice and dirt, which may reach a very high grade, and has sometimes been mistaken for Addison's disease.

(*f*) In rare instances there is deep discoloration of the skin in melanotic cancer, so deep and general that it has been confounded with *melasma suprarenale.*

(*g*) In certain cases of exophthalmic goitre abnormal pigmentation occurs.

(*h*) In a few rare instances the pigmentation in scleroderma may be general and deep.

(*i*) In the face there may be an extraordinary degree of pigmentation due to innumerable small black comedones. If not seen in a very good light, the face may suggest argyria. Pigmentation of an advanced grade may occur in chronic ulcer of the stomach and in dilatation of the organ.

(*j*) Argyria could scarcely be mistaken, and yet I was consulted in a case in which the diagnosis of Addison's disease had been made by several good observers.

(*k*) Arsenic when taken for many months may cause a most intense pigmentation of the skin.

(*l*) With arterio-sclerosis and chronic heart-disease there may be marked melanoderma.

(*m*) In pernicious anæmia the pigmentation may be extreme, most commonly due to the prolonged administration of arsenic.

(*n*) There is a form of deep pigmentation, usually in women, which persists for years without change and without any special impairment of health. I have met with two cases; in one the pigmentation was a little more leaden than is usual in Addison's disease; in both the condition had lasted some years.

(*o*) In ochronosis there may be a deep melanotic pigmentation of the face and hands.

In any case of unusual pigmentation these various conditions must be sought for; the diagnosis of Addison's disease is scarcely justifiable without the asthenia. In many instances it is difficult early in the disease to arrive at a definite conclusion. The occurrence of fainting fits, of nausea, and gastric irritability are important indications. As the lesion of the capsules is almost always tuberculous, in doubtful cases the tuberculin test may be used. In two of my cases, robust, healthy men with pigmentation and gastric symptoms, the reaction was obtained.

Prognosis.—The disease is usually fatal. The cases in which the bronzing is slight or does not occur run a more rapid course. There are occasionally acute cases which, with great weakness, vomiting, and diarrhœa, prove fatal in a few weeks. In a few cases the disease is much prolonged, even to six or ten years. In rare instances recovery has taken place, and periods of improvement, lasting many months, may occur.

Treatment.—When asthenia appears the patient should be confined to bed and sudden efforts and muscular exercise should not be allowed. Fatal syncope may at any time occur. In three of my cases death was sudden. For the debility arsenic and strychnia are useful; for the diarrhœa large doses of bismuth, and for the irritability of the stomach creosote, hydrocyanic acid, ice, and champagne. The diet should be light and nutritious. As the disease is nearly always tuberculous an open air treatment may be carried out. Tuberculin may be tried, particularly if the case is seen early.

Operation has been suggested. The lesion is usually localized, and nowadays it should not be a difficult matter to remove the diseased glands; but, so far as we know, in animals this is always a fatal procedure, and in any case, unless there were supernumerary adrenals and a considerable portion of the extracapsular chromaffin intact, the operation would be useless.

Adrenal Therapy.—Evidently the relation of Addison's disease to the adrenals is not quite the same as that of myxœdema to the thyroid gland, in which the insufficiency is promptly and permanently relieved by the administration of preparations of the thyroid. The tuberculous nature of the lesions in most of the cases of Addison's disease is in itself an obstacle, and there is usually widespread cicatricial involvement of the sympathetic system. There is now a large series of cases treated with various preparations, but only a very few with satisfactory results. In only two of my patients was there marked improvement. In one, which I have reported, all the severer symptoms disappeared, the pigmentation cleared up, and the patient died subsequently of an acute infection, which apparently had nothing to do with the disease. The adrenals were found sclerotic but not tuberculous. The dried gland may be given in doses of from 5 to 20 grains (0.3 to 1.3 gm.) three times a day. There are also liquid extracts. Epinephrin may also be used and when the blood pressure is low it can be given systematically, carefully testing its effects.

2. OTHER AFFECTIONS OF THE SUPRARENAL GLANDS

Hyperplasia of the cortex has been met with in defective development of the genitals. Enlargement is not uncommon in chronic nephritis and in arterio-sclerosis. The latter has been attributed to the overactivity of the gland. Hypertrophy with tumor has also been associated with a remarkable precocious development of the sexual organs. When one gland is diseased the other may be enlarged. In cases of disease of both glands the chromaffin tissues along the aorta and in the sympathetic system have been found hypertrophied.

Hypoplasia.—There is an interesting association of absence of the adrenals or absence of the medulla with anomalies of the brain, particularly anencephaly. It has been suggested that chronic hypoplasia associated with insufficiency of the internal secretion is responsible for the low blood pressure in the specific fevers and in conditions of debility. Some have attributed the "white line," the anæmic vaso-motor skin reflex, to adrenal insufficiency, but, in any case, it is too common to be of much import.

Hæmorrhage.—Acute hæmorrhagic adrenalitis presents a picture somewhat resembling acute pancreatitis—a sudden onset with pain, vomiting, profound prostration and death within a few days. In other cases convulsions occur or the patient falls into a typhoid state with profound asthenia. In children the disease may be associated with purpura, both cutaneous and visceral.

Tumors.—Both carcinoma and sarcoma have been described. They are very apt to undergo fatty degeneration and hæmorrhage, so that they may form very large cysts. In children excessive development of the genitals with hair and fat has been found, as noted by Bullock and Sequeira, who have collected a number of cases. On this account a suggestion has been made that the adrenal cortex has an hormonic internal secretion which influences sexual development. Robert Hutchison has described a remarkable syndrome in children of adrenal tumor, exophthalmos, and cranial tumors; and William Pepper (tertius) has described a form characterized by rapid growth, diffuse involvement of the liver, and great distention of the abdomen without ascites or jaundice.

II. DISEASES OF THE THYMUS GLAND

While probably an organ of internal secretion the thymus in structure has little resemblance to the other ductless glands, with the exception of the epiphysis cerebri, and must be classed as an epithelial rather than as a lymphoid organ (Pappenheimer).

At birth the thymus gland weighs about 12 grams; from the first to the fifth year about 23 grams; from the sixth to the tenth year about 26 grams; from the eleventh to the fifteenth year about 37½ grams, and from the sixteenth to the twentieth year about 25½ grams, after which it undergoes a gradual atrophy (Hammar). Involution not taking place, a "persistent thymus" remains.

The function of the gland is not known. Friedleben, whose remarkable monograph (1858) is a storehouse of all knowledge on the subject, found no ill effects from extirpation, but this has not been confirmed. There is an obscure relationship between the thymus and the sexual glands. After castration N. Patton found persistency and hypertrophy of the gland. A disturbance of the normal development of the bones, particularly in ossification, also occurs (Basch) and there is an increase in the excitability of the nerves. The nature of the internal secretion is unknown. Many experiments have been made with extract from the gland, but without definite results.

1. HYPERTROPHY OF THE THYMUS

The size of the gland varies so greatly that it is not easy to define the limits between persistency and enlargement. Between the manubrium sterni and the vertebral column in an infant of eight months the distance is only 2.2 cm. (Jacobi), so that it is easy to understand how an enlarged gland may induce what Warthin calls "thymic tracheostenosis." There would appear to be, as this author suggests, three groups of cases:

(*a*) Thymic stridor, either congenital or developing soon after birth, varying in intensity and aggravated by crying and coughing.

(*b*) Thymic asthma, sometimes known as Copp's or Miller's asthma, which is an exaggerated and more persistent form of the stridor. While much dispute exists as to this form, there can be no doubt as to its occurrence, as there are cases, those reported by Siegel and König, for example, in which complete relief has followed removal of the gland. Olivier has collected 39 cases of thymectomy with 24 recoveries.

(c) Lastly, in a few cases sudden death has been met with, usually in connection with the condition of lymphatism about to be described.

Persistence of the gland has been met with in many affections, such as Graves' disease, Addison's disease, acromegaly, myasthenia gravis, rickets, etc. Many observers have regarded the association of an enlargement with Graves' disease as more than accidental and as a sort of compensatory process.

2. ATROPHY OF THE THYMUS

This is met with accidentally in children who show no special pathological changes, especially as Ruhräh has shown, in marasmus and the chronic wasting disorders of children.

Of other morbid conditions met with, hæmorrhages are not uncommon. Many mediastinal tumors originate in the remnants of the thymus; dermoid tumors and cysts have also been met with; tuberculosis and syphilis of the gland are occasionally seen.

The condition described by Dubois, met with sometimes in the subjects of congenital syphilis, in which there are fissure like cavities in the gland filled with a purulent fluid, is stated by Chiari and by Dudgeon to be a post mortem softening.

3. STATUS THYMICO-LYMPHATICUS

(*Lymphatism*)

Definition.—A condition in children of hyperplasia of the lymphatic tissues and of the thymus, in association with a flabby, fat overgrowth of the body and hypoplasia of the heart and blood vessels.

The subjects of lymphatism, as this condition has been called, have a lowered resistance, and are liable to sudden death from trifling and apparently inadequate causes. The so-called "thymic death" has been much discussed. In young infants who have been found dead in bed, or who have been suddenly attacked with dyspnœa and cyanosis and died in a few minutes, the thymus gland has been found enlarged. Paltauf increased our knowledge of this condition when he described (in 1889) a *lymphatic constitution,* in which there was hyperplasia of the general lymphatic apparatus, enlargement of the thymus and of the spleen, with a fat, flabby state of the body.

Pathology.—The children have a well-developed panniculus adiposus, are often large for their age, and with relatively large heads. There are hyperplasia of the lymphatic apparatus and structures of the tonsillar ring, moderate enlargement of the external and internal lymph glands, and hyperplasia of the solitary and agminated follicles of the small and large intestines. In the moderately enlarged spleen the Malphigian bodies may stand out very prominently, and if anæmic look like large tubercles. The thymus may measure as much as 10 cm. in length, is swollen and soft, and on section exudes a milky white fluid. The bone marrow has been found hyperplastic, and in young adults the yellow is replaced by the red marrow. A small heart, small aorta and peripheral vessels have been found, and sometimes an associated condition of rickets.

Symptoms.—The subjects of lymphatism are usually fat, often anæmic and flabby, but are regarded as in good health. It is usually met with in children, but the condition may persist beyond puberty, and is seen in the flabby young adults with pasty complexions, large heads, and slender skeletons.

What has called special attention to the condition is the tragedy of sudden death following trifling causes—as the prick of a hypodermic needle, a sudden plunge into cold water, but much more often in anæsthesia, either by ether or chloroform, when an amount has been given, not itself lethal. Possibly, too, some of the sudden deaths of convalescents from infectious fevers are from this cause, and the remarkable cases of sudden death during bathing, or of persons who have fallen into the water, and though immediately rescued were dead. Two explanations have been offered of this sudden death: first, that it is due to mechanical pressure of the enlarged thymus on the trachea. This is not likely, as the majority of these cases have shown no previous signs of thymic asthma, and in only one of Blumer's 9 cases was there any evidence of this. The other view is that it is a toxæmia from an overproduction of the internal secretion of the thymus and of the lymph glands.

Diagnosis.—Suspected cases should be carefully examined before trifling operations. The enlargement of the superficial glands of the tonsillar tissues and of the spleen is easily determined. A persistence of the thymus is indicated by an area of dulness at the upper part, and particularly to the left of the sternum merging with the cardiac flatness and which shifts upward with extreme retraction of the head and neck (Boggs). A distinct bulging may be seen, or the top of the gland may be felt in the episternal notch. The X-ray picture may show a definite shadow. With the laryngoscope a narrowing of the windpipe may be seen. A careful blood count should always be made, as there may be a marked lymphocytosis. It is not easy to determine the existence of vascular hypoplasia.

Treatment.—Lymphatism is a condition out of which the child gradually grows. A general tonic treatment with iron and arsenic should be given. A large thymus causing compression should be removed. Treatment by the X-ray is often successful.

III. DISEASES OF THE THYROID GLAND

1. CONGESTION

At puberty, in girls, often at the onset of menstruation, the gland enlarges; in certain women the neck becomes fuller at each menstruation, and it was an old idea that the gland enlarged at or after defloration. The slight enlargement at puberty may persist for months and cause uneasiness, but, as a rule, it disappears completely. I do not remember a single instance in which the goitre has remained, though, of course, such a possibility has to be considered. From mechanical causes, as tight collars, repeated crying, or prolonged use of the voice, the gland may swell for a short time.

2. THYROIDITIS

Etiology.—Inflammation of the gland, which is nearly always secondary to some infection, may be simple or purulent. It has been met with most frequently in typhoid fever, small-pox, measles, pneumonia, rheumatic fever, and mumps. Epidemics of thyroiditis have been reported. It is a rare disease in ordinary hospital practice, and did not occur in one of our series of 1,500 cases of typhoid fever.

Symptoms.—The whole gland may be involved, or only one lobe. There are swelling, pain on pressure, redness over the affected part, and, when suppuration occurs, softening or fluctuation. Often the acute inflammation subsides spontaneously. Myxœdema has followed destruction of the entire gland by acute suppuration.

A remarkable sclerotic thyroiditis has been described by Riedel and is sometimes called after his name. It is important, as, in the rapidity of its evolution and in the production of a diffuse tumor involving the whole gland, the clinical picture may resemble cancer. The gland becomes firmly fixed to the surrounding parts and serious effects may be produced by compression of the trachea and of the recurrent laryngeal nerves. The cut section of the gland is white and smooth, and microscopically consists of a dense fibrous tissue.

3. TUMORS OF THE THYROID

Of these the most important are:

(*a*) Infective granulomata—tuberculosis, actinomycosis, and syphilis. Cases are very rarely met with. Swelling of the gland has been seen in the recent syphilitic infection, and gummata may occur in the congenital form.

(*b*) Adenomata, simple or malignant. The latter may cause extensive metastases, as in the case reported by Hayward, in which tumors resembling thyroid tissue occurred in the lungs and various bones.

(*c*) Cancer and sarcoma, which are rare, have a surgical interest.

4. ABERRANT AND ACCESSORY THYROIDS

In various places, from the root of the tongue to the arch of the aorta, fragments of thyroidal tissue have been found. These aberrant portions of the gland are very apt to enlarge and undergo cystic degeneration. In the mediastinum they may form large tumors, and in the pleura I have seen an accessory cystic thyroid occupy the upper portion, and a case was reported by F. A. Packard, in which the cystic gland filled nearly the entire side. The so-called lingual thyroid is not uncommon, varying in size from a hemp seed to a pea, usually free in the deep muscles of the tongue, or attached to the hyoid bone. When enlarged the lingual goitre may form a tumor of considerable size. The true thyroid gland has been absent, and removal of the lingual goitre has been followed by myxœdema.

5. GOITRE

(*Struma, Bronchocele*)

Definition.—A chronic enlargement of the thyroid gland, of unknown origin, occurring sporadically or endemically.

Distribution.—Goitre, on the whole, is rare in the United States; it is perhaps most common in the region of the Great Lakes. In an investigation in Michigan, Dock found a large number of cases and the disease is not very uncommon in Lower Canada. In England it is common in certain regions; the Thames valley, the Dales, Derbyshire, Sussex, and Hampshire. It is very prevalent about Oxford and the upper Thames valley. In Switzerland, in the mountains of Germany and Austria, the mountainous districts of France, and in the Pyrenees the disease is very prevalent. In regions of Central Asia, in the Abyssinian mountains, and in the Himalayas there are many foci of the disease.

Etiology.—The disease is rarely congenital except in very goitrous districts. Cases are most common at or about puberty, and the tendency diminishes after the twentieth year. Women are much more frequently attacked than men, in a proportion of 6 or 8 to 1.

In its endemic form the disease occurs at every latitude and in every altitude, in valleys and in plains, and in various climates. It seems to be much less prevalent by the seashore.

The cause is obscure. The water in goitrous districts is hard, rich in lime and magnesia, poor in iodine, and (so Rédin affirms of the Swiss waters) with a high degree of radio-activity. Others speak of a "miasma" of the soil which gets into the drinking water. McCarrison in Kashmir found that the specific agent could be killed by boiling the water and that it did not pass a Berkefeld filter. He produced goitre in himself and in others by the daily consumption of the residue of the filter, but the residue when boiled was harmless. The disease was transmitted to goats who drank water contaminated by goitre patients. There are "goitre springs" and "goitre wells." These and other facts strongly suggest a specific organism; and this view is supported by the remarkable outbreaks of acute goitre in schools, lasting for a few months and disappearing. In one such outbreak 161 boys among 350 and 245 girls among 381 were attacked (Guillaume).

Morbid Anatomy.—Usually the whole gland is involved, but one lobe only may be attacked. When the enlargement is uniform, and the appearance of the gland natural, it is spoken of as parenchymatous goitre; when the blood vessels are very large, vascular goitre. In both forms there is an increase in the colloid material of the follicles. Degenerations of various kinds are common, particularly cystic, in which there are many large and small cavities with colloid contents. In some of these cystic forms there are papillary ingrowths into the alveoli. Sometimes the cysts contain blood and extensive hæmorrhages occur in the gland.

Symptoms.—When small a goitre is not inconvenient, but when large pressure symptoms may cause the patient to seek relief. The windpipe may be flattened from pressure, usually of an enlarged isthmus, or it is narrowed by circular compression. The symptoms are more or less marked stridor and cough, which may persist for years without special aggravation. They may be present with very large glands, or with the small encircling goitre, or with the goitre which passes deeply beneath the sternum. Pressure on the recurrent nerves may cause attacks of dyspnœa, particularly at night, and the voice may be altered. Pressure on the vagus is not common. Sometimes there is difficulty in swallowing, and the veins of the neck may be compressed. The heart is often involved, either from pressure on the vagi, or there is dilatation of the organ associated with dyspnœa. This is sometimes spoken of as the "goitre heart" in contra-distinction to the cardiac condition in Graves' disease.

Prognosis.—Many cases in the young get well; too often in goitrous districts the tumor persists. It may disappear on leaving the district. Many cases get well without medical treatment, but when pressure symptoms occur surgery gives relief.

Treatment.—In goitrous districts the drinking water should be boiled. Iodine in some form is used extensively, and often is curative. Its effect is to stimulate the gland to healthy action. In young people 2 to 5 grains (0.13 to 0.3 gm.) of potassium or sodium iodide may be given daily. Iodine injections into the gland have been used but are not advisable. Iodine may be applied externally as an ointment (5 per cent.). The X-rays have been tried with success. When the gland is large, surgical measures must be resorted to.

6. HYPOTHYROIDISM

(*Cretinism and Myxœdema*)

Definition.—A constitutional affection due to the loss of function of the thyroid gland, characterized clinically by a myxœdematous condition of the subcutaneous tissues and mental failure, and anatomically by atrophy of the thyroid gland.

History.—As early as 1859 Schiff had noted that in the dog removal of the gland was followed by certain symptoms. Gull described "A cretinoid change in women," and in the eighties the observations of Ord and other English physicians separated a well defined clinical entity called "myxœdema."

Kocher (in 1883) reported that 30 of his first 100 thyroidectomies had been followed by a very characteristic picture, to which he gave the name "cachexia strumipriva," an observation which had already been made in the previous year by the Reverdins, who also had recognized the relation of this change to the disease known as "myxœdema." The researches of Horsley, and the elaborate investigation of the Committee of the Clinical Society of London, made it clear that the changes following complete removal of the gland, the so-called cachexia strumipriva, myxœdema, and the sporadic cretinism, were one and the same disease, due to the loss of the function of the thyroid gland. Schiff and Horsley demonstrated that animals could be saved by the transplantation of the glands. Lastly came the discovery of George Murray and Howitz that feeding with the thyroid extract replaced the gland function, and cured the disease. The activity of the gland is in some way connected with the metabolism of iodine. Baumann determined the presence of this body in the secretion of the thyroid as an organic combination which he called iodothyrin, not to be confounded with the simple extract of the gland, which is usually called thyreoidin.

The outcome of a host of researches has been the recognition of the enormous importance of the internal secretion of the gland, which is essential for the normal growth of the body in childhood, and for the maintenance of the proper metabolism of the epidermic tissues and of the brain.

Clinical Forms.—There are three groups of cases—cretinism, myxœdema proper, and operative myxœdema. To Felix Simon is due the credit of recognizing that these were one and the same condition and all due to loss of function of the thyroid gland.

CRETINISM.—Two forms are recognized—the sporadic and the endemic. In the *sporadic* form the gland may be congenitally absent, or is atrophied after one of the specific fevers, or the condition develops with goitre. The disease is not very uncommon. I was able to collect the histories of 58 cases in a few years in the United States and Canada. It is more common in females than in males—35 in my series.

Morbid Anatomy.—Absence of the gland, or complete fibrous atrophy, is the common condition. Goitre with any trace of gland tissue is rare. In the sporadic form sometimes the hypophysis and thymus have been found enlarged. Arrest of development, a brachycephalic skull in the endemic, and a doliocephalic in the sporadic form, are the chief skeletal changes.

Symptoms.—In the congenital cases the condition is rarely recognized before the infant is six or seven months old. Then it is noticed that the child does not grow so rapidly and is not bright mentally. The tongue looks large and hangs out of the mouth. The hair may be thin and the skin very dry. Usually by the end of the first year and during the second year the signs become very marked. The face is large, looks bloated, the eyelids are puffy and swollen; the alæ nasi are thick, the nose looks depressed and flat. Dentition is delayed, and the teeth which appear decay early. The abdomen is swollen, the legs are thick and short, and the hands and feet are undeveloped and pudgy. The face is pale and sometimes has a waxy, sallow tint. The fontanelles remain open; there is much muscular weakness, and the child can not support itself. In the supraclavicular regions there are large pads of fat. The child does not develop mentally and may lapse into a state of imbecility.

In cases in which the atrophy of the gland follows a fever the condition may not come on until the fourth or fifth year, or later. This is really, as Parker determined, a juvenile myxœdema. In a few of the sporadic forms cretinism develops with an existing goitre. It may retard development, bodily and mental, without ever progressing to complete imbecility.

ENDEMIC CRETINISM.—This occurs wherever goitre is very prevalent, as in parts of Switzerland, Savoy, Tyrol, and the Pyrenees. It formerly prevailed in parts of England. I know of no centres in the United States or Canada. The clinical features of the disease are the same as in the sporadic form, stunted growth and feeble mind, plus goitre. To some poison in the water—mineral or organic—the thyroid changes have been attributed, but whatever the toxic agent may be, it is the interference with the function of the gland that leads to the cretinous change in the body.

The *diagnosis* is very easy after one has seen a case, or good illustrations.

Infants a year or so old sometimes become flabby, lose their vivacity, or show a protuberant abdomen, and lax skin with slight cretinoid appearance. These milder forms, as they have been termed, are probably due to transient functional disturbance in the gland.

Myxœdema of Adults (*Gull's Disease*).—Women are much more frequently affected than men—in a ratio of 6 to 1. The disease may affect several members of a family, and it may be transmitted through the mother. In some instances there has been first the appearance of exophthalmic goitre. Though occurring most commonly in women, it seems to have no special relation to the catamenia or to pregnancy; the symptoms of myxœdema may disappear during pregnancy or may develop post partum. Myxœdema and exophthalmic goitre may occur in sisters. It is not so common in America as in England. In sixteen years I saw only 10 cases in Baltimore, 7 of which were in the hospital. C. P. Howard has collected 100 American cases, of which 86 were in women. The symptoms of this form, as given by Ord, are marked increase in the general bulk of the body, a firm, inelastic swelling of the skin, which does not pit on pressure; dryness and roughness, which tend with the swelling to obliterate in the face the lines of expression; imperfect nutrition of the hair; local tumefaction of the skin and subcutaneous tissues, particularly in the supraclavicular region. The physiognomy is altered in a remarkable way: the features are coarse and broad, the lips thick, the nostrils broad and thick, and the mouth is enlarged. Over the cheeks, sometimes the nose, there is a reddish patch. There is a striking slowness of thought and of movement. The memory becomes defective, the patients grow irritable and suspicious, and there may be headache. In some instances there are delusions and hallucinations, leading to a final condition of dementia. The gait is heavy and slow. The temperature may be below normal. The functions of the heart, lungs, and abdominal organs are normal. Hæmorrhage sometimes occurs. Albuminuria is sometimes present, more rarely glycosuria. Death is usually due to some intercurrent disease, most frequently tuberculosis (Greenfield). The thyroid gland is diminished in size and may become completely atrophied and converted into a fibrous mass. The subcutaneous fat is abundant, and in one or two instances a great increase in the mucin has been found. The larynx is also involved.

The course of the disease is slow but progressive, and extends over ten or fifteen years. A condition of acute and temporary myxœdema may develop in connection with enlargement of the thyroid in young persons. Myxœdema may follow exophthalmic goitre. In other instances the symptoms of the two diseases have been combined. I have reported a case in which a young man became bloated and increased in weight enormously during three months, then had tachycardia with tremor and active delirium, and died within six months of the onset of the symptoms.

Operative Myxœdema; Cachexia Strumipriva.—Horsley showed that complete removal of the thyroid in monkeys was followed by the production of a condition similar to that of myxœdema and sometimes associated with spasms or tetanoid contractures, and followed by apathy and coma. An identical condition sometimes follows extirpation of the thyroid in man. The disease follows only a certain number of total and a much smaller proportion of partial removals of the thyroid gland. Of 408 cases, in 69 the operative myxœdema occurred (Kocher). If a small fragment of the thyroid remains, or if there are accessory glands, which in animals are very common, the symptoms do not develop. Operative myxœdema is very rare in America. A few years ago I was able to find only two cases, one of which, McGraw's, referred to in previous editions of this work, has since been cured.

The *diagnosis* of myxœdema is easy, as a rule. The general aspect of the patient—the subcutaneous swelling and the pallor—suggests Bright's disease, which may be strengthened by the discovery of tube casts and of albumin in the urine; but the solid character of the swelling, the exceeding dryness of the skin, the yellowish white color, the low temperature, the loss of hair, and the dull, listless mental state should suffice to differentiate the two conditions. In dubious cases not too much stress should be laid upon the supraclavicular swellings. There may be marked fibro-fatty enlargements in this situation in healthy persons, the supraclavicular pseudo-lipomata of Verneuil.

Treatment.—The patients suffer in cold and improve greatly in warm weather. They should therefore be kept at an even temperature, and should, if possible, move to a warm climate during the winter months. Repeated warm baths with shampooing are useful. Our art has made no more brilliant advance than in the cure of these disorders due to disturbed function of the thyroid gland. That we can to-day rescue children otherwise doomed to helpless idiocy—that we can restore to life the hopeless victims of myxœdema—is a triumph of experimental medicine for which we are indebted very largely to Victor Horsley and to his pupil Murray. Transplantation of the gland was first tried; then Murray used an extract subcutaneously. Hector Mackenzie in London and Howitz in Copenhagen introduced the method of feeding. We now know that the gland, taken either fresh, or as the watery or glycerin extract, or dried and powdered, is equally efficacious in a majority of all the cases of myxœdema in infants or adults. Many preparations are now on the market, but it makes little difference how the gland is administered. The dried powdered gland and the glycerin extract are most convenient. It is well to begin with the powdered gland, 1 grain (0.065 gm.) three times a day, of the Parke Davis preparation, or one of the Burroughs and Welcome tablets. The dose may be increased gradually until the patient takes 10 or 15 grains (0.6 gm. to 1 gm.) in the day. In many cases there are no unpleasant symptoms; in others there are irritation of the skin, restlessness, rapid pulse, and delirium; in rare instances tonic spasms, the condition to which the term *thyroidism* is applied. The results, as a rule, are most astounding—unparalleled by anything in the whole range of curative measures. Within six weeks a poor, feeble-minded, toad-like caricature of humanity may be restored to mental and bodily health. Loss of weight is one of the first and most striking effects; one of my patients lost over 30 pounds within six weeks. The skin becomes moist, the urine is increased, the perspiration returns, the temperature rises, the pulse rate quickens, and the mental torpor lessens. Ill effects are rare. Two or three cases with old heart lesions have died during or after the treatment; in one instance a temporary condition of Graves' disease was induced.

The treatment, as Murray suggests, must be carried out in two stages—one, early, in which full doses are given until the cure is effected; the other, the permanent use of small doses sufficient to preserve the normal metabolism.

In the cases of cretinism it seems to be necessary to keep up the treatment indefinitely. I have seen several instances of remarkable relapse follow the cessation of the use of the extract.

7. HYPERTHYROIDISM; EXOPHTHALMIC GOITRE

(*Graves', Basedow's, or Parry's Disease*)

Definition.—A disease characterized by goitre, exophthalmos, tachycardia, and tremor, associated with a perverted or hyperactive state of the thyroid gland.

Historical Note.—In the posthumous writings of Caleb Hillier Parry (1825) is a description of 8 cases of Enlargement of the Thyroid Gland in Connection with Enlargement or Palpitation of the Heart. In the first case, seen in 1786, he also described the exophthalmos: "The eyes were protruded from their sockets, and the countenance exhibited an appearance of agitation and distress, especially in any muscular movement." The Italians claim that Flajani described the disease in 1800. I have not been able to see his original account, but Moebius states that it is meagre and inaccurate, and bears no comparison with that of Parry. If the name of any physician is to be associated with the disease, undoubtedly it should be that of the distinguished old Bath physician. Graves described the disease in 1835 and Basedow in 1840.

Etiology.—*Age*—In Sattler's collection of 3,477 cases only 184 were under the age of sixteen.

Sex—In England and America the proportion of females is greatly in excess, as much probably as 20 to 1, but in Sattler's collected cases from the literature the ratio was 5.4 to 1, which would indicate marked differences in different countries.

A strong *family predisposition* may exist and five or six members may be affected. *Fright* is a rare cause. Various depressive influences, such as worry, nervous strain, disappointment in love, illnesses, and mental shocks, as well as dread of the disease itself, may have an important influence.

Pathology.—The disease is regarded by some as a pure neurosis, in favor of which are urged the onset after a profound emotion, the absence of lesions, and the cure which has followed in a few cases after operations upon the nose. Of late the views of Moebius and Greenfield have prevailed, that exophthalmic goitre is primarily a disease of the thyroid gland (*hyperthyroidism*), in antithesis to myxœdema (*athyroidism*). The clinical contrast between these two diseases is most suggestive—the increased excitability of the nervous system, the flushed, moist skin, the vascular erythism in the one; the dull apathy, the low temperature, slow pulse, and dry skin of the other. The changes in the gland in exophthalmic goitre are, as shown by Greenfield, those of an organ in active evolution—viz., increased proliferation, with the production of newly formed tubular spaces and absorption of the colloid material which is replaced by a more mucinous fluid. The thyroid extract given in excess produces symptoms not unlike those of Parry's disease—tachycardia, tremor, headache, sweating, and prostration. Beclère has reported a case in which exophthalmos developed after an overdose. Use of the thyroid extract usually aggravates the symptoms of exophthalmic goitre. The most successful line of treatment has been that directed to diminish the bulk of the goitre. These are some of the considerations which favor the view that the symptoms are due to disturbed function of the thyroid gland, probably to hypersecretion of materials which induce a sort of chronic intoxication. Myxœdema may develop in the late stages, and there are transient œdema and in a few cases scleroderma, which indicate that the nutrition of the skin is involved.

Anatomical Changes.—In rare instances the thyroid gland has been stated to be normal. In the majority of cases there is active hyperplasia of the gland, with enlarged and newly formed follicles, and an increase in the lymphoid tissue of the gland stroma. Involuntary and regressive changes are common; the hyperplasia may cease and the gland returns to the colloid state. Finally, in certain cases, atrophy of the cell elements takes place.

The iodine content of the gland bears a direct relationship to the amount of colloid; the gland in hyperplasia has the lowest percentage, the pure colloid glands the highest.

Symptoms.—Acute and chronic forms may be recognized. In the acute form the disease may arise with great rapidity. In a patient of J. H. Lloyd's, of Philadelphia, a woman, aged thirty-nine, who had been considered perfectly healthy, but whose friends had noticed that for some time her eyes looked rather large, was suddenly seized with intense vomiting and diarrhœa, rapid action of the heart, and great throbbing of the arteries. The eyes were prominent and staring and the thyroid gland was found much enlarged and soft. The gastro-intestinal symptoms continued, the pulse became more rapid, the vomiting was incessant, and the patient died on the third day of the illness. Only the abdominal and thoracic organs could be examined and no changes were found. I saw two rapidly fatal cases at the Philadelphia Hospital, one of which, under F. P. Henry's care, had marked cerebral symptoms. The acute cases are not always associated with delirium.

More frequently the onset is gradual and the disease is chronic. There are four characteristic symptoms of the disease—tachycardia, exophthalmos, enlargement of the thyroid, and tremor.

Tachycardia.—Rapid heart action is only one of a series of remarkable vascular phenomena in the disease. The pulse rate at first may be not more than 95 or 100, but when the disease is established it may be from 140 to 160, or even higher. Irregularity is not common, except toward the close. In a well developed case the visible area of cardiac pulsation is much increased, the action is heaving and forcible, and the shock of the heart sounds is well felt. The large arteries at the root of the neck throb forcibly. There is visible pulsation in the peripheral arteries. The capillary pulse is readily seen, and there are few diseases in which one may see at times with greater distinctness the venous pulse in the veins of the hand. The throbbing pulsation of the arteries may be felt even in the finger tips. Vascular erythema is common—the face and neck are flushed and there may be a widespread erythema of the body and limbs. On auscultation murmurs are usually heard over the heart, a loud apex systolic and loud bruits at the base and over the manubrium. The sounds of the heart may be very intense. In rare instances they may be heard at some distance from the patient; according to Graves, as far as four feet. Attacks of acute dilatation of the heart may occur with dyspnœa, cough, and a frothy bloody expectoration.

Exophthalmos.—A characteristic facial aspect is given to Graves' disease by the staring expression, caused in part by protrusion of the eyeballs, but more particularly by retraction of the lids exposing the scleræ above and below the corneæ. The exophthalmos, which may be unilateral, usually follows the vascular disturbance. The protrusion may become very great and the eye may even be dislocated from the socket, or both eyes may be destroyed by panophthalmitis, a condition present in one of Basedow's cases. The vision is normal. Graefe noted that when the eyeball is moved downward the upper lid does not follow it as in health. This is known as Graefe's sign. The palpebral aperture is wider than in health, owing to spasm or retraction of the upper lid (Stellwag's sign). The patient winks less frequently than in health. There is marked tremor of the lids and they contract spasmodically in advance of the elevating eyeball. Moebius has called attention to the lack of convergence of the two eyes. Changes in the pupils and in the optic nerves are rare. Pulsation of the retinal arteries is common.

Enlargement of the thyroid is the rule. It may be general or in only one lobe, and is rarely so large as in ordinary goitre. It may be absent. The swelling is firm, but elastic. There are rarely pressure signs. The vessels are usually much dilated, and the whole gland may be seen to pulsate. A thrill may be felt on palpation and on auscultation a loud systolic murmur, or more commonly a *bruit de diable*. A double murmur is common and is pathognomonic (Guttmann).

Tremor is the fourth cardinal symptom, and was really first described by Basedow. It is involuntary, fine, about eight to the second. It is of great importance in the diagnosis of the early cases.

Other symptoms are anæmia, emaciation, and slight fever. Attacks of vomiting and diarrhœa may occur. The latter may be very severe and distressing, recurring at intervals. The greatest complaint is of the forcible throbbing in the arteries, often accompanied with unpleasant flushes of heat and profuse perspirations. An erythematous flushing is common. Pruritus may be a severe and persistent symptom. Multiple telangiectases have been described. Solid, infiltrated œdema is not uncommon. It may be transitory. A remarkable myxœdematous state may supervene. Pigmentary changes are very common. They may be patchy or generalized. The coexistence of scleroderma and Graves' disease has been frequently noticed. Irritability of temper, change in disposition, and great mental depression have been described. An important complication is acute mania, in which the patient may die in a few days. Weakness of the muscles is not uncommon, particularly a feeling of "giving way" of the legs. If the patient holds the head down and is asked to look up without raising the head, the forehead remains smooth and is not wrinkled, as in a normal individual (Joffroy). A feature of interest noted by Charcot is the great diminution in the electrical resistance, which may be due to the saturation of the skin with moisture owing to the vaso-motor dilatation (Hirt). Bryson has noted the fact that the chest expansion may be greatly diminished. The emaciation may be extreme. Glycosuria and albuminuria are not infrequent complications. True diabetes may occur.

The course of the disease is usually chronic, lasting several years. After persisting for six months or a year the symptoms may disappear. There are remarkable instances in which the symptoms have come on with great intensity, following fright, and have disappeared again in a few days.

Prognosis.—Statistics are misleading as only the severe cases come under hospital treatment. Sattler estimates the mortality at 11 per cent. In Hale White's series it was 84 in 214 cases. In the hands of Kocher and the Mayos the mortality from operation is below 4 per cent. and some 70 per cent. of cases are claimed to have been cured.

Diagnosis.—Few diseases are so easily recognized. The difficulty is with the partially developed forms, *formes frustes*, which are not uncommon. The nervous state, the tremor, and tachycardia may be the only features, or there may be slight swelling of the thyroid with tremor alone. The greatest difficulty arises in the cases of hysterical tremor with rapid heart action. Doubtful cases may be tested by the careful administration of iodine internally, as patients with hyperthyroidism show a marked intolerance, even to small doses. A differential count of the leucocytes shows an increase in the mononuclears.

Treatment.—(*a*) The disease is serious enough to warrant strong measures systematically carried out; much valuable time is lost in trying various remedies. The patient should be in bed, at absolute rest, and see very few persons. To quiet the heart's action the icebag may be continuously applied through the day, and veratrum viride, aconite, or strophanthus given in full doses. Ergot, belladonna, phosphate of soda, small doses of opium, and many other remedies are recommended, and in some instances I have seen benefit from the belladonna and the phosphate of soda. Electricity may be helpful.

(*b*) *Serum Therapy.*—Two methods are employed: feeding with the milk of dethyroidized goats, introduced by Lanz, which is obtainable as a substance called rodagen. Good results have been reported by Mackenzie and others. Beebe, on the other hand, uses the serum of animals into which human thyroid extract has been injected. Excellent results have been obtained, but the method has the danger associated with the use of foreign sera.

(*c*) *Surgical Treatment.*—Removal of part of the thyroid gland offers the best hope of permanent cure. It is remarkable with what rapidity all the symptoms may disappear after partial thyroidectomy. A second operation may be necessary in severe cases. The results obtained by the brothers Mayo and by Kocher give a remarkable percentage of recoveries. The operation under cocaine may be done with safety when the condition of the heart and the extreme tachycardia do not contraindicate it. Tying of the arteries and exothyropexia are also recommended. Excision of the superior cervical ganglia of the sympathetic has one beneficial result, viz., the production of slight ptosis, which obviates the staring character of the exophthalmos.

Marked benefit has followed the use of the X-rays in a few cases.

IV. DISEASES OF THE PARATHYROID GLANDS

The parathyroid bodies occur, as a rule, in two pairs on either side of the lateral lobes of the thyroid gland; small ovoid structures from 6 to 8 mm. in length. Some observers regard them as simply supplementary to the thyroid, without a special function; others believe that they have an important internal secretion supplementing that of the thyroid gland and controlling calcium metabolism.

The studies of Gley, Halsted, and others leave no question as to the importance of these glands. Following their removal in animals there are twitching, spasms of the voluntary muscles, gradual paralysis with dyspnœa, and death from exhaustion. These sometimes disappear when a saline extract of the parathyroid is injected into a vein, or if the parathyroid glands are fed or transplanted. The association of tetany with the disturbance of the function of the thyroid seems to be definitely established. MacCallum has shown the importance of the function of these glands in controlling calcium metabolism, and it is possible that in impoverishment of the tissues in this ingredient is to be sought the cause of the great excitability of the nervous system and of tetany.

These studies have thrown great light upon various spasmodic disorders of children, and some have gone so far as to embrace such conditions as laryngismus, infantile convulsions, and tetany under the term "spasmophilia" (Heubner).

These glands have also hormonic relations, as yet not thoroughly understood, with the other ductless glands, and have some influence on carbohydrate metabolism.

The definite association of the glands with tetany is sufficient warrant for treating this disease here.

TETANY

Definition.—An affection characterized by bilateral, chronic, or intermittent spasms of the extremities, with gradually increasing irritability of the nerves.

Etiology.—The following groups are made by Frankl-Hochwart:

(*a*) Tetany of Adults.—(1) Epidemic tetany, also known as rheumatic tetany, idiopathic workman's tetany, or shoemaker's cramp. In certain parts of the Continent of Europe the disease has prevailed widely, particularly in the winter season. Von Jacksch, who has described an epidemic form occurring in young men of the working classes, sometimes with slight fever, regards the disease as infectious. This form is acute, lasting only two or three weeks, and rarely proving fatal.

(2) Tetany of gastric and intestinal disorders, as dyspepsia, gastrectasis, diarrhœa, and helminthiasis. The form associated with dilatation of the stomach is rare, not more than 30 cases having been reported.

(3) Tetany of the acute infectious diseases (typhoid, cholera, influenza, measles, scarlatina, etc.). In some typhoid epidemics many cases have occurred.

(4) Tetany following poisoning from chloroform, morphia, ergot, lead, alcohol, and uræmia. Isolated examples of each have been reported.

(5) Tetany may also develop during pregnancy or recur in successive pregnancies. From its occurrence in nursing women, Trousseau called it "nurse's contracture."

(6) Tetany following removal of the thyroid gland is probably due to a removal of the parathyroid bodies at the same time.

(7) Tetany may complicate other nervous disorders, as Basedow's disease, cerebral tumor, cysts of the cerebellum, and syringomyelia.

(*b*) Tetany in Children.—Tetany bears a definite relation to gastro-intestinal disorders, acute infections, and rickets in childhood.

Mild cases of tetany are not uncommon in children, particularly in connection with rickets and gastro-intestinal disorders. The other forms are not common, either in the United States or in England. Campbell Howard reported from my clinic 8 cases of tetany, 4 accompanying dilatation of the stomach, 2 with hyperacidity without dilatation, 1 with chronic diarrhœa, and 1 occurring in connection with repeated pregnancies and lactation.

Morbid Anatomy.—It is now well established that the tetany following extirpation of the thyroid gland is due to coincident removal of the parathyroids; and the observations of MacCallum suggest that, occurring spontaneously, it is associated with insufficiency of the parathyroids, which appear to control calcium metabolism. Absence or perversion of the parathyroid secretion leads to impoverishment of the tissues in calcium, and to hyperexcitability of the nerves.

Symptoms.—In cases associated with general debility or in children with rickets the spasm is limited to the hands and feet. The fingers are bent at the metacarpo-phalangeal joint, extended at the terminal joints, pressed close together, and the thumb is contracted in the palm of the hand. The wrist is flexed, the elbows are bent, and the arms are folded over the chest. In the lower limbs the feet are extended and the toes adducted. The muscles of the face and neck are less commonly involved, but in severe cases there may be trismus, and the angles of the mouth are drawn out. The skin of the hands and feet is sometimes tense and œdematous. The spasms are usually paroxysmal and last for a variable time. In children the attack may pass off in a few hours. In some of the more severe chronic cases in adults the stiffness and contracture may continue or even increase for many days, and the attack may last as long as two weeks. In the acute cases the temperature may be elevated and the pulse quickened. In the severe paroxysms there may be involvement of the muscles of the back and of the thorax, inducing dyspnœa and cyanosis. Certain additional features, valuable in diagnosis, are present.

Trousseau's symptom: "So long as the attack is not over, the paroxysms may be reproduced at will. This is effected by simply compressing the affected parts, either in the direction of their principal nerve trunks or over their blood vessels, so as to impede the venous or arterial circulation."

Chvostek's symptom is shown in the remarkable increase in the mechanical excitability of the motor nerves. A slight tap, for example, in the course of the facial nerve will throw the muscles to which it is distributed into active contraction. Erb has shown that the electrical irritability of the motor nerves, especially to the galvanic current, is also greatly increased, and Hofmann has demonstrated the heightened excitability of the sensory nerves, the slightest pressure on which may cause paræsthesia in the region of distribution.

Diagnosis.—The disease is readily recognized. It is a mistake to call instances of carpo-pedal spasm of children true tetany. It is common to find in rickety children or in cases of severe gastro-intestinal catarrh a transient spasm of the fingers or even of the arms. By many authors these are considered cases of mild tetany, and there are all grades in rickety children between the simple carpo-pedal spasm and the condition in which the four extremities are involved; but it is well, I think, to limit the term *tetany* to the more severe affection.

With true tetanus the disease is scarcely ever confounded, as the commencement of the spasm in the extremities, the attitude of the hands, and the etiological factors are very different. Hysterical contractures are usually unilateral.

Treatment.—In the case of children the condition with which the tetany is associated should be treated. Baths and cold sponging are recommended and often relieve the spasm as promptly as in child-crowing. Bromide of potassium may be tried. In severe cases chloroform inhalations may be given. Massage, electricity, and the spinal icebag have also been used with success. Cases, however, may resist all treatment, and the spasms recur for many years. The thyroid extract should be tried. Gottstein reports relief in a case of long standing, and Bramwell reports one case of operative tetany and one of the idiopathic form successfully treated in this way.

In gastric tetany, especially when due to dilatation of the stomach, the mortality is high, and recovery without operative interference is rare: of 27 cases collected by Riegel, 16 terminated fatally. Cunningham collected 8 cases treated surgically, with a mortality of 37.5 per cent., as compared with 70 per cent. treated by medical means. Regular, systematic lavage with large quantities of saline or mildly antiseptic solutions is sometimes beneficial.

The administration of calcium is frequently effective. It may be given as calcium lactate in doses of 15 grains (1 gm.) every three or four hours. In severe cases much larger amounts may be given.

V. DISEASES OF THE SPLEEN

1. GENERAL REMARKS.

Though a ductless gland, the spleen is not known to have an internal secretion, and its functions are as yet ill understood. It is not an organ essential to life. In the fetus it takes part in the formation of the red blood corpuscles, and as it contains hæmatoblasts, it is possible that in the adult this function may be exercised to some extent, particularly in cases of severe anæmia.

Hæmolysis is generally believed to be its special function, a view—not held by all physiologists—based upon the presence of a large percentage of organic compounds of iron, the deposit in the organ of blood pigments in various diseases, the presence of many macrophages containing red blood corpuscles, and upon the evidence, after removal of the spleen, of compensatory hæmolysis in many newly formed hæmo-lymph glands (Warthin).

Removal of the spleen, an operation practised by the ancients in the belief that it improved the wind of runners, is not, as a rule, followed by serious effects. There may be slight eosinophilia and temporary anæmia, and later there is usually slight leucocytosis, with relative increase of the lymphocytes.

In infections the organ enlarges and micro-organisms are present in large numbers. It has been supposed to play some part in the processes of immunity and phagocytosis goes on actively in the organ. In experimental anæmia caused by various hæmolytic agents the spleen enlarges, and in these conditions Bunting and Norris found evidence of vicarious blood formation. Chronic enlargement of the spleen may be present with very little disturbance of health. Attacks of anæmia sooner or later occur, and consecutive fibrosis may occur in the liver with jaundice and ascites (Banti's disease).

2. MOVABLE SPLEEN

Movable or wandering spleen is seen most frequently in women the subjects of enteroptosis. It may be present without signs of displacement of other organs. It may be found accidentally in individuals who present no symptoms whatever. In other cases there are dragging, uneasy feelings in the back and side. All grades are met with, from a spleen that can be felt completely below the margin of the ribs to a condition in which the tumor-mass impinges upon the pelvis; indeed, the organ has been found in an inguinal hernia! In the large majority of all cases the spleen is enlarged. Sometimes it appears that the enlargement has caused relaxation of the ligaments; in other instances the relaxation seems congenital, as movable spleens have been found in different members of the same family. Possibly traumatism may account for some of the cases. Apart from the dragging, uneasy sensations and the worry in nervous patients, wandering spleen causes very few serious symptoms. Torsion of the pedicle may produce a very alarming and serious condition, leading to great swelling of the organ, high fever, or even to necrosis. A young woman was admitted to my colleague Kelly's ward with a tumor supposed to be ovarian, but which proved to be a wandering, moderately enlarged spleen. She was transferred to the medical ward, where she had suddenly very great pain in the abdomen, a large swelling in the left flank, and much tenderness. Halsted operated and found an enormously enlarged spleen in a condition of necrosis, adherent to the adjacent parts and to the abdominal wall. He laid it open freely, and large necrotic masses of spleen tissue discharged for some time. She made a good recovery.

The *diagnosis* of a wandering spleen is usually easy unless the organ becomes fixed and is deformed by adhesions and perisplenitis. The shape of the organ and the sharp margin with the notches are the points to be specially noted.

The *treatment* of the condition is important. Occasionally the organ may be kept in position by a properly adapted belt and a pad under the left costal margin. Removal of the displaced organ has been advised and carried out in many cases, and nowadays it is not a very serious operation. It is, however, as a rule unnecessary. In two cases of enlarged spleen under my care, with great mobility, causing much discomfort and uneasiness, Halsted completely relieved the condition by replacing the spleen, packing it in position with gauze, and allowing firm adhesions to take place. Both these patients were seen more than eighteen months after the operation and the organ had remained in position.

3. RUPTURE OF THE SPLEEN

This is of interest in connection with the spontaneous rupture in cases of acute enlargement during typhoid fever or malaria, which is very rare. Rupture of a malarial spleen may follow a blow, or a fall, or an exploratory puncture. In India and in Mauritius rupture of the spleen is stated to be very common. Fatal hæmorrhage may follow puncture of a swollen spleen with a hypodermic needle. Occasionally the rupture results from the breaking of an infarct or of an abscess. The symptoms are those of hæmorrhage into the peritoneum, and the condition demands immediate laparotomy.

4. INFARCT, ABSCESS AND CYSTS OF THE SPLEEN

Emboli in the splenic arteries causing *infarcts* may be either infective or simple. They are seen most frequently in ulcerative endocarditis and in septic conditions. Infarcts may also follow the formation of thrombi in the branches of the splenic artery in cases of fever. They are not very infrequent in typhoid. In a few instances the infarcts have followed thrombosis in the splenic veins. They are chiefly of pathological interest. The infarct of the spleen may be suspected in cases of septicæmia or pyæmia when there are pain in the splenic region, tenderness on pressure, and slight swelling of the organ; on several occasions I have heard a well-marked peritoneal friction rub. Occasionally in the infective infarcts large *abscesses* are formed, and in rare instances the whole organ may be converted into a sac of pus.

Tumors of the spleen, hydatid and other *cysts* of the organ, and *gummata* are rare conditions of anatomical interest. In Hodgkin's disease the organ may be enlarged and smooth, or irregular from the presence of nodular tumors.

Cysts are rare; I have seen but two, one an echinococcus, and the other a double cyst of the hilus. The latter apparently are very common, and probably arise from a hæmatoma subcapsular or in the hilus. They have been successfully removed. Very small cysts are not infrequent in connection with polycystic disease of the liver and the kidneys. A dermoid cyst has been described. The diagnosis of cysts is not often made; the mass is usually irregular in the region of the spleen, but the splenic outlines are marked. In the case I saw with two cysts at the hilus, the tumor was very movable, very irregular, and I urged operation on the grounds of mechanical discomfort, and increase in size. In a recent paper Musser stated that there have been 21 operations, all successful, in cysts of this sort.

5. PRIMARY SPLENOMEGALY WITH ANÆMIA

(*Splenic Anæmia, Banti's Disease*)

Definition.—A primary disease of the spleen of unknown origin, characterized by progressive enlargement, attacks of anæmia, a tendency to hæmorrhage, and in some cases a secondary cirrhosis of the liver, with jaundice and ascites. That the spleen itself is the seat of the disease is shown by the fact that complete recovery follows its removal.

History.—The name "splenic anæmia" was applied to a group of cases by Griesinger in 1866. H. C. Wood, in 1871, described cases as the splenic form of pseudo-leukæmia. The real study of the disease was initiated by Banti in 1883. In France the condition was called "primitive splenomegaly," and many different types of the disease have been described. Here we shall deal only with the form referred to in the definition as splenic anæmia and Banti's disease.

Etiology.—In the majority of cases the enlargement of the spleen comes on without any recognizable cause. In a few of my cases malaria has been present, but in the greater number the first thing noticed has been the mechanical inconvenience of the big spleen. Males are more frequently attacked than females. It is a disease of young and middle life, the majority of cases occurring before the fortieth year. It is also met with in young children. Many of the cases of infantile splenic anæmia of von Jaksch and of the Italian writers belong to this disease.

Morbid Anatomy.—The spleen is greatly enlarged, coming perhaps next to the size of the leukæmic organ. It is very firm, the capsule is thickened, the texture of the gland very tough and firm, and the whole in a state of advanced fibrosis. Banti has described a proliferation of the endothelial cells of the venous sinuses of the pulp, and he believes there are very characteristic histological changes.

The blood vessels in the neighborhood of the spleen may be very large, particularly the vasa brevia, and the splenic vein itself and the portal vein may be enormously dilated, and show atheroma and calcification. The lymphatic glands are not involved. Hyperplasia of the bone marrow has been found, but no other changes of special importance.

The cases of the Gaucher type, primitive endothelioma of the spleen, do not belong in this group.

Symptoms.—The disease is extraordinarily chronic; seven of my cases had a longer duration than ten years. Usually the first feature to attract attention is:

Splenomegaly.—The enlargement is uniform, smooth, painless, usually reaches to the navel, very often to the anterior superior spine, and the organ may occupy the whole of the left half of the abdomen. It may exist for years without any symptoms other than the inconvenience caused by the distention of the abdomen. Following an infarct pain may be present.

Anæmia.—Sooner or later the patients become anæmic. The attack may develop with rapidity, and in children a severe and even fatal form may follow in a few weeks. More commonly the pallor is gradual and the patient may come under observation for the first time with swelling of the feet, shortness of breath, and all the signs of advanced anæmia. The blood picture is, as a rule, that of a secondary anæmia with a very low color index and a marked leucopenia. The red blood corpuscles may fall as low as two million and in an average of a series of uncomplicated cases the leucocyte count was under 3,500 per c. mm. There are no special changes in the differential count. Following a severe hæmorrhage there may be a rise in the leucocytes. Some patients have permanent slight anæmia of the secondary type; others remain very well except for recurring attacks of anæmia, of great severity, which may be independent of hæmorrhage.

The question whether the anæmia splenica infantum of von Jaksch and the Italian writers is the same malady has been much discussed. There are cases in which enlargement of the spleen without obvious cause has been followed by a rapidly progressing anæmia with marked leucopenia. A very suggestive thing is that in a case in a child, with a blood count below one million reds, removal of the spleen was followed by complete recovery.

Hæmorrhages.—Bleeding, usually hæmatemesis, may be a special feature of the disease and may occur for many years. One of my patients had recurring attacks for twelve years, and one at the London Hospital, noted by R. Hutchison, for fifteen years. In such cases the diagnosis of ulcer of the stomach may be made. The bleeding may be of great severity. On several occasions one of my patients was brought into the hospital completely exsanguine; in two the hæmorrhage proved directly fatal; in a third the hæmorrhage proved fatal ten days after a successful removal of the spleen. The bleeding comes, as a rule, from œsophageal varices. Melæna may be present. Hæmaturia occurred in one of my cases; purpura is not uncommon.

Ascites.—Usually a terminal event, it may be due to the enlarged spleen itself or to secondary cirrhosis of the liver. When due to the liver, it is associated with slight jaundice.

Jaundice.—Icterus has been a rare symptom in my cases. Enlargement of the spleen may persist for many years without any consecutive change in the liver. One patient has splenomegaly with repeated hæmorrhages and has now (1912) had more than twelve years of good health after splenectomy. Slight jaundice may persist for years, sometimes with enlargement of the liver, in others with distinct reduction in its volume, and in either case with a progressive cirrhosis—the features to which Banti called special attention.

Course of the Disease.—It is extraordinarily chronic. A patient may for ten or twelve years have a large spleen causing no inconvenience, then an attack of anæmia may occur, from which recovery gradually takes place; or the first symptom may be ascites or a severe hæmorrhage from the stomach. As a rule, the anæmia becomes more or less chronic, with marked exacerbations, and in the later stages jaundice with ascites develops.

Diagnosis.—Here may be mentioned a series of forms of splenomegaly which differ essentially from the splenic anæmia, and in which, so far as we know, the condition of the spleen is not primary.

SPLENOMEGALY WITH ACHOLURIC JAUNDICE.—This type, first described by Minkowski and sometimes called after his name, is usually a familial form, often hereditary. It is consistent with good health throughout life, and there may be no symptoms. Characteristic features are: (*a*) its familial form; (*b*) chronic enlargement of the spleen; (*c*) good health; (*d*) chronic slight jaundice; (*e*) presence of urobilin in the urine, but absence of bile pigment. In a few instances gall stone colic has been present, due to the presence of small calculi. Chauffard showed that the red blood corpuscles in these cases have an increased fragility, the cause of which is unknown, but this is an essential feature in the hæmolytic jaundice. In the familial form good health is the rule, but in the acquired form the patient often becomes anæmic and is very ill. Cures have been reported after splenectomy.

SPLENOMEGALY OF THE GAUCHER TYPE (*Primary Endothelioma of the Spleen*).—In a dozen or more cases the enlarged spleen has retained its form and presents on section a grayish red appearance, with whitish spots or streaks; but histologically shows large cells from 20 to 40 μ in size, filling the alveolar spaces. The nature of this affection, first described by Gaucher in 1882, has been much discussed. The general opinion now is that of Stengel, that it is a type of new growth, an endothelioma; in any case, it differs entirely from the splenic anæmia.

SPLENOMEGALY ASSOCIATED WITH PRIMARY PYLETHROMBOSIS.—Cases have been reported of enlarged spleen in connection with phlebitis of the splenic and portal veins, and clinically such cases closely resemble Banti's disease. The spleen is very large and there are jaundice and ascites with moderate anæmia. The recognition of the pylethrombosis is only made post mortem.

HEPATIC SPLENOMEGALY.—Three varieties of cirrhosis of the liver may lead to great enlargement of the spleen with anæmia and a symptom-complex resembling that of splenic anæmia.

(*a*) *Alcoholic Cirrhosis.*—With recurring hæmorrhages, a consecutive anæmia, ascites, and an unusually large spleen, the condition may simulate closely the last stage of splenic anæmia. The history, particularly the late appearance of the hepatic changes, may be the most important point. In the cases in which I have been in doubt the difficulty has arisen from an imperfect history and from the presence of recurring hæmorrhages.

(*b*) *Syphilitic Cirrhosis.*—Great enlargement of the spleen may follow gummous hepatitis, either congenital or acquired. Toward the close the picture is very similar to Banti's disease—slight jaundice, ascites, big spleen, recurring hæmorrhages, and marked anæmia. Signs of other syphilitic lesions and the irregular nodular liver may suggest the diagnosis.

(*c*) In a few cases of hypertrophic cirrhosis, as in Hanot's form and in hæmochromatosis, the spleen may be greatly enlarged, and in the late stages, when ascites and hæmorrhages occur, the clinical picture may be like that of splenic anæmia.

SPLENOMEGALY IN PERNICIOUS ANÆMIA.—Sometimes the spleen is greatly enlarged in this disease, reaching to the navel, but, as a rule, the lower blood count, the high color index, the large number of nucleated red blood corpuscles, and the clinical course enable one to make the diagnosis.

TROPICAL SPLENOMEGALY.—Kala-azar has been considered elsewhere and can be distinguished by the presence of the Leishman-Donovan bodies in the splenic blood. There are big spleens with anæmia in the Tropics which are not Kala-azar, and the experience of some of the physicians in Cairo indicates that some of these, at any rate, are of the ordinary splenic anæmia type, in which removal of the organ cures the disease.

Treatment.—In the first stage with simple splenomegaly nothing is indicated; the patients, as a rule, look very well. For the anæmia the usual measures may be adopted, and the patient gets gradually better. The ultimate outlook is bad, and there is only one radical cure—removal of the spleen. This has now been done in a sufficiently large number of cases to determine its value. Of 6 of my cases 3 have recovered; one is alive more than 12 years after the operation, another between 6 and 7. One died on the table from hæmorrhage, a second from shock, and a third died ten days after from a rupture of the œsophageal varix. Armstrong of Montreal has collected 32 cases operated upon with 9 deaths. The fact that removal of the spleen is followed by complete recovery, even after the appearance of the jaundice and of chronic anæmia, is the best proof that the source of the trouble is in this organ itself, and is one of the best warrants for the recognition of the disease as a separate clinical entity.

VI. DISEASES OF THE PITUITARY BODY

The hypophysis cerebri consists of two lobes, (*a*) an anterior lobe, originating from the roof of the pharynx and composed of large granular epithelial cells arranged in columns surrounded by large venous spaces into which their secretion discharges; and (*b*) a smaller posterior lobe which arises from the floor of the third ventricle and is composed (1) of a central neuroglial portion (pars nervosa) and (2) an investment of epithelial cells (pars intermedia). The secretion of the posterior lobe is supposed by some to find its way into the cerebro-spinal fluid.

Complete experimental removal of the gland is fatal (Paulesco). Partial removal leads, in young animals, to a stunting of growth, to adiposity and failure of sexual development, in adult animals to adiposity and genital dystrophy (Cushing).

Modern knowledge of the functions of the gland began with the studies of Marie on the relation of the pituitary gland to acromegaly and gigantism. Then Schäfer and Oliver discovered that injection of an extract of the gland caused a rise in the blood pressure. Since these two cardinal observations an enormous amount of work has been done, and we are beginning to appreciate the remarkable influence of this small structure upon the processes of development and metabolism. Briefly, the anterior lobe influences growth and development, and is necessary to life; the posterior lobe influences the metabolism of the carbohydrates and fats.

Disturbances in the function of the pituitary gland are not clearly grouped, as in the thyroid, into the effects of deficiency and excess, though one can usually differentiate states of hyper- and hypopituitarism. The hypophysis appears to be closely related to other glands of internal secretion and, as is well known, involvement of any member of the series causes a physiological readjustment in the activity of the others. Owing to the situation of the gland it is very liable to feel the effect of pressure in neighboring or even in distant lesions, so that disturbance of function may be due not only to a primary involvement, but to secondary compression. As a result of his experimental work and studies of clinical cases Cushing prefers to group the conditions associated with disturbance of the function of the gland under the term "dyspituitarism" and recognizes a number of groups:

(*a*) Cases of tumor growth showing signs of distortion of neighboring structures, and also the constitutional effects of altered glandular activity. The X-rays show changes in the configuration of the pituitary fossa; there are pressure signs on the adjacent cranial nerves, bi-temporal hemianopia, optic atrophy, and occulomotor palsies. Uncinate fits are not unusual. Epistaxis is common and cerebro-spinal rhinorrhœa may occur in rare cases. The constitutional effects vary from primary over-activity to glandular underactivity.

(*b*) Cases in which the neighborhood manifestations are pronounced but the constitutional features are slight. The characteristic regional signs of tumor are marked, but there may be slight or very transient evidence of disturbed glandular activity, perhaps only disturbed carbohydrate metabolism with adiposity.

(*c*) Cases in which the neighborhood manifestations are absent or slight, though the glandular symptoms are unmistakable. The gland is not so large as to cause regional symptoms. There are skeletal changes on the side of overgrowth or undergrowth. Disturbance of carbohydrate metabolism is a matter of modified posterior lobe activity, whether occurring as a lowering of the assimilation limit, which is so often associated with the early stages of acromegaly, or a great increase in tolerance, such as characterizes all grades of hypopituitarism. In posterior lobe insufficiency there are a tendency to the deposition of fat, a subnormal temperature, drowsiness, slow pulse, dry skin, loss of hair, and an extraordinary high tolerance for sugars. Most of the cases of acromegaly fall in this group and show at first evidences of hyperpituitarism, and later of insufficiency. In the adult, adiposity, high sugar tolerance, subnormal temperature, psychic manifestations, and sexual infantilism of the reversive type indicate hypopituitarism and may exist without the regional symptoms of tumor (Cushing).

(*d*) Hypophysial symptoms may be shown by patients with internal hydrocephalus from any cause, probably by interference with the passage of the posterior lobe secretion into the cerebro-spinal fluid, and this obstructive dyspituitarism may result from any lesion, inflammatory or neoplastic, in the neighborhood of the third ventricle.

These are the most important of the groups to which Cushing refers, but there are also cases with manifestations indicating involvement of other internal secretions together with that of the hypophysis, and a large group in which transient hypophysial symptoms occur, as, in pregnancy, cranial injuries and infectious diseases.

It is quite clear that disturbances in the function of the pituitary gland may lead to remarkable changes in growth; *hyperpituitarism* may lead to gigantism, when the process antedates ossification of the epiphyses—the Launois type; to acromegaly when it is of later date; *hypopituitarism* to adiposity, with skeletal and sexual infantilism when the process originates in childhood—the Frölich type; to adiposity and sexual infantilism of the reversive type when originating in the adult.

Much has been done to clear the subject, but much remains, particularly to clear up the relations of the various types of infantilism which have been described—the Lorain, the Brissaud, the pancreatic, the intestinal—to the different internal secretions. One condition is important enough to merit separate consideration, the one differentiated clearly by Marie and known as acromegaly. (The student is referred to Hastings Gilford's "Disorders of Post-natal Growth," to Vincent's "Innere Secretion," *Ergeb. d. Phys.*, IX and X, and to Cushing's work, "The Pituitary Gland and Its Disorders," J. B. Lippincott Co., 1912.)

ACROMEGALY

Definition.—A dystrophy characterized by increase in size of the face and extremities associated with perverted function of the pituitary gland.

The essence of the disease is a hyperpituitarism which, if it antedates ossification of the epiphyses, leads to gigantism, and in the adult leads to overgrowth of the skeleton and other changes which we know as acromegaly.

Etiology.—It is a rare disease, and rather more frequent in women. It affects particularly persons of large size. Twenty per cent. of acromegalics are above six feet in height when the symptoms begin, and fully 40 per cent. of giants are acromegalics (Sternberg). Trauma, the infections, and emotional shock have preceded the onset of the disease.

Pathology.—Practically all of the cases show changes in the pituitary gland, hyperplasia, adenoma, fibroma, or sarcoma, causing distention of the sella turcica and, in the late stages, pressure on surrounding structures; the symptoms of the disease are in part due to disturbance of the function of the gland, and in part to the pressure on the adjacent parts.

The bones show the most striking changes; there is a general enlargement of the extremities, but the skeleton on the whole is more or less affected. The enlargement, due to a periosteal growth, is most evident in the hands and feet. The bones of the face are always involved. The orbital arches, frontal prominences, zygoma, malar, and nasal bones are all increased in size, the lower jaw is elongated, thickened, and the teeth separated. The X-ray picture shows very characteristic changes in the sella turcica. The skin and subcutaneous tissues are thickened, so that the enlargement of the extremities is not altogether bony, and the hypertrophy is seen in the soft parts of the face as well.

The brain has been found large, but the most important changes are those due to pressure at the base. The internal organs have been found enlarged, and in Osborne's case the heart weighed 2 lbs. 9 oz.

Symptoms.—As already mentioned, when the pituitary gland is involved in tumor growth, which is the common condition in acromegaly, the symptoms may be grouped into those due to the mechanical effects and those associated with perversion of the secretion of the gland.

(*a*) Regional Symptoms.—Headache is common, usually frontal. Somnolence has been noted in many cases, and in one of my patients was the first symptom. Ocular features occur in a large proportion of the cases, bitemporal hemianopia, optic atrophy, and, in the late stages, pressure on the third nerve and the abducens. One eye only may be affected. Exophthalmos may occur. Deafness is not infrequent. Irritability of temper, marked change in the disposition, great depression, and progressive dementia have been noted. Epistaxis and rhinorrhœa may be present.

(*b*) Symptoms due to the perversion of the internal secretion itself form the striking features of the disease. The patient's friends first notice a gradual increase in the features, which become heavy and thick; or the patient himself may notice that he takes a larger size of hat, or with the progressive enlargement of the hands a larger size of gloves. The enlargement of the extremities does not interfere with their free use.

The hypertrophy is general, involving all the tissues, and gives a curious spadelike character to the hands. The lines on the palms are much deepened. The wrists may be enlarged, but the arms are rarely affected. The feet are involved like the hands and are uniformly enlarged. The big toe, however, may be much larger in proportion. The nails are usually broad and large, but there is no curving, and the terminal phalanges are not bulbous. The head increases in volume, but not as much in proportion as the face, which becomes much elongated and enlarged in consequence of the increase in the size of the superior and inferior maxillary bones. The latter in particular increases greatly in size, and often projects below the upper jaw. The alveolar processes are widened and the teeth are often separated. The soft parts also increase in size, and the nostrils are large and broad. The eyelids are sometimes greatly thickened, and the ears enormously hypertrophied. The tongue in some instances becomes greatly enlarged. Late in the disease the spine may be affected and the back bowed—kyphosis. The bones of the thorax may slowly and progressively enlarge. With this gradual increase in size the skin of the hands and face may appear normal. Sometimes it is slightly altered in color, coarse, or flabby, but it has not the dry, harsh appearance of the skin in myxœdema. The muscles are sometimes wasted.

Also associated with disturbance of the function of the gland is the diabetes noticed in many cases, which is common in the early stages; in the advanced stages there is an extraordinary high tolerance for sugar. Symptoms on the part of other ductless glands are common. Goitre is of frequent occurrence. Amenorrhœa is the earliest symptom in women. Impotence is common in advanced cases in men.

The various symptoms of the disease are now readily explained with the knowledge we possess of the functions of the gland, which have already been discussed.

Treatment.—The use of extracts of the gland has been extensively tried. Possibly now with our better knowledge of the functions of the different parts we shall arrive at a more intelligent organo-therapy. Unquestionably glandular therapy should only be used when the condition has passed into its ultimate stage of glandular insufficiency—a stage which is indicated usually by an increased sugar tolerance.

Surgical treatment has been carried out in a number of cases following Schloffer's suggestion. Doubtless the chief surgical indication is to give relief to the local pressure symptoms when there is marked glandular enlargement. The tumor or glandular struma may be reached by a transphenoidal or a subtemporal route. Partial removal of the growth or the evacuation of a cyst under favorable circumstances may save the optic nerves from complete pressure atrophy.

VII. INFANTILISM

Definition.—The failure of the appearance of the primary and secondary sexual characteristics, together with the retention of mental and bodily conditions of childhood.

Etiology.—It is not possible at present to make a satisfactory classification either of the causes or of the cases of infantilism—in some no cause is evident, in others the failure in development has followed obvious disease, and there are cases directly dependent upon loss of some internal secretion.

I. **Cachectic infantilism** is by no means uncommon, as any serious chronic malady may delay sexual development. For example, the children affected with hookworm disease may reach the age of 20 or older before the change from the infantile to the adult state. Syphilis is a very common cause. In regions in which malaria is very prevalent delayed sexual development is not uncommon in children, and we see it not infrequently in cases of congenital heart disease. There is also a toxic infantilism due to the slow and prolonged action of alcohol and tobacco.

II. Idiopathic Infantilism (*So-called Lorain Type*).—"In this variety the figure is so small that, at first sight, it looks like that of a child. When the patient is stripped, however, his outlines are seen to be those of an adult, and not those of childhood. The head is proportionately small, and the trunk well formed; for the shoulders are broad compared to the hips, and the bony prominences and the muscles stand out distinctly. We have before us a miniature man (or woman, as the case may be), and not one who has retained the characteristics of childhood beyond the proper time. There is, indeed, no growth of facial, pubic or axillary hair, yet the genital organs, though small, are well shaped and quite large enough for the size of the body. The intelligence in both sexes is generally normal" (John Thomson).

The cause of this form is yet unknown, but it is probably associated with perversion of the pituitary secretions. It has also been called an "angioplastic infantilism," in the belief that it was due to a defect of development of the vascular system.

III. The Hormonic Type.—Here we are on safer ground, as we know definitely of several varieties directly dependent upon changes in the ductless glands. The most important of these are:

(*a*) Thyroidal or Cretinoid Infantilism.—This form has already been described.

(*b*) The Frölich type, dystrophia adiposo-genitalis, associated with a tumor of the pituitary region, is characterized by great obesity and genital hypoplasia. The symptoms are due to a secretory deficit, for they are capable of experimental reproduction by partial glandular extirpation in animals (Cushing). There are adult and infantile types, just as there are in myxœdema; in the former the individual becomes fat and the sexual organs revert to the preadolescent state. The *Brissaud type* is in all probability due to hypopituitarism. A round, chubby face, under-developed skeleton, prominent abdomen, large layer of fat over the whole body, rudimentary sexual organs, no growth of hair except on the head, and absence of the second dentition, are some of the prominent features of this form, which Brissaud attributed to hypothyroidism, but which appears more likely to be due to dyspituitarism.

(*c*) Pancreatico-intestinal Type.—Bramwell, Herter, Freedman, and others have reported cases of infantilism associated with intestinal changes. Bramwell thought the pancreas was at fault, and his cases improved remarkably under treatment with pancreatic extract. In Herter's case there were looseness of the bowels, often fatty stools, and a change in the flora of the intestine with a rise in the ethereal sulphates in the urine.

IV. Progeria.—Under this term Hastings Gilford has described a condition in children of incomplete development (infantilism) with premature decay. The facial appearance, the attitude, the loss of hair, wasting of the skin, are those of old age, and post mortem the most extensive fibroid changes in the organs, particularly in the arteries and kidneys. The condition is probably associated with unknown changes in the internal secretions.

SECTION XI

DISEASES OF THE NERVOUS SYSTEM

A. GENERAL INTRODUCTION

The Neurone.—ITS STRUCTURE.—The nervous system is a combination of an immense number of units called neurones and all having an essentially similar structure. Each is composed of a receptive cell body and of conducting elements—namely, protoplasmic processes or dendrites, and the axis-cylinder process or axone. The dendrites conduct impulses toward the cell body (cellulipetal conduction) and the axones conduct them away from the cell (cellulifugal conduction). Depending upon whether the axones conduct impulses in a direction away from or toward the cerebrum they are called efferent or afferent. The axis-cylinder process gives off at varying intervals lateral branches called collaterals, running at right angles to the process, and these, and finally the axis-cylinder process itself, split up at their terminations into many fine fibres, forming the end brushes. These, known as arborizations, surround the body of one or more of the many other cells, or interlace with their protoplasmic processes. Thus, the terminals of the axone of one neurone are related to the dendrites and cell bodies of other neurones by contact or by concrescence.

FUNCTION OF THE NEURONE.—As already stated, the function of the neurone is to conduct nervous impulses. Reduced to its simplest form, the mode of action may be represented by two cells, one of which, reacting to the environment, conducts impulses inward, whereas the other, awakened by this afferent impulse, conducts an impulse outward. This reflex response Marshall Hall showed to be the fundamental principle of action of the nervous system. The environment acts on the afferent neurones through special sense organs, so that a variety of afferent impulses, olfactory, visual, auditory, gustatory, tactile, painful, thermic, muscular, visceral, and vascular, may be originated. The efferent neurones convey impulses outward to non-nervous tissues, to the skeletal, visceral, and vascular muscles and to the secretory glands, whose activities may thus be augmented or inhibited. The more important reflex centres lie in the bulbo-spinal axis. The situation of the vascular and respiratory centres in the bulb makes it the vital centre of the body. In the spinal cord the location of many reflex centres, particularly those for the muscle tendons and for some of the viscera, is represented in the table on page 898. The visceral mechanism is almost wholly regulated by the bulbo-spinal axis, and its reactions are usually unperceived. Only in conditions of disease do the visceral reflexes "rise into consciousness," and it is at such times that the referred pains and areas of tenderness are produced in the skin-fields of the spinal segments corresponding to the centre for registration of the visceral reflex.

Degeneration and Regeneration of the Neurone.—The nutrition of the neurone depends in large part upon the condition of the cell body, and this in turn upon the activity of the nucleus. If the cell is injured in any manner the processes degenerate, or the processes separated from the cell degenerate. Though the nerve cells cease to multiply soon after birth, they nevertheless retain remarkable powers of growth and repair. Injury to the cell body may not be recovered from, but if the axone be severed and degeneration take place in consequence, it may under favorable circumstances be replaced by sprouts from the central stump, and its function be regained. Bethe and others believe that the peripheral section, independently of the cell body, has the power of regeneration. It is probable, however, that both factors play a part in the regeneration—namely, the down growth of the axone from the central end of the divided nerve as well as the changes in the periphery, which are most marked in the cells of the sheath of Schwann.

Cell Systems.—The cell bodies of the neurones are collected more or less closely together in the gray matter of the brain and spinal cord and in the ganglia of the peripheral nerves. Their processes, especially the axis-cylinder processes, run for the most part in the white tracts of the brain and spinal cord and in the peripheral nerves. In this way the different parts of the central nervous system are brought into relation with each other and with the rest of the body. Furthermore, the axis-cylinder processes arising from cells subserving similar functions are collected together into bundles or tracts, and though in many cases the course of these tracts and the functions which they possess are extremely complicated and as yet have not been completely unravelled, nevertheless some of them are simple and fairly well understood. By the study of the degenerations that have resulted from injury or from the toxins of certain diseases which possess an affinity for one or another of these individual tracts or systems, it has been possible to trace the course of certain of them through the nervous system. Fortunately for the clinician, the best understood and the simplest system in its arrangement is that which conveys motor impulses from the cortex to the periphery—the so-called pyramidal tract.

The Motor System.—Motor impulses starting in the left side of the brain cause contractions of muscles on the right side of the body, and those from the right side of the brain in muscles of the left side of the body. Leaving out of consideration some few exceptions, it may be stated as a general rule that the motor path is crossed, and that the crossing takes place in the upper segment (Figs. 10 and 11). Every muscular movement, even the simplest, requires the activity of many neurones. In the production of each movement special neurones are brought into play in a definite combination, and acting in this combination specific movement is the result. In other words, all the movements of the body are represented in the central nervous system by combinations of neurones—that is, they are localized. Muscular movements are localized in every part of the motor path, so that in cases of disease of the nervous system a study of the motor defect often enables one to fix upon the site of the process, and it would be hard to over-estimate the importance of a thorough knowledge of such localization. A voluntary motor impulse starting

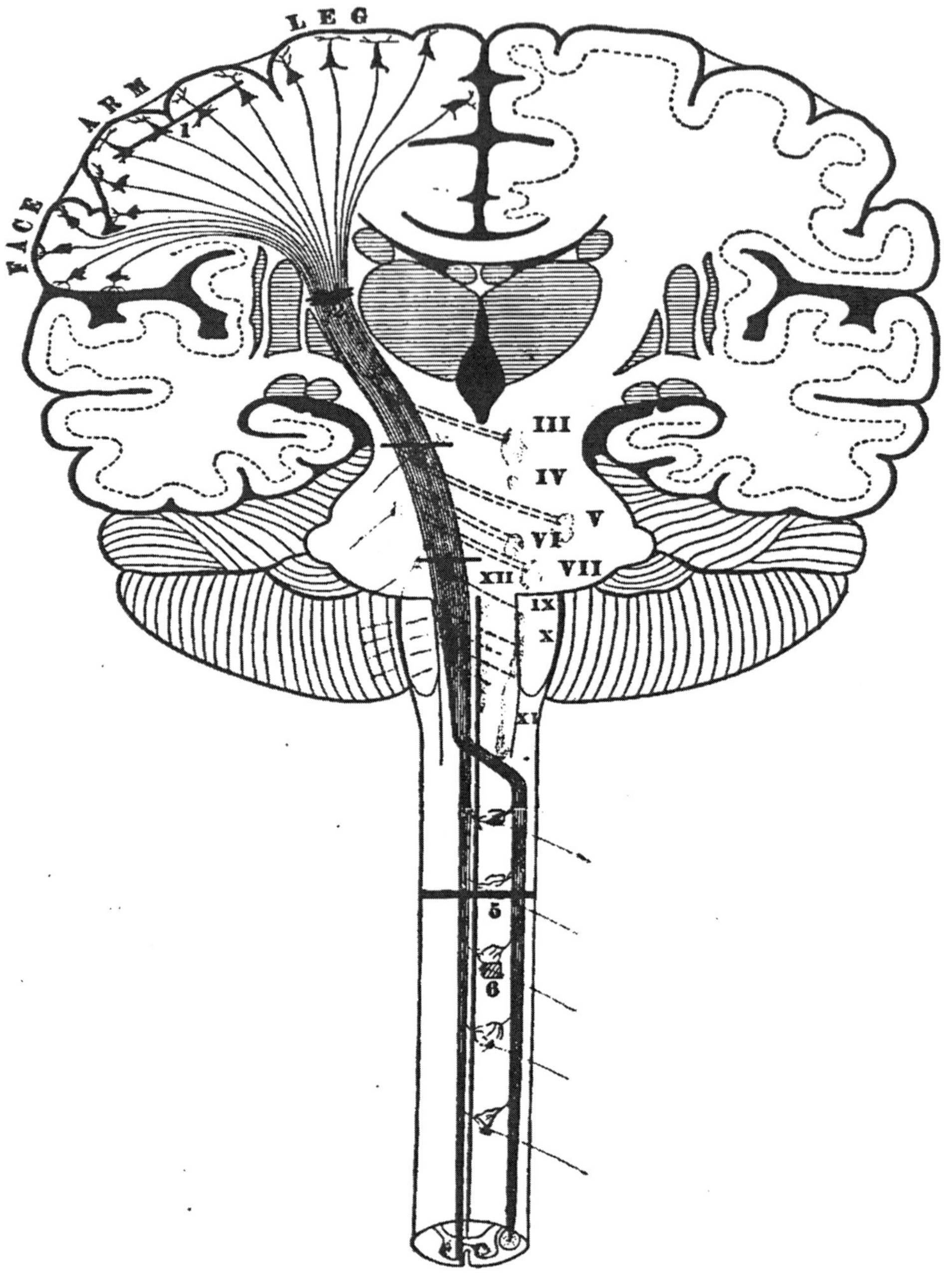

FIG. 10.—DIAGRAM OF MOTOR PATH FROM LEFT BRAIN. The upper segment is black, the lower red. The nuclei of the motor cerebral nerves are shown in red on the right side; on the left side the cerebral nerves of that side are indicated. A lesion at 1 would cause upper segment paralysis in the arm of the opposite side—cerebral monoplegia; at 2, upper segment paralysis of the whole opposite side of the body—hemiplegia; at 3, upper segment paralysis of the opposite face, arm, and leg, and lower segment paralysis of the eye muscles on the same side—crossed paralysis; at 4, upper segment paralysis of opposite arm and leg, and lower segment paralysis of the face and the external rectus on the same side—crossed paralysis; at 5, upper segment paralysis of all muscles below lesion, and lower segment paralysis of muscles represented at level of lesion—spinal paraplegia; at 6, lower segment paralysis of muscles localized at seat of lesion—anterior poliomyelitis. (Van Gehuchten, modified.)

from the brain cortex must pass through at least two neurones before it can reach the muscles, and we therefore speak of the motor tract as being composed of two segments—an upper and a lower.

THE LOWER MOTOR SEGMENT.—The neurones of the lower segment have the cell bodies and their protoplasmic processes in the different levels of the ventral horns of the spinal cord and in the motor nuclei of the cerebral nerves. The axis-cylinder processes of the lower motor neurones leave the spinal cord in the ventral roots and run in the peripheral nerves, to be distributed to all the muscles of the body, where they end in arborizations in the motor end plates. These neurones are direct—that is, their cell bodies, their processes, and the muscles in which they end are all on the same side of the body.

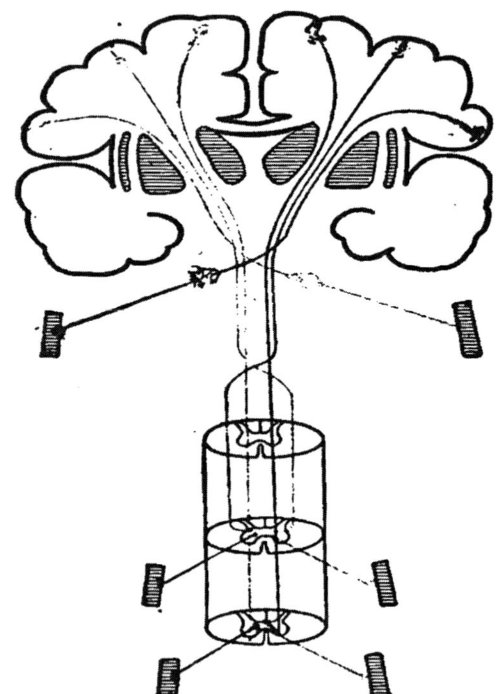

FIG. 11.—DIAGRAM OF MOTOR PATH FROM EACH HEMISPHERE, SHOWING THE CROSSING OF THE PATH, WHICH TAKES PLACE IN THE UPPER SEGMENT BOTH FOR THE CRANIAL AND SPINAL NERVES. (Van Gehuchten, colored.)

The ventral roots of the spinal cord are collected, from above down, into small groups, which, after joining with the dorsal roots of the same level of the cord, leave the spinal canal between the vertebræ as the spinal nerves. That part of the cord from which the roots forming a single spinal nerve arise is called a segment, and corresponds to the nerve which arises from it and not to the vertebra to which it may be opposite. With the exception of the cervical region, in which all the nerve roots but the eighth emerge from above the vertebræ, the roots of each segment for the remainder of the cord leave the spinal canal below the vertebra of corresponding number, and consequently, owing to the fact that during growth the bony canal lengthens much more than the cord itself, the more tailward one goes the greater is the discrepancy in position between each spinal segment and its particular vertebra. This must be borne in mind when determining upon the site of a lesion known to occupy a given segment, for it may lie far above the vertebra of like number and name. A chart has been prepared from numerous measurements by Reid showing the level of the various segments of the cord in relation to the spines of the vertebræ. The axis-cylinder processes which go to make up any one peripheral nerve do not necessarily arise from the same segment of the spinal cord; in fact, most peripheral nerves contain processes from several often quite widely separated segments. Most of the long striped muscles, furthermore, having originated in the embryo from more than one myatome, are innervated from more than one segment.

Our knowledge of the localization of the muscular movements in the gray matter of the lower motor segment is far from complete, but enough is known to aid materially in determining the site of a spinal lesion. The following table, in which is included for each of the spinal segments the centres of representation for the more important skeletal muscles, the main reflex centres, and the main location of the segmental skin-field, has been prepared from the studies of Starr, Edinger, Wichmann, Sherrington, Bolk, and others:

LOCALIZATION OF THE FUNCTIONS IN THE SEGMENTS OF THE SPINAL CORD

SEGMENT.	STRIPED MUSCLES.	REFLEX.	SKIN-FIELDS (CF. FIGS. 16 AND 17).
I, II and III C.	Splenius capitis. Hyoid muscles. Sterno-mastoid. Trapezius. Diaphragm (C III–V). Levator scapulæ (C III–V).	Hypochondrium (?). Sudden inspiration produced by sudden pressure beneath the lower border of ribs (diaphragmatic).	Back of head to vertex. Neck (upper part).
IV C.	Trapezius. Diaphragm. Levator scapulæ. Scaleni (C IV–T I). Teres minor. Supraspinatus. Rhomboid.	Dilatation of the pupil produced by irritation of neck. Reflex through the sympathetic (C IV–T I).	Neck (lower part to second rib). Upper shoulder.
V C.	Diaphragm. Teres minor. Supra and infra spinatus (C V–VI). Rhomboid. Subscapularis. Deltoid. Biceps. Brachialis anticus. Supinator longus (C V–VII). Supinator brevis (C V–VII). Pectoralis (clavicular part). Serratus magnus.	Scapular (C V–T I). Irritation of skin over the scapula produces contraction of the scapular muscles. Supinator longus and biceps. Tapping their tendons produces flexion of forearm.	Outer side of shoulder and upper arm over deltoid region.
VI C.	Teres minor and major Infraspinatus. Deltoid. Biceps. Brachialis anticus. Supinator longus. Supinator brevis. Pectoralis (clavicular part). Serratus magnus (C V–VIII). Coraco-brachialis. Pronator teres. Triceps (outer and long heads). Extensors of wrist (C VI–VIII).	Triceps. Tapping elbow tendon produces extension of forearm. Posterior wrist. Tapping tendons causes extension of hand (C VI–VII).	Outer side of forearm, front and back. Outer half of hand (?).
VII C.	Teres major. Subscapularis. Deltoid (posterior part). Pectoralis major (costal part). Pectoralis minor. Serratus magnus. Pronators of wrist. Triceps. Extensors of wrist and fingers. Flexors of wrist. Latissimus dorsi (C VI–VIII).	Scapulo-humeral. Tapping the inner lower edge of scapula causes adduction of the arm. Anterior wrist. Tapping anterior tendons causes flexion of wrist (C VII–VIII).	Inner side and back of arm and forearm. Radial half of the hand.

Localization of the Functions in the Segments of the Spinal Cord *(Continued)*

Segment.	Striped Muscles.	Reflex.	Skin-Fields (cf. Figs. 16 and 17).
VIII C.	Pectoralis major (costal part). Pronator quadratus. Flexors of wrist and fingers. Latissimus. Radial lumbricales and interossei.	Palmar. Stroking palm causes closure of fingers.	Forearm and hand, inner half.
I T.	Lumbricales and interossei. Thenar and hypothenar eminences (C VII–T I).		Upper arm, inner half.
II to XII T.	Muscles of back and abdomen. Erectores spinæ (T I–LV). Intercostals (T I–T XII). Rectus abdominis (T V-T XII). External oblique (T V–XII). Internal oblique (T VII–L I). Transversalis (T VII–L I).	Epigastric. Tickling mammary region causes retraction of epigastrium (T IV–VII). Abdominal. Stroking side of abdomen causes retraction of belly (T IX–XII).	Skin of chest and abdomen in oblique dorso-ventral zones. The nipple lies between the zone of T IV and T V. The umbilicus lies in the field of T X.
I L.	Lower part of external and internal oblique and transversalis. Quadratus lumborum (L I–II). Cremaster. Psoas major and minor (?).	Cremasteric. Stroking inner thigh causes retraction of scrotum (L I–II).	Skin over lowest abdominal zone and groin.
II L.	Psoas major and minor. Iliacus. Pectineus. Sartorius (lower part). Flexors of knee (Remak). Adductor longus and brevis.		Front of thigh.
III L.	Sartorius (lower part). Adductors of thigh. Quadriceps femoris (L II-L IV). Inner rotators of thigh. Abductors of thigh.	Patellar tendon. Tapping tendon causes extension of leg. "Knee-jerk."	Front and inner side of thigh.
IV L.	Flexors of knee (Ferrier). Quadriceps femoris. Adductors of thigh. Abductors of thigh. Extensors of ankle (tibalis anticus). Glutei (medius and minor).	Gluteal. Stroking buttock causes dimpling in fold of buttock (L IV–V).	Mainly inner side of thigh and leg to ankle.
V L.	Flexors of knee (ham-string muscles) (L IV–S II). Outward rotators of thigh. Glutei. Flexors of ankle (gastrocnemius and soleus) (L IV–S II). Extensors of toes (L IV–S I). Peronæi.		Back of leg, and part of foot.

Localization of the Functions in the Segments of the Spinal Cord (*Continued*)

Segment.	Striped Muscles.	Reflex.	Skin-Fields (cf. Figs. 16 and 17).
I to II S.	Flexors of ankle (L V–S II). Long flexor of toes (L V–S II). Peronæi. Intrinsic muscles of foot.	Foot reflex. Extension of Achilles tendon causes flexion of ankle (S I–II). Ankle-clonus. Plantar. Tickling sole of foot causes flexion of toes or extension of great toe and flexion of others.	Back of thigh, leg, and foot; outer side.
III to V S.	Perineal muscles. Levator and sphincter ani (S I–III).	Vesical and anal reflexes.	Skin over sacrum and buttock. Anus. Perineum. Genitals.

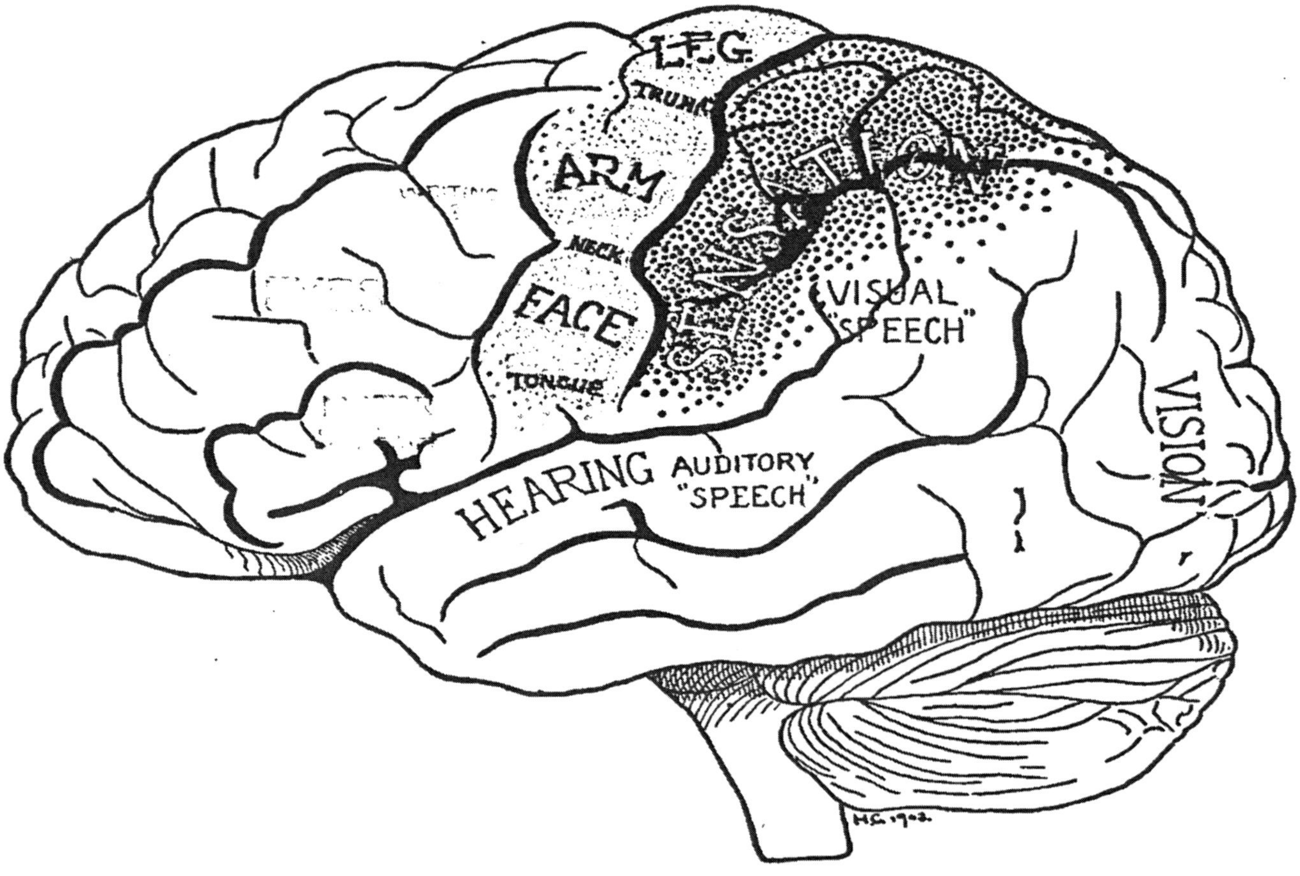

Fig. 12.—Diagrammatic Representation of Cortical Localization in the Left Hemisphere, Showing the Speech Centres. The motor areas determined by unipolar faradic excitation of the anthropoid cortex (Sherrington and Grünbaum) are here shown stippled in red and lie anterior to the Rolandic fissure. The sensory areas presumably lie posterior to this fissure and are roughly indicated in blue without accurate delineation. Lying as it does on the upper surface of the hemisphere, the leg area should not be visible on a lateral view such as is given here.

The Upper Motor Segment and Motor Areas of the Cortex.—The cell bodies of the upper motor neurones are found in the brain cortex lying for the most part in a strip anterior to the fissure of Rolando, and it is in this region that we find the movements of the body again represented.

The clinical studies of Hughlings Jackson, the experiments of Hitzig and Fritsch and of Ferrier, and the anatomical studies of tract myelinization by Flechsig laid the foundation for the great mass of most excellent work which has been done upon this subject. We owe much to Victor Horsley and his associates for their careful researches in this direction. True motor responses are elicited only by stimulation *anterior* to the Rolandic fissure; practically no point over the ascending frontal convolution fails to respond to stimulation. There is but slight extension of the motor cortex on to the paracentral lobule of the mesial surface of the brain. Movements are obtainable not only from the exposed part of the convolution, but also from its hidden surface to the very depths of the Rolandic sulcus. There is an area of representation for the trunk between the centres for the leg and arm, and also for the neck between those of the arm and face. The superior and inferior genua are the landmarks which indicate the situation of these small areas of representation for trunk and neck. These results have in large measure been confirmed by Cushing by unipolar electrical stimulation of the human cortex in a number of brain cases. From above down the motor areas occur in the following order: leg, trunk, arm, neck, head (Fig. 12). Those of the leg and arm occupy the upper half of the convolution, and that for the head, including movements of the face, jaws, tongue, and larynx, the lower half.

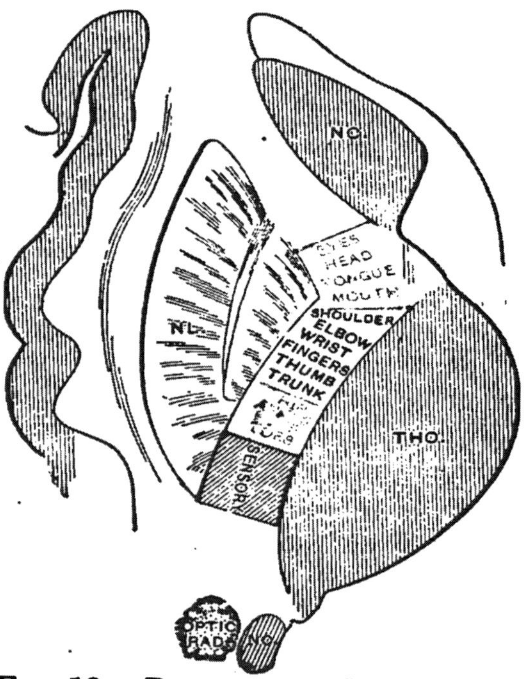

Fig. 13.—Diagram of Motor and Sensory Representation in the Internal Capsule. NL., Lenticular nucleus. NC., Caudate nucleus. THO., Optic thalamus. The motor paths are red and black, the sensory are blue.

The speech centres are indicated in the diagram (Fig. 12) in accordance with the generally accepted views: that for motor speech occupies the posterior part of the left third frontal or Broca's convolution. It is a disputed point whether or not there is a separate centre presiding over the movements employed in writing. Some have assumed such a centre to be present in the second frontal convolution as indicated on the diagram. The conjugate movement of head and eyes to the opposite side has commonly been found in apes to follow stimulation of the external surface of the frontal lobe. Similarly movements of the eyes may be elicited from the occipital cortex, but probably none of these reactions are comparable to the more simple movements through the pyramidal tract which follow stimulation of the ascending frontal convolution.

The axis-cylinder processes of the upper motor neurones after leaving the gray matter of the motor cortex pass into the white matter of the brain and form part of the corona radiata. They converge and pass between the basal ganglia in the internal capsule. Here the motor axis-cylinders are collected into a compact bundle—the pyramidal tract—occupying the knee and anterior two-thirds of the posterior limb of the internal capsule. The order in which the movements of the opposite side of the body are represented at this level, as learned from experimental observations on apes, is given in Fig. 13.

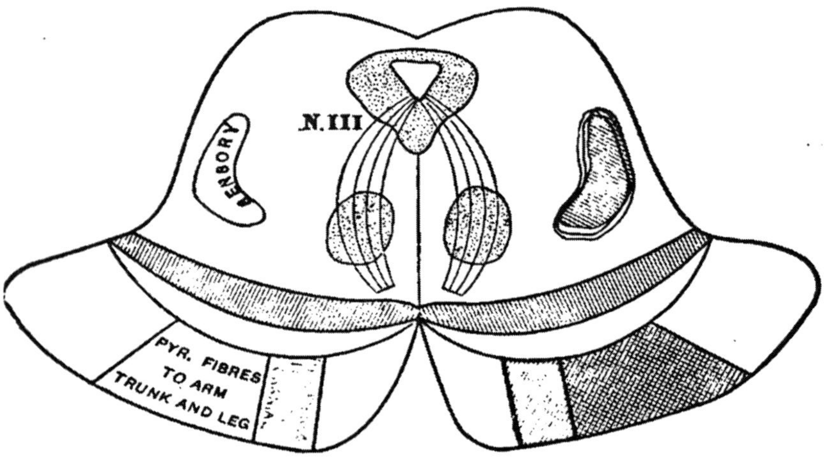

FIG. 14.—Diagram of Motor and Sensory Paths in Crura.

After passing through the internal capsule the fibres of the pyramidal tract leave the hemisphere by the crus, of which they occupy about the middle three-fifths (Fig. 14). The movements of the tongue and lips are represented nearest the middle line.

As soon as the tract enters the crus, some of its axis-cylinder processes leave it and cross the middle line to end in arborizations about the ganglion cells in the nucleus of the third nerve on the opposite side; and in this way, as the pyramidal tract passes down, it gives off at different levels fibres which end in the nuclei of all the motor cerebral nerves on the opposite side of the body. Some fibres, however, go to the nuclei of the same side. From the crus the pyramidal tract runs through the pons and forms in the medulla oblongata the pyramid, which gives its name to the tract. At the lower part of the medulla, after the fibres going to the cerebral nerves have crossed the middle line, a large proportion of the remaining fibres cross, decussating with those from the opposite pyramid, and pass into the opposite side of the spinal cord, forming the crossed pyramidal tract of the lateral column (fasciculus cerebrospinalis lateralis) (Fig. 15, 1). The smaller number of fibres which do not at this time cross descend in the ventral column of the same side, forming the

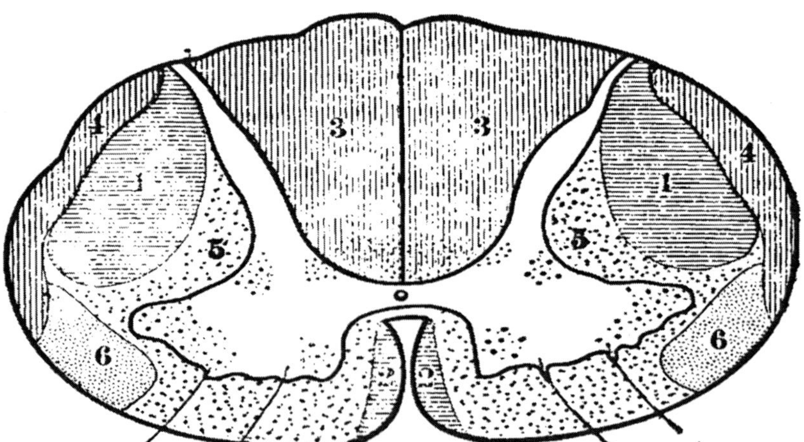

FIG. 15.—DIAGRAM OF CROSS-SECTION OF THE SPINAL CORD, SHOWING MOTOR, RED, AND SENSORY, BLUE, PATHS. 1, Lateral pyramidal tract. 2, Ventral pyramidal tract. 3, Dorsal columns. 4, Direct cerebellar tract. 5, Ventro-lateral ground bundles. 6, Ventro-lateral ascending tract of Gowers. (Van Gehuchten, colored.)

direct pyramidal tract, or Türck's column (fasciculus cerebro-spinalis ventralis) (Fig. 15, 2).

At every level of the spinal cord axis-cylinder processes leave the crossed pyramidal tract to enter the ventral horns and end about the cell bodies of the lower motor neurones. The tract diminishes in size from above downward. The fibres of the direct pyramidal tract cross at different levels in the ventral white commissure, and also, it is believed, end about cells in the ventral horns on the opposite side of the cord. This tract usually ends about the middle of the thoracic region of the cord.

The Sensory System.—The path for sensory conduction is more complicated than the motor path, and in its simplest form is composed of at least three sets of neurones, one above the other. The cell bodies of the lowest neurones are in the ganglia, on the dorsal roots of the spinal nerves, and the ganglia of the sensory cerebral nerves. These ganglion cells have a special form, having apparently but a single process, which, soon after leaving the cell, divides in a T-shaped manner, one portion running into the central nervous system and the other to the periphery of the body. Embryological and comparative anatomical studies have made it seem probable that the peripheral sensory fibre, the process which conducts toward the cell, represents the protoplasmic processes, while that which conducts away from the cell is the axis-cylinder process. In the peripheral sensory nerves we have, then, the dendrites of the lower sensory neurones. These start in the periphery of the body from their various specialized end organs. The axis-cylinder processes leave the ganglia and enter the spinal cord by the dorsal roots of the spinal nerves. After entering the cord each axis-cylinder process divides into an ascending and a descending branch, which run in the dorsal fasciculi. The descending branch runs but a short distance, and ends in the gray matter of the same side of the cord. It gives off a number of collaterals, which also end in the gray matter. The ascending branch may end in the gray matter soon after entering, or it may run in the dorsal fasciculi as far as the medulla, to end about the nuclei there. In any case it does not cross the middle line. The lower sensory neurone is direct.

The cells about which the axis-cylinder processes and their collaterals of the lower sensory neurone end are of various kinds. They are known as sensory neurones of the second order. In the first place, some of them end about the cell bodies of the lower motor neurones, forming the path for reflexes. They also end about cells whose axis-cylinder processes cross the middle line and run to the opposite side of the brain. In the spinal cord these cells are found in the different parts of the gray matter, and their axis-cylinder processes run in the opposite ventro-lateral ascending tract of Gowers (Fig. 15, 6) and in the ground bundles (fasciculus lateralis proprius and fasciculus ventralis proprius).

In the medulla the nuclei of the dorsal fasciculi (nucleus fasciculi gracilis and nucleus fasciculi cuneati) contain for the most part cells of this character. Their axis-cylinder processes, after crossing, run toward the brain in the medial lemniscus or bundle of the fillet; certain of the longitudinal bundles in the formatio reticularis also represent sensory paths from the spinal cord and medulla toward higher centres. The fibres of the medial lemniscus or fillet do not, however, run directly to the cerebral cortex. They end about cells in the ventro-lateral portion of the optic thalamus, and the tract is continued on by way of another set of neurones, which send processes to end in the cortex of the posterior central and perietal convolutions. This is the most direct path of sensory conduction, but by no means the only one. The peripheral sensory neurones may also end about cells in the cord whose axones run but a short distance toward the brain before ending again in the gray matter, and the path, if path it can be called, is made up of a series of these superimposed neurones. The gray matter of the cord itself is also believed to offer paths of sensory conduction. All these paths reach the tegmentum and optic thalamus, and thence are distributed to the cortex along with the other sensory paths. There may also be paths of sensory conduction through the cerebellum by way of the direct cerebellar tract and Gowers' bundle.

From this short summary it is evident that the possible paths for the conduction of afferent impulses are many, and become more complex as the various tracts approach the brain where our knowledge of them is somewhat indefinite. The anatomical arrangement of the two lower orders of sensory neurones is, however, sufficiently well understood to be of great clinical value. We have seen in the case of the motor neurones that the distribution of the peripheral nerves to the muscles, owing largely to the interlacing into plexuses of the neurones from the various spinal units, is quite different from that of the ventral roots themselves, and the same rule holds true for the peripheral nerve and dorsal root distribution for the cutaneous areas. The cutaneous fields corresponding to the peripheral nerves are well known, and although our knowledge of the exact site and outline of some of the segmental skin-fields, represented by the dorsal roots, is less accurately established, nevertheless they are sufficiently well understood to be of aid in determining the segmental level of spinal cord and of dorsal root lesions. Information concerning the topography in the adult of these skin units or dermatomes has been obtained from various sources; from morphological studies; from anatomical dissections; from physiological experimentation, particularly in Sherrington's hands; from the study of anæsthesias in clinical cases after traumatic injuries to the cord, and from Head's studies of the distribution of the cutaneous lesions in herpes zoster, and of the areas of referred pain and tenderness in visceral disease. The diagrams on pages 906 and 907 embody the results of many of these observations.

The cutaneous sensory impressions are in man conducted toward the brain, probably on the opposite side of the cord—that is, the path crosses to the opposite side soon after entering the cord. Muscular sense, on the other hand, is conducted on the same side of the cord in the fasciculus of Goll, to cross above by means of the axones of sensory neurones of the second order in the medulla.

Sensory Areas of the Brain.—Head and Holmes believe that there are two sensory centres—one in the optic thalamus, the other in a considerable area of the cerebral cortex. The thalamus plays a three-fold part in the fate of sensory impulses. Here all the afferent paths terminate; secondly, it contains a mass of gray matter which forms the centre for certain fundamental elements of sensation, particularly those capable of evoking pleasure and discomfort and consciousness of changes of state. Thirdly, in the lateral part of the thalamus is the centre through which the cortex influences the essential thalamic centre, controlling and checking its activity. On their way from the periphery to the cortex afferent impulses pay toll to the co-ordinate mechanisms of the spinal cord and the cerebellum. At the thalamic junction they are re-grouped to act upon the two terminal centres. One of these, the essential organ of the optic thalamus, responds to all those elements which evoke consciousness of an internal change in state, more particularly pleasure and discomfort. Sensory impulses, then, pass by way of the internal capsule to the cortex, and these authors hold that in the main five groups of sensory impulses are distributed in this way: (1) those underlying postural recognition and the appreciation of passive movement and weight; (2) the impulses underlying the recognition of tactile differences; (3) those upon which depends the recognition of size and space; (4) those which enable us to localize the spot stimulated; and (5) thermal impulses.

These afferent materials are combined in the cortex with each other and with other sense impressions in intellectual processes. The cortical area concerned is that situated between the pre-central fissure and the occipital lobe.

The paths for the conduction of the stimuli which underlie the special senses are given in the section upon the cerebral nerves, and it is only necessary here to refer to what is known of the cortical representation of these senses.

Visual impressions are localized in the occipital lobes. The primary visual centre is on the mesial surface in the cuneus, especially about the calcarine fissure, and here are represented the opposite visual half-fields. Some authors believe that there is another higher centre on the outer surface of the occipital lobe, in which the vision of the opposite eye is chiefly represented. However this may be, most authors hold that the angular gyrus of the left hemisphere is a part of the brain in which are stored the memories of the meaning of letters, words, figures, and, indeed, of all seen objects. This is designated as the visual speech centre on the diagram (Fig. 12).

Auditory impressions are localized for the most part in the first temporal convolution and the transverse temporal gyri, and it is in this region in the left hemisphere that the memories of the meanings of heard words and sounds are stored. Musical memories are localized somewhat in front of those for words. The cortical centres for smell include a part of the base of the frontal lobe, the uncus, and perhaps the gyrus hippocampi. The centres for taste are supposed to be situated near those for smell, but we possess as yet no definite information about them.

Topical Diagnosis.—The successful diagnosis of the position of a lesion in the nervous system depends upon a careful and exhaustive examination into all the symptoms that are present, and then endeavoring with the help of anatomy and physiology to determine the place, a disturbance at which might produce these symptoms.

The abnormalities of motion are usually the most important localizing symptoms, both on account of the ease with which they can be demonstrated, and also because of the comparative accuracy of our knowledge of the motor path.

Lesions in any part of the motor path cause disturbances of motion. If destructive, the function of the part is abolished, and as the result there is *paralysis.* If, on the other hand, the lesion is an irritative one, the structures are thrown into abnormal activity, which produces *abnormal muscular con-*

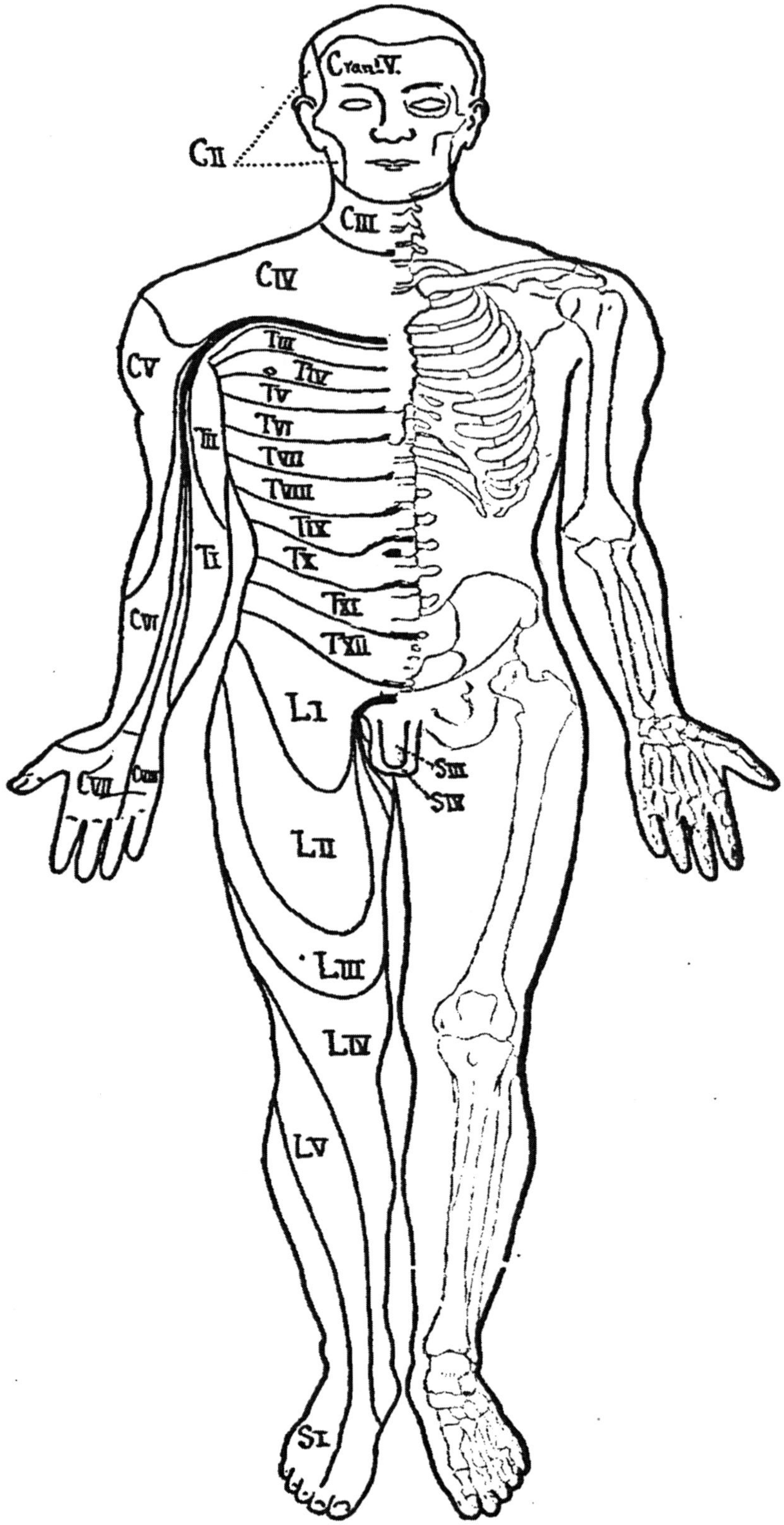

FIG. 16.—ANTERIOR ASPECT OF THE SEGMENTAL SKIN-FIELDS OF THE BODY, COMBINED FROM THE STUDIES OF HEAD, KOCHER, STARR, THORBURN, EDINGER, SHERRINGTON, WICHMANN, SEIFFER, BOLK, CUSHING, AND OTHERS. Heavy lines represent levels of fusion of dermatomes and the preaxial and postaxial lines of the limbs.

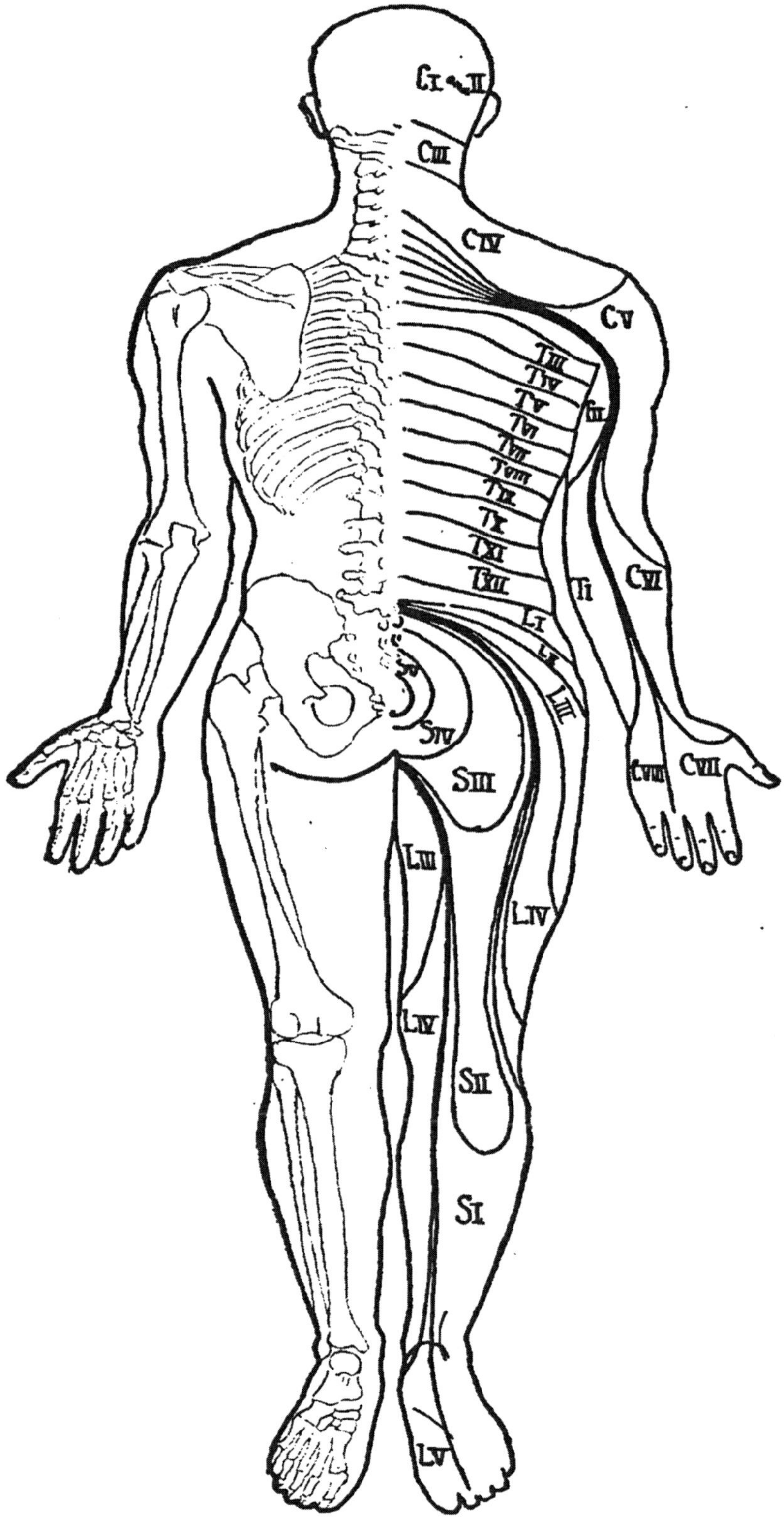

FIG. 17.—POSTERIOR ASPECT OF THE SEGMENTAL SKIN-FIELDS OF THE BODY.

traction. The character of the paralysis or of the abnormal muscular contraction varies with lesions of the upper and lower segment, the variations depending, first, upon the anatomical position of the two segments; and, secondly, upon the symptoms which are the result of secondary degeneration in each of the segments.

(*a*) Lesions of the Lower or Spino-muscular Segment.—*Destructive Lesions.*—It has been stated above that the nutrition of all parts of a neurone depends upon their connection with its healthy cell body; and if the cell body be injured, its processes undergo degeneration, or if a portion of a process be separated from the cell body, that part degenerates along its whole length. This so-called secondary degeneration plays a very important rôle in the symptomatology.

In the lower motor segment the degeneration not only affects the axis-cylinder processes which run in the peripheral nerves, but also the muscle fibres in which the axis-cylinder processes end. The degeneration of the nerves and muscles is made evident, first by the muscles becoming smaller and flabby, and, secondly, by change in their reaction to electrical stimulation. The degenerated nerve gives no response to either the galvanic or the faradic current, and the muscle does not respond to faradic stimulation, but reacts in a characteristic manner to the galvanic current. The contraction, instead of being sharp, quick, lightning-like, as in that of a normal muscle, is slow and lazy, and is often produced by a weaker current, and the anode-closing contraction may be greater than the cathode-closing contraction. This is the reaction of degeneration, but it is not always present in the classical form. The essential feature is the slow, lazy contraction of the muscle to the galvanic current, and when this is present the muscle is degenerated.

The myotatic irritability, or muscle reflex, and the muscle tonus depend upon the integrity of the reflex arc, of which the lower motor segment is the efferent limb, and in a paralysis due to lesion of this segment the muscle reflexes (tendon reflexes) are abolished and there is a diminished muscular tension.

Lower segment paralyses have for their characteristics degenerative atrophy with the reaction of degeneration in the affected muscles, loss of their reflex excitability, and a diminished muscular tension. These are the general characteristics, but the anatomical relations of this segment also give certain peculiarities in the distribution of the paralyses which help to distinguish them from those which follow lesions of the upper segment, and which also aid in determining the site of the lesion in the lower segment itself. The cell bodies of this segment are distributed in groups, from the level of the peduncles of the brain throughout the whole extent of the spinal cord to its termination opposite the second lumbar vertebra, and their axis-cylinder processes run in the peripheral nerves to every muscle in the body; so that the component parts are more or less widely separated from each other, and a local lesion causes paralysis of only a few muscles or groups of muscles, and not of a whole section of the body, as is the case where lesions affect the upper segment. The muscles which are paralyzed indicate whether the disease is in the peripheral nerves or spinal cord; for, as we have seen above, the muscles are represented differently in the peripheral nerves and in the spinal cord. Sensory symptoms, which may accompany the paralysis, are often of great assistance in making a local diagnosis. Thus, in a paralysis with the characteristics of a lesion of the lower motor segment, if the paralyzed muscles are all supplied by one nerve, and the anæsthetic area of the skin is supplied by that nerve, it is evident that the lesion must be in the nerve itself. On the other hand, if the muscles paralyzed are not supplied by a single nerve, but are represented close together in the spinal cord, and the anæsthetic area corresponds to that section of the cord (see table), it is equally clear that the lesion must be in the cord itself or in its nerve roots.

Irritative Lesions of the Lower Motor Segment.—Lesions of this segment cause comparatively few symptoms of irritation. The fibrillary contractions which are so common in muscles undergoing degeneration are probably due to stimulation of the cell bodies in their slow degeneration, as in progressive muscular atrophy, or to irritation of the axis-cylinder processes in the peripheral nerves, as in neuritis. Lesions which affect the motor roots as they leave the central nervous system may cause spasmodic contractions in the muscles supplied by them. Certain convulsive paroxysms, of which laryngismus stridulus is a type, and to which the spasms of tetany also belong, are believed to be due to abnormal activity in the lower motor centres. These are the "lowest level fits" of Hughlings Jackson. Certain poisons, as strychnia and that of tetanus, act particularly upon these centres.

The lower motor segment may be involved in all diseases involving the peripheral nerves in cerebral and spinal meningitis, in injuries, in hæmorrhages and tumors of the medulla and cord or their membranes, in lesions of the gray matter of the segment, in anterior poliomyelitis, progressive muscular atrophy, bulbar paralysis, ophthalmoplegia, syringomyelia, etc.

(*b*) Lesions of the Upper Motor Segment.—*Destructive lesions* cause paralysis, as in the lower motor segment, and here again the secondary degeneration which follows the lesion gives to the paralysis its distinctive characteristics. In this case the paralysis is accompanied by a spastic condition, shown in an exaggeration of muscle reflex and an increase in the tension of the muscle. It is not accurately known how the degeneration of the pyramidal fibres causes this excess of the muscle reflex. The usual explanation is that under normal circumstances the upper motor centres are constantly exerting a restraining influence upon the activity of the lower centres, and that when the influence ceases to act, on account of disease of the pyramidal fibres, the lower centres take on increased activity, which is made manifest by an exaggeration of the muscle reflex.

We have seen that the neurones composing each segment of the motor path are to be considered as nutritional units, and therefore the secondary degeneration in the upper segment stops at the beginning of the lower. For this reason the muscles paralyzed from lesions in the upper segment do not undergo degenerative atrophy, nor do they show any marked change in their electrical reactions.

The separate parts of the upper motor segment lie much more closely together than do those of the lower segment, and therefore a small lesion may cause paralysis in many muscles. This is more particularly true in the internal capsule, where all the axis-cylinder processes of this segment are collected into a compact bundle—the pyramidal tract. A lesion in this region usually causes paralysis of most of the muscles on the opposite side of the body—that is, hemiplegia. The pyramidal tract continues in a compact bundle, giving off fibres to the motor nuclei at different levels; a lesion anywhere in its course is followed by paralysis of all the muscles whose spinal centres are situated below the lesion. When the disease is above the decussation, the paralysis is on the opposite side of the body; when below, the paralyzed muscles are on the same side as the lesion. Above the internal capsule the path is somewhat more separated, and in the cortex the centres for the movements of the different sections of the body are comparatively far apart, and a sharply localized lesion in this region may cause a more limited paralysis, affecting a limb or a segment of a limb—the cerebral monoplegias; but even here the paralysis is not confined to an individual muscle or group of muscles, as is commonly the case in lower segment paralysis (see Fig. 10 and explanation).

To sum up, the paralyses due to lesions of the upper motor segment are widespread, often hemiplegic; the paralyzed muscles are spastic (the tendon reflexes exaggerated), they do not undergo degenerative atrophy, and they do not present the degenerative reaction to electrical stimulation.

There is an exception to the above statement—that is, in the paralyses which follow a complete transverse lesion of the spinal cord. Here the limbs are of course completely paralyzed, but instead of being spastic they are flaccid and the deep reflexes are absent. The muscles react normally to electricity. There is no satisfactory explanation of the loss of the reflexes under these conditions.

Irritative Lesions of the Upper Motor Segment.—Our knowledge of such lesions is confined for the most part to those acting on the motor cortex. The abnormal muscular contractions resulting from lesions so situated have as their type the localized convulsive seizures classed under Jacksonian or cortical epilepsy, which are characterized by the convulsion beginning in a single muscle or group of muscles and involving other muscles in a definite order, depending upon the position of their representation in the cortex. For instance, such a convulsion, beginning in the muscles of the face, next involves those of the arm and hand, and then the leg. The convulsion is usually accompanied by sensory phenomena and followed by a weakness of the muscles involved.

A majority of lesions of the motor cortex are both destructive and irritative—i. e., they destroy the nerve cells of a certain centre, and either in their growth or by their presence throw into abnormal activity those of the surrounding centres.

The upper motor segment is involved in nearly all the diseases of the brain and spinal cord, especially in injuries, tumors, abscesses, and hæmorrhages; transverse lesions of the cord; syringomyelia, progressive muscular atrophy, bulbar paralysis, etc. One lesion often involves both the upper and the lower motor segments, and there is paralysis in the different parts of the body, with the characteristics of each. Such a combination enables us in many cases to make an accurate local diagnosis.

Lesions in the optic path and in the different speech centres also give localizing symptoms, which should always be looked for.

(*c*) LESIONS OF THE SENSORY PATH.—Here again the lesion may be either irritative or destructive. *Irritative lesions* cause abnormal subjective sensory impressions—paræsthesia, formication, a sense of cold or constriction, and pain of every grade of intensity. The character of the sensory symptoms gives very little indication as to the position of the irritating process. Intense pain is, as a rule, a symptom of a lesion in the peripheral sensory neurones, but it may be caused by a disease of the sensory path within the central nervous system.

The exact distribution of symptoms gives more accurate data, for if they are confined to the distribution of a peripheral nerve or of a spinal segment the indication is plain. If one side of the body is more or less completely affected, the lesion is somewhere within the brain, etc.

Destructive Lesions.—A complete destruction of the sensory paths from any part of the body would of course deprive that part of sensation in all its qualities. This occurs most frequently from injury to the peripheral sensory neurones within the peripheral nerves, and the area of anæsthesia depends upon the nerve injured. Complete transverse lesion of the cord causes complete anæsthesia below the injury.

Unilateral lesions of the cord, medulla, dorsal part of the pons, tegmentum, thalamus, internal capsule, and cortex cause disturbances of sensation on the opposite side of the body; here again the extent of the defect more than its character helps us to determine the position of the lesion. Hemianæsthesia involving the face as well as the rest of the body can only occur above the place where the sensory paths from the fifth nerve have crossed the middle line on their way to the cortex. This is in the upper part of the pons. From this point to where they leave the internal capsule the sensory paths are in fairly close relation, and are at times involved in a very small lesion. Above the internal capsule the paths diverge quickly, and for this reason only an extensive lesion can involve them all, and in lesions of this part we are more apt to have the sensory disturbances confined to one or another region of the body. Unilateral lesions of the thalamus, pons, medulla, and cord usually cause sensory disturbances on the same side of the body, as well as those on the opposite side. These are due to the involvement of the sensory paths as they enter the central nervous system at or a little below the site of the lesion and before the axones of the sensory neurones of the second order have crossed the middle line. The area of disturbed sensation on the same side is limited to the distribution of one or more spinal segments and often indicates accurately the position and extent of the diseased process. As a rule, destructive lesions of the central nervous system do not involve all the paths of sensory conduction, and the loss of sensation is not complete. It is often astonishing how very slight the sensory disturbances are which result from an extensive lesion. Sensation may be diminished in all of its qualities, or, what is more common, certain qualities may be affected while others are normal. These cases of dissociation of sensation, or so-called elective sensory paralysis, have been much studied of late. Thus, the sense of pain and temperature may be lost while that of touch remains normal, as is often the case in diseases of the spinal cord, or there may be simply a loss of the muscular sense and of the stereognostic sense (the complex sensory impression which enables one to recognize an object placed in the hand), as occurs frequently from lesions of the cortex. Occasionally pain sensation persists with loss of tactile and thermic sensations. Almost every other combination has been described. It is the distribution more than the character of the sensory defect that is of importance, and often the distribution gives but uncertain indication of the position of the lesion. The combination of the sensory defect with different forms of paralysis gives the most certain diagnostic signs.

B. SYSTEM DISEASES

I. INTRODUCTION

There are certain diseases of the nervous system which are confined, if not absolutely, still in great part, to definite tracts (combinations of neurones) which subserve like functions. These tracts are called *systems,* and a disease which is confined to one of them is a *system disease.* If more than one system is involved, the process is called a combined system disease. Just what diseases should be classed under these names has given rise to much discussion but to very little agreement. We can not speak positively; our knowledge is as yet not sufficiently accurate, either in regard to the exact limits of the systems themselves, or to the nature and extent of the morbid process in the several diseases.

It may be said that the nervous system is composed of two great systems of neurones, the afferent or sensory system and the efferent or motor system, and the connections between them. (See General Introduction.)

Locomotor ataxia is a disease confined at its onset to the afferent system, and progressive muscular atrophy is one of the efferent system. Representing typical system diseases as we now understand them, they have been taken as the basis of the classification. Several theories have been advanced to explain why a disease should be limited to a definite system of neurones. One view is based upon the idea that in certain individuals one or the other of these systems has an innate tendency to undergo degeneration; another assumes that neurones with a similar function have a similar chemical construction (which differs from that of neurones with a different function), and this is taken to explain why a poison circulating in the blood should show a selective action for a single functional system of neurones.

In the afferent tract locomotor ataxia stands alone as a system disease, and we now believe that herpes zoster is an inflammation of the dorsal root ganglia and stands in the same relation to tabes that acute anterior poliomyelitis does to chronic progressive muscular atrophy. In the efferent tract progressive (central) muscular atrophy is the chief representative, as in it the whole motor path is more or less involved. Theoretically, primary lateral sclerosis is a disease confined to the upper segment of the efferent tract, while chronic anterior poliomyelitis involves the lower segment of the tract.

In connection with locomotor ataxia, general paralysis is considered on account of their frequent association and as they are but different expressions of one and the same morbid process; and with progressive (central) muscular atrophy, the other forms of muscular atrophy are considered as a matter of convenience. In other instances, too, diseases are arranged in positions to which they might not be entitled, had a rigid classification of system diseases been maintained.

II. DISEASES OF THE AFFERENT OR SENSORY SYSTEM

1. LOCOMOTOR ATAXIA

(*Tabes Dorsalis; Posterior Spinal Sclerosis*)

Definition.—An affection characterized clinically by sensory disturbances, incoördination, trophic changes, and involvement of the special senses, particularly the eyes. Anatomically there are found degenerations of the root fibres of the dorsal columns of the cord, of the dorsal roots, and at times of the spinal ganglia and peripheral nerves. Degenerations have been described in the brain, particularly the cortex cerebri, in the ganglion cells of the cord, and in the endogenous fibres of the dorsal columns.

Etiology.—It is a widespread disease, more frequent in cities than in the country. The relative proportion may be judged from the fact that of 16,562 cases in the neurological dispensary of the Johns Hopkins Hospital there were 201 cases of locomotor ataxia. Males are attacked more frequently than females, the proportion being nearly 10 to 1. The disease, although uncommon in the negro, is seen in them more frequently than some authors state. It is a disease of adult life, the great majority of cases occurring between the thirtieth and fiftieth years. Occasionally cases are seen in young men, and it may occur in children with hereditary syphilis. Syphilis is the important cause. In the Johns Hopkins Hospital the percentage, as found by Thomas, was 63.1. Erb's figures are most striking—of 300 cases of tabes in private practice, 89 per cent. had had syphilis. Moebius goes so far as to say, "The longer I reflect upon it, the more firmly I believe that tabes never originates without syphilis," and recent results of cases tested with the Wassermann reaction bear out this statement.

Contributing causes are excessive fatigue, overexertion, injury, exposure to cold and wet, and sexual excesses. There are instances in which the disease has closely followed severe exposure. Trauma has been noted in a few cases. Alcoholic excess does not seem to predispose to the disease. There are now a good many cases on record of the existence of the disease in both husband and wife, and a few in which the children were also affected.

Morbid Anatomy and Pathology.—Posterior spinal sclerosis, although the most obvious gross change, is now no longer, as in Romberg's time, an adequate description of the condition. The dorsal fibres are of two kinds, those with their cell bodies outside the cord in the spinal ganglia, the so-called exogenous, or root fibres, and those which arise from cells within the cord, the endogenous fibres. These two sets occupy fairly well-determined regions, and a study of early cases of tabes has shown that it is the exogenous or root fibres that are first affected. The fibres of the dorsal roots enter the cord in two divisions, an external and an internal; the former is composed of fibres of small calibre, which, in the cord, make up Lissauer's tract, and occupy the space between the apex of the dorsal cornua and the periphery of the cord, and really do not form part of the dorsal columns. They are short, soon entering the gray matter, and do not seem to be affected, or only slightly so, in early cases.

The larger fibres enter the cord by the internal division, just medial to the cornua, in what is known as the root entry zone. Some enter the gray matter of the spinal cord almost directly and others after a longer course, while still others run in the cord to the medulla, to end in the nuclei of the dorsal columns. As the fibres of every spinal nerve enter the cord between the dorsal cornua and the nerve fibres which have entered lower down, the fibres from each root are successively pushed more and more toward the median line, and so in the cervical cord the fasciculi of Goll are largely composed of long fibres derived from the sacral and lumbar roots.

That it is the coarse dorsal root fibres which are first affected in tabes is generally admitted, but there is much divergence of opinion as to the character and location of the initial process.

Nageotte calls attention to the frequency of a transverse, interstitial neuritis of the dorsal roots just after they have left the ganglia and are still surrounded by the dura, and he believes that it is this neuritis which is the primary lesion in tabes. Obersteiner and Redlich have laid great stress on the presence of an inflammation of the pia mater over the dorsal aspect of the cord, which involves the root fibres as they pass through. They point out that it is just here that the dorsal roots are most vulnerable, for at this point—that is, while surrounded by the pia—they are almost completely devoid of their myelin sheaths. Changes in the blood-vessels of the cord, of the pia, and of the nerve roots have been described in early tabes, and Marie and Guillain have advanced the belief that the changes in the cord are due to an affection (syphilis) of the posterior lymphatic system which is confined to the dorsal columns of the cord, the pia mater over them, and the dorsal roots. For them the changes in the nervous system are only apparently radicular or systemic.

With the Marchi stain, degeneration of the root fibres in the root-entry zone is a constant finding. This change is radicular in the sense that it varies in intensity with the different roots and is most marked in the sacral and lumbar regions. The degeneration is not found in the dorsal roots, but begins within the cord just beyond where the root fibres lose their neurolemma and their myelin sheaths. Degenerated fibres may be traced into the dorsal gray matter and among the ganglion cells of the columns of Clarke. The long columns which ascend the cord also degenerate.

In more advanced cases, in addition to the lesion described above, there are degeneration of the dorsal roots and some alteration of the cells in the spinal ganglia. The fibres distal to the ganglia are practically normal, although at times the sensory fibres, at the periphery of a limb, show degeneration. Within the cord, the exogenous fibres are diseased as already described; there is also degeneration in the endogenous system of fibres. Optic atrophy is frequently found. The other cranial nerves, especially the fifth with its ganglion, have been found degenerated.

The disease occasionally spreads beyond the sensory system in the cord, and in advanced cases the cells in the ventral horns may be degenerated in association with muscular atrophy. Mott very generally found more or less marked changes in the pyramidal fibres; these he believed to be evidence of changes in the cerebral cortex. Degeneration of the cortex may exist, but even in cases where the mental symptoms are absent, or very mild, similar though slight changes have been described, just as in general paralysis, without marked tabetic symptoms, there may be degeneration of the dorsal columns.

The close association, or even identity, of tabes and general paralysis will be considered later.

Symptoms.—These are best considered under three stages—the incipient stage, the ataxic stage, and the paralytic stage.

INCIPIENT STAGE.—This is sometimes called the pre-ataxic stage. The manner in which tabes makes its onset differs very widely in the different cases, and mistakes in diagnosis are often made early in the disease. The following are the most characteristic initial symptoms:

Pains, usually of a sharp stabbing character; hence, the term lightning pains. They last for only a second or two and are most common in the legs or about the trunk, and tend to follow dorsal root areas. They dart from place to place. At times they are associated with a hot burning feeling and often leave the affected area painful to pressure, and occasionally herpes may follow. The intensity of the pain varies from a sore, burning feeling of the skin to a pain so intense that, were it not for momentary duration, it would exceed human endurance. They occur at irregular intervals, and are prone to follow excesses or to come on when health is impaired. When typical, these pains are practically pathognomonic of the condition. The gastric crises and other crises may occur. Paræsthesia may also be among the first symptoms—numbness of the feet, tingling, etc.—and at times a sense of constriction about the body.

Ocular Symptoms.—(*a*) Optic atrophy. This occurs in about 10 per cent. of the cases, and is often an early and even the first symptom. There is a gradual loss of vision, which in a large majority of cases leads to total blindness. (*b*) Ptosis, which may be double or single. (*c*) Paralysis of the external muscles of the eye. This may be of a single muscle or occasionally of all the muscles of the eye. The paralysis is often transient, the patient merely complaining that he saw double for a certain period. (*d*) Argyll-Robertson pupil, in which there is loss of the iris reflex to light but contraction during accommodation. The pupils are often very small—spinal myosis.

Bladder Symptoms.—The first warning of the disease which the patient has may be a certain difficulty in emptying the bladder. Incontinence of urine occurs only at a later stage of the disease. Decrease in sexual desire and power may also be an early symptom.

Trophic Disturbances.—These usually occur later in the disease, but at times they are very early symptoms, and it is not very infrequent to have one's attention called to the trouble by the presence of a perforating ulcer or of a characteristic Charcot's joint.

Loss of the Deep Reflexes.—This early and most important symptom may occur years before the development of ataxia. Even alone it is of great moment, since it is very rare to meet with individuals in whom the knee and ankle jerks are normally absent. The combination of loss of either of these with one or more of the symptoms mentioned above, especially with the lightning pains and ptosis or Argyll-Robertson pupil, is practically diagnostic. These reflexes gradually decrease, and one may be lost before the other, or disappear first in one leg.

These are the most common symptoms of the initial stage of tabes and may persist for years without the development of incoördination. The patient may look well and feel well, and be troubled only by occasional attacks of lightning pains or of one of the other subjective symptoms. Moebius goes so far as to state that the typical Argyll-Robertson pupil means either tabes or general paralysis, and that paralysis of the external muscles of the eye developing in adults is of almost equal importance, especially if it develops painlessly.

The time between the syphilitic infection and the occurrence of the first symptoms of locomotor ataxia varies within wide limits. About one-half the cases occur between the sixth and fifteenth year, but many begin even later than this.

The disease may never progress beyond this stage, and when optic atrophy develops early and leads to blindness, ataxia rarely, if ever, supervenes, but the mental symptoms of paresis not infrequently follow, a sequence which must be kept in mind. There is a sort of antagonism between the ocular symptoms and the progress of the ataxia. Charcot laid considerable stress upon this, and both Dejerine and Spiller have since emphasized the point.

Ataxic Stage.—*Motor Symptoms.*—The ataxia is believed to be due to a disturbance or loss of the afferent impulses from the muscles, joints, and deep tissues, and a disturbance of the muscle sense itself can usually be demonstrated. It develops gradually. One of the first indications to the patient is inability to get about readily in the dark or to maintain his equilibrium when washing his face with the eyes shut. When the patient stands with the feet together and the eyes closed, he sways and has difficulty in maintaining his position (Romberg's symptom), and he may be quite unable to stand on one leg. He does not start off promptly at the word of command. On turning quickly he is apt to fall. He descends stairs with more difficulty than he ascends them. Gradually the characteristic ataxic gait develops. The patient, as a rule, walks with a stick, the eyes are directed to the ground, the body is thrown forward, and the legs are wide apart. In walking, the leg is thrown out violently, the foot is raised too high and is brought down in a stamping manner with the heel first, or the whole sole comes in contact with the ground. Ultimately the patient may be unable to walk without the assistance of two canes. This gait is very characteristic, and unlike that seen in any other disease. The incoördination is not only in walking, but in the performance of other movements. If the patient is asked, when in the recumbent posture, to touch one knee with the other foot, the irregularity of the movement is very evident. Incoördination of the arms is less common, but usually develops in some grade. It may in rare instances exist before the incoördination of the legs. It may be tested by asking the patient to close his eyes and to touch the tip of the nose or the tip of the ear with the finger, or with the arms thrust out to bring the tips of the fingers together. The incoördination may early be noticed by a difficulty which the patient experiences in buttoning his collar or in performing one of the ordinary routine acts of dressing.

One of the most striking features of the disease is that with marked incoordination there is but little loss of muscular power. The grip of the hands may be strong and firm, the power of the legs, tested by trying to flex them, may be unimpaired, and their nutrition, except toward the close, may be unaffected.

There is a remarkable muscular relaxation (hypotonia) which enables the joints to be placed in positions of hyperextension and hyperflexion. It gives sometimes a marked backward curve to the legs.

Sensory Symptoms.—The lightning pains may persist. They vary greatly in different cases. Some patients are rendered miserable by the frequent occurrence of the attacks; others escape altogether. In addition, common symptoms are tingling, pins and needles, particularly in the feet, and areas of hyperæsthesia or of anæthesia. The patient may complain of a change in the sensation in the soles of the feet, as if cotton was interposed between the floor and the skin. Sensory disturbances occur less frequently in the hands. Objective sensory disturbances can usually be demonstrated, and, indeed, almost every variety of sensory disturbance has been described. Bands of a moderate grade of anæsthesia about the chest are not uncommon; they are apt to follow the distribution of spinal segments. The most marked disturbances are usually found on the legs. Retardation of the sense of pain is common, and a pin prick on the foot is first felt as a simple tactile impression, and the sense of pain is not perceived for a second or two or may be delayed for as much as ten seconds. The pain felt may persist. A curious phenomenon is the loss of the power of localizing the pain. For instance, if the patient is pricked on one limb he may say that he feels it on the other (allocheiria), or a pin prick on the foot may be felt on both feet. The muscular sense which is usually affected early, becomes much impaired and the patient no longer recognizes the position in which his limbs are placed. This may be present in the pre-ataxic stage.

Reflexes.—As mentioned, the loss of the knee and ankle jerks is one of the earliest symptoms of the disease. Occasionally a case is found in which they are retained, and anatomically it has been shown that in these cases the lumbar segments were little if at all involved. The skin reflexes may at first be increased, but later are usually involved with the deep reflexes.

Special Senses.—The eye symptoms noted above may be present, but, as mentioned, ataxia is rare with atrophy of the optic nerve.

Deafness may occur, due to lesion of the auditory nerve. There may also be attacks of vertigo. Olfactory symptoms are rare.

Visceral Symptoms.—Among the most remarkable sensory disturbances are the tabetic crises, severe paroxysms of pain referred to various viscera; thus, laryngeal, gastric, nephric, rectal, urethral, and clitoral crises have been described. The most common are the gastric and laryngeal. Gastric crises may occur early and persist as the most prominent feature. Starr found them as the first symptom 18 times in 450 cases. The onset is usually sudden, with pain of a severe burning, twisting type in the epigastrium, radiating to the back and behind the sternum. Vomiting follows the pain, and may be quite independent of food. Pallor, sweating, cold extremities, and a small pulse are associated, and in rare instances death occurs in collapse. The attacks are not unlike and are probably of the same nature as the so-called abdominal angina pectoris. The blood pressure may be very high, as reported by Barker, and it seems not improbable that the condition is associated with angiospasm in the territory of the gastric and mesenteric vessels. No special change may be found at autopsy. In the laryngeal crises there may be true spasm with dyspnœa and noisy inspiration. A patient may die in the attack. There are also nasal crises, associated with sneezing fits.

The sphincters are frequently involved. Early in the disease there may be a retardation or hesitancy in making water. Later there is retention, and cystitis may occur. Unless great care is taken the inflammation may extend to the kidneys. Constipation is extremely common. Later in the disease the sphincter ani is weakened. The sexual power is usually lost in the ataxic stage.

Trophic Changes.—Skin rashes, such as herpes, œdema, or local sweating, may develop in the course of the lightning pains. Alteration in the nails may occur. A perforating ulcer may develop on the foot, usually beneath the great toe. A perforating buccal ulcer has also been described. Onychia may prove very troublesome.

Arthropathies (Charcot's Joints).—Anatomically there are: (1) enlargement of the capsule with thickening of the synovial membranes and increase in the fluids; (2) slight enlargement of the ends of the bones, with slight exostoses; (3) a dull velvety appearance of the cartilages, with atrophy in places (V. E. Henderson). The knees are most frequently involved. The spine is affected in rare instances. Recurring trauma is an important element in the causation, but trophic disturbances have a strong influence in the etiology. A striking feature is the absence of pain. Suppuration may occur, also spontaneous fractures. Among other trophic disturbances may be mentioned atrophy of the muscles, which is usually a late manifestation, but may be localized and associated with neuritis. In any very large collection of cases many instances of atrophy are found, due either to involvement of the ventral horns or to peripheral neuritis.

Aneurism is found in many cases, in as high as 20 per cent. of some series.

Cerebral Symptoms.—Hemiplegia may develop at any stage of the disease, more commonly when it is well advanced. It may be due to hæmorrhagic softening in consequence of disease of the vessels or to progressive cortical changes. Hemianæsthesia is sometimes present. Very rarely the hemiplegia is due to coarse syphilitic disease.

Dementia paralytica frequently exists with tabes; indeed, we have come to regard these two diseases as simply different localizations of the same morbid process. In other instances melancholia, dementia, or paranoia occur.

Paralytic Stage.—After persisting for an indefinite number of years the patient gradually loses the power of walking and becomes bedridden or paralyzed. In this condition he is very likely to be carried off by some intercurrent affection, such as pyelo-nephritis, pneumonia, or tuberculosis.

The Course of the Disease.—A patient may remain in the pre-ataxic stage for an indefinite period; and the loss of knee-jerk and the gray atrophy of the optic nerves may be the sole indication of the true nature of the disease. In such cases incoördination rarely develops. In a majority of cases the progress is slow, and after six or eight years, sometimes less, the ataxia is well developed. The symptoms may vary a good deal; thus, the pains, which may have been excessive at first, often lessen. The disease may remain stationary for years; then exacerbations occur and it makes rapid progress. Occasionally the process seems to be arrested. There are instances of what may be called acute ataxia, in which, within a year or even less, the incoördination is marked, and the paralytic stage may develop within a few months. The disease itself rarely causes death, and after becoming bedridden the patient may live for fifteen or twenty years.

Diagnosis.—In the initial stage the lightning pains are almost distinctive, and when combined with any of the other signs are quite so. The association of progressive atrophy of the optic nerves with loss of knee-jerk is also characteristic. The early ocular palsies are of the greatest importance. A squint, ptosis, or the Argyll-Robertson pupil may be the first symptom, and may exist with the loss only of the knee-jerk. Loss of the knee-jerk alone, however, does occasionally occur in healthy individuals. A history of preceding syphilis lends added weight to the symptoms, and its presence or absence may be of the utmost importance in determining the diagnosis. The Wassermann reaction is present in a large proportion of all cases, and a study of the spinal fluid may be a help in doubtful cases (see General Paresis).

The diseases most likely to be confounded with locomotor ataxia are: (*a*) Peripheral Neuritis.—The steppage gait of arsenical, alcoholic, or diabetic paralysis is quite unlike that of locomotor ataxia. In these forms there is a paralysis of the feet, and the leg is lifted high in order that the toes may clear the floor. The use of the word *ataxia* in this connection should no longer be continued. In the rare cases in which the muscle sense nerves are particularly affected and in which there is true ataxia, the absence of the lightning pains and eye symptoms and the history will suffice in a majority of cases to make the diagnosis clear. In diphtheritic paralysis the early loss of the knee-jerk and the associated eye symptoms may suggest tabes, but the history, the existence of paralysis of the throat, and the absence of pains render a diagnosis easy.

(*b*) Ataxic Paraplegia.—Marked incoördination with spastic paralysis is characteristic of the condition which Gowers has termed ataxic paraplegia. In a majority of the cases this affection is distinguished also by the absence of pains and of eye symptoms, but it may be a manifestation of the cord lesions in tabo-paralysis.

(*c*) Cerebral Disease.—In diseases of the brain involving the afferent tracts ataxia is at times a prominent symptom. It is usually unilateral or limited to one limb; this, with the history and the associated symptoms, excludes tabes.

(*d*) Cerebellar Disease.—The cerebellar incoördination has only a superficial resemblance to that of locomotor ataxia, and is more a disturbance of equilibrium than a true ataxia; the knee-jerk is usually present, there are no lightning pains, no sensory disturbances; while, on the other hand, there are headache, optic neuritis, and vomiting.

(*e*) Acute syphilitic affections involving the dorsal columns of the cord may be associated with incoördination and resemble tabes very closely. In a case under my care, the gait was characteristic and Romberg's symptom was present. The knee-jerk, however, was retained and there were no ocular symptoms. The condition had developed within three months, and there was a well-marked history of syphilis. Under large doses of iodide of potassium the ataxia and other symptoms completely disappeared.

(*f*) General Paresis.—Even though these two diseases are so nearly allied and often associated, it is of very great practical importance to determine, when possible, whether the type is to be spinal or cerebral, for, in the great majority of cases, when this is established, it does not change. The difficulty arises in the premonitory stage, when ocular changes and abnormalities of sensation and the deep reflexes may be the only symptoms. At this stage any alteration in the mental characteristics is of the utmost significance. (See General Paresis.) Loss of the deep reflexes and lightning pains speak for tabes; active reflexes, with ocular changes, especially optic atrophy, are suggestive of paresis.

(*g*) VISCERAL CRISES and NEURALGIC SYMPTOMS may lead to error, and in middle-aged men with severe, recurring attacks of gastralgia it is always well to bear in mind the possibility of tabes, and to make a careful examination of the eyes and of the knee-jerk.

Prognosis.—Complete recovery can not be expected, but arrest of the process is not uncommon and a marked amelioration of the symptoms is frequent. Optic-nerve atrophy, one of the most serious events in the disease, has this hopeful aspect—that incoördination rarely follows and the progress of the spinal symptoms may be arrested. On the other hand, mental symptoms are more likely to follow. The optic atrophy itself is occasionally checked. On the whole, the prognosis in tabes is bad. The experience of such men as Weir Mitchell, Charcot, and Gowers is distinctly opposed to the belief that locomotor ataxia is ever completely cured. There is more hope now that in very early cases coming on soon after infection the course may be arrested by salvarsan. Death is usually from some cardio-vascular complication; next in frequency from tuberculosis and pneumonia (Burr).

Treatment.—To arrest the progress and to relieve, if possible, the symptoms are the objects which the practitioner should have in view. A quiet, well-regulated method of life is essential. It is not well, as a rule, for a patient to give up his occupation so long as he is able to keep about and perform ordinary work, provided there is no evident mental change. I know tabetics who have for years conducted large businesses, and there have been several notable instances in our profession of men who have risen to distinction in spite of the existence of this disease. Excesses of all sorts, more particularly *in baccho et venere*, should be carefully avoided. A man in the pre-ataxic stage should not marry.

Care should be taken in the diet, particularly if gastric crises have occurred. To secure arrest of the disease many remedies have been employed. Salvarsan in small repeated doses (0.2 gm.) should be tried in early cases, though the published results have not, on the whole, been satisfactory. Neither mercury nor the iodide of potassium has anything like the same influence over the tabetic lesions that they have over the ordinary syphilitic processes. However, when the syphilis is comparatively recent, when symptoms develop within two years of the primary infection, the disease may be arrested by mercury and iodide of potassium. The French authors have recently spoken much more hopefully of the benefit of anti-syphilitic treatment in early cases of tabes, and it is well to give the patient the benefit of salvarsan and a thorough course of mercurial inunctions and iodide of potassium. Of remedies which may be tried and are believed by some writers to retard the progress, the following are recommended: Arsenic in full doses, nitrate of silver in quarter-grain doses, Calabar bean, ergot, and the preparations of gold.

For the pains, complete rest in bed, as advised by Weir Mitchell, and counter-irritation to the spine (either blisters or the thermo-cautery) may be employed. The severe spells which come on particularly after excesses of any kind are often promptly relieved by a hot bath or by a Turkish bath. For the severe recurring attacks of lightning pains spinal cocainization may be tried. A prolonged course of nitrate of silver seems in some cases to allay the pains and lessen the liability to the attacks. Antipyrin and antifebrin may be employed, and occasionally do good, but their analgesic powers in this disease have been greatly overrated. Cannabis indica is sometimes useful. In the severe paroxysms of pain hypodermics of morphia or of cocaine must be used. The use of morphia should be postponed as long as possible. Electricity is of very little benefit. For the severe attacks of gastralgia morphia is also required. Gastro-enterostomy has been performed, the solar plexus has been stretched, and the dorsal spinal nerve roots of the seventh, eighth, ninth, and tenth have been divided with good results. The laryngeal crises are rarely dangerous. An application of cocaine may be made during the spasm, or a few whiffs of chloroform may be given, or nitrite of amyl. In all cases of tabes with increased arterial tension the prolonged use of nitroglycerin, given in increasing doses until the physiological effect is produced, is of great service in allaying the neuralgic pains and diminishing the frequency of the crises. Its use must be guarded when there is aortic insufficiency. The special indication is increased tension. The bladder symptoms demand constant care. When the organ can not be perfectly emptied the catheter should be used, and the patient may be taught its use and how to keep it thoroughly sterilized.

Frenkel's method of re-education often helps the patient to regain to a considerable extent the control of the voluntary movements which he has lost. By this method the patient is first taught, by repeated systematic efforts, to perform simple movements; from this he goes to more and more complex movements. The treatment should be directed and supervised by a trained teacher, as the result depends upon the skill of the teacher quite as much as upon the perseverance of the patient.

2. GENERAL PARALYSIS OF THE INSANE AND TABO-PARALYSIS

(*Dementia Paralytica; General Paresis*)

As has been said in the last section, the belief in the essential identity of general paralysis and tabes has gained more and more ground and has much in its favor. Mott says: "I maintain that etiologically and pathogenetically there is *one tabes* which may begin in the brain (especially in certain regions), or in the spinal cord in certain regions, or in the peripheral nervous structures connected with vision, or in nervous structures connected with the viscera, constituting, therefore, different types, any of which may be present or be associated with one or all of the others." Fournier has taken practically the same view and describes them together under the heading *Les Affections Parasyphilitiques.*

It is undoubted that most cases of tabes run their course with practically no mental symptoms, and that cases of general paralysis may never present symptoms that suggest tabes. For practical purposes we are forced to keep the distinction clearly in mind, and for this reason it seems best, at least for the present, to consider them separately.

There is, however, a group of cases in which the symptoms of the two diseases are associated in every combination. The name "tabo-paralysis" has been given to these cases.

General Paralysis

Definition.—A chronic, progressive disease of the brain and its meninges, associated with psychical and motor disturbances, finally leading to dementia and paralysis.

Etiology.—As in tabes, the important factor is syphilis, which is antecedent in both conditions in practically all cases. Males are affected much more frequently than females. It occurs chiefly between the ages of thirty and fifty-five, although it may begin in childhood as the result of congenital syphilis. An overwhelming majority of the cases are in married people, and not infrequently both husband and wife are affected, or one has paresis and the other tabes. Statistics show that it is more common in the lower classes of society, but in America in general medical practice the disease is certainly more common in the well-to-do classes. Heredity is a more important factor here than in tabes, although its influence is not great. An important predisposing cause is "a life absorbed in ambitious projects with all its strongest mental efforts, its long-sustained anxieties, deferred hopes, and straining expectation" (Mickle). The habits of life so frequently seen in active business men in our large cities, and well expressed by the phrase "burning the candle at both ends," strongly predispose to the disease.

Morbid Anatomy.—The dura is often thickened, and its inner surface may show the various forms of hypertrophic pachymeningitis. The pia is cloudy, thickened, and adherent to the cortex. The cerebro-spinal fluid is increased in the meningeal spaces, especially in the meshes of the pia, and at times to such an extent as to resemble cysts. The brain is small, and weighs less than normal. The convolutions are atrophied, especially in the anterior and middle lobes. In acute cases the brain may be swollen, hyperæmic, and œdematous. The brain cortex is usually red, and, except in advanced cases, it may not be atrophied, the atrophy of the hemispheres being at the expense of the white matter. The lateral ventricles are dilated to compensate for the atrophy of the brain, and the ependyma may be granular. The fourth ventricle is more constantly dilated, with granulations of its floor covering the calamus scriptorius, a condition seldom seen in any other affection.

The disease process is diffuse, and affects practically all parts of the brain, but its intensity varies greatly, even in adjoining areas. As a rule, the cortex of the frontal and central convolutions and the gray matter about the ventricles are most affected.

In many cases changes are present in the spinal cord and peripheral nerves. There are the typical tabetic changes described in the preceding section. There may be degeneration of the pyramidal systems of fibres secondary to the cortical changes. Most commonly there is a combination of these two processes. Foci of hæmorrhages, and softening dependent upon coarse vascular changes, are not infrequently found, but are not typical of the disease.

There are various views as to the nature of the changes. The vascular theory is that from an inflammatory process starting in the sheaths of the arterioles there is a diffuse parenchymatous degeneration with atrophic changes in the nerve cells and neuroglia. The syphilitic toxin causes degeneration in the nervous tissues with secondary changes in the neuroglia and vascular systems. The spirochætes are found in the nervous tissues.

Symptoms.—PRODROMAL STAGE.—This is of variable duration, and is characterized by a general mental state which finds expression in symptoms trivial in themselves but important in connection with others. Irritability, inattention to business amounting sometimes to indifference or apathy, and sometimes a *change in character,* marked by acts which may astonish the friends and relatives, may be the first indications. There may be unaccountable fatigue after moderate physical or mental exertion. Instead of apathy or indifference there may be an extraordinary degree of physical and mental restlessness. The patient is continually planning and scheming, or may launch into extravagances and speculation of the wildest character. A common feature at this period is the display of an unbounded egoism. He boasts of his personal attainments, his property, his position in life, or of his wife and children. Following these features are important indications of moral perversion, manifested in offences against decency or the law, many of which acts have about them a suspicious effrontery. Forgetfulness is common, and may be shown in inattention to business details and in the minor courtesies of life. At this period there may be no motor phenomena. The onset of the disease is usually insidious, although cases are reported in which epileptiform or apoplectiform seizures were the first symptoms. Among the early motor features are tremor of the tongue and lips in speaking, slowness of speech and hesitancy. Inequality of the pupils, the Argyll-Robertson pupil, optic atrophy, and changes in the deep reflexes may precede the occurrence of mental symptoms for years.

SECOND STAGE.—This is characterized in brief by mental exaltation or excitement and a progress in the motor symptoms. "The intensity of the excitement is often extreme, acute maniacal states are frequent; incessant restlessness, obstinate sleeplessness, noisy, boisterous excitement, and blind, uncalculating violence especially characterize such states" (Lewis). It is at this stage that the delusion of grandeur becomes marked and the patient believes himself to be possessed of countless millions or to have reached the most exalted sphere possible in profession or occupation. This expansive delirium, as it is called, is, however, not characteristic, as was formerly supposed, of paralytic dementia. Besides, it does not always occur, but in its stead there may be marked melancholia or hypochondriasis, or, in other instances, alternate attacks of delirium and depression.

The facies has a peculiar stolidity, and in speaking there is marked tremulousness of the lips and facial muscles. The tongue is also tremulous, and may be protruded with difficulty. The speech is slow, interrupted, and blurred. Writing becomes difficult on account of unsteadiness of the hand. Letters, syllables, and words may be omitted. The subject matter of the patient's letters gives valuable indications of the mental condition. In many instances the pupils are unequal, irregular, sluggish, sometimes large. Important symptoms in this stage are apoplectiform seizures and paralysis. There may be slight syncopal attacks in which the patient turns pale and may fall. Some of these are *petit mal.* In the true apoplectiform seizure the patient falls suddenly, becomes unconscious, the limbs are relaxed, the face is flushed, the breathing stertorous, the temperature increased, and death may occur. Epileptic seizures are more common than the apoplectiform. There may be a definite aura. The attack usually begins on one side and may not spread. There may be twitchings either in the facial or brachial muscles. Typical Jacksonian epilepsy may occur. Recurring attacks of aphasia are not uncommon, and paralysis, either monoplegic or hemiplegic, may follow these epileptic seizures, or may come on with great suddenness and be transient. In this stage the gait becomes impaired, the patient trips readily, has difficulty in going up or down stairs, and the walk may be spastic or occasionally tabetic. This paresis may be progressive. The deep reflexes are usually increased, but may be lost. Bladder or rectal symptoms gradually develop. The patient becomes helpless, bedridden, and completely demented, and unless care is taken may suffer from bedsores. Death occurs from exhaustion or from some intercurrent affection. The spinal cord features of dementia paralytica may come on with or precede the mental troubles. There are cases in which one is in doubt for a time whether the symptoms indicate tabes or dementia paralytica, and it is well to bear in mind that every feature of pre-ataxic tabes may exist in the early stage of general paresis.

Tabo-paralysis

Emphasis has been laid on the probable identity of the processes underlying tabes and dementia paralytica, the spinal cord in the first case receiving the full force of the attack, and the brain in the second. It has been thought that stress is the factor which determines the location of the process, and that men whose occupations require much bodily exercise would be apt to have tabes, while those whose activities are largely mental would suffer from paresis. Usually when the cord symptoms are pronounced the symptoms from the brain remain in abeyance, and the reverse is also true. There are exceptions to this, and cases of well marked tabes may later show the typical symptoms of paresis, but even then the ataxia, if it is not of too high a grade, often improves.

Optic atrophy, when it occurs in the pre-ataxic stage of tabes, usually indicates that the ataxia will never be pronounced, but unfortunately it is frequently followed by the occurrence of mental symptoms. Mott believes that about 50 per cent. of his asylum cases of tabo-paralysis had had preceding optic atrophy. Its occurrence is therefore of grave significance. The mental symptoms may be delayed for many years.

The *symptom complex* of tabo-paralysis is made up of a combination of the symptoms of the two conditions, and varies greatly. It may begin as tabes with lightning pains, bladder symptoms, Argyll-Robertson pupil, loss of the deep reflexes, etc., to have the mental symptoms added later; or, on the other hand, cord symptoms may come on after the patient has shown marked mental changes. In a number of cases the symptoms are from the first so combined that the name tabo-paralysis is at once applicable. Absent knee-jerks, ocular palsies, or pupillary symptoms may precede the breakdown for many years, but none of them have so grave a significance in regard to the mental state as has optic atrophy. Other types of alienation may interrupt the course of tabes, and the mistake must not be made of regarding them all as general paralysis. In such instances the mind may become clear and remain so to the end.

Diagnosis.—The recognition of general paralysis in the earliest stage is extremely difficult, as it is often impossible to decide that the slight alteration in conduct is anything more than one of the moods or phases to which most men are at times subject. The following description by Folsom is an admirable presentation of the diagnostic characters of the early stage of the disease: "It should arouse suspicion if, for instance, a strong, healthy man, in or near the prime of life, distinctly not of the 'nervous,' neurotic, or neurasthenic type, shows some loss of interest in his affairs or impaired faculty of attending to them; if he becomes varyingly absent-minded, heedless, indifferent, negligent, apathetic, inconsiderate, and, although able to follow his routine duties, his ability to take up new work is, no matter how little, diminished; if he can less well command mental attention and concentration, conception, perception, reflection, judgment; if there is an unwonted lack of initiative, and if exertion causes unwonted mental and physical fatigue; if the emotions are intensified and easily change, or are excited readily from trifling causes; if the sexual instinct is not reasonably controlled; if the finer feelings are even slightly blunted; if the person in question regards with a placid apathy his own acts of indifference and irritability and their consequences, and especially if at times he sees himself in his true light and suddenly fails again to do so; if any symptoms of cerebral vaso-motor disturbances are noticed, however vague or variable."

There are cases of cerebral syphilis which closely simulate dementia paralytica. The mode of onset is important, particularly since paralytic symptoms are usually early in syphilis. The affection of the speech and tongue is not present. Epileptic seizures are more common and more liable to be cortical or Jacksonian in character. The expansive delirium is rare. While symptoms of general paresis are not common in connection with the development of gummata or definite gummatous meningitis, there are, on the other hand, instances of paresis following closely upon the syphilitic infection. Post mortem in such cases there may be nothing more than a general arterio-sclerosis and diffuse meningo-encephalitis, which may present nothing distinctive, but the lesions, nevertheless, may be caused by the syphilitic virus. Cases also occur in which typical syphilitic lesions are combined with the ordinary lesions of dementia paralytica. There are certain forms of lead encephalopathy which resemble general paresis, and, considering the association of plumbism with arterio-sclerosis, it is not unlikely that the anatomical substratum of the disease may result from this poison. Tumor may sometimes simulate progressive paresis, but in the former the signs of general increase of the intracranial pressure are usually present. The Wassermann reaction in the blood or spinal fluid is nearly constant.

Cytodiagnosis.—The study of the cellular elements suspended in the cerebro-spinal fluid has come to be an important diagnostic measure, particularly in tabes and paresis. In both of these affections spinal lymphocytosis is the rule and is usually associated with a marked albumin reaction—the normal fluid containing no albumin, or at most minute traces, and a negligible number of formed elements. It is simply the expression of a subacute or chronic inflammatory process, just as polymorphonuclear leukocytosis is characteristic of an acute process. It is, however, first and foremost the syphilitic triad—tabes, paresis, and cerebro-spinal lues—which is suggested by lymphocytosis in the spinal fluid. Positive reactions, cytological and chemical, are among the earliest somatic symptoms, and may therefore clear up obscure cases of tabes and paresis, just at the time when diagnosis is most difficult.

Prognosis.—The disease rarely ends in recovery. As a rule the progress is slowly downward and the case terminates in a few years, although it is occasionally prolonged ten or fifteen years.

Treatment.—Salvarsan in small repeated doses may be tried in early cases, after which large doses of iodide of potassium and a mercurial course should be given. Careful nursing and the orderly life of an asylum are the only measures necessary in a great majority of the cases. For sleeplessness and the epileptic seizures bromides may be used. Prolonged remissions, which are not uncommon, are often erroneously attributed to the action of remedies. Active treatment in the early stage by wet-packs, cold to the head, and systematic massage has been followed by temporary improvement.

3. ACUTE POSTERIOR GANGLIONITIS

(*Herpes Zoster*)

Definition.—An acute disease with localization in the cerebral ganglia and in the ganglia of the posterior nerve roots, associated with a vesicular inflammation of the skin of the corresponding cutaneous areas.

Distribution.—Herpes most frequently occurs in the region of the dorsal roots and extends in the form of a half girdle, on which account the names "zona" and "zoster" have been given. The trigeminal region is very often involved, particularly the first branch. Common forms also are the herpes sterno-nuchalis, cervico-subclavicularis and dorso-ulnaris.

Pathology.—Bärensprung first showed that there was involvement of the spinal ganglia. The exhaustive studies of Head and Campbell show that the primary disease is an acute hæmorrhagic inflammation of the ganglia of the posterior nerve roots and of the homologous cranial ganglia. It is analogous to acute anterior polio-myelitis. There are inflammatory foci, hæmorrhage in and destruction of certain of the ganglion cells leading to degeneration of the axis-cylinders. In herpes facialis accompanying pneumonia W. T. Howard has shown that similar lesions are demonstrable in the Gasserian ganglion, and Hunt has found the same changes in the otic ganglion in herpes auricularis. It is met with in the acute infections, particularly pneumonia, malaria, and cerebro-spinal fever. Epidemics have been described. Micro-organisms have been found in the cerebro-spinal fluid.

Symptoms.—In ordinary zona there is often a slight prodromal period in which the patient feels ill, has moderate fever, and pain in the side, sometimes of such severity as to suggest pleurisy. On the third or fourth day the rash appears. The characteristic group of vesicles has a segmental distribution limited to one side of the body. One or more of the adjoining skin fields is usually affected. With involvement of the cervical, lumbar, or sacral ganglion the zonal or girdle form of the vesicular crop is naturally lost owing to the distortion of the skin fields from the growth of the limbs. The typical zonal form is only seen in involvement of the thoracic ganglia. Groups of vesicles are regularly arranged on the hyperæmic skin, at first filled with a clear or sometimes bloody serum, which later becomes purulent. The crop varies greatly, and the individual vesicles may be superficial, in which case they leave no scar, or they may be deep and in healing leave superficial scars. By far the most serious form is that seen in the upper division of the fifth. The fever may be high and the eruption very profuse with great swelling and much pain. I have seen several cases of permanent disfigurement from the scarring.

It seems not improbable, as Chauffard suggests, that there may be extension of the disease from the posterior ganglia to the neighboring meninges as there may be pains down the spine, the girdle sensation, exaggerated knee-jerks, the Kernig sign, and lymphocytosis in the cerebro-spinal fluid.

Complications.—Perhaps the most serious of these is that occasionally seen in ophthalmic zoster, when there is intense inflammation of the conjunctiva and cornea with consecutive pan-ophthalmitis and destruction of the eye, of which I have seen one instance.

In a few cases the eruption becomes gangrenous. Swelling of the lymph glands has been noted. A bilateral distribution has occurred. A generalized herpes zoster is occasionally seen with a widespread vesicular rash on the face, neck, trunk, and thighs. A facial paralysis may develop during or after ophthalmic or cervical herpes. I have seen swelling of the parotid gland on the same side. In rare cases paralysis of the extremities has occurred. By far the most distressing complication is *post-zonal neuralgia.* After recovery from the herpes, hot burning sensations are not uncommon in the cutaneous distribution. In other instances, particularly in old people, the pain persists and for years may be a terrible affliction resisting all measures of treatment. Gowers speaks of suicide in despair, one instance of which came under my notice.

Treatment.—Care should be taken to protect the vesicles; a one per cent. cocaine ointment with lanolin carefully applied on lint gives relief to the pain. In very severe involvement of the ophthalmic division of the fifth nerve the greatest care should be taken to keep the conjunctiva clean. For the severe post-zonal neuralgia, injections into the spinal cord have been tried, and in cases of great severity the posterior nerve roots may be cut.

III. DISEASES OF THE EFFERENT OR MOTOR TRACT

A. OF WHOLE TRACT

1. PROGRESSIVE (CENTRAL) MUSCULAR ATROPHY

(*Poliomyelitis Anterior Chronica; Amyotrophic Lateral Sclerosis; Progressive Bulbar Paralysis*)

Definition.—A disease characterized by a chronic degeneration of the motor tract, usually of the whole, but at times limited to the lower segment. Associated with it is a progressive atrophy of the muscles, with more or less spastic rigidity.

Three affections, as a rule described apart, belong together in this category: (*a*) Progressive muscular atrophy of spinal origin; (*b*) amyotrophic lateral sclerosis; and (*c*) progressive bulbar paralysis. A slow atrophic change in the motor neurones is the anatomical basis, and the disease is one of the whole motor path, involving, in many cases, the cortical, bulbar, and spinal centres. There may be simple muscular atrophy with little or no spasm, or progressive wasting with marked spasm and great increase in the reflexes. In others, there are added symptoms of involvement of the motor nuclei in the medulla—a glosso-labio-laryngeal paralysis; while in others, again, with atrophy (especially of the arms), a spastic condition of the legs and bulbar phenomena, tremors develop and signs of cortical lesion. These various stages may be traced in the same case.

For convenience, bulbar paralysis will be considered separately, and here are taken together *progressive muscular atrophy* and *amyotrophic lateral sclerosis.*

The disease is known as the Aran-Duchenne type of progressive muscular atrophy and as Cruveilhier's palsy, after the French physician who early described it. Luys and Lockhart Clarke first demonstrated that the cells of the ventral horns of the spinal cord were diseased. Charcot separated two types—one with simple wasting of the muscles, due, he believed, to degeneration confined to the ventral horns (and to this he restricted the name progressive muscular atrophy—type, Aran-Duchenne); the other, in which there was spastic paralysis of the muscles followed by atrophy. As the anatomical basis for this he assumed a primary degeneration of the pyramidal tracts and a secondary atrophy of the ventral horns. To this he gave the name of amyotrophic lateral sclerosis. There is but little evidence, however, to show that any such sharp distinction can be made between these two diseases, and Leyden and Gowers regard them as identical.

Etiology.—The cause of the disease is unknown. It is more frequent in males than in females. It affects adults, usually after the thirtieth year, though occasionally younger persons are attacked. A majority of all cases of progressive muscular atrophy under twenty five years of age belong to the dystrophies. Cold, wet, exposure, fright, and mental worries are mentioned as possible causes. Certain cases follow injury. Hereditary influences are present in some cases. The rare form which occurs in infancy usually affects several members of the same family. Hereditary and family influences, however, play but a small part in the etiology, and in this it is in contrast to progressive neural muscular atrophy and the dystrophies. Yet, in the Farr family, which I recorded some years ago, in which thirteen members were affected in two generations, with the exception of two, the cases occurred or proved fatal above the age of forty, and the late onset speaks rather for a central affection. The spastic form may develop late in life—after seventy—as a senile change.

Morbid Anatomy.—The essential anatomical change is a slow degeneration of the motor path, involving particularly the lower motor neurones. The upper neurones are also involved, either first, simultaneously, or at a later period. Associated with the degeneration in the cells of the ventral horns there is a degenerative atrophy of the muscles. The following are the important anatomical changes: (*a*) The gray matter of the cord shows the most marked alteration. The large ganglion cells of the ventral horns are atrophied, or, in places, have entirely disappeared, the neuroglia is increased, and the medullated fibres are much decreased. The fibres of the ventral nerve-roots passing through the white matter are wasted. (*b*) The ventral roots outside of the cord are also atrophied. (*c*) The muscles affected show degenerative atrophy, and the inter-muscular branches of the motor nerves are degenerated. (*d*) The degeneration of the gray matter is rarely confined to the cord, but extends to the medulla, where the nuclei of the motor cerebral nerves are found extensively wasted. (*e*) In a majority of all the cases there is sclerosis in the ventro-lateral white tracts, the lateral pyramidal tracts particularly are diseased, but the degeneration is not confined to them, but extends into the ventro-lateral ground bundles. The direct cerebellar and the ventro-lateral ascending tracts are spared. The degeneration in the pyramidal tracts extends toward the brain to different levels, and in several cases has been traced to the motor cortex, the cells of which have been found degenerated. In the medulla the medial longitudinal fasciculus has been found diseased. (*f*) In those cases in which no sclerosis has been found in the pyramidal tracts there has been a sclerosis of the ventro-lateral ground bundle (short tracts).

Symptoms.—Irregular pains may precede the onset of the wasting, and cases may be treated for chronic rheumatism. The hands are usually first affected, and there is difficulty in performing delicate manipulations. The muscles of the ball of the thumb waste early, then the interossei and lumbricales, leaving marked depressions between the metacarpal bones. Ultimately the contraction of the flexor and extensor muscles and the extreme atrophy of the thumb muscles, the interossei, and lumbricales produce the claw-hand —*main en griffe* of Duchenne. The flexors of the forearm are usually involved before the extensors. In the shoulder-girdle the deltoid is first affected; it may waste even before the other muscles of the upper extremity. The trunk muscles are gradually attacked; the upper part of the trapezius long remains unaffected. Owing to the feebleness of the muscles which support it, the head tends to fall forward. The platysma myoides is unaffected and often hypertrophies. The arms and the trunk muscles may be much atrophied before the legs are attacked. The face muscles are attacked late. Ultimately the intercostal and abdominal muscles may be involved, the wasting proceeds to an extreme grade, and the patient may be actually "skin and bone," and, as "living skeletons," the cases are not uncommon in "museums" and "side-shows." Deformities and contractures result, and lordosis is almost always present. A curious twitching of the muscles (fibrillation) is a common symptom, and may occur in muscles which are not yet attacked. It is a most important symptom, but is not, as was formerly supposed, a characteristic feature. The irritability of the muscles is increased. Sensation is unimpaired, but the patient may complain of numbness and coldness of the affected limbs. The galvanic and faradic irritability of the muscles progressively diminishes and may become extinct, the galvanic persisting for the longer time. In cases of rapid wasting and paralysis the reaction of degeneration may be obtained. The excitability of the nerve trunks may persist after the muscles have ceased to respond. The loss of power is usually proportionate to the wasting.

The foregoing description applies to the group of cases in which the atrophy and paralysis are flaccid—*atonic,* as Gowers calls it. In other cases, those which Charcot describes as amyotrophic lateral sclerosis, spastic paralysis precedes the wasting. This *tonic* atrophy first involves the arms and then the legs. The reflexes are greatly increased. It is one of the rare conditions in which a jaw clonus may be obtained. The most typical condition of spastic paraplegia may be produced. On starting to walk, the patient seems glued to the ground and makes ineffectual attempts to lift the toes; then four or five short, quick steps are taken on the toes with the body thrown forward; and finally he starts off, sometimes with great rapidity. Some of the patients can walk up and down stairs better than on the level. The wasting is never so extreme as in the atonic form, and the loss of power may be out of proportion to it. The sphincters are unaffected. Sexual power may be lost early. Cases are met with which correspond accurately to the clinical picture given by Charcot of amyotrophic lateral sclerosis. These are not very common, and it is much more usual to have a combination of the two types. A flaccid atrophic paralysis with increased reflexes is often met with. These differences depend upon the relative extent of the involvement of the upper and lower motor segments and the time of the involvement of each. The condition may be unilateral.

As the degeneration extends upward an important change takes place from the occurrence of bulbar symptoms, which may, however, precede the spinal manifestations. The lips, tongue, face, pharynx, and larynx may be involved. The lips may be affected and articulation impaired for years before serious symptoms occur. In the final stage there may be tremor, the memory fails, and a condition of dementia supervenes.

Gowers gives the following useful classification of the varieties of this affection: (1) Atonic atrophy, becoming extreme; (2) muscular weakness with spasm, but without wasting or with only slight wasting; and (3) atonic atrophy, rarely extreme in degree, with exaggeration of the reflexes. These conditions may "coexist in every degree and combination—between universal atonic atrophy on the one hand and universal spastic paralysis without wasting on the other."

Diagnosis.—Progressive (central) muscular atrophy begins, as a rule, in adult life, without hereditary or family influences (the early infantile form being an exception), and usually affects first the muscles of the thumb, and gradually involves the interossei and lumbricales. Fibrillary contractions are common, electrical changes occur, and the deep reflexes are usually increased. These characteristics are usually sufficient to distinguish it from the other forms of muscular wasting.

In syringo-myelia the symptoms may be very similar to those in the spastic form of muscular atrophy. The sensory disturbances in the former disease, as a rule, make the diagnosis clear, but when these are absent or but little developed it may be very difficult or even impossible to distinguish the diseases.

Treatment.—The disease is incurable. The downward progress is slow but certain, though in a few cases a temporary arrest may take place. With a history of syphilis, mercury and iodide of potassium may be tried, and Gowers recommends courses of arsenic and the hypodermic injection of strychnine. Probably the most useful means is systematic massage, particularly in the spastic cases.

Bulbar Paralysis (Glosso-labio-laryngeal Paralysis)

When the disease affects the motor nuclei of the medulla first or early, it is called bulbar paralysis, but it has practically no independent existence, as the spinal cord is sooner or later involved.

Symptoms.—The disease usually begins with slight defect in the speech, and the patient has difficulty in pronouncing the dentals and linguals. The paralysis starts in the tongue, and the superior lingual muscle gradually becomes atrophied, and finally the mucous membrane is thrown into transverse folds. In the process of wasting the fibrillary tremors are seen. Owing to the loss of power in the tongue, the food is with difficulty pushed back into the pharynx. The saliva also may be increased, and is apt to accumulate in the mouth. When the lips become involved the patient can neither whistle nor pronounce the labial consonants. The mouth looks large, the lips are prominent, and there is constant drooling. The food is masticated with difficulty. Swallowing becomes difficult, owing partly to the regurgitation into the nostrils, partly to the involvement of the pharyngeal muscles. The muscles of the vocal cords waste and the voice becomes feeble, but the laryngeal paralysis is rarely so extreme as that of the lips and tongue.

The **course** of the disease is slow but progressive. Death often results from an aspiration pneumonia, sometimes from choking, more rarely from involvement of the respiratory centres. The mind usually remains clear. The patient may become emotional. In a majority of the cases the disease is only part of a progressive atrophy, either simple or associated with a spastic condition. In the later stage of amyotrophic lateral sclerosis the bulbar lesions may paralyze the lips long before the pharynx or larynx becomes affected.

The **diagnosis** of the disease is readily made, either in the acute or chronic form. The involvement of the lips and tongue is usually well marked, while that of the palate may be long deferred. A condition has been described, however, which may closely simulate bulbar paralysis. This is the so-called *pseudo-bulbar* form or bulbar palsy of cerebral origin. Bilateral disease of the motor cortex in the lower part of the ascending frontal convolution, or about the knee of the internal capsule, may cause paralysis of the lips and tongue and pharynx, which closely simulates a lesion of the medulla. Sometimes the symptoms appear on one side, but in many instances they develop suddenly on both sides. A bilateral lesion has usually been found, but in several instances the disease was unilateral.

The so-called *acute bulbar paralysis* may be due to (*a*) hæmorrhagic or embolic softening in the pons and medulla; (*b*) acute inflammatory softening, analogous to polio-myelitis, occurring occasionally as a post-febrile affection. It has occasionally followed diphtheria, and occurred after severe electric shocks of high voltage. It usually comes on very suddenly, hence the term apoplectiform. The symptoms in this form may correspond closely to those of an advanced case of chronic bulbar paralysis. The sudden onset and the associated symptoms make the diagnosis easy. In these acute cases there may be loss of power in one arm, or hemiplegia, sometimes alternate hemiplegia, with paralysis on one side of the face and loss of power on the other side of the body. (*c*) In epidemics of polio-myelitis cases occur with acute bulbar symptoms.

2. PROGRESSIVE NEURAL MUSCULAR ATROPHY

This form, known also as the peroneal type, or by the names of the men who have described it most accurately—namely, Charcot, Marie, and Tooth—

occurs either as a hereditary or as a family affection. It usually begins in early childhood, affecting first the muscles of the feet and the peroneal group; as a result of the weakening of these muscles, club-foot, either pes equinus or pes equino-varus, occurs. In rare instances the disease may begin in the hands, but the upper limbs, as a rule, are not affected for some years after the legs are attacked, and the trouble then begins in the small muscles of the hand. Sensory disturbances are frequently present and form important diagnostic features. Fibrillary contractions and twitchings also occur. The electrical reactions are altered; there is either a loss or a very great decrease of the excitability, which can be demonstrated not only in the atrophic muscles, but also in muscles and nerves which are apparently normal.

This form seems to stand between the central muscular atrophy and the muscular dystrophies. Occurring in families and beginning in early life, it resembles the latter, but it is more like the former in that fibrillary contractions and muscular twitchings are common, that the small muscles of the hand are apt to be involved, and that electrical changes are present. In the prominence of sensory symptoms it differs from both. In cases of acquired double club-foot this disease should be suspected.

3. THE MUSCULAR DYSTROPHIES

(*Dystrophia muscularis progressiva,* Erb)

Definition.—Muscular wasting, with or without an initial hypertrophy, beginning in various groups of muscles, usually progressive in character, and dependent on primary changes in the muscles themselves. A marked hereditary disposition is met with in the disease.

Etiology.—No etiological factors of any moment are known other than heredity. The influence may show itself by true heredity—the disease occurring in two or more generations—or several members of the same generation may be affected, showing a family tendency. Many members of the same family may be attacked through several generations. Males, as a rule, are more frequently affected than females. The disease is usually transmitted through the mother, though she may not herself be affected. As many as 20 or 30 cases have been described in five generations. In Erb's cases 44 per cent. showed no heredity. The disease usually sets in before puberty, but may be as late as the twentieth or twenty-fifth year, or in some instances even later.

Symptoms.—The first symptom noticed is, as a rule, clumsiness in the movements of the child, and on examination certain muscles or groups of muscles seem to be enlarged, particularly those of the calves. The extensors of the leg, the glutei, the lumbar muscles, the deltoid, triceps and infraspinatus, are the next most frequently involved, and may stand out with great prominence. The muscles of the neck, face, and forearm rarely suffer. Sometimes only a portion of a muscle is involved. With this hypertrophy of some muscles there is wasting of others, particularly the lower portion of the pectorals and the latissimus dorsi. The attitude when standing is very characteristic. The legs are far apart, the shoulders thrown back, the spine is greatly curved, and the abdomen protrudes. The gait is waddling and awkward. In getting up from the floor the position assumed, so well known now through Gowers' figures, is pathognomonic. The patient first turns over in the all-fours position and raises the trunk with his arms; the hands are then moved along the ground until the knees are reached; then with one hand upon a knee he lifts himself up, grasps the other knee, and gradually pushes himself into the erect posture, as it has been expressed, by climbing up his legs. The striking contrast between the feebleness of the child and the powerful looking pseudo-hypertrophic muscles is very characteristic. The enlarged muscles may, however, be relatively very strong.

The course of the disease is slow, but progressive. Wasting proceeds and finally all traces of the enlarged condition of the muscles disappear. At this late period distortions and contractions are common.

The muscles of the shoulder-girdle are nearly always affected early in the disease, causing a symptom upon which Erb lays great stress. With the hands under the arms, when one endeavors to lift the patient, the shoulders are raised to the level of the ears, and one gets the impression as though the child were slipping through. These "loose shoulders" are very characteristic. The abnormal mobility of the shoulder blades gives them a winged appearance, and makes the arms seem much longer than usual when they are stretched out.

There are no sensory symptoms. The atrophic muscles do not show the reaction of degeneration except in extremely rare instances.

Clinical Forms.—A number of different types have been described, depending upon the age at the onset, the muscles first affected, the occurrence of hypertrophy, the prominence of heredity, etc. But Erb has shown that there is no sharp division between these different forms, and classes them all under the name of *dystrophia muscularis progressiva*. For convenience of description he subdivides the disease into two large groups:

I. Those cases which occur in childhood.

II. The cases occurring in youth and adult life.

The first division is subdivided into (1) the hypertrophic and (2) the atrophic form.

Under the hypertrophic form, which is the pseudo-hypertrophic muscular paralysis of authors, he thinks it is useful to distinguish between the cases in which (*a*) the enlarged muscles have undergone lipomatosis—i. e., pseudo-hypertrophy—from those (*b*) in which there is a real hypertrophy.

The atrophic form also includes two subclasses: (*a*) Those cases in which the muscles of the face are involved early; this corresponds to the infantile form of Duchenne—the Landouzy-Dejerine type. (*b*) Those cases in which the face is not involved. They may be grouped as follows:

I. *Dystrophia muscularis progressiva infantum.*
  1. Hypertrophic form.
    (*a*) With pseudo-hypertrophy.
    (*b*) With real hypertrophy.
  2. Atrophic form.
    (*a*) With primary involvement of the face (infantile form of Duchenne).
    (*b*) Without involvement of the face.

II. *Dystrophia muscularis progressiva juvenum vel adultorum* (Erb's juvenile form).

Morbid Anatomy.—According to Erb, the disease consists in a change in the muscles themselves. At first the muscle fibres hypertrophy, and become round; the nuclei increase, and the muscle fibres may become fissured. At the same time there is a slight increase in the connective tissue. Sooner or later the muscle fibres begin to atrophy, and the nuclei become greatly increased. Vacuoles and fissures appear, and the fibres finally become completely atrophic, the connective tissue becoming markedly increased. Fat may be deposited in the connective tissue to such an extent as to cause hypertrophic lipomatosis—pseudo-hypertrophy. The different stages of these changes may be found in a single muscle at the same time.

The nervous system has very generally been found to be without demonstrable lesions, but in certain cases changes in the cells of the ventral horns have been described.

Diagnosis.—The muscular dystrophies can usually be distinguished readily from the other forms of muscular atrophy.

(*a*) In the cerebral atrophy loss of power usually precedes the atrophy, which is either of a monoplegic or hemiplegic type.

(*b*) From progressive (central) muscular atrophy the distinctions are plainly marked. This form begins in the small muscles of the hand, a situation rarely, if ever, affected by the dystrophies, which involve first those of the calves, the trunk, the face, or the shoulder-girdle. In the central atrophy the reaction of degeneration is present and fibrillary twitchings occur in both the atrophied and non-atrophied muscles. In many cases, in addition to the wasting in the arms, there is a spastic condition in the legs and increase in the reflexes. The central atrophies come on late in life; the dystrophies develop, as a rule, early. In the progressive muscular dystrophies heredity plays an important rôle, which in the central form is quite subsidiary. In the rare cases of early infantile spinal muscular atrophy occurring in families the symptoms are so characteristic of a central disease that the diagnosis presents no difficulty.

(*c*) In the neuritic muscular atrophies, whether due to lead or to trauma, the general characters and the mode of onset are distinctive. In the cases of multiple neuritis seen for the first time at a period when the wasting is marked there is often difficulty, but the absence of family history and the distribution are important features. Moreover, the paralysis is out of proportion to the atrophy. Sensory symptoms may be present, and in the cases in which the legs are chiefly involved there is usually the *steppage* gait so characteristic of peripheral neuritis.

(*d*) Progressive neural muscular atrophy. Here heredity is also a factor, and the disease usually begins in early life, but the distribution of atrophy and paralysis, which in this affection is at first confined to the periphery of the extremities, helps to distinguish it from the dystrophies; while the occurrence of sensory symptoms, fibrillary contractions, and the marked decrease in the electrical excitability usually make the distinction clear.

The outlook in the primary muscular dystrophies is bad. The wasting progresses uniformly, uninfluenced by treatment. Erb holds that by electricity and massage the progress is occasionally arrested. The general health should be carefully looked after, moderate exercise allowed, frictions with oil applied to the muscles, and when the patient becomes bedfast, as is inevitable sooner or later, care should be taken to prevent contractures in awkward positions.

The forms of progressive muscular wasting—progressive (central) muscular atrophy, progressive neural muscular atrophy, and the muscular dystrophies—have been considered as distinct diseases, but possibly the distinction may not be so sharp as we believe. Certain cases occur which seem not to belong to any one of the forms, but to stand between them. The changes in the muscles which were thought to be characteristic of the dystrophies have been found in the other forms. The central form occurs as a family disease in infancy, and the nervous system has been found diseased in the dystrophies.

B. SYSTEM DISEASES OF THE UPPER MOTOR SEGMENT

The question of an uncomplicated primary degeneration of the upper motor neurones has not been decided. Cases with a clinical picture corresponding to this lesion are not uncommon, and they may persist for a long time without change. Unfortunately the cases which have come to autopsy have shown various conditions. In only two or three has the disease been so nearly confined to the pyramidal tract that they can be used as an argument for the independence of this condition. The cases of Minkowski, Dreschfeld, and Strümpell are not absolutely conclusive, as they are not quite pure, although they go far to prove that a degeneration in the pyramidal tract may be uncomplicated, at least for a long time. The same may be said for the group of cases described by Bernhardt and Strümpell under the name hereditary spastic spinal paralysis, in which the extensive systemic degeneration of the pyramidal tracts is combined with slight degeneration in other tracts of the cord.

1. SPASTIC PARALYSIS OF ADULTS

(*Tabes dorsalis spasmodique; Primary Lateral Sclerosis*)

Definition.—A gradual loss of power with spasm of the muscles of the body, the lower extremities being first and most affected, unaccompanied by muscular atrophy, sensory disturbance, or other symptoms. The pathological anatomy is undetermined, but a systemic degeneration of the pyramidal tracts is assumed.

Symptoms.—The general symptoms of spastic paraplegia in adults are very distinctive. The patient complains of feeling tired, of stiffness in the legs, and perhaps of pains of a dull aching character in the back or in the calves. There may be no definite loss of power, even when the spastic condition is well established. In other instances there is definite weakness. The stiffness is felt most in the morning. In a well developed case the gait is most characteristic. The legs are moved stiffly and with hesitation, the toes drag and catch against the ground, and, in extreme cases, when the ball of the foot rests upon the ground a distinct clonus develops. The legs are kept close together, the knees touch, and in certain cases the adductor spasm may cause cross-legged progression. On examination, the legs may at first appear tolerably supple, perhaps flexed and extended readily. In other cases the rigidity is marked, particularly when the limbs are extended. The spasm of the adductors of the thigh may be so extreme that the legs are separated with the greatest difficulty. In cases of this extreme rigidity the patient usually loses the power of walking. The nutrition is well maintained, the muscles may be hypertrophied. The reflexes are greatly increased. The slightest touch upon the patellar tendon produces an active knee-jerk. The rectus clonus and the ankle clonus are easily obtained. In some instances the slightest touch may throw the legs into violent clonic spasm, the condition to which Brown-Séquard gave the name of spinal epilepsy. The superficial reflexes are also increased. The arms may be unaffected for years, but occasionally they become weak and stiff at the same time as the legs.

The course of the disease is progressively downward. Years may elapse before the patient is bedridden. Involvement of the sphincters, as a rule, is late; occasionally, however, it is early. The sensory symptoms rarely progress, and the patients may retain their general nutrition and enjoy excellent health. Ocular symptoms are rare.

Diagnosis.—The diagnosis, so far as the clinical picture is concerned, is readily made, but it is often very difficult to determine accurately the nature of the underlying pathological condition. A history of syphilis is present in many of the cases. Cases which have run a fairly typical clinical course upon coming to autopsy have been found to have been due to very different conditions—transverse myelitis, multiple sclerosis, cerebral tumor, etc. General paralysis of the insane may begin with symptoms of spastic paraplegia, and Westphal believed that it was only in relation to this disease that a primary sclerosis of the pyramidal tracts ever occurred. In any case the diagnosis of primary systemic degeneration of the pyramidal tract is, to say the least, doubtful.

Treatment.—Not much can be done to check the progress of the disease. Division of the posterior nerve roots is permissible when the motor weakness is due chiefly to the spasticity. A number of cases have been operated upon successfully. The same practice has been followed in the spasticity with bilateral athetosis.

2. SPASTIC PARALYSIS OF INFANTS—SPASTIC DIPLEGIA—BIRTH PALSIES

(*Paraplegia cerebralis spastica* (*Heine*); *Little's Disease*)

In this condition there is a paralysis with spasm of all extremities, dating from or shortly succeeding birth, more rarely following the fevers or an attack of convulsions. The legs are usually more involved than the arms; there is no wasting, no disturbance of sensation. The reflexes are increased. The mental condition is usually much disturbed. The patients are often imbeciles or idiots, helpless in mind and body. Ataxic and athetoid movements of the most exaggerated kind may occur.

While only a limited number of cases of infantile hemiplegia are congenital, on the other hand, in spastic diplegia and paraplegia a large proportion of the cases results from injury at birth. The arms may be so slightly affected as to make it difficult to determine whether it is a case of diplegia or paraplegia. The disease usually dates from birth, and a majority of the children are born in first labors or are forceps cases, and are at birth asphyxiated blue babies. In feet presentations there may be laceration or tearing of the cerebro-spinal membranes. Premature birth is also given as a cause.

Morbid Anatomy.—The birth palsies which ultimately induce the spastic diplegias or paraplegias are most frequently the result of meningeal hæmorrhage. The importance of this condition has been shown by the studies of Litzmann and Sarah J. McNutt. The bleeding may come from the veins, or from the longitudinal sinus. The hæmorrhage has in many cases been greatest over the motor areas, and in these cases the intelligence may suffer but little; with a more extensive hæmorrhage, especially when it implicates the frontal lobes, any grade of amentia may be occasioned. It seems probable that the sclerosis found in these cases may result from compression by the blood clot. In other instances the condition may be due to a fetal meningo-encephalitis. In 16 autopsies collected in the literature, in which the patients died at ages varying from two to thirty, the anatomical condition was either a diffuse atrophy, which was most common, or porencephalus. From the fact that certain of the patients are born prematurely, before the pyramidal tracts are developed, it has been assumed by some that a non-development of these tracts is the cause of the disease. In others the fibres have been few in number and incompletely myelinized. This hypothesis has been urged by Marie, who limits the name spastic paraplegia to that group of the infantile cases in which there is no evidence of involvement of the brain—intellectual disturbances, epilepsy, etc., and it is in these cases that he believes the pyramidal tracts have remained undeveloped.

Symptoms.—At first nothing abnormal may be noticed about the child. In some instances there have been early and frequent convulsions; then at the age when the child should begin to walk it is noticed that the limbs are not used readily, and on examination a stiffness of the legs and arms is found. Even at the age of two the child may not be able to sit up, and often the head is not well supported by the neck muscles. The rigidity, as a rule, is more marked in the legs, and there is an adductor spasm. When supported on the feet, the child either rests on its toes and the inner surface of the feet, with the knees close together, or the legs may be crossed. The stiffness of the upper limbs varies. It may be scarcely noticeable or the rigidity may be as marked as in the legs. When the spastic condition affects the arms as well as the legs, we speak of the condition as diplegia; when the legs alone are involved, as paraplegia. There seems to be no sufficient reason for considering them separately. The spasticity is probably due to interruption of the cortico-spinal fibres which exercise an inhibitory influence on the cells of the anterior horns. Constant irregular movements of the arms are not uncommon. The child has great difficulty in grasping an object. The spasm and weakness may be more evident on one side than the other. The mental condition is, as a rule, defective and convulsive seizures are common.

Associated with the spastic paralysis are two allied conditions of considerable interest, characterized by spasm and disordered movements. A child with spastic diplegia may present, in an unusual degree, irregular movements of the muscles. In attempting to grasp an object the fingers may be thrown out in a stiff, spasmodic, irregular manner, or there may be constant irregular movements of the shoulders, arms, and hands, with slight incoördination of the head. Cases of this description have been described as *chorea spastica,* and they may be difficult to separate from multiple sclerosis and from Friedreich's ataxia.

A still more remarkable condition is that of *bilateral athetosis,* in which there is a combination of spasm more or less marked with the most extraordinary bizarre movements of the muscles. The condition, as a rule, dates from infancy. The patient may not be able to walk. The head is turned from side to side; there are continual irregular movements of the face muscles, and the mouth is drawn and greatly distorted. The extremities are more or less rigid, particularly in extension. On the slightest attempt to move, often spontaneously, there are extraordinary movements of the arms and legs, particularly of the arms, somewhat like athetosis, though much more exaggerated. The patients are often unable to help themselves on account of these movements. The reflexes are increased. The mental condition is variable. The patient may be idiotic, but in 3 of the 6 cases which I have seen the patients were intelligent. Massalongo, who has carefully studied this condition, describes 3 cases in one family. I have collected 53 cases from the literature, 33 of which occurred in males and 20 in females.

Treatment.—Little can be done for these children when the symptoms are extreme. In the milder cases patient training may do much to better the mental state when feeble-mindedness accompanies the motor palsies. Exercises and massage should be given for the spastic muscles, and in many instances tenotomies and tendon transplantations may be helpful in improving the usefulness particularly of the lower extremities. Division of the posterior nerve roots is of great use in certain cases. On the view that most of these cases date back to an intracranial hæmorrhage during parturition, it is reasonable to suppose that an immediate operation with the removal of the cortical clot—for the effusion of blood is usually on the surface of the hemisphere—might ward off the disastrous consequences of compression on the infant's brain. Cases, with asphyxia and convulsions after difficult labors, have been operated upon soon after birth by Cushing and others, and cortical clots have been removed. In some cases there has been a complete restoration to health and the usual spastic sequels have not occurred.

3. HEREDITARY SPASTIC PARAPLEGIA

(*Hereditary Spastic Spinal Paralysis; Family form of Spastic Spinal Paralysis*)

It is a family affection and only occasionally are the ascendants affected. There are several forms:

1. The pure spastic paraplegia—Strümpell's type—in which two or more members of a family are attacked. Trunk, arms, and brain are not affected.

2. Mixed forms: (*a*) with features of multiple sclerosis as described by Cestan and Guillain; (*b*) amyotrophic lateral sclerosis type, with the added feature of atrophy; (*c*) forms resembling Friedreich's ataxia and the hereditary cerebellar ataxia; (*d*) forms resembling cerebral diplegia.

In a majority of the cases the disease begins in children between the seventh and the fifteenth years. It may not occur until the twentieth year. Two, three, or four members of a family are affected. Beginning in the legs with characteristic spastic gait and all the features of an ordinary spinal paralysis, the disease may extend and affect the arms, or there are added the symptoms of multiple sclerosis or of one of the other above-named affections. Boys are more often affected than girls, 88 to 51, in the cases collected by Deléarde and Minet.

The pathology of the disease is still under discussion.

Amaurotic Family Idiocy (*Sachs' Disease*).—A remarkable form of infantile paralysis has been described by Sachs, Peterson, and Hirsch. The disease is one which involves the entire gray matter of the central nervous system. The symptoms as summarized by Sachs are: (1) Psychic disturbances that appear in early life (first or second year) and progress to total idiocy. (2) Paresis, and ultimately complete paralysis of the extremities, which may be either flaccid or spastic. (3) Increased, decreased, or normal tendon reflexes. (4) Partial, followed by total blindness (macular changes, with subsequent atrophy of the optic nerve). (5) Marasmus and death, usually before the second year. (6) Distinct familial type. Occasional symptoms are nystagmus, strabismus, hyperacusis, or impairment of hearing. The pathological changes are primitive type of the cerebral convolutions, macrogyria, degenerative changes in the large pyramidal cells, absence of the tangential fibres, and decrease of the fibres of the white matter. The blood-vessels are normal. There is also degeneration of the pyramidal columns of the cord. Of 27 cases collected by Sachs, 17 occurred in six families; all in Hebrews.

4. ERB'S SYPHILITIC SPINAL PARALYSIS

Erb has described a symptom group under the term syphilitic spinal paralysis, to which much attention has been given. The points upon which he lays stress are a very gradual onset with a development finally of the features of a spastic paresis; the tendon reflexes are greatly increased, but the muscular rigidity is slight in comparison with the exaggerated deep reflexes. There is rarely much pain, and the sensory disturbances are trivial, but there may be paræsthesia and the girdle sensation. The bladder and rectum are usually involved, and there is sexual failure or impotence. And, lastly, improvement is not infrequent. A majority of instances of spastic paralysis of adults not the result of slow compression of the cord are associated with syphilis and belong to this group.

Erb believes the lesion to be a special form of transverse myelitis, but perhaps it should be classed, with the system diseases, under the name toxic spastic spinal paralysis.

5. SECONDARY SPASTIC PARALYSIS

Following any lesion of the pyramidal tract there may be a spastic paralysis; thus, in a transverse lesion of the cord, whether the result of slow compression (as in caries), chronic myelitis, the pressure of tumor, chronic meningo-myelitis, or multiple sclerosis, degeneration takes place in the pyramidal tracts, below the point of disease. The legs soon become stiff and rigid, and the reflexes increase. Bastian has shown that in compression paraplegia if the transverse lesion is complete, the limbs may be flaccid, without increase in the reflexes—*paraplégie flasque* of the French. The condition of the patient in these secondary forms varies very much. In chronic myelitis or in multiple sclerosis he may be able to walk about, but with a characteristic spastic gait. In the compression myelitis, in fracture, or in caries, there may be complete loss of power with rigidity.

It may be difficult or even impossible to distinguish these cases from those of primary spastic paralysis. Reliance is to be placed upon the associated symptoms; when these are absent no definite diagnosis as to the cause of the spastic paralysis can be given.

6. HYSTERICAL SPASTIC PARAPLEGIA

There is no spinal cord disease which may be so accurately mimicked as spastic paraplegia. In the hysterical form there is wasting, the sensory symptoms are not marked, the loss of power is not complete, and there is not that extensor spasm so characteristic of organic disease. The reflexes are, as a rule, increased. The knee-jerk is present, and there may be a well developed ankle clonus. Gowers calls attention to the fact that it is usually a spurious clonus, "due to a half-voluntary contraction in the calf muscles." A true clonus does occur, however, and there may be the greatest difficulty in determining whether or not the case is one of hysterical paraplegia. The hysterical contracture will be considered later.

C. SYSTEM DISEASES OF THE LOWER MOTOR SEGMENT

1. CHRONIC ANTERIOR POLIO-MYELITIS

(*Progressive Muscular Atrophy—Aran-Duchenne*)

This disease has been considered as one of the types making up the progressive (central) muscular atrophies. In certain rare cases the process is confined to the lower motor segment. They, however, differ so little clinically from many of the cases in which the pyramidal tracts are involved that it seems better to make no sharp distinction between them. The same may be said of chronic bulbar paralysis.

2. OPHTHALMOPLEGIA

This disease is at times due to a chronic degeneration of the nuclei of the motor nerves of the eyeballs, and so is a system disease of the lower motor segment. It is treated of in connection with the other ocular palsies for the sake of simplicity and because all ophthalmoplegias are not due to nuclear disease.

3. ACUTE POLIO-MYELITIS

(*Infantile Spinal Paralysis, Heine-Medin Disease*)

The epidemic form of this affection has been considered with the infectious diseases. The sporadic cases are very probably, although not surely, due to the same infection. They present the same clinical picture and need no further consideration.

4. ACUTE AND SUBACUTE POLIO-MYELITIS IN ADULTS

An acute polio-myelitis in adults, the exact counterpart of the disease in children, is recognized. Many of the cases represent the sporadic form of polio-myelitis. A certain number of the cases described under this heading have been multiple neuritis; but the suddenness of onset, the rapid wasting, and the marked reaction of degeneration are thought by some to be distinguishing features. Multiple neuritis may, however, set in with rapidity; there may be great wasting and the reaction of degeneration is sometimes present. The time element alone may determine the true nature. Recovery in a case of extensive multiple paralysis from polio-myelitis will certainly be with loss of power in certain groups of muscles; whereas, in multiple neuritis the recovery, while slow, may be perfect.

The subacute form, the *paralysie générale spinale antérieure subaiguë* of Duchenne, is in all probability a peripheral palsy. The paralysis usually begins in the legs with atrophy of the muscles, then the arms are involved, but not the face. Sensation, as a rule, is not involved.

5. ACUTE ASCENDING (LANDRY'S) PARALYSIS

Definition.—An ascending flaccid paralysis, beginning in the legs, rapidly extending to the trunk and arms, and finally involving the muscles of respiration. Sensation and electrical reactions are normal, and there is retention of sphincter control.

Etiology and Pathology.—The disease occurs most commonly in males between the twentieth and thirtieth years. It has sometimes followed the specific fevers. As already mentioned, there is a form of the epidemic polio-myelitis which has an acute course and a clinical picture similar to Landry's paralysis; but it is not likely, as has been suggested, that this disease always represents the sporadic variety. Many of the common pathogenic organisms may, especially in patients debilitated by disease, give rise to symptoms of acute ascending paralysis. Thus, the typhoid bacillus may produce clinically an acute ascending paralysis. The most careful studies have not solved the problem of this remarkable disease. There are two views: First, that it is a peripheral neuritis. Spiller in a rapidly fatal case found destructive changes in the peripheral nerves and corresponding alterations in the cell bodies of the ventral horns. He suggests that the toxic agent acts on the lower motor neurones as a whole, and that possibly the reason why no lesions were found in some of the cases is that the more delicate histological methods were not used. Buzzard has isolated a micrococcus (*M. thecalis*) in pure culture in one case, and found the organism in large numbers in the tissues outside the spinal dura. Secondly, that it is a functional disorder without a recognizable anatomical basis.

Symptoms.—Weakness of the legs, gradually progressing, often with tolerable rapidity, is the first symptom. In some cases within a few hours the paralysis of the legs becomes complete. The muscles of the trunk are next affected, and within a few days, or even less in more acute cases, the arms are also involved. The neck muscles are next attacked, and finally the muscles of respiration, deglutition, and articulation. The reflexes are lost, but the muscles neither waste nor show electrical changes. The sensory symptoms are variable; in some cases tingling, numbness, and hyperæsthesia have been present. In the more characteristic cases sensation is intact and the sphincters are uninvolved. Enlargement of the spleen, which occurred in the only two cases in my wards, has been noticed in several other cases. The course of the disease is variable. It may prove fatal in less than two days. Other cases persist for a week or for two weeks. In a large proportion of the cases the disease is fatal. One patient was kept alive for 41 days by artificial respiration (C. L. Greene).

Diagnosis.—The diagnosis is difficult, particularly from certain forms of multiple neuritis, and if we include in Landry's paralysis the cases in which sensation is involved distinction between the two affections is impossible. We apparently have to recognize the existence of a rapidly advancing motor paralysis without involvement of the sphincters, without wasting or electrical changes in the muscles, without trophic lesions, and without fever—features sufficient to distinguish it from either the acute central myelitis or the polio-myelitis anterior. It is doubtful, however, whether these characters always suffice to enable us to differentiate the cases of multiple neuritis. The cases of acute polio-myelitis with the picture of an acute ascending paralysis should not be difficult to recognize during the progress of an epidemic.

IV. COMBINED SYSTEM DISEASES

When the disease is not confined within the limits of either the afferent or efferent systems, but affects both, it is known as a *combined system disease.* Some authors contend that the diseases usually classed under this head are not really system diseases, but are diffuse processes. This is the view taken by Leyden and Goldscheider, who limit the term system disease to locomotor ataxia and progressive muscular atrophy.

In certain cases of locomotor ataxia which have run a fairly typical course there may be found after death, besides the anatomical picture corresponding to this disease, a moderate degeneration of the pyramidal tracts and of the ventral horns. In progressive muscular atrophy, on the other hand, there may be degeneration in the dorsal columns. During life these secondary involvements of other systems may or may not be accompanied by demonstrable symptoms, and when such do occur they make their appearance late in the disease.

There is another group of cases in which from the very first the symptoms point to an involvement of both the afferent and efferent systems, and it is to these that the term primary combined system disease is usually limited.

1. ATAXIC PARAPLEGIA

This name is applied by Gowers to a disease characterized clinically by a combination of ataxia and spastic paraplegia, and anatomically by involvement of the dorsal and lateral columns.

The disease is most common in middle aged males. Exposure to cold and traumatism have been occasional antecedents. In striking contrast to ordinary tabes a history of syphilis is rarely to be obtained.

The anatomical features are a sclerosis of the dorsal columns, which is not more marked in the lumbar region and not specially localized in the root zone of the cuneate fasciculi. The involvement of the lateral columns is diffuse, not always limited to the pyramidal tracts, and there may be an annular sclerosis. Marie believes that in many cases the distribution of the sclerosis is due to the arterial supply and not to a true systematic degeneration, the vessels involved being branches of the dorsal spinal artery.

The *symptoms* are well defined. The patient complains of a tired feeling in the legs, not often of actual pain. The sensory symptoms of true tabes are absent. An unsteadiness in the gait gradually comes on with progressive weakness. The reflexes are increased from the outset, and there may be well marked ankle clonus. Rigidity of the legs comes on slowly, but it is rarely extreme as in the uncomplicated cases of lateral sclerosis. From the start incoördination is a well characterized feature, and the difficulty of walking in the dark, or swaying when the eyes are closed, may, as in true tabes, be the first symptom to attract attention. In walking the patient uses a stick, keeps the eyes fixed on the ground, the legs far apart, but the stamping gait, with elevation and sudden descent of the feet, is not often seen. The incoordination may extend to the arms. Sensory symptoms are rare, but Gowers calls attention to a dull, aching pain in the sacral region. The sphincters usually become involved. Eye symptoms are rare. Late in the disease mental symptoms may occur, similar to those of general paresis.

In well marked cases the *diagnosis* is easy. The combination of marked incoördination with retention of the reflexes and more or less spasm are characteristic features. The absence of ocular and sensory symptoms is an important point.

2. PRIMARY COMBINED SCLEROSIS (PUTNAM)

The studies of J. J. Putnam, Dana, Bastianelli, Risien Russell, Collier, and Batten have separated from among the lesions of the cord a fairly well defined disease, characterized anatomically by a diffuse degeneration, often in discrete patches. The dorsal and lateral columns are constantly involved, chiefly in the thoracic and cervical regions. The nerve roots and the gray matter show no changes. The lesions have the "appearance of a non-systemic primary neurone degeneration, not dependent upon antecedent inflammation" (E. W. Taylor).

Of Putnam's 50 cases, 31 were women, all but 5 above thirty years old. A majority of the patients were of small stature and slender frame, and in many there had been a general lack of vigor and a chronic pallor and debility; 7 presented profound anæmia. There was no luetic history. The relation of this group to anæmia is interesting. Russell, Batten, and Collier make three groups: (1) cases of profound anæmia (and one may add of cachexia), in which during life no symptoms were present, but in which there were found combined scleroses of the cord post mortem; (2) cases of progressive pernicious anæmia, in which spinal symptoms have occurred; (3) cases of chronic sclerosis of the cord, in which there occurs, as a secondary feature, a severe anæmia.

The *symptoms* are both sensory and motor. The onset is usually with numbness in the extremities, progressive loss of strength, and emaciation. Paraplegia gradually develops, before which there have been, as a rule, spastic symptoms with exaggerated knee-jerk. The arms are affected less than the legs. Mental symptoms suggestive of dementia paralytica may occur toward the close.

3. HEREDITARY ATAXIA

(*Friedreich's Ataxia*)

In 1861 Friedreich reported 6 cases of a form of hereditary ataxia, and the affection has usually gone by his name. Unfortunately, *paramyoclonus multiplex* is also called Friedreich's disease; so it is best, if his name is used in connection with this affection, to term it Friedreich's ataxia. It is a very different disease in many respects from ordinary tabes. It may or may not be hereditary. It is really a family disease, several brothers and sisters being, as a rule, affected. The 143 cases analyzed by Griffith occurred in 71 unrelated families. In his series inheritance of the disease itself occurred in only 33 cases. Various influences in the parents have been noted; alcoholism in only 7 cases. Syphilis has rarely been present. Of the 143 cases, 86 were males and 57 females. The disease sets in early in life, and in Griffith's series 15 occurred before the age of two years, 39 before the sixth year, 45 between the sixth and tenth, 20 between the eleventh and fifteenth, 18 between the sixteenth and twentieth, and 5 between the twentieth and twenty-fifth years.

The *morbid anatomy* shows an extensive sclerosis of the dorsal and lateral columns of the spinal cord. The periphery and the cerebellar tracts are usually involved. The observations of Dejerine and Letulle are of special interest, since they seem to indicate that the change in this disease is a neurogliar (ectodermal) sclerosis, differing entirely from the ordinary spinal sclerosis. According to this view, Friedreich's disease is a gliosis of the dorsal columns due to developmental errors; but the question is still unsettled.

Symptoms.—The ataxia differs somewhat from the ordinary form. The incoördination begins in the legs, but the gait is peculiar. It is swaying, irregular, and more like that of a drunken man. There is not the characteristic stamping gait of the true tabes. Romberg's symptom may or may not be present. The ataxia of the arms occurs early and is very marked; the movements are almost choreiform, irregular, and somewhat swaying. In making any voluntary movement the action is overdone, the prehension is clawlike, and the fingers may be spread or overextended just before grasping an object. The hand frequently moves about an object for a moment and then suddenly pounces upon it. There are irregular, swaying movements of the head and shoulders, some of which are choreiform. There is present in many cases what is known as static ataxia, that is to say, ataxia of quiet action. It occurs when the body is held erect or when a limb is extended—irregular, oscillating movements of the head and body or of the extended limb.

Sensory symptoms are not usually present. The deep reflexes are lost early in the disease, and, next to the ataxia, this is the most constant and important symptom. The skin reflexes are usually normal, and the pupillary reflex to light is practically never affected.

Nystagmus is a characteristic symptom. Atrophy of the optic nerve rarely occurs. A striking feature is early deformity of the feet. There is talipes equinus, and the patient walks on the outer edge of the feet. The big toe is flexed dorsally on the first phalanx. Scoliosis is very common.

Trophic lesions are rare. As the disease advances paralysis comes on and may ultimately be complete. Some of the patients never walk.

Disturbance of speech is common. It is usually slow and scanning; the expression is often dull; the mental power is, as a rule, maintained, but late in the disease becomes impaired.

Diagnosis.—The diagnosis of the disease is not difficult when several members of a family are affected. The onset in childhood, the curious form of incoördination, the loss of knee-jerks, the early talipes equinus, the position of the great toe, the scoliosis, the nystagmus, and scanning speech make up an unmistakable picture. The disease is often confounded with chorea, with the ordinary form of which it has nothing in common. With hereditary chorea it has certain similarities, but usually this disease does not set in until after the thirtieth year.

The affection lasts for many years and is incurable. Care should be taken to prevent contractures.

Cerebellar Type

There is a form of hereditary ataxia, described by Marie as *cerebellar heredo-ataxia,* which starts later in life, after the age of twenty, with disability in the legs, but the gait is less ataxic than "groggy." The knee-jerks are retained, and a spastic condition of the legs ultimately develops. There is no scoliosis, nor does club-foot develop. Sanger Brown's cases, 25 in one family, and J. H. Neff's, 13, appear to belong to this type. The cerebellum has been found atrophied in 2 cases.

4. PROGRESSIVE INTERSTITIAL HYPERTROPHIC NEURITIS OF INFANTS

Under this imposing title Dejerine and Sottas described a rare and interesting affection. It is a family disease, and begins in early life. The symptoms are those typical of locomotor ataxia, to which is added progressive muscular atrophy, with involvement of the face and a hypertrophy and hardening of the peripheral nerves. As the name indicates, it is an interstitial hypertrophic neuritis with secondary involvement of the dorsal columns of the cord. This disease has been associated with progressive neural muscular atrophy, but Dejerine has shown that it is quite distinct.

5. TOXIC COMBINED SCLEROSIS

Certain poisons cause changes in the lateral and dorsal columns of the cord that resemble those of the combined system diseases. They have been demonstrated in pellagra and in ergotism. In pernicious anæmia and many chronic wasting diseases these scleroses occur, and are believed to be due to the action of poisons produced within the system.

C. DIFFUSE DISEASES OF THE NERVOUS SYSTEM

I. AFFECTIONS OF THE MENINGES

DISEASES OF THE DURA MATER

(*Pachymeningitis*)

Pachymeningitis Externa.—CEREBRAL.—Hæmorrhage often occurs as a result of fracture. Inflammation of the external layer of the dura is rare. Caries of the bone, either extension from middle-ear disease or due to syphilis, is the principal cause. In the syphilitic cases there may be a great thickening of the inner table and a large collection of pus between the dura and the bone. Occasionally the pus is infiltrated between the two layers of the dura mater or may extend through and cause a dura-arachnitis.

The symptoms of external pachymeningitis are indefinite. In the syphilitic cases there may be a small sinus communicating with the exterior. Compression symptoms may occur with or without paralysis.

SPINAL.—An acute form may occur in syphilitic affections of the bones, in tumors, and in aneurism. The symptoms are those of a compression of the cord. A chronic form is much more common, and is a constant accompaniment of tuberculous caries of the spine. The internal surface of the dura may be smooth, while the external is rough and covered with caseous masses. The entire dura may be surrounded, or the process may be confined to the ventral surface.

Pachymeningitis Interna.—This occurs in three forms: (1) Pseudo-membranous, (2) purulent, and (3) hæmorrhagic. The first two are unimportant. Pseudo-membranous inflammation of the lining membrane of the dura is not usually recognized, but a most characteristic example of it came under my observation as a secondary process in pneumonia. Purulent pachymeningitis may follow an injury, but is more commonly the result of extension from inflammation of the pia. It is remarkable how rarely pus is found between the dura and arachnoid membranes.

HÆMORRHAGIC PACHYMENINGITIS

(*Hæmatoma of the Dura Mater*)

Cerebral Form.—This remarkable condition, first described by Virchow, is very rare in general medical practice. During ten years no instance of it came under my observation at the Montreal General Hospital. On the other hand, in the post-mortem room of the Philadelphia Hospital, which received material from a large almshouse and asylum, the cases were not uncommon, and within three months I saw four characteristic examples, three of which came from the medical wards. The frequency of the condition in asylum work may be gathered from the fact that in 1,185 post mortems at the Government Hospital for the Insane, Washington, to June 30, 1897, there were 197 cases with "a true nec-membrane of internal pachymeningitis" (Blackburn). Of these cases, 45 were chronic dementia, 37 were general paresis, 30 senile dementia, 28 chronic mania, 28 chronic melancholia, 22 chronic epileptic insanity, 6 acute mania, and 1 case imbecility. Forty-two of the cases were in persons over seventy years of age.

It has also been found in profound anæmia and other diseases of the blood and of the blood vessels, and is said to have followed certain of the acute fevers. Herter called attention to the not infrequent occurrence of the lesion in badly nourished cachectic children.

The morbid anatomy is interesting. Virchow's view that the delicate vascular membrane precedes the hæmorrhage is undoubtedly correct. Practically we see one of three conditions in these cases: (*a*) subdural vascular membranes, often of extreme delicacy; (*b*) simple subdural hæmorrhage; (*c*) a combination of the two, vascular membrane and blood clot. Certainly the vascular membrane may exist without a trace of hæmorrhage—simply a fibrous sheet of varying thickness, permeated with large vessels, which may form beautiful arborescent tufts. On the other hand, there are instances in which the subdural hæmorrhage is found alone, but it is possible that in some of these at least the hæmorrhage may have destroyed all trace of the vascular membrane. In some cases a series of laminated clots are found, forming a layer from 3 to 5 mm. in thickness. Cysts may occur within this membrane. The source of the hæmorrhage is probably the dural vessels. Huguenin and others hold that the bleeding comes from the vessels of the pia mater, but certainly in the early stage of the condition there is no evidence of this; on the other hand, the highly vascular subdural membrane may be seen covered with the thinnest possible sheeting of clot, which has evidently come from the dura. The subdural hæmorrhage is usually associated with atrophy of the convolutions, and it is held that this is one reason why it is so common in the insane, especially in dementia paralytica and dementia senilis. We meet with the condition also in phthisis and various cachectic conditions in which the cerebral wasting is as common and almost as marked as in cases of insanity. König found in 135 cases of hæmorrhagic pachymeningitis from the Berlin Pathological Institute that 23 per cent. accompanied phthisis. Atrophy, however, may not be the only factor.

The symptoms are indefinite, or there may be none at all, especially when the hæmorrhages are small or have occurred very gradually, and the diagnosis can not be made with certainty. Headache has been a prominent symptom in some cases, and when the condition exists on one side there may be hemiplegia. The most helpful symptoms for diagnosis, indicating that the hæmorrhage in an apoplectic attack is meningeal, are (1) those referable to increased intracranial pressure (slowing and irregularity of the pulse, vomiting, coma, contracted pupils, reacting to light slowly or not at all) and (2) paresis and paralysis, gradually increasing in extent, accompanied by symptoms which point to a *cortical* origin. Extensive bilateral disease may, however, exist without any symptoms whatever.

Spinal Form.—The spinal *pachymeningitis interna,* described by Charcot and Joffroy, involves chiefly the cervical region (*P. cervicalis hypertrophica*). The space between the cord and the dura is occupied by a firm, concentrically arranged, fibrinous growth, which is seen to have developed within, not outside of, the dura mater. It is a condition anatomically identical with the hæmorrhagic pachymeningitis interna of the brain. The cord is usually compressed; the central canal may be dilated—hydromyelus—and there are secondary degenerations. The nerve roots are involved in the growth and are damaged and compressed. The extent is variable. It may be limited to one segment, but more commonly involves a considerable portion of the cervical enlargement. The disease is chronic, and in some cases presents a characteristic group of symptoms. There are intense neuralgic pains in the course of the nerves whose roots are involved. They are chiefly in the arms and in the cervical region, and vary greatly in intensity. There may be hyperæsthesia with numbness and tingling; atrophic changes may develop, and there may be areas of anæsthesia. Gradually motor disturbances appear; the arms become weak and the muscles atrophied, particularly in certain groups, as the flexors of the hand. The extensors, on the other hand, remain intact, so that the condition of claw-hand is gradually produced. The grade of the atrophy depends much upon the extent of involvement of the cervical nerve roots, and in many cases the atrophy of the muscles of the shoulders and arms becomes extreme. The condition is one of cervical paraplegia, with contractures, flexion of the wrist, and typical *main en griffe.* Usually before the arms are greatly atrophied there are the symptoms of what the French writers term the second stage—namely, involvement of the lower extremities and the gradual production of a spastic paraplegia, which may develop several months after the onset of the disease, and is due to secondary changes in the cord.

The disease runs a chronic course, lasting, perhaps, two or more years. In a few instances, in which symptoms pointed definitely to this condition, recovery has taken place. The disease is to be distinguished from amyotrophic lateral sclerosis, syringomyelia, and tumors. From the first it is separated by the marked severity of the initial pains in the neck and arms; from the second by the absence of the sensory changes characteristic of syringomyelia. From certain tumors it is very difficult to distinguish; in fact, the fibrinous layers form a tumor around the cord.

The condition known as *hæmatoma* of the dura mater may occur at any part of the cord, or, in its slow, progressive form—pachymeningitis hæmorrhagica interna—may be limited to the cervical region and produce the symptoms just mentioned. It is sometimes extensive, and may coexist with a similar condition of the cerebral dura. Cysts may occur filled with hæmorrhagic contents.

DISEASES OF THE PIA MATER

(*Acute Cerebro-spinal Leptomeningitis*)

Etiology.—Under cerebro-spinal fever and tuberculosis the two most important forms of meningitis have been described. Other conditions with which meningitis is associated are: (1) *The acute fevers,* more particularly pneumonia, erysipelas, and septicæmia; less frequently small-pox, typhoid fever, scarlet fever, measles, influenza, etc. (2) *Injury or disease of the bones of the skull.* In this group by far the most frequent cause is necrosis of the petrous portion of the temporal bone in chronic otitis. (3) *Extension from disease of the nose.* Meningitis has followed perforation of the skull in sounding the frontal sinuses, suppurative disease of these sinuses, and necroses of the cribriform plate. As mentioned under cerebro-spinal fever, the infection is thought to be possible through the nose. (4) As a *terminal infection* in chronic nephritis, arterio-sclerosis, heart disease, gout, and the wasting diseases of children.

The following etiological table of the chief acute forms of meningitis may be useful to the student:

Acute Leptomeningitis.	Primary.	1. Of cerebro-spinal fever.	(*a*) Sporadic. (*b*) Epidemic.	Diplococcus intracellularis.
		2. Pneumococcic.	Meninges involved alone or in a general pneumococcus infection.	Pneumococcus.
	Secondary.	1. Tuberculous	....	Bacillus tuberculosis.
		2. Pneumococcic.	(*a*) Secondary to pneumonia, endocarditis, etc. (*b*) Secondary to disease or injury of cranium or its fossæ.	Pneumococcus.
		3. Pyogenic.	(*a*) Following local disease of cranium or a local infection elsewhere. (*b*) Terminal infection in various chronic maladies.	Various forms of staphylococci and streptococci.
		4. Miscellaneous acute infections.	In typhoid fever, influenza, diphtheria, gonorrhœa, anthrax, actinomycosis, and other acute diseases.	Typhoid bacillus, influenza bacillus, diphtheria bacillus, gonococcus, etc.

Morbid Anatomy.—The basal or cortical meninges may be chiefly attacked. The degree of involvement of the spinal meninges varies. In the form associated with pneumonia and ulcerative endocarditis the disease is bilateral and usually limited to the cortex. In extension from disease of the ear it is often unilateral and may be accompanied with abscess or with thrombosis of the sinuses. In the non-tuberculous form in children, in the meningitis of chronic Bright's disease, and in cachectic conditions the base is usually involved. In the cases secondary to pneumonia the effusion beneath the arachnoid may be very thick and purulent, completely hiding the convolutions. The ventricles also may be involved, though in these simple forms they rarely present the distention and softening which are so frequent in the tuberculous meningitis. For a more detailed description the student is referred to the sections on cerebro-spinal fever and tuberculous meningitis.

Symptoms.—The clinical features of meningitis have already been described at length in the diseases just referred to, and I shall here give a general summary. Cortical meningitis is not to be recognized by any symptoms or set of symptoms from a condition which may be produced by the poison of many of the specific fevers. In the cases of so-called cerebral pneumonia, unless the base is involved and the nerves affected, the disease is unrecognizable, since identical symptoms may be produced by intense engorgement of the meninges. In typhoid fever, in which meningitis is very rare, the twitchings, spasms, and retractions of the neck are almost invariably associated with cerebro-spinal congestion, not with meningitis. Actual meningitis does, however, occur in typhoid fever, and typhoid bacilli may be present in the exudate.

A knowledge of the etiology gives a very important clew. Thus, in middle-ear disease the development of high fever, delirium, vomiting, convulsions, and retraction of the head and neck would be extremely suggestive of meningitis or abscess. Headache, which may be severe and continuous, is the most common symptom. While the patient remains conscious this is usually the chief complaint, and even when semicomatose he may continue to groan and to place his hand on his head. In the fevers, particularly in pneumonia, there may be no complaint of headache. Delirium is frequently early, and is most marked when the fever is high. Convulsions are less common in simple than in tuberculous meningitis. They were not present in a single instance in the cases which I have seen in pneumonia, ulcerative endocarditis, or septicæmia. In the simple meningitis of children they may occur. Epileptiform attacks which come and go are highly characteristic of direct irritation of the cortex. Rigidity and spasm or twitchings of the muscles are more common. Stiffness and retraction of the muscles of the neck are important symptoms; but they are by no means constant, and are most frequent when the inflammation is extensive on the meninges of the cervical cord. There may be trismus, gritting of the teeth, or spastic contraction of the abdominal muscles. Vomiting is a common symptom in the early stages, particularly in basilar meningitis. Constipation is usually present. In the late stages the urine and fæces may be passed involuntarily. Optic neuritis is rare in the meningitis of the cortex, but is not uncommon when the base is involved. Leube lays stress on the hyperæsthesia of the skin and muscles, especially of the muscles of the neck and calves.

Important symptoms are due to lesions of the nerves at the base. Strabismus or ptosis may occur. The facial nerve may be involved, producing slight paralysis, or there may be damage to the fifth nerve, producing anæsthesia and, if the Gasserian ganglion is affected, trophic changes in the cornea. The pupils are at first contracted, subsequently dilated, and perhaps unequal. The reflexes in the extremities are often accentuated at the beginning of the disease; later they are diminished or entirely abolished. Herpes is common, particularly in the epidemic form.

Fever is present, moderate in grade, rarely rising above 103°. In the non-tuberculous leptomeningitis of debilitated children and in Bright's disease there may be little or no fever. The pulse may be increased in frequency at first, though this is unusual. One of the striking features of the disease is the slowness of the pulse in relation to the temperature, even in the early stages. Subsequently it may be irregular and still slower. The very rapid emaciation which often occurs is doubtless to be referred to a disturbance of the cerebral influence upon metabolism. Kernig's sign has been described under cerebro-spinal fever. There may be a concomitant reflex of one leg when passive flexion is made of the other (Brudzinksi's sign); and when the neck is bent forward there is flexion of the legs both at the knees and hips. Lumbar puncture is exceedingly valuable for diagnosis. It may be that a turbid fluid indicates an acute non-tuberculous meningitis. At first the fluid may be only opalescent. A close relationship exists between the severity of the symptoms, the height of the pyrexia, and the degree of turbidity (Connal). As a rule a preponderance of polynuclear leucocytes is present with the meningococcus or the pyogenic organisms; a mononuclear exudate is characteristic of tuberculosis. It is to be remembered that in tuberculous meningitis the fluid is usually clear; in only one of 69 cases was it opalescent (Connal).

Treatment.—There are no remedies which in any way control the course of acute meningitis. An ice-bag should be applied to the head and, if the subject is young and full blooded, general or local depletion may be practised. Absolute rest and quiet should be enjoined. When disease of the ear is present, a surgeon should be early called in consultation, and if there are symptoms of meningo-encephalitis which can in any way be localized trephining should be practised. An occasional saline purge will do more to relieve the congestion than blisters and local depletion. The warm baths, as recommended by Aufrecht and described under cerebro-spinal fever, should be given every three hours. It is possible that recovery may follow in the primary pneumococcus form (Netter). If counter-irritation is deemed essential, the thermo-cautery may be lightly applied to the back of the neck. Large doses of the perchloride of iron, iodide of potassium, and mercury are recommended by some authors. Hexamethylenamine in doses of 60 grains (4 gm.) daily may be tried, as Crowe has shown that it is excreted in the cerebro-spinal fluid and controls the growth of organisms in the meninges.

The application of an ice-cap, attention to the bowels and stomach, and keeping the fever within moderate limits by sponging are the necessary measures in a disease recognized as almost invariably fatal, in which also the cases of recovery are extremely doubtful. Lumbar puncture may be used as a therapeutic measure.

The **posterior basic meningitis** of Gee, Lees, and Bartow is the sporadic form of cerebro-spinal fever and has been already described.

Meningism.—Sometimes spoken of as the syndrome of Dupré, this is a condition in which there are symptoms of meningitis, but post mortem the characteristic pathological changes are not present. It is practically the condition described formerly as meningeal irritation, and is seen most frequently in the acute fevers of children, particularly in pneumonia and typhoid fever, sometimes in alcoholism and in middle-ear disease.

Chronic Leptomeningitis.—This is rarely seen apart from syphilis or tuberculosis, in which the meningitis is associated with the growth of the granulomata in the meninges and about the vessels. The symptoms in such cases are extremely variable, depending entirely upon the situation of the growth. The epidemic meningitis may run a very chronic course, but of all forms the posterior basic may be the most protracted, as cases have been described with a duration of a year or more. Quincke's *meningitis serosa* is considered with hydrocephalus.

II. SCLEROSES OF THE BRAIN

General Remarks.—The supporting tissue of the central nervous system is the neuroglia, derived from the ectoderm, with distinct morphological and chemical characters. The meninges are composed of true connective tissue derived from the mesoderm, a little of which enters the brain and cord with the blood-vessels. The neuroglia plays the chief part in pathological processes within the central nervous system, but changes in the connective tissue elements may also be important. A convenient division of the cerebro-spinal scleroses is into degenerative, inflammatory, and developmental forms.

The *degenerative scleroses* comprise the largest and most important subdivision, in which provisionally the following groups may be made: (*a*) The common secondary degeneration which follows when nerve fibres are cut off from their trophic centres; (*b*) toxic forms, among which may be placed the scleroses from lead and ergot, and, most important of all, the scleroses of the dorsal columns, due in such a large proportion of cases to the virus of syphilis; (*c*) the sclerosis associated with change in the smaller arteries and capillaries, which is met with as a senile process in the convolutions.

The *inflammatory scleroses* embrace a less important and less extensive group, comprising secondary forms which follow irritative inflammation about tumors, foreign bodies, hæmorrhages, and abscess. Possibly a similar change may follow the primary, acute encephalitis, which Strümpell holds is the initial lesion in the cortical sclerosis which is so commonly found post mortem in infantile hemiplegia.

The *developmental scleroses* are believed to be of a purely neurogliar character, and embrace the new growth about the central canal in syringomyelia and, according to recent French writers, the sclerosis of the dorsal columns in Friedreich's ataxia.

Anatomically we meet with the following varieties:

Miliary sclerosis is a term which has been applied to several different conditions. Gowers mentions a case in which there were grayish red spots at the junction of the white and gray matters, and in which the neuroglia was increased. There is also a condition in which, on the surface of the convolutions, there are small nodular projections, varying from a half to five or more millimetres in diameter.

Diffuse sclerosis, which may involve an entire hemisphere, or a single lobe, in which case the term *sclérose lobaire* has been applied to it by the French. It is not an important condition in general medical practice, but occurs most frequently in idiots and imbeciles. In extensive cortical sclerosis of one hemisphere the ventricle is usually dilated. The symptoms of this condition depend upon the region affected. There may be a considerable extent of sclerosis without symptoms or without much mental impairment. In a majority of cases there is hemiplegia or diplegia with imbecility or idiocy.

Tuberous Sclerosis.—In this remarkable form, which is also known as hypertrophic sclerosis, there are on the convolutions areas, projecting beyond the surface, of an opaque white color and exceedingly firm. The sclerosis may not disturb the symmetry of the convolution, but simply cause a great enlargement, increase in the density, and a change in the color.

These three forms are not of much practical interest except in asylum and institution work. The fourth variety forms a well characterized disease of considerable importance, namely, multiple sclerosis.

Multiple (Insular: Disseminated) Sclerosis (*Sclérose en plaques.*)—Definition.—A chronic affection of the brain and cord, characterized by localized areas in which the nerve elements are more or less replaced by neuroglia. This may occur in the brain or cord alone, more commonly in both.

Etiology.—The cause is unknown. Kahler, Marie, and others assign great importance to the infectious diseases, particularly scarlet fever. Injury has occasionally preceded the onset. It is most common in young persons and in females. Several members in a family may be attacked.

Morbid Anatomy.—The sclerotic areas are widely distributed through the brain and cord, and cases limited to either part alone are almost unknown. The grayish red areas are scattered indifferently through the white and gray matter (E. W. Taylor). The patches are most abundant in the neighborhood of the ventricles, and in the pons, cerebellum, basal ganglia, and the medulla. The cord may be only slightly involved or there may be very many areas throughout its length. The cervical region is apt to be most affected. The nerve roots and the branches of the cauda equina are often attacked. Histologically in the sclerosed patches there is a degeneration of the medullary sheaths, with the persistence for some time of the axis-cylinders. These naked axis-cylinders are thought by some to be new formed nerve fibres. Accompanying this there is marked proliferation of the neuroglia, the fibres of which are denser and firmer. Secondary degeneration, although relatively slight, does occur.

SYMPTOMS.—The onset is slow and the disease is chronic. Feebleness of the legs with irregular pains and stiffness are among the early symptoms. Indeed, the clinical picture may be that of spastic paraplegia with great increase in the reflexes. The following are the most important features:

(*a*) *Volitional Tremor or So-called Intention Tremor.*—There is no paralysis of the arms, but on attempting to pick up an object there is trembling or rapid oscillation. A patient may be unable to lift even a glass of water to the mouth. The tremor may be marked in the legs, and in the head, which shakes as he walks. When the patient is recumbent the muscles may be perfectly quiet. On attempting to raise the head from the pillow, trembling at once comes on. (*b*) *Scanning Speech.*—The words are pronounced slowly and separately, or the individual syllables may be accentuated. This staccato or syllabic utterance is a common feature. (*c*) *Nystagmus,* a rapid oscillatory movement of both eyes, is more common in multiple sclerosis than any other affection of the nervous system.

Sensation is unaffected in a majority of the cases. Optic atrophy may occur early, but is usually partial, rarely leading to complete blindness. The sphincters, as a rule, are unaffected until the last stages. Mental debility is not uncommon. Remarkable remissions occur in the course of the disease, in which for a time all the symptoms may improve. Vertigo is common, and there may be sudden apoplectiform attacks, such as occur in general paresis. The presence of the extensor plantar reflex (Babinski sign) and the absence of the abdominal reflexes are common.

The symptoms, on the whole, are extraordinarily variable, corresponding to the very irregular distribution of the nodules.

DIAGNOSIS.—The diagnosis in well marked cases is easy. Volitional tremor, scanning speech, and nystagmus form a characteristic symptom-group. With this there is usually more or less spastic weakness of the legs. Paralysis agitans, certain cases of general paresis, and occasionally hysteria may simulate the disease very closely. If the case is not seen until near the end the diagnosis may be impossible. Buzzard holds that of all organic diseases of the nervous system disseminated sclerosis in its early stages is that which is most commonly taken for hysteria. The points to be relied upon in the differentiation are, in order of importance, optic atrophy, the nystagmus, the bladder disturbances, when present, and the volitional tremor. The tremor in hysteria is not volitional. Unilateral cases are recorded.

Pseudo-sclerosis—the Westphall-Strümpell disease—is a rare condition simulating multiple sclerosis and not often distinguished from it during life. Mental changes are more pronounced, the tremor is more exaggerated, the nystagmus not always present, and the gait more ataxic. It sets in earlier, sometimes in the first decade, and in a majority of the cases no lesions have been found post mortem.

The PROGNOSIS is unfavorable. Ultimately, the patient, if not carried off by some intercurrent affection, becomes bedridden.

TREATMENT.—No known treatment has any influence on the progress of sclerosis of the brain. Neither the iodides nor mercury have the slightest effect, but a prolonged course of nitrate of silver or arsenic may be tried. The X-rays have been used with success (Raymond).

D. DIFFUSE AND FOCAL DISEASES OF THE SPINAL CORD

I. TOPICAL DIAGNOSIS

From the symptoms presented by a spinal cord lesion it is possible to determine more or less accurately not only the segmental level but also the transverse extent of the segmental involvement. The effects of an injury or of disease may be circumscribed and involve the gray matter of the segment or the tracts running through it; it may be more extensive and involve the cord in a given level in its entire transverse extent; finally, there are cases in which only one lateral half of the cord is implicated. It is well for the student to have a definite routine to follow in making his examinations, for each factor may be helpful in determining the site and character of the lesion. Some of the more important points to observe are the following: (1) *subjective sensations,* particularly the character and seat of pain, if any be present, such as the radiating pains of dorsal root compression; (2) the patient's *attitude,* as the position of the arms in cervical lesions, the character of the respiration, whether diaphragmatic, etc.; (3) *motor symptoms,* the groups of paralyzed muscles and their electrical reaction; (4) the *sensory symptoms,* including tests for tactual, thermic, and dolorous impressions, for muscle sense, bone sensation, etc.; (5) the condition of the *reflexes,* both the tendon and the skin reflexes as well as those for the pupil, the bladder and rectum, etc.; (6) the surface temperature and condition of moisture or dryness of the skin, which gives an indication of *vaso-motor* paralysis. The table on pages 898-900 and the figures on pages 906 and 907 will be useful while making an examination.

Focal Lesions.—We have seen that a lesion involving a definite part of the gray matter of the spinal cord, owing to destruction of the cell bodies of the lower motor neurones and consequent degeneration of their axis-cylinder processes, is accompanied by a loss of power to perform certain definite movements. Thus a disease, such as anterior poliomyelitis, may give as its only symptom a characteristic flaccid paralysis, and the seat of the lesion is revealed by the muscles involved. If from injury or disease a lesion involves more than the gray matter and, for example, if the neighboring fibres of the pyramidal tract be affected there may be in addition a spastic paralysis of the muscles whose centres lie in the lower levels of the cord. The degree of such a paralysis depends upon the intensity of the lesion of the pyramidal tract and may vary from a slight weakness in dorsal flexion of the ankle to an absolute paralysis of all the muscles below the lesion. Again, if the afferent tracts of the cord are affected sensory symptoms may be added to the motor palsy. There may be disturbances of pain and temperature sense alone or touch also may be affected. This, however, is more rare except in serious lesions. The upper border of disturbed sensation often indicates most clearly the level of the disease, especially when this is in the thoracic region where the corresponding level of motor paralysis is not easily demonstrated. It is unusual for cutaneous anæsthesia in organic lesions of the cord to extend above the level of the second rib and the tip of the shoulder, for this represents the lower border of the skin-field of the fourth cervical (see sensory charts), and as the chief centre for the diaphragm lies in this segment, a lesion at this level sufficiently serious to cause sensory disturbances would probably occasion motor paralyses as well and would entirely shut off the movements necessary for respiration. It is to be noted that the demonstrable upper border of the anæsthetic field may not quite reach that which represents the level of the lesion. This is due to the functional overlapping of the segmental skin-fields (Sherrington) and applies more to touch than to pain and temperature. There is often a narrow zone of hyperæsthesia above the anæsthetic region.

Complete Transverse Lesions.—When the transverse lesion is total and the lower part of the cord is cut off entirely from above, there is complete sensory and motor paralysis to the segmental level of the injury, and the tendon reflexes, whose centres lie below, are lost instead of being exaggerated, as they are apt to be in case the lesion is a focal one. The symptomatology of total transverse lesions in man has thus been given by Collier. (1) Total flaccid paralysis of muscles below the level of the lesion. (Spastic paralysis indicates that the lesion is incomplete.) (2) Permanent abolition of the knee-jerk and other deep reflexes supplied by the lower segments of the cord. (3) A rapid wasting of the paralyzed muscles with a loss of the faradic excitability. (4) The sphincters lose their tone and there is dribbling of urine. (5) There is total anæsthesia to the level of the lesion (the zone of hyperæsthesia is rarer). (6) The only sign of self-action remaining is in the occasional presence, though in reduced degree, of certain skin reflexes such as the plantar reflex with its dorsal flexor response in the great toe.

Unilateral Lesions.—The motor symptoms, which follow lesions limited to one lateral half of the cross section of the spinal cord, are confined to one side of the body; they are on the same side as the lesion. At the level of the lesion, owing to destruction of cell bodies of the lower system of neurones, there will be found flaccid paralysis and atrophy of those muscles whose centres of innervation happen to lie at this level. Owing to degeneration of the pyramidal tract, the muscles whose centres be at lower levels are also paralyzed, but they retain their normal electrical reactions, become spastic, and do not atrophy to any great degree.

The sensory symptoms are peculiar. On the side of the lesion corresponding to the segment or segments of the cord involved there is a zone of anæsthesia to all forms of sensation. Below this there is no loss in the perception of pain, temperature, or touch. Indeed, hyperæsthesia has been described. Muscle sense is disturbed, and the ability to appreciate the size, consistency, weight, and shape of an object. On the side opposite to the lesion and nearly up to its level there is complete loss of perception for pain and temperature and there may be some dulling of tactile sense as well.

The following table, slightly modified from Gowers, illustrates the distribution of these symptoms in a complete hemi-lesion of the cord:

Cord

Zone of cutaneous hyperæsthesia. Zone of cutaneous anæsthesia. Lower segment type of paralysis with atrophy.	Lesion.	
Upper segment type of paralysis. Hyperæsthesia of skin. Muscular sense and allied sensations impaired. Reflex action first lessened and then increased. Surface temperature raised.		Muscular power normal. Loss of sensibility of skin to pain and temperature. Muscular sense normal. Reflex action normal. Temperature same as that above lesion.

This combination of symptoms was first recognized by Brown-Séquard, after whom it has been named. It is common in syphilitic diseases of the cord, tumors and stab-wounds, and is not infrequently associated with syringomyelia and hæmorrhages into the cord. It is only in exceptional cases, of course, that the lesion is absolutely limited to the hemi-section of the cord and the symptoms consequently may vary somewhat in degree.

II. AFFECTIONS OF THE BLOOD VESSELS

1. CONGESTION

Apart from actual myelitis, we rarely see post mortem evidences of congestion of the spinal cord, and, when we do, it is usually limited either to the gray matter or to a definite portion of the organ. The white matter is rarely found congested, even when inflamed. The gray matter often has a reddish pink tint, but rarely a deep reddish hue, except when myelitis is present. If we know little anatomically of conditions of congestion of the cord, we know less clinically, for there are no features in any way characteristic of it.

2. ANÆMIA

So, too, with this state. There may be extreme grades of anæmia of the cord without symptoms. In chlorosis, for example, there are rarely symptoms pointing to the cord, and there is no reason to suppose that such sensations as heaviness in the limbs and tingling are especially associated with anæmia.

Profound anæmia of the cord follows ligature of the aorta. In experiments made in Welch's laboratory by Herter it was found that within a few moments after the application of the ligature to the aorta paraplegia came on. Paralysis of the sphincters occurred, but less rapidly. Observations made by Halsted on occlusion of the abdominal aorta in dogs have shown that paraplegia occurs in a large percentage of cases, many of which, however, may recover as the collateral circulation is established. In the fatal cases Gilman found extensive alterations in the cell bodies of the lower part of the cord with degenerations. This condition is of interest in connection with the occasional rapid development of a paraplegia after profuse hæmorrhage, usually from the stomach or uterus. It may come on at once or at the end of a week or ten days, and is probably due to an anatomical change in the nerve elements similar to that produced in Herter's experiments. The degeneration of the dorsal columns of the cord in pernicious anæmia has already been described.

3. EMBOLISM AND THROMBOSIS

Blocking of the spinal arteries by emboli rarely occurs. It may be produced experimentally, and Money found that it was associated with choreiform movements. Thrombosis of the smaller vessels in connection with endarteritis plays an important part in many of the acute and chronic changes in the cord.

4. ENDARTERITIS

It is remarkable how frequently in persons over fifty the arteries of the spinal cord are found sclerotic. The following forms may be met with: (1) A nodular peri-arteritis or endarteritis associated with syphilis and sometimes with gummata of the meninges; (2) an arteritis obliterans, with great thickening of the intima and narrowing of the lumen of the vessels, involving chiefly the medium and larger-sized arteries. Miliary aneurisms or aneurisms of the larger vessels are rarely found in the spinal cord.

5. HÆMORRHAGE INTO THE SPINAL MEMBRANES; HÆMATORRHACHIS

In meningeal apoplexy, as it is called, the blood may lie between the dura mater and the spinal canal—extra-meningeal hæmorrhage—or within the dura mater—intra-meningeal hæmorrhage.

Extra-meningeal hæmorrhage occurs usually as a result of traumatism. The exudation may be extensive without compression of the cord. The blood comes from the large plexuses of veins which may surround the dura. The rupture of an aneurism into the spinal canal may produce extensive and rapidly fatal hæmorrhage.

Intra-meningeal hæmorrhage is a less frequent result of trauma, but in general is perhaps rather more common. It is rarely extensive from causes acting directly on the spinal meninges themselves. Scattered hæmorrhages are not infrequent in the acute infectious fevers, and I have twice, in malignant small-pox, seen much extravasation. Bleeding may occur also in death from convulsive disorders, such as epilepsy, tetanus, and strychnia poisoning, and has been recorded in association with difficult parturition. The most extensive hæmorrhages occur in cases in which the blood comes from rupture of an aneurism at the base of the brain, either of the basilar or vertebral artery. In ventricular apoplexy the blood may pass from the fourth ventricle into the spinal meninges. In cranial fractures, particularly those of the base of the skull, the resultant hæmorrhage almost always finds its way into the subarachnoid space about the cord and may be demonstrated by the withdrawal of bloody fluid by a lumbar puncture. The procedure is of considerable diagnostic value. On the other hand, hæmorrhage into the spinal meninges may possibly ascend into the brain.

Symptoms.—The symptoms in moderate grades may be slight and indefinite. In the non-traumatic cases the hæmorrhage may either come on suddenly or after a day or two of uneasy sensations along the spine. As a rule, the onset is abrupt, with sharp pain in the back and symptoms of irritation in the course of the nerves. There may be muscular spasms, or paralysis may come on suddenly, either in the legs alone or both in the legs and arms. In some instances the paralysis develops more slowly and is not complete. There is no loss of consciousness, and there are no signs of cerebral disturbance. The clinical picture naturally varies with the site of the hæmorrhage. If in the lumbar region, the legs alone are involved, the reflexes may be abolished, and the action of the bladder and rectum is impaired. If in the thoracic region, there is more or less complete paraplegia, the reflexes are usually retained, and there are signs of disturbance in the thoracic nerves, such as girdle sensations, pains, and sometimes eruption of herpes. In the cervical region the arms as well as the legs may be involved; there may be difficulty in breathing, stiffness of the muscles of the neck, and occasionally pupillary symptoms.

The prognosis depends much upon the cause of the hæmorrhage. Recovery may take place in the traumatic cases, and in those associated with the infectious diseases.

6. HÆMORRHAGE INTO THE SPINAL CORD; HÆMATOMYELIA

Most frequently a result of traumatism, intraspinal hæmorrhage is naturally more common in males, and during the active period of life. Cases have been known to follow cold or exposure; it occurs also in tetanus and other convulsive diseases, and hæmorrhage may be associated with tumors, with syringomyelia or myelitis. A direct injury to the spine, however, from blows or from falls, is by far the most common cause. Thorburn was among the first to point out that acute flexure of the neck, often without attendant fracture or dislocation of the vertebræ, was a form of accident that most commonly preceded these hæmorrhages. The level of the lesion, for this reason, is most frequently in the lower cervical region.

Anatomical Condition.—The extent of the hæmorrhage may vary from a small focal extravasation to one which finds its way in columnar fashion a considerable distance up and down the cord. The bleeding primarily takes place into the gray matter, and this as a rule suffers most, but the surrounding medullated tracts may be thinned out and lacerated. In a case which occurred at the Montreal General Hospital under Wilkins the hæmorrhage occupied a position opposite the region of the fifth and sixth cervical nerves, and on transverse section the cord was occupied by a dark red clot measuring 12 by 5 mm., around which the white substance formed a thin, ragged wall. The clot could be traced upward as far as the second cervical, and downward as far as the fourth thoracic segment.

Symptoms.—As one side of the cord is usually involved more than the other, a type of the Brown-Séquard syndrome is common. The symptoms are sudden in onset, and leave the patient with hyperæsthesia and a paralysis which becomes spastic and is most marked on one side, while anæsthesia, chiefly to pain and temperature, is most marked on the opposite side of the body. Often a most distressing hyperæsthesia, usually a "pins and needles" sensation, may be present for many days, but there is rarely any acute pain of the radiating or root type. As hæmatomyelia is most frequent in the lower cervical region, in addition to the symptoms just mentioned a brachial type of palsy is commonly seen, with flaccid and atrophic paralysis of the muscles innervated from the lowest cervical and first thoracic segments. The hæmorrhage may occur in segments farther down the cord, the lumber enlargement being affected next in frequency to the lower cervical. The segmental level of the paralysis necessarily would vary accordingly.

The condition may prove rapidly fatal, particularly if the extravasation is bilateral and extends high enough in the cord to involve the centres for the diaphragm. More frequently there is a more or less complete recovery with a residual palsy of the upper extremity and a partial anæsthesia, corresponding to the level of the lesion, and some spasticity of the leg.

Diagnosis.—The diagnosis of the traumatic cases is comparatively easy, and it is important to recognize them, as they are often needlessly subjected to operation under the belief that they are instances of acute compression. The residual symptoms in old cases may closely simulate those seen in syringomyelia.

Treatment.—Absolute rest is important and the patient should be disturbed as little as possible. Special care must be given the skin to prevent bed-sores and to the bladder to prevent cystitis. Treatment of the paralyzed parts should not be begun for six weeks after the hæmorrhage, when electricity, gentle massage, and passive movements are indicated.

III. COMPRESSION OF THE SPINAL CORD

(*Compression Myelitis*)

Definition.—Interruption of the functions of the cord by slow compression.

Etiology.—Caries of the spine, new growths, aneurism, and parasites are the important causes of slow compression. Caries, or Pott's disease, as it is usually called, after the surgeon who first described it, is in the great majority of instances a tuberculous affection. Pressure paralysis from this cause is often associated with angular curvature, but in a large proportion of all the cases the involvement of the cord is due to pachymeningitis externa, to abscess, or in rare cases to direct spicules of bone. There may be a tuberculous pachymeningitis without caries. The paraplegia in Pott's disease may occur without any spinal deformity. These are very difficult cases to recognize, and they are usually associated with pressure of tuberculous material inside the dura. In a few rare cases the paraplegia may be due to a secondary myelitis. In a few cases it is due to syphilis and occasionally to extension of disease from the pharynx. It is most common in early life, but may occur after middle age.

It may follow trauma. Compression occasionally results from aneurism of the thoracic aorta or the abdominal aorta, in the neighborhood of the cœliac axis. Malignant growths frequently cause a compression paraplegia. A retroperitoneal sarcoma or the lymphadenomatous growths of Hodgkin's disease may invade the vertebræ. More commonly, however, the involvement is secondary to scirrhus of the breast. Of parasites, the echinococcus and the cysticercus occasionally occur in the spinal canal.

Symptoms.—These may be considered as they affect the bones, the nerves, and the cord.

VERTEBRAL.—In malignant diseases and in aneurism erosion of the bodies may take place without producing any deformity of the spine. Fatal hæmorrhage may follow erosion of the vertebral artery. In caries, on the other hand, it is the rule to find more or less deformity, amounting often to angular curvature. The compression of the cord, however, is rarely if ever the direct result of this bony kyphosis but is due to the thickening of the dura and the presence of caseous and inflammatory products between this membrane and the bodies of the diseased vertebræ. The spinous processes of the affected vertebræ are tender on pressure, and pain follows jarring movements or twisting of the spine. There may be extensive tuberculous disease without much deformity, particularly in the cervical region. In the case of aneurism or tumor pain is a constant and agonizing feature.

NERVE-ROOT SYMPTOMS.—These result from compression of the nerve roots as they pass out between the vertebræ. In caries, even when the disease is extensive and the deformity great, radiating pains from compression involvement of the roots are rare. Pains are more common in cancer of the spine secondary to that of the breast, and in such cases may be agonizing. There may be acutely painful areas—the *anæsthesia dolorosa*—in regions of the skin which are anæsthetic to tactile and painful impressions. Trophic disturbances may occur, particularly herpes. Pressure on the ventral roots may give rise to wasting of the muscles supplied by the affected nerves. This is most noticeable in disease of the cervical or lumbar regions.

CORD SYMPTOMS.—(*a*) *Cervical Region.*—Not infrequently the caries is high up between the axis and the atlas or between the latter and the occipital bone. In such instances a retropharyngeal abscess may be present, giving rise to difficulty in swallowing. There may be spasm of the cervical muscles, the head may be fixed, and movements may either be impossible or cause great pain. In a case of this kind in the Montreal General Hospital movement was liable to be followed by transient, instantaneous paralysis of all four extremities, owing to compression of the cord. In one of these attacks the patient died.

In the lower cervical region there may be signs of interference with the cilio-spinal centre and dilatation of the pupils. Occasionally there is flushing of the face and ear of one side or unilateral sweating. Deformity is not so common, but healing may take place with the production of a callus of enormous breadth, with complete rigidity of the neck.

(*b*) *Thoracic Region.*—The deformity is here more marked and pressure symptoms are more common. The time of onset of the paralysis varies very much. It may be an early symptom, even before the curvature is manifest, and it is noteworthy that Pott first described the disease that bears his name as "a palsy of the lower limbs which is frequently found to accompany a curvature of the spine." More commonly the paralysis is late, occurring many months after the curvature has developed. The paraplegia is slow in its development; the patient at first feels weak in the legs or has disturbance of sensation, numbness, tingling, pins and needles. The girdle sensation may be marked, or severe pains in the course of the intercostal nerves. Motion is, as a rule, more quickly lost than sensation. The paraplegia is usually of the spastic type, with exaggeration of the reflexes. Bastian's symptom—abolition of the reflexes—is rarely met with in compression from caries as the transverse nature of the lesion is rarely complete. The paraplegia may persist for months, or even for more than a year, and recovery still be possible.

(*c*) *Lumbar Region.*—In the lower dorsal and lumbar regions the symptoms are practically the same, but the sphincter centres are involved and the reflexes are not exaggerated.

Diagnosis.—The X-ray picture is of first importance. Caries is by far the most frequent cause of slow compression of the cord, and when there are external signs the recognition is easy. There are cases in which the exudation in the spinal canal between the dura and the bone leads to compression before there are any signs of caries, and if the root symptoms are absent it may be extremely difficult to arrive at a diagnosis. Janeway has called attention to persistent lumbago as a symptom of importance in masked Pott's disease, particularly after injury. Brown-Séquard's paralysis is more common in tumor and in injuries than in caries. Pressure on the nerve roots, too, is less frequent in caries than in malignant disease. The cervical form of pachymeningitis also produces a pressure paralysis. Pressure from secondary carcinoma is naturally suggested when spinal symptoms follow within a few years after an operation for cancer of the breast. In paraplegia following tumor of the vertebra secondary to cancer of the breast, and in the erosion of the spine by retroperitoneal growths, the suffering is most intense. The condition has been well termed *paraplegia dolorosa.* I have seen two cases in which the breast tumor had not been recognized.

Treatment.—In compression by aneurism or metastatic tumors the condition is hopeless. In the former the pains are often not very severe, but in the latter morphia is always necessary. On the other hand, compression by caries is often successfully relieved even after the paralysis has persisted for a long period. When caries is recognized early, rest and support to the spine by the various methods now used by surgeons may do much to prevent the onset of paraplegia. When paralysis has occurred, rest with extension gives the best hope of recovery. It is to be remembered that restoration may occur after compression of the cord has lasted for many months, or even more than a year. Cases have been cured by recumbency alone, enforced for weeks or months; the extradural and inflammatory products are absorbed and the caries heals. In earlier days brilliant results were obtained in these cases by suspension, a method introduced by J. K. Mitchell in 1826, and pursued with remarkable success by his son, Weir Mitchell. In recent years the suspension methods in the erect posture have been largely superseded by those of hyperextension during recumbency with the application of plaster jackets to hold the body and spine immovable in the improved position. Forcible correction of the deformity under anæsthesia as sometimes advocated is not to be recommended; but the gentler partial corrections, perhaps repeated several times with a few weeks' interval, often lead to a rapid disappearance of paralyses through the lessening of the angular deformity of the vertebra. In protracted cases, after these methods have been given a fair trial, laminectomy may become advisable, and has in many instances been successful in relieving paralyses when bloodless methods have failed.

The general treatment of caries is that of tuberculosis—fresh air, good food, cod-liver oil, and arsenic.

IV. LESIONS OF THE CAUDA EQUINA AND CONUS MEDULLARIS

The spinal cord extends only to the second lumbar vertebra. Injury, tumors, and caries at or below this level involve not the cord itself, but the bundle of nerves known as the cauda equina and the terminal portion of the cord, the conus medullaris. Much attention has been given to lesions of this part. Fractures and dislocations are common in the lumbo-sacral region, tumors not infrequently involve the filaments of the cauda equina, and some of the nerves are often entangled in the cicatrix of a spina bifida.

A lesion limited to the conus medullaris is rare. A myelitis or a focal hæmatomyelia may be limited to this site with symptoms referable to a lesion of the lowest sacral segments—anæsthesia over the buttocks, perineum, and genitalia, paralysis of the levator ani and the vesical and anal sphincters. Such a focalized lesion has been known to follow a lumbar puncture made between the first and second lumbar vertebræ.

In a fracture or dislocation of the first lumbar vertebra the conus medullaris may be compressed together with the lowest sacral nerves given off from it. It is rare, however, in traumatic cases for the tip of the cord to suffer injury alone without simultaneous involvement of the nerve roots comprising the cauda equina from the second lumbar down. In fracture or dislocation of the fifth lumbar vertebra the sacral roots may alone be involved. Thus in a case which I have reported the patient fell from a bridge and had paralysis of the legs and of the bladder and rectum. When seen sixteen years after the injury, there was slight weakness, with wasting of the left leg; there was complete loss of the function in the ano-vesical and genital centres with anæsthesia in a strip at the back part of the thigh (in the distribution of the small sciatic), and of the perineum, scrotum, and penis. The urethra was also insensitive.

It is sometimes very difficult to differentiate between a lesion, possibly at the first lumbar vertebra, involving the lower part of the spinal cord and one in the sacral region which compromises those peripheral nerves of the cauda equina that are given off from the same segment. This is particularly so in the case of tumors, for in fractures or caries there may be some palpable indication of the seat of trouble. In cauda equina lesions, however, pressure upon the nerve roots is supposed to affect motion much more markedly than sensation, and this discrepancy may be helpful since in the cord lesions themselves the motor and sensory disturbances are more apt to have a correspondingly segmental distribution.

The table and figures given in the general introduction will be found useful in determining the nerve fibres and segments involved in these cases of injury of the cauda equina.

V. TUMORS OF THE SPINAL CORD AND ITS MEMBRANES

Morbid Anatomy.—New growths may grow in the cord or in its membranes, or may extend into them from the spine. These invading growths are the more common and have been touched upon in a previous section. Here the primary spinal growths only will be considered.

Schlesinger's tabulation of 400 cases shows that meningeal tumors are considerably more common than medullary or true cord tumors. Solitary tubercles are by far the most frequent medullary growths. The meningeal tumors may be either intra- or extradural and the intradural sarcomata or fibromata—it is often difficult to tell under which of these terms they should be classified—are by far the most common. This is important because these particular growths remain for a long time non-infiltrating and offer most favorable opportunities for surgical treatment. In the extradural space echinococcus cysts are in some countries frequently found. They are usually multiple, and, indeed, most of the other forms of tumor may be multiple. A lipoma, psammoma, myxoma, neuroma, and other varieties of growth may be met with. Gummata and gliosarcomata are not infrequent and usually involve both the cord and the meninges.

Tumors are more commonly situated on the lateral and dorsal surfaces of the cord, but there is no level of the spine in which they may not occur.

The effects of tumor on the functions of the cord are varied. Slow compression is usually produced by growths external to the cord, and it is remarkable what a high grade of compression the cord will bear without serious interference with its functions. In cases of prolonged interruption of function ascending and descending degenerations occur. Tumors developing within the cord may lead to syringomyelia.

Symptoms.—These will naturally vary a good deal with the segment involved and with the degree of pressure and the extent of implication of the nerve roots. Neuralgic pains which persist over a particular territory, and a slowly progressive paralysis which may at first suggest a Brown-Séquard syndrome, should always make one suspect a spinal growth.

The symptoms of the commoner intradural tumors are as follows: Radiating (root) pains from the level of the lesion; segmental atrophy from pressure on the ventral horns; weakness of the leg, going on to paralysis, at first only on the side occupied by the growth, and due to pyramidal tract involvement; sensory disturbances on the opposite side, first affecting pain and temperature sense; with increase of symptoms the crossed type of paralysis is lost and motor palsy occurs on both sides with great increase of reflexes; even in advanced cases the sensory paralysis rarely becomes quite complete, since some tactual transmission from the lower sacral segments usually persists; spasmodic, painful, jerking movements of the lower extremities are very characteristic of the advanced cases. These symptoms will vary naturally with the character of the growth, its segmental level, place of origin, and other factors, but in no other disease is there the same coincidence of a gradual compression paraplegia and persistent radiating pain. In some cases pain may be elicited by deep pressure alongside the spinous processes at the level of the growth, and the patient, by sudden exertion, or by straining, coughing, or sneezing, may greatly increase it.

Diagnosis.—When constant and severe root pains are associated with a progressive paralysis, the diagnosis may be easily made. Caries may cause identical symptoms, but the radiating pains are rarely so severe. Cervical meningitis simulates tumor very closely, and in reality produces identical effects, but the very slow progress and the bilateral character from the outset may be sufficient to distinguish it. In chronic transverse myelitis the symptoms, according to Gowers, may resemble tumor very closely and present radiating pains, a sense of constriction, and progressive paralysis. Syringomyelia, too, may give a similar picture. A radiogram may be of diagnostic aid in case the vertebræ are infiltrated by the growth.

The nature of the tumor can rarely be indicated with precision. With a marked syphilitic history gumma may naturally be suspected, or, with coexisting tuberculous disease, a solitary tubercle.

Treatment.—If the possibility of syphilitic infection is present the iodide of potassium should be given in large and increasing doses. For the severe pains counter-irritation is sometimes beneficial, particularly the thermo-cautery; morphia is, however, often necessary. A successful laminectomy offers the only hope of relief in case the lesion prove to be non-syphilitic. Since Horsley's first brilliant operation there have been scores of cases of successful extirpation of spinal cord tumors. The intradural fibrosarcomata are the most favorable cases and complete restoration of function in the cord may follow the removal of the tumor. In the infiltrating growths the nerve roots may be divided, or, as has been suggested, even the cord itself sectioned for the relief of the agonizing pain, but ultimate cure is hopeless in malignant growths of this character.

VI. SYRINGOMYELIA

Definition.—A gliomatous new growth about the central canal of the spinal cord, with cavity formation.

Etiology and Morbid Anatomy.—Syringomyelia must be distinguished from dilatation of the central canal—hydromyelus—slight grades of which are not very uncommon either as a congenital condition or as a result of the pressure of tumors. The cavity of syringomyelia has a variable extent in the cord, sometimes running the entire length, but in many cases involving only the cervical and thoracic regions or a more limited area. It is usually in the dorsal portion of the cord and may extend only into one dorsal cornu. The transverse section may be oval or circular or narrow and fissure like. It varies at different levels. The condition is now regarded as a *gliosis,* a development of embryonal neurogliar tissue in which hæmorrhage or degeneration takes place with the formation of cavities.

Of 190 cases, 133 were in men, 57 in women (Schlesinger). A large majority of the cases begin before the thirtieth year. The disease has been met with in three members of the same family.

Symptoms.—The clinical features are extremely complex. In the classical form there are irregular pains, chiefly in the cervical region; muscular atrophy comes on, which may be confined to the arms, or sometimes extends to the legs. The reflexes are increased and a spastic condition develops in the legs. Ultimately the clinical picture may be that of an amyotrophic lateral sclerosis. The tactile sensation is usually normal and the muscular sense is retained, but painful and thermic sensations are not recognized, or there may be in rare instances complete anæsthesia of the skin and of the mucous membranes. This combination of loss of painful and thermic sensations with paralysis of an amyotrophic type is characteristic, but not pathognomonic of the disease. The special senses are usually intact and the sphincters uninvolved. Trophic troubles are not uncommon. Owing to the loss of the pain and heat sensations, the patients are apt to injure themselves. Scoliosis also may be present. The loss of painful and thermic impressions is due to the fact that these pass to the brain in the peri-ependymal gray matter, particularly that portion in the dorsal roots, which is almost constantly involved in syringomyelia. The tactile sensation is retained because the postero-lateral columns are uninvolved.

Schlesinger, in his monograph, recognizes the following types: (1) With the classical features above described, which may begin in the cervical or lumbar regions; (2) a motor type, with the picture of an amyotrophic or a spastic paralysis—the sensation may be undisturbed for years; (3) with predominant sensory features, simulating hysterical hemiplegia, or with general pain and temperature anæsthesia; (4) with pronounced trophic disturbances—to this type belong the cases described as Morvan's disease, an affection characterized by neuralgic pains, cutaneous anæsthesia, and painless, destructive whitlows; and (5) the tabetic type, either a combination of the symptoms of tabes in the lower, and of syringomyelia in the upper extremities, or a pure tabetic symptom-complex, due to invasion of the dorsal columns by the gliosis. Arthropathies occur in about 10 per cent. of the cases.

Diagnosis.—In typical cases the diagnosis is easy. The combination of an amyotrophic paralysis, the picture of progressive muscular atrophy of the Aran-Duchenne type, with retention of tactile and loss of thermic and painful sensation, is probably pathognomonic of the disease. Of affections with which it may be confounded, anæsthetic leprosy is the most important, since the anæsthesia and the wasting may closely simulate it; but, as a rule, in leprosy trophic changes are more or less marked. There is often loss of phalanges and there is no characteristic dissociation of sensory impressions.

Treatment.—This is unsatisfactory, but in a few cases the X-rays have given great relief, particularly to the stiffness.

VII. ACUTE MYELITIS

Etiology.—Acute myelitis results from many causes, and may affect the cord in a limited or extended portion—the gray matter chiefly, or the gray and white matter together. It is met with: (*a*) As an independent affection following exposure to cold, or exertion, and leading to rapid loss of power with the symptoms of an acute ascending paralysis. (*b*) As a sequel of the infectious diseases, such as small-pox, typhus, measles, and gonorrhœa. (*c*) As a result of traumatism, either fracture of the spine or very severe muscular effort. Concussion without fracture may produce it, but this is rare. Acute myelitis, for instance, scarcely ever follows railway accidents. (*d*) In diseases of the bones of the spine, either caries or cancer. This is a more common cause of localized acute transverse myelitis than of the diffuse affection. (*e*) In disease of the cord itself, such as tumors and syphilis; in the latter, either in association with gummata, in which case it is usually a late manifestation; or it may follow within a year or eighteen months of the primary affection.

Morbid Anatomy.—In localized acute myelitis affecting white and gray matter, as met with after accident or an acute compression, the cord is swollen, the pia injected, the consistence greatly reduced, and on incising the membrane an almost diffluent material may escape. In less intense grades, on section at the affected area, the distinction between the gray and white matter is lost, or is extremely indistinct. The chief features have already been described in discussing the epidemic form.

Histologically the nerve fibres are much swollen and irregularly distorted, the axis-cylinders are beaded, the myelin droplets are abundant, and the laminated bodies known as corpora amylacea may be seen. Changes in the blood vessels are striking; the smaller veins are distended and may show varicosities. The perivascular lymph spaces contain numerous leucocytes, and the smaller arteries themselves are frequently the seat of hyaline thrombi. The ganglion cells are swollen and irregular in outline, the protoplasm is extremely granular and vacuolated, and the nuclei, though usually invisible, may show signs of division, and the processes of the cells are not seen. The acute, inflammatory, hyperæmic or red softening is succeeded by stages in which the affected area becomes more yellow from gradual alteration of the blood pigment, and finally white in color from the advancing fatty degeneration. In cases of compression myelitis, a sclerosis may gradually be produced with the anatomical picture of a chronic diffuse myelitis.

Symptoms.—(*a*) Acute Diffuse Myelitis.—This form is in the epidemic poliomyelitis, or occurs in connection with syphilis or one of the infectious diseases, or is seen in a typical manner in the extension from injuries or from tumor. The onset, though scarcely so abrupt as in hæmorrhage, may be sudden; a person may be attacked on the street and have difficulty in getting home. In some instances, the onset is preceded by pains in the legs or back, or a girdle sensation is present. It may be marked by chills, occasionally by convulsions; fever is usually present from the beginning—at first sight, but subsequently it may become high.

The *motor* functions are rapidly lost, sometimes as quickly as in Landry's ascending paralysis. The paraplegia may be complete, and, if the myelitis extends to the cervical region, there may be impairment of motion, and ultimately complete loss of power in the upper extremities as well. The sensation is lost, but there may at first be hyperæsthesia. The reflexes in the initial stage are increased, but in acute central myelitis, unless limited in extent to the thoracic and cervical regions, the reflexes are usually abolished. The rectum and bladder are paralyzed. Trophic disturbances are marked; the muscles waste rapidly; the skin is often congested, and there may be localized sweating. The temperature of the affected limbs may be lowered. Acute bed-sores may occur over the sacrum or on the heels, and sometimes a multiple arthritis is present. In these acute cases the general symptoms become greatly aggravated, the pulse is rapid, the tongue becomes dry; there is delirium, the fever increases, and may reach 107° or 108° F.

The course of the disease is variable. In very acute cases death follows in from five to ten days. The cases following the infectious diseases, particularly the fevers and sometimes syphilis, may run a milder course.

The *diagnosis* of this variety of acute myelitis is rarely difficult. In common with the acute ascending paralysis of Landry, and with certain cases of multiple neuritis, it presents a rapid and progressive motor paralysis. From the former it is distinguished by the more marked involvement of sensation, the trophic disturbances, the paralysis of bladder and rectum, the rapid wasting, the electrical changes, and the fever. From acute cases of multiple neuritis it may be more difficult to distinguish, as the sensory features in these cases may be marked, though there is rarely, if ever, in multiple neuritis complete anæsthesia; the wasting, moreover, is more rapid in myelitis. The bladder and rectum are rarely involved—though in exceptional cases they may be—and, most important of all, the trophic changes, the development of bullæ, bed-sores, etc., are not seen in multiple neuritis.

(*b*) Acute Transverse Myelitis.—The symptoms naturally differ with the situation of the lesion.

(1) Acute transverse myelitis in the *thoracic region,* the most common situation, produces a very characteristic picture. The symptoms of onset are variable. There may be initial pains or numbness and tingling in the legs. The paralysis may set in quickly and become complete within a few days; but more commonly it is preceded for a day or two by sensations of pain, heaviness, and dragging in the legs. The paralysis of the lower limbs is usually complete, and if at the level, say, of the sixth thoracic vertebra, the abdominal muscles are involved. Sensation may be partially or completely lost. At the onset there may be numbness, tingling, or even hyperæsthesia in the legs. At the level of the lesion there is often a zone of hyperæsthesia, which is discovered by passing a test tube containing hot water along the spine, when the sensation of warmth changes to one of actual pain. A girdle sensation may occur early, and when the lesion is in this situation it is usually felt between the ensiform and umbilical regions. The reflex functions are variable. There may at first be abolition of the reflexes; subsequently, those which pass through the segments lower than the one affected may be exaggerated and the legs may take on a condition of spastic rigidity. It does not always happen, however, that the reflexes are increased here, for in a total transverse lesion of the cord they are usually entirely lost, as first pointed out by Bastian. That this is not due to the preliminary shock is shown by the fact that the abolition of the reflexes may be permanent. The muscles become extremely flabby, waste, and lose their faradic excitability, and the sphincters lose their tone. The temperature of the paralyzed limbs is variable. It may at first rise, then fall and become subnormal. Lesions of the skin are not uncommon, and bed-sores are apt to form. There is at first retention of urine and subsequently spastic incontinence. If the lumbar centres are involved, there are

from the outset vesical symptoms. The urine is alkaline in reaction and may rapidly become ammoniacal. The bowels are constipated and there is usually incontinence of the fæces. Some writers attribute the cystitis associated with transverse myelitis to disturbed trophic influence.

The course of complete transverse myelitis depends a good deal upon its cause. Death may result from extension. Segments of the cord may be completely and permanently destroyed, in which case there is persistent paraplegia. The pyramidal fibres below the lesion undergo the secondary degeneration, and there is an ascending degeneration of the dorsal median columns. If the lower segments of the cord are involved the legs may remain flaccid. In some instances a transverse myelitis of the thoracic region involves the ventral horns above and below the lesion, producing flaccidity of the muscles, with wasting, fibrillar contractions, and the reaction of degeneration. More commonly, however, in the cases which last many months there is more or less rigidity of the muscles with spasm or persistent contraction of the flexors of the knee.

(2) *Transverse Myelitis of the Cervical Region.*—If the lesion is at the level of the sixth or seventh cervical nerves, there is paralysis of the upper extremities, more or less complete, sometimes sparing the muscles of the shoulder. Gradually there is loss of sensation. The paralysis is usually complete below the point of lesion, but there are rare instances in which the arms only are affected, the so-called cervical paraplegia. In addition to the symptoms already mentioned there are several which are more characteristic of transverse myelitis in the cervical region, such as the occurrence of vomiting, hiccough, and slow pulse, which may sink to 20 or 30, pupillary changes—myosis—sometimes attacks of dysphagia, dyspnœa, or syncope.

Treatment of Acute Myelitis.—In the rapidly advancing form due either to a diffuse inflammation in the gray matter or to transverse myelitis, the important measures are scrupulous cleanliness, care and watchfulness in guarding against bed-sores, the avoidance of cystitis, either by systematic catheterization or, if there is incontinence, by a carefully adjusted bed urinal, or the use of antiseptic cotton-wool repeatedly changed. In an acute onset in a healthy subject the spine may be cupped. Counter-irritation is of doubtful advantage. Chapman's ice-bag is sometimes useful. No drugs have the slightest influence upon an acute myelitis, except in subjects with well-marked syphilis, in which case mercury and potassium iodide should be given energetically. Tonic remedies, such as quinine, arsenic, and strychnia, may be used in the later stages. When the muscles have wasted, massage is beneficial in maintaining their nutrition. The patient should make every effort to perform muscular movements himself and thus aid improvement. Electricity should not be used in the early stages of myelitis. It is of no value in the transverse myelitis in the thoracic region with retention of the nutrition in the muscles of the leg.

E. DIFFUSE AND FOCAL DISEASES OF THE BRAIN

I. TOPICAL DIAGNOSIS

Only certain regions of the brain give localizing symptoms. These are the cortical motor centres and the associated sensory centres, the speech centres, the centres for the special senses, and the tracts which connect these cortical areas with each other and with other parts of the nervous system.

The following is a brief summary of the effects of lesions from the cortex to the spinal cord:

The Cerebral Cortex.—(*a*) *Destructive lesions* of the motor cortex cause *paralysis* in the muscles of the opposite side of the body. The paralysis is at first flaccid, but the spastic condition subsequently develops. The extent of the paralysis depends upon that of the lesion. It is apt to be limited to the muscles of the head or of an extremity, giving rise to the cerebral monoplegias. One group of muscles may be much more affected than others, especially in lesions of the highly differentiated area for the upper extremity. It is uncommon to find all the muscle groups of an extremity equally involved in cortical monoplegia. In small bilateral symmetrical lesions monoplegia of the tongue may result without paralysis of the face. A lesion may involve centres lying close together or overlapping one another, thus producing associated monoplegias—e. g., paralysis of the face and arm, or of the arm and leg, but not of the face and leg without involvement of the arm. Very rarely the whole motor cortex is involved, causing paralysis of the opposite side—cortical hemiplegia. Usually in such instances there is marked recovery, so that only a monoplegia persists.

Adjoining and posterior to the motor area is believed to be the region of the cortex in which the impulses concerned in general bodily sensation (cutaneous sensibility, muscle sense, visceral sensations) first arrive (the somæsthetic area). Combined with the muscular weakness there is usually some disturbance of sensations, particularly of those of the muscular sense. In lesions of the superior parietal lobe the stereognostic sense is very often affected. For example, when a coin or a knife is placed in the hand of the affected limb, the patient's eyes being closed, it is not recognized, owing to inappreciation of the form and consistence of the object, and this even though the slightest tactile stimulus applied to the fingers or surface of the hand is felt and may be correctly localized. The sense of touch, pain, and temperature may be lowered, but usually not markedly unless the superior and inferior parietal lobules are involved in subcortical lesions. Paræsthesias and vaso-motor disturbances are common accompaniments of paralyses of cortical origin.

(*b*) *Irritative lesions* cause localized spasms. The most varied muscle groups corresponding to particular movement forms may be picked out. If the irritation be sudden and severe, typical attacks of Jacksonian epilepsy may occur. These convulsions are often preceded and accompanied by subjective sensory impressions. Tingling or pain, or a sense of motion in the part, is often the *signal symptom* (Seguin), and is of great importance in determining the seat of the lesion.

When lesions are often both destructive and irritative, there are combinations of the symptoms produced by each. For instance, certain muscles may be paralyzed, and those represented near them in the cortex may be the seat of localized convulsions, or the paralyzed limb itself may be at times subject to convulsive spasms, or muscles which have been convulsed may become paralyzed. The close observation of the sequence of the symptoms in such cases often makes it possible to trace the progress of a lesion involving the motor cortex. In these cases the most frequent cause is a developing tumor, though sometimes local thickenings of the membranes of the brain, small abscesses, minute hæmorrhages, or fragments of a fractured skull must be held responsible.

In another section lesions involving the centres for the special senses are considered, and we shall simply refer to them here. The symptoms caused by lesions of the speech centres will be described under aphasia, and it is only necessary to note here the near situation of the motor speech area (Broca's centre) in the left inferior frontal convolution to the centres for the face and tongue on that side, and the nearness of the supposed centre for writing to that of the hand and arm, and to state that motor aphasia is often associated with paralysis of the right side of the face and the right arm. Accompanying the paralysis, following a Jacksonian fit, of the right face or arm there is often a transient motor aphasia.

According to Flechsig, the sensori-motor centres are limited to tolerably circumscribed areas in the cortex, which differ from other portions in that they are provided with projection fibres which connect them with lower centres. The remaining areas of the cortex, amounting, he believes, to about two-thirds of the whole, are devoid of projection fibres and are concerned entirely in associative activities. These latter areas, the "association centres" of Flechsig, are three in number: (1) The anterior association centre, including the whole of the frontal lobe in front of the somæsthetic area; (2) the middle association centre, corresponding to the cortex of the island of Reil; and (3) the large, posterior association centre, including the præcuneus, the superior and inferior parietal lobules, the supramarginal and angular gyri, and the whole of the temporal and occipital lobes except the auditory and visual sensory areas.

Flechsig attributes the higher psychic functions, especially those connected with the personality of the individual, to the anterior association centres, while the intellectual activities which have to do with knowledge of the external world he believes correspond to the functions of the large posterior association centre. Whether these views be true, and, if so, in how far they may be applied practically in the localization of diseases, especially of the mind, the future has to decide.

Centrum Semiovale.—Lesions in this part may involve either projection fibres (motor or sensory) or association fibres. If involvement of the motor path cause paralysis, this has the distribution of a cortical palsy when the lesion is near the cortex, and of a paralysis due to a lesion of the internal capsule when it is near that region. These lesions of the motor fibres may be associated with symptoms due to interruption in the other systems of fibres running in the centrum semiovale; there may be sensory disturbances—hemianæsthesia and hemianopia—and if the lesion is in the left hemisphere one of the different forms of aphasia may accompany the paralysis.

Corpus Callosum.—This may be congenitally absent without symptoms. An acute lesion involving a large portion of the corpus callosum may, however, yield symptoms suggestive of its localization in this region. In the case recorded by Reinhard, in which the situation of the lesion was suspected ante mortem, there was a disturbance of equilibration (without vertigo) and of the synergetic movements of both halves of the body. The autopsy revealed a gliosarcoma which had destroyed the posterior three-fourths of the corpus callosum. In Bristowe's 4 cases there existed, as symptoms common to all, pain in the head and partial or complete hemiplegia, with gradual extension of the paralysis to the opposite side of the body. Toward the end of life there were disturbance of speech, difficulty in deglutition, incontinence of urine and fæces, and dementia. Here the symptoms have in them nothing that can be looked upon as pathognomonic; indeed, many of the phenomena were doubtless dependent upon involvement of the projection and association fibres of the centrum semiovale.

In animals in which the corpus callosum has been cut experimentally progressive emaciation has been mentioned as a characteristic phenomenon.

Internal Capsule (Fig. 13).—Through this pass within a rather narrow area all, or nearly all, of the projection fibres (both motor and sensory) which are connected with the cerebral cortex. It is divided into an anterior limb, a knee, and a posterior limb, the latter consisting of a thalamo-lenticular portion (its anterior two-thirds) and a retro-lenticular portion (its posterior third). In considering the effects of a given focal lesion involving the fibres of the internal capsule, it is not to be forgotten that the relations of the two limbs of the capsule to one another and to the knee vary considerably in different horizontal planes. Much of the confusion in the bibliography is dependent upon neglect to describe the horizontal level of the lesion, as well as its situation in an antero-posterior direction. The principal bundle passing through the anterior limb of the capsule is that which connects the frontal gyri and the medial bundle in the base of the peduncle (crus) with the nuclei of the pons. These fibres are centrifugal, and innervate chiefly the lower motor nuclei governing bilaterally innervated muscles, especially those of the eyes, head, neck, and probably those of the mouth, tongue, and larynx. In lower horizontal planes these fibres are situated near the knee of the capsule. It is the region of the knee of the capsule which transmits especially the fibres passing from the cerebral cortex to the nuclei of the facial, hypoglossal, and third nerves. The path which supplies the nuclei governing the muscles used in speech passes through the knee.

The pyramidal tract goes through the thalamo-lenticular portion of the capsule. The motor fibres are arranged according to definite muscle groups, or rather movement forms, those for the movements of the arm being anterior to those for the leg. The number of fibres for a given muscle group corresponds rather to the degree of complexity of the movements than to the size of the muscles concerned. Thus the areas for the fingers and toes are relatively large.

The fibres to the somæsthetic area of the cortex—that is, those from the centro-lateral group of nuclei of the thalamus and the tegmental radiations—carrying impulses concerned in general bodily sensation, pass upward through the posterior part of the thalamo-lenticular portion of the capsule. Some of these fibres pass through the anterior two-thirds of the posterior limb alongside of the fibres of the pyramidal tract.

Through the retro-lenticular portion of the posterior limb, opposite the posterior third of the lateral surface of the thalamus, pass (1) the fibres carrying impulses concerned in the sensations of the opposite visual field (optic radiation from the lateral geniculate body to the visual sense area in the occipital cortex; (2) the fibres carrying impulses concerned in auditory sensations (radiation from the medial geniculate body to the auditory sense area in the cortex of the temporal lobe); (3) the fibres (probably centrifugal) connecting the cortex of the temporal lobe with the nuclei of the pons.

With this preliminary knowledge concerning the internal capsule, it is not difficult to understand the symptoms which result when it is diseased.

Since here all the fibres of the upper motor segment are gathered together in a compact bundle, a lesion in this region is apt to cause complete hemiplegia of the opposite side, followed later by contractures; and if the lesion involves the hinder portion of the posterior limb there is also hemianæsthesia, including even the special senses (Fig. 13). As a rule, however, lesions of the internal capsule do not involve the whole structure. The disease usually affects mainly either the anterior or posterior portions, and even in instances in which at first the symptoms point to total involvement there is a disappearance often of a large part of the phenomena after a short time. Thus, when the pyramidal tract is destroyed (lesion of the thalamo-lenticular portion of the capsule) the arm may be affected more than the leg, or *vice versa*. The facial paralysis is usually slight, though if the lesion be well forward in the capsule the paralysis of the face and tongue may be marked.

Hemianæsthesia alone without involvement of the motor fibres, due to disease of the capsule, is rare. There is usually also at least partial paralysis of the leg. When the retro-lenticular portion of the capsule is destroyed the hemianæsthesia is accompanied by hemianopsia, disturbances of hearing, and sometimes of smell and taste. The occurrence of hemianæsthesia with pain, hemichorea, marked tremor, or hemiathetosis—thalamic syndrome—after a capsular hemiplegia points to the involvement of the thalamus or of the hypothalamic region.

Charcot and others have described cases in which as a result of disease of the internal capsule there has been paralysis of the face and leg without involvement of the arm. In such instances the lesion is linear, extending from the posterior part of the anterior limb of the internal capsule backward and lateralward to the leg region in the posterior limb of the capsule, the region for the arm escaping.

Capsular lesions when pure are not usually accompanied by aphasic symptoms, alexia, or agraphia. A "subcortical" motor aphasia may result if the lesion is bilateral, as in pseudo-bulbar paralysis, or if on the left side it is so extensive as to destroy the fibres connecting Broca's convolution with the opposite hemisphere, as well as the pyramidal fibres on the same side.

Crura (Cerebral Peduncles).—From this level through the pons, medulla, and cord the upper and lower motor segments are represented, the first by the fibres of the pyramidal tracts and by the fibres which go from the cerebral cortex to the nuclei of the cerebral nerves, the latter by the motor nuclei and the nerve fibres arising from them. Lesions often affect both motor segments, and produce paralyses having the characteristics of each. Thus a single lesion may involve the pyramidal tract and cause a spastic paralysis on the opposite side of the body, and also involve the nucleus or the fibres of one of the cerebral nerves, and so produce a lower segment paralysis on the same side as the lesion—crossed paralysis. In the crus the third and fourth cerebral nerves run near the pyramidal tract, and a lesion of this region is apt to involve them or their nuclei, causing partial paralysis of the muscles of the eye on the same side as the lesions, combined with a hemiplegia of the opposite side (Fig. 10, 3).

The optic tract also crosses the crus and may be involved, giving hemianopsia in the opposite halves of the visual fields.

If the tegmentum be the seat of a lesion which does not involve the base of the peduncle (or pes) there may be disturbances of cutaneous and muscular sensibility, ataxia, disturbances of hearing, or oculo-motor paralysis. An oculo-motor paralysis of one side, accompanied by a hemiataxia of the opposite side, appears to be especially characteristic of a tegmental lesion.

Corpora Quadrigemina.—Anatomical studies point to the view that the superior colliculus (anterior quadrigeminal body) represents the most important subcortical central organ for the control of the eye-muscle nuclei. This is supported to a certain extent by clinical evidence, though as yet but few cases have been carefully studied. Sight is only slightly, if at all, disturbed when the superior colliculus is destroyed. The pupil is usually widened, and the pupillary reaction, both to light and on accommodation, interfered with. Apparently actual paralysis of the eye muscles does not occur unless the nucleus of the third nerve ventral to the aqueduct be also injured.

The inferior colliculus (posterior quadrigeminal body), on the other hand, has been shown by anatomical study to be an important way-station in the auditory conduction-path. A large part of the lateral lemniscus ends in its nucleus, and from it emerge medullated fibres which pass through the brachium quadrigeminum inferius to the medial geniculate body. Thence a large bundle runs through the retro-lenticular portion of the internal capsule to the auditory sense area in the cortex of the temporal lobe.

Weinland has collected 19 cases of tumors of the corpora quadrigemina from the bibliography; in 9 of these auditory disturbances were especially noted. Since the central auditory path of each side receive impulses from both ears, lesion of the colliculus on one side may dull the hearing on both sides, though the opposite ear is usually the more defective. Lesion of the inferior colliculus may be accompanied by disturbance of mastication, owing to paralysis of the descending (mesencephalic) root of the trigeminus. The fourth nerve may also be involved. The ataxia which sometimes accompanies lesions of the corpora quadrigemina is probably to be referred to disturbance in conduction in the medial lemniscus.

Pons and Medulla Oblongata.—Lesions involving the pyramidal tract, together with any one of the motor cerebral nerves of this region, cause crossed paralysis. A lesion in the lower part of the pons is apt to cause a lower-segment paralysis of the face on the same side (destruction of the nucleus of the facial nerve or of its root fibres) and a spastic paralysis of the arm and leg on the opposite side (injury to pyramidal tract) (Fig. 10, 4). The abducens, the motor part of the trigeminus, and the hypoglossus nerves may also be paralyzed in the same manner. When the central fibres to the nucleus of the hypoglossus are involved a peculiar form of anarthria results. If the nucleus itself be diseased, swallowing is interfered with.

When the sensory fibres of the fifth nerve are interrupted, together with the sensory tract (the medial lemniscus or fillet) for the rest of the body, which has already crossed the middle line, there is a crossed sensory paralysis—i. e., disturbed sensation in the distribution of the fifth on the side of the lesion, and of all the rest of the body on the opposite side.

A paralysis of the external rectus muscle of one eye and of the internal rectus of the other eye (conjugate paralysis of the muscles which turn the eyes to one side), in the absence of a "forced position" of the eyeballs, is highly characteristic of certain lesions of the pons. In such cases the internal rectus may still be capable of functioning on convergence, or when the eye to which it belongs is tested independently of that in which the external rectus is paralyzed. This form of paralysis is found, as a rule, only when the lesion lies just in front of the abducens or involves the nucleus itself, or includes, besides the root fibres of the abducens, that portion of the formatio reticularis that lies between them and the fasciculus longitudinalis medialis (von Monakow). The cases of conjugate paralysis just referred to may be complicated by other disturbances of the eye-muscle movements, in which case the interpretation of the symptoms may be rendered difficult. The facial nerve is often involved in these paralyses.

In lesions of the pons the patient often has a tendency to fall toward the side on which the lesion is, probably on account of implication of the middle peduncle of the cerebellum (brachium pontis). Still more frequent is the simple motor hemi-ataxia consequent upon lesion of the medial lemniscus, and perhaps of longitudinal bundles in the formatio reticularis. This is often accompanied by a dissociated sensory disturbance, pain and temperature being affected, while touch remains normal. The muscular sense may also be involved. Only when the lesion is very extensive are there disturbances of hearing (involvement of the lateral lemniscus or corpus trapezoideum).

The symptoms produced by involvement of the different cerebral nerves will be considered in detail in another section.

Cerebellum.—The functions of this part of the brain are still under consideration. Luciani, whose monograph is exhaustive, regards it as "an end organ, directly or indirectly related to certain peripheral sensory organs and in direct efferent relationship with certain ganglia of the cerebro-spinal axis, and indirectly with the motor apparatus in general. It is functionally homogeneous, each part exercising the functions of the whole, but having special relations to the muscles of the corresponding side of the body" (Krauss).

Lesions of the lateral lobes affect the corresponding side of the body, while lesions of the middle lobe (vermis) affect both sides. Partial removal is followed by transient muscular weakness; complete removal by extreme incoordination. Its one important function would appear to be the coördination of the muscular movements.

In monkeys the symptoms differ much at different periods after the operation. During the first five or six days irritation phenomena predominate. According to Luciani, there are asthenia, atony of the muscles, and astasia on the side of the body operated upon. The animal can not stand or walk. All these symptoms may gradually disappear in the course of a few months.

The experiments of Risien Russell do not entirely confirm the observations of Luciani. In the first place, the occurrence of asthenia is not constant, and as to atony, while the patellar tendon reflexes are sometimes absent, they are, as a rule, intact in pure cerebellar lesions. There may be even muscular rigidity instead of atony. Russell's experiments make it seem likely that the cerebellar hemisphere of one side exercises constantly an inhibitory effect upon the activities of the cerebral hemisphere of the opposite side (probably by way of the brachium conjunctivum). Thus, after removal of one cerebellar hemisphere, he found that movements of the arm and leg could be caused by a faradic stimulation of the contralateral motor area, much milder than that necessary to stimulate the homolateral motor area. The epileptic seizures following the administration of absinthe were far greater on the side of ablation. It is not impossible that the explanation of the epileptiform attacks by no means rare in cerebellar disease is here to be sought.

W. C. Krauss has analyzed the lesions and symptoms in 100 cases of disease of this part. The morbid conditions were as follows: Sarcoma in 22 cases; tubercle in 22; glioma in 18; abscess in 10; tumor of unspecified origin in 13; cyst in 7; and 1 case each of softening, endothelioma, cyst and sarcoma, cancer, gumma, fibroma, and hæmorrhage. The left lobe was affected 32 times, the right lobe 32 times, and the middle lobe 17 times. Thus, tumor constituted by far the most important affection. There may be no symptoms whatever if it is in one hemisphere only and does not involve the middle lobe. There are instances not only of complete absence of one whole hemisphere from arrest of growth, but also of extensive bilateral disease, which throughout life has yielded no noticeable symptoms. Only when lesions are comparatively sudden do the symptoms resemble the early experimental states in animals. Other portions of the brain appear to be able to take on the functions normally performed by the cerebellum. The most common symptoms in tumor of the cerebellum are as follows:

Vertigo, which is more constant in this than in affections of any other region of the brain. Some believe this to be due to involvement of the nervus vestibularis or its nuclei of termination, by means of which the semicircular canals are connected with the cerebellum. The symptom was present in 48 of the cases of Krauss' collection, not reported in 43. The vertigo appears to be entirely independent of the ataxia. Though most frequently associated, either symptom may be present without the other. The vertigo of cerebellar disease is often associated with the feeling that objects are revolving about the body, or that the body itself is moving. *Headache* was present in 83 cases. *Vomiting* occurred in 69 cases, not reported in 23. *Optic neuritis* was found in 66 cases, not reported in 23. It is apt to appear early, and is probably brought about by the obstructive internal hydrocephalus that commonly results from subtentorial growths through pressure on the aqueductus cerebri.

Of symptoms which are designated as more particularly cerebellar, *ataxia,* particularly of the homolateral limbs, is the most important. In cerebellar ataxia the gait is irregular and staggering, often zigzag, and in attempting to walk the patient sways to and fro like a drunken man (*démarche d'ivresse* of the French writers). As a rule, the patient walks and tends to fall toward the affected side, but the rule is not certain. The ataxia of cerebellar disease is to be sharply differentiated from the ataxia of tabes dorsalis, from cortical ataxia, and probably from the ataxia accompanying diseases of the tegmental portion of the pons and cerebral peduncle. Cerebellar ataxia is both static and dynamic. The opening or closing of the eyes has less influence than in spinal ataxia. Very important for differential diagnosis is the fact that when the patient lies in bed movements tolerably well coördinated can be carried out.

The coarse nature of the incoördination distinguishes cerebellar ataxia from that due to lesion of the cerebral cortex. In the latter the finer movements (buttoning, etc.) are especially apt to be involved, and there is usually hemi-paresis or mono-paresis, and often disturbance of muscular sense and of the stereognostic sense (von Monakow). Cerebellar ataxia may depend upon the withdrawal of the influence of the cerebellum upon the cerebrum. Babinski has pointed out that the affected limb, although ataxic, may be held in a given position more steadily than normal, and also that repeated movements can not be as quickly performed on the affected as on the normal side (dys-diado-chokinesia).

Paresis, especially of the homolateral trunk muscles, manifest in an inability to perform the movements of bending, erection, and lateral flexion of the trunk, may be present. Risien Russell holds that the paralysis is "probably directly due to the withdrawal of the cerebellar influence from the muscles." A peculiar attitude of the head has been described, in which the face looks upward and is turned away from the side occupied by the growth. Deficiency in power of the limbs on the same side is frequent.

Other less constant but suggestive symptoms are neuralgic pains in the region of the neck and occiput; blocking of the venæ Galeni and dilatation of the lateral ventricles, causing in children hydrocephalus; pressure on the mid-brain, pons, or medulla oblongata, producing paralysis of the cerebral nerves (most commonly the sixth cranial), rhythmical contractions of the head or extremities, nystagmus (particularly when looking toward the side of the lesion), tremor, anarthria, auditory or visual disturbances. There may be glycosuria, and bilateral rigidity from pressure on the motor paths. Sudden death may occur.

The reflexes, though variable, are apt to be increased on the side of the lesion, and if internal hydrocephalus develops they may be exaggerated on both sides. When the cerebellar disease involves other structures directly, or indirectly through action at a distance, the reflexes may be abolished.

Symptoms of general mental disturbance may accompany cerebellar disease, but they are not characteristic. There are often irritability, enfeebled memory, and toward the end sopor and coma.

II. APHASIA

Speech disorders give important information as to the position of lesions of the nervous system, and it is for this reason that they are considered here.

The studies of Boulliaud, Dax, Broca, Bastian, Kussmaul, Lichtheim, Marie, and others have done much to widen our knowledge of this very difficult subject. The student is referred to the works of these authors, and especially to the monograph of Moutier.

As in all other voluntary movements speech requires not only a motor but a sensory apparatus, and we have, as composing the speech mechanism, a sensory or receptive part as well as a motor or emissive part. These two parts are associated with the higher centres underlying the intellectual process, and are controlled by them.

The muscles which are used in the production of articulate speech are many and widely distributed; thus, the respiratory muscles, the muscles of the larynx, the pharynx, the tongue, the lips, and those which move the jaws are all brought into play during speech. These muscles are all active in other less complicated movements; for instance, respiration, crying, sucking, etc., and these comparatively simple movements are represented in the gray matter of the lower motor segment in the pons, medulla, and spinal cord. The association of neurones upon which these movements depend is made during fetal life, and is in good working order at the time of birth.

As the child's brain grows and takes control of the spinal centres through the medium of the pyramidal tracts, other more complex movements are developed and special neurones are set apart for this purpose. There is, then, a re-representation (Hughlings Jackson) of the finer movements of these muscles in the upper motor segment. They are localized in the central convolutions about the lower part of the Rolandic fissure. All these muscles except those of the tongue and lips are used bilaterally, and so their movements on each side of the body are represented on both sides of the brain.

This group of movements, which are in part congenital and in part acquired during the early months of life, is that from which the delicate movements of articulate speech are developed. The structures upon which these movements depend make the *primary* or *elementary speech mechanism*.

The cortical centres are in the lower third of the central convolution on both sides of the brain. They are bilaterally acting centres, and a lesion limited to either one should not produce marked or permanent defects in speech. This is true for the right side, but on the left Broca's convolution and the insula are so closely situated that they are usually injured at the same time, and motor aphasia results. The path from the cortical centres is made up of the motor fibres which go to the nuclei of the pons and medulla, and in the internal capsule is situated near the knee. As in the cortex, a unilateral lesion here causes only slight disturbances of speech due to difficult articulation, following weakness of the opposite side of the face and tongue. On the left side, if the lesion is so near the cortex as to involve the fibres which connect Broca's convolution with the primary speech mechanism, *subcortical motor aphasia* is produced. Bilateral lesions (usually in the internal capsule, but at times in the cortex) cause speechlessness, with paralysis of the muscles of articulation—pseudo-bulbar paralysis. To these speech defects Bastian gives the name aphemia.

The lower segment of the primary speech mechanism is made up of the motor nuclei in the medulla, etc., and the peripheral nerves arising from them. Lesions here, if extensive enough—as, for instance, in progressive bulbar paralysis—may cause speechlessness—anarthria (Bastian); but usually they are more limited, giving various disturbances of articulation.

The Auditory Speech Centre.—As the child learns to speak there is developed in the cortex of the brain an association of centres which takes control of the primary speech mechanism. The child is constantly hearing objects called by names, and he learns to associate certain sounds with the look, feel, taste, etc., of certain things. When he hears such a sound he gets a more or less clear mental picture of the object, or, in other words, he has developed certain auditory memories. These memories of the sounds of words are stored in what is called the *auditory speech centre*. This centre, which in the majority of people is the controlling speech centre, is situated on the left side in right-handed people, and on the right side in those who are left-handed. The afferent impressions arising in the ears reach the transverse gyri of the temporal lobes, those from each ear going to both sides of the brain. From each of these primary auditory centres impulses are sent to the auditory speech centre in the temporal lobe of the left hemisphere. The exact location of this so-called centre is not accurately determined, but it is thought to occupy the first and perhaps part of the second temporal convolutions. Marie in his work on aphasia denies all speech centres, but places the cortical region, which has to do with the intellectual processes underlying language, rather vaguely in the left temporo-parietal lobe. This he designates "Wernicke's zone," a lesion of which alone can produce aphasia. The child endeavors, and by repeated efforts learns, to make the sounds that he hears, and he first becomes able to repeat words, then to speak voluntarily. To do this, he has had to learn certain very delicate movements, and so there has been developed under the control of the auditory speech centres a special motor centre for speech in which these movements are localized.

The Motor Speech Centre.—This was placed by Broca, and those who immediately followed him, in the posterior part of the left third frontal convolution. It is around this—Broca's centre—that the discussion started by Marie has been most heated. Marie and his followers deny that this portion of the brain has anything to do with speech, and insist that the so-called motor aphasia is merely a "combination of aphasia" (of which they admit but one type, that due to lesions of Wernicke's zone) with anarthria. Anarthria they think of as a speech disturbance without any intellectual defect, due to a lesion of their lenticular zone, an ill-defined area in the centre of the brain.

Marie's position has been much discussed, and many excellent observers have come to the rescue of the old view which accepts Broca's convolution as the motor speech centre. The recent studies of cases of apraxia, which seem to have determined a centre in the left frontal lobe for certain purposive movements, as in the use of objects, gestures, etc., have lent support to the importance of Broca's convolution.

The motor speech centres and the corresponding area in the right brain are connected either directly by special motor fibres with the bulbar nuclei, or, as is more probable, indirectly, through the medium of the cortical centres of the primary speech mechanism in the lower part of the Rolandic region on both sides.

The speech centres are in close connection with the rest of the brain cortex, and in this way they take part in the general mental activities, of which, indeed, the speech processes form a large part. Some authors have assumed that the several sensory elements which go to make a concept are brought together in a special region of the brain, and here, as it were, united by a name. This is called "the centre for concepts," or "naming centre" (Broadbent), but most writers have followed Bastian in considering that the supposition of such a centre is unnecessary.

The mechanism which has been described is that which is developed in uneducated people and in children before they have learned to read and write, and is of primary importance in all speech processes. As the child learns to read he associates certain visual impressions with the speech memories he has already acquired, and he then adds to his concepts the visual memories of written or printed symbols. These memories are stored in the visual speech centre.

The Visual Speech Centre.—This is placed by nearly all authors in the angular and supramarginal convolutions on the left side, where it is believed visual impressions from both occipital lobes are combined in speech memories. Von Monakow denies such a special centre, but holds that visual speech memories are dependent upon the direct connection of the general visual centres in both occipital lobes with the speech sphere. That speech defects result from injury to the angular and supramarginal convolutions, he admits; but he thinks these are due to an interruption of fibre tracts which lie beneath and not to a destruction of a cortical centre. The distinction is, therefore, of more theoretical than practical importance. Marie includes this region in his Wernicke's zone.

In learning to write, the child develops certain delicate movements of the arm and hand, and thus acquires another method of externalizing his speech activities. Whether or not this requires the development of a separate writing centre, apart from the general Rolandic arm centre, or is brought about by an evolution of the latter through the medium of Broca's convolution, is a vexed question. Gordinier has recorded a remarkable case of total agraphia, with no sensory or motor speech aphasia, in which a tumor occupying the foot of the second left frontal convolution was found at autopsy. Agraphia is a special form of apraxia. The movements of writing are learned under the influence of visual impressions in association with the other speech memories, although there is a more direct path, which is used in copying unknown characters. Just as the movements of articulate speech are constantly under the control of auditory memories, so are the movements of writing regulated by visual memories; but in this case the other speech memories are of great importance.

With the development of the associations which underlie reading and writing, the speech mechanism may be said to be complete, although its activities are capable of practically endless extension, as when music or foreign languages are learned.

It will be seen that the cortical speech centres—the speech sphere of the French—occupy the part of the brain near the Sylvian fissure, and that they all receive their blood from the Sylvian artery. Speaking broadly, the posterior part of this region is sensory and the anterior is motor. The sensory areas are near the optic radiation and the motor are near the general motor tracts, and so, with lesions of the posterior part, hemianopia is apt to be associated with the speech disturbance while hemiplegia occurs with disease of the anterior areas. These associations often help to distinguish a sensory from a motor aphasia, but each type has special characteristics which must be studied.

Auditory Aphasia.—Most people in mentally recalling words do so by means of their auditory speech memories—i. e., they think of the sound of the words, and, in voluntary speech, it is probable that the will acts on the motor centre indirectly through the auditory centre. This centre is also necessary for reading in such persons. There are certain persons, however, in whom the mental processes are carried on by visual memories, and in these rare "visuals" the visual speech centres take the predominant place in speech usually occupied by the auditory centres.

Complete abolition of all the auditory speech memories by destruction of the first temporal convolution causes the most extensive disturbances of speech. Such a person is unable to comprehend speech, either spoken or printed. Voluntary speech is much disturbed, and although at first he may talk, his speech is nothing but a jargon of misplaced words, and he soon becomes speechless. Writing is also lost, and he can neither repeat words nor write at dictation. He may be able to copy.

Lesions are often only partial, and the resultant disturbance may be simply a difficulty in speech due to the loss of nouns or to the transposition of words (paraphasia), the writing showing the same defect. The patient usually understands what he hears and reads, and can repeat words and write at dictation. This is the condition Bastian calls "amnesia verbalis." The condition may be so pronounced that voluntary speech and writing are nearly lost, even when the auditory memories can still be aroused by new afferent impressions and he is able to understand what is said to him and what he reads. He can usually repeat and read aloud.

The afferent paths, which reach the auditory speech centre from the two primary auditory centres, may be destroyed. A lesion to do this must be in the white matter beneath the first temporal convolution on the left side. Such a lesion would block all auditory impressions coming to the centre, and the patient would not be able to understand anything that was said to him, could not repeat words nor write from dictation. As the cortical centres are not disturbed, and the auditory speech memories are still present, there is no disturbance of voluntary speech or writing, and the patient can read perfectly. This is pure word-deafness or subcortical sensory aphasia.

Visual Aphasia.—Destruction of the visual centre in the angular and supramarginal convolutions causes a loss of the visual speech memories, and the patient is unable to read printed or written characters. He is unable to write—i. e., there is agraphia—and he can not copy. His understanding of spoken words is good, and voluntary speech is normal or only slightly paraphasic.

A subcortical lesion involving the afferent fibres going to the visual speech centre causes pure word-blindness (subcortical alexia)—i. e., there is inability to understand written or printed words. Voluntary speech and writing are good. The patient can not read his own writing except by aid of muscle-sense impression, in retracing the letters, either voluntarily or passively. Associated with this is always hemianopia.

Word-deafness and word-blindness are often combined, and at times it is not only the tracts that connect the primary auditory and visual centres with the speech spheres, but also those which associate them with the other sensory centres in the formation of concepts, that are diseased. In this case the patient has lost not only his auditory and visual speech memories, but also all of his memories which have to do with hearing and sight, and he has mind-deafness and mind-blindness—i. e., he is unable to recognize objects when he hears or when he sees them. Further than this, there may be a dissociation of all the sensory centres from each other or from the higher psychical centre, which is practically the same thing, in which case the patient is entirely unable to recognize objects and to use them properly—i. e., he has sensory aphasia or agnosia.

Motor Aphasia.—Lesions of the motor speech zone, possibly in rare cases of Broca's convolution alone, more commonly of a wider area, cause loss of the power of speech. The patient may be absolutely dumb, or he may have retained one or two words or phrases, which is believed to be due to the activity of the corresponding region of the right brain. He will make no effort to repeat words. His mind is comparatively clear, and he understands what is said to him, but reads poorly. He has not a clear mental picture of words. This is tested by asking him to squeeze the observer's hand or to make expiratory efforts as many times as there are syllables in a well-known name.

Voluntary writing is usually lost in cortical motor aphasia, and many authors believe that writing movements are controlled from this centre. Others, who believe that there is a special writing centre, contend that a lesion strictly limited to the motor speech centre would not cause agraphia, and cite cases which seem to support their view. If there is much disturbance of internal speech, writing must be impaired.

Subcortical motor aphasia is described as due to the destruction of the fibres which join Broca's convolution to the primary speech mechanism. Lesions which have produced this type of aphasia have been in the white matter of the left hemisphere near Broca's convolution. These would be within Marie's lenticular zone. There is complete loss of the power of speech without any disturbance of internal speech. The patient's mental processes are not disturbed, and he can write perfectly if the hand is not paralyzed.

Cases of aphasia are rarely simple, and it is often impossible to classify them accurately. The problems involved are, in reality, exceedingly complicated, and the student must not for a moment suppose that cases are as straightforward as the various diagrams at first sight would appear to indicate. A majority of them are very complex, but with patience the diagnosis of the different varieties can often be worked out. The following tests should be applied in each case of aphasia, after the presence or absence of paralysis has been determined and whether the patient is right-handed or left-handed: (1) The power of recognizing the nature, uses, and relations of objects—i. e., whether agnosia and apraxia are present or not; (2) the power to recall the name of familiar objects seen, smelled, or tasted, or of a sound when heard, or of an object touched; (3) the power to understand spoken words; (4) the capability of understanding printed or written language; (5) the power of appreciating and understanding music; (6) the power of voluntary speech—in this it is to be noted particularly whether he misplaces words or not; (7) the power of reading aloud and of understanding what he reads; (8) the power to write voluntarily and of reading what he has written; (9) the power to copy; (10) the power to write at dictation; and (11) the power of repeating words.

The *medico-legal aspects* of aphasia are of great importance. No general principle can be laid down, but each case must be considered on its merits.

Langdon, in reviewing the whole question, concludes: "Sanity established, any legal document should be recognized when it can be proved that the person making it can understand fully its nature by any receptive channel (viz., hearing, vision, or muscular sense), and can, in addition, express assent or dissent with certainty to proper witnesses, whether this expression be by spoken speech, written speech, or pantomime."

PROGNOSIS AND TREATMENT OF APHASIA

In young persons the outlook is good, and the power of speech is gradually restored apparently by the development of other portions of the brain. The opposite hemisphere often takes part in this. In adults the condition is less hopeful, particularly in the cases of complete motor aphasia with right hemiplegia. The patient may remain speechless, though capable of understanding everything, and attempts at re-education may be futile. Partial recovery may occur, and the patient may be able to talk, but misplaces words. In sensory aphasia the condition may be only transient, and the different forms rarely persist alone without impairment of the powers of expression.

The education of an aphasic person requires the greatest care and patience, particularly if, as so often happens, he is emotional and irritable. It is best to begin by the use of detached letters, and advance, not too rapidly, to words of only one syllable. Children often make rapid progress, but in adults failure is only too frequent, even after the most painstaking efforts. In the cases of right hemiplegia with aphasia the patient may be taught to write with the left hand.

III. AFFECTIONS OF THE BLOOD VESSELS

1. CEREBRAL CIRCULATION

There is much that is still indefinite in the physiology of the circulation of the brain, but that which is known is of the greatest practical moment to the physician.

The brain receives blood from the internal carotid arteries, the vertebrals, and, to some extent, from the spinal arteries. These anastomose soon after entering the skull to form the circle of Willis. The extent of this intercommunication is subject to considerable variation, which may be of extreme importance in pathological conditions. Collected by the veins, the blood is emptied into large venous sinuses, which are, to a great extent, protected from pressure changes by the skull and dura mater.

The cerebro-spinal fluid is collected in the meningeal spaces and fills the interstices between the convolutions, etc. Under normal conditions there is but a small quantity of this fluid within the skull, which is entirely filled with brain, blood, and the cerebro-spinal fluid. Practically a closed box, with contents uninfluenced by atmospheric pressure, the quantity of blood within the skull under normal circumstances is almost constant, for the brain substance itself can not be compressed, so that the only increase or decrease is that which compensates for the small quantity of cerebro-spinal fluid that can pass between the cranial and spinal cavities.

Although the quantity of blood does not change materially, its rapidity of flow may, and does, show marked variations, and thus the relation between arterial and venous blood is subject to change. The circulation within the skull not only differs from the circulation in other parts in its freedom from the effects of atmospheric pressure, but apparently it is not under local vaso-motor control and is in an organ that can only expand slightly. Although nerve fibres have been demonstrated in the walls of the small arteries of the brain, it has not been proved that they cause dilatation or contraction under influences from the vaso-motor centres; indeed, there is little experimental evidence that speaks for, and much that speaks against, this view.

Under ordinary circumstances, the circulation of the brain follows passively the general bodily conditions. When anything increases the force with which the blood enters the skull—i. e., when blood pressure is raised, either by increase in the heart's action or by general vaso-motor effects—more blood passes through the brain in a given time, and it is, as it were, flooded with blood. This active hyperæmia must occur under many circumstances, but it is doubtful whether it causes any symptoms; in fact, it is difficult to see how it, in itself, can do anything but good.

Although without direct vaso-motor control, the circulation of the brain is regulated by the action of the vaso-motor centre on the splanchnic areas and skin. This centre itself shares with the respiratory and cardiac centres the same circulatory conditions as prevail throughout the brain.

Consciousness depends upon a due blood supply to the brain, particularly to the cortex, and life itself depends upon the circulation in the medullary centres. When the blood circulating about these centres is poor in oxygen—i. e., when there is a lack of arterial blood—the arterioles within the splanchnic and skin areas contract under vaso-motor influences, the blood pressure is raised, and the blood enters the brain with unusual force and supplies the capillaries with arterial blood. The extent to which this regulating mechanism can counteract an obstruction to the circulation through these centres has been well shown experimentally by Harvey Cushing. When the general intracranial pressure was raised to arterial blood pressure, instead of the circulation being blocked and the animal dying from anæmia of the brain, as has been stated, he showed that the vaso-motor centres responded with a sufficient rise of blood pressure to overcome the impediment, and so restore the circulation. With every repeated increase of intracranial pressure, there was an answering rise of blood pressure, until, at the end of the experiment, the brain was acting under an intracranial pressure much above the arterial pressure of the animal at the beginning of the experiment, and this pressure had been correspondingly raised to a startling extent. The interesting clinical deductions which Cushing draws from this experiment will be referred to under cerebral hæmorrhage.

When this regulating mechanism is disturbed, serious results may follow. The ordinary fainting fit is an example: Under the influence of emotion the vaso-motor centre is inhibited, and, in consequence, the abdominal blood vessels become dilated, blood pressure falls, and the heart is no longer able to drive the blood back to itself against the force of gravity; the blood accumulates in the abdominal veins, the heart empties, cerebral circulation fails, and unconsciousness occurs. A similar condition may follow the sudden removal of something that has caused pressure on the abdominal vessels for a considerable time, as the withdrawal of the ascitic fluid. In this case the vaso-motor control influences have not been called on for some time, and the centre itself has taken part in the general weakened condition of the individual, so that, when a sudden demand is made upon it to compensate for the accustomed external support to the blood vessels, it is entirely unable to respond, and the blood collects in the splanchnic vessels, the patient becomes unconscious and may die, having bled to death into his own veins.

While under ordinary circumstances the vaso-motor mechanism and the tonicity of the muscles of the abdominal walls compensate perfectly for the change from the horizontal to the upright position—i. e., for the effect of gravity upon the column of venous blood from the heart to the feet, in asthenic states, as after severe illness, the compensation may be very imperfect. When such is the case, if the patient stands, or, at times, even if he sits up in bed, his heart beats more rapidly, he becomes giddy and may faint. The change in the pulse rate, with a change in position, is a fair indication of the vaso-motor control, for the heart itself endeavors to make up for this incompetence.

Chloroform and, to a less extent, ether tend to induce vaso-motor paralysis, and this is the reason why position is such an important factor in the safety of patients during anæsthesia. The splanchnic circulation, under these circumstances, may, to a certain extent, be supported by bandaging the legs and abdomen and elevating the foot of the bed. Crile's pneumatic operating suit, in which the patient is encased below the chest in an inflatable suit, by means of which pressure on the peripheral and abdominal vessels may be varied, is an attempt to establish an artificial vaso-constructor system under the control of the operator, which can compensate for the paralyzing effects of the anæsthetic, and obviate the necessity of considering position.

The heart itself may become weak from various causes and so be unable to keep the brain properly supplied with arterial blood. The extreme example of this is paralysis of the heart muscles from failure of the coronary circulation, which is immediately followed by unconsciousness and death. In Stokes-Adams disease the cerebral symptoms, attacks of unconsciousness, convulsions, and apoplectiform seizures are due to cerebral anæmia, caused by the temporary cessation of the ventricular systole. When the chest is forcibly compressed the heart may be unable to fill itself with blood, and so unconsciousness, or even death, may follow from failure of the cerebral circulation.

Respiration is an essential part of circulation; this is true not only in the primary sense, that it is through this function that venous is changed into arterial blood, but also in a more truly mechanical sense. With every inspiration the blood is sucked into the heart from the veins, and the descent of the diaphragm, by increasing the pressure on the abdominal veins, tends to force the blood into the heart. During expiration the entrance of the blood into the heart is impeded by the increase in the intra-thoracic pressure. Respiration has direct, but slight, influence upon the blood pressure within the arteries.

The circulation within the skull is very intimately related to respiration. The blood from the brain sinuses passes through the jugular veins directly into the superior vena cava and the columns of blood appear to be uninterrupted by competent valves, so that every change of pressure in the cava is transmitted directly to the sinuses and veins of the brain. Intracranial pressure has been shown to be equal to venous blood pressure within the sinuses and to follow every change in this. The brain dilates with each pulse-beat, but relatively much more with each expiration. In expiration intrathoracic pressure is increased, and this causes an increase in the pressure within the cava, the jugular, and the brain sinuses. The blood is, as it were, dammed back, venous congestion occurs, intracranial pressure rises, and the brain receives less arterial blood, and the symptoms of cerebral anæmia may follow. Under ordinary conditions these effects are not so pronounced or protracted as to cause marked symptoms, but at times they may be, as when a crying child holds his breath until he becomes unconscious. Here the difficulty which the heart has in filling itself with blood under increased thoracic pressure is also a factor. When the superior vena cava is alone obstructed, as by pressure from a tumor, there may be not the slightest disturbance of the functions. This depends upon the freedom of the cranio-vertebral venous anastomosis, and other paths which allow the blood to reach the heart through the inferior vena cava. Strong respiratory efforts against an obstruction may change intrathoracic pressure very greatly. In forced expiration with the glottis closed, the normal negative pressure becomes markedly positive and may far exceed the normal pressure on the intrathoracic veins, while if the glottis be closed and a strong inspiratory effort be made the pressure may fall far below atmospheric pressure. Intracranial hæmorrhages not infrequently take place during a strong effort with the breath held as when straining at stool, or when lifting a heavy weight, or during a severe coughing spell, all conditions in which, among other things, the flow of the venous blood from the brain to the heart is impeded, and in consequence of which intracranial circulatory conditions are altered in the direction of a rise of venous and capillary pressure. The importance of preventing, as far as possible, any obstruction to respiration during the course of apoplexy will be referred to in a subsequent paragraph.

The venous outlets from the skull are so large and the anastomoses are so free that they must all be obstructed to cause any marked anæmia of the brain, and for this reason thrombosis or ligature of one of the sinuses is not necessarily followed by any symptoms. If all the veins in the neck are compressed, as by a tight band or strong flexion of the neck, the circulation may be impeded to a considerable extent, and this is of definite importance under pathological conditions.

Any one of the arteries may be tied before entering the skull, with but little danger, owing to the freedom of the anastomosis in the circle of Willis, but, as this is subject to variation, the closure should be made slowly. With this precaution, both carotids may be tied if an interval be allowed between the operations.

Obliteration of an artery beyond the circle of Willis is always followed by a disturbance of function of the part of the brain supplied by that artery, and is considered under Embolism and Thrombosis.

2. HYPERÆMIA AND ANÆMIA

Less and less stress is now laid on active hyperæmia as a cause of symptoms. As Leube suggests, the symptoms usually referred to active hyperæmia in the infectious diseases, or in association with hypertrophy of the heart accompanying disease of the kidney, are due to the action of toxic agents rather than to changes in the circulation. On the other hand, venous stasis and anæmia of the brain must be a very potent cause of head symptoms. The uncertainty which exists is largely due to the fact that the condition of the blood vessels as seen within the skull after death may bear no relation to that which held sway during life.

The anatomical condition of the brain in anæmia is very striking. The membranes are pale, only the large veins are full, the small vessels over the gyri are empty, and an unusual amount of cerebro-spinal fluid is present. On section both the gray and white matter look extremely pale and the cut surface is moist. Very few *puncta vasculosa* are seen.

The effects of sudden anæmia of the brain are well illustrated by the ordinary fainting fit, and have been described above.

Symptoms.—When the symptoms are the result of hæmorrhage, there are drowsiness, giddiness, inability to stand; flashes of light, dark spots before the eyes, and noises in the ears; the respiration becomes hurried; the skin is cool and covered with sweat; the pupils are dilated, there may be vomiting, headache, or delirium, and gradually, if the bleeding continues, consciousness is lost and death may occur with convulsions. In the more chronic forms of brain anæmia, such as result from the gradual impoverishment of the blood, as in protracted illness or in starvation, the condition known as irritable weakness results. Mental effort is difficult, the slightest irritation is followed by undue excitement, the patient complains of giddiness and noises in the ears, or there may be hallucinations or delirium. These symptoms are met with in an extreme grade as a result of prolonged starvation, and a very similar condition is seen in certain cases of arterio-sclerosis where the brain is poorly nourished.

An interesting set of symptoms, to which the term *hydrencephaloid* was applied by Marshall Hall, occurs in the debility produced by prolonged diarrhœa in children. The child is in a semi-comatose condition with the eyes open, the pupils contracted, and the fontanelle depressed. In the earlier period there may be convulsions. The coma may gradually deepen, the pupils become dilated, and there may be strabismus and even retraction of the head, symptoms which closely simulate those of basilar meningitis.

3. ŒDEMA OF THE BRAIN

Pathology.—In the pathology of brain lesions œdema formerly played a rôle almost equal in importance to congestion. It occurs under the following conditions: In general atrophy of the convolutions, in which case the œdema is represented by an increase in the cerebro-spinal fluid and in that of the meshes of the pia. In extreme venous dilatation from obstruction, as in mitral stenosis or in tumors, there may be a condition of congestive œdema, in which, in addition to great filling of the blood vessels, the substance of the brain itself is unusually moist. The most acute œdema is a local process found around tumors and abscesses. The symptoms of compression following concussion or contusion, as shown by Cannon, are frequently attributable to cerebral œdema due to change in osmotic pressure. An intense infiltration, local or general, may occur in Bright's disease, and to it, as Traube suggested, certain of the uræmic symptoms may be due.

Anatomical Changes.—The anatomical changes are not unlike those of anæmia. When the œdema follows progressive atrophy, the fluid is chiefly within and beneath the membranes. The brain substance is anæmic and moist, and has a wet, glistening appearance, which is very characteristic. In some instances the œdema is more intense and local, and the brain substance may look infiltrated with fluid. The amount of fluid in the ventricles is usually increased.

Symptoms.—The symptoms are in great part those of lessened blood flow, and are not well defined. As just stated, some of the cerebral features of uræmia may depend upon it. Cases have been reported by Raymond, Tenneson, and Dercum, in which unilateral convulsions or paralysis have occurred in connection with chronic Bright's disease, and in which the condition appeared to be associated with œdema of the brain. The older writers laid great stress upon an apoplexia serosa, which may really have been a general œdema of the brain. Inasmuch as the instances in which œdema of the brain occurs are often those in which there is also intoxication, or anæmia, or both, it is probably impossible to say at the bedside definitely which of these possible factors is responsible for the symptoms in a given case.

4. CEREBRAL HÆMORRHAGE

The bleeding may come from branches of either of the two great groups of cerebral vessels—the *basal,* comprising the circle of Willis and the central arteries passing from it and from the first portion of the cerebral arteries, or the *cortical group,* the anterior, middle, and the posterior cerebral vessels. In a majority of the cases the hæmorrhage is from the central branches, more particularly from those which are given off by the middle cerebral arteries in the anterior perforated spaces, and which supply the corpora striata and internal capsules. One of the largest of these branches which passes to the third division of the lenticular nucleus and to the anterior part of the internal capsule, the lenticulo-striate artery of Duret, is so frequently involved in hæmorrhage that it has been called by Charcot *the artery of cerebral hæmorrhage.* Hæmorrhages from this and from the lenticulo-thalamic artery include more than 60 per cent. of all cerebral hæmorrhages. The bleeding may be into the substance of the brain, to which alone the term cerebral apoplexy is applied, or into the membranes, in which case it is termed meningeal hæmorrhage; both, however, are usually included under the terms intracranial or cerebral hæmorrhage.

Etiology.—The conditions which produce degeneration of the blood vessels play the important part:

AGE.—The liability increases with each decade. H. M. Thomas, in his analysis of the United States Census Report for 1907, states that the greatest number of cases occurred in the seventh and eighth decades. Cerebral hæmorrhage may be congenital. One of the only recorded instances is that which I reported in a six-month fetus of a woman dead of typhoid fever. The clot was in the left hemisphere and had broken into the ventricle. Apart from meningeal hæmorrhage, which is common as a result of the accidents of birth, hæmorrhage is rare in children, and we had no instance at the Johns Hopkins Hospital during my term of service. Before the fifth decade hæmorrhage is rare; then in the fifth and sixth decades cases progressively increase in number.

SEX.—There is a marked preponderance of males.

RACE.—In the United States the death rate from apoplexy and paralysis in the Report of 1906 was 88.7 per 100,000 of the population. In England and Wales in 1909 the deaths from apoplexy were 502 per million living. Both apoplexy and paralysis seem to be much more prevalent among the negroes.

HEREDITY.—Formerly thought to be a very important factor, heredity influences the incidence in rendering members of families in which the blood vessels degenerate early more liable to cerebral hæmorrhage. What was formerly known as the apoplectic habitus, or build, is still spoken of, by which we mean a stout, plethoric person of medium size with a short neck.

SPECIAL FACTORS.—Individuals with progressive renal disease and consecutive arterio-sclerosis and hypertrophy of the heart are particularly liable to cerebral hæmorrhage. The causes of arterio-sclerosis, such as alcohol, immoderate eating, prolonged muscular exertion, syphilis, chronic lead poisoning, and gout, are antecedents in many cases. Endocarditis may lead indirectly to apoplexy by causing embolism and aneurism of the vessels of the brain. Cerebral hæmorrhage occurs occasionally in the specific fevers and in such profound alterations of the blood as are met with in leukæmia.

The actual exciting cause is not always evident. The attacks may be sudden without any preliminary symptoms. In other instances violent exertion, particularly straining efforts or overaction of the heart in emotion, may cause a rupture. Many cases occur during sleep. Some instances follow slight trauma. The records of University College Hospital analyzed by Ernest Jones indicate that in none of 123 cases did the attack come on through excessive bodily effort.

Morbid Anatomy.—DIRECT CHANGES.—The lesions causing apoplexy are almost invariably in the cerebral arteries, in which the following changes may lead directly to it:

(*a*) The production of miliary aneurisms, rupture of which is the most common cause of cerebral hæmorrhage. The origin of the miliary aneurisms is disputed. Charcot thought they resulted from changes in the *adventitia* (periarteritis). Others find the primary change in the *intima*. The weight of opinion at present, however, is on the side of the view that the *media* is first degenerated. They occur most frequently on the central arteries, but also on the smaller branches of the cortical vessels. On section of the brain substance they may be seen as localized, small dark bodies, about the size of a pin's head. Sometimes they are seen in numbers upon the arteries when carefully withdrawn from the anterior perforated spaces. According to Charchot and Bouchard, who have described them, they are most frequent in the central ganglia. In apoplexy after the fortieth year if sought for they are rarely missed. The actual miliary aneurism, which by its rupture has occasioned the hæmorrhage, may be difficult to find, but if one pours water carefully on the area of hæmorrhage, or, better still, submerges the apoplectic mass for a time, it will usually be found possible to do so, and even to find the hole in its wall.

(*b*) Aneurism of the branches of the circle of Willis. These are by no means uncommon, and will be considered subsequently.

(*c*) Endarteritis and periarteritis in the cerebral vessels most commonly lead to apoplexy by the production of aneurisms, either miliary or coarse. There are instances in which the most careful search fails to reveal anything but diffuse degeneration of the cerebral vessels, particularly of the smaller branches; so that we must conclude that spontaneous rupture may occur without the previous formation of aneurism.

(*d*) Increased permeability of the walls of the vessels may account for hæmorrhages by *diapedesis* without actual rupture. Such hæmorrhages are not uncommon in cases of contracted kidney, grave anæmia, and various infections and intoxications.

(*e*) In persons over sixty the hemiplegia may depend upon small areas of softening in the gray matter—the *lacunæ* of Marie—areas varying in size from a pin's head to a pea or a small bean, grayish red in tint. The lenticular nucleus is particularly apt to be involved. The blood vessels are always diseased.

The hæmorrhage may be meningeal, cerebral, or intraventricular.

Meningeal hæmorrhage may be outside the dura, between this membrane and the bone, or between the dura and arachnoid, or between the arachnoid and the pia mater. The following are the chief causes of this form of hæmorrhage: Fracture of the skull, in which case the blood usually comes from the lacerated meningeal vessels, sometimes from the torn sinuses. In these cases the blood is usually outside the dura or between it and the arachnoid. The next most frequent cause is rupture of aneurisms on the larger cerebral vessels. The blood is usually subarachnoid. An intracerebral hæmorrhage may burst into the meninges. A special form of meningeal hæmorrhage is found in the new-born, associated with injury during birth. And lastly, meningeal hæmorrhage may occur in the constitutional diseases and fevers. The blood may be in a large quantity at the base; in cases of ruptured aneurism, particularly, it may extend into the cord or upon the cortex. Owing to the greater frequency of the aneurisms in the middle cerebral vessels, the Sylvian fissures are often distended with blood.

Intracerebral hæmorrhage is most frequent in the neighborhood of the corpus striatum, particularly toward the outer section of the lenticular nucleus. The hæmorrhage may be small and limited to the lenticular body, the thalamus, and the internal capsule, or it may extend to the insula. Hæmorrhages confined to the white matter—the centrum semiovale—are rare. Localized bleeding may occur in the crura or in the pons. Hæmorrhage into the cerebellum is not uncommon, and usually comes from the superior cerebellar artery. The extravasation may be limited to the substance or may rupture into the fourth ventricle.

Ventricular Hæmorrhage.—This is rarely primary, coming from the vessels of the plexuses or of the walls. More often it is secondary, following hæmorrhage into the cerebral substance. It is not infrequent in early life and may occur during birth. Of 94 cases collected by Edward Sanders, 7 occurred during the first year, and 14 under the twentieth year. In the cases which I have seen in adults it has almost always been caused by rupture of a vessel in the neighborhood of the caudate nucleus. The blood may be found in one ventricle only, but more commonly it is in both lateral ventricles, and may pass into the third ventricle and through the aqueduct of Sylvius into the fourth ventricle, forming a complete mould in blood of the ventricular system. In these cases the clinical picture may be that of *"apoplexie foudroyante."*

Subsequent Changes.—The blood gradually changes in color, and ultimately the hæmoglobin is converted into the reddish brown hæmatoidin. Inflammation occurs about the apoplectic area, limiting and confining it, and ultimately a definite wall may be produced, inclosing a cyst with fluid contents. In other instances a cyst is not formed, but the connective tissue proliferates and leaves a pigmented scar. In meningeal hæmorrhage the effused blood may be gradually absorbed and leave only a staining of the membranes. In other cases, particularly in infants, when the effusion is cortical and abundant, there may be localized wasting of the convolutions and the production of a cyst in the meninges. Possibly porencephaly may arise in this way. Secondary degeneration follows, varying in character according to the location of the hæmorrhage and the actual damage done by it to nerve cells or their medullated axones. Thus, in persons dying some years after a cerebral apoplexy which has produced hemiplegia (lesion of the motor area in the cortex or of the pyramidal tract leading from it), the degeneration may be traced through the cerebral peduncle, the ventral part of the pons, the pyramids of the medulla, the fibres of the direct pyramidal tract of the cord of the same side, and the fibres of the crossed pyramidal tract on the opposite side. After hæmorrhages in the middle and inferior frontal gyri there follows degeneration of the frontal cerebro-cortico-pontal path, going through the anterior limb of the internal capsule and the medial portion of the basis pedunculi to the nuclei pontis; also degeneration of the fibres connecting the nucleus medialis thalami and the anterior part of the nucleus lateralis thalami with the cortex.

When the temporal gyri or their white matter are destroyed by a hæmorrhage the lateral segment of the basis pedunculi degenerates. Cerebellar hæmorrhage, especially if it injure the nucleus dentatus, may lead to degeneration of the brachium conjunctivum.

There may be slow degeneration in the lemniscus medialis, extending as far as the nuclei on the opposite side of the medulla oblongata, after hæmorrhages in the central gyri, hypothalamic region, or dorsal part of the pons. Hæmorrhages destroying the occipital cortex, or subcortical hæmorrhages injuring the optic radiations, occasion slow degeneration (cellulipetal) of the radiations from the lateral geniculate body, and after a time cause marked atrophy or even disappearance of its ganglion cells.

Symptoms.—These may be divided into primary, or those connected with the onset, and secondary, or those which develop later, after the early manifestations have passed away.

Primary Symptoms.—Premonitory indications are rare. As a rule, the patient is seized while in full health or about the performance of some every day action, occasionally an action requiring strain or extra exertion. Now and then instances are found in which there are sensations of numbness or tingling or pains in the limbs, or even choreiform movements in the muscles of the opposite side, the so-called prehemiplegic chorea. In other cases temporary disturbances of vision and of associated movements of the eye-muscles have been noted, but none of the prodromata of apoplexy (the so-called "warnings") are characteristic. The onset of the apoplexy, as the symptoms of cerebral hæmorrhage are usually called, varies greatly. There may be sudden loss of consciousness and complete relaxation of the extremities. In such instances the name *apoplectic stroke* is particularly appropriate. In other cases the onset is more gradual and the loss of consciousness may not occur for a few minutes after the patient has fallen, or after the paralysis of the limbs is manifest. In the typical apoplectic attack the condition is as follows: There is deep unconsciousness; the patient can not be roused. The face is injected, sometimes cyanotic, or of an ashen gray hue. The pupils vary; usually they are dilated, sometimes unequal, and always, in deep coma, inactive. If the hæmorrhage be so located that it can irritate the nucleus of the third nerve the pupils are contracted (hæmorrhages into the pons or ventricles). The respirations are slow, noisy, and accompanied with stertor. Sometimes the Cheyne-Stokes rhythm may be present. The chest movements on the paralyzed side may be restricted, in rare instances on the opposite side. The cheeks are often blown out during expiration, with spluttering of the lips. The pulse is usually full, slow, and of increased tension. The temperature may be normal, but is often found subnormal, and, as in a case reported by Bastian, may sink below 95°. In cases of basal hæmorrhage the temperature, on the other hand, may be high. The urine and fæces are usually passed involuntarily. Convulsions are not common. It may be difficult to decide whether the condition is apoplexy associated with hemiplegia or sudden coma from other causes. An indication of hemiplegia may be discovered in the difference in the tonus of the muscles on the two sides. If the arm or the leg is lifted, it drops "dead" on the affected side, while on the other it falls more slowly. The lack of muscular tone of the paralyzed limb may be determined by inspection. In this condition the muscle mass of the thigh acts like a semi-fluid sac and takes the shape determined by gravity. In a patient lying or sitting on a firm support, the thigh of the paralyzed limb is broadened or flattened, while that on the normal side has a more rounded contour. Rigidity also may be present. In watching the movements of the facial muscles in the stertorous respiration it will be seen that on the paralyzed side the relaxation permits the cheek to be blown out in a more marked manner. The head and eyes may be turned strongly to one side—conjugate deviation. In such an event the turning is *toward* the side of the hæmorrhage.

In other cases, in which the onset is not so abrupt, the patient may not lose consciousness, but in the course of a few hours there is loss of power, unconsciousness gradually develops, and deepens into profound coma. This is sometimes termed ingravescent apoplexy. The attack may occur during sleep. The patient may be found unconscious, or wakes to find that the power is lost on one side. Small hæmorrhages in the territory of the central arteries may cause hemiplegia without loss of consciousness. In old persons the hemiplegia may be slight and follow a transient loss of consciousness, and is usually most marked in the leg, which is dragged. It may be quite slight ond difficult to make out. It is associated with other senile changes. This is the form very often due to the presence of lacunar softening.

Usually within forty eight hours after the onset of an attack, sometimes within from two to six hours, there are febrile reaction and more or less constitutional disturbance associated with inflammatory changes about the hæmorrhage and absorption of the blood. The period of inflammatory reaction may continue for from one week to two months. The patient may die in this reaction, or, if consciousness has been regained, there may be delirium or recurrence of the coma. At this period the so-called early rigidity may develop in the paralyzed limbs. The so-called trophic changes may occur, such as sloughing or the formation of vesicles. The most serious of these is the sloughing eschar of the lower part of the back, or on the paralyzed side, which may appear within forty eight hours of the onset and is usually of grave significance. The congestion at the bases of the lungs so common in apoplexy is regarded by some as a trophic change.

Conjugate Deviation.—In a right hemiplegia the eyes and head may be turned to the left side; that is to say, the eyes look toward the cerebral lesion. This is almost the rule in the conjugate deviation of the head and eyes which occurs early in hemiplegia. When, however, convulsions or spasm occur or the state of so-called early rigidity in hemiplegia, the conjugate deviation of the head and eyes may be in the opposite direction; that is to say, the eyes look away from the lesion and the head is rotated toward the convulsed side. This symptom may be associated with cortical lesions, particularly, according to some authors, when in the neighborhood of the supramarginal and angular gyri. It may also occur in a lesion of the internal capsule or in the pons, but in the latter situation the conjugate deviation is the reverse of that which occurs in other cases, as the patient looks away from the lesion, and in spasm or convulsion looks toward the lesion.

Hemiplegia.—In cases in which consciousness is restored and the patient improves, a unilateral paralysis may persist due to the destruction of the motor area or the pyramidal tract in any part of its course. Hemiplegia is complete when it involves face, arm, and leg, or partial when it involves only one or other of these parts. This may be the result of a lesion (*a*) of the motor cortex; (*b*) of the pyramidal fibres in the corona radiata and in the internal capsule; (*c*) of a lesion in the cerebral peduncle; or (*d*) in the pons Varolii. The situation of the lesions and their effects are given in Fig. 18. Hæmorrhage is perhaps the most common cause, but tumors and spots of softening may also induce it. The special details of the hemiplegia may here be considered. The face (except in lesions in the lower part of the pons) is involved on the same side as the arm and leg. This results from the fact that the facial muscles stand in precisely the same relation to the cortical centres as those of the arm and leg, the fibres of the upper motor segment of the facial nerve from the cortex decussating just as do those of the nerves of the limbs. The signs of the facial paralysis are usually well marked. There may be a slight difficulty in elevating the eyebrows or in closing the eye on the paralyzed side, or in rare cases the facial paralysis is complete, but the movements may be present with emotion, as laughing or crying. The facial paralysis is partial, involving only the lower portion of the nerve, so that the orbicularis oculi and the frontalis muscles are much less involved than the lower branch. The hypoglossal nerve also is involved. In consequence, the patient can not put out the tongue straight, but it deviates toward the paralyzed side, inasmuch as the genio-hyo-glossus of the sound side is unopposed. In a few cases the protrusion is toward the side of the lesion, a fact not easily explained in the present state of our knowledge of the nervous control of the tongue. With right hemiplegia there may be aphasia. Even without marked aphasia difficulty in speaking and slowness are common.

The arm is, as a rule, more completely paralyzed than the leg. The loss of power may be absolute or partial. In severe cases it is at first complete. In others, when the paralysis in the face and arm is complete, that of the leg is only partial. The face and arm may alone be paralyzed, while the leg escapes. Less commonly the leg is more affected than the arm, and the face may be only slightly involved.

Certain muscles escape in hemiplegia, particularly those associated in symmetrical movements, as those of the thorax and abdomen, a fact which Broadbent explains by supposing that as the spinal nuclei controlling these movements on both sides constantly act together they may, by means of this intimate connection, be stimulated by impulses coming from only one side of the brain. Hughlings Jackson pointed out that in quiet respiration the muscles on the paralyzed side acted more strongly than the corresponding muscles, but that in forced respiration the reverse condition was true. The degree of permanent paralysis after a hemiplegic attack varies much in different cases. When the restitution is partial, it is always certain groups of muscles which recover rather than others. Thus in the leg the residual paralysis concerns the flexors of the leg and the dorsal flexors of the foot—i. e., the muscles which are active in the second period of walking, shortening the leg, and bringing it forward while it swings. The muscles which lift the body when the foot rests upon the ground, those used in the first period of walking, include the extensors of the leg and the plantar flexors of the foot. These "lengtheners" of the leg often recover almost completely in cases in which the paralysis is due to lesions of the pyramidal tract. In the arms the residual paralysis usually affects the muscle groups which oppose the thumb, those which rotate the arm outward, and the openers of the hand.

As a rule, there is at first no wasting of the paralyzed limbs.

Crossed Hemiplegia.—A paralysis in which there is loss of function in a cerebral nerve on one side with loss of power (or of sensation) on the opposite side of the body is called a crossed or alternate hemiplegia. It is met with in lesions, commonly hæmorrhage, in the crus, the pons, and the medulla (Figs. 18, 12 and 13).

(*a*) *Crus.*—The bleeding may extend from vessels supplying the corpus striatum, internal capsule, and optic thalamus, or the hæmorrhage may be primarily in the crus. In the classical case of Weber, on section of the lower part of the left crus, an oblong clot 15 mm. in length lay just below the medial and inferior surface. The characteristic features of a lesion in this locality are paralysis of arm, face, and leg of the opposite side, and oculo-motor paralysis of the same side—the syndrome of Weber. Sensory changes may also be present. Hæmorrhage into the tegmentum is not necessarily associated with hemiplegia, but there may be incomplete paralysis of the oculo-motor nerve, with disturbance of sensation and ataxia on the opposite side of the body. The optic tract or the lateral geniculate body lying on the lateral side of the crus may be compressed, in which event there will be hemianopia.

(*b*) *Pons and Medulla.*—Lesions may involve the pyramidal tract and one

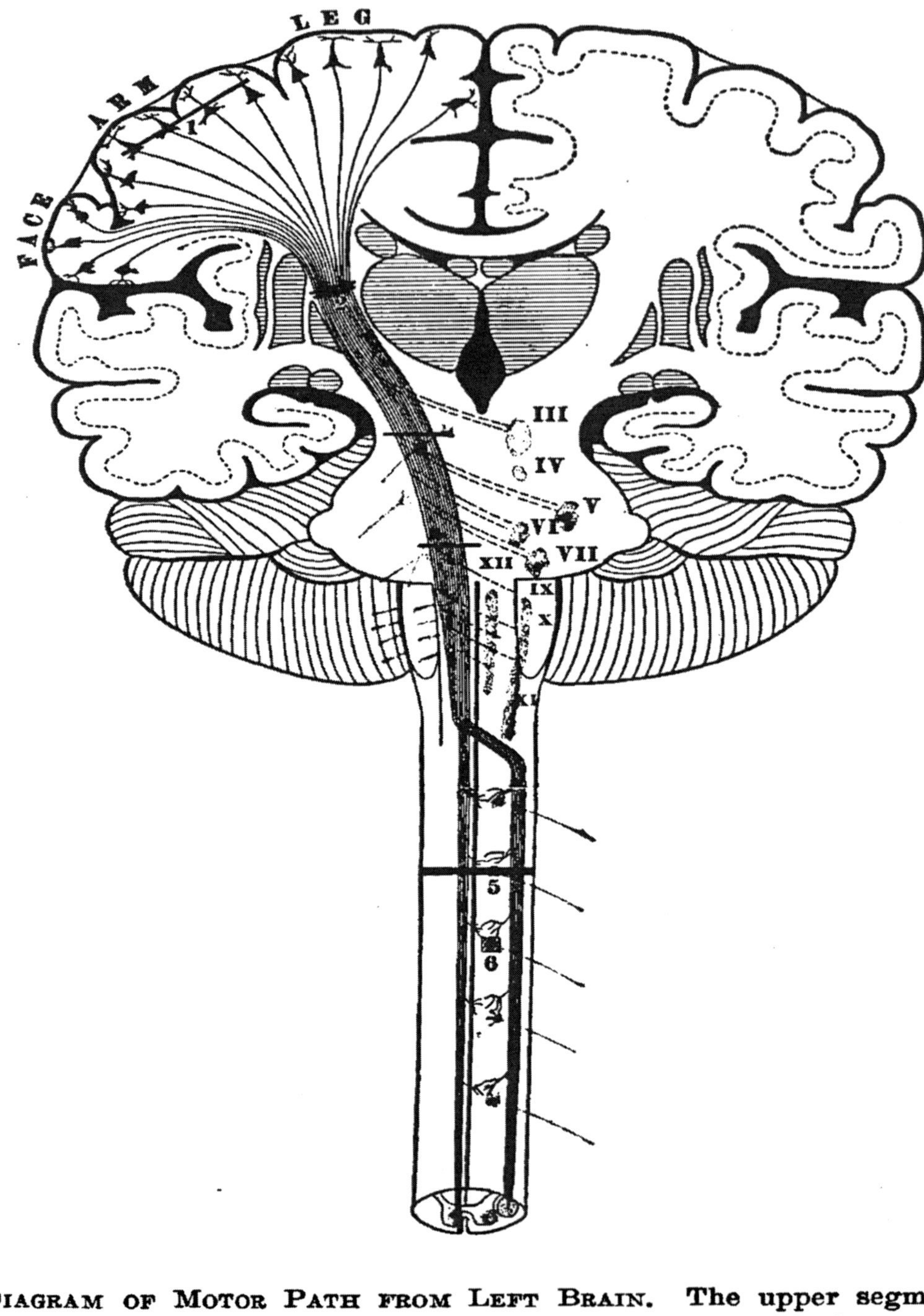

Fig. 18.—Diagram of Motor Path from Left Brain. The upper segment is black, the lower red. The nuclei of the motor cerebral nerves are shown on the right side; on the left side the cerebral nerves of that side are indicated. A lesion at 1 would cause upper segment paralysis in the arm of the opposite side—cerebral monoplegia; at 2, upper segment paralysis of the whole opposite side of the body—hemiplegia; at 3 (in the crus), upper segment paralysis of the opposite face, arm, and leg, and lower segment paralysis of the eye-muscles on the same side—crossed paralysis; at 4 (in the lower part of the pons), upper segment paralysis of the opposite arm and leg, and lower segment paralysis of the face and external rectus on the same side—crossed paralysis; at 5, upper segment paralysis of all muscles represented below lesion, and lower segment paralysis of muscles represented at level of lesion—spinal paraplegia; at 6, lower segment paralysis of muscles localized at seat of lesion—anterior poliomyelitis. (Van Gehuchten, modified.)

or more of the cerebral nerves. If at the lower aspect of the pons, the facial nerve may be involved, causing paralysis of the face on the same side and hemiplegia on the opposite side. The fifth nerve may be involved, with the fillet (the sensory tract), causing loss of sensation in the area of distribution of the fifth on the same side as the lesion and loss of sensation on the opposite side of the body. The sensory disturbance here is apt to be dissociated, of the syringomyelic type, affecting particularly the sense of pain and temperature.

Sensory Disturbances Resulting from Cerebral Hæmorrhage.—These are variable. Hemianæsthesia may coexist with hemiplegia, but in many instances there is only slight numbing of sensation. When the hemianæsthesia is marked, it is usually the result of a lesion in the internal capsule involving the retrolenticular portion of the posterior limb. In C. L. Dana's study of sensory localization he found that anæsthesia of organic cortical origin was always limited or more pronounced in certain parts, as the face, arm, or leg, and was generally incomplete. Total anæsthesia was either of functional or subcortical origin. Marked anæsthesia was much more common in softening than in hæmorrhage. Complete hemianæsthesia is certainly rare in hæmorrhage. Disturbance of the special senses is not common. Hemianopia may exist on the same side as the paralysis, and there may be diminution in the acuteness of the senses of hearing, taste, and smell. Gowers thinks that homonymous hemianopia of the halves of the visual fields opposite to the lesion is very frequent shortly after the onset, though often overlooked.

Psychic disturbances, variable in nature and degree, may result from cerebral hæmorrhage.

The Reflexes in Apoplectic Cases.—During the apoplectic coma all the reflexes are abolished, but immediately on recovery of consciousness they return, first on the non-hemiplegic side, later, sometimes only after weeks, on the paralyzed side. As to the time of return, especially of the patellar reflexes, marked differences are observable in individual cases. The deep reflexes later are increased on the paralyzed side, and ankle clonus may be present. Plantar stimulation usually gives an extensor response in the great toe (Babinski's reflex). This may occur very early and is an important indication of the paralyzed side. The other superficial reflexes are usually diminished. The sphincters are not affected.

The *course* of the disease depends upon the situation and extent of the lesion. If slight, the hemiplegia may disappear completely within a few days or a few weeks. In severe cases the rule is that the leg gradually recovers before the arm, and the muscles of the shoulder girdle and upper arm before those of the forearm and hand. The face may recover quickly.

Except in the very slight lesions, in which the hemiplegia is transient, changes take place which may be grouped as

Secondary Symptoms.—These correspond to the chronic stage. In a case in which little or no improvement takes place within eight or ten weeks it will be found that the paralyzed limbs undergo certain changes. The leg, as a rule, recovers enough power to enable the patient to get about, although the foot is dragged. Occasionally a recurrence of severe symptoms is seen, even without a new hæmorrhage having taken place. In both arm and leg the condition of *secondary contraction* or *late rigidity* comes on and is always most marked in the upper extremity. The arm becomes permanently flexed at the elbow and resists all attempts at extension. The wrist is flexed upon the forearm and the fingers upon the hand. The position of the arm and hand is very characteristic. There is frequently, as the contractures develop, a great deal of pain. In the leg the contracture is rarely so extreme. The loss of power is most marked in the muscles of the foot and, to prevent the toes from dragging, the knee in walking is much flexed, or more commonly the foot is swung round in a half circle.

The reflexes are at this stage greatly increased. These contractures are permanent and incurable, and are associated with a secondary descending sclerosis of the motor path. There are instances, however, in which rigidity and contracture do not occur, but the arm remains flaccid, the leg having regained its power. This *hémiplégie flasque* of Bouchard is found most commonly in children. Among other secondary changes in late hemiplegia may be mentioned the following: Tremor of the affected limbs, post-paralytic chorea, the mobile spasm known as athetosis, arthropathies in the joints of the affected side, and muscular atrophy. Athetosis and post-hemiplegic chorea will be considered in the hemiplegia of children. The cool surface and thin glossy skin of a hemiplegic limb are familiar to all. A word may here be said upon the subject of muscular atrophy of cerebral origin.

As a rule, atrophy is not a marked feature in hemiplegia, but in some instances it does occur. It has been thought to be due in some cases to secondary alterations in the gray matter of the ventral horns; but atrophy may follow as a direct result of the cerebral lesion, the ventral horns remaining intact. In Quincke's case atrophy of the arm followed the development of a glioma in the anterior central convolution. The gray matter of the ventral horns was normal. These atrophies are most common in cortical lesions involving the domain of the third main branch of the Sylvian artery, and in central lesions involving the lenticulo-thalamic region. Their explanation is not clear. The wasting of cerebral origin, which occurs most frequently in children, and leads to hemiatrophy of the muscles along with stunted growth of the bones and joints, is to be sharply separated from the hemiatrophy of the muscles of the adult following within a relatively short time upon the hemiplegia.

Diagnosis.—There are three groups of cases which offer increasing difficulty in recognition.

(1) Cases in which the onset is gradual, a day or two elapsing before the paralysis is fully developed and consciousness completely lost, are readily recognized, though it may be difficult to determine whether the lesion is due to thrombosis or to hæmorrhage.

(2) In the sudden apoplectic stroke in which the patient rapidly loses consciousness the difficulty in diagnosis may be still greater, particularly if the patient is in deep coma when first seen.

The first point to be decided is the existence of hemiplegia. This may be difficult, although, as a rule, even in deep coma the limbs on the paralyzed side are more flaccid and drop instantly when lifted; whereas on the non-paralyzed side the muscles retain some degree of tonus. The reflexes may be decreased or lost on the affected side ond there may be conjugate deviation of the head and eyes. Rigidity in the limbs on one side is in favor of a hemiplegic lesion. It is practically impossible in a majority of these cases to say whether the lesion is due to hæmorrhage, embolism, or thrombosis.

(3) Large hæmorrhage into the ventricles or into the pons may produce sudden loss of consciousness with complete relaxation, so that the condition may simulate coma from uræmia, diabetes, alcoholism, opium poisoning, or epilepsy.

The previous history and the mode of onset may give valuable information. In epilepsy convulsions have preceded the coma; in alcoholism there is a history of constant drinking, while in opium poisoning the coma develops more gradually; but in many instances the difficulty is practically very great, and on more than one occasion I have seen mortifying post mortem disclosures under these circumstances. With diabetic coma the breath often smells of acetone. In ventricular hæmorrhage the coma is sudden and comes on rapidly. The hemiplegic symptoms may be transient, quickly giving place to complete relaxation. Convulsions occur in many cases, and may be the very symptom to lead astray—as in a case of ventricular hæmorrhage which occurred in a puerperal patient, in whom, naturally enough, the condition was thought to be uræmic. Rigidity is often present. In hæmorrhage into the pons convulsions are frequent. The pupils may be strongly contracted, conjugate deviation may occur, and the temperature is apt to rise rapidly. The contraction of the pupils in pontine hæmorrhage naturally suggests opium poisoning. The difference in temperature in the two conditions is a valuable diagnostic point. The apoplectiform seizures of general paresis have usually been preceded by abnormal mental symptoms, and the associated hemiplegia is seldom permanent.

It may be impossible at first to give a definite diagnosis. In admissions to hospitals or in emergency cases the physician should be particularly careful about the following points: The examination of the head for injury or fracture; the urine should be tested for albumin, examined for sugar, and studied microscopically; a careful examination should be made of the limbs with reference to their degree of relaxation or the presence of rigidity, and the condition of the reflexes; the state of the pupils should be noted and the temperature taken. The odor of the breath (alcohol, acetone, chloroform, etc.) should be remarked. The most serious mistakes are made in the case of patients who are drunk at the time of the attack, a combination by no means uncommon in the class of patients admitted to hospital. Under these circumstances the case may erroneously be looked upon as one of alcoholic coma. It is best to regard each case as serious and to bear in mind that this is a condition in which, above all others, mistakes are common.

Prognosis.—From cortical hæmorrhage, unless very extensive, the recovery may be complete without a trace of contracture. This is more common when the hæmorrhage follows injury than when it results from disease of the arteries. Infantile meningeal hæmorrhage, on the other hand, is a condition which may produce idiocy or spastic diplegia.

Large hæmorrhages into the corona radiata, and especially those which rupture into the ventricles, rapidly prove fatal.

The hemiplegia which follows lesions of the internal capsule, the result of rupture of the lenticulo-striate artery, is usually persistent and followed by contracture. When the retro-lenticular fibres of the internal capsule are involved there may be hemianæsthesia, and later, especially if the thalamus be implicated, hemichorea or athetosis. In any case of cerebral apoplexy the following symptoms are of grave omen: persistence or deepening of the coma during the second and third day; rapid rise in temperature within the first forty-eight hours after the initial fall. In the reaction which takes place on the second or third day the temperature usually rises, and its gradual fall on the third or fourth day with return of consciousness is a favorable indication. The rapid formation of bed-sores, particularly the malignant decubitus of Charcot, is a fatal indication. The occurrence of albumin and sugar, if abundant, in the urine is an unfavorable symptom.

When consciousness returns and the patient is improving, the question is anxiously asked as to the paralysis. The extent of this can not be determined for some weeks. With slight lesions it may pass off entirely. If persistent at the end of a month some grade of permanent palsy is certain to remain, and gradually the late rigidity supervenes.

5. EMBOLISM AND THROMBOSIS

(Cerebral Softening)

Embolism.—The embolus usually enters the carotid, rarely the vertebral artery. In the great majority of cases it comes from the left heart and is either a vegetation of a fresh endocarditis or, more commonly, of a recurring endocarditis, or from the segments involved in an ulcerative process. Less often the embolus is a portion of a clot which has formed in the auricular appendix. Portions of clot from an aneurism, thrombi from atheroma of the aorta, or from the territory of the pulmonary veins, may also cause blocking of the branches of the circle of Willis. In the puerperal condition cerebral embolism is not infrequent. It may occur in women with heart disease, but in other instances the heart is uninvolved, and the condition has been thought to be associated with the development of heart clots, owing to increased coagulability of the blood. A majority of cases of embolism occur in heart disease, 89 per cent. (Saveliew). Cases are rare in the acute endocarditis of rheumatic fever, chorea, and febrile conditions. It is much more common in the secondary recurring endocarditis which attacks old sclerotic valves. The embolus most frequently passes to the left middle cerebral artery, as it enters the left carotid oftener than the right because of the more direct course of the blood in the former. The posterior cerebral and the vertebral are less often affected. A large plug may lodge at the bifurcation of the basilar. Embolism of the cerebellar vessels is rare.

Embolism occurs more frequently in women, owing, no doubt, to the greater frequency of mitral stenosis. Contrary to this general statement, Newton Pitt's statistics of 79 cases at Guy's Hospital indicate, however, that males are more frequently affected; as in this series there were 44 males and 35 females. Saveliew gives 54 per cent. in women.

Thrombosis.—Clotting of blood in the cerebral vessels occurs (1) about an embolus, (2) as the result of a lesion of the arterial wall (either endarteritis with or without atheroma or, particularly, the syphilitic arteritis), (3) in aneurisms, both coarse and miliary, and (4) very rarely as a direct result of abnormal conditions of the blood. Thrombosis occasionally follows ligation of the carotid artery. The thrombosis is most common in the middle cerebral and in the basilar arteries. According to Kolisko, softening of limited areas, sufficient to induce hemiplegia, may be caused by sudden collapse of certain cerebral arteries from cardiac weakness.

Anatomical Changes.—Degeneration and softening of the territory supplied by the vessels are the ultimate result in both embolism and thrombosis. Blocking in a terminal artery may be followed by infarction, in which the territory may either be deeply infiltrated with blood (hæmorrhagic infarction) or be simply pale, swollen, and necrotic (anæmic infarction). Gradually the process of softening proceeds, the tissue is infiltrated with serum and is moist, the nerve fibres degenerate and become fatty. The neuroglia is swollen and œdematous. The color of the softened area depends upon the amount of blood. The hæmoglobin undergoes gradual transformation, and the early red color may give place to yellow. Formerly much stress was laid upon the difference between *red, yellow,* and *white* softening. The red and yellow are seen chiefly on the cortex. Sometimes the red softening is particularly marked in cases of embolism and in the neighborhood of tumors. The gray matter shows many punctiform hæmorrhages—capillary apoplexy. There is a variety of yellow softening—the *plaques jaunes*—common in elderly persons, which occurs in the gray matter of the convolutions. The spots are from 1 to 2 cm. in diameter, sometimes are angular in shape, the edges cleanly cut, and the softened area is represented by either a turbid, yellow material, or in some instances there is a space crossed by fine trabeculæ, in the meshes of which there is fluid. White softening occurs most frequently in the white matter, and is seen best about tumors and abscesses. Inflammatory changes are common in and about the softened areas. When the embolus is derived from an infected focus, as in ulcerative endocarditis, suppuration may follow. The final changes vary very much. The degenerated and dead tissue elements are gradually but slowly removed, and if the region is small may be replaced by a growth of connective tissue and the formation of a scar. If large, the resorption results in the formation of a cyst. It is surprising for how long an area of softening may persist without much change.

The position and extent of the softening depend upon the obstructed artery. An embolus which blocks the middle cerebral at its origin involves not only the arteries to the anterior perforated space, but also the cortical branches, and in such a case there is softening in the neighborhood of the corpus striatum, as well as in part of the region supplied by the cortical vessels. The freedom of anastomosis between these branches varies a good deal. Thus, there are instances of embolism of the middle cerebral artery in which the softening has involved only the territory of the central branches, in which case blood has reached the cortex through the anterior and posterior cerebrals. When the middle cerebral is blocked (as is perhaps oftenest the case) beyond the point of origin of the central arteries, one or other of its branches is usually most involved. The embolus may lodge in the vessel passing to the third frontal convolution, or in the artery of the ascending frontal or ascending parietal; or it may lodge in the branch passing to the supramarginal and angular gyri, or it may enter the lowest branch which is distributed to the upper convolutions of the temporal lobe. These are practically terminal arteries, and instances frequently occur of softening limited to a part, at any rate, of the territory supplied by them. Some of the most accurate focalizing lesions are produced in this way.

Symptoms.—Extensive thrombotic softening may exist without any symptoms. It is not uncommon in the post mortem examination of the bodies of elderly persons to find the *plaques jaunes* scattered over the convolutions. So, too, softening may take place in the "silent" regions, as they are termed, without exciting any symptoms. When the central or cortical branches of the middle cerebral arteries are involved the symptoms are similar to those of hæmorrhage from the same arteries. Permanent or transient hemiplegia results. When the central arteries are involved the softening in the internal capsule is commonly followed by permanent hemiplegia. There are certain peculiarities associated with embolism and with thrombosis respectively.

In *embolism* the patient is usually the subject of heart trouble, or there exist some of the conditions already mentioned. The onset is sudden, without premonitory symptoms but sometimes with intense headache. When the embolus blocks the left middle cerebral artery the hemiplegia is associated with aphasia. In *thrombosis,* on the other hand, the onset is more gradual; the patient has previously complained of headache, vertigo, tingling in the fingers; the speech may have been embarrassed for some days; the patient has had loss of memory or is incoherent, or paralysis begins at one part, as the hand, and extends slowly, and the hemiplegia may be incomplete or variable. Abrupt loss of consciousness is much less common, and when the lesion is small consciousness is retained. Thus, in thrombosis due to syphilitic disease, the hemiplegia may come on gradually without the slightest disturbance of consciousness.

The hemiplegia following thrombosis or embolism has practically the characteristics, both primary and secondary, described under hæmorrhage.

The following may be the effects of blocking the different vessels: (*a*) *Vertebral.*—The left branch is more frequently plugged. The effects are involvement of the nuclei in the medulla and symptoms of acute bulbar paralysis. It rarely occurs alone; more commonly with

(*b*) Blocking of the *basilar artery.* When this is entirely occluded, there may be bilateral paralysis from involvement of both motor paths. Bulbar symptoms may be present; rigidity or spasm may occur. The temperature may rise rapidly. The symptoms, in fact, are those of apoplexy of the pons.

(*c*) The *posterior cerebral* supplies the occipital lobe on its medial surface and the greater part of the temporo-sphenoidal lobe. If the main stem be thrombosed there is hemianopia with sensory aphasia. Localized areas of softening may exist without symptoms. Blocking of the main occipital branch (arteria occipitalis of Duret), or of the arteria calcarina, passing to the cuneus may be followed by hemianopia. Hemianæsthesia may result from involvement of the posterior part of the internal capsule. Not infrequently symmetrical thrombosis of the occipital arteries of the two sides occurs, as in Förster's well-known case. Still more frequent is the occurrence of thrombosis of a branch of the posterior cerebral of one hemisphere and a branch of the middle cerebral of the other. It is in such cases that the most pronounced instances of apraxia are met with.

(*d*) *Internal Carotid.*—The symptoms are variable. As is well known, the vessel is in a majority of cases ligated without risk. In other instances transient hemiplegia follows; in others again the hemiplegia is permanent. These variations depend on the anastomoses in the circle of Willis. If these are large and free, no paralysis follows, but in cases in which the posterior communicating and the anterior communicating vessels are small or absent the paralysis may persist. In No. 7 of my Elwyn series of cases of infantile hemiplegia, the woman, aged twenty four, when six years old, had the right carotid ligated for abscess following scarlet fever, with the result of permanent hemiplegia. Blocking of the internal carotid within the skull by thrombosis or embolism is followed by hemiplegia, coma, and usually death. The clot is rarely confined to the carotid itself, but spreads into its branches and may involve the ophthalmic artery.

(*e*) *Middle Cerebral.*—This is the vessel most commonly involved, and, as already mentioned, if plugged before the central arteries are given off, permanent hemiplegia usually follows from softening of the internal capsule. Blocking of the branches beyond this point may be followed by hemiplegia, which is more likely to be transient, involves chiefly the arm and face, and if the lesion be on the left side is associated with aphasia. There may be plugging of the individual branches passing to the inferior frontal (producing typical motor aphasia if the disease be on the left side), to the anterior and posterior central gyri (usually causing total hemiplegia), to the supramarginal and angular gyri (giving rise, if the thrombosis be on the left side, probably without exception to the so-called visual aphasia (alexia), usually also to right-sided hemionopsia), or to the temporal gyri (in which event with left-sided thrombosis word-deafness results).

(*f*) *Anterior Cerebral.*—No symptoms may follow, and even when the branches which supply the paracentral lobule and the top of the ascending convolutions are plugged the branches from the middle cerebral are usually able to effect a collateral circulation in these parts. Monoplegia of the leg may, however, result. Hebetude and dullness of intellect may occur with obstruction of the vessel.

There is unquestionably greater freedom of communication in the cortical branches of the different arteries than is usually admitted, although it is not possible, for example, to inject the posterior cerebral through the middle cerebral, or the middle cerebral from the anterior; but the absence of softening in some instances in which smaller branches are blocked shows how complete may be the compensation, probably by way of the capillaries. The dilatation of the collateral branches may take place very rapidly; thus a patient with chronic nephritis died about twenty four hours after the hemiplegic attack. There were recent vegetations on the mitral valve and an embolus in the right middle cerebral artery just beyond the first two branches. The central portion of the hemisphere was swollen and œdematous. The right anterior cerebral was greatly dilated, and by measurement its diameter was found to be nearly three times that of the left.

Treatment of Cerebral Hæmorrhage and of Softening.—The chief difficulty in deciding upon a method of treatment is to determine whether the apoplexy is due to hæmorrhage or to thrombosis or embolism. The patient should be placed in bed, with his head moderately elevated and the neck free. He should be kept absolutely quiet. If there are dyspnœa, stertor, and signs of mechanical obstruction to respiration, he should be turned on his side, as recommended by Bowles. This procedure also lessens the liability to congestion of the lungs. If the signs of intracranial hæmorrhage are certain, and if the arterial tension is high, measures may be taken for its reduction. Of these the most rapid and satisfactory is venesection, which in many cases seems to do good. However, as Cushing has shown experimentally, a rapid and increasing rise of arterial tension usually indicates an endeavor of the vasomotor centres to counteract an increasing intracranial pressure, in this case due to a continuing hæmorrhage. The indication under these circumstances is the relief of the intracranial pressure by craniotomy and removal of the clot, if this is possible. This is particularly applicable in subdural hæmorrhage. Horsley and Spencer have recently, on experimental grounds, recommended the practice, formerly employed empirically, of compression of the carotid, particularly in the ingravescent form; or even, in suitable cases, passing a ligature round the vessel. An ice-bag may be placed on the head and hot bottles to the feet. The bowels should be freely opened, either by calomel, elaterium, or elaterin. Counter-irritation to the neck or to the feet is not necessary. Catheterization of the bladder may be necessary, especially if the patient remains long unconscious.

Special care should be taken to avoid bed-sores; and if bottles are used to the feet, they should not be too hot, since blisters may be readily caused by a much lower temperature than in health. In the fever of reaction aconite may be indicated, but should be cautiously used. Stimulants are not necessary, unless the pulse becomes feeble and signs of collapse supervene. No digitalis is to be given. During recovery the patient should be still kept entirely at rest, even in the mildest attacks remaining in bed for at least fourteen days. The ice-bag should still be kept to the head. The diet should be light and no medicine other than some placebo should be administered, at least during the first month after the hæmorrhage. Attention should be paid to the position occupied by the paralyzed limb or limbs, which if swollen may be wrapped in cotton batting or flannel.

The treatment of *softening* from thrombosis or embolism is very unsatisfactory. Venesection is not indicated, as it lowers the tension and rather promotes clotting. If, as is often the case, the heart's action is feeble and irregular, stimulants and small doses of digitalis may be given with, if necessary, ether or ammonia. The bowels should be kept open, but it is not well to purge actively, as in hæmorrhage.

In the thrombosis which follows syphilitic disease of the arteries, and which is met with most frequently in men between twenty and forty (in whom the hemiplegia often sets in without loss of consciousness), the iodide of potassium should be freely used, giving from 20 to 30 grains (1.3 to 2 gm.) three times a day, or, if necessary, larger doses. If the syphilis has been recent, mercurials by inunction are also indicated. Practically these are the only cases of hemiplegia in which we see satisfactory results from treatment.

Very little can be done for the hemiplegia which remains. The damage is too often irreparable and permanent, and it is very improbable that iodide of potassium, or any other remedy, hastens in the slightest degree Nature's dealing with the blood clot.

The paralyzed limbs may be gently rubbed once or twice a day, and this should be systematically carried out, in order to maintain the nutrition of the muscles and to prevent, if possible, contractures. The massage should not, however, be begun until at least ten days after the attack. The rubbing should be *toward* the body, and should not be continued for more than fifteen minutes at a time. After the lapse of a fortnight, or in severe cases a month, the muscles may be stimulated by the faradic current; faradic stimulation alternating with massage, especially if applied to the antagonists of the muscles which ordinarily undergo contracture, is of very great service, even in cases where there can be but little hope of any return of voluntary movement. When contractures occur, electricity properly applied at intervals may still be of some benefit along with the passive movements and frictions, and it has been suggested that tendon transplantation, or indeed cross suture of nerves, may cause some improvement.

In a case of complete hemiplegia the friends should at the outset be frankly told that the chances of full recovery are slight. Power is usually restored in the leg sufficient to enable the patient to get about, but in the majority of instances the finer movements of the hand are permanently lost. The general health should be looked after, the bowels regulated, and the secretions of the skin and kidneys kept active. In permanent hemiplegia in persons above the middle period of life, more or less mental weakness is apt to follow the attack, and the patient may become irritable and emotional.

And, lastly, when hemiplegia has persisted for more than three months and contractures have developed, it is the duty of the physician to explain to the patient, or to his friends, that the condition is past relief, that medicines and electricity will do no good, and that there is no possible hope of cure.

6. ANEURISM OF THE CEREBRAL ARTERIES

Miliary aneurisms are not included, but reference is made only to aneurism of the larger branches. The condition is not uncommon. There were 12 instances in my first 800 autopsies in Montreal. This is a considerably larger proportion than in Newton Pitt's collection from Guy's Hospital, 19 times in 9,000 inspections.

Etiology.—Males are more frequently affected than females. Of my 12 cases 7 were males. The disease is most common at the middle period of life. One of my cases was a lad of six. Pitt describes one at the same age. The chief causes are (*a*) endarteritis, either simple or syphilitic, which leads to weakness of the wall and dilatation; and (*b*) embolism. These aneurisms are often found with endocarditis. Pitt, in his study of the subject, concludes that it is exceptional to find cerebral aneurism unassociated with fungating endocarditis. The embolus disappears, and dilatation follows the secondary inflammatory changes in the coats of the vessel.

Morbid Anatomy.—The middle cerebral branches are most frequently involved. In my 12 cases the distribution on the arteries was as follows: Internal carotid, 1; middle cerebral, 5; basilar, 3; anterior communicating, 3. Except in one case they were saccular and communicated with the lumen of the vessel by an orifice smaller than the circumference of the sac. In the 154 cases which make up the statistics of Lebert, Durand, and Bartholow the middle cerebral was involved in 44, the basilar in 41, internal carotid in 23, anterior cerebral in 14, posterior communicating in 8, anterior communicating in 8, vertebral in 7, posterior cerebral in 6, inferior cerebellar in 3 (Gowers). The size of the aneurism varies from that of a pea to that of a walnut. The hæmorrhage may be entirely meningeal with very slight laceration of the brain substance, but the bleeding may be, as Coats has shown, entirely within the substance.

Symptoms.—The aneurism may attain considerable size and cause no symptoms. In a majority of the cases the first intimation is the rupture and the fatal apoplexy. Distinct symptoms are most frequently caused by aneurism of the internal carotid, which may compress the optic nerve or the commissure, causing neuritis or paralysis of the third nerve. A murmur may be audible on auscultation of the skull. Aneurism in this situation may give rise to irritative and pressure symptoms at the base of the brain or to hemianopia. In the remarkable case reported by Weir Mitchell and Dercum an aneurism compressed the chiasma and produced bilateral temporal hemianopia.

Aneurism of the vertebral or of the basilar may involve the nerves from the fifth to the twelfth. A large sac at the termination of the basilar may compress the third nerves or the crura.

The diagnosis is, as a rule, impossible. The larger sacs produce the symptoms of tumor, and their rupture is usually fatal.

7. ENDARTERITIS

In no group of vessels do we more frequently see chronic degenerative changes than in those of the circle of Willis. The condition occurs as:

Arterio-sclerosis, producing localized or diffused thickening of the intima with the formation of atheromatous patches or areas of calcification. In the later stages, as seen in elderly people, the arteries of the circle of Willis may be dilated, stiff, or almost universally calcified.

Syphilitic Endarteritis.—As already mentioned under the section of syphilis, gummatous endarteritis is specially prone to attack the cerebral vessels. It has in itself no specific characters—that is to say, it is impossible in given sections to pick out an endarteritis syphilitica from an ordinary endarteritis obliterans. On the other hand, as already stated, the nodular periarteritis is never seen except in syphilis.

8. THROMBOSIS OF THE CEREBRAL SINUSES AND VEINS

The condition may be primary or secondary. Lebert (1854) and Tonnele were among the first to recognize the condition clinically.

Primary thrombosis of the sinuses and veins is rare. It occurs (*a*) in children, particularly during the first six months of life, usually in connection with diarrhœa. Gowers believes that it is of frequent occurrence, and that thrombosis of the veins is not an uncommon cause of infantile hemiplegia.

(*b*) In connection with chlorosis and anæmia, the so-called *autochthonous sinus-thrombosis.* Of 82 cases of thrombosis in chlorosis, 78 were in the veins and 32 in the cerebral sinuses. The longitudinal sinus is most frequently involved. The thrombosis is usually associated with venous thromboses in other parts of the body, and the patients die, as a rule, in from one to three weeks, but both Bristowe and Buzzard report recoveries.

(*c*) In the terminal stages of cancer, phthisis, and other chronic diseases thrombosis may gradually occur in the sinuses and cortical veins. To the coagulum developing in these conditions the term marantic thrombus is applied.

Secondary thrombosis is much more frequent and follows extension of inflammation from contiguous parts to the sinus wall. The common causes are disease of the internal ear, fracture, compression of the sinuses by tumor, or suppurative disease outside the skull, particularly erysipelas, carbuncle, and parotitis. In secondary cases the lateral sinus is most frequently involved. Of 57 fatal cases in which ear disease caused death with cerebral lesions, there were 22 in which thrombosis existed in the lateral sinuses (Pitt). Tuberculous caries of the temporal bone is often directly responsible. The thrombus may be small, or may fill the entire sinus and extend into the internal jugular vein. In more than one half of these instances the thrombus was suppurating. The disease spreads directly from the necrosis on the posterior wall of the tympanum. According to Voltolini, the inflammation extends by way of the petroso-mastoid canal. It is not so common in disease of the mastoid cells.

Symptoms.—*Primary thrombosis* of the longitudinal sinus may occur without exciting symptoms and is found accidentally at the post mortem. There may be mental dullness with headache. Convulsions and vomiting may occur. In other instances there is nothing distinctive. In the chlorosis cases the head symptoms have, as a rule, been marked. Ball's patient was dull and stupid, had vomiting, dilatation of the pupils, and double choked disks. Slight paresis of the left side occurred. An interesting feature in this case was the development of swelling of the left leg. In the cases reported by Andrews, Church, Tuckwell, Isambard Owen, and Wilks the patients had headache, vomiting, and delirium. Paralysis was not present. In Douglas Powell's case, with similar symptoms, there was loss of power on the left side. Bristowe reports a case of great interest in an anæmic girl of nineteen, who had convulsions, drowsiness, and vomiting. Tenderness and swelling developed in the position of the right internal jugular vein, and a few days later on the opposite side. The diagnosis was rendered definite by the occurrence of phlebitis in the veins of the right leg. The patient recovered.

The onset of such symptoms as have been mentioned in an anæmic or chlorotic girl should lead to the suspicion of cerebral thrombosis. In infants the diagnosis can rarely be made. Involvement of the cavernous sinus may cause œdema about the eyelids or prominence of the eyes.

In the *secondary thrombi* the symptoms are commonly those of septicæmia. For instance, in over 70 per cent. of Pitt's cases the mode of death was by pulmonary pyæmia. This author draws the following important conclusions: (1) The disease spreads oftener from the posterior wall of the middle ear than from the mastoid cells. (2) The otorrhœa is generally of some standing, but not always. (3) The onset is sudden, the chief symptoms being pyrexia, rigors, pains in the occipital region and in the neck, associated with a septicæmic condition. (4) Well-marked optic neuritis may be present. (5) The appearance of acute local pulmonary mischief or of distant suppuration is almost conclusive of thrombosis. (6) The average duration is about three weeks, and death is generally from pulmonary pyæmia. The chief points in the diagnosis may be gathered from these statements.

Associated with thrombosis of the lateral sinus there may be venous stasis and painful œdema behind the ear and in the neck. The external jugular vein on the diseased side may be less distended than on the opposite side, since owing to the thrombus in the lateral sinus the internal jugular vein is less full than on the normal side, and the blood from the external jugular can flow more easily into it.

Treatment.—In marantic individuals roborants and stimulants are indicated. The position assumed in bed should favor both the arterial and venous circulation. The clothing should not restrict the neck, and care should be taken to avoid *bending* of the neck. The internal administration of potassium iodide and calomel has been recommended in the autochthonous forms, but no treatment is likely to be of any avail.

The secondary forms, especially those following upon disease of the middle ear, are often amenable to operation, and, especially recently, many lives have been saved by surgical intervention after extensive sinus thrombosis.

9. HEMIPLEGIA IN CHILDREN

Etiology.—Of 135 cases, 60 were in boys and 75 in girls. Right hemiplegia occurred in 79, left in 56. In 15 cases the condition was said to be congenital.

In a great majority the disease sets in during the first or second year; thus of the total number of cases, 95 were under two. Cases above the fifth year are rare, only 10 in my series. Neither alcoholism nor syphilis in the parents appears to play an important rôle in this affection. Difficult or abnormal labor is responsible for certain of the cases, particularly injury with the *forceps.* Trauma, such as falls or puncturing wounds, is more rare. The condition followed ligation of the common carotid in one case.

Infectious diseases. All the authors lay special stress upon this factor. In 19 cases in my series the disease came on during or just after one of the specific fevers. I saw one case in which during the height of vaccination convulsions occurred, followed by hemiplegia. The organism of anterior poliomyelitis (Heine-Medin disease) is probably responsible for a considerable share of the cases. In a great majority the disease sets in with a convulsion, in which the child may remain for several hours or longer, and after recovery the paralysis is noticed.

Morbid Anatomy.—In an analysis which I have made of 90 autopsies reported in the literature, the lesions may be grouped under three headings:

(*a*) Embolism, thrombosis, and hæmorrhage, comprising 16 cases, in 7 of which there was blocking of a Sylvian artery, and in 9 hæmorrhage. A striking feature in this group is the advanced age of onset. Ten of the cases occurred in children over six years old.

(*b*) Atrophy and sclerosis, comprising 50 cases. The wasting is either of groups of convolutions, an entire lobe, or the whole hemisphere. The meninges are usually closely adherent over the affected region, though sometimes they look normal. The convolutions are atrophied, firm, and hard, contrasting strongly with the normal gyri. The sclerosis may be diffuse and widespread over a hemisphere, or there may be nodular projections—the hypertrophic sclerosis. Some of the cases show remarkable unilateral atrophy of the hemisphere. In one of my cases the atrophied hemisphere weighed 169 grams and the normal one 653 grams. The brain tissue may be a mere shell over a dilated ventricle.

(*c*) Porencephalus, which was present in 24 of the 90 autopsies. This term was applied by Heschel (1868) to a loss of substance in the form of cavities and cysts at the surface of the brain, either opening into and bounded by the arachnoid, and even passing deeply into the hemisphere, or reaching to the ventricle. In the study by Audrey of 103 cases of porencephalus, hemiplegia was mentioned in 68 cases.

Practically, then, in infantile hemiplegia cortical sclerosis and porencephalus are the important anatomical conditions. The primary change in the majority of these cases is still unknown. Porencephalus may result from a defect in development or from hæmorrhage at birth. The etiology is clear in the limited number of cases of hæmorrhage, embolism, and thrombosis, but there remains the large group in which the final change is sclerosis and atrophy. What is the primary lesion in these instances? The clinical history shows that in nearly all these cases the onset is sudden, with convulsions—often with slight fever. Strümpell believes that this condition is due to an inflammation of the gray matter—polioencephalitis. A certain number of the cases represent the cerebral sporadic form of epidemic polio-myeloencephalitis. The clinical picture of cases described in the Swedish and other epidemics is identical with that with which we are only too familiar in this disease.

Symptoms.—(*a*) The Onset.—The disease may set in suddenly without spasms or loss of consciousness. In more than half the cases the child is attacked with partial or general convulsions and loss of consciousness, which may last from a few hours to many days. This is one of the most striking features in the disease. Fever is usually present. The hemiplegia, noticed as the child recovers consciousness, is generally complete. Sometimes the paralysis is not complete at first, but occurs after subsequent convulsions. The right side is more frequently affected than the left. The face is commonly not involved.

(*b*) Residual Symptoms.—In some cases the paralysis gradually disappears and leaves scarcely a trace as the child grows up. The leg, as a rule, recovers more rapidly and more fully than the arm, and the paralysis may be scarcely noticeable. In a majority of cases, however, there is a characteristic hemiplegic gait. The paralysis is most marked in the arm, which is usually wasted; the forearm is flexed at right angles, the hand is flexed, and the fingers are contracted. Motion may be almost completely lost; in other instances the arm can be lifted above the head. Late rigidity, which almost always develops, is the symptom which suggested the name *hemiplegia spastica cerebralis* to Heine, the orthopædic surgeon, who first accurately described these cases. It is, however, not constant. The limbs may be quite relaxed even years after the onset. The reflexes are usually increased. In several instances, however, I have known them to be absent. Sensation, as a rule, is not disturbed.

Aphasia is a not uncommon symptom, and occurred in 16 cases of my series.

Mental Defects.—One of the most serious consequences of infantile hemiplegia is the failure of mental development. A considerable number of these cases drift into the institutions for feeble minded children. Three grades may be distinguished—idiocy, which is most common when the hemiplegia has existed from birth; imbecility, which often increases with the development of epilepsy; and feeble mindedness, a retarded rather than an arrested development.

Epilepsy.—Of the cases in my series, 41 were subjects of convulsive seizures, one of the most distressing sequels of the disease. The seizures may be either transient attacks of *petit mal,* true Jacksonian fits, beginning in and confined to the affected side, or general convulsions.

Post-hemiplegic Movements.—It was in cases of this sort that Weir Mitchell first described the post-hemiplegic movements. They are extremely common, and were present in 34 of my series. There may be either slight tremor in the affected muscles, or incoördinate choreiform movements—the so-called post-hemiplegic chorea—or, lastly,

Athetosis.—In this condition, described by Hammond, there are remarkable spasms of the paralyzed extremities, chiefly of the fingers and toes, and in rare instances of the muscles of the mouth. The movements are involuntary and somewhat rhythmical; in the hand, movements of adduction or abduction and of supination and pronation follow each other in orderly sequence. There may be hyperextension of the fingers, during which they are spread wide apart. This condition is much more frequent in children than in adults. In the latter it may be combined with hemianæsthesia, and the lesion is not cortical, but basic, in the neighborhood of the thalamus. The movements are sometimes increased by emotion. They usually persist during sleep.

Treatment.—The possibility of injury to the brain in protracted labor and in forceps cases should be borne in mind by the practitioner. The former entails the greater risk. In infantile hemiplegia the physician at the outset sees a case of ordinary convulsions, perhaps more protracted and severe than usual. These should be checked as rapidly as possible by the use of the bromides, the application of cold or heat, and a brisk purge. During convulsions chloroform may be administered with safety even to the youngest children. When the paralysis is established not much can be hoped from medicines. In only rare instances does the paralysis entirely disappear. When the recovery is partial the "residual paralysis" is similar to that seen in other lesions of the upper motor segment. Thus in the lower extremity it is the flexors of the leg and the dorsal flexors of the foot which are most often permanently paralyzed (Wernicke). The indications are to favor the natural tendency to improve by maintaining the general nutrition of the child, to lessen the rigidity and contractures by massage and passive motion, and if necessary to correct deformities by mechanical or surgical measures. Much may be done by careful manipulation and rubbing and the application of a proper apparatus. In children the aphasia usually disappears. The epilepsy is a distressing and obstinate symptom, for which a cure can rarely be anticipated. Prolonged periods of quiescence are, however, not uncommon. In the Jacksonian fits the bromides rarely do good, unless there is much irritability and excitement. Operative measures in favorable cases of this particular form of epilepsy may often prove beneficial in reducing the number and severity of the seizures, but it is very unusual for them to be completely or permanently checked. The liability to feeble mindedness is the most serious outlook in the infantile cerebral palsies. In many cases the damage is irreparable, and idiocy and imbecility result. With patient training and with care many of the children reach a fair measure of intelligence and self-reliance.

IV. TUMORS, INFECTIONS, GRANULOMATA, AND CYSTS OF THE BRAIN

The following are the most common varieties of new growths within the cranium:

Infectious Granulomata.—(*a*) *Tubercle,* which may form large or small growths, usually multiple. Tuberculosis of the glands or bones may be coexistent, but the tuberculous disease of the brain may occur in the absence of other clinically recognizable tuberculous lesions. The disease is most frequent early in life. Three-fourths of the cases occur under twenty, and one-half of the patients are under ten years of age (Gowers). Of 300 cases of tumor in persons under nineteen collected from various sources by Starr, 152 were tubercle. The nodules are most numerous in the cerebellum and about the base.

(*b*) *Syphiloma* is most commonly found on the cortex cerebri or about the pons. The tumors are superficial, attached to the arteries or the meninges, and rarely grow to a large size, although they may do so. They may be multiple. A gummatous meningitis of the base is common and in this process the oculomotor nerves are often affected. The motor nerves of the eye are particularly prone to syphilitic infiltration, and ptosis and the ordinary forms of squint are common. It is common for the pituitary body to be involved with symptoms suggestive of diabetes insipidus.

Tumors.—(*c*) *Glioma and Neuroglioma.*—These vary greatly in appearance. They may be firm and hard, almost like an area of sclerosis, and are not sharply defined from the surrounding brain substance. They may be soft and very vascular, and hæmorrhages are common. They persist remarkably for many years. Klebs has called attention to the occurrence of elements in them not unlike ganglion-cells. Tumors of this character may contain the "Spinnen" or spider cells; enormous spindle-shaped cells with single large nuclei; cells like the ganglion-cells of nerve-centres with nuclei and one or more processes; and translucent, band-like fibres, tapering at each end, which result from a vitreous or hyaline transformation of the large spindle-cells. A separate type is also recognizable, in which the cells resemble the ependymal epithelium.

(*d*) *Fibrosarcoma* (endothelioma) occurs most commonly in the membranes covering the hemispheres or brain stem, and for a long time may cause injury by its compression effects alone. Tumors of this kind are particularly common in the cerebello-pontine recess. When sarcoma originates in the brain substance it may become one of the largest and most diffusely infiltrating of intracranial growths. When meningeal in origin, it is the form of tumor most amenable to surgical treatment.

(*e*) *Carcinoma* not infrequently is secondary to cancer in other parts. It is seldom primary. Occasionally cancerous tumors have been found in symmetrical parts of the brain.

(*f*) Other varieties occur, such as fibroid growths, which usually develop from the membranes; bony tumors, which grow sometimes from the falx, psammona, cholesteatoma, and angioma. Fatty tumors are occasionally found on the corpus callosum.

Cysts.—These occur between the membranes and the brain, as a result of hæmorrhage or of softening. Porencephalus is a sequel of congenital atrophy or of hæmorrhage, or may be due to a developmental defect. Hydatid cysts have been referred to in the section on parasites. An interesting variety of cyst is that which follows severe injury to the skull in early life. Gliomata often undergo cystic degeneration. Dermoid cyst has been described.

Site.—A majority of all tumors occur in the cerebrum and especially in the centrum ovale. The cerebellum, pons, and membranes are next most often involved. Glioma is more common in the hemispheres and grows slowly. It is usually single. Tubercles are usually multiple. Secondary sarcoma and carcinoma are often mutiple.

Symptoms.—GENERAL.—The following are the most important: *Headache,* either dull, aching, and continuous, or sharp, stabbing, and paroxysmal. It may be diffused over the entire head; sometimes it is limited to the back or front. When in the back of the head it may extend down the neck (especially in tumors in the posterior fossa), and when in the front it may be accompanied with neuralgic pains in the face. Occasionally the pain may be very localized and associated with tenderness on pressure.

Choked disk (optic neuritis) occurs in four fifths of all the cases (Gowers). It should be looked for in every patient presenting cerebral symptoms, for it may be present in high degree without impairment of vision. Loss of visual acuity usually indicates that optic atrophy has set in. It is usually double, but occasionally is found in only one eye. A growth may develop slowly and attain considerable size without producing optic neuritis. On the other hand, it may occur with a very small tumor, when this tumor is so situated as to cause internal hydrocephalus. J. A. Martin, from an extensive analysis of the literature with reference to the localizing value, concludes: When there is a difference in the amount of the neuritis in each eye it is more than twice as probable that the tumor is on the side of the most marked neuritis. It is constant in tumors of the corpora quadrigemina, present in 89 per cent. of cerebellar tumors, and absent in nearly two thirds of the cases of tumor of the pons, medulla, and of the corpus callosum. It is least frequent in cases of tuberculous tumor; most common in cases of glioma and cystic tumors.

Paton and Holmes, who reported upon the eyes of 700 cases of cerebral tumor, concluded that the essential feature of the associated optic neuritis is œdema, and in 60 eyes examined histologically the one unfailing change was acute œdema, the origin of which they attribute to the venous engorgement.

Vomiting is a common feature and, with headache and optic neuritis, makes up the characteristic clinical picture of cerebral tumor. An important point is the absence of definite relation to the meals. A chemical examination shows that the vomiting is independent of digestive disturbances. It may be very obstinate, particularly in growths of the cerebellum and the pons.

Giddiness is often an early symptom. The patient complains of vertigo on rising suddenly or on turning quickly.

Mental Disturbance.—The patient may act in an odd, unnatural manner, or there may be stupor and heaviness. The patient may become emotional or silly, or there are symptoms resembling hysteria.

Convulsions, either general and resembling true epilepsy or localized (Jacksonian) in character. Seizures beginning with a gustatory or olfactory aura are particularly common with tumors originating in the infundibular region. There may be *slowing of the pulse,* as in all cases of increased intracranial pressure.

LOCALIZING SYMPTOMS.—Focal symptoms often occur, but it must not be forgotten that these may be *indirectly* produced. The smaller the tumor and the less marked the general symptoms of cerebral compression the more likely is it that any focal symptoms occurring are of *direct* origin.

(*a*) *Central Motor Area.*—The symptoms are either irritative or destructive in character. Irritation in the lower third may produce spasm in the muscles of the face, in the angle of the mouth, or in the tongue. The spasm with tingling may be strictly limited to one muscle group before extending to others, and this Seguin terms the *signal symptom.* The middle third of the motor area contains the centres controlling the arm, and here, too, the spasm may begin in the fingers, in the thumb, in the muscles of the wrist, or in the shoulder. In the upper third of the motor areas the irritation may produce spasm beginning in the toes, in the ankles, or in the muscles of the leg. In many instances the patient can determine accurately the point of origin of the spasm, and there are important sensory disturbances, such as numbness and tingling, which may be felt first at the region affected.

In all cases it is important to determine, first, the point of origin, the *signal symptom;* second, the order or march of the spasm; and third, the subsequent condition of the parts first affected, whether it is a state of paresis or anæsthesia.

Destructive lesions in the motor zone cause paralysis, which is often preceded by local convulsive seizures; there may be a monoplegia, as of the leg, and convulsive seizures in the arm, often due to irritation in these centres. Tumors in the neighborhood of the motor area may cause localized spasms and subsequently, as the centres are invaded by the growth, paralysis occurs. When tumors are situated in the left hemisphere the speech mechanism is apt to be involved if the transverse temporal gyrus or the third frontal convolution and their connecting path are implicated.

(*b*) *Prefrontal Region.*—Neither motor nor sensory disturbance may be present. The general symptoms are often well marked. The most striking feature of growths in this region is mental torpor and gradual imbecility. Particularly when the left side is involved mental characteristics may be greatly altered. In its extension downward the tumor may involve on the left side the lower frontal convolution and produce aphasia, or in its progress backward cause irritative or destructive lesions of the motor area. Exophthalmos on the side of the tumor may occur and be helpful in diagnosis.

(*c*) Tumors in the *parieto-occipital lobe,* particularly on the right side, may grow to a large size without causing any symptoms. There may be word-blindness and mind-blindness when the left angular gyrus and its underlying white matter are involved, and paraphasia. Astereognosis may accompany growths in the superior parietal region.

(*d*) Tumors of the *occipital lobe* produce hemianopia, and a bilateral lesion may produce blindness. Tumors in this region on the left hemisphere may be associated with word-blindness and mind-blindness. In all cases of tumor a careful study should be made of the fields of vision. In addition to the lateral hemianopia there may be remarkable visual hallucinations, and in tumors of the left occipital lobe dissociation of the color sense and inability to find the proper colors of various objects presented.

(*e*) Tumors in the *temporal lobe* may attain a large size without producing symptoms. In their growth they involve the lower motor centres. On the left side involvement of the transverse temporal gyri (auditory sense area) may be associated with word-deafness.

(*f*) Tumors growing in the neighborhood of the *basal ganglia* produce hemiplegia from involvement of the internal capsule. Limited growths in either the nucleus caudatus or the nucleus lentiformis of the corpus striatum do not necessarily cause paralysis. Tumors in the thalamus opticus may also, when small, cause no symptoms, but, increasing, they may involve the fibres of the sensory portion of the internal capsule, producing hemianopia and sometimes hemianæsthesia. Growths in this situation are apt to cause early optic neuritis, and, growing into the third ventricle, may cause a distention of the lateral ventricles. What has been termed the thalamic syndrome may be present—hemianæsthesia to pain, touch and temperature, with the loss of deep sensibility. With this there may be a very remarkable type of pain, involving the hand and arm and the foot and leg, on the affected side, a sense of burning discomfort rather than sharp pain. Ataxic features are usually present and astereognosis. Motor hemiplegia may be present, and it is unaccompanied by contractures (Dana).

Growths in the *corpora quadrigemina* are rarely limited, but most commonly involve the crura cerebri as well. Ocular symptoms are marked. The pupil reflex is lost and there is nystagmus. In the gradual growth the third nerve is involved as it passes through the crus, in which case there will be oculo-motor paralysis on one side and hemiplegia on the other, a combination almost characteristic of unilateral disease of the crus.

(*g*) Tumors of the *pons* and *medulla*. The symptoms are chiefly those of pressure upon the nerves emerging in this region. In disease of the pons the nerves may be involved alone or with the pyramidal tract. Of 52 cases analyzed by Mary Putnam Jacobi, there were 13 in which the cerebral nerves were involved alone, 13 in which the limbs were affected, and 26 in which there were hemiplegia and involvement of the nerves. Twenty-two of the latter had what is known as alternate paralysis—i. e., involvement of the nerves on one side and of the limbs on the opposite side. In 4 cases there were no motor symptoms. In tuberculosis (or syphilis) a growth at the inferior and inner aspects of the crus may cause paralysis of the third nerve on one side, and of the face, tongue, and limbs on the opposite side (syndrome of Weber). A tumor growing in the lower part of the pons usually involves the sixth nerve, producing internal strabismus, the seventh nerve, producing facial paralysis, and the auditory nerve, causing deafness. Conjugate deviation of the eyes to the side opposite that on which there is facial paralysis also occurs. When the motor cerebral nerves are involved the paralyses are of the peripheral type (lower segment paralyses).

Tumors of the *medulla* may involve the cerebral nerves alone or cause in some instances a combination of hemiplegia with paralysis of the nerves. Paralyses of the nerves are helpful in topical diagnosis, but the fact must not be overlooked that one or more of the cerebral nerves may be paralyzed as a result of a much increased general intracranial pressure. Signs of irritation in the ninth, tenth, and eleventh nerves are usually present, and produce difficulty in swallowing, irregular action of the heart, irregular respiration, vomiting, and sometimes retraction of the head and neck. The hypoglossal nerve is least often affected. The gait may be unsteady or, if there is pressure on the cerebellum, ataxic. Occasionally there are sensory symptoms, numbness, and tingling. Toward the end convulsions may occur.

(*h*) Tumors of the *cerebellum* may be latent, but they usually give rise to very characteristic symptoms, headache in the occipital region, giddiness, incoordination, but there is nothing definite in the direction of the swaying, and early optic neuritis. They may be intracerebellar or extracerebellar.

Tumors or enlargements of the *pituitary gland* itself, or growths from a congenital *anlage* in its neighborhood which implicate the pituitary gland secondarily, are very common. The congenital tumors arise presumably from developmental faults, and show either a teratomatous character or are solid or cystic tumors with squamous epithelium, often attaining adamantine characteristics. The most common tumor is a so-called struma (malignant adenoma) of the gland proper. There are characteristic signs of pressure upon the neighborhood structures, bitemporal hemianopia being a frequent though not invariable feature. These lesions may occur in patients who have suffered from acromegaly, or in those who show signs of glandular deficiency or dyspituitarism, and in whom there may or may not be suggestive acromegalic tendencies. The X-rays are most useful in diagnosis.

Diagnosis.—From the general symptoms alone the existence of tumor may be determined, for the combination of headache, optic neuritis, and vomiting is distinctive. As pointed out by R. T. Williamson, progressive hemiplegia, without other symptoms, a paralysis, which gradually becomes more marked day by day and week by week, is almost pathognomic, even in the absence of optic neuritis, headache, and vomiting. The two exceptions to this rule appear to be in cerebral abscess, and in rare instances a polioencephalitis. It must not be forgotten that severe headache and neuro-retinitis may be caused by Bright's disease. The localization must be gathered from the consideration of the symptoms above detailed and from the data given in the section on Topical Diagnosis of Diseases of the Brain. Mistakes are most likely to occur in connection with uræmia, hysteria, vascular lesions, abscess, serous meningitis, hydrocephalus, and general paralysis; but careful consideration of all the circumstances of the case usually enables the practitioner to avoid error.

Prognosis.—Syphilitic tumors alone are amenable to medical treatment. Tuberculous growths occasionally cease to grow and become calcified. The gliomata and fibromata, particularly when the latter grow from the membranes, may last for years. I have described a case of small, hard glioma, in which the Jacksonian epilepsy persisted for fourteen years. Hughlings Jackson has reported cases of glioma in which the symptoms lasted for over ten years. The more rapidly growing sarcomata usually prove fatal in from six to eighteen months. Death may be sudden, particularly in growths near the medulla;

more commonly it is due to coma in consequence of gradual increase in the intracranial pressure.

Treatment.—(*a*) Medical.—A Wassermann test of the blood and cerebrospinal fluid should always be made before antiluetic measures are instituted. It must not be overlooked that vigorous treatment with potassium iodide often causes a temporary amelioration of pressure symptoms due to a glioma, so that the therapeutic test is not entirely a dependable one. If syphilis is proved the iodide of potassium and mercury should be given. Salvarsan is sometimes given in repeated small doses. Nowhere do we see more brilliant therapeutical effects than in certain cases of cerebral gummata. The iodide should be given in increasing doses. In tuberculous tumors the outlook is less favorable, though instances of cure are reported, and there is post mortem evidence to show that the solitary tuberculous tumors may undergo changes and become obsolete. A general tonic treatment is indicated in these cases. The headache usually demands prompt treatment. The iodide of potassium in full doses sometimes gives marked relief. An ice-cap for the head or, in the occipital headache, the application of the Paquelin cautery may be tried. The bromides are not of much use in the headache from this cause, and, as the last resort, morphia must be given. For the convulsions bromide of potassium is of little service.

(*b*) Surgical.—Scores of tumors of the brain have now been successfully removed. Though the percentage of cases in which total enucleation is possible is doubtless small, yet in all cases marked amelioration of the pressure symptoms is possible by modern surgical measures. It is important that they should be instituted early, even in the absence of localizing symptoms, for the sake of preserving vision. The most advantageous cases are the localized fibromata and sarcomata growing from the dura and only compressing the brain substance. Of late years there have been numerous successful operations with removal of growths from the cerebellum and cerebello-pontine recess. The safety with which the exploratory operation can be made warrants it in all doubtful cases. For two objects the so-called decompression operation may be performed, to relieve the headache, which it sometimes does promptly and permanently, and to save sight. It is now very generally practised by surgeons, and the reduction of the greatly increased intracranial pressure may cause the choked disk to subside and the risk of subsequent atrophy is much diminished.

V. INFLAMMATION OF THE BRAIN

1. ACUTE ENCEPHALITIS

A focal or diffuse inflammation of the brain substance, usually of the gray matter (poliencephalitis), is met with (*a*) as a result of trauma; (*b*) in certain intoxications, alcohol, food poisoning, and gas poisoning; (*c*) following the acute infections; and (*d*) as one of the varieties of the poliomyelo-encephalitis (Heine-Medin disease). The anatomical features are those of an acute hæmorrhagic poliencephalitis, corresponding in histological details with acute polio-myelitis. Focal forms are seen in ulcerative endocarditis, in which the gray matter may present deeply hæmorrhagic areas, firmer than the surrounding tissue. In the fevers there may be more extensive regions, involving two or three convolutions. This acute hæmorrhagic poliencephalitis superior is thought by Strümpell to be the essential lesion in infantile hemiplegia, and it seems probable that many of the cases represent the sporadic form (cerebral variety of the Heine-Medin disease). Localizing symptoms are usually present, though they may be obscured in the severity of the general infection. The most typical encephalitis accompanies the meningitis in cerebro-spinal fever.

In acute mania, in delirium tremens, in chorea insaniens, in the maniacal form of exophthalmic goitre, and in the so-called cerebral forms of the malignant fevers the gray cortex is deeply congested, moist, and swollen, and with the recent finer methods of research will probably show changes which may be classed as encephalitis.

The *symptoms* are not very definite. In severe forms they are those of an acute infection; some cases have been mistaken for typhoid fever. The onset may be abrupt in an individual apparently healthy. Other cases have occurred in the convalescence from the fevers, particularly influenza. One of J. J. Putnam's cases followed mumps. The general symptoms are those which accompany all severe acute affections of the brain—headache, somnolence, coma, delirium, vomiting, etc. The local symptoms are very varied, depending on the extent of the lesions, and may be irritative or paralytic. Usually fatal within a few weeks, cases may drag on for weeks or months and recover, generally with paralysis.

2. ABSCESS OF THE BRAIN

Definition.—Purulent encephalitis with abscess formation the result of infection by micro-organisms.

Etiology.—Suppuration of the brain substance is rarely if ever primary, but results, as a rule, from extension of inflammation from neighboring parts or infection from a distance through the blood. The question of idiopathic brain abscess need scarcely be considered, though occasionally instances occur in which it is extremely difficult to assign a cause. There are three important etiological factors.

(*a*) *Trauma.* Falls upon the head or blows, with or without abrasion of the skin. More commonly it follows fracture or punctured wounds. In this group meningitis is frequently associated with the abscess. As Bergmann says, simple trauma or concussion can never produce abscess but organisms may enter through a laceration of the base opening one of the many sinuses.

(*b*) By far the most important infective foci are those which arise in *direct extension from disease of the middle ear,* of the *mastoid cells,* or of the *frontal sinuses.* From the roof of the mastoid antrum the infection readily passes to the sigmoid sinus and induces an infective thrombosis. In other instances the dura becomes involved, and a subdural abscess is formed, which may readily involve the arachnoid or the pia mater. In another group the inflammation extends along the lymph spaces, or the thrombosed veins, into the substance of the brain and causes suppuration. Macewen thinks that without local areas of meningitis the infective agents may be carried through the lymph and blood channels into the cerebral substance. Infection which extends from the roof of the tympanic cavity is most likely to be followed by abscess in the temporal lobe, while infection extending from the mastoid cells causes most frequently sinus thrombosis and cerebellar abscess.

(*c*) *In septic processes.* Abscess of the brain is not often found in pyæmia. In ulcerative endocarditis multiple foci of suppuration are common. Localized bone disease and suppuration in the liver are occasional causes. Certain inflammations in the lungs, particularly bronchiectasis, as already referred to in connection with Schörstein's researches, may be followed by abscess. It is an occasional complication of empyema. Abscess of the brain may follow the specific fevers. Bristowe has called attention to its occurrence as a sequel of influenza. The largest number of cases occur between the twentieth and fortieth years, and the condition is more frequent in men than in women. Holt has collected 25 cases in children under five years of age, the chief causes of which were otitis media and trauma.

Morbid Anatomy.—The abscess may be solitary or multiple, diffuse or circumscribed. Practically any one of the different varieties of pyogenic bacteria may be concerned. The bacteriological examination often shows a mixture of different varieties. Occasionally cultures are sterile, owing to death of the bacteria. In the acute, rapidly fatal cases following injury the suppuration is not limited; but in long standing cases the abscess is inclosed in a definite capsule, which may have a thickness of from 2 to 5 mm. The pus varies much in appearance, depending upon the age of the abscess. In early cases it may be mixed with reddish *débris* and softened brain matter, but in the solitary encapsulated abscess the pus is distinctive, having a greenish tint, an acid reaction, and a peculiar odor, sometimes like that of sulphuretted hydrogen. The brain substance surrounding the abscess is usually œdematous and infiltrated. The size varies from that of a walnut to that of a large orange. There are cases on record in which the cavity has occupied the greater portion of a hemisphere. Multiple abscesses are usually small. In four fifths of all cases the abscess is solitary. Suppuration occurs most frequently in the cerebrum, and the temporal lobe is more often involved than other parts, and always on the side of the ear disease. The cerebellum is the next most common seat, particularly in connection with ear disease.

Symptoms.—Following injury or operation the disease may run an *acute* course, with fever, headache, delirium, vomiting, and rigors. The symptoms are those of suppurative meningo-encephalitis, and it may be very difficult to determine, unless there are localizing symptoms, whether there is really suppuration in the brain substance. In the cases following ear disease the symptoms may at first be those of meningeal irritation. There may be irritability, restlessness, severe headache, and aggravated earache. Other striking symptoms, particularly in the more prolonged cases, are drowsiness, slow cerebration, vomiting, and optic neuritis. In the chronic form of brain abscess which may follow injury, otorrhœa, or local lung trouble, there may be a latent period ranging from one or two weeks to several months, or even a year or more. In the "silent" regions, when the abscess becomes encapsulated there may be no symptoms whatever during the latent period. During all this time the patient may be under careful observation and no suspicion be aroused of the existence of suppuration. Then severe headache, vomiting, and fever set in, perhaps with a chill. So, too, after a blow upon the head or a fracture the symptoms of the lesion may be transient, and months afterward cerebral symptoms of the most aggravated character may develop.

The localization of the lesion is often difficult. If situated in or near the motor region there may be convulsions or paralysis, and it is to be remembered that an abscess in the temporal lobe may compress the lower part of the pre-central convolution and produce paralysis of the arm and face, and on the left side cause aphasia. A large abscess may exist in the frontal lobe without causing paralysis, but in these cases there is almost always some mental dullness. In the temporal lobe, the common seat, there may be no focalizing symptoms. So also in the parieto-occipital region; though here early examination may lead to the detection of hemianopia. In abscess of the cerebellum vomiting is common. If the middle lobe is affected there may be staggering —cerebellar incoördination. Localizing symptoms in the pons and other parts are still more uncertain.

Diagnosis.—In the acute cases there is rarely any doubt. A consideration of possible etiological factors is of the highest importance. The history of injury followed by fever, marked cerebral symptoms, the onset of rigors, delirium, and perhaps paralysis, make the diagnosis certain. In chronic ear disease, such cerebral symptoms as drowsiness and torpor, with irregular fever, supervening upon the cessation of a discharge, should excite the suspicion of abscess. Cases in which suppurative processes exist in the orbit, nose, or naso-pharynx, or in which there has been subcutaneous phlegmon of the head or neck, a parotitis, a facial erysipelas, or tuberculous or syphilitic disease of the bones of the skull, should be carefully watched, and immediately investigated should cerebral symptoms appear. It is particularly in the chronic cases that difficulties arise. The symptoms resemble those of tumor of the brain; indeed, they are those of tumor plus fever. Choked disk, however, so commonly associated with tumor, is very frequently absent in abscess of the brain. In a patient with a history of trauma or with localized lung or pleural trouble, who for weeks or months has had slight headache or dizziness, the onset of a rapid fever, especially if it be intermittent and associated with rigors, intense headache, and vomiting, points strongly to abscess. The pulse rate in cases of cerebral abscess is usually accelerated, but cases are not rare in which it is slowed. Macewen lays stress upon the value of percussion of the skull as an aid in diagnosis. The note, which is uniformly dull, becomes much more resonant when the lateral ventricles are distended in cerebellar abscess and in conditions in which the venæ Galeni are compressed.

It is not always easy to determine whether the meninges are involved with the abscess. Often in ear disease the condition is that of meningo-encephalitis. Sometimes in association with acute ear disease the symptoms may simulate closely cerebral meningitis or even abscess. Indeed, Gowers states that not only may these general symptoms be produced by ear disease, but even distinct optic neuritis.

Treatment.—A remarkable advance has been made of late years in dealing with these cases, owing to the impunity with which the brain can be explored. In ear disease free discharge of the inflammatory products should be promoted and careful disinfection practiced. The treatment of injuries and fractures comes within the scope of the surgeon. The acute symptoms, such as fever, headache, and delirium, must be treated by rest, an ice-cap, and, if necessary, local depletion. In all cases, when a reasonable suspicion exists of the occurrence of abscess, the brain should be explored. The cases following ear disease, in which the suppuration is in the temporal lobe or in the cerebellum, offer the most favorable chances of recovery. The localization can rarely be made accurately in these cases, and the operator must be guided more by general anatomical and pathological knowledge. In cases of injury the trephine should be applied over the seat of the blow or the fracture. In ear disease the suppuration is most frequent in the temporal lobe or in the cerebellum, and the operation should be performed at the points most accessible to these regions. Crowe's discovery of the secretion of hexamethylenamine into the cerebro-spinal fluid suggests its administration in every case in which meningeal infection is threatened or has occurred.

VI. HYDROCEPHALUS

Definition.—A condition, congenital or acquired, in which there is a great accumulation of fluid within the ventricles of the brain.

The term hydrocephalus has also been applied to the collection of fluid between the cortex of the brain and the skull, known in this situation as *hydrocephalus externus* or *hydrocephalus ex vacuo,* a condition common in cases of atrophy of the brain substance, met with in old age, after hæmorrhages, softenings, or scleroses, in lingering and cachectic diseases, as cancer, chronic nephritis, chronic alcoholism, and sometimes in rickets. Occasionally the disease is caused by meningeal cysts. A true dropsy, however, of the arachnoid sac probably does not occur.

The cases may be divided into three groups—idiopathic internal hydrocephalus (serous meningitis), congenital or infantile, and secondary or acquired.

Serous Meningitis (Quincke) (*Idiopathic Internal Hydrocephalus; Angio-neurotic Hydrocephalus*).—This remarkable form, described by Quincke, is very important, since a knowledge of the condition may explain very anomalous and puzzling cases. It is an ependymitis causing a serous effusion into the ventricles, with distention and pressure effects. It may be compared to the serous exudates in the pleura or in synovial membranes. It is not certain that the process is inflammatory, and Quincke likens it to the angio-neurotic œdema of the skin. In very acute cases the ependyma may be smooth and natural looking; in more chronic cases it may be thickened and sodden. The exudate does not differ from the normal, and if on lumbar puncture a fluid is removed of a specific gravity above 1.009, with albumin above two tenths per cent., the condition is more likely to be hydrocephalus from stasis, secondary to tumor, etc.

Both children and adults are affected, the latter more frequently. In the acute form the condition is mistaken for tuberculous or purulent meningitis. There are headache, retraction of the neck, and signs of increased intracranial pressure, choked disks, slow pulse, etc. Fever is usually absent, but I have seen one case with recurring paroxysms of fever, and Morton Prince has described a similar one. In both the exudate was clear and the ependyma not acutely inflamed. Quincke has reported cases of recovery. In the chronic form the symptoms are those of tumor—general, such as headache, slight fever, somnolence, and delirium; and local, as exophthalmos, optic neuritis, spasms, and rigidity of muscles and paralysis of the cerebral nerves. Remarkable exacerbations occur, and the symptoms vary in intensity from day to day. Recovery may follow after an illness of many weeks, and some of the reported cases of disappearance of all symptoms of brain tumor belong in this category.

Congenital Hydrocephalus.—The enlarged head may obstruct labor; more frequently the condition is noticed some time after birth. The cause is unknown. It has occurred in several members of the same family.

The anatomical condition in these cases offers no clew to the nature of the trouble. The lateral ventricles are enormously distended, but the ependyma is usually clear, sometimes a little thickened and granular, and the veins large. The choroid plexuses are vascular, sometimes sclerotic, but often natural looking. The third ventricle is enlarged, the aqueduct of Sylvius dilated, and the fourth ventricle may be distended. The quantity of fluid may reach several litres. It is limpid and contains a trace of albumin and salts. The changes in consequence of this enormous ventricular distention are remarkable. The cerebral cortex is greatly stretched, and over the middle region the thickness may amount to no more than a few millimetres without a trace of the sulci or convolutions. The basal ganglia are flattened. The skull enlarges, and the circumference of the head of a child of three or four years may reach 25 or even 30 inches. The sutures widen, Wormian bones develop in them, and the bones of the cranium become exceedingly thin. The veins are marked beneath the skin. A fluctuation wave may sometimes be obtained, and Fisher's brain murmur may be heard. The orbital plates of the frontal bone are depressed, causing exophthalmos, so that the eyeballs can not be covered by the eyelids. The small size of the face, widening somewhat above, is striking in comparison with the enormously expanded skull.

Convulsions may occur. The reflexes are increased, the child learns to walk late, and ultimately in severe cases the legs become feeble ond sometimes spastic. Sensation is much less affected than motility. Choked disk is not uncommon. The mental condition is variable; the child may be bright, but, as a rule, there is some grade of imbecility. The congenital cases usually die within the first four or five years. The process may be arrested and the patient may reach adult life. Cases of this sort are not very uncommon. Even when extreme, the mental faculties may be retained, as in Bright's celebrated patient, Cardinal, who lived to the age of twenty-nine, and whose head was translucent when the sun was shining behind him. Care must be taken not to mistake the rachitic head for hydrocephalus.

Acquired Chronic Hydrocephalus.—This is stated to be occasionally primary (idiopathic)—that is to say, it comes on spontaneously in the adult without observable lesion. Dean Swift is said to have died of hydrocephalus, but this seems very unlikely. It is based upon the statement that "he (Mr. Whiteway) opened the skull and found much water in the brain," a condition no doubt of *hydrocephalus ex vacuo,* due to the wasting associated with his prolonged illness and paralysis. In nearly all cases there is either a tumor at the base of the brain or in the third ventricle, which compresses the venæ Galeni. The passage from the third to the fourth ventricle may be closed, either by a tumor or by parasites. More rarely the foramen of Magendie, through which the ventricles communicate with the cerebro-spinal meninges, becomes closed by meningitis. Chronic inflammations of the ependyma may in similar fashion block the foramina of exit of the ventricular fluid. There may be unilateral hydrocephalus from closure of one of the foramina of Monro. In cerebro-spinal fever, particularly in the sporadic form, the foramina of exit of the fluid may be occluded, with great distention of the ventricles. These conditions, occurring in adults, may produce the most extreme hydrocephalus without any enlargement of the head. Even when the tumor begins early in life there may be no expansion of the skull. In the case of a girl aged sixteen, blind from her third year, the head was not unusually large, the ventricles were enormously distended, and in the Rolandic region the brain substance was only 5 mm. in thickness. A tumor occupied the third ventricle. In a case of cholesteatoma of the floor of the third ventricle, in which the symptoms persisted at intervals for eight or nine years, the ventricles were enormously distended without enlargement of the skull. In other instances the sutures separate and the head gradually enlarges.

The symptoms of hydrocephalus in the adult are curiously variable. In the first case mentioned there were early headaches and gradual blindness; then a prolonged period in which she was able to attend to her studies. Headaches again supervened, the gait became irregular and somewhat ataxic. Death occurred suddenly. In the other case there were prolonged attacks of coma with a slow pulse, and on one occasion the patient remained unconscious for more than three months. Gradually progressing optic neuritis without focalizing symptoms, headache, and attacks of somnolence or coma are suggestive symptoms. These cases of acquired chronic hydrocephalus can not be certainly diagnosed during life, though in certain instances the condition may be suspected. They simulate tumor very closely.

Treatment.—Very little can be done to relieve hydrocephalus. Medicines are powerless to cause the absorption of the fluid. In the meningitis serosa Quincke advises the use of mercury. Many operative procedures have been devised, tapping of the ventricles, lumbar puncture, making communications between the ventricles and the subarachnoid spaces, into the extracranial tissues, or into the retro-peritoneal tissues and through the body of the fifth lumbar vertebra; and Cushing has practiced an anastomosis by means of a transplanted vein between the external jugular and the subdural space. Bramann claims beneficial results from puncture of the corpus callosum.

F. DISEASES OF THE PERIPHERAL NERVES

I. NEURITIS

(*Inflammation of the Bundles of Nerve Fibres*)

Neuritis may be *localized* in a single nerve, or *general,* involving a large number of nerves, in which case it is usually known as *multiple neuritis* or *polyneuritis.*

Etiology.—*Localized neuritis* arises from (*a*) cold, which is a very frequent cause, as, for example, in the facial nerve. This is sometimes known as rheumatic neuritis. (*b*) Traumatism—wounds, blows, direct pressure on the nerves, the tearing and stretching which follow a dislocation or a fracture, and the hypodermic injection of ether. Under this section come also the professional palsies, due to pressure in the exercise of certain occupations. (*c*) Extension of inflammation from neighboring parts, as in a neuritis of the facial nerve due to caries in the temporal bone, or in that met with in syphilitic disease of the bones, disease of the joints, and occasionally in tumors.

Multiple neuritis has a very complex etiology, the causes of which may be classified as follows: (*a*) The poisons of infectious diseases, as in leprosy, diphtheria, typhoid fever, small-pox, scarlet fever, and occasionally in other forms; (*b*) the organic poisons, comprising the diffusible stimulants, such as alcohol and ether, bisulphide of carbon and naphtha, and the metallic bodies, such as lead, arsenic, and mercury; (*c*) cachectic conditions, such as occur in anæmia, cancer, tuberculosis, or marasmus from any cause; (*d*) the endemic neuritis or beri-beri; and (*e*) lastly, there are cases in which none of these factors prevail, but the disease sets in suddenly after overexertion or exposure to cold.

Morbid Anatomy.—In neuritis due to the extension of inflammation the nerve is usually swollen, infiltrated, and red in color. The inflammation may be chiefly perineural or it may pass into the deeper portion—*interstitial* neuritis—in which form there is an accumulation of lymphoid elements between the nerve bundles. The nerve fibres themselves may not appear involved, but there is an increase in the nuclei of the sheath of Schwann. The myelin is fragmented, the nuclei of the internodal cells are swollen, and the axis-cylinders present varicosities or undergo granular degeneration. Ultimately the nerve fibres may be completely destroyed and replaced by a fibrous connective tissue in which much fat is sometimes deposited—the *lipomatous neuritis* of Leyden.

In other instances the condition is termed *parenchymatous* neuritis, in which the changes are like those met with in the secondary or Wallerian degeneration, which follows when the nerve fibre is cut off from the cell body of the neurone to which it belongs. The medullary substance and the axis-cylinders are chiefly involved, the interstitial tissue being but little altered or only affected secondarily. The muscles connected with the degenerated nerves usually show marked atrophic changes, and in some instances the change in the nerve sheath appears to extend directly to the interstitial tissue of the muscles—the *neuritis fascians* of Eichhorst.

Symptoms.—LOCALIZED NEURITIS.—As a rule, the constitutional disturbances are slight. The most important symptom is pain of a boring or stabbing character, usually felt in the course of the nerve and in the parts to which it is distributed. The nerve itself is sensitive to pressure, probably, as Weir Mitchell suggests, owing to the irritation of its nervi nervorum. The skin may be slightly reddened or even œdematous over the seat of the inflammation. Mitchell has described increase in the temperature and sweating in the affected region, and such atrophic disturbances as effusion into the joints and herpes. The function of the muscle to which the nerve fibres are distributed is impaired, motion is painful, and there may be twitchings or contractions. The tactile sensation of the part may be somewhat deadened, even when the pain is greatly increased. In the more chronic cases of local neuritis, such, for instance, as follow the dislocation of the humerus, the localized pain, which at first may be severe, gradually disappears, though some sensitiveness of the brachial plexus may persist for a long time, and the nerve cords may be felt to be swollen and firm. The pain is variable—sometimes intense and distressing; at others not causing much inconvenience. Numbness and formication may be present and the tactile sensation may be greatly impaired. The motor disturbances are marked. Ultimately there is extreme atrophy of the muscles. Contractures may occur in the fingers. The skin may be reddened or glossy, the subcutaneous tissue œdematous, and the nutrition of the nails may be defective. In the rheumatic neuritis subcutaneous fibroid nodules may develop.

A neuritis limited at first to a peripheral nerve may extend upward—the so-called ascending or migratory neuritis—and involve the larger nerve trunks, or even reach the spinal cord, causing subacute myelitis (Gowers). The condition is rarely seen in the neuritis from cold, or in that which follows fevers; but it occurs most frequently in traumatic neuritis.

J. K. Mitchell, in his monograph on injuries of nerves, concludes that the larger nerve trunks are most susceptible, and that the neuritis may spread either up or down, the former being the most common. The paralysis secondary to visceral disease, as of the bladder, may be due to an ascending neuritis. The inflammation may extend to the nerves of the other side, either through the spinal cord or its membranes, or without any involvement of the nerve-centres, the so-called sympathetic neuritis. The electrical changes in localized neuritis vary a great deal, depending upon the extent to which the nerve is injured. The lesion may be so slight that the nerve and the muscles to which it is distributed may react normally to both currents; or it may be so severe that the typical reaction of degeneration develops within a few days—i. e., the nerve does not respond to stimulation by either current, while the muscle reacts only to the galvanic current and in a peculiar manner. The contraction caused is slow and lazy, instead of sharp and quick as in the normal muscle, and the AC contraction is usually stronger than the KC contraction. Between these two extremes there are many different grades, and a careful electrical examination is most important as an aid to diagnosis and prognosis.

The duration varies from a few days to weeks or months. A slight traumatic neuritis may pass off in a day or two, while the severer cases, such as follow unreduced dislocation of the humerus may persist for months or never be completely relieved.

Multiple Neuritis.—The following are the most important groups of cases:

(a) *Acute Febrile Polyneuritis.*—The attack follows exposure to cold or overexertion, or, in some instances, comes on spontaneously. The onset resembles that of an acute infectious disease. There may be a definite chill, pains in the back and limbs or joints, so that the case may be thought to be rheumatic fever. The temperature rises rapidly and may reach 103° or 104° F. There are headache, loss of appetite, and the general symptoms of acute infection. The limbs and back ache. Intense pain in the nerves, however, is by no means constant. Tingling and formication are felt in the fingers and toes, and there is increased sensitiveness of the nerve trunks or of the entire limb. Loss of muscular power, first marked, perhaps, in the legs, gradually comes on and extends with the features of an ascending paralysis. In other cases the paralysis begins in the arms. The extensors of the wrists and the flexors of the ankles are early affected, so that there is foot and wrist drop. In severe cases there is general loss of muscular power, producing a flabby paralysis, which may extend to the muscles of the face and to the intercostals, and respiration may be carried on by the diaphragm alone. The muscles soften and waste rapidly. There may be only hyperæsthesia with soreness and stiffness of the limbs; in some cases, increased sensitiveness with anæsthesia; in other instances the sensory disturbances are slight. The Argyll-Robertson pupil may be present and the pupils may be unequal. Involvement of the cranial nerves is rare, but the oculo-motor, the facial, and the fifth have been involved. The vagus may be attacked and the quickening of the pulse is usually attributed to this cause. Involvement of the bladder and rectum is rare, but it does occur in undoubted cases and does not necessarily mean involvement of the cord. The clinical picture is not to be distinguished, in many cases, from Landry's paralysis; in others, from the subacute myelitis of Duchenne.

The course is variable. In the most intense forms the patient may die in a week or ten days, with involvement of the respiratory muscles or from paralysis of the heart. As a rule, in cases of moderate severity, after persisting for five or six weeks, the condition remains stationary and then slow improvement begins. The paralysis in some muscles may persist for many months and contractures may occur from shortening of the muscles, but even when this occurs the outlook is, as a rule, good, although the paralysis may have lasted for a year or more.

(*b*) *Recurring Multiple Neuritis.*—Under the term *polyneuritis recurrens* Mary Sherwood has described from Eichhorst's clinic 2 cases in adults—in one case involving the nerves of the right arm, in the other both legs. In one patient there were three attacks, in the other two, the distribution in the various attacks being identical.

(*c*) *Alcoholic Neuritis.*—This, perhaps the most important form of multiple neuritis, was graphically described in 1822 by James Jackson, Sr., of Boston. Wilks recognized it as alcoholic paraplegia, but the starting point of the recent researches on the disease dates from the observations of Dumenil, of Rouen. It occurs most frequently in women, particularly in steady, quiet tipplers. Its appearance may be the first revelation to the physician or to the family of habits of secret drinking. The onset is usually gradual, and may be preceded for weeks or months by neuralgic pains and tingling in the feet and hands. Convulsions are not uncommon. Fever is rare. The paralysis gradually sets in, at first in the feet and legs, and then in the hands and forearms. The extensors are affected more than the flexors, so that there is wrist-drop and foot-drop. The paralysis may be thus limited and not extend higher in the limbs. In other instances there is paraplegia alone, while in the most extreme cases all the extremities are involved. In rare instances the facial muscles and the sphincters are also affected. The sensory symptoms are very variable. There are cases in which there are numbness and tingling only, without great pain. In other cases there are severe burning or boring pains, the nerve trunks are sensitive, and the muscles are sore when grasped. The hands and feet are frequently swollen and congested, particularly when held down for a few moments. The cutaneous reflexes, as a rule, are preserved. The deep reflexes are usually lost.

The course of these alcoholic cases is, as a rule, favorable, and after persisting for weeks or months improvement gradually begins, the muscles regain their power, and even in the most desperate cases recovery may follow. The extensors of the feet may remain paralyzed for some time, and give to the patient a distinctive walk, the so-called *steppage* gait, characteristic of peripheral neuritis. It is sometimes known as the pseudo-tabetic gait, although in reality it could not well be mistaken for the gait of ataxia. The foot is thrown forcibly forward, the toe lifted high in the air so as not to trip upon it. The entire foot is slapped upon the ground as a flail. It is an awkward, clumsy gait, and gives the patient the appearance of constantly stepping over obstacles. Among the most striking features of alcoholic neuritis are the mental symptoms. Delirium is common, and there may be hallucinations with extravagant ideas, resembling somewhat those of general paralysis. In some cases the picture is that of ordinary delirium tremens, but the most peculiar and almost characteristic mental disorder is that so well described by Wilks, in which the patient loses all appreciation of time and place, and describes with circumstantial details long journeys which, he says, he has recently taken, or tells of persons whom he has just seen. This is the so-called Korsakoff's syndrome.

(*d*) *Multiple Neuritis in the Infectious Diseases.*—This has been already referred to, particularly in diphtheria, in which it is most common. The peripheral nature of the lesion in these instances has been shown by post mortem examination. The outlook is usually favorable and, except in diphtheria, fatal cases are uncommon. Multiple neuritis in tuberculosis, diabetes, and syphilis is of the same nature, being probably due to toxic materials absorbed into the blood.

(*e*) *The Metallic Poisons.*—Neuritis from arsenic may follow: (1) The medicinal use particularly of Fowler's solution. I have reported a case of Hodgkin's disease in which general neuritis was caused by ℥ j ʒ ij of the solution. In chorea a good many cases have been reported. Changes in the nails are not uncommon, chiefly the transverse ridging. In one case in my wards, of a young woman who had taken rough-on-rats, there were remarkable white lines—the leuconychia—running across the nails, without any special ridging. C. J. Aldrich finds that this is not uncommon in chronic arsenical poisoning. (2) The accidental contamination of food or drink. Chrome yellow may be used to color cakes, as in the cases recorded by D. D. Stewart. A remarkable epidemic of neuritis occurred in the Midland Counties of England, which was traced to the use of beer containing small quantities of arsenic, a contamination from the sulphuric acid used in making glucose. Reynolds, who studied these cases, believes that most of the instances of neuritis in drinkers are arsenical, but admits that the slight cases may be due to the alcohol itself. Pigmentation of the skin is an important distinguishing sign. The general features have been referred to under arsenical poisoning. Lead is a much more frequent cause. Neuritis has followed the use of mercurial inunctions. Zinc is a rare cause. I saw a case with Urban

Smith which followed the use of two grains of the sulpho-carbolate taken daily for three years. Tea, coffee, and tobacco are mentioned as rare causes.

(*f*) *Endemic neuritis, beri-beri,* has been considered elsewhere.

Anæsthesia Paralysis.—Here perhaps may most appropriately be considered the forms of paralysis following the use of anæsthetics, or of too long-continued compression during operations. Much has been written in the past few years upon this subject. There are two groups of cases:

(*a*) During an operation the nerves may be compressed, either the brachial plexus by the humerus or the musculo-spiral by the table. The pressure most frequently occurs when the arm is elevated alongside the head, as in laparotomy done in the Trendelenburg position, or held out from the body, as in breast amputations. Instances of paralysis of the crural nerves by leg-holders are also reported. The too firm application of a tourniquet may be followed by a severe paralysis.

(*b*) Paralysis from cerebral lesions during etherization. In one of Garrigues' cases paralysis followed the operation, and at the autopsy, seven weeks later, softening of the brain was found. Apoplexy or embolism may occur during anæsthesia. In Montreal a cataract operation was performed on an old man. He did not recover from the anæsthetic; I found post mortem a cerebral hæmorrhage. A man was admitted to the Philadelphia Hospital, completely comatose, who on the previous day had been given ether for a minor operation. He never recovered consciousness, but remained deeply comatose, with great muscular relaxation, low temperature, 97.5°, and noisy respirations; he died two days later. There was, unfortunately, no autopsy. Epileptic convulsions may occur during the anæsthesia, and may even prove fatal. The possibility has to be considered of paralysis from loss of blood in prolonged operations, though I have no personal knowledge of any such cases.

And, lastly, a paralysis might result from the toxic effects of the ether in a very protracted administration.

Diagnosis.—The electrical condition in multiple neuritis is thus described by Allen Starr: "The excitability is very rapidly and markedly changed; but the conditions which have been observed are quite various. Sometimes there is a simple diminution of excitability, and then a very strong faradic or galvanic current is needed to produce contractions. Frequently all faradic excitability is lost and then the muscles contract to a galvanic current only. In this condition it may require a very strong galvanic current to produce contraction, and thus far it is quite pathognomonic of neuritis. For in anterior polio-myelitis, where the muscles respond to galvanism only, it does not require a strong current to cause a motion until some months after the invasion.

"The action of the different poles is not uniform. In many cases the contraction of the muscle when stimulated with the positive pole is greater than when stimulated with the negative pole, and the contractions may be sluggish. Then the reaction of degeneration is present. But in some cases the normal condition is found and the negative pole produces stronger contractions than the positive pole. A loss of faradic irritability and a marked decrease in the galvanic irritability of the muscle and nerve are therefore important symptoms of multiple neuritis."

There is rarely any difficulty in distinguishing the alcohol cases. The combination of wrist and foot drop with congestion of the hands and feet, and the peculiar delirium already referred to, are quite characteristic. The rapidly advancing cases with paralysis of all extremities, often reaching to the face and involving the sphincters, are more commonly regarded as of spinal origin, but the general opinion seems to point strongly to the fact that all such cases are peripheral. The less acute cases, in which the paralysis gradually involves the legs and arms with rapid wasting, simulate closely and are usually confounded with the subacute atrophic spinal paralysis of Duchenne. The diagnosis from locomotor ataxia is rarely difficult. The *steppage* gait is entirely different from that of tabes. There is rarely positive incoördination. The patient can usually stand well with the eyes closed. Foot-drop is not common in locomotor ataxia. The lightning pains are absent and there are usually no pupillary symptoms. The etiology, too, is of moment. The patient is recovering from a paralysis which has been more extensive, or from arsenical poisoning, or he has diabetes.

Treatment.—Rest in bed is essential. In the acute cases with fever the salicylates and antipyrin are recommended. To allay the intense pain morphia or the hot applications of lead water and laudanum are often required. Great care must be exercised in treating the alcoholic form, and the physician must not allow himself to be deceived by the statements of the relatives. It is sometimes exceedingly difficult to get a history of spirit drinking. In the alcoholic form it is well to reduce the stimulants gradually. If there is any tendency to bed-sores an air-bed should be used or the patient placed in a continuous bath. Gentle friction of the muscles may be applied from the outset, and in the later stages, when the atrophy is marked and the pains have lessened, massage is probably the most reliable means at our command. Contractures may be gradually overcome by passive movements and extension. Often with the most extreme deformity from contracture, recovery is, in time, still possible. The interrupted current is useful when the acute stage is passed.

Of internal remedies, strychnia is of value and may be given in increasing doses. Arsenic also may be employed, and if there is a history of syphilis the iodide of potassium and mercury may be given.

II. NEUROMATA

Tumors situated on nerve fibres may consist of nerve substance proper, the true neuromata, or of fibrous tissue, the false neuromata. The true neuroma usually contains nerve fibres only, or in rare instances ganglion cells. Cases of ganglionic or medullary neuroma are extremely rare; some of them, as Lancereaux suggests, are undoubtedly instances of malformation of the brain substance. In other instances the tumor is, in all probability, a glioma with cells closely resembling those of the central nervous system. The growths are often intermediate in their anatomical structure between the true and the false.

Plexiform Neuroma.—In this remarkable condition the various nerve cords may be occupied by many hundreds of tumors. The cases are often hereditary and usually congenital. The tumors may occur in all the nerves of the body, and, as numbers of them may be made out on palpation, the diagnosis is usually easy. One of the most remarkable cases is that described by Prudden, the specimens of which are in the medical museum of Columbia College, New York. There were over 1,182 distinct tumors distributed on the nerves of the body. These tumors rarely are painful, but may cause symptoms through pressure on neighboring structures.

Generalized Neuro-fibromatosis: von Recklinghausen's Disease.—Special attention was first directed to this particular form of multiple neuroma by von Recklinghausen in 1882. The disease presents four essential features:

(*a*) Soft, fibrous nodules, some sessile, others pedunculated, varying greatly in size and number, are scattered over the surface of the body. These subcutaneous growths at times may be diffuse and reach an enormous size, producing a condition called "Elephantiasis Neuromatosa."

(*b*) Tumors resembling those of plexiform neuroma may be present on any part of the nerve trunks from their central origin to the periphery. Their variable situation may lead to a variety of symptoms, more especially as they may arise from the nerve roots within the spinal canal or cranium. Superficial painful nodules may also be present.

(*c*) Patches of brownish pigmentation of the skin, either as small spots or large areas, are always present. Congenital nævi are a frequent accompaniment of the disease.

(*d*) There are many variable sensory or motor phenomena resulting from the presence of the nerve tumors, but peculiar mental changes, with loss of intellectual power and sometimes difficulty in speaking, are especially characteristic of the disease.

Three generations have been affected. A sarcomatous change has been present in some tumors, and in a few cases associated brain tumors, as gliomata, have been present. The tumors are believed to originate in the sheath of Schwann, in confirmation of which is the interesting point that the optic and olfactory nerves which are devoid of this sheath have never been found affected with neuromatosis.

The prognosis depends on the possibility of successful removal of such tumors as are causing greatest inconvenience.

"Tubercula Dolorosa."—Multiple neuromata may especially affect the terminal cutaneous branches of the sensory nerves and lead to small subcutaneous painful nodules, often found on the face, breast, or about the joints. They may be associated with tumors of the nerve trunks.

"Amputation Neuromata."—These bulbous swellings may form on the central ends of nerves which have been divided in injuries or operations. They are especially common after amputations. They are due to the tangled coil of axis-cylinder processes growing down from the central stump in an effort to reach their former end structures. They are very painful and usually require surgical removal, but often recur.

III. DISEASES OF THE CEREBRAL NERVES

OLFACTORY NERVES AND TRACTS

The functions of the olfactory nerves may be disturbed at their origin, in the nasal mucous membrane, at the bulb, in the course of the tract, or at the centres in the brain. The disturbances may be manifested in subjective sensations of smell, complete loss of the sense, and occasionally in hyperæsthesia.

Subjective Sensations; Parosmia.—Hallucinations of this kind are found in the insane and in epilepsy. The aura may be represented by an unpleasant odor, described as resembling chloride of lime, burning rags, or feathers. In a few cases with these subjective sensations tumors have been found in the hippocampi. In rare instances, after injury of the head, the sense is perverted—odors of the most different character may be alike, or the odor may be changed, as in a patient noted by Morell Mackenzie, who for some time could not touch cooked meat, as it smelt to her exactly like stinking fish.

Increased sensitiveness (hyperosmia) occurs chiefly in nervous, hysterical women, in whom it may sometimes be developed so greatly that, like a dog, they can recognize the difference between individuals by the odor alone.

Anosmia; Loss of the Sense of Smell.—This may be produced by: (*a*) Affections of the origin of the nerves in the mucous membrane, which is perhaps the most frequent cause. It is by no means uncommon in association with chronic nasal catarrh and polypi. In paralysis of the fifth nerve, the sense of smell may be lost on the affected side, owing to interference with the secretion.

It is doubtful whether the cases of loss of smell following the inhalations of very foul or strong odors should come under this or under the central division.

(*b*) Lesions of the bulbs or of the tracts. In falls or blows, in caries of the bones, and in meningitis or tumor, the bulbs or the olfactory tracts may be involved. After an injury to the head the loss of smell may be the only symptom. Mackenzie notes a case of a surgeon who was thrown from his gig and lighted on his head. The injury was slight, but the anosmia which followed was persistent. In locomotor ataxia the sense of smell may be lost, possibly owing to atrophy of the nerves.

(*c*) Lesions of the olfactory centres. There are congenital cases in which the structures have not been developed. Cases have been reported by Beevor, Hughlings Jackson, and others, in which anosmia has been associated with disease in the hemisphere.

To test the sense of smell the pungent bodies, such as ammonia, which act upon the fifth nerve, should not be used, but such substances as cloves, peppermint, and musk. This sense is readily tested as a routine matter in brain cases by having two or three bottles containing the essential oils. In all instances a rhinoscopic examination should be made, as the condition may be due to local, not central causes. The *treatment* is unsatisfactory even in the cases due to local lesions in the nostrils.

OPTIC NERVE AND TRACT

(1) *Lesions of the Retina*

These are of importance to the physician, and information of the greatest value may be obtained by a systematic examination of the eye grounds. Only a brief reference can here be made to the more important of the appearances.

Retinitis.—This occurs in certain general affections, more particularly in Bright's disease, syphilis, leukæmia, and anæmia. The common feature in all these states is the occurrence of hæmorrhage and the development of opacities. There may also be a diffuse cloudiness due to effusion of serum. The hæmorrhages are in the layer of nerve fibres. They vary greatly in size and form, but often follow the course of vessels. When recent the color is bright red, but they gradually change and old hæmorrhages are almost black. The white spots are due either to fibrinous exudate or to fatty degeneration of the retinal elements, and occasionally to accumulation of leucocytes or to a localized sclerosis of the retinal elements. The more important of the forms of retinitis to be recognized are:

ALBUMINURIC RETINITIS, which occurs in chronic nephritis, particularly in the interstitial or contracted form. The percentage of cases affected is from 15 to 25. There are instances in which these retinal changes are associated with the granular kidney at a stage when the amount of albumin may be slight or transient; but in all such instances it will be found that there is a marked arterio-sclerosis. Gowers recognizes a degenerative form (most common), in which, with the retinal changes, there may be scarcely any alteration in the disk; a hæmorrhagic form, with many hæmorrhages and but slight signs of inflammation; and an inflammatory form, in which there is much swelling of the retina and obscuration of the disk. It is noteworthy that in some instances the inflammation of the optic nerve predominates over the retinal changes, and one may be in doubt for a time whether the condition is really associated with the renal changes or dependent upon intracranial disease.

SYPHILITIC RETINITIS.—In the acquired form this is less common than choroiditis. In inherited syphilis *retinitis pigmentosa* is sometimes met with.

RETINITIS IN ANÆMIA.—It has long been known that a patient may become blind after a large hæmorrhage, either suddenly or within two or three days, and in one or both eyes. Occasionally the loss may be permanent and complete. In some of these instances a neuro-retinitis has been found, probably sufficient to account for the symptoms. In the more chronic anæmias, particularly in the pernicious form, retinitis is common, as determined first by Quincke.

In MALARIA retinitis or neuro-retinitis may be present, as noted by Stephen Mackenzie. It is seen only in the chronic cases with anæmia, and in my experience is not nearly so common proportionately as in pernicious anæmia.

LEUKÆMIC RETINITIS.—In this affection the retinal veins are large and distended; there is also a peculiar retinitis, as described by Liebreich. It is not very common. There are numerous hæmorrhages and white or yellow areas, which may be large and prominent. In one of my cases the retina post mortem was dotted with many small, opaque, white spots, looking like little tumors, the larger of which had a diameter of nearly 2 mm.

Retinitis is also found occasionally in diabetes, in purpura, in chronic lead poisoning, and sometimes as an idiopathic affection.

Functional Disturbances of Vision.—(*a*) Toxic Amaurosis.—This occurs in uræmia and may follow convulsions or come on independently. The condition, as a rule, persists only for a day or two. This form of amaurosis occurs in poisoning by lead, alcohol, and occasionally by quinine. It seems more probable that the poisons act on the centres and not on the retina.

(*b*) Tobacco Amblyopia.—The loss of sight is usually gradual, equal in both eyes, and affects particularly the centre of the field of vision. The eye-grounds may be normal, but occasionally there is congestion of the disks. On testing the color fields a central scotoma for red and green is found in all cases. Ultimately, if the use of tobacco is continued, organic changes may develop with atrophy of the disk.

(*c*) Hysterical Amaurosis.—More frequently this is loss of acuteness of vision—amblyopia—but the loss of sight in one or both eyes may apparently be complete. The condition will be mentioned subsequently under hysteria.

(*d*) Night-blindness—nyctalopia—the condition in which objects are clearly seen during the day or by strong artificial light, but become invisible in the shade or in twilight, and *hemeralopia,* in which objects can not be clearly seen without distress in daylight or in a strong artificial light, but are readily seen in a deep shade or in twilight, are functional anomalies of vision which rarely come under the notice of the physician. It may occur in epidemic form.

(*e*) Retinal hyperæsthesia is sometimes seen in hysterical women, but is not found frequently in actual retinitis. I have seen it once, however, in albuminuric retinitis, and once, in a marked degree, in a patient with aortic insufficiency, in whose retinæ there were no signs other than the throbbing arteries.

(2) *Lesions of the Optic Nerve*

Optic Neuritis (*Papillitis; Choked Disk*).—In the first stage there is congestion of the disk and the edges are blurred and striated. In the second stage the congestion is more marked; the swelling increases, the striation also is more visible. The physiological cupping disappears and hæmorrhages are not uncommon. The arteries present little change, the veins are dilated, and the disk may swell greatly. In slight grades of inflammation the swelling gradually subsides and occasionally the nerve recovers completely. In instances in which the swelling and exudate are very great the subsidence is slow, and when it finally disappears there is complete atrophy of the nerve. The retina not infrequently participates in the inflammation, which is then a neuro-retinitis.

This condition is of the greatest importance in diagnosis. It may exist in its early stages without any disturbance of vision, and even with extensive papillitis the sight may for a time be good.

Optic neuritis is seen occasionally in anæmia and lead poisoning, more commonly in Bright's disease as neuro-retinitis. It occurs occasionally as a primary idiopathic affection. The frequent connection with intracranial disease, particularly tumor, makes its presence of great value to practitioners. The nature of the growth is without influence. In over 90 per cent. of such instances the papillitis is bilateral. It is also found in meningitis, either the tuberculous or the simple form. In meningitis it is easy to see how the inflammation may extend down the nerve sheath. In the case of tumor, however, it is probable that mechanical conditions, especially the venous stasis, are alone responsible for the œdematous swelling. It often subsides very rapidly after a palliative craniectomy has been performed.

Optic Atrophy.—This may be: (*a*) A primary affection. There is an hereditary form, in which the disease has developed in all the males of a family shortly after puberty. A large number of the cases of primary atrophy are associated with spinal disease, particularly locomotor ataxia. Other causes which have been assigned for the primary atrophy are cold, sexual excesses, diabetes, the specific fevers, methyl alcohol, and lead.

(*b*) Secondary atrophy results from cerebral diseases, pressure on the chiasma or on the nerves, or, most commonly of all, as a sequence of papillitis.

The ophthalmoscopic appearances are different in the cases of primary and secondary atrophy. In the former the disk has a gray tint, the edges are well defined, and the arteries look almost normal; whereas in the consecutive atrophy the disk has a staring opaque white aspect, with irregular outlines, and the arteries are very small.

The symptom of optic atrophy is loss of sight, proportionate to the damage in the nerve. The change is in three directions: "(1) Diminished acuity of vision; (2) alteration in the field of vision; and (3) altered perception of color" (Gowers). The outlook in primary atrophy is bad.

(3) *Affections of the Chiasma and Tract.*

At the chiasma the optic nerves undergo partial decussation. Each optic tract, as it leaves the chiasma, contains nerve fibres which originate in the retinæ of both eyes. Thus, of the fibres of the right tract, part have come through the chiasma without decussating from the temporal half of the right retina, the other and larger portion of the fibres of the tract have decussated in the chiasma, coming as they do from the left optic nerve and the nasal half of the retina on the left side. The fibres which cross are in the middle portion of the chiasma, while the direct fibres are on each side. The following are the most important changes which ensue in lesions of the tract and of the chiasma:

Unilateral Affection of Tract.—If on the right side, this produces loss of function in the temporal half of the retina on the right side, and in the nasal half of the retina on the left side, so that there is only half vision, and the patient is blind to objects on the left side. This is termed homonymous hemianopia or lateral hemianopia. The fibres passing to the right half of each retina being involved, the patient is blind to objects in the left half of each visual field. The hemianopia may be partial and only a portion of the half field may be lost. The unaffected visual fields may have the normal extent, but in some instances there is considerable reduction. When the left half of one field and the right half of the other, or *vice versa*, are blind, the condition is known as heteronymous hemianopia.

Disease of the Chiasma.—(*a*) A lesion involves, as a rule, chiefly the central portion, in which the decussating fibres pass which supply the inner or nasal halves of the retinæ, producing in consequence loss of vision in the outer half of each field, or what is known as temporal hemianopia.

(*b*) If the lesion is more extensive it may involve not only the central portion, but also the direct fibres on one side of the commissure, in which case there would be total blindness in one eye and temporal hemianopia in the other.

(*c*) Still more extensive disease is not infrequent from pressure of tumors in this region, the whole chiasma is involved, and total blindness results. The different stages in the process may often be traced in a single case from temporal hemianopia, then complete blindness in one eye with temporal hemianopia in the other, and finally complete blindness.

(*d*) A limited lesion of the outer part of the chiasma involves only the direct fibres passing to the temporal halves of the retinæ and inducing blindness in the nasal field, or, as it is called, nasal hemianopia. This, of course, is extremely rare. Double nasal hemianopia may occur as a manifestation of tabes and in tumors involving the outer fibres of each tract.

(4) *Affections of the Tract and Centres*

The optic tract crosses the crus (cerebral peduncle) to the hinder part of the optic thalamus and divides into two portions, one of which (the lateral root) goes to the pulvinar of the thalamus, the lateral geniculate body, and to the anterior quadrigeminal body (superior colliculus). From these parts, in which the lateral root terminates, fibres pass into the posterior part of the internal capsule and enter the occipital lobe, forming the fibres of the optic radiation, which terminate in and about the cuneus, the region of the visual perceptive centre. The fibres of the medial division of the tract pass to the medial geniculate body and to the posterior quadrigeminal body. The medial root contains the fibres of the commissura inferior of v. Gudden, which are believed to have no connection with the retinæ. It is still held by some physiologists that the cortical visual centre is not confined to the occipital lobe alone, but embraces the occipito-angular region.

A lesion of the fibres of the optic path anywhere between the cortical centre and the chiasma will produce hemianopia. The lesion may be situated: (*a*) In the optic tract itself. (*b*) In the region of the thalamus, lateral geniculate body, and the corpora quadrigemina, into which the larger part of each tract enters. (*c*) A lesion of the fibres passing from the centres just mentioned to the occipital lobe. This may be either in the hinder part of the internal capsule or the white fibres of the optic radiation. (*d*) Lesion of the cuneus. Bilateral disease of the cuneus may result in total blindness. (*e*) There is clinical evidence to show that lesion of the angular gyrus may be associated with visual defect, not so often hemianopia as crossed amblyopia, dimness of vision in the opposite eye, and great contraction in the field of vision. Lesions in this region are associated with mind-blindness, a condition in which there is failure to recognize the nature of objects.

The effects of lesions in the optic nerve in different situations from the retinal expansion to the brain cortex are as follows: (1) Of the optic nerve—total blindness of the corresponding eye; (2) of the optic chiasma, either temporal hemianopia, if the central part alone is involved, or nasal hemianopia, if the lateral region of each chiasma is involved; (3) lesion of the optic tract between the chiasma and the lateral geniculate body produces lateral hemianopia; (4) lesion of the central fibres of the nerve between the geniculate

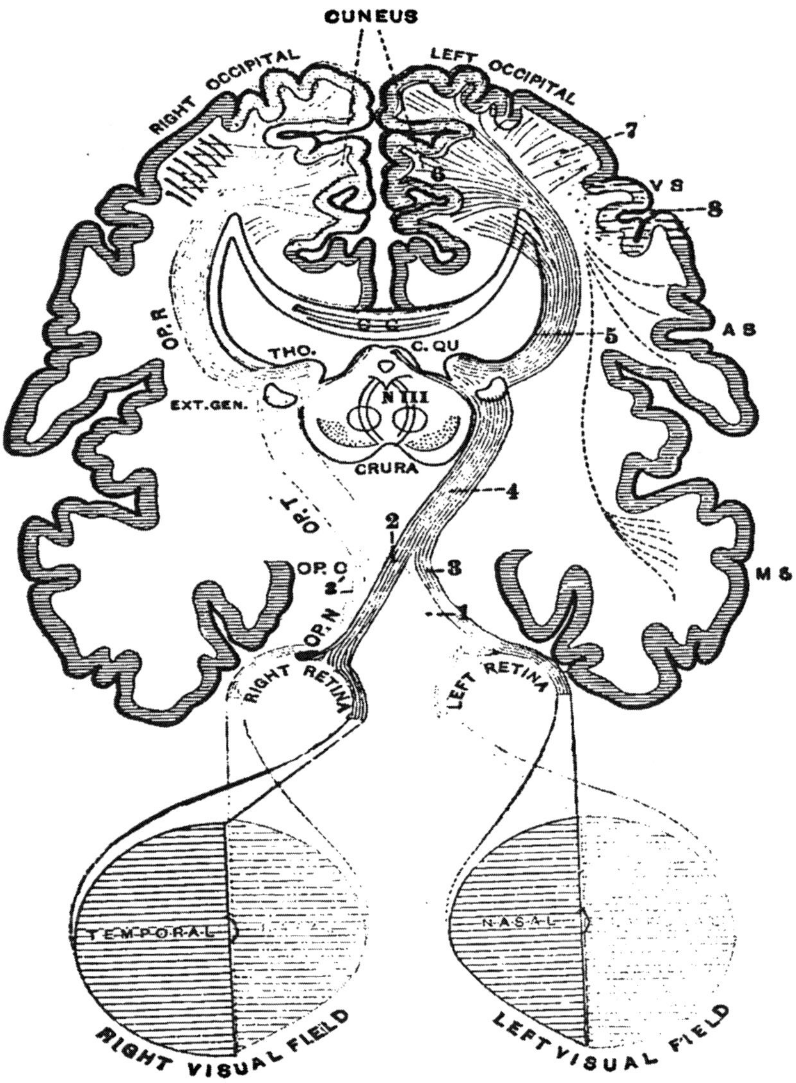

Fig. 19.—Diagram of Visual Paths. (From Vialet, modified.) OP. N., Optic nerve. OP. C., Optic chiasm. OP. T., Optic tract. OP. R., Optic radiations. EXT. GEN., External geniculate body. THO., Optic thalamus. C. QU., Corpera quadrigemina. C. C., Corpus callosum. V. S., Visual speech centre. A. S., Auditory speech centre. M. S., Motor speech centre. A lesion at 1 causes blindness of that eye; at 2, bi-temporal hemianopia; at 3, nasal hemianopia. Symmtrical lesions at 3 and 3′ would cause bi-nasal hemianopia; at 4, hemianopia of both eyes, with hemianopic pupillary inaction; at 5 and 6, hemianopia of both eyes, pupillary reflexes normal; at 7, amblyopia, especially of opposite eye; at 8, on left side, word-blindness.

bodies and the cerebral cortex produces lateral hemianopia; (5) lesion of the cuneus causes lateral hemianopia; and (6) lesion of the angular gyrus may be associated with hemianopia, sometimes crossed amblyopia, and the condition known as mind-blindness. (See Fig. 19, with accompanying explanation.)

Diagnosis of Lesions of the Optic Nerve and Tract.—Having determined the presence of hemianopia, the question arises as to the situation of the lesion, whether in the tract between the chiasma and the geniculate bodies or in the central portion of the fibres between these bodies and the visual centres. This can be determined in some cases by the test known as Wernicke's *hemiopic pupillary inaction.* The pupil reflex depends on the integrity of the retina or receiving membrane, on the fibres of the optic nerve and tract which transmit the impulse, and the nerve-centre at the termination of the optic tract which receives the impression and transmits it to the third nerve along which the motor impulses pass to the iris. If a bright light is thrown into the eye and the pupil reacts, the integrity of this reflex arc is demonstrated. It is possible in cases of lateral hemianopia so to throw the light into the eye that it falls upon the blind half of the retina. If when this is done the pupil contracts, the indication is that the reflex arc above referred to is perfect, by which we mean that the optic nerve fibres from the retinal expansion to the centre, the centre itself, and the third nerve are uninvolved. In such a case the conclusion would be justified that the cause of the hemianopia was central; that is, situated beyond the geniculate body, either in the fibres of the optic radiation or in the visual cortical centres. If, on the other hand, when the light is carefully thrown on the hemiopic half of the retina the pupil remains inactive, the conclusion is justifiable that there is interruption in the path between the retina and the nucleus of the third nerve, and that the hemianopia is not central, but dependent upon a lesion situated in the optic tract. This test of Wernicke's is sometimes difficult to obtain. It is best performed as follows: "The patient being in a dark or nearly dark room with the lamp or gas-light behind his head in the usual position, I bid him look over to the other side of the room, so as to exclude accommodative iris movements (which are not necessarily associated with the reflex). Then I throw a faint light from a plane mirror or from a large concave mirror, held well out of focus, upon the eye and note the size of the pupil. With my other hand I now throw a beam of light, focussed from the lamp by an ophthalmoscopic mirror, directly into the optical centre of the eye; then laterally in various positions, and also from above and below the equator of the eye, noting the reaction at all angles of incidence of the ray of light" (Seguin).

The significance of hemianopia varies. There is a functional hemianopia associated with migraine and hysteria. In a considerable proportion of all cases there are signs of organic brain disease. In a certain number of instances of slight lesions of the occipital lobe hemichromatopsia has been observed. The homonymous halves of the retina as far as the fixation point are dulled, or blind for colors. Hemiplegia is common, in which event the loss of power and blindness are on the same side. Thus, a lesion in the left hemisphere involving the motor tract produces right hemiplegia, and when the fibres of the optic radiation are involved in the internal capsule there is also lateral hemianopia, so that objects in the field of vision to the right are not perceived. Hemianæsthesia is not uncommon in such cases, owing to the close association of the sensory and visual tracts at the posterior part of the internal capsule. Certain forms of aphasia also occur in many of the cases.

The optic aphasia of Freund may be mentioned here. The patient, after an apoplectic attack, though able to recognize ordinary objects shown to him, is unable to name them correctly. If he be permitted to touch the object he may be able to name it quickly and correctly. Freund's optic aphasia differs from mind-blindness, since in the latter affection the objects seen are not recognized. Optic aphasia, like word-blindness, never occurs alone, but is always associated with hemianopia, or mind-blindness, and often also with word-deafness. In the cases which have thus far come to autopsy there has always been a lesion in the white matter of the occipital lobe on the left side.

MOTOR NERVES OF THE EYEBALL

Third Nerve (*Nervus oculomotorius*).—The nucleus of origin of this nerve is situated in the floor of the aqueduct of Sylvius; the nerve passes through the crus at the side of which it emerges. Passing along the wall of the cavernous sinus, it enters the orbit through the sphenoidal fissure and supplies, by its superior branch, the levator palpebræ superioris and the superior rectus, and by its inferior branch the internal and inferior recti muscles and the inferior oblique. Branches pass to the ciliary muscle and the constrictor of the iris. Lesions may affect the nucleus or the nerve in its course and cause either paralysis or spasm.

PARALYSIS.—A nuclear lesion is usually associated with disease of the centres for the other eye muscles, producing a condition of general ophthalmoplegia. More commonly the nerve itself is involved in its course, either by meningitis, gummata, or aneurism, or is attacked by a neuritis, as in diphtheria and locomotor ataxia. Complete paralysis of the third nerve is accompanied by the following symptoms:

Paralysis of all the muscles, except the superior oblique and external rectus, by which the eye can be moved outward and a little downward and inward. There is divergent strabismus. There is ptosis or drooping of the upper eyelid, owing to paralysis of the levator palpebræ. The pupil is usually dilated. It does not contract to light, and the power of accommodation is lost. The most striking features of this paralysis are the external strabismus, with diplopia or double vision, and the ptosis. In very many cases the affection of the third nerve is partial. Thus the levator palpebræ and the superior rectus may be involved together, or the ciliary muscles and the iris may be affected and the external muscles may escape.

There is a remarkable form of recurring oculo-motor paralysis affecting chiefly women, and involving all the branches of the nerve. In some cases the attacks have come on at intervals of a month; in others a much longer period has elapsed. The attacks may persist throughout life. They are sometimes associated with pain in the head and sometimes with migraine. Mary Sherwood has collected from the literature 23 cases.

PTOSIS is a common and important symptom in nervous affections. We may here briefly refer to the conditions under which it may occur: (*a*) A congenital, incurable form, which is frequently seen; (*b*) the form associated with definite lesion of the third nerve, either in its course or at its nucleus. This may come on with paralysis of the superior rectus alone or with paralysis of the internal and inferior recti as well. (*c*) There are instances of complete or partial ptosis associated with cerebral lesions without any other branch of the third nerve being paralyzed. The exact position of the cortical centre or centres is as yet unknown. (*d*) Hysterical ptosis, which is double and occurs with other hysterical symptoms. (*e*) Pseudo-ptosis, due to affection of the sympathetic nerve, is associated with symptoms of vaso-motor palsy, such as elevation of the temperature on the affected side with redness and œdema of the skin. Contraction of the pupil exists on the same side and the eyeball appears rather to have shrunk into the orbit. (*f*) In idiopathic muscular atrophy, when the face muscles are involved, there may be marked bilateral ptosis. And, lastly, in weak, delicate women there is often to be seen a transient ptosis, particularly in the morning.

Among the most important of the symptoms of the third-nerve paralysis are those which relate to the ciliary muscle and iris.

Cycloplegia, paralysis of the ciliary muscle, causes loss of the power of accommodation. Distant vision is clear, but near objects can not be properly seen. In consequence the vision is indistinct, but can be restored by the use of convex glasses. This may occur in one or in both eyes; in the latter case it is usually associated with disease in the nuclei of the nerve. Cycloplegia is an early and frequent symptom in diphtheritic paralysis and occurs also in tabes.

Iridoplegia, or paralysis of the iris, occurs in three forms (Gowers):

(*a*) *Accommodation iridoplegia,* in which the pupil does not diminish in size during the act of accommodation. To test for this the patient should look first at a distant and then at a near object in the same line of vision.

(*b*) *Reflex Iridoplegia.*—The path for the iris reflex is along the optic nerve and tract to its termination, then to the nucleus of the third nerve, and along the trunk of this nerve to the ciliary ganglion, and so through the ciliary nerves to the eyes. Each eye should be tested separately, the other one being covered. The patient should look at a distant object in a dark part of the room; then a light is brought suddenly in front of the eye at a distance of three or four feet, so as to avoid the effect of accommodation. Loss of this iris reflex with retention of the accommodation contraction is known as the Argyll-Robertson pupil.

(*c*) *Loss of the Skin Reflex.*—If the skin of the neck is pinched or pricked the pupil dilates reflexly, the afferent impulses being conveyed along the cervical sympathetic. Erb pointed out that this skin reflex is lost usually in association with the reflex contraction, but the two are not necessarily conjoined. In iridoplegia the pupils are often small, particularly in spinal disease, as in the characteristic small pupils of tabes—spinal myosis. Iridoplegia may coexist with a pupil of medium size.

Inequality of the pupils—anisocoria—is not infrequent in progressive paresis and in tabes. It may also occur in perfectly healthy individuals.

Spasm.—Occasionally in meningitis and in hysteria there is spasm of the muscles supplied by the third nerve, particularly the internal rectus and the levator palpebræ. The clonic rhythmical spasm of the eye muscles is known as *nystagmus,* in which there is usually a bilateral, rhythmical, involuntary movement of the eyeballs. The condition is met with in many congenital and acquired brain lesions, in albinism, and sometimes in coal miners.

Fourth Nerve (*Nervus trochlearis*).—This supplies the superior oblique muscle. In its course around the outer surface of the crus and in its passage into the orbit it is liable to be compressed by tumors, by aneurism, or in the exudation of basilar meningitis. Its nucleus in the upper part of the fourth ventricle may be involved by tumors or undergo degeneration with the other ocular nuclei. The superior oblique muscle acts in such a way as to direct the eyeball downward and rotate it slightly. The paralysis causes defective downward and inward movement, often too slight to be noticed. The head is inclined somewhat forward and toward the sound side, and there is double vision when the patient looks down.

Sixth Nerve (*Nervus abducens*).—This nerve emerges at the junction of the pons and medulla, then, passing forward, it enters the orbit and supplies the external rectus muscle. Owing to its long course and exposed position it is more commonly injured than any other cranial nerve. It is affected by meningitis at the base, by gummata or other tumors, and sometimes by cold. There is internal strabismus, and the eye can not be turned outward. Diplopia occurs on looking toward the paralyzed side.

"When the nucleus is affected there is, in addition to paralysis of the external rectus, inability of the internal rectus of the opposite eye to turn that eye inward. As a consequence of this the axes of the eyes are kept parallel, and both are conjugately deviated to the opposite side, away from the side of lesion. The reason of this is that the nucleus of the sixth nerve sends fibres up in the pons to that part of the nucleus of the opposite third nerve which supplies the internal rectus. We thus have paralysis of the internal rectus without the nucleus of the third nerve being involved, owing to its receiving its nervous impulses for parallel movement from the sixth nucleus of the opposite side. As the sixth nucleus is in such proximity to the facial nerve in the substance of the pons, it is frequently found that the whole of the face on the same side is paralyzed, and gives the electrical reaction of degeneration, so that with a lesion of the *left* sixth nucleus there is conjugate deviation of both eyes to the *right*—i. e., paralysis of the left external and the right internal rectus, and sometimes complete paralysis of the *left* side of the face" (Beevor).

General Features of Paralysis of the Motor Nerves of the Eye.—Gowers divides them into five groups:

(*a*) *Limitation of Movement.*—Thus, in paralysis of the external rectus, the eyeball can not be moved outward. When the paralysis is incomplete the movement is deficient in proportion to the degree of the palsy.

(*b*) *Strabismus.*—The axes of the eyes do not correspond. Thus, paralysis of the internal rectus causes a divergent squint; of the external rectus, a convergent squint. At first this is evident only when the eyes are moved in the direction of the action of the weak muscle, but may become constant by the contraction of the opposing muscle. The deviation of the axis of the affected eye from parallelism with the other is called the primary deviation.

(*c*) *Secondary Deviation.*—If, while the patient is looking at an object, the sound eye is covered, so that he fixes the object looked at with the affected eye only, the sound eye is moved still further in the same direction—e. g., outward, when there is paralysis of the opposite internal rectus. This is known as secondary deviation. It depends upon the fact that, if two muscles are acting together, when one is weak and an effort is made to contract it, the increased effort—innervation—acts powerfully upon the other muscle, causing an increased contraction.

(*d*) *Erroneous Projection.*—"We judge of the relation of external objects to each other by the relation of their images on the retina; but we judge of their relation to our own body by the position of the eyeball as indicated to us by the innervation we give to the ocular muscles" (Gowers). With the eyes at rest in the mid-position, an object at which we are looking is directly opposite our face. Turning the eyes to one side, we recognize that object in the middle of the field or to the side of this former position. We estimate the degree by the amount of movement of the eyes, and when the object moves and we follow it we judge of its position by the amount of movement of the eyeballs. When one ocular muscle is weak the increased innervation gives the impression of a greater movement of the eye than has really taken place. The mind, at the same time, receives the idea that the object is further on one side than it really is, and in an attempt to touch it the finger may go beyond it. As the equilibrium of the body is in a large part maintained by a knowledge of the relation of external objects to it obtained by the action of the eye muscles, this erroneous projection resulting from paralysis disturbs the harmony of these visual impressions and may lead to giddiness—ocular vertigo.

(*e*) *Double Vision.*—This is one of the most disturbing features of paralysis of the eye muscles. The visual axes do not correspond, so that there is a double image—diplopia. That seen by the sound eye is termed the true image; that by the paralyzed eye, the false. In simple or homonymous diplopia the false image is "on the same side of the other as the eye by which it is seen." In crossed diplopia it is on the other side. In convergent squint the diplopia is simple; in divergent it is crossed.

Ophthalmoplegia.—Under this term is described a chronic progressive paralysis of the ocular muscles. Two forms are recognized—ophthalmoplegia *externa* and ophthalmoplegia *interna.* The conditions may occur separately or together and are described by Gowers under nuclear ocular palsy.

Ophthalmoplegia externa.—The condition is one of more or less complete palsy of the external muscles of the eyeball, due usually to a slow degeneration in the nuclei of the nerves, but sometimes to pressure of tumors or to basilar meningitis. It is often, but not necessarily, associated with ophthalmoplegia interna. Of 62 cases analyzed by Siemerling in only 11 could syphilis be positively determined. The levator muscles of the eyelids and the superior recti are first involved, and gradually the other muscles, so that the eyeballs are fixed and the eyelids droop. There is sometimes slight protrusion of the eyeballs. The disease is essentially chronic and may last for many years. It is found particularly in association with general paralysis, locomotor ataxia, and in progressive muscular atrophy. Mental disorders were present in 11 of the 62 cases. With it may be associated atrophy of the optic nerve and affections of other cerebral nerves. Occasionally, as noted by Bristowe, it may be functional.

Ophthalmoplegia interna.—Jonathan Hutchinson applied this term to a progressive paralysis of the internal ocular muscles, causing loss of pupillary action and the power of accommodation. When the internal and external muscles are involved the affection is known as total ophthalmoplegia, and in a majority of the cases the two conditions are associated. In some instances the internal form may depend upon disease of the ciliary ganglion.

While, as a rule, ophthalmoplegia is a chronic process, there is an acute form associated with hæmorrhagic softening of the nuclei of the ocular muscles. There is usually marked cerebral disturbance. It was to this form that Wernicke gave the name poliencephalitis superior.

Treatment of Ocular Palsies.—It is important to ascertain, if possible, the cause. The forms associated with locomotor ataxia are obstinate, and resist treatment. Occasionally, however, a palsy, complete or partial, may pass away spontaneously. The group of cases associated with chronic degenerative changes, as in progressive paresis and bulbar paralysis, is little affected by treatment. On the other hand, in syphilitic cases, mercury and iodide of potassium are indicated and are often beneficial. Arsenic and strychnia, the latter hypodermically, may be employed. In any case in which the onset is acute, with pain, hot fomentations and counter-irritation or leeches applied to the temple give relief. The direct treatment by electricity has been extensively employed, but probably without any special effect. The diplopia may be relieved by the use of prisms, or it may be necessary to cover the affected eye with an opaque glass.

FIFTH NERVE

(*Nervus trigeminus*)

Etiology.—Paralysis may result from: (*a*) Disease of the pons, particularly hæmorrhage or patches of sclerosis. (*b*) Injury or disease at the base of the brain. Fracture rarely involves the nerve; on the other hand, meningitis, acute or chronic, and caries of the bone are not uncommon causes. (*c*) The branches may be affected as they pass out—the first division by tumors pressing on the cavernous sinus or by aneurism; the second and third divisions by growths which invade the spheno-maxillary fossa. (*d*) Primary neuritis, which is rare.

Symptoms.—(*a*) Sensory Portion.—Disease of the fifth nerve may cause loss of sensation in the parts supplied, including the half of the face, the corresponding side of the head, the conjunctiva, the mucosa of the lips, tongue, hard and soft palate, and of the nose of the same side. The anæsthesia may be preceded by tingling or pain. The muscles of the face are also insensible and the movements may be slower. The sense of smell is interfered with, owing to dryness of the mucous membrane. There may be disturbance of the sense of taste. The salivary, lachrymal, and buccal secretions may be lessened, and the teeth may become loose. Unless properly guarded from injury an ulcerative inflammation of the eye may follow. This was formerly supposed to be due to nutritional changes from paralysis of so-called trophic nerve fibres. This idea has of late years been overthrown by the large number of cases in which the Gasserian ganglion has been removed for obstinate neuralgia without consequent inflammation of the eye. Herpes may occur in the region supplied by the nerve, usually the upper branch, and is associated with much pain, which may be peculiarly enduring, lasting for months or years (Gowers). In herpes zoster with the neuritis there may be slight enlargement of the cervical glands. (See under Neuralgia for Tic Douloureux.)

(*b*) Motor Portion.—The inability to use the muscles of mastication on the affected side is the distinguishing feature of paralysis of this portion of the nerve. It is recognized by placing the finger on the masseter and temporal muscles, and, when the patient closes the jaw, the feebleness of their contraction is noted. If paralyzed, the external pterygoid can not move the jaw toward the unaffected side; and when depressed, the jaw deviates to the paralyzed side. The motor paralysis of the fifth nerve is almost invariably a result of involvement of the nerve after it has left the nucleus. Cases, however, have been associated with cortical lesions. The cortical motor centre for the trigeminus, or for movements effecting closure of the jaw, lies below that for movements of the face at the lower part of the anterior central convolution.

Spasm of the Muscles of Mastication.—Trismus, the masticatory spasm of Romberg, may be tonic or clonic, and is either an associated phenomenon in general convulsions or, more rarely, an independent affection. In the tonic form the jaws are kept close together—lock-jaw—or can be separated only for a short space. The muscles of mastication can be seen in contraction and felt to be hard; the spasm is often painful. This tonic contraction is an early symptom in tetanus, and is sometimes seen in tetany. A form of this tonic spasm occurs in hysteria. Occasionally trismus follows exposure to cold, and is said to be due to reflex irritation from the teeth, the mouth, or caries of the jaw. It may also be a symptom of organic disease due to irritation near the motor nucleus of the fifth nerve.

Clonic spasm of the muscles supplied by the fifth occurs in the form of rapidly repeated contractions, as in "chattering teeth." This is rare apart from general conditions, though cases are on record, usually in women late in life, in whom this isolated clonic spasm of the muscles of the jaw has been found. In another form of clonic spasm sometimes seen in chorea there are forcible single contractions. Gowers mentions an instance of its occurrence as an isolated affection.

(*c*) Gustatory.—Complete or partial loss of the sense of taste over the anterior two-thirds of the tongue has been supposed by some to follow paralysis of the fifth nerve. There are two views concerning the course of the fibres that carry gustatory impulse from this part of the tongue. According to some they take a devious path, passing with the chorda tympani to the geniculate ganglion, thence by the great superficial petrosal nerve to Meckel's ganglion, and this they leave to reach the maxillary nerve, which they follow through the trigeminal nerve to the brain. A study of clinical cases of disease of the fifth nerve has led to this view. It seems more probable, however, from the fact that a large number of the trigeminal neurectomies are not followed by loss of taste, that the fibres pass to the brain directly from the geniculate ganglion by the nervus intermedius of Wrisberg. Possibly there may be more than one course for these fibres.

The *diagnosis* of disease of the trifacial nerve is rarely difficult. It must be remembered that the preliminary pain and hyperæsthesia are sometimes mistaken for ordinary neuralgia. The loss of sensation and the palsy of the muscles of mastication are readily determined.

Treatment.—When the pain is severe morphia may be required and local applications are useful. If there is a suspicion of syphilis, appropriate treatment should be given. Faradization is sometimes beneficial.

FACIAL NERVE

Paralysis (*Bell's Palsy*).—ETIOLOGY.—The facial or seventh may be paralyzed by (*a*) lesions of the cortex—supranuclear palsy; (*b*) lesions of the nucleus itself; or (*c*) involvement of the nerve trunk in its tortuous course within the pons and through the wall of the skull.

(*a*) *Supranuclear paralysis,* due to lesion of the cortex or of the facial fibres in the corona radiata or internal capsule, is, as a rule, associated with hemiplegia. It may be caused by tumors, abscess, chronic inflammation, or softening in the cortex or in the region of the internal capsule. It is distinguished from the peripheral form by well marked characters—the persistence of the normal electrical excitability of both nerves and muscles and the frequent absence of involvement of the upper branches of the nerve, so that the orbicularis palpebrarum, frontalis, and corrugator muscles are spared. In rare instances these muscles are paralyzed. In this form the voluntary movements are more impaired than the emotional. Isolated paralysis—monoplegia facialis—due to involvement of the cortex or of the fibres in their path to the nucleus, is uncommon. In the great majority of cases supranuclear facial paralysis is part of a hemiplegia. Paralysis is on the same side as that of the arm and leg because the facial muscles bear precisely the same relation to the cortex as the spinal muscles. The nuclei of origin on either side of the middle line in the medulla are united by decussating fibres with the cortical centre on the opposite side (see Fig. 18). A few fibres reach the nucleus from the cerebral cortex of the same side, and this uncrossed path may innervate the upper facial muscles.

(*b*) The *nuclear paralysis* caused by lesions of the nerve centres in the medulla is not common alone; but is seen occasionally in tumors, chronic softening, and hæmorrhage. It may be involved in anterior polio-myelitis. In diphtheria this centre may also be attacked. The symptoms are practically similar to those of an affection of the nerve fibre itself—infranuclear paralysis.

(*c*) *Involvement of the Nerve Trunk.*—Paralysis may result from:

(1) Involvement of the nerve as it passes through the pons—that is, between its nucleus in the floor of the fourth ventricle and the point of emergence in the postero-lateral aspect of the pons. The specially interesting feature in connection with involvement of this part is the production of what is called alternating or *crossed paralysis,* the face being involved on the same side as the lesion, and the arm and leg on the opposite side, since the motor path is involved above the point of decussation in the medulla (Fig. 18). This occurs only when the lesion is in the lower section of the pons. A lesion in the upper half of the pons involves the fibres not of the outgoing nerve on the same side, but of the fibres from the hemispheres before they have crossed to the nucleus of the opposite side. In this case there would of course be, as in hemiplegia, paralysis of the face and limbs on the side opposite to the lesion. The palsy, too, would resemble the cerebral form, involving only the lower fibres of the facial nerve.

(2) The nerve may be involved at its point of emergence by tumors, particularly by the cerebello-pontine growths, by gummata, meningitis, or occasionally it may be injured in fracture of the base.

(3) In passing through the Fallopian canal the nerve may be involved in disease of the ear, particularly by caries of the bone in otitis media. This is a common cause in children. I have seen two instances follow otitis in puerperal fever.

(4) As the nerve emerges from the styloid foramen it is exposed to injuries and blows which not infrequently cause paralysis. The fibres may be cut in the removal of tumors in this region, or the paralysis may be caused by pressure of the forceps in an instrumental delivery.

(5) Exposure to cold is the most common cause of facial paralysis (Bell's palsy), inducing a neuritis of the nerve within the Fallopian canal. Reik believes that in most of these cases there is an acute otitis media from which the nerve is involved.

(6) Syphilis is not an infrequent cause, and the paralysis may appear early with the secondary symptoms.

(7) It may occur in association with herpes.

Facial diplegia is a rare condition occasionally found in affections at the base of the brain, lesions in the pons, simultaneous involvement of the nerves in ear-disease, and in diphtheritic paralysis. Disease of the nuclei or symmetrical involvement of the cortex might also produce it. It may occur as a congenital affection. H. M. Thomas has described two cases in one family.

Symptoms.—In the peripheral facial paralysis all the branches of the nerve are involved. The face on the affected side is immobile and can neither be moved at will nor participate in any emotional movements. The skin is smooth and the wrinkles are effaced, a point particularly noticeable on the forehead of elderly persons. The eye can not be closed, the lower lid droops, and the eye waters. On the affected side the angle of the mouth is lowered, and in drinking the lips are not kept in close apposition to the glass, so that the liquid is apt to run out. In smiling or laughing the contrast is most striking, as the affected side does not move, which gives a curious unequal appearance to the two sides of the face. The eye can not be closed nor can the forehead be wrinkled. In long standing cases, when the reaction of degeneration is present, if the patient tries to close the eyes while looking fixedly at an object the lids on the sound side close firmly, but on the paralyzed side there is only a slight inhibitory droop of the upper lid, and the eye is turned upward and outward by the inferior oblique. On asking the patient to show his upper teeth, the angle of the mouth is not raised. In all these movements the face is drawn to the sound side by the action of the muscles. Speaking may be slightly interfered with, owing to the imperfection in the formation of the labial sounds. Whistling can not be performed. In chewing the food, owing to the paralysis of the buccinator, particles collect on the affected side. The paralysis of the nasal muscles is seen on asking the patient to sniff. Owing to the fact that the lips are drawn to the sound side, the tongue, when protruded, looks as if it were pushed to the paralyzed side; but on taking its position from the incisor teeth, it will be found to be in the middle line. The reflex movements are lost in this peripheral form. It is usually stated that the palate is partially paralyzed on the same side and that the uvula deviates. Both Gowers and Hughlings Jackson deny the existence of this involvement in the great majority of cases, and Horsley and Beevor have shown that these parts are innervated by the accessory nerve to the vagus.

The *sensory functions* of the facial nerve, to which much attention has been paid of late by Cushing, Mills and others, are ministered to by the geniculate ganglion, the intermediary nerve of Wrisberg, and the chorda tympani, which last has chiefly gustatory functions. It seems likely that deep sensibility with sense of pressure, position and passive movement runs in a separate afferent system in the motor nerve of the face. Cutaneous sensibility, both epicritic, by which we localize light touch, and protopathic, by which we recognize degrees of heat and cold, is not ministered to by the facial nerve proper. There are observations that would indicate, however, that the anterior part of the tongue and possibly a little strip of the skin of the auricle have a vestigial supply from this nerve.

When the nerve is involved within the canal between the genu and the origin of the chorda tympani, the sense of taste is lost in the anterior part of the tongue on the affected side. When the nerve is damaged outside the skull the sense of taste is unaffected. Hearing is often impaired in facial paralysis, most commonly by preceding ear disease. The paralysis of the stapedius muscle may lead to increased sensitiveness to musical notes. Herpes is sometimes associated with facial paralysis. Pain is not common, but there may be neuralgia about the ear. The face on the affected side may be swollen.

The *electrical reactions,* which are those of a peripheral palsy, have considerable importance from a prognostic standpoint. Erb's rules are as follows: If there is no change, either faradic or galvanic, the prognosis is good and recovery takes place in from fourteen to twenty days. If the faradic and galvanic excitability of the nerve is only lessened and that of the muscle increased to the galvanic current and the contraction formula altered (the contraction sluggish AC<KC), the outlook is relatively good and recovery will probably take place in from four to six weeks; occasionally in from eight to ten. When the reaction of degeneration is present—that is, if the faradic and galvanic excitability of the nerves and the faradic excitability of the muscles are lost and the galvanic excitability of the muscle is quantitatively increased and qualitatively changed, and if the mechanical excitability is altered —the prognosis is relatively unfavorable and the recovery may not occur for two, six, eight, or even fifteen months.

COURSE.—The course of facial paralysis is usually favorable. The onset in the form following cold is very rapid, developing perhaps within twenty-four hours, but rarely is the paralysis permanent. Now and again the paralysis never disappears; after four years I have seen only slight recovery. Recurring attacks have been described; Sinkler mentions five. On the other hand, in the paralysis from injury, as by a blow on the mastoid process, the condition may remain. When permanent, the muscles are entirely toneless. In some instances contracture develops as the voluntary power returns, and the natural folds and the wrinkles on the affected side may be deepened, so that on looking at the face one at first may have the impression that the affected side is the sound one. This is corrected at once on asking the patient to smile, when it is seen which side of the face has the most active movement.

Aretæus noted the difficulty sometimes experienced in determining which side was affected until the patient spoke or laughed.

Diagnosis.—The diagnosis of facial paralysis is usually easy. The distinction between the peripheral and central form is based on facts already mentioned.

Treatment.—In the cases which result from cold and are probably due to neuritis within the bony canal, hot applications first should be made; subsequently the thermo-cautery may be used lightly at intervals of a day or two over the mastoid process, or small blisters applied. If the ear is diseased, free discharge for the secretion should be obtained. The galvanic current may be employed to keep up the nutrition of the muscles. The positive pole should be placed behind the ear, the negative one along the zygomatic and other muscles. The application can be made daily for a quarter of an hour and the patient can readily be taught to make it himself before a looking glass. Massage in the course of the nerve and of the muscles of the face is also useful. A course of iodide of potassium may be given even when there is no indication of syphilis.

In those cases in which the nerve has been destroyed by an injury, during an operation or from disease, and when there has been no evidence of returning function after keeping up the electric treatment for a few months, a nerve anastomosis should be performed. For this purpose either the spinal accessory or the hypoglossal nerve may be used. Though the normal conditions may never be completely regained after such an operation, the motor power will be largely restored to the paralyzed muscles and the obtrusive deformity greatly lessened. This procedure, based on the results of physiological experimentation, makes one of the most striking of modern operations.

Spasm.—The spasm may be limited to a few or involve all the muscles innervated by the facial nerve, and may be unilateral or bilateral.

It is known also by the name of mimic spasm or of convulsive tic. Several different affections are usually considered under the name of facial or mimic spasm, but we shall here speak only of the simple spasm of the facial muscles, either primary or following paralysis, and shall not include the cases of habit spasm in children, or the *tic convulsif* of the French.

Gowers recognizes two classes—one in which there is an organic lesion, and an idiopathic form. It is thought to be due also to reflex causes, such as the irritation from carious teeth or the presence of intestinal worms. The disease usually occurs in adults, whereas the habit spasm and the *tic convulsif* of the French, often confounded with it, are most common in children. True mimic spasm occasionally comes on in childhood and persists. In the case of a school-mate the affection was marked as early as the eleventh or twelfth year and still continues. When the result of organic disease, there has usually been a lesion of the centre in the cortex, as in the case reported by Berkley, or pressure on the nerve at the base of the brain by aneurism or tumor.

Symptoms.—The spasm may involve only the muscles around the eye—blepharospasm—in which case there is constant, rapid, quick action of the orbicularis palpebrarum, which, in association with photophobia, may be tonic in character. More commonly the spasm affects the lateral facial muscles with those of the eye, and there is constant twitching of the side of the face with partial closure of the eye. The frontalis is rarely involved. In aggravated cases the depressors of the angle of the mouth, the levator menti, and the platysma myoides are affected. This spasm is confined to one side of the face in a majority of cases, though it may extend and become bilateral. It is increased by emotional causes and by voluntary movements of the face. As a rule, it is painless, but there may be tender points over the course of the fifth nerve, particularly the supraorbital branch. Tonic spasm of the facial muscle may follow paralysis, and is said to result occasionally from cold.

The outlook in facial spasm is always dubious. A majority of the cases persist for years and are incurable.

TREATMENT.—Sources of irritation should be looked for and removed. When a painful spot is present over the fifth nerve, blistering or the application of the thermo-cautery may relieve it. Hypodermic injections of strychnia may be tried, but are of doubtful benefit. Weir Mitchell recommends the freezing of the cheek for a few minutes daily or every second day with the spray, and this, in some instances, is beneficial. Often the relief is transient; the cases return, and at every clinic may be seen half a dozen or more of such patients who have run the gamut of all measures without material improvement. Severe cases may require surgical interference. The nerve may be divided near the stylomastoid foramen and an anastomosis made between it and the spinal accessory.

AUDITORY NERVE

The eighth, known also as *portio mollis* of the seventh pair, passes from the ear through the internal auditory meatus, and in reality consists of two separate nerves—the cochlear and vestibular roots. These two roots have entirely different functions, and may therefore be best considered separately. The cochlear nerve is the one connected with the organ of Corti, and is concerned in hearing. The vestibular nerve is connected with the vestibule and semicircular canals, and has to do with the maintenance of equilibrium.

The Cochlear Nerve

The cortical centre for hearing is in the temporo-sphenoidal lobe. Primary disease of the auditory nerve in its centre or intracranial course is uncommon. More frequently the terminal branches are affected within the labyrinth.

Affection of the Cortical Centre.—The superior temporal gyrus represents the centre for hearing. In man destruction of this gyrus on the left side results in word-deafness, which may be defined as an inability to understand the meaning of words, though they may still be heard as sounds. The central auditory path extending to the cortical centre from the terminal nuclei of the cochlear nerve may be involved and produce deafness. This may result from involvement of the lateral lemniscus, from the presence of a tumor in the corpora quadrigemina, especially if it involve the posterior quadrigeminal bodies, from a lesion of the internal geniculate body, or it may be associated with a lesion of the internal capsule.

Lesions of the nerve at the base of the brain may result from the pressure of tumors, meningitis (particularly the cerebro-spinal form), hæmorrhage, or traumatism. A primary degeneration of the nerve may occur in locomotor ataxia. Primary disease of the terminal nuclei of the cochlear nerve (nucleus nervi cochlearis dorsalis and nucleus nervi cochlearis ventralis) is rare. By far the most interesting form results from epidemic cerebro-spinal meningitis, in which the nerve is frequently involved, causing permanent deafness. In young children the condition results in deaf-mutism.

Internal Ear.—In a majority of the cases associated with auditory nerve symptoms the lesion is in the internal ear, either primary or the result of extension of disease of the middle ear. Two groups of symptoms may be produced—hyperæsthesia and irritation, and diminished function or nervous deafness.

(*a*) Hyperæsthesia and Irritation.—This may be due to altered function of the centre as well as of the nerve ending. True hyperæsthesia—hyperacusis—is a condition in which sounds, sometimes even those inaudible to other persons, are heard with great intensity. It occurs in hysteria and occasionally in cerebral disease. As already mentioned, in paralysis of the stapedius low notes may be heard with intensity. In dysæsthesia, or dysacusis, ordinary sounds cause an unpleasant sensation, as commonly happens in connection with headache, when ordinary noises are badly borne.

Tinnitus aurium is a term employed to designate certain subjective sensations of ringing, roaring, tickling, and whirring noises in the ear. It is a very common and often a distressing symptom. It is associated with many forms of ear disease and may result from pressure of wax on the drum. It is rare in organic disease of the central connections of the nerve. Sudden intense stimulation of the nerve may cause it. A form not uncommonly met with in medical practice is that in which the patient hears a continual *bruit* in the ear, and the noise has a systolic intensification, usually on one side. I have twice been consulted by physicians for this condition under the belief that they had an internal aneurism. A systolic murmur may be heard occasionally on auscultation. It occurs in conditions of anæmia and neurasthenia. Subjective noises in the ear may precede an epileptic seizure and are sometimes present in migraine. In whatever form tinnitus exists, though slight and often regarded as trivial, it occasions great annoyance and often mental distress, and has even driven patients to suicide.

The *diagnosis* is readily made; but it is often extremely difficult to determine upon what condition the tinnitus depends. The relief of constitutional states, such as anæmia, neurasthenia, or gout, may result in cure. A careful local examination of the ear should always be made. One of the most worrying forms is the constant clicking, sometimes audible many feet away from the patient, and due probably to clonic spasm of the muscles connected with the Eustachian tube or of the levator palati. The condition may persist for years unchanged, and then disappear suddenly. The pulsating forms of tinnitus, in which the sound is like that of a systolic *bruit*, are almost invariably subjective, and it is very rare to hear anything with the stethoscope. It is to be remembered that in children there is a systolic brain murmur, best heard over the ear, and in some instances appreciable in the adult.

(*b*) Diminished Function or Nervous Deafness.—In testing for nervous deafness, if the tuning fork can not be heard when placed near the meatus, but the vibrations are audible by placing the foot of the tuning fork against the temporal bone, the conclusion may be drawn that the deafness is not due to involvement of the nerve. The vibrations are conveyed through the temporal bone to the cochlea and vestibule. The watch may be used for the same purpose, and if the meatus is closed and the watch is heard better in contact with the mastoid process than when opposite the open meatus, the deafness is probably not nervous. Disturbance of the function of the auditory nerve is not a very frequent symptom in brain disease, but in all cases the function of the nerve should be carefully tested.

The Vestibular Nerve

The most frequent symptoms met with in association with disease of the vestibular nerve and its central connections are vertigo, nystagmus, and loss of coördination of the muscles of the head, neck, and eyes.

Auditory Vertigo—Ménière's Disease.—In 1861 Ménière, a French physician, described an affection characterized by noises in the ear, vertigo (which might be associated with loss of consciousness), vomiting, and, in many cases, progressive loss of hearing. Bárány, of Vienna, has thrown much light on this subject. He groups the conditions in which the labyrinth may be affected under the following heads: (*a*) Acute infectious diseases, influenza, cerebro-spinal meningitis, mumps, etc. (*b*) Chronic infectious diseases, syphilis particularly. (*c*) Constitutional conditions and auto-intoxications. Hæmorrhage into the labyrinth (in leukæmia, purpura hæmorrhagica, pernicious anæmia); chlorosis, thyroid intoxications, arterio-sclerosis, etc. (*d*) Tumors and diseases of the central nervous system; tumors of the acoustic nerve, cerebellum, pons, and fourth ventricle, meningitis, cerebellar abscess, multiple sclerosis, tabes, etc. (*e*) Traumatic injuries, fracture of the base, etc. (*f*) Hereditary degenerative diseases and malformations of the internal ear. (*g*) Intoxications, alcohol, nicotine, quinine, salicylic acid group, arsenic (salvarsan?).

Symptoms.—The attack usually sets in suddenly with a buzzing noise in the ears and the patient feels as if he was reeling or staggering. He may feel himself to be reeling, or the objects about him may seem to be turning, or the phenomena may be combined. The attack is often so abrupt that the patient falls, though, as a rule, he has time to steady himself by grasping some neighboring object. Consciousness is generally maintained, but may be momentarily lost. Ocular symptoms are usually present. Jerking of the eyeballs, or nystagmus, occurs. The patient becomes pale and nauseated, a clammy sweat breaks out on the face, and vomiting may follow. The duration of the attack varies greatly. At times it may be very short, but it usually causes the patient to lie quietly for some time, as any movement of the head brings on another attack.

Labyrinthine vertigo is usually paroxysmal, coming on at irregular intervals, sometimes of weeks or months; or several attacks may occur in a day.

The disturbances of equilibrium, including the vertigo, are dependent upon a disturbance of the functions of the vestibular nerve or of the organs with which this nerve is connected, either in its peripheral distribution or by means of its central connection. The auditory symptoms often accompanying it are doubtless always due to involvement of the cochlear nerve or its peripheral or central connections.

Diagnosis.—The combination of tinnitus with giddiness, with or without gastric disturbance, is sufficient to establish a diagnosis. There are other forms of vertigo from which it must be distinguished. The form known as gastric vertigo, which is associated with dyspepsia and occurs most commonly in persons of middle age, is, as a rule, readily distinguished by the absence of tinnitus or evidences of disturbance in the function of the auditory nerve. This variety of vertigo is much less common than Trousseau's description would lead us to believe. It is important to note the close connection of vertigo with ocular defects.

The cardio-vascular vertigo, one of the most common forms, occurs in cases of valvular disease, particularly aortic insufficiency, and as frequently in arterio-sclerosis.

Aural vertigo must be carefully distinguished from attacks of *petit mal*, or, indeed, of definite epilepsy. It is rare in *petit mal* to have noises in the ear or actual giddiness, but in the aura preceding an epileptic attack the patient may feel giddy. Giddiness and transient loss of consciousness may be associated with organic disease of the brain, more particularly with tumor. Vomiting also may be present. A careful investigation will usually lead to a correct diagnosis. Bárány's special tests for the functional activity of the vestibular nerve are of great use in the hands of a skilled observer, particularly his caloric test (irrigation of the external meatus with cold or warm water, and observing its effect on the production of nystagmus).

Prognosis.—The outlook in Ménière's disease is uncertain. While many cases recover completely, in others deafness results and the attacks recur at shorter intervals. In aggravated cases the patient constantly suffers from vertigo, and may even be confined to his bed.

Treatment.—Bromide of potassium, in 20 grain (1.3 gm.) doses three times a day, is sometimes beneficial. If there is a history of syphilis the iodides should be administered. The salicylates are recommended, and Charcot advises quinine to cinchonism. In cases in which there is increase in the arterial tension nitroglycerin may be given, at first in very small doses, but increasing gradually. It is not specially valuable in Ménière's disease, but in the cases of giddiness in middle aged men and women associated with arterio-sclerosis it sometimes acts very satisfactorily. Correction of errors of refraction is sometimes followed by prompt relief of the vertigo.

Endemic Paralytic Vertigo.—In parts of Switzerland and France there is a remarkable form of vertigo described by Gerlier, which is characterized by attacks of paretic weakness of the extremities, falling of the eyelids, remarkable depression, but with retention of consciousness. It occurs also in northern Japan, where Miura says it develops paroxysmally among the farm laborers of both sexes and all ages. It is known there as *kubisagari*.

GLOSSO-PHARYNGEAL NERVE

(*Nervus glossopharyngeus*)

The ninth nerve contains both motor and sensory fibres and is also a nerve of the special sense of taste to the tongue. It supplies, by its motor branches, the stylo-pharyngeus and the middle constrictor of the pharynx. The sensory fibres are distributed to the upper part of the pharynx.

Symptoms.—Of nuclear disturbance we know very little. The pharyngeal symptoms of bulbar paralysis are probably associated with involvement of the nuclei of this nerve. Lesion of the nerve trunk itself is rare, but it may be compressed by tumors or involved in meningitis. Disturbance of the sense of taste may result from loss of function of this nerve, in which case it is chiefly in the posterior part of the tongue and soft palate.

The general disturbances of the sense of taste may here be briefly referred to. Loss of the sense of taste—*ageusia*—may be caused by disturbance of the peripheral end organs, as in affections of the mucosa of the tongue. This is very common in the dry tongue of fever or the furred tongue of dyspepsia, under which circumstances, as the saying is, everything tastes alike. Strong irritants, too, such as pepper, tobacco, or vinegar, may dull or diminish the sense of taste. Complete loss may be due to involvement of the nerves either in their course or in the centres. Perversion of the sense of taste—*parageusis*—is rarely found, except as an hysterical manifestation and in the insane. Increased sensitiveness is still more rare. There are occasional subjective sensations of taste, occurring as an aura in epilepsy or as part of the hallucinations in the insane.

To test the sense of taste the patient's eyes should be closed and small quantities of various substances applied to the protruded tongue. The sensation should be perceived before the tongue is withdrawn. The following are the most suitable tests: For bitterness, quinine; for sweetness, a strong solution of sugar or saccharin; for acidity, vinegar; and for the saline test, common salt. One of the most important tests is the feeble galvanic current, which gives the well-known metallic taste.

PNEUMOGASTRIC NERVE

(*Nervus vagus*)

The tenth nerve has an important and extensive distribution, supplying the pharynx, larynx, lungs, heart, œsophagus, and stomach. The nerve may be involved at its nucleus along with the spinal accessory and the hypoglossal, forming what is known as bulbar paralysis. It may be compressed by tumors or aneurism, or in the exudation of meningitis, simple or syphilitic. In its course in the neck the trunk may be involved by tumors or in wounds. It has been tied in ligature of the carotid, and has been cut in the removal of deep-seated tumors. The trunk may be attacked by neuritis.

The affections of the vagus are best considered in connection with the distribution of the separate nerves.

Pharyngeal Branches.—In combination with the glosso-pharyngeal the branches from the vagus form the pharyngeal plexus, from which the muscles and mucosa of the pharynx are supplied. In *paralysis* due to involvement of this either in the nuclei, as in bulbar paralysis, or in the course of the nerve, as in diphtheritic neuritis, there is difficulty in swallowing and the food is not passed on into the œsophagus. If the nerve on one side only is involved the deglutition is not much impaired. In these cases the particles of food frequently pass into the larynx, and, when the soft palate is involved, into the posterior nares.

Spasm of the pharynx is always a functional disorder, usually occurring in hysterical and nervous people. Gowers mentions a case of a gentleman who could not eat unless alone, on account of the inability to swallow in the presence of others from spasm of the pharynx. This spasm is a well marked feature in hydrophobia, and it occurs also in pseudo-hydrophobia.

Laryngeal Branches.—The superior laryngeal nerve supplies the mucous membrane of the larynx above the cords and the crico-thyroid muscle. The inferior or recurrent laryngeal curves around the arch of the aorta on the left side and the subclavian artery on the right passes along the trachea and supplies the mucosa below the cords and all the muscles of the larynx except the crico-thyroid and the epiglottidean. Experiments have shown that these motor nerves of the pneumogastric are all derived from the spinal accessory. The remarkable course of the recurrent laryngeal nerves renders them liable to pressure by tumors within the thorax, particularly by aneurism. The following are the most important forms of paralysis:

(*a*) Bilateral Paralysis of the Abductors.—In this condition the posterior crico-arytenoids are involved and the glottis is not opened during inspiration. The cords may be close together in the position of phonation, and during inspiration may be brought even nearer together by the pressure of air, so that there is only a narrow chink through which the air whistles with a noisy stridor. This dangerous form of laryngeal paralysis occurs occasionally as a result of cold, or may follow a laryngeal catarrh. The posterior muscles have been found degenerated when the others were healthy. The condition may be produced by pressure upon both vagi, or upon both recurrent nerves. As a central affection it occurs in tabes and bulbar paralysis, but may be seen also in hysteria. The characteristic symptoms are inspiratory stridor with unimpaired phonation. Possibly, as Gowers suggests, many cases of so-called hysterical spasm of the glottis are in reality abductor paralysis.

(*b*) Unilateral Abductor Paralysis.—This frequently results from the pressure of tumors or involvement of one recurrent nerve. Aneurism is by far the most common cause, though on the right side the nerve may be involved in thickening of the pleura. The symptoms are hoarseness or roughness of the voice, such as is so common in aneurism. Dyspnœa is not often present. The cord on the affected side does not move in inspiration. Subsequently the adductors may also become involved, in which case the phonation is still more impaired.

(*c*) Adductor Paralysis.—This results from involvement of the lateral crico-arytenoid and the arytenoid muscle itself. It is common in hysteria, particularly of women, and causes the hysterical aphonia, which may come on suddenly. It may result from catarrh of the larynx or from overuse of the voice. In laryngoscopic examination it is seen, on attempting phonation, that there is no power to bring the cords together.

(*d*) Spasm of the Muscles of the Larynx.—In this the adductor muscles are involved. It is not an uncommon affection in children, and has already been referred to as laryngismus stridulus. Paroxysmal attacks of laryngeal spasm are rare in the adult, but cases are described in which the patient, usually a young girl, wakes at night in an attack of intense dyspnœa, which may persist long enough to produce cyanosis. Liveing states that they may replace attacks of migraine. They occur in a characteristic form in locomotor ataxia, forming the so-called laryngeal crises. There is a condition known as spastic aphonia, in which, when the patient attempts to speak, phonation is completely prevented by a spasm.

Disturbance of the sensory nerves of the larynx is rare.

(*e*) ANÆSTHESIA may occur in bulbar paralysis and in diphtheritic neuritis —a serious condition, as portions of food may enter the windpipe. It is usually associated with dysphagia and is sometimes present in hysteria. Hyperæsthesia of the larynx is rare.

Cardiac Branches.—The cardiac plexus is formed by the union of branches of the vagi and of the sympathetic nerves. The vagus fibres subserve motor, sensory, and probably trophic functions.

MOTOR.—The fibres which inhibit, control, and regulate the cardiac action pass in the vagi. Irritation may produce slowing of the action. Czermak could slow or even arrest the heart's action for a few beats by pressing a small tumor in his neck against one pneumogastric nerve, and it is said that the same can be produced by forcible bilateral pressure on the carotid canal. There are instances in which persons appear to have had voluntary control over the action of the heart. Cheyne mentions the case of Colonel Townshend, "who could die or expire when he pleased, and yet by an effort or somehow come to life again, which it seems he had sometimes tried before he had sent for us." Retardation of the heart's action has also followed accidental ligature of one vagus. Irritation of the nuclei may also be accompanied with a neurosis of this nerve. On the other hand, when there is complete paralysis of the vagi, the inhibitory action may be abolished and the acceleratory influences have full sway. The heart's action is then greatly increased. This is seen in some instances of diphtheritic neuritis and in involvement of the nerve by tumors, or its accidental removal or ligature. Complete loss of function of one vagus, however, may not be followed by any symptoms.

SENSORY symptoms on the part of the cardiac branches are very varied. Normally, the heart's action proceeds regularly without the participation of consciousness, but the unpleasant feelings and sensations of palpitation and pain are conveyed to the brain through this nerve. How far the fibres of the pneumogastric are involved in angina it is impossible to say. The various disturbances of sensation are described under the cardiac neuroses.

Pulmonary Branches.—We know very little of the pulmonary branches of the vagi. The motor fibres are stated to control the action of the bronchial muscles, and it has long been held that asthma may be a neurosis of these fibres. The various alterations in the respiratory rhythm are probably due more to changes in the centre than in the nerves themselves.

Gastric and Œsophageal Branches.—The muscular movements of these parts are presided over by the vagi and vomiting is induced through them, usually reflexly, but also by direct irritation, as in meningitis. Spasm of the œsophagus generally occurs with other nervous phenomena. Gastralgia may sometimes be due to cramp of the stomach, but is more commonly a sensory disturbance of this nerve, due to direct irritation of the peripheral ends, or is a neuralgia of the terminal fibres. Hunger is said to be a sensation aroused by the pneumogastric, and some forms of nervous dyspepsia probably depend upon disturbed function of this nerve. The severe gastric crises which occur in locomotor ataxia are due to central irritation of the nuclei.

SPINAL ACCESSORY NERVE

(*Nervus accessorius*)

Paralysis.—The smaller or internal part of this nerve joins the vagus and is distributed through it to the laryngeal muscles. The larger external part is distributed to the sterno-mastoid and trapezius muscles.

The nuclei of the nerve, particularly of the accessory part, may be involved in bulbar paralysis. The nuclei of the external portion, situated as they are in the cervical cord, may be attacked in progressive degeneration of the motor nuclei of the cord. The nerve may be involved in the exudation of meningitis, or be compressed by tumors, or in caries. The *symptoms* of paralysis of the accessory portion which joins the vagus have already been given in the account of the palsy of the laryngeal branches of the pneumogastric. Disease or compression of the external portion is followed by paralysis of the sterno-mastoid and of the trapezius on the same side. In paralysis of one sterno-mastoid the patient rotates the head with difficulty to the opposite side, but there is no torticollis, though in some cases the head is held obliquely. As the trapezius is supplied in part from the cervical nerves, it is not completely paralyzed, but the portion which passes from the occipital bone to the acromion is functionless. The paralysis of the muscle is well seen when the patient draws a deep breath or shrugs the shoulders. The middle portion of the trapezius is also weakened, the shoulder droops a little, and the angle of the scapula is rotated inward by the action of the rhomboids and the levator anguli scapulæ. Elevation of the arm is impaired, for the trapezius does not fix the scapula as a point from which the deltoid can work.

In progressive muscular atrophy we sometimes see bilateral paralysis of these muscles. Thus, if the sterno-mastoids are affected, the head tends to fall back; when the trapezii are involved, it falls forward, a characteristic attitude of the head in many cases of progressive muscular atrophy. Gowers suggests that lesions of the accessory in difficult labor may account for those cases in which during the first year of life the child has great difficulty in holding up the head. In children this drooping of the head is an important symptom in cervical meningitis, the result of caries.

The TREATMENT of the condition depends much upon the cause. In the central nuclear atrophy but little can be done. In paralysis from pressure the symptoms may gradually be relieved. The paralyzed muscles should be stimulated by electricity and massage.

Accessory Spasm (*Torticollis; Wryneck*).—The forms of spasm affecting the cervical muscles are best considered here, as the muscles supplied by the accessory are chiefly, though not solely, responsible for the condition. The following forms may be described in this section:

(*a*) CONGENITAL TORTICOLLIS.—This condition, also known as fixed torticollis, depends upon the shortening and atrophy of the sterno-mastoid on one side. It occurs in children and may not be noticed for several years on account of the shortness of the neck, the parents often alleging that it has only recently come on. It affects the right side almost exclusively. A remarkable circumstance in connection with it is the existence of facial asymmetry noted by Wilks, which appears to be an essential part of this congenital form. In congenital wryneck the sterno-mastoid is shortened, hard and firm, and in a condition of more or less advanced atrophy. This must be distinguished from the local thickening in the sterno-mastoid due to rupture, which may occur at the time of birth and produce an induration or muscle callus. Although the sterno-mastoid is almost always affected, there are rare cases in which the fibrous atrophy affécts the trapezius. This form of wryneck in itself is unimportant, since it is readily relieved by tenotomy, but Golding-Bird states that the facial asymmetry persists, or, indeed, may, as shown by photographs in my case, become more evident. With reference to the pathology of the affection, Golding-Bird concludes that the facial asymmetry and the torticollis are integral parts of one affection which has a central origin, and is the counterpart in the head and neck of infantile paralysis with talipes in the foot.

(*b*) Spasmodic Wryneck.—Two varieties of this spasm occur, the tonic and the clonic, which may alternate in the same case; or, as is most common, they are separate and remain so from the outset. The disease is most frequent in adults and, according to Gowers, more common in females. In America it is certainly more frequent in males. In females it may be an hysterical manifestation. There may be a marked neurotic family history, but it is usually impossible to fix upon any definite etiological factor. Some cases have followed cold; others a blow. Brissaud has described what he calls mental torticollis. It is usually met with in neurasthenic patients and in elderly persons, and consists of a clonic spasm of the rotators of the head.

The *symptoms* are well defined. In the tonic form the contracted sterno-mastoid draws the occiput toward the shoulder of the affected side; the chin is raised, and the face rotated to the other shoulder. The sterno-mastoid may be affected alone or in association with the trapezius. When the latter is implicated the head is depressed still more toward the same side. In long-standing cases these muscles are prominent and very rigid. There may be some curvature of the spine, the convexity of which is toward the sound side. The cases in which the spasm is clonic are much more distressing and serious. The spasm is rarely limited to a single muscle. The sterno-mastoid is almost always involved and rotates the head so as to approximate the mastoid process to the inner end of the clavicle, turning the face to the opposite side and raising the chin. When with this the trapezius is affected, the depression of the head toward the same side is more marked. The head is drawn somewhat backward; the shoulder, too, is raised by its action. According to Gowers, the splenius is associated with the sterno-mastoid about half as frequently as the trapezius. Its action is to incline the head and rotate it slightly toward the same side. Other muscles may be involved, such as the scalenus and platysma myoides; and in rare cases the head may be rotated by the deep cervical muscles, the rectus and obliquus. There are cases in which the spasm is bilateral, causing a backward movement—the retro-collic spasm. This may be either tonic or clonic, and in extreme cases the face is horizontal and looks upward.

These clonic contractions may come on without warning, or be preceded for a time by irregular pains or stiffness of the neck. The jerking movements recur every few moments, and it is impossible to keep the head still for more than a minute or two. In time the muscles undergo hypertrophy and may be distinctly larger on one side than the other. In some cases the pain is considerable; in others there is simply a feeling of fatigue. The spasms cease during sleep. Emotion, excitement, and fatigue increase them. The spasm may extend from the muscles of the neck and involve those of the face or the arms.

The disease varies much in its course. Cases occasionally get well, but the great majority of them persist, and, even if temporarily relieved, the disease frequently recurs. The affection is usually regarded as a functional neurosis, but it is possibly due to disturbance of the cortical centres presiding over the muscles.

Treatment.—Temporary relief is sometimes obtained; a permanent cure is exceptional. Various drugs have been used, but rarely with benefit. Occasionally, large doses of bromide will lessen the intensity of the spasm. Morphia, subcutaneously, has been successful in some reported cases, but there is the great danger of establishing the morphia habit. Galvanism may be tried. Counter-irritation is probably useless. Fixation of the head mechanically can rarely be borne by the patient. These obstinate cases fall ultimately into the hands of the surgeon, and the operations of stretching, division, and excision of the accessory nerve and division of the muscles have been tried. Temporary relief may follow, but, as a rule, the condition returns. Risien Russell thinks that resection of the posterior branches of the upper cervical nerves is most likely to give relief, and this has been done by Keen and others.

(*c*) The NODDING SPASM of children may here be mentioned as involving chiefly the muscles innervated by the accessory nerve. It may be a simple trick, a form of habit spasm, or a phenomenon of epilepsy (E. nutans), in which case it is associated with transient loss of consciousness. A similar nodding spasm may occur in older children. In women it sometimes occurs as an hysterical manifestation, commonly as part of the so-called salaam convulsion.

HYPOGLOSSAL NERVE

This is the motor nerve of the tongue and for most of the muscles attached to the hyoid bone. Its cortical centre is probably the lower part of the anterior central gyrus.

Paralysis.—(*a*) CORTICAL LESION.—The tongue is often involved in hemiplegia, and the paralysis may result from a lesion of the cortex itself, or of the fibres as they pass to the medulla. It does not occur alone and is considered with hemiplegia. There is this difference, however, between the cortical and other forms, that the muscles on both sides of the tongue may be more or less affected but do not waste, nor are their electrical reactions disturbed.

(*b*) NUCLEAR and INFRA-NUCLEAR lesions of the hypoglossal result from slow progressive degeneration, as in bulbar paralysis or in locomotor ataxia; occasionally there is acute softening from obstruction of the vessels. The nuclei of both nerves are usually affected together, but may be attacked separately. Trauma and lead poisoning have also been assigned as causes. The fibres may be damaged by a tumor, and at the base by meningitis; or the nerve is sometimes involved in the condylar foramen by disease of the skull. It may be involved in its course in a scar, as in Birkett's case, or compressed by a tumor in the parotid region. As a result, there is loss of function in the nerve fibres and the tongue undergoes atrophy on the affected side. It is protruded toward the paralyzed side and may show fibrillary twitching.

The *symptoms* of involvement of one hypoglossal, either at its centre or in its course, are those of unilateral paralysis and atrophy of the tongue. When protruded, it is pushed toward the affected side, and there are fibrillary twitchings. The atrophy is usually marked and the mucous membrane on the affected side is thrown into folds. Articulation is not much impaired in the unilateral affection. There is a remarkable triad of symptoms, to which Hughlings Jackson first called attention—unilateral hemi-atrophy of the tongue, loss of power in the palate muscle, with paralysis of the larynx on the same side. When the disease is bilateral, the tongue lies almost motionless in the floor of the mouth; it is atrophied, and can not be protruded. Speech and mastication are extremely difficult and deglutition may be impaired. If the seat of the disease is above the nuclei, there may be little or no wasting. The condition is seen in progressive bulbar paralysis and occasionally in progressive muscular atrophy.

The *diagnosis* is readily made and the situation of the lesion can usually be determined, since when supra-nuclear there is associated hemiplegia and no wasting of the muscles of the tongue. Nuclear disease is only occasionally unilateral; most commonly bilateral and part of a bulbar paralysis. It should be borne in mind that the fibres of the hypoglossal may be involved within the medulla after leaving their nuclei. In such a case there may be paralysis of the tongue on one side and paralysis of the limbs on the opposite side, and the tongue, when protruded, is pushed toward the sound side.

Spasm.—This rare affection may be unilateral or bilateral. It is most frequently a part of some other convulsive disorder, such as epilepsy, chorea, or spasm of the facial muscles. In some cases of stuttering, spasm of the tongue precedes the explosive utterance of the words. It may occur in hysteria, and is said to follow reflex irritation in the fifth nerve. The most remarkable cases are those of paroxysmal clonic spasm, in which the tongue is rapidly thrust in and out, as many as forty or fifty times a minute. The prognosis is usually good.

IV. DISEASES OF THE SPINAL NERVES

CERVICAL PLEXUS

Occipito-cervical Neuralgia.—This involves the nerve territory supplied by the occipitalis major and minor, and the auricularis magnus nerves. The pains are chiefly in the back of the head and neck and in the ear. The condition may follow cold and is sometimes associated with stiffness of the neck or torticollis. Unless connected with it there exists disease of the bones or unless it is due to pressure of tumors, the outlook is usually good. There are tender points midway between the mastoid process and the spine and just above the parietal eminence, and between the sterno-mastoid and the trapezius. The affection may be due to direct pressure in carrying heavy weights.

Affections of the Phrenic Nerve.—Paralysis may follow a lesion in the anterior horns at the level of the third and fourth cervical nerves, or may be due to compression of the nerve by tumors or aneurism. More rarely paralysis results from neuritis, diphtheritic or saturnine.

When the diaphragm is paralyzed respiration is carried on by the intercostal and accessory muscles. When the patient is quiet and at rest little may be noticed, but the abdomen retracts in inspiration and is forced out in expiration. On exertion or even on attempting to move there may be dyspnœa. If the paralysis sets in suddenly there may be dyspnœa and lividity, which is usually temporary (W. Pasteur). Intercurrent attacks of bronchitis seriously aggravate the condition. Difficulty in coughing, owing to the impossibility of drawing a full breath, adds greatly to the danger of this complication.

When the phrenic nerve is paralyzed on one side the paralysis may be scarcely noticeable, but careful inspection shows that the descent of the diaphragm is much less on the affected side.

The *diagnosis* of paralysis is not always easy, particularly in women, who habitually use this muscle less than men, and in whom the diaphragmatic breathing is less conspicuous. Immobility of the diaphragm is not uncommon, particularly in diaphragmatic pleurisy, in large effusions, and in extensive emphysema. The muscle itself may be degenerated and its power impaired.

Owing to the lessened action of the diaphragm, there is a tendency to accumulation of blood at the bases of the lungs, and there may be impaired resonance and signs of œdema. As a rule, however, the paralysis is not confined to this muscle, but is part of a general neuritis or an anterior poliomyelitis, and there are other symptoms of value in determining its presence. The outlook is usually serious. Pasteur states that of 15 cases following diphtheria only 8 recovered. The treatment is that of the neuritis or poliomyelitis.

Hiccough.—Here may, perhaps, best be considered this remarkable symptom, caused by intermittent, sudden contraction of the diaphragm. The mechanism, however, is complex, and while the afferent impressions to the respiratory centre may be peripheral or central the efferent are distributed through the phrenic nerve to the diaphragm, causing the intermittent spasm, and through the laryngeal branches of the vagus to the glottis, causing sudden closure as the air is rapidly inspired. There are various groups:

(*a*) Inflammatory, seen particularly in affections of the abdominal viscera, gastritis, peritonitis, hernia, internal strangulation, appendicitis, suppurative pancreatitis, and in the severe forms of typhoid fever.

(*b*) Irritative, as in the direct stimulation of the diaphragm when very hot substances are swallowed, in disease of the œsophagus near the diaphragm, and in many conditions of gastric and intestinal disorder, more particularly those associated with flatus.

(*c*) Specific, or, perhaps more properly, *idiopathic*, in which no evident causes are present. In these cases there is usually some constitutional taint, as gout, diabetes, or chronic Bright's disease. I have seen several instances of obstinate hiccough in the later stages of chronic interstitial nephritis.

(*d*) Neurotic, cases in which the primary cause is in the nervous system; hysteria, epilepsy, shock, or cerebral tumors. Of these cases the hysterical are, perhaps, the most obstinate.

The TREATMENT is often very unsatisfactory. Sometimes in the milder forms a sudden reflex irritation will check it at once. Readers of Plato's Symposium will remember that the physician Eryximachus recommended to Aristophanes, who had hiccough from eating too much, either to hold his breath (which for trivial forms of hiccough is very satisfactory) or to gargle with a little water; but if it still continued, "tickle your nose with something and sneeze; and if you sneeze once or twice even the most violent hiccough is sure to go." The attack must have been of some severity, as it is stated subsequently that the hiccough did not disappear until Aristophanes had resorted to the sneezing.

Ice, a teaspoonful of salt and lemon juice, or salt and vinegar, or a teaspoonful of raw spirits may be tried. When the hiccough is due to gastric irritation, lavage is sometimes promptly curative. I saw a case of a week's duration cured by a hypodermic injection of gr. 1/8 (0.008 gm.) of apomorphia. In obstinate cases the various antispasmodics have been used in succession. Pilocarpine has been recommended. The ether spray on the epigastrium may be promptly curative. Hypodermics of morphia, inhalations of chloroform, the use of nitrite of amyl and of nitroglycerin have been beneficial in some cases. Galvanism over the phrenic nerve, or pressure on the nerves, applied between the heads of the sterno-cleido-mastoid muscles may be used. Strong traction upon the tongue may give immediate relief. Of all measures morphia used freely is the best.

BRACHIAL PLEXUS

Cervical Rib Pressure.—Symptoms from pressure of this anomaly are by no means rare. It is usually bilateral, but the rib may be much longer on one side than on the other. The rib may be short and straight with the subclavian artery and brachial plexus in front of it, or longer and curved with the subclavian artery on its upper surface in a groove, in which case the artery is lengthened and elevated in the neck. Only about 5 or 10 per cent. of the cases have any trouble. The symptoms are either from pressure on the artery or on the nerve. The pulsation of the abnormally high artery may be mistaken for aneurism. In a few rare instances aneurism has occurred at the site of the pressure, and there have been cases of thrombosis with gangrene of the finger tips. I have seen three cases in which on exertion the arm became swollen, red and hot with numbness and tingling, but when quiet and at rest there was no inconvenience.

Affections of the nerves are more frequent and important. Pain is common, corresponding, as a rule, to the distribution of the eighth cervical and first dorsal roots, extending along the ulnar border of the forearm to the wrist or fingers. In other cases there is marked pressure on the brachial plexus with partial paralysis and wasting of the intrinsic muscles of the hand. There may be anæsthesia or hyperæsthesia of the inner aspect of the arm and the ulnar half of the hand. In a few instances there has been pressure on the cervical sympathetic nerve.

The condition is, as a rule, readily recognized, sometimes by palpation, always with the X-ray picture.

Combined Paralysis.—The plexus may be involved in the supraclavicular region by compression of the nerve trunks as they leave the spine, or by tumors and other morbid processes in the neck. Below the clavicle lesions are more common and result from injuries following dislocation or fracture, sometimes from neuritis. A cervical rib may lead to a pressure paralysis of the lower cord of the plexus. A not infrequent form of injury in this region follows falls or blows on the neck, which by lateral flexion of the head and depression of the shoulder seriously stretch the plexus. The entire plexus may be ruptured and the arm be totally paralyzed. The rupture may occur anywhere between the vertebræ and the clavicle, and involve all the cords of the plexus, or only the upper ones. The so-called "obstetrical palsy," due to drawing apart of the head and the shoulder during delivery, is an instance of this sort of injury. In these cases, however, the rupture of the plexus is usually only a partial one, involving its upper cord alone, so that the deltoid, biceps, supra- and infra-spinati, brachialis anticus, and supinator longus muscles may alone be affected. When the entire plexus has been ruptured a complete motor and sensory paralysis of the arm is produced. The roots may even be torn away from the spinal cord. The pupil will then be contracted on the side of the injury, and the arm hang from the body like a flail. Another common cause of lesion of the brachial plexus is luxation of the head of the humerus, particularly the subcoracoid form.

A primary neuritis of the brachial plexus is rare. More commonly the process is an ascending neuritis from a lesion of a peripheral branch, involving first the radial or ulnar nerves, and spreading upward to the plexus, producing gradually complete loss of power in the arm.

Lesions of Individual Nerves of the Plexus.—(*a*) LONG THORACIC NERVE.—*Serratus paralysis* follows injury to this nerve in the neck, usually by direct pressure in carrying loads, and is very common in soldiers. It may be due to a neuritis following an acute infection or exposure. Isolated serratus paralysis is rare. It usually occurs in connection with paralysis of other muscles of the shoulder girdle, as in the myopathies and in progressive muscular atrophy. Concomitant trapezius paralysis is the most frequent. In the isolated paralysis there is little or no deformity with the hands hanging by the sides. There are slight abnormal obliquity of the posterior border of the scapula and prominence of the inferior angle, but when, as so commonly happens, the middle part of the trapezius is also paralyzed the deformity is marked. The shoulder is at a lower level, the inferior angle of the scapula is displaced inward and upward, and the superior angle projects upward. When the arms are held out in front at right angles to the body the scapula becomes winged and stands out prominently. The arm can not, as a rule, be raised above the horizontal. The outlook of the cases due to injury or to neuritis is good.

(*b*) CIRCUMFLEX NERVE.—This supplies the deltoid and the teres minor. The nerve is apt to be involved in injuries, in dislocations, bruising by a crutch, or sometimes by extension of inflammation from the joint. Occasionally the paralysis arises from a pressure neuritis during an illness. As a consequence of loss of power in the deltoid, the arm can not be raised. The wasting is usually marked and changes the shape of the shoulder. Sensation may also be impaired in the skin over the muscle. The joint may be relaxed and there may be a distinct space between the head of the humerus and the acromion.

(*c*) Musculo-spiral Paralysis; Radial Paralysis.—This is one of the most common of peripheral palsies, and results from the exposed position of the musculo-spiral nerve. It is often bruised in the use of the crutch, by injuries of the arm, blows, or fractures. It is frequently injured when a person falls asleep with the arm over the back of a chair, or by pressure of the body upon the arm when a person is sleeping on a bench or on the ground. It may be paralyzed by sudden violent contraction of the triceps. It is sometimes involved in a neuritis from cold, but this is uncommon in comparison with other causes. The paralysis of lead poisoning is the result of involvement of certain branches of this nerve.

A lesion when high up involves the triceps, the brachiális anticus, and the supinator longus, as well as the extensors of the wrist and fingers. Naturally, in lesions just above the elbow the arm muscles and the supinator longus are spared. The most characteristic feature of the paralysis is the wrist-drop and the inability to extend the first phalanges of the fingers and thumb. In the pressure palsies the supinators are usually involved and the movements of supination can not be accomplished. The sensations may be impaired, or there may be marked tingling, but the loss of sensation is rarely so pronounced as that of motion.

The affection is readily recognized, but it is sometimes difficult to say upon what it depends. The sleep and pressure palsies are, as a rule, unilateral and involve the supinator longus. The paralysis from lead is bilateral and the supinators are unaffected. Bilateral wrist-drop is a very common symptom in many forms of multiple neuritis, particularly the alcoholic; but the mode of onset and the involvement of the legs and arms are features which make the diagnosis easy. The duration and course of the musculo-spiral paralyses are very variable. The pressure palsies may disappear in a few days. Recovery is the rule, even when the affection lasts for many weeks. The electrical examination is of importance in the prognosis, and the rules laid down under paralysis of the facial nerve hold good here.

The treatment is that of neuritis.

(*d*) Ulnar Nerve.—The motor branches supply the ulnar half of the deep flexor of the fingers, the muscles of the little finger, the interossei, the adductor and the inner head of the short flexor of the thumb, and the ulnar flexor of the wrist. The sensory branches supply the ulnar side of the hand—two and a half fingers on the back, and one and a half fingers on the front. Paralysis may result from pressure, usually at the elbow joint, although the nerve is here protected. Possibly the neuritis in the ulnar nerve in some cases of acute illness may be due to this cause. Gowers mentions the case of a lady who twice had ulnar neuritis after confinement. Owing to paralysis of the ulnar flexor of the wrist, the hand moves toward the radial side; adduction of the thumb is impossible; the first phalanges can not be flexed, and the others can not be extended. In long standing cases the first phalanges are overextended and the others strongly flexed, producing the claw-hand; but this is not so marked as in the progressive muscular atrophy. The loss of sensation corresponds to the sensory distribution just mentioned.

(*e*) Median Nerve.—This supplies the flexors of the fingers except the ulnar half of the deep flexors, the abductor and the flexors of the thumb, the two radial lumbricales, the pronators, and the radial flexor of the wrist. The sensory fibres supply the radial side of the palm and the front of the thumb, the first two fingers and half the third finger, and the dorsal surfaces of the same three fingers.

This nerve is seldom involved alone. Paralysis results from injury and occasionally from neuritis. The signs are inability to pronate the forearm beyond the mid-position. The wrist can be flexed only toward the ulnar side; the thumb can not be opposed to the tips of fingers. The second phalanges can not be flexed on the first; the distal phalanges of the first and second fingers can not be flexed; but in the third and fourth fingers this action can be performed by the ulnar half of the flexor profundus. The loss of sensation is in the region corresponding to the sensory distribution already mentioned. The wasting of the thumb muscles, which is usually marked in this paralysis, gives to it a characteristic appearance.

LUMBAR AND SACRAL PLEXUSES

Lumbar Plexus.—The lumbar plexus is sometimes involved in growths of the lymph glands, in psoas abscess, and in disease of the bones of the vertebræ. When paralyzed the *obturator nerve* is occasionally injured during parturition. When paralyzed the power is lost over the abductors of the thigh and one leg can not be crossed over the other. Outward rotation is also disturbed. The *anterior crural nerve* is sometimes involved in wounds or in dislocation of the hip-joint, less commonly during parturition, and sometimes by disease of the bones and in psoas abscess. The special symptoms of affection of this nerve are paralysis of the extensors of the knee with wasting of the muscles, anæsthesia of the antero-lateral parts of the thigh and of the inner side of the leg to the big toe. This nerve is sometimes involved early in growths about the spine, and there may be pain in its area of distribution. Loss of the power of abducting the thigh results from paralysis of the *gluteal nerve*, which is distributed to the gluteus medius and minimus muscles.

External Cutaneous Nerve.—A peculiar form of sensory disturbance, confined to the territory of this nerve, was first described by Bernhardt in 1895, and a few months later by Roth, who gave it the name of *meralgia parœsthetica*. The disease is probably due to a neuritis which seems to originate in that part of the nerve where it passes under Poupart's ligament, just internal to the anterior superior iliac spine. The nerve is usually tender on pressure at this point. The disease is more common in men. Musser and Sailer in 1900 collected 99 cases, of which 75 were in men. A large number of the cases are attributable to direct traumatism or to simple pressure on the nerve by the aponeurotic canal through which it passes. Pregnancy is among the more common causes in women. The sensory disturbances consist of various forms of paræsthesia located over the outer side of the thigh, oftentimes with some actual diminution in the acuity of sense perception. The symptoms in varying intensity may persist for years, and the discomfort in some cases be so great, and so much exaggerated even by the mere touch of the clothing, that patients may be greatly incapacitated thereby. Excision of the nerve as it passes under Poupart's ligament has given good results.

Sacral Plexus.—The sacral plexus is frequently involved in tumors and inflammations within the pelvis and may be injured during parturition. Neuritis is common, usually an extension from the sciatic nerve.

Goldthwaite calls attention to the fact that the lumbo-sacral articulation varies very greatly in its stability, and actual displacement of the bones may result with separation of the posterior portion of the intervertebral disc. The cauda equina, or the nerve roots, may be compressed. With displacement on one side the spine is rotated and the articular process of the fifth is drawn into the spinal canal, with such narrowing that paraplegia may result, and he reports a remarkable case in which the paralysis came on during the application of a plaster jacket. Weakness of the joints or the partial displacements may cause irritation of the nerves inside and outside the canal with resulting bilateral sciatica.

Of the branches, the *sciatic nerve,* when injured at or near the notch, causes paralysis of the flexors of the legs and the muscles below the knee, but injury below the middle of the thigh involves only the latter muscles. There is also anæsthesia of the outer half of the leg, the sole, and the greater portion of the dorsum of the foot. Wasting of the muscles frequently follows, and there may be trophic disturbances. In paralysis of one sciatic the leg is fixed at the knee by the action of the quadriceps extensor and the patient is able to walk.

Paralysis of the *small sciatic nerve* is rarely seen. The gluteus maximus is involved and there may be difficulty in rising from a seat. There is a strip of anæsthesia along the back of the middle third of the thigh.

External Popliteal Nerve.—Paralysis involves the peronæi, the long extensor of the toes, tibialis anticus, and the extensor brevis digitorum. The ankle can not be flexed, resulting in a condition known as foot-drop, and as the toes can not be raised the whole leg must be lifted, producing the characteristic *steppage* gait seen in so many forms of peripheral neuritis. In long-standing cases the foot is permanently extended and there is wasting of the anterior tibial and peroneal muscles. The loss of sensation is in the outer half of the front of the leg and on the dorsum of the foot.

Internal Popliteal Nerve.—When paralyzed, plantar flexion of the foot and flexion of the toes are impossible. The foot can not be adducted, nor can the patient rise on tiptoe. In long standing cases talipes calcaneus follows and the toes assume a claw-like position from secondary contracture, due to over-extension of the proximal and flexion of the second and third phalanges.

SCIATICA

This is, as a rule, a neuritis either of the sciatic nerve or of its cords of origin. It may in some instances be a functional neurosis or neuralgia.

It occurs most commonly in adult males. A history of rheumatism or of gout is present in many cases. Exposure to cold, particularly after heavy muscular exertion, or a severe wetting are not uncommon causes. Within the pelvis the nerves may be compressed by large ovarian or uterine tumors, by lymphadenomata, by the fetal head during labor; occasionally lesions of the hip-joint induce a secondary sciatica. More commonly, however, the condition is due to chronic arthritis of the spinal column. The condition of the nerve has been examined in a few cases, and it has often been seen in the operation of stretching. It is, as a rule, swollen, reddened, and in a condition of interstitial neuritis. The affection may be most intense at the sciatic notch or in the nerve about the middle of the thigh.

Symptoms.—Of the symptoms, pain is the most constant and troublesome. The onset may be severe, with slight pyrexia, but, as a rule, it is gradual, and for a time there is only slight pain in the back of the thigh, particularly in certain positions or after exertion. Soon the pain becomes more intense and, instead of being limited to the upper portion of the nerve, extends down the thigh, reaching the foot and radiating over the entire distribution of the nerve. The patient can often point out the most sensitive spots, usually at the notch or in the middle of the thigh; and on pressure these are exquisitely painful. The pain is described as gnawing or burning, and is usually constant, but in some instances is paroxysmal, and often worse at night. On walking it may be very great; the knee is bent and the patient treads on the toes, so as to relieve the tension on the nerve. In protracted cases there may be much wasting of the muscles, but the reaction of degeneration can seldom be obtained. In these chronic cases cramp may occur and fibrillar contractions. Herpes may develop, but this is unusual. In rare instances the neuritis ascends and involves the spinal cord.

Duration and Course.—The duration and course are extremely variable. As a rule, it is an obstinate affection, lasting for months, or even, with slight remissions, for years. Relapses are not uncommon, and the disease may be relieved in one nerve only to appear in the other. In the severer forms the patient is bedridden, and such cases prove among the most distressing and trying which the physician is called upon to treat.

Diagnosis.—In the diagnosis it is important, in the first place, to determine whether the disease is primary, or secondary to some affection of the pelvis or of the spinal cord. A careful rectal examination should be made, and, in women, pelvic tumor should be excluded. Lumbago may be confounded with it. Affections of the hip-joint are easily distinguished by the absence of tenderness in the course of the nerve and the sense of pain on movement of the hip-joint or on pressure in the region of the trochanter. There are instances of sacro-iliac disease in which the patient complains of pain in the upper part of the thigh, which may sometimes radiate; but careful examination will readily distinguish between the affections. Pressure on the nerve trunks of the cauda equina, as a rule, causes bilateral pain and disturbances of sensation, and, as double sciatica is rare, these circumstances always suggest lesion of the nerve roots. Between the severe lightning pains of tabes and sciatica the differences are usually well defined. It is not to be forgotten that in a certain number of cases of so-called rheumatic sciatica the condition is a myositis, or, as Gowers calls it, a fibrositis. There is no tenderness along the course of the sciatic nerve, but there is pain in the gluteal region, with disability and Lasègue's sign, i. e., inability to extend the leg completely when the thigh is flexed on the abdomen.

Treatment.—The spinal column should be carefully and systematically examined, for numerous cases have been relieved by orthopædic procedures. The pelvic organs should also be investigated. Constitutional conditions, such as rheumatism and gout, should receive appropriate treatment. In a few cases with pronounced rheumatic history, which come on acutely with fever, the salicylates seem to do good. In other instances they are quite useless. If there is a suspicion of syphilis, the iodide of potassium should be employed, and in gouty cases salines.

Rest in bed with fixation of the limb by means of a long splint is a most valuable method of treatment in many cases, one upon which Weir Mitchell has specially insisted. I have known it to relieve, and in some instances to cure, obstinate and protracted cases which had resisted all other treatment. Hydrotherapy is sometimes satisfactory, particularly the warm baths or the mud baths. Many cases are relieved by a prolonged residence at one of the thermal springs. Antipyrin, antifebrin, and quinine are of doubtful benefit.

Local applications are more beneficial. The hot iron or the thermo-cautery or blisters relieve the pain temporarily. Deep injections into the nerves give great relief and may be necessary for the pain. It is best to use cocaine at first, in doses of from an eighth to a quarter of a grain (0.008 to 0.016 gm.). If the pain is unbearable morphia may be used, but it is a dangerous remedy in sciatica and should be withheld as long as possible. The disease is so protracted, so liable to relapse, and the patient's *morale* so undermined by the constant worry and the sleepless nights, that the danger of contracting the morphia habit is very great. On no consideration should the patient be permitted to use the hypodermic needle himself. It is remarkable how promptly, in some cases, the injection of distilled water into the nerve will relieve the pain. Acupuncture may also be tried; the needles should be thrust deeply into the most painful spot for a distance of about 2 inches, and left for from fifteen to twenty minutes. The injection of chloroform into the nerve has also been recommended.

Electricity is an uncertain remedy. Sometimes it gives prompt relief; in other cases it may be used for weeks without the slightest benefit. It is most serviceable in the chronic cases in which there is wasting of the legs, and should be combined with massage. The galvanic current should be used; a flat electrode should be placed over the sciatic notch, and a smaller one used along the course of the nerve and its branches. In very obstinate cases nerve-stretching may be employed. It is sometimes successful; but in other instances the condition recurs and is as bad as ever.

G. GENERAL AND FUNCTIONAL DISEASES

I. PARALYSIS AGITANS

(*Parkinson's Disease; Shaking Palsy*)

Definition.—A chronic affection of the nervous system, characterized by muscular weakness, tremors, and rigidity.

Etiology.—Men are more frequently affected than women. It rarely occurs under forty, but instances have been reported in which the disease began about the twentieth year. It is by no means an uncommon affection. Direct heredity is rare, but the patients often belong to families in which there are other nervous affections. Among exciting causes may be mentioned exposure to cold and wet, and business worries and anxieties. In some instances the disease has followed directly upon severe mental shock or trauma. Cases have been described after the specific fevers. Malaria is believed by some to be an important factor, but of this there is no satisfactory evidence.

Morbid Anatomy.—No constant lesions have been found. The similarity between certain of the features of Parkinson's disease and those of old age suggests that the affection may depend upon a premature senility of certain regions of the brain. Our organs do not age uniformly, but in some, owing to hereditary disposition, the process may be more rapid than in others. "Parkinson's disease has no characteristic lesions, but, on the other hand, it is not a neurosis. It has for anatomical basis the lesions of cerebro-spinal senility, which only differ from those of true senility in their early onset and greater intensity" (Dubief). The important changes are doubtless in the cerebral cortex. No special changes have been found in the organs of internal secretion.

Symptoms.—The disease begins gradually, usually in one or other hand, and the tremor may be either constant or intermittent. With this may be associated weakness or stiffness. At first these symptoms may be present only after exertion. Although the onset is slow and gradual in nearly all cases, there are instances in which it sets in abruptly after fright or trauma. When well established the disease is very characteristic, and the diagnosis can be made at a glance. The four prominent symptoms are tremor, weakness, rigidity, and the attitude.

TREMOR.—This may be in the four extremities or confined to hands or feet; the head is not so commonly affected. The tremor is usually marked in the hands, and the thumb and forefinger display the motion made in the act of rolling a pill. At the wrist there are movements of pronation and supination, and, though less marked, of flexion and extension. The upper-arm muscles are rarely involved. In the legs the movement is most evident at the ankle-joint, and less in the toes than in the fingers. Shaking of the head is less frequent, but does occur, and is usually vertical, not rotatory. The rate of oscillation is about five per second. Any emotion exaggerates the movement. The attempt at a voluntary movement may check the tremor (the patient may be able to thread a needle), but it returns with increased intensity. The tremors cease, as a rule, during sleep, but persist when the muscles are not in use. The writing of the patient is tremulous and zigzag.

WEAKNESS.—Loss of power is present in all cases, and may occur even before the tremor, but is not very striking, as tested by the dynamometer, until the late stages. The weakness is greatest where the tremor is most developed. The movements, too, are remarkably slow. There is rarely complete loss of power.

RIGIDITY may early be expressed in a slowness and stiffness in the voluntary movements, which are performed with some effort and difficulty, and all the actions of the patient are deliberate. This rigidity is in all the muscles, and leads ultimately to the characteristic attitude.

ATTITUDE AND GAIT.—The head is bent forward, the back is bowed, and the arms are held away from the body and are somewhat flexed at the elbow-joints. The face is expressionless, and the movements of the lips are slow.

The eyebrows are elevated, and the whole expression is immobile or mask-like, the so-called Parkinson's mask. The voice, as pointed out by Buzzard, is apt to be shrill and piping, and there is often a hesitancy in beginning a sentence; then the words are uttered with rapidity, as if the patient was in a hurry. This is sometimes in striking contrast to the scanning speech of insular sclerosis. The fingers are flexed and in the position assumed when the hand is at rest; in the late stages they can not be extended. Occasionally there is overextension of the terminal phalanges. The hand is usually turned toward the ulnar side and the attitude somewhat resembles that of advanced cases of rheumatoid arthritis. In the late stages there are contractures at the elbows, knees, and ankles. The movements of the patient are characterized by great deliberation. He rises from the chair slowly in the stooping attitude, with the head projecting forward. In attempting to walk the steps are short and hurried, and, as Trousseau remarks, he appears to be running after his centre of gravity. This is termed festination or propulsion, in contradistinction to a peculiar gait observed when the patient is pulled backward, when he makes a number of steps and would fall over if not prevented—retropulsion.

The REFLEXES are normal in most cases, but in a few they are exaggerated.

Of SENSORY disturbances Charcot has noted abnormal alterations in the temperature sense. The patient may complain of subjective sensations of heat, either general or local—a phenomenon which may be present on one side only and associated with an actual increase of the surface temperature, as much as 6° F. (Gowers). In other instances, patients complain of cold. Localized sweating may be present. The skin, especially of the forehead, may be thickened. The mental condition rarely shows any change.

VARIATIONS IN THE SYMPTOMS.—The tremor may be absent, but the rigidity, weakness, and attitude are sufficient to make the diagnosis. The disease may be hemiplegic in character, involving only one side or even one limb. Usually these are but stages of the disease.

Diagnosis.—In well developed cases the disease is recognized at a glance. The attitude, gait, stiffness, and mask-like expression are points of as much importance as the oscillations, and usually serve to separate the cases from senile and other forms of tremor. Disseminated sclerosis develops earlier, and is characterized by the nystagmus, and the scanning speech, and does not present the *attitude* so constant in paralysis agitans. Yet Schultze and Sachs have reported cases in which the signs of multiple sclerosis have been associated with those of paralysis. The hemiplegic form might be confounded with post-hemiplegic tremor, but the history, the mode of onset, and the greatly increased reflexes would be sufficient to distinguish the two. The Parkinsonian face is of great importance in the diagnosis of the obscure and anomalous forms.

The disease is incurable. Periods of improvement may occur, but the tendency is for the affection to proceed progressively downward. It is a slow, degenerative process and the cases last for years.

Treatment.—There is no method which can be recommended as satisfactory in any respect. Arsenic, opium, hyoscine, and the extract of the parathyroid gland may be tried and sometimes give relief, but are not curative. The friends should be told frankly that the disease is incurable, and that nothing can be done except to attend to the physical comforts of the patient. Regulated and systematized exercises should be carried out.

OTHER FORMS OF TREMOR

Simple Tremor.—This is occasionally found in persons in whom it is impossible to assign any cause. It may be transient or persist for an indefinite time. It is often extremely slight, and is aggravated by all causes which lower the vitality.

Hereditary Tremor.—C. L. Dana has reported remarkable cases of hereditary tremor. It occurred in all the members of one family, and beginning in infancy continued without producing any serious changes.

Senile Tremor.—With advancing age tremulousness during muscular movements is extremely common, but is rarely seen under seventy. It is always a fine tremor, which begins in the hands and often extends to the muscles of the neck, causing slight movement of the head.

Toxic tremor is seen chiefly as an effect of tobacco, alcohol, lead, or mercury; more rarely in arsenical or opium poisoning. In elderly men who smoke much it may be entirely due to the tobacco. One of the commonest forms of this is the alcoholic tremor, which occurs only on movement and has considerable range. Lead tremor is considered under lead poisoning, of which it constitutes a very important symptom.

Hysterical tremor, which usually occurs under circumstances which make the diagnosis easy, will be considered in the section on hysteria.

II. ACUTE CHOREA

(Sydenham's Chorea; St. Vitus's Dance)

Definition.—A disease chiefly affecting children, characterized by irregular, involuntary contraction of the muscles, a variable amount of psychical disturbance, and a remarkable liability to acute endocarditis.

Etiology.—Sex.—Of 554 cases which I analyzed from the Philadelphia Infirmary for Diseases of the Nervous System, 71 per cent. were in females and 29 per cent. in males. Of 808 Johns Hopkins Hospital cases, 71.2 per cent. were females (Thayer and Thomas).

Age.—The disease is most common between the ages of five and fifteen. Of 522 cases, 380 occurred in this period; 84.5 per cent. in Thayer and Thomas' series. It is rare among the negroes and native races of America. Only 25 of the Johns Hopkins Hospital cases were in negroes. The cases are most numerous when the mean relative humidity is excessive and the barometric pressure low (Lewis).

Rheumatism.—A casual relationship between rheumatism and chorea has been claimed by many since the time of Bright. The English and French writers maintain the closeness of this connection; on the other hand, German authors, as a rule, regard the connection as by no means very close. Of the 554 cases, in 15.5 per cent. there was a history of rheumatism in the family. In 88 cases, 15.8 per cent., there was a history of articular swelling, acute or subacute. In 33 cases there were pains, sometimes described as rheumatic, in various parts, but not associated with joint trouble. Adding these to those with manifest articular trouble, the percentage is raised to nearly 21. It is rather remarkable that in our Baltimore series the percentage with a history of rheumatism was the same—21.6.

We find two groups of cases in which acute arthritis is present in chorea. In one, the arthritis antedates by some months or years the onset of the chorea, and does not recur before or during the attack. In the other group, the chorea sets in with or follows immediately upon the acute arthritis. In some instances it is impossible to decide whether the joint symptoms or the movements have appeared first. It is difficult to differentiate the cases of irregular pains without definite joint affection. It is probable that many of them are rheumatic, and yet I think it would be a mistake to regard as such all cases in children in which there are complaints of vague pains in the bones or muscles—so-called growing pains. It should never be forgotten, however, that a slight articular swelling may be the sole manifestation of rheumatic fever in a child—so slight, indeed, that the disease may be entirely overlooked.

Heart-disease.—Endocarditis is believed by some writers to be the cause of the disease. The particles of fibrin and vegetations from the valves pass as emboli to the cerebral vessels. On this view, which we shall discuss later, chorea is the result of an embolic process occurring in the course of a rheumatic endocarditis.

Infectious Diseases.—Scarlet fever with arthritic manifestations may be a direct antecedent. Sturges states that a history of previous whooping-cough occurs more frequently in choreic than in other children, but I find no evidence of this in the Infirmary records. With the exception of rheumatic fever, there is no intimate relationship between chorea and the acute diseases incident to childhood. It may be noted in contrast to this that the so-called canine chorea is a common sequel of distemper. Chorea has been known to develop in the course of an acute pyæmia, and to follow gonorrhœa and puerperal fever.

Anæmia is less often an antecedent than a sequence of chorea, and though cases develop in children who are anæmic and in poor health, this is by no means the rule. Chorea may develop in chlorotic girls at puberty.

Pregnancy.—A choreic patient may become pregnant; more frequently the disease occurs during pregnancy; sometimes it develops post partum. Buist, of Dundee, has tabulated carefully 226 cases: in 6 the chorea preceded the pregnancy; in 105 it occurred during the pregnancy; in 31 in recurrent pregnancies; 45 cases terminated fatally, and in 16 cases the chorea developed post partum. The alleged frequency in illegitimate primiparæ is not borne out by his figures. Beginning in the first three months were 108 cases, in the second three months 70 cases, in the last three months 25 cases. The disease is often severe, and maniacal symptoms may develop.

A tendency to the disease is found in certain families. In 80 cases there was a history of attacks of chorea in other members. In one instance both mother and grandmother had been affected. High-strung, excitable, nervous children are especially liable to the disease. *Fright* is considered a frequent cause, but in a large majority of the cases no close connection exists between the fright and the onset of the disease. Occasionally the attack sets in at once. Mental worry, trouble, a sudden grief, or a scolding may apparently be the exciting cause. The strain of *education,* particularly in girls during the third hemidecade, is a most important factor in the etiology of the disease. Bright, intelligent, active minded girls from ten to fourteen, ambitious to do well at school, often stimulated in their efforts by teachers and parents, form a large contingent of the cases of chorea in hospital and private practice. Sturges has called special attention to this *school-made* chorea as one serious evil in our modern method of forced education. *Imitation,* which is mentioned as an exciting cause, is extremely rare, and does not appear to have influenced the onset in a single case in the Infirmary records.

The disease may rapidly follow an injury or a slight surgical operation. Reflex irritation was believed to play an important rôle in the disease, particularly the presence of worms or genital irritation; but I have met with no instance in which the disease could be attributed to either of these causes. Local spasm, particularly of the face—the habit chorea of Mitchell—may be associated with irritation in the nostrils and adenoid growths in the vault of the pharynx, as pointed out by Jacobi.

It has been claimed by Stevens that *ocular defects* lie at the basis of many cases of chorea, and that with the correction of these the irregular movements disappear. The investigations of De Schweinitz show that ocular defects do not occur in greater proportion in choreic than in other children. A majority of the cases in which operation has been followed by relief have been instances of *tic,* local or general.

Morbid Anatomy and Pathology.—No constant lesions have been found in the nervous system in acute chorea. Vascular changes, such as hyaline transformation, exudation of leucocytes, minute hæmorrhages, and thrombosis of the smaller arteries, have been described.

Embolism of the smaller cerebral vessels has been found, and there are on record 7 cases of embolism of the central artery of the retina (H. M. Thomas). Based on the presence of emboli, Kirkes and others have supported what is known as the embolic theory of the disease. Endocarditis is by far the most frequent lesion in Sydenham's chorea. With no disease, not excepting rheumatism, is it so constantly associated. I collected from the literature the records of 73 autopsies; there were 62 with endocarditis.* The endocarditis is usually of the simple variety, but the ulcerative form has occasionally been described.

We are still far from a solution of all the problems connected with chorea. Unfortunately, the word has been used to cover a series of totally diverse disorders of movement, so that there are still excellent observers who hold that chorea is only a symptom, and is not to be regarded as an etiological unit. The chorea of childhood, the disease which Sydenham described, presents, however, characteristics so unmistakable that it must be regarded as a definite, substantive affection. Some regard it as *a functional brain disorder* affecting the nerve centres controlling the motor apparatus, an instability of the nerve cells, brought about, one supposes by hyperæmia, another by anæmia, a third by psychical influences, a fourth by irritation, central or peripheral. Of the actual nature of this derangement we know nothing, nor, indeed, whether the changes

---

* Osler, "Chorea and Choreiform Affections."

are primary and the result of a faulty action of the cortical cells or whether the impulses are secondarily disturbed in their course down the motor path. The predominance of the disease in females, and its onset at a time when the education of the brain is rapidly developing, are etiological facts which Sturges has urged in favor of the view that chorea is an expression of functional instability of the nerve centres.

The *embolic theory* originally advanced by Kirkes has a solid basis of fact, but it is not comprehensive enough, as all of the cases can not be brought within its limits. There are instances without endocarditis and without, so far as can be ascertained, plugging of cerebral vessels; and there are also cases with extensive endocarditis in which the histological examination of the brain, so far as embolism is concerned, was negative. In favor of the embolic view is the experimental production in animals of chorea by Rosenthal, and later by Money, by injecting fine particles into the carotids.

Lately, as indeed might be expected, chorea has been regarded as an *infectious disease.* Nothing definite has yet been determined. In favor of this view it has been urged, as it is impossible to refer the chorea to endocarditis or the endocarditis in all cases to rheumatism, that both have their origin in a common cause, some infectious agent, which is capable also, in persons predisposed, of exciting articular disease. Cases have been reported in scarlet fever with arthritic manifestations, in puerperal fever, and rheumatism, also after gonorrhœa, and such facts are suggestive at least of the association of the disease with infective processes. Possibly, as has been suggested by some writers, the paralytic condition associated with chorea may be analogous to those which occur in typhoid and certain of the infectious diseases. On the other hand, there are conditions extremely difficult to harmonize with this view. The prominent psychical element is certainly one of the most serious objections, since there can be no doubt that ordinary chorea may rapidly follow a fright or a sudden emotion.

Symptoms.—Three groups of cases may be recognized—the mild, severe, and maniacal chorea.

Mild Chorea.—In this the affection of the muscles is slight, the speech is not seriously disturbed, and the general health not impaired. Premonitory symptoms are shown in restlessness and inability to sit still, a condition well characterized by the term "fidgets." There are emotional disturbances, such as crying spells, or sometimes night terrors. There may be pains in the limbs and headache. Digestive disturbances and anæmia may be present. A change in the temperament is frequently noticed, and a docile, quiet child may become cross and irritable. After these symptoms have persisted for a week or more the characteristic involuntary movements begin, and are often first noticed at the table, when the child spills a tumbler of water or upsets a plate. There may be only awkwardness or slight incoördination of voluntary movements, or constant irregular clonic spasms. The jerky, irregular character of the movements differentiates them from almost every other disorder of motion. In the mild cases only one hand, or the hand and face, are affected, and it may not spread to the other side.

In the second grade, the *severe form,* the movements become general and the patient may be unable to get about or to feed or undress herself, owing to the constant, irregular, clonic contractions of the various muscle groups

The speech is also affected, and for days the child may not be able to talk. Often with the onset of the severer symptoms there is loss of power on one side or in the limb most affected.

The third and most extreme form, the so-called maniacal chorea, or *chorea insaniens,* is truly a terrible disease, and may develop out of the ordinary form. These cases are more common in adult women and may develop during pregnancy.

Chorea begins, as a rule, in the hands and arms, then involves the face, and subsequently the legs. The movements may be confined to one side—hemichorea. The attack begins oftenest on the right side, though occasionally it is general from the outset. One arm and the opposite leg may be involved. In nearly one-fourth of the cases speech is affected; this may amount only to an embarrassment or hesitancy, but in other instances it becomes an incoherent jumble. In very severe cases the child will make no attempt to speak. The inability is in articulation rather than in phonation. Paroxysms of panting and of hard expiration may occur, or odd sounds may be produced. As a rule the movements cease during sleep.

Paralysis.—A prominent symptom is muscular weakness, usually no more than a condition of paresis. The loss of power is slight, but the weakness may be shown by an enfeebled grip or by a dragging of the leg or limping. In his original account Sydenham refers to the "unsteady movements of one of the legs, which the patient drags." There may be extreme paresis with but few movements—the paralytic chorea of Todd. Occasionally a local paralysis or weakness remains after the attack.

Mutism is an interesting feature; for weeks the child may not say a word. It is more common in severe cases, but is not marked by special choreic unrest of the muscles of speech; it is probably a motor weakness. Complete recovery follows.

It is doubtful whether choreic spasms extend to the muscles of organic life. The rapid action and disturbed rhythm of the heart present nothing peculiar to the disease, and there is no support for the view that irregular contractions occur in the papillary muscles.

HEART SYMPTOMS.—*Neurotic.*—As so many of the subjects of chorea are nervous girls, it is not surprising that a common symptom is a rapidly acting heart. Irregularity is not so special a feature in chorea as rapidity. The patients seldom complain of pain about the heart.

Hæmic Murmurs.—With anæmia and debility, not uncommon associates of chorea in the third or fourth week, we find a corresponding cardiac condition. The impulse is diffuse, perhaps wavy in thin children. The carotids throb visibly, and in the recumbent posture there may be pulsation in the cervical veins. On auscultation a systolic murmur is heard at the base, perhaps, too, at the apex, soft and blowing in quality.

Endocarditis.—As in rheumatism, so in chorea, acute valvulitis rarely gives evidence of its presence by symptoms. It must be sought, and clinical experience has shown that it is usually associated with murmurs at one or other of the cardiac orifices.

For the guidance of the practitioner these statements may be made:

(*a*) In thin, nervous children a systolic murmur of soft quality is extremely common at the base, with accentuation of the second sound, particularly at the second left costal cartilage, and is probably of no moment.

(*b*) A systolic murmur of maximum intensity at the apex, and heard also along the left sternal margin, is not uncommon in anæmic, enfeebled states, and does not necessarily indicate either endocarditis or insufficiency.

(*c*) A murmur of maximum intensity at the apex, with rough quality, and transmitted to the axilla or angle of the scapula, indicates an organic lesion of the mitral valve, and is usually associated with enlargement of the heart.

(*d*) When in doubt it is much safer to trust to the evidence of eye and hand than to that of the ear. If the apex beat is in the normal position, and the area of dulness not increased vertically or to the right of the sternum, there is probably no serious valvular disease.

(*e*) The endocarditis of chorea is almost invariably of the simple or warty form, and in itself is not dangerous; but it is apt to lead to those sclerotic changes in the valve which produce incompetency. Of 140 patients examined more than two years after the attack, I found the heart normal in 51; in 17 there was functional disturbance, and 72 presented signs of organic heart-disease.

(*f*) Pericarditis is an occasional complication of chorea, usually in cases with well-marked rheumatism.

In an analysis of the cases at the Johns Hopkins Hospital, Thayer found evidence of involvement of the heart in 25 per cent. of the out-patients and in more than 50 per cent. of the cases in the wards. Cardiac involvement was more common in the cases with a history of rheumatism, and was much more frequent in the relapses.

SENSORY DISTURBANCES.—Pain in the affected limbs is not common. Occasionally there is soreness on pressure. There are cases, usually of hemichorea, in which pain in the limbs is a marked symptom. Weir Mitchell has spoken of these as *painful choreas.* Tender points along the lines of emergence of the spinal nerves or along the course of the nerves of the limbs are rare.

PSYCHICAL DISTURBANCES are common, though in a majority of the cases slight in degree. Irritability of temper, marked wilfulness, and emotional outbreaks may indicate a complete change in the character of the child. There is deficiency in the powers of concentration, the memory is enfeebled, and the aptitude for study is lost. Rarely there is progressive impairment of the intellect with termination in actual dementia. Acute melancholia has been described. Hallucinations of sight and hearing may occur. Patients may behave in an odd and strange manner and do all sorts of meaningless acts. By far the most serious manifestation of this character is the maniacal delirium, occasionally associated with the very severe cases—*chorea insaniens.* Usually the motor disturbance in these cases is aggravated, but it has been overlooked and patients have been sent to an asylum.

The psychical element in chorea is apt to be neglected by the practitioner. It is always a good plan to tell the parents that it is not the muscles alone of the child which are affected, but that the general irritability and change of disposition, so often found, really form part of the disease.

The condition of the REFLEXES in chorea is usually normal. Trophic lesions rarely occur in chorea unless, as some writers have done, we regard the joint troubles as arthropathies occurring in the course of a cerebro-spinal disease.

Fever, usually slight, was present in all but one of 110 cases treated in my wards (Thayer). H. A. Hare states that in monochorea the temperature on the affected side may be elevated; but this is not an invariable rule. Endocarditis may occur with little if any rise in temperature; but, on the other hand, with an acute arthritis, severe endocarditis or pericarditis, and in the cases of maniacal chorea, the fever may range from 102° to 104°.

Cutaneous Affections.—The pigmentation, which is not uncommon, is due to the arsenic. Herpes zoster occasionally occurs. Certain skin eruptions, usually regarded as rheumatic in character, are not uncommon. Erythema nodosum has been described and I have seen several cases with a purpuric urticaria. There may, indeed, be the more aggravated condition of rheumatic purpura, known as Schönlein's *peliosis rheumatica.* Subcutaneous fibrous nodules, which have been noted by English observers in many cases of chorea, associated with rheumatism, are extremely rare in the United States.

Duration and Termination.—From eight to ten weeks is the average duration of an attack of moderate severity. Chronic chorea rarely follows the minor disease which we have been considering. The cases described under this designation in children are usually instances of cerebral sclerosis or Friedreich's ataxia; but occasionally an attack which has come on in the ordinary way persists for months or years, and recovery ultimately takes place. A slight grade of chorea, particularly noticeable under excitement, may persist for months in nervous children.

The tendency of chorea to recur has been noticed by all writers since Sydenham first made the observation. Of 410 cases analyzed for this purpose, 240 had one attack, 110 had two attacks, 35 three attacks, 10 four attacks, 12 five attacks, and 3 six attacks. The recurrence is apt to be vernal.

Recovery is the rule in children. The statistics of out-patient departments are not favorable for determining the mortality. A reliable estimate is that of the Collective Investigation Committee of the British Medical Association, in which 9 deaths were reported among 439 cases, about 2 per cent.

The paralysis rarely persists. Mental dulness may be present for a time, but usually passes away; permanent impairment of the mind is an exceptional sequence.

Diagnosis.—There are few diseases which present more characteristic features, and in a majority of instances the nature of the trouble is recognized at a glance; but there are several affections in children which may simulate and be mistaken for it.

(*a*) *Multiple and diffuse cerebral sclerosis.* The cases are often mistaken for ordinary chorea, and have been described in the literature as *chorea spastica.* There are doubtless chronic changes in the cortex. As a rule, the movements are readily distinguishable from those of true chorea, but the simulation is sometimes very close; the onset in infancy, the impaired intelligence, increased reflexes and in some instances rigidity, and the chronic course of the disease separate them sharply from true chorea.

(*b*) *Friedreich's ataxia.* Cases of this well-characterized disease were formerly classed as chorea. The slow, irregular, incoördinate movements, the scoliosis, the scanning speech, the early talipes, the nystagmus, and the family character of the disease are points which should render the diagnosis easy.

(*c*) In rare cases the paralytic form of chorea may be mistaken for *polio-*

myelitis or, when both legs are affected, for paraplegia of spinal origin; but this can be the case only when the choreic movements are very slight.

(*d*) *Hysteria* may simulate chorea minor most closely, and unless there are other manifestations it may be impossible to make a diagnosis. Most commonly, however, the movements in the so-called hysterical chorea are rhythmic and differ entirely from those of ordinary chorea.

(*e*) As mentioned above, the *mental symptoms* in maniacal chorea may mask the true nature of the disease and patients have even been sent to the asylum.

Treatment.—Abnormally bright, active minded children belonging to families with pronounced neurotic taint should be carefully watched from the ages of eight to fifteen and not allowed to overtax their mental powers. So frequently in children of this class does the attack of chorea date from the worry and stress incident to school examinations that the competition for prizes or places should be emphatically forbidden.

The treatment of the attack consists largely in attention to hygienic measures, with which alone, in time, a majority of the cases recover. Parents should be told to scan gently the faults and waywardness of choreic children. The psychical element, strongly developed in so many cases, is best treated by quiet and seclusion. The child should be confined to bed in the recumbent posture, and mental as well as bodily quiet enjoined. In private practice this is often impossible, but with well-to-do patients the disease is always serious enough to demand the assistance of a skilled nurse. Toys and dolls should not be allowed at first, for the child should be kept amused without excitement. The rest allays the hyper-excitability and reduces to a minimum the possibility of damage to the valve segments should endocarditis exist. Time and again have I seen very severe cases which had resisted treatment for weeks outside a hospital become quite and the movements subside after two or three days of absolute rest in bed.

The child should be kept apart from other children and, if possible, from other members of the family, and should see only those persons directly concerned with the nursing of the case. In the latter period of the disease daily rubbings may be resorted to with great benefit.

The medical treatment of the disease is unsatisfactory; with the exception of arsenic, no remedy seems to have any influence in controlling the progress of the affection. Without any specific action, it certainly does good in many cases, probably by improving the general nutrition. It is conveniently given in the form of Fowler's solution, and the good effects are rarely seen until maximum doses are taken. It may be given as Martin originally advised (1813); he began "with five drops and increased one drop every day, until it might begin to disagree with the stomach or bowels." When the dose of 15 minims is reached, it may be continued for a week, and then again increased, if necessary, every day or two, until physiological effects are manifest. On the occurrence of these the drug should be stopped for three or four days. The practice of resuming the administration with smaller doses is rarely necessary, as tolerance is usually established and we can begin with the dose which the child was taking when the symptoms of saturation occurred. I have frequently given as much as 25 minims three times a day. Usually the signs of saturation are trivial but plain, but in very rare instances more serious symptoms develop. A fatal arsenical neuritis followed in the case of a child, aged eight, who took seven drops of Fowler's solution three times a day for ten days, then stopped for a week, and then took seven drops three times a day for fourteen days (Cary Gamble).

Of other medicines sedatives are useful in the severe attacks. Chloral is the most useful and may be begun in doses of five grains (0.3 gm.), gradually increased if necessary. Sodium bromide in the same dosage may be added. Belladonna has been found useful in some cases.

For its tonic effect electricity is sometimes useful; but it is not necessary as a routine treatment. The question of gymnastics is an important one. Early in the disease, when the movements are active, they are not advisable; but during convalescence carefully graduated exercises are undoubtedly beneficial. It is not well, however, to send a choreic child to a school gymnasium, as the stimulus of the other children and the excitement of the romping, violent play are very prejudicial.

Other points in treatment may be mentioned. Food should be simple and some children do best on a milk diet, the amount being rapidly increased. It is important to regulate the bowels and to attend carefully to the digestive functions. For the anæmia so often present preparations of iron are indicated.

In the severe cases with incessant movements, sleeplessness, dry tongue, and delirium, the important indication is to procure rest, for which purpose chloral may be freely given, and, if necessary, morphia. Chloroform inhalations may be necessary to control the intensity of the paroxysms, but the high rate of mortality in this class of cases illustrates how often our best endeavors are fruitless. The wet pack is sometimes very soothing and should be tried. As these patients are apt to sink rapidly into a low typhoid state with heart weakness, a supporting treatment is required from the outset.

Cases are found now and then which drag on from month to month without getting either better or worse and resist all mòdes of treatment. In such cases a combination of suggestion and passive movements, followed by voluntary movements under control, and later simple exercises, may be useful. Change of air and scene is sometimes followed by rapid improvement, and in these cases the treatment by rest and seclusion should always be given a full trial.

In all cases care should be taken to examine the nostrils, and glaring ocular defects should be properly corrected either by glasses or, if necessary, by operation.

After the child has recovered from the attack, the parents should be warned that return of the disease is by no means infrequent, and is particularly liable to follow overwork at school or debilitating influences of any kind. These relapses are apt to occur in the spring. Sydenham advised purging in order to prevent the vernal recurrence of the disease.

III. OTHER AFFECTIONS DESCRIBED AS CHOREA

Chorea Major: Pandemic Chorea.—The common name, St. Vitus's dance, applied to chorea has come to us from the middle ages, when under the influence of religious fervor there were epidemics characterized by great excitement, gesticulations, and dancing. For the relief of these symptoms, when excessive, pilgrimages were made, and, in the Rhenish provinces, particularly to the Chapel of St. Vitus in Zebern. Epidemics of this sort occurred also during the nineteenth century, and descriptions of them among the early settlers in Kentucky have been given by Robertson and Yandell. It was unfortunate that Sydenham applied the term chorea to an affection in children totally distinct from this chorea major, which is in reality an hysterical manifestation under the influence of religious excitement.

Habit Spasm (*Habit Chorea*); **Convulsive Tic** (of the French).—Two groups of cases may be recognized under the designation of habit spasm—one in which there are simply localized spasmodic movements, and the other in which, in addition to this, there are explosive utterances and psychical symptoms, a condition to which French writers have given the name *tic convulsif*.

(*a*) HABIT SPASM.—This is found chiefly in childhood, most frequently in girls from seven to fourteen years of age (Mitchell). In its simplest form there is a sudden, quick contraction of certain of the facial muscles, such as rapid winking or drawing of the mouth to one side, or the neck muscles are involved and there are unilateral movements of the head. The head is given a sudden, quick shake, and at the same time the eyes wink. A not infrequent form is the shrugging of one shoulder. The grimace or movement is repeated at irregular intervals, and is much aggravated by emotion. A short inspiratory sniff is not an uncommon symptom. The cases are found most frequently in children who are "out of sorts," or who have been growing rapidly, or who have inherited a tendency to neurotic disorders. Allied to or associated with this are some of the curious tricks of children. A boy at my clinic was in the habit every few moments of putting the middle finger into the mouth, biting it, and at the same time pressing his nose with the forefinger. Hartley Coleridge is said to have had a somewhat similar trick, only he bit his arm. In all these cases the habits of the child should be examined carefully, the nose and vault of the pharynx thoroughly inspected, and the eyes accurately tested. As a rule the condition is transient, and after persisting for a few months or longer gradually disappears. Occasionally a local spasm persists—twitching of the eyelids, or the facial grimace.

(*b*) IMPULSIVE TIC (GILLES DE LA TOURETTE'S DISEASE).—This remarkable affection, often mistaken for chorea, more frequently for habit spasm, is really a psychosis allied to hysteria, though in certain of its aspects it has the features of monomania. The disease begins, as a rule, in young children, occurring as early as the sixth year, though it may develop after puberty. There is usually a markedly neurotic family history. The special features of the complaint are:

(1) Involuntary muscular movements, usually affecting the facial or brachial muscles, but in aggravated cases all the muscles of the body may be involved and the movements may be extremely irregular and violent.

(2) Explosive utterances, which may resemble a bark or an inarticulate cry. A word heard may be mimicked at once and repeated over and over again, usually with the involuntary movements. To this the term *echolalia* has been applied. A much more distressing disturbance in these cases is *coprolalia,* or the use of bad language. A child of eight or ten may shock its

mother and friends by constantly using the word *damn* when making the involuntary movements, or by uttering all sorts of obscene words. Occasionally actions are mimicked—*echokinesis.*

(3) Associated with some of these cases are curious mental disturbances; the patient becomes the subject of a form of obsession or a fixed idea. In other cases the fixed idea takes the form of the impulse to touch objects, or it is a fixed idea about words—onomatomania—or the patient may feel compelled to count a number of times before doing certain actions—arithmomania.

The disease is well marked and readily distinguished from ordinary chorea. The movements have a larger range and are explosive in character. Tourette regards the coprolalia as the most distinctive feature of the disease. The prognosis is doubtful. I have, however, known recovery to follow.

Saltatory Spasm (*Latah; Myriachit; Jumpers*).—Bamberger has described a disease in which when the patient attempted to stand there were strong contractions in the leg muscles, which caused a jumping or springing motion. This occurs only when the patient attempts to stand. The affection has occurred in both men and women, more frequently in the former, and the subjects have usually shown marked neurotic tendencies. In many cases the condition has been transitory; in others it has persisted for years. Remarkable affections similar to this in certain points occur as a sort of epidemic neurosis. One of the most striking of these occurs among the "jumping Frenchmen" of Maine and Canada. As described by Beard and Thornton, the subjects are liable on any sudden emotion to jump violently and utter a loud cry or sound, and will obey any command or imitate any action without regard to its nature. The condition of echolalia is present in a marked degree. The "jumping" prevails in certain families.

A very similar disease prevails in parts of Russia and in Java and Borneo, where it is known by the names of myriachit and latah, the chief feature of which is mimicry by the patient of everything he sees or hears.

Chronic Chorea (*Huntington's Chorea*).—This is an affection characterized by irregular movements, disturbance of speech, and gradual dementia. It is frequently hereditary. Irving W. Lyon described it in 1863 as *chronic hereditary chorea* and traced the disease through five generations. Huntington, of Pomeroy, Ohio, at the time a practitioner on Long Island, gave, in 1872, in three brief paragraphs the salient points in connection with the disease—namely, the hereditary nature, the association with psychical troubles, and the late onset—between the thirtieth and fortieth years. The disease is not uncommon in the United States. Under the term chronic chorea may be grouped the hereditary form and the cases which come on without family disposition, either at middle life or, more commonly, in the aged—senile chorea. It is doubtful whether the cases in children with chronic choreiform movements, often with mental weakness and spastic condition of the legs, should go into this category.

The hereditary character of the disease is very striking; it has been traced through four or five generations. Huntington's father and grandfather, also physicians, had treated the disease in the family which he described. Osborn, of East Hampton, tells me that the disease still continues to recur in certain families described by Huntington, as it has done, so it is said, for fully two centuries. An identical affection occurs without any hereditary disposition. The age of onset is late, rarely before the thirtieth or the thirty-fifth year.

The symptoms are very characteristic. The irregular movements are usually first seen in the hands, and the patient has slight difficulty in performing delicate manipulations or in writing. When well established the movements are disorderly, irregular, incoördinate rather than choreic, and have not the sharp, brusque motion of Sydenham's chorea. In the face there are slow, involuntary grimaces. In a well-developed case the gait is irregular, swaying, and somewhat like that of a drunken man. The speech is slow and difficult the syllables are badly pronounced and indistinct, but not definitely staccato. The mental impairment leads finally to dementia. The anatomical condition is a chronic diffuse cortical encephalitis not unlike that in general paralysis.

Rhythmic or Hysterical Chorea.—This is readily recognized by the rhythmical character of the movements. It may affect the muscles of the abdomen, producing the salaam convulsion, or involve the sterno-mastoid, producing a rhythmical movement of the head, or the psoas, or any group of muscles. In its orderly rhythm it resembles the canine chorea.

IV. INFANTILE CONVULSIONS

(*Eclampsia*)

Convulsive seizures similar to those of epilepsy are not infrequent in children and in adults. The fit may indeed be identical with epilepsy, from which the condition differs in that when the cause is removed there is no tendency for the fits to recur. Occasionally, however, the convulsions in children continue and develop into true epilepsy.

Etiology.—A convulsion in a child may be due to many causes, all of which lead to an unstable condition of the nerve centres, permitting sudden, excessive, and temporary nervous discharges. The following are the most important of them:

(1) *Debility,* resulting usually from gastro-intestinal disturbance. Convulsions frequently supervene toward the close of an attack of entero-colitis and recur, sometimes proving fatal. The death-rate in children from eclampsia rises steadily with that of gastro-intestinal disorders (Morris J. Lewis).

(2) *Peripheral Irritation.*—Dentition alone is rarely a cause of convulsions, but is often one of several factors in a feeble, unhealthy infant. The greatest mortality from convulsions is during the first six months, before the teeth have really cut through the gums. Other irritative causes are the overloading of the stomach with indigestible food. It has been suggested that some of these cases are toxic, owing to the absorption of poisonous ptomaines. Worms, to which convulsions are so frequently attributed, probably have little influence. Among other sources possible are phimosis and otitis.

(3) *Rickets.*—The observation of Sir William Jenner upon the association of rickets and convulsions has been amply confirmed. The spasms may be laryngeal, the so-called child-crowing, which, though convulsive in nature, can scarcely be reckoned under eclampsia. The influence of this condition is more apparent in Europe than in the United States, although rickets is a com-

mon disease, particularly among the colored people. Spasms, local or general, in rickets are probably associated with the condition of debility and malnutrition and with cranio-tabes.

(4) *Fever.*—In young children the onset of the infectious diseases is frequently with convulsions, which often take the place of a chill in the adult. It is not known upon what they depend. Scarlet fever, measles, and pneumonia are most often preceded by convulsions.

(5) *Congestion of the Brain.*—That extreme engorgement of the blood-vessels may produce convulsions is shown by their occasional occurrence in severe whooping-cough, but their rarity in this disease really indicates how small a part mechanical congestion plays in the production of fits.

(6) *Severe convulsions* usher in or accompany many of the serious diseases of the nervous system in children. In more than 50 per cent. of the cases of infantile hemiplegia the affection follows severe convulsions. They less frequently precede a spinal paralysis. They occur with meningitis, tuberculous or simple, and with tumors and other lesions of the brain.

And, lastly, convulsions may occur immediately after birth and persist for weeks or months. In such instances there has probably been meningeal hæmorrhage or serious injury to the cortex.

The most important question is the relation of convulsions in children to true epilepsy. In Gowers' figures of 1,450 cases of epilepsy, the attacks began in 180 during the first three years of life. Of 460 cases of epilepsy in children which I have analyzed, in 187 the fits began within the first three years. Of the total list the greatest number, 74, was in the first year. In nearly all these instances there was no interruption in the convulsions. That convulsions in early infancy are necessarily followed by epilepsy in after life is certainly a mistake.

Symptoms.—The attack may come on suddenly without any warning; more commonly it is preceded by a stage of restlessness, accompanied by twitching and perhaps grinding of the teeth. It is rarely so complete in its stages as true epilepsy. The spasm begins usually in the hands, most commonly in the right hand. The eyes are fixed and staring or are rolled up. The body becomes stiff and breathing is suspended for a moment or two by tonic spasm of the respiratory muscles, in consequence of which the face becomes congested. Clonic convulsions follow, the eyes are rolled about, the hands and arms twitch, or are fixed and extended in rhythmical movements, the face is contorted, and the head is retracted. The attack gradually subsides and the child sleeps or passes into a state of stupor. Following indigestion the attack may be single, but in rickets and intestinal disorders it is apt to be repeated. Sometimes the attacks follow each other with great rapidity, so that the child never rouses but dies in a deep coma. If the convulsion has been limited chiefly to one side there may be slight paresis after recovery, or in instances in which the convulsions usher in infantile hemiplegia, when the child arouses, one side is completely paralyzed. During the fit the temperature is often raised. Death rarely occurs from the convulsion itself, except in debilitated children or when the attacks recur with great frequency. In the so-called hydrocephaloid state in connection with protracted diarrhœa convulsions may close the scene.

Diagnosis.—Coming on when the subject is in full health, the attack is probably due either to an overloaded stomach, to some peripheral irritation, or occasionally to trauma. Setting in with high fever and vomiting, it may indicate the onset of an exanthem, or occasionally be the primary symptom of encephalitis, or whatever the condition is which causes infantile hemiplegia. When the attack is associated with debility and with rickets the diagnosis is easily made. The carpopedal spasms and pseudo-paralytic rigidity which are often associated with rickets, laryngismus stridulus, and the hydrocephaloid state are usually confined to the hands and arms and are intermittent and usually tonic. The convulsions associated with tumor or those which follow infantile hemiplegia are usually at first Jacksonian in character. After the second year convulsive seizures which come on irregularly without apparent cause and recur while the child is apparently in good health, are likely to prove true epilepsy.

Prognosis.—Convulsions play an important part in infantile mortality. In Morris J. Lewis's table of deaths in children under ten, 8.5 per cent. were ascribed to convulsions. In chronic diarrhœa convulsions are usually of ill omen. Those ushering in fevers are rarely serious, and the same may be said of the fits associated with indigestion and peripheral irritation.

Treatment.—Every source of irritation should be removed. If associated with indigestible food, a prompt emetic should be given, followed by an enema. The teeth should be examined, and if the gum is swollen, hot, and tense, it may be lanced; but never if it looks normal. When seen at first, if the paroxysm is severe, no time should be lost by giving a hot bath, but chloroform should be given at once, and repeated if necessary. A child is so readily put under chloroform and with such a small quantity that this procedure is quite harmless and saves much valuable time. The practice is almost universal of putting the child into a warm bath, and if there is a fever the head may be douched with cold water. The temperature of the bath should not be above 95° or 96°. The very hot bath is not suitable, particularly if the fits are due to indigestion. After the attack an ice-cap may be placed upon the head. If there is much irritability, particularly in rickets and in severe diarrhœa, small doses of opium will be found efficacious. When the convulsions recur after the child comes from under the influence of chloroform it is best to place it rapidly under the influence of opium, which may be given as morphia hypodermically, in doses of from one-twenty-fifth to one-thirtieth of a grain (0.0026 to 0.0022 gm.) for a child of one year. Other remedies recommended are chloral by enema, in 5 grain (0.3 gm.) doses, and nitrite of amyl. After the attack has passed the bromides are useful, of which 5 to 8 grains (0.3 to 0.5 gm.) may be given in a day to a child a year old. Recurring convulsions, particularly if they come on without special cause, should receive the most thorough and careful treatment with bromides. When associated with rickets the treatment should be directed to improving the general condition.

V. EPILEPSY

Definition.—An affection of the nervous system characterized by attacks of unconsciousness, with or without convulsions.

The transient loss of consciousness without convulsive seizures is known as *petit mal;* the loss of consciousness with general convulsive seizures is known as *grand mal.* Localized convulsions, occurring usually without loss of consciousness, are known as epileptiform, or more frequently as Jacksonian or cortical epilepsy.

Etiology.—AGE.—In a large proportion of all cases the disease begins before puberty. Of the 1,450 cases observed by Gowers, in 422 the disease began before the tenth year, and three-fourths of the cases began before the twentieth year. Of 460 cases of epilepsy in children which I have analyzed the age of onset in 427 was as follows: First year, 74; second year, 62; third year, 51; fourth year, 24; fifth year, 17; sixth year, 18; seventh year, 19; eighth year, 23; ninth year, 17; tenth year, 27; eleventh year, 17; twelfth year, 18; thirteenth year, 15; fourteenth year, 21; fifteenth year, 34. Arranged in hemidecades the figures are as follows: From the first to the fifth year, 229; from the fifth to the tenth year, 104; from the tenth to the fifteenth year, 95. These figures illustrate in a striking manner the early onset of the disease in a large proportion of the cases. It is well always to be suspicious of epilepsy beginning in adult life, for in a majority of such cases the convulsions are due to a local lesion.

SEX.—No special influence appears to be discoverable in this relation, certainly not in children. Of 433 cases in my tables, 232 were males and 203 were females, showing a slight predominance of the male sex. After puberty unquestionably, if a large number of cases are taken, the males are in excess.

HEREDITY.—Much stress has been laid upon this by many authors as an important predisposing cause, and the statistics collected give from 9 to over 40 per cent. Gowers gives 35 per cent. for his cases, which have special value apart from other statistics embracing large numbers of epileptics in that they were collected by him in his own practice. In other figures it appears to play a minor rôle. In my list there were only 31 cases in which there was a history of marked neurotic taint, and only 3 in which the mother herself had been epileptic. In the Elwyn cases, as might be expected, the percentage is larger. Of the 126 there was in 32 a family history of nervous derangement of some sort, either paralysis, epilepsy, marked hysteria, or insanity. Spratling found 16 per cent. among 2,523 cases.

While, then, it may be said that direct inheritance is comparatively uncommon, yet the children of neurotic families in which neuralgia, insanity, and hysteria prevail are more liable to fall victims to the disease.

Chronic alcoholism in the parents is regarded by many as a potent predisposing factor in the production of epilepsy. Echeverria has analyzed 572 cases bearing upon this point and divided them into three classes, of which 257 cases could be traced directly to alcohol as a cause; 126 cases in which there were associated conditions, such as syphilis and traumatism; 189 cases in which the alcoholism was probably the result of the epilepsy. Figures equally strong are given by Martin, who in 150 insane epileptics found 83 with a marked history of parental intemperance. Spratling found 15 per cent. with marked alcoholic history in the parents.

Syphilis.—This in the parents is probably less a predisposing than an actual cause of epilepsy, which is the direct outcome of local cerebral manifestations. There is no reason for recognizing a special form of syphilitic epilepsy. On the other hand, convulsive seizures due to acquired syphilitic disease of the brain are very common.

Alcohol.—Severe epileptic convulsions may occur in steady drinkers.

Of exciting causes fright is believed to be important, but is less so, I think, than is usually stated. Trauma is present in a certain number of instances. An important group depends upon a local disease of the brain existing from childhood, as seen in the post-hemiplegic epilepsy. Occasionally cases follow the infectious fevers. Masturbation has been stated to be a special cause, but its influence is probably overrated. A large group of convulsive seizures allied to epilepsy are due to some toxic agent, as in lead poisoning and in uræmia.

Reflex Causes.—Eye strain, dentition, and worms, the irritation of a cicatrix, some local affection, such as adherent prepuce, or a foreign body in the ear or the nose, are given as causes. In some of these cases the fits cease after the removal of the cause, so that there can be no question of the association between the two. In others the attacks persist. Genuine cases of reflex epilepsy are, I believe, rare. A remarkable instance of it occurred at the Philadelphia Infirmary for Diseases of the Nervous System in the case of a man with a testis in the inguinal canal, pressure upon which would cause a typical fit. Removal of the organ was followed by cure.

Cardio-vascular epilepsy is usually a manifestation of advanced arteriosclerosis, and is associated with slow pulse (see Stokes-Adams Disease). There may be palpitation and uneasy sensations about the heart prior to the attack. The passage of a gall-stone or the removal of pleuritic fluid may induce a fit. Indigestion and gastric troubles are extremely common in epilepsy, and in many instances the eating of indigestible articles seems to precipitate an attack. And lastly, epileptic seizures may occur in old people without obvious cause.

Symptoms.—(*a*) Grand Mal.—Preceding the fits there is usually a localized sensation, known as an *aura,* in some part of the body. This may be somatic, in which the feeling comes from some particular region in the periphery, as from the finger or hand, or is a sensation felt in the stomach or about the heart. The peripheral sensations preceding the fit are of great value, particularly those in which the aura always occurs in a definite region, as in one finger or toe. It is the equivalent of the signal symptom in a fit from a brain tumor. The varieties of these sensations are numerous. The epigastric sensations are most common. In these the patient complains of an uneasy sensation in the epigastrium or distress in the intestines, or the sensation may not be unlike that of heartburn and may be associated with palpitation These groups are sometimes known as pneumogastric auræ or warnings.

Of psychical auræ one of the most common, as described by Hughlings Jackson, is the vague, dreamy state, a sensation of strangeness or sometimes of terror. The auræ may be associated with special senses; of these the most common are the visual, consisting of flashes of light or sensations of color; less commonly, distinct objects are seen. The auditory auræ consist of noises in the ear, odd sounds, musical tones, or occasionally voices. Olfactory and gustatory auræ, unpleasant tastes and odors, are rare.

Occasionally the fit may be preceded not by an aura, but by certain movements; the patient may turn round rapidly or run with great speed for a few minutes, the so-called epilepsia procursiva. In one of the Elwyn cases the lad stood on his toes and twirled with extraordinary rapidity, so that his features were scarcely recognizable. It is stated that the pulse sometimes stops just before the fit. The studies of Gibson and Good show that no alteration in the pulse occurred up to the point of clonic convulsions, and there was no lowering of the general blood pressure suggesting anæmia of the brain. At the onset of the attack the patient may give a loud scream or yell, the so-called epileptic cry. The patient drops as if shot, making no effort to guard the fall. In consequence of this epileptics frequently injure themselves, cutting the face or head or burning themselves. In the attack, as described by Hippocrates, "the patient loses his speech and chokes, and foam issues from the mouth, the teeth are fixed, the hands are contracted, the eyes distorted, he becomes insensible, and in some cases the bowels are affected. And these symptoms occur sometimes on the left side, sometimes on the right, and sometimes on both." The fit may be described in three stages:

(1) *Tonic Spasm.*—The head is drawn back or to the right, and the jaws are fixed. The hands are clinched and the legs extended. This tonic contraction affects the muscles of the chest, so that respiration is impeded and the initial pallor of the face changes to a dusky or livid hue. The muscles of the two sides are unequally affected, so that the head and neck are rotated or the spine is twisted. The arms are usually flexed at the elbows, the hand at the wrist, and the fingers are tightly clinched in the palm. This stage lasts only a few seconds, and then the clonic stage begins.

(2) *Clonic Stage.*—The muscular contractions become intermittent; at first tremulous or vibratory, they gradually become more rapid and the limbs are jerked and tossed about violently. The muscles of the face are in constant clonic spasm, the eyes roll, the eyelids are opened and closed convulsively. The movements of the muscles of the jaw are very forcible and strong, and it is at this time that the tongue is apt to be caught between the teeth and lacerated. The cyanosis, marked at the end of the tonic stage, gradually lessens. A frothy saliva, which may be blood stained, escapes from the mouth. The fæces and urine may be discharged involuntarily. The duration of this stage is variable. It rarely lasts more than one or two minutes. The contractions become less violent and the patient gradually sinks into the condition of coma.

(3) *Coma.*—The breathing is noisy or even stertorous, the face congested, but no longer intensely cyanotic. The limbs are relaxed and the unconsciousness is profound. After a variable time the patient can be aroused, but if left alone he sleeps for some hours and then awakes, complaining only of slight headache or mental confusion. If the attack has been severe, petechial hæmorrhages may be scattered over the neck and chest. In the case of a young man in good health in a severe convulsion both sub-conjunctival spaces were entirely filled with blood, and free blood oozed from them (Walter James). Hæmoptysis is a rare sequel.

(4) *Status Epilepticus.*—This is the climax of the disease, in which attacks occur in rapid succession, and the patient does not recover consciousness. The pulse, respiration, and temperature rise in the attack. It is a serious condition, and often proves fatal.

After the attack the reflexes are sometimes absent; more frequently they are increased and the ankle clonus can usually be obtained. The state of the urine is variable, particularly as regards the solids. The quantity is usually increased after the attack, and albumin is not infrequently present.

(5) *Post-epileptic symptoms* are of great importance. The patient may be in a trance-like condition, in which he performs actions of which subsequently he has no recollection. More serious are the attacks of mania, in which the patient is often dangerous and sometimes homicidal. It is held by good authorities that an outbreak of mania may be substituted for the fit. And, lastly, the mental condition of an epileptic patient is often seriously impaired, and profound defects are common.

(6) *Paralysis,* which rarely follows the epileptic fit, is usually hemiplegic and transient. Slight disturbances of speech also may occur; in some instances, forms of sensory aphasia.

The attacks may occur at night, and a person may be epileptic for years without knowing it. As Trousseau truly remarks, when a person tells us that in the night he has incontinence of urine and awakes in the morning with headache and mental confusion, and complains of difficulty in speech owing to the fact that he has bitten his tongue, if also there are purpuric spots on the skin of the face and neck, the probability is very strong indeed that he is subject to nocturnal epilepsy.

(*b*) Petit Mal.—This is epilepsy without the convulsions. The attack consists of transient unconsciousness, which may come on at any time, accompanied or unaccompanied by a feeling of faintness and vertigo. Suddenly, for example, at the dinner table, the subject stops talking and eating, the eyes become fixed, and the face slightly pale. Anything which may have been in the hand is usually dropped. In a moment or two consciousness is regained and the patient resumes conversation as if nothing had happened. In other instances there is slight incoherency or the patient performs some almost automatic action. He may begin to undress himself and on returning to consciousness find that he has partially disrobed. He may rub his beard or face, or may spit about in a careless way. In other attacks the patient may fall without convulsive seizures. A definite aura is rare. Though transient, unconsciousness and giddiness are the most constant manifestations of *petit mal;* there are many other equivalent manifestations, such as sudden jerkings in the limbs, sudden tremor, or a sudden visual sensation. Gowers mentions no less than seventeen different manifestations of *petit mal.* Occasionally there are cases in which the patient has a sensation of losing his breath and may even get red in the face.

After the attack the patient may be dazed for a few seconds and perform certain automatic actions, which may seem to be volitional. As mentioned, undressing is a common action, but all sorts of odd actions may be performed, some of which are awkward or even serious. One of my patients after an attack was in the habit of tearing anything he could lay hands on, particularly books. Violent actions have been committed and assaults made, frequently giving rise to questions which come before the courts. This condition has been termed masked epilepsy, or *epilepsia larvata.*

In a majority of the cases of *petit mal* convulsions finally occur, at first slight, but ultimately the *grand mal* becomes well developed, and the attacks may then alternate.

(*c*) Jacksonian Epilepsy.—This is also known as cortical, symptomatic, or partial epilepsy. It is distinguished from the ordinary epilepsy by the important fact that consciousness is retained or is lost late. The attacks are usually the result of irritative lesions in the motor zone, though there are probably also sensory equivalents of this motor form. In a typical attack the spasm begins in a limited muscle group of the face, arm, or leg. The zygomatic muscles, for instance, or the thumb may twitch, or the toes may first be moved. Prior to the twitching the patient may feel a sensation of numbness or tingling in the part affected. The spasm extends and may involve the muscles of one limb only or of the face. The patient is conscious throughout and watches, often with interest, the march of the spasm.

The onset may be slow, and, as in a case which I have reported, there may be time for the patient to place a pillow on the floor, so as to be as comfortable as possible during the attack. The spasms may be localized for years, but there is a great risk that the partial epilepsy may become general. The condition is due, as a rule, to an irritative lesion in the motor zone. Thus of 107 cases analyzed by Roland, there were 48 of tumor, 21 instances of inflammatory softening, 14 instances of acute and chronic meningitis, and 8 cases of trauma. The remaining instances were due to hæmorrhage or abscess, or were associated with sclerosis cerebri. Two other conditions may be mentioned, which may cause typical Jacksonian epilepsy—namely, uræmia and progressive paralysis of the insane. A considerable number of the cases of Jacksonian epilepsy are found in children following hemiplegia, the so-called posthemiplegic epilepsy. The convulsions usually begin on the affected side, either in the arm or leg, and the fit may be unilateral and without loss of consciousness. Ultimately they become more severe and general.

Diagnosis.—In *major epilepsy* the suddenness of the attack, the abrupt loss of consciousness, the order of the tonic and clonic spasm, and the relaxation of the sphincters at the height of the attack are distinctive features. The convulsive seizures due to uræmia are epileptic in character and usually readily recognized by the existence of greatly increased tension and the condition of the urine. Practically in young adults hysteria causes the greatest difficulty, and may closely simulate true epilepsy. The table on page 1085, from Gowers' work, draws clearly the chief differences between them.

Recurring epileptic seizures in a person over thirty who has not had previous attacks is always suggestive of organic disease. According to H. C. Wood, whose opinion is supported by that of Fournier, in 9 cases out of 10 the condition is due to syphilis.

Petit mal must be distinguished from attacks of syncope, and the vertigo of Ménière's disease, of a cardiac lesion, and of indigestion. In these cases there is no actual loss of consciousness, which forms a characteristic though not an invariable feature of *petit mal.*

Jacksonian epilepsy has features so distinctive and peculiar that it is at once recognized. It is, however, by no means easy always to determine upon what the spasm depends. Irritation in the motor centres may be due to a great variety of causes, among which tumors and localized meningo-encephalitis are the most frequent; but it must not be forgotten that in uræmia localized epilepsy may occur. The most typical Jacksonian spasms also are not infrequent in general paresis of the insane.

	Epileptic	Hysteroid
Apparent cause..........	none.	emotion.
Warning................	any, but especially unilateral or epigastric auræ.	palpitation, malaise, choking, bilateral foot aura.
Onset..................	always sudden.	often gradual.
Scream.................	at onset.	during course.
Convulsion.............	rigidity followed by "jerking," rarely rigidity alone.	rigidity or "struggling," throwing about of limbs or head, arching of back.
Biting.................	tongue.	lips, hands, or other people and things.
Micturition............	frequent.	never.
Defecation.............	occasional.	never.
Talking................	never.	frequent.
Duration...............	a few minutes.	more than ten minutes, often much longer.
Restraint necessary.....	to prevent accident.	to control violence.
Termination............	spontaneous.	spontaneous or induced (water, etc.).

Prognosis.—This may be given to-day in the words of Hippocrates: "The prognosis in epilepsy is unfavorable when the disease is congenital, and when it endures to manhood, and when it occurs in a grown person without any previous cause. . . . The cure may be attempted in young persons, but not in old." W. A. Turner concludes that of cases beginning under ten years few are arrested, whereas of those beginning at puberty the opposite is true. Cases beginning between the twentieth and thirty-fifth years give few arrests. After thirty-five the outlook is good.

Death during the fit rarely occurs, but it may happen if the patient falls into the water or if the fit comes on while he is eating. Occasionally the fits seem to stop spontaneously. This is particularly the case in the epilepsy in children which has followed the convulsions of teething or of the fevers. Frequency of the attacks and marked mental disturbance are unfavorable indications. Hereditary predisposition is apparently of no moment in the prognosis. The outlook is better in males than in females. The post-hemiplegic epilepsy is rarely arrested. Of the cases coming on in adults, those due to syphilis and to local affections of the brain allow a more favorable prognosis.

Treatment.—General.—In the case of children the parents should be made to understand from the outset that epilepsy in the great majority of cases is an incurable affection, so that the disease may interfere as little as possible with the education of the child. The subjects need firm but kind treatment. Indulgence and yielding to caprices and whims are followed by weakening of the moral control, which is so necessary in these cases. The disease does not incapacitate a person for all occupation. It is much better for epileptics to have some definite pursuit. There are many instances in which they have been persons of extraordinary mental and bodily vigor, as, for example, Julius Cæsar and Napoleon. One of the most distressing features in epilepsy is the gradual mental impairment which follows in a certain number of cases. If such patients become extremely irritable or show signs of violence they should be placed under supervision in an asylum. Marriage should be forbidden to epileptics. During the attack a cork or bit of rubber should be placed between the teeth and the clothes should be loosened. The patient should be in the recumbent posture. As the attack usually passes off with rapidity, no special treatment is necessary, but in cases in which the convulsion is prolonged a few whiffs of chloroform or nitrite of amyl or a hypodermic of a quarter of a grain of morphia may be given.

Dietetic.—The old authors laid great stress upon regimen in epilepsy. The important point is to give the patient a light diet at fixed hours, and on no account to permit overloading of the stomach. Meat should not be given more than once a day. There are cases in which animal food seems injurious. A strict vegetable diet has been warmly recommended. The patient should not go to sleep until the completion of gastric digestion.

Medicinal.—The bromides are the only remedies which have a special influence upon the disease. Either the sodium or potassium salt may be given. Sodium bromide is probably less irritating and is better borne for a long period. It may be given in milk, in which it is scarcely tasted. In all instances the dilution should be considerable. In adults it is well taken in soda water or in some mineral water. The dose for an adult should be from half a drachm to a drachm and a half (2 to 6 gm.) daily. As Seguin recommends, it is often best to give but a single dose daily, about four to six hours before the attacks are most likely to occur. For instance, in the case of nocturnal epilepsy a drachm should be given an hour or two after the evening meal. If the attack occurs early in the morning, the patient should take a full dose when he awakes. When given three times a day it is less disturbing after meals. Each case should be carefully studied to determine how much bromide should be used. The individual susceptibility varies and some patients require more than others. Fortunately, children take the drug well and stand proportionately larger doses than adults. Saturation is indicated by certain unpleasant effects, particularly drowsiness, mental torpor, and gastric and cardiac distress. Loss of palate reflex is one of the earliest indications that the system is under the influence of the bromides, and is a condition which should be attained. A very unpleasant feature is the development of acne, which, however, is no indication of bromism. Seguin states that the tendency to this is much diminished by giving the drug largely diluted in alkaline waters and administering from time to time full doses of arsenic. To be effectual the treatment should be continued for a prolonged period and the cases should be incessantly watched in order to prevent bromism. The medicine should be continued for at least two years after the cessation of the fits; indeed, Seguin recommends that the reduction of the bromides should not be begun until the patient has been three years without any manifestations. Written directions should be given to the mother or to the friends of the patient, and he should not himself be held responsible for the administration of the medicine. A book should be provided in which the daily number of attacks and the amount of medicine taken should be noted. The addition of belladonna to the bromide is warmly recommended by Black, of Glasgow. In very obstinate cases Flechsig uses opium, 5 or 6 grains (0.35 gm.), in three doses daily; then at the end of six weeks opium is stopped and the bromides in large amounts, 75 to 100 grains (4 to 6 gm.) daily, are used for two months.

Among other remedies which have been recommended as controlling epilepsy are chloral, cannabis indica, zinc, nitroglycerin, and borax. Nitroglycerin is sometimes advantageous in *petit mal,* but is not of much service in the major form. To be beneficial it must be given in full doses, from 2 to 5 drops of the 1 per cent. solution, and increased until the physiological effects are produced. Calcium lactate in 20 grain (1.3 gm.) doses daily has been highly recommended. Counter-irritation is rarely advisable. When the aura is very definite and constant in its onset, as from the hand or from the toe, a blister about the part or a ligature tightly applied may stop the oncoming fit. In children, care should be taken that there is no source of peripheral irritation. In boys, adherent prepuce may occasionally be the cause. The irritation of teething, the presence of worms, and foreign bodies in the ears or nose have been associated with epileptic seizures.

The subjects of a chronic and, in most cases, a hopelessly incurable disease, epileptic patients form no small portion of the unfortunate victims of charlatans and quacks, who prescribe to-day, as in the time of the father of medicine, "purifications and spells and other illiberal practices of like kind."

SURGICAL.—In Jacksonian epilepsy the propriety of surgical interference is universally granted. It is questionable, however, whether in the epilepsy following hemiplegia, considering the anatomical condition, it is likely to be of any benefit. In idiopathic epilepsy, when the fit starts in a certain region —the thumb, for instance—and the signal symptom is invariable, the centre controlling this part may be removed. Operation in the traumatic epilepsy, in which the fit follows fracture, is much more hopeful.

The operation, *per se,* appears in some cases to have a curative effect. Thus of 50 cases of trephining for epilepsy in which nothing abnormal was found to account for the symptoms, 25 were reported as cured and 18 as improved. The operations have not been always on the skull, and White has collected an interesting series in which various surgical procedures have been resorted to, often with curative effect, such as ligation of the carotid artery, castration, tracheotomy, excision of the superior cervical ganglia, incision of the scalp, circumcision, etc.

VI. MIGRAINE

(*Hemicrania; Sick Headache*)

Definition.—A paroxysmal affection characterized by severe headache, usually unilateral, and often associated with disorders of vision.

Etiology.—Heredity plays an important rôle in 90 per cent. of cases according to Möbius. Women and members of neurotic families are most frequently attacked. Many distinguished men have been its victims, and the astronomer Airy gave a classical account of his case. The nature of the disease is unknown, and many views have been entertained:

(*a*) That it is a toxæmia from disorder of the intestinal digestion, from disturbed uric acid output, or from some self-manufactured poison.

(*b*) That it is a vasomotor affection with spasm of the arteries, in favor of which are the facts that in the attack the temporal arteries on the affected side may be felt to be small, the retinal arteries may sometimes be seen in spasm, and sclerosis of the arteries on the same side is found in a certain number of cases of hemicrania. A still more striking confirmation is the temporary paralysis which may be associated with an attack of monoplegic or hemiplegic character. Mitchell Clarke has reported a history of recurring motor paralysis in eleven members in three generations of the same family. The characteristic visual phenomena preceded the unilateral headache, especially the hemiopia. In most of the attacks the hemiplegia was on the right side. It lasted from a few hours to a day and disappeared completely, leaving no damage. It is difficult to explain such cases except on the view of a transient spasm of the arteries.

(*c*) Others regard the affection as of reflex origin arising from a refractive error in the eyes, or from troubles in the nose or sexual organs.

(*d*) The disease has been attributed to transient plugging of the foramen of Monro with increased pressure in the ventricles (Spitzner).

The majority of cases begin early in life, and Sinclair refers to a case in a child of two years. Many circumstances bring on the attack: a powerful emotion of any sort, mental or bodily fatigue, digestive disturbances, or the eating of some particular article of food. The paroxysmal character is one of the most striking features of the attacks which may occur on the same day every week, every fortnight, or every month. Headaches of the migraine type may occur for years in connection with chronic nephritis, and it is well to remember that attacks may occur in connection with tumors and other lesions of the base of the brain.

Symptoms.—Premonitory signs are present in many cases, and the patient can tell when an attack is coming on. Remarkable prodromata have been described, particularly in connection with vision. Apparitions may appear—visions of animals, such as mice, dogs, etc. Transient hemianopia or scotoma may be present. In other instances there is spasmodic action of the pupil on the affected side, which dilates and contracts alternately, the condition known as *hippus*. Frequently the disturbance of vision is only a blurring, or there are balls of light, or zigzag lines, or the so-called fortification spectra (teichopsia), which may be illuminated with gorgeous colors. Disturbances of the other senses are rare. Numbness of the tongue and face and occasionally of the hand may occur with tingling. More rarely there are cramps or spasms in the muscles of the affected side. Transient aphasia has also been noted, which may be intermittent. Some patients show marked psychical disturbance, either excitement or, more commonly, mental confusion or great depression. Dizziness occurs in some cases. The headache follows a short time after the prodromal symptoms have appeared. It is cumulative and expansile in character, beginning as a localized small spot, which is generally constant either on the temple or forehead or in the eyeball. It is usually described as of a penetrating, sharp, boring character. The pain gradually spreads and involves the entire side of the head, sometimes the neck, and may pass into the arm. In some cases both sides are affected. Nausea and vomiting are common symptoms. If the attack comes on when the stomach is full vomiting usually gives relief. Vasomotor symptoms may be present. The face, for instance, may be pale, and there may be a marked difference between the two sides. Subsequently the face and ear on the affected side may become a burning red from the vaso-dilator influences. The pulse may be slow. The temporal artery on the affected side may be firm and hard, and in a condition of arterio-sclerosis—a fact which has been confirmed anatomically by Thoma. Few affections are more prostrating than migraine, and during the paroxysm the patient may scarcely be able to raise the head from the pillow. The slightest noise or light aggravates the condition.

The duration of the entire attack is variable. The severer forms usually incapacitate the patient for at least three days. In other instances the entire attack is over in a day. The disease recurs for years, and in cases with a marked hereditary tendency may persist throughout life. In women the attacks often cease after the climacteric, and in men after the age of fifty. Two of the greatest sufferers I have known, who had recurring attacks every few weeks from early boyhood, now have complete freedom.

Treatment.—The patient is usually aware of the causes which precipitate an attack. Avoidance of excitement, regularity in the meals, and moderation in diet are important rules. I have known cases greatly benefited by a strict vegetable diet. The treatment should be directed toward the removal of the conditions upon which the attacks depend. In children much may be done by watchfulness and care on the part of the mother in regulating the bowels and watching the diet of the child. Errors of refraction should be adjusted. On no account should such children be allowed to compete in school for prizes. A prolonged course of bromides sometimes proves successful. If anæmia is present, iron and arsenic should be given. When the arterial tension is increased a course of nitroglycerin may be tried. Not too much, however, should be expected of the preventive treatment of migraine. In a very large proportion of the cases the headaches recur in spite of all we (including the refractionists) can do. Herter advised, so soon as the patient has any intimation of the attack, to wash out the stomach with water at 105°, and to give a brisk saline cathartic. Irrigation of the colon with hot saline solution is sometimes of value if done at the onset. Alkaline water should be taken freely by mouth. During the paroxysm the patient should be kept in bed and absolutely quiet. If the patient feels faint and nauseated a small cup of hot, strong coffee or 20 drops of chloroform give relief. Cannabis indica is probably the most satisfactory remedy. Seguin recommends a prolonged course of the drug. Antipyrin, antifebrin, and phenacetin have been much used of late. When given early, at the very outset of the paroxysm, they are sometimes effective. Small, repeated doses are more satisfactory. Of other remedies, caffeine, in 5-grain doses of the citrate, nux vomica, and ergot have been recommended. Electricity does not appear to be of much service.

Ophthalmoplegic Migraine.—This term was applied by Charcot to a special form in which there is weakness or paralysis of one or more eye muscles, with or after a migraine attack. The oculo-motor nerve is usually involved. Ptosis, loss of certain movements, and double vision are the common features, which may persist for some days. Local causes, especially syphilis, should be excluded before the diagnosis is established. The treatment is the same as for migraine.

VII. NEURALGIA

Definition.—A painful affection of the nerves, due either to functional disturbance of their central or peripheral extremities or to neuritis in their course.

Etiology.—Members of neuropathic families are most subject to the disease. It affects women more than men. Children are rarely attacked. Of all causes debility is the most frequent. It is often the first indication of an enfeebled nervous system. The various forms of anæmia are frequently associated with neuralgia. It may be a prominent feature at the onset of certain acute diseases, particularly typhoid fever. Malaria has been thought to be a potent cause, but it has not been shown that neuralgia is more frequent in malarial districts, and the error has probably arisen from regarding periodicity as a special manifestation of paludism. It occasionally occurs in malarial cachexia. Exposure to cold is a cause in very susceptible persons. Reflex irritation, particularly from carious teeth, and disease of the antrum and frontal sinuses are common causes of neuralgia of the fifth nerve. The disease occurs sometimes in gout, lead poisoning, and diabetes. Persistent neuralgia may be a feature of latent Bright's disease.

Symptoms.—Before the onset of the pain there may be uneasy sensations, sometimes tingling in the part which will be affected. The pain is localized to a certain group or division of nerves, usually affecting one side. The pain is not constant, but paroxysmal, and is described as stabbing, burning, or darting in character. The skin may be exquisitely tender in the affected region, particularly over certain points along the course of the nerve, the so-called tender points. Movements, as a rule, are painful. Trophic and vaso-motor changes may accompany the paroxysm; the skin may be cool, and subsequently hot and burning; occasionally local œdema or erythema occurs. More remarkable still are the changes in the hair, which may become blanched (canities), or even fall out. Fortunately, such alterations are rare. Twitchings of the muscles, or even spasms, may be present during the paroxysm. After lasting a variable time—from a few minutes to many hours—the attack subsides. Recurrence may be at definite intervals—every day at the same hour, or at intervals of two, three, or even seven days. Occasionally the paroxysms develop only at the catamenia. This periodicity is quite as marked in non-malarial as in malarial regions.

CLINICAL VARIETIES, DEPENDING ON THE NERVE ROOTS AFFECTED

Trigeminal Neuralgia; Tic Douloureux.—A distinction must be drawn between the minor and major neuralgias of the fifth cranial nerve. The former may merely be symptomatic of the involvement of one or another of its peripheral branches in some disease process—the pressure of a tumor, carious teeth, or a neuritis due to the proximity of suppurative processes in the bony sinuses, etc. There may be referred neuralgic pains in this area from morbid processes within the cranium, or from visceral disease elsewhere. A painful neuralgia may follow an attack of zoster in any division of the fifth nerve.

The typical *tic douloureux, epileptiform neuralgia,* or "*neuralgia quinti major,*" as it has been called, is probably a primary affection of the Gasserian ganglion. The disease starts in middle life, without obvious cause, as a simple neuralgia in one of the trigeminal branches, and from a particular spot the pain radiates through the course of one of the nerves, most often the upper branch. The pain is of sudden onset, violent and paroxysmal in character. There are periods of remission, which at first may extend over several months, and in which the paroxysms do not occur, but these intervals of release shorten after each successive attack. The attacks themselves are of ever increasing severity and longer duration. The pain finally invades the territory of adjoining nerves and ultimately, after years, may extend over the entire trigeminal distribution. Though by sympathy there may be pain outside of the fifth nerve area, particularly in the occipital region, in true tic douloureux the pain remains limited to the distribution of one trigeminal nerve, and probably never becomes bilateral. In advanced cases the paroxysms follow one another rapidly and without assignable cause, and in the intervals the patient may never be quite free from pain. They are inaugurated by almost any form of external stimulus, by a draught of air, by movement of the facial muscles or of the tongue in speaking, by touching the skin, particularly over those points from which the pain seems to take its origin, by the act of swallowing, especially when the pain involves the mucous membrane field of distribution of the nerve. It is not a self-limited disease. In some instances the neuralgia reaches such a frightful intensity that it renders the patient's life insupportable. In former years suicide was not an uncommon consequence.

Cervico-occipital neuralgia involves the posterior branches of the first four cervical nerves, particularly the inferior occipital, at the emergence of which there is a painful point about half-way between the mastoid process and the first cervical vertebra. It may be caused by cold, and these nerves are often affected in cervical caries. Surgical measures may be required if the pain is severe. Krause has devised an operation for division and evulsion of the affected nerves.

Cervico-brachial neuralgia involves the sensory nerves of the brachial plexus, particularly in the cubital division. When the circumflex nerve is involved the pain is in the deltoid. The pain is most commonly about the shoulder and down the course of the ulnar nerve. There is usually a marked tender point upon this nerve at the elbow. This form rarely follows cold, but more frequently results from rheumatic affections of the joints, and trauma.

Neuralgia of the phrenic nerve is rare. It is sometimes found in pleurisy and in pericarditis. The pain is chiefly at the lower part of the thorax on a line with the insertion of the diaphragm, and here may be painful points on deep pressure. Full inspiration is painful, and there is great sensitiveness on coughing or in the performance of any movement by which the diaphragm is suddenly depressed.

Intercostal Neuralgia.—Next to the *tic douloureux* this is the most important form. It is most frequent in women and very common in hysteria. Post-zoster neuralgias are common in this situation. The possibility of spinal disease, of tumor, caries, or aneurism must always be borne in mind.

Lumbar Neuralgia.—The affected nerves are the posterior fibres of the lumbar plexus, particularly the ilio-scrotal branch. The pain is in the region of the iliac crest, along the inguinal canal, in the spermatic cord, and in the scrotum or labium majus. The affection known as irritable testis, probably a neuralgia of this nerve, may be very severe and accompanied by syncopal sensations.

Coccydynia.—This is regarded as a neuralgia of the coccygeal plexus.

It is most common in women, and is aggravated by the sitting posture. It is very intractable, and may necessitate the removal of the coccyx, an operation, however, which is not always successful. Neuralgias of the nerves of the leg have already been considered.

Neuralgias of the Nerves of the Feet.—Many of these cases accompany varying degrees of flat-foot. The condition is brought about by weakness or fatigue of the muscles supporting the arches of the foot, which consequently settle until the strain of the superimposed body-weight falls upon the ligamentous and aponeurotic attachments between the metatarsal and tarsal bones. Rest, massage, exercises, and orthopædic measures are indicated.

PAINFUL HEEL.—Both in women and men there may be about the heel severe pains which interfere seriously with walking—the pododynia of S. D. Gross. There may be little or no swelling, no discoloration, and no affection of the joints. Some cases follow a gonococcus infection and are due to a bony spur.

PLANTAR NEURALGIA.—This is often associated with a definite neuritis, such as follows typhoid fever, and has been seen in an aggravated form in caisson disease (Hughes). The pain may be limited to the tips of the toes or to the ball of the great toe. Numbness, tingling, and hyperæsthesia or sweating may occur with it. In typhoid fever it is not uncommon for patients to complain of great sensitiveness in the toes.

METATARSALGIA.—Thomas G. Morton's "painful affection of the fourth metatarso-phalangeal articulation" is a peculiar and very trying disorder, seen most frequently in women, and usually in one foot. Morton regards it as due to a pinching of the metatarsal nerve. The condition usually requires operation. The red, painful neuralgia—erythromelalgia—is described under the vaso-motor and trophic disturbances.

Visceral Neuralgias.—The more important of these have already been referred to in connection with the cardiac and the gastric neuroses. They are most frequent in women, and are constant accompaniments of neurasthenia and hysteria. The pains are most common in the pelvic region, particularly about the ovaries. Nephralgia is of great interest, for, as has already been mentioned, the symptoms may closely simulate those of stone.

TREATMENT OF NEURALGIA

In general, causes of reflex irritation should be carefully removed. The neuralgia, as a rule, recurs unless the general health improves; so that tonic and hygienic measures of all sorts should be employed. Often a change of air or surroundings will relieve a severe neuralgia. I have known obstinate cases to be cured by a prolonged residence in the mountains, with an out-of-door life and plenty of exercise. A strict vegetable diet will sometimes relieve the neuralgia or headache of a gouty person. Of general remedies, iron is often a specific in the cases associated with chlorosis and anæmia. Arsenic, too, is very beneficial in these forms, and should be given in ascending doses. The value of quinine has been much overrated. It probably has no more influence than any other bitter tonic, except in the rare instances in which the neuralgia is definitely associated with malarial poisoning. Strychnine, cod-liver oil, and phosphorus are also advantageous. Of remedies for the pain, antipyrin, antifebrin, and phenacetin should first be tried, for they are sometimes of service. Morphia should be given with great caution, and only after other remedies have been tried in vain. On no consideration should the patient be allowed to use the hypodermic syringe. Gelsemium is highly recommended. Of nerve stimulants, valerian and ether, which often act well together, may be given. Alcohol is a valuable though dangerous remedy, and should not be ordered for women. In the minor form of trigeminal neuralgia nitroglycerin in large doses may be tried. Dana has seen good results follow rest with large doses of strychnia given hypodermically. Aconitin in doses of one two-hundredth of a grain (0.00032 gm.) may be tried.

Of local applications, the thermo-cautery is invaluable, particularly in zona and the more chronic forms of neuralgia. Acupuncture may be used. Chloroform liniment, camphor and chloral, menthol, the oleates of morphia, atropia, and belladonna used with lanolin may be tried. Freezing over the tender point with ether spray is sometimes successful. The continuous current may be used. The sponges should be warm, and the positive pole should be placed near the seat of the pain. The strength of the current should be such as to cause a slight tingling or burning, but not pain.

For the trigeminal neuralgia cutting of the nerves and removal of the Gasserian ganglion are practised. Alcohol injections into the nerve trunks have been extensively used, and in some hands with excellent results. The nerve fibres are destroyed with total loss of the function of the nerve until regeneration occurs. Wilfred Harris has destroyed the Gasserian ganglion by injecting alcohol into it through the foramen ovale. One of his patients treated in this way thirteen months before has remained perfectly well, and the fifth nerve area is completely anæsthetic. Removal of the ganglion is very satisfactory in skilled hands. Cushing has operated on 130 cases with two deaths, both cases early in the series.

VIII. PROFESSIONAL SPASMS; OCCUPATION NEUROSES

The continuous and excessive use of the muscles in performing a certain movement may be followed by an irregular, involuntary spasm or cramp, which may completely check the performance of the action. The condition is found most frequently in writers, hence the term writer's cramp or scrivener's palsy; but it is also common in piano and violin players and in telegraph operators. The spasms occur in many other persons, such as milkmaids, weavers, and cigarette-rollers.

The most common form is writer's cramp, which is much more frequent in men than in women. Of 75 cases of impaired writing power reported by Poore, all of the instances of undoubted writer's cramp were in men. Morris J. Lewis states that in the United States, in the telegrapher's cramp, women, who are employed a great deal in telegraphy, are much less frequently affected (only 4 out of 43 cases). An investigation by H. Theodore Thompson and J. Sinclair into telegraphist cramp in England shows that the disease is rare, only 13 cases among between 7,000 and 8,000 employees. Persons of a nervous temperament are more liable to the disease. Occasionally it follows slight injury.

Gowers states that in a majority of the cases a faulty method of writing has been employed, using either the little finger or the wrist as the fixed point. Persons who write with the middle of the forearm or the elbow as the fixed point are rarely affected.

No anatomical changes have been found. The most reasonable explanation of the disease is that it results from a deranged action of the nerve centres presiding over the muscular movements involved in the act of writing, a condition which has been termed irritable weakness. "The education of centres which may be widely separated from each other for the performance of any delicate movement is mainly accomplished by lessening the lines of resistance between them, so that the movement, which was at first produced by a considerable mental effort, is at last executed almost unconsciously. If, therefore, through prolonged excitation, this lessened resistance be carried too far, there is an increased and irregular discharge of nerve energy, which gives rise to spasm and disordered movement. According to this view, the muscular weakness is explained by an impairment of nutrition accompanying that of function, and the diminished faradic excitability by the nutritional disturbance descending the motor nerves" (Gay).

Symptoms.—These may be described under five heads (Lewis).

(*a*) Cramp or Spasm.—This is often an early symptom and most commonly affects the forefinger and thumb; or there may be a combined movement of flexion and adduction of the thumb, so that the pen may be twisted from the grasp and thrown to some distance. Weir Mitchell has described a lock-spasm, in which the fingers become so firmly contracted upon the pen that it can not be removed.

(*b*) Paresis and Paralysis.—This may occur with the spasm or alone. The patient feels a sense of weakness and debility in the muscles of the hand and arm and holds the pen feebly. Yet in these circumstances the grasp of the hand may be strong and there may be no paralysis for ordinary acts.

(*c*) Tremor.—This is most commonly seen in the forefinger and may be a premonitory symptom of atrophy. It is not an important symptom, and is rarely sufficient to produce disability.

(*d*) Pain.—Abnormal sensations, particularly a tired feeling in the muscles, are very constantly present. Actual pain is rare, but there may be irregular shooting pains in the arm. Numbness or soreness may exist. If, as sometimes happens, a subacute neuritis develops, there may be pain over the nerves and numbness or tingling in the fingers.

(*e*) Vaso-motor Disturbances.—These may occur in severe cases. There may be hyperæsthesia. Occasionally the skin becomes glossy, or there is a condition of local asphyxia resembling chilblains. In attempting to write, the hand and arm may become flushed and hot and the veins increased in size. Early in the disease the electrical reactions are normal, but in advanced cases there may be diminution of faradic and sometimes increase in the galvanic irritability.

Diagnosis.—A well marked case of writer's cramp or palsy could scarcely be mistaken for any other affection. Care must be taken to exclude the existence of any cerebro-spinal disease, such as progressive muscular atrophy or hemiplegia. The physician is sometimes consulted by nervous persons who fancy they are becoming subject to the disease and complain of stiffness or weakness without displaying any characteristic features.

Prognosis.—The course of the disease is usually chronic. If taken in time and if the hand is allowed perfect rest, the condition may improve rapidly, but too often there is a strong tendency to recurrence. The patient may learn to write with the left hand, but this also may after a time be attacked.

Treatment.—Various prophylactic measures have been advised. As mentioned, it is important that a proper method of writing be adopted. Gowers suggests that if all persons wrote from the shoulder writer's cramp would practically not occur. Various devices have been invented for relieving the fatigue, but none of them are very satisfactory. The use of the type-writer has diminished very much the frequency of scrivener's palsy. Rest is essential. No measures are of value without this. Massage and manipulation, when combined with systematic gymnastics, give the best results. The patient should systematically practise the opposite movements to those concerned in the cramp. This muscle training often gives good results. Poore recommends the galvanic current applied to the muscles, which are at the same time rhythmically exercised. In very obstinate cases the condition remains incurable. I saw a few years ago a distinguished gynæcologist who had had writer's cramp twenty years before, and who had tried all sorts of treatment, including Wolff's method, without any avail. He still has it in aggravated form, but he can do all the finer manipulations of operative work without any difficulty.

The nutrition of the patients is apt to be much impaired, and cod-liver oil, strychnia, and other tonics will be found advantageous. Local applications are of little benefit. Tenotomy and nerve stretching have been abandoned.

IX. HYSTERIA

Definition.—A disorder, chiefly of young women, in which emotional states control the body, leading to perversion of mental, sensory, motor and secretory functions.

Etiology.—Many and diverse views have prevailed since the Greeks ascribed the disease to the vague desires and wanderings of the womb, after which they named it.

Charcot and his followers regarded hysteria as a psychosis, in which morbid states are induced by ideas. The capability of responding to suggestion is the test of its existence. It is a disturbance in the sphere of personality, in which the emotions have an exaggerated influence on the sensory, motor and secretory functions.

Babinski, in a modification of this view, holds that hysteria is a mental condition with certain primary phenomena and certain secondary accidental symptoms. The essence of the primary features is that they may be produced by suggestion, and they may be made to disappear by persuasion (pithiatism). The primary symptoms include such features as hemi-anæsthesia, paralysis, contractures, etc.; secondary features, as for example muscular atrophy, are directly dependent upon the primary and cannot themselves be induced by suggestion.

In the Breuer-Freud theory, now the vogue, we return to the days of Aretæus, who originated (?) the views of sexual hysteria and believed the womb, "like an animal within an animal" and altogether erratic, caused all sorts of trouble in its wanderings. Freud's view is thus analyzed by Jelliffe in his article in my "System of Medicine," Vol. VII., page 817: "There develop usually on a constitutional basis, in the period before puberty, definite sexual activities which are mostly of a perverse nature. These activities do not, as a rule, lead to a definite neurosis up to the time of puberty, which in the psychic sphere appears much earlier than in the body, but sexual phantasy maintains a perverse constellated direction by reason of the infantile sexual activities. On constitutional (affect) grounds the increased fantasy of the hysteric leads to the formation of complexes which are not taken up by the personality and by reason of shame or disgust remain buried. There, therefore, results a conflict between the characteristic normal libido and the sexual repressions of these buried infantile perversions. These conflicts give rise to the hysterical symptoms. It is in his contributions to the sexual theory that Freud develops his later thoughts of the sexual origin of the hysterical reaction. By sexual it is important to remember that Freud is not speaking of sensual.

"The significance of Freud's theory is the tracing of every case to sexual traumata during early childhood. Sexual experiences differ, however, from ordinary experiences—the latter have a tendency to fade out, while the idea of the former grows with increasing sexual maturity. There results a disproportionate capacity for increased reaction which takes place in the subconscious. This is the cause of the mischief.

"There must be, however, a connecting link between the infantile sexual traumata and the later manifestations. This connection Freud finds in the so-called 'hysterical fancies.' These are the day-dreams of erotic coloring, wish-gratifications, originating in privation and longing. These fancies hark back to the original traumatic moment, and, either originating in the subconscious or shortly becoming conscious, are transformed into hysterical symptoms. They constitute a defence of the ego against the revival, as reminiscences, of the repressed traumatic experiences of childhood" (White).

The affection is most common in women, and usually appears first about the time of puberty, but the manifestations may continue until the menopause, or even until old age. Men, however, are by no means exempt, and hysteria in the male is not rare. It occurs in all races, but is much more prevalent, particularly in its severer forms, in members of the Latin race. In England and the United States the milder grades are common, but the graver forms are rare in comparison with the frequency with which they are seen in France.

Children under twelve years of age are not very often affected, but the disease may be well marked as early as the fifth or sixth year. One of the saddest chapters in the history of human deception, that of the Salem witches, might be headed *hysteria in children,* since the tragedy resulted directly from the hysterical pranks of girls under twelve years of age.

Of predisposing causes, two are important—heredity and education. The former acts by endowing the child with a mobile, abnormally sensitive nervous organization. We see cases most frequently in families with marked neuropathic tendencies, the members of which have suffered from neuroses of various sorts. Education at home too often fails to inculcate habits of self control. A child grows to girlhood with an entirely erroneous idea of her relations to others, and accustomed to have every whim gratified and abundant sympathy lavished on every woe, however trifling; she reaches womanhood with a moral organization unfitted to withstand the cares and worries of every-day life. At school, between the ages of twelve and fifteen, the most important period in her life, when the vital energies are absorbed in the rapid development of the body, she is often cramming for examinations and cooped in close school rooms for six or eight hours daily. The result too frequently is an active, bright mind in an enfeebled body, ill adapted to subserve the functions for which it was framed, easily disordered, and prone to react abnormally to the ordinary stimuli of life. Among the more direct influences are emotions of various kinds, fright occasionally, more frequently love affairs, grief, and domestic worries. Physical causes less often bring on hysterical outbreaks, but they may follow directly upon an injury or develop during the convalescence from an acute illness or be associated with disease of the generative organs.

Symptoms.—A useful division is into the convulsive and non-convulsive varieties.

Convulsive Hysteria.—(*a*) *Minor Forms.*—The attack, commonly following emotional disturbance, sets in suddenly or may be preceded by symptoms, called by the laity "hysterical," such as laughing and crying alternately, or a sensation of constriction in the neck, or of a ball rising in the throat—the *globus hystericus.* Sometimes, preceding the convulsive movements, there may be painful sensations arising from the pelvic, abdominal, or thoracic regions. From the description these sensations resemble auræ. They become more intense with the rising sensation of choking in the neck and difficulty in getting breath, and the patient falls into a more or less violent convulsion. The fall is not sudden, as in epilepsy, but the subject goes down, as a rule, easily, often picking a soft spot, like a sofa or an easy-chair, and in the movements apparently exercises care to do herself no injury. Yet at the same time she appears to be quite unconscious. The movements are clonic and disorderly, while the head and arms are thrown about in an irregular manner. The paroxysm after a few minutes slowly subsides, then the patient becomes emotional, and gradually regains consciousness. When questioned the patient may confess to having some knowledge of the events which have taken place, but, as a rule, has no accurate recollection. During the attack the abdomen may be much distended with flatus, and subsequently a large amount of clear urine may be passed. These attacks vary greatly in character. There may be scarcely any movements of the limbs, but after a nerve storm the patient sinks into a torpid, semi-unconscious condition, from which she is roused with great difficulty. In some cases from this state the patient passes into a condition of catalepsy.

(*b*) *Major Forms; Hystero-epilepsy.*—Typical instances passing through the various phases are very rare in the United States and in England. The attack is initiated by certain prodromata, chiefly minor hysterical manifestations, either foolish or unseemly behavior, excitement, sometimes dyspeptic symptoms with tympanites, or frequent micturition. Areas of hyperæsthesia may at this time be marked, the so-called hysterogenic spots so elaborately described by Richet. These are usually symmetrical and situated over the upper dorsal vertebra, and in front in a series of symmetrically placed spots on the chest and abdomen, the most marked being those in the inguinal regions over the ovaries. Painful sensations or a feeling of oppression and a *globus* rising in the throat may be complained of prior to the onset of the convulsion, which, according to French writers, has four distinct stages: (1) Epileptoid condition, which closely simulates a true epileptic attack with tonic spasm (often leading to opisthotonos), grinding of the teeth, congestion of the face, followed by clonic convulsions, gradual relaxation, and coma. (2) Succeeding this is the period which Charcot has termed *clownism,* in which there is an emotional display and a remarkable series of contortions or of cataleptic poses. (3) Then in typical cases there is a stage in which the patient assumes certain attitudes expressive of the various passions—ecstasy, fear, beatitude, or erotism. (4) Finally consciousness returns and the patient enters upon a stage in which she may display very varied symptoms, chiefly manifestations of a delirium with the most extraordinary hallucinations. Visions are seen, voices heard, and conversations held with imaginary persons. In this stage patients will relate with the utmost solemnity imaginary events, and make extraordinary and serious charges against individuals. This sometimes gives a grave aspect to these seizures, for not only will the patient at this stage make and believe the statements, but when recovery is complete the hallucination sometimes persists. After an attack a patient may remain for days in a state of lethargy or trance.

NON-CONVULSIVE FORMS.—So complex and varied is the clinical picture of hysteria that various manifestations are best considered according to the systems which are involved.

(*a*) *Disorders of Motion.*—(1) *Paralysis.*—These may be hemiplegic, paraplegic, or monoplegic. Hysterical diplegia is extremely rare. The paralysis either sets in abruptly or gradually, and may take weeks to attain its full development. *There is no type or form of organic paralysis which may not be simulated in hysteria.* Sensation is either lessened or lost on the affected side. The hysterical paraplegia is more common than hemiplegia. The loss of power is not absolute; the legs can usually be moved, but do not support the patient. The reflexes may be increased, though the knee-jerk is often normal. A spurious ankle clonus may sometimes be present. The feet are usually extended and turned inward in the equino-varus position. The muscles do not waste and the electrical reactions are normal. Other manifestations, such as paralysis of the bladder or aphonia, are usually associated with the hysterical paraplegia. Hysterical monoplegias may be facial, crural, or brachial. A condition of ataxia sometimes occurs with paresis. The incoördination may be a marked feature, and there are usually sensory manifestations.

(2) *Contractures and Spasms.*—The hysterical contractures may attack almost any group of voluntary muscles and be of the hemiplegic, paraplegic, or monoplegic type. They may come on suddenly or slowly, persist for months or years, and disappear rapidly. The contracture is most commonly seen in the arm, which is flexed at the elbow and wrist, while the fingers tightly grasp the thumb in the palm of the hand; more rarely the terminal phalanges are hyperextended as in athetosis. It may occur in one or in both legs, more commonly in one. The ankle clonus is present; the foot is inverted and the toes are strongly flexed. These cases may be mistaken for lateral sclerosis and the

difficulty in diagnosis may really be very great. The spastic gait is very typical, and with the exaggerated knee-jerk and ankle clonus the picture may be characteristic. Other forms of contracture may be in the muscles of the hip, shoulder, or neck; more rarely in those of the jaws—hysterical trismus—or in the tongue. Remarkable indeed are the local contractures in the diaphragm and abdominal muscles, producing a phantom tumor, in which just below and in the neighborhood of the umbilicus is a firm, apparently solid growth. According to Gowers, this is produced by relaxation of the recti and a spasmodic contraction of the diaphragm, together with inflation of the intestines with gas and an arching forward of the vertebral column. They are apt to occur in middle-aged women about the menopause, and are frequently associated with the symptoms of spurious pregnancy—*pseudo-cyesis*. The resemblance to a tumor may be striking, and I have known skilful diagnosticians to be deceived. The only safeguard is to be found in complete anæsthesia, when the tumor entirely disappears. Mitchell has reported an instance of a phantom tumor in the left pectoral region just above the breast, which was tender, hard, and dense.

Rhythmic Hysterical Spasm.—The movements may be of the arm, either flexion and extension, or, more rarely, pronation and supination. Clonic contractions of the sterno-cleido-mastoid or of the muscles of the jaws or of the rotatory muscles of the head may produce rhythmic movements of these parts. The spasm may be in one or both psoas muscles, lifting the leg in a rhythmic manner eight or ten times in a minute. In other instances the muscles of the trunk are affected, and every few moments there is a bowing movement—salaam convulsions—or the muscles of the back may contract, causing strong arching of the vertebral column and retraction of the head.

Tremor may be a purely hysterical manifestation, occurring either alone or with paralysis and contracture. It most commonly involves the hands and arms; more rarely the head and legs. The movements are small and quick. In the type described by Rendu the tremor may or may not persist during repose, but it is increased or provoked by volitional movements. Volitional or intentional tremor may exist, simulating closely the movements of insular sclerosis. Buzzard states that many instances of this disease in young girls are mistaken for hysteria.

(*b*) *Disorders of Sensation.*—*Anæsthesia* is most common, and usually confined to one half of the body. It may not be noticed by the patient. Usually it is accurately limited by the middle line and involves the mucous surfaces and deeper parts. The conjunctiva, however, is often spared. There may be hemianopia. This symptom may come on slowly or follow a convulsive attack. Sometimes the various sensations are dissociated and the anæsthesia may be only to pain and to touch. The skin of the affected side is usually pale and cool, and a pin-prick may not be followed by blood. With the loss of feeling there may be loss of muscular power. Curious trophic changes may be present, as in an interesting case of Weir Mitchell's, in which there was unilateral swelling of the hemiplegic side.

By metallotherapy, the application of certain metals, the anæsthesia or analgesia can be transferred to the other side of the body. It has been shown, however, that this phenomenon may be caused by the electro-magnet and by wood and various other agents, and is an effect of suggestion.

Hyperæsthesia.—Increased sensitiveness and pains occur in various parts of the body. One of the most frequent complaints is of pain in the head, usually over the sagittal suture, less frequently in the occiput. This is described as agonizing, and is compared to the driving of a nail into the part; hence the name *clavus hystericus.* Neuralgias are common. Hyperæsthetic areas, the hysterogenic points, exist on the skin of the thorax and abdomen, pressure upon which may cause minor manifestations or even a convulsive attack. Increased sensitiveness exists in the ovarian region, but is not peculiar to hysteria. Pain in the back is an almost constant complaint of hysterical patients. The sensitiveness may be limited to certain spinous processes, or it may be diffuse. In hysterical women the pains in the abdomen may simulate those of gastralgia and of gastric ulcer, or the condition may be almost identical with that of peritonitis; more rarely the abdominal pains closely resemble those of appendix disease.

Special Senses.—Disturbances of taste and smell are not uncommon and may cause a good deal of distress. Of ocular symptoms, retinal hyperæsthesia is the most common, and the patients always prefer to be in a darkened room. Retraction of the field of vision is common and usually follows a convulsive seizure. It may persist for years. The color perception may be normal even with complete anæsthesia. Hysterical deafness may be complete and may alternate or come on at the same time with hysterical blindness. Hysterical amaurosis may occur in children. One must carefully distinguish between functional loss of power and simulation.

(*c*) *Visceral Manifestations.*—*Respiratory Apparatus.*—Of disturbances in the respiratory rhythm, the most frequent, perhaps, is an exaggeration of the deeper breath, which is taken normally every fifth or sixth inspiration, or there may be a "catching" breathing, such as is seen when cold water is poured over a person. In hysterical dyspnœa there is no special distress and the pulse is normal. In what is known as the syndrome of Briquet there are shortness of breath, suppression of the voice, and paralysis of the diaphragm. The anhelation is extreme. In rare instances there is bradypnœa. Among laryngeal manifestations aphonia is frequent and may persist for months or even years without other special symptoms of the disease. Spasm of the muscles may occur with violent inspiratory efforts and great distress, and may even lead to cyanosis. Hiccough, or sounds resembling it, may be present for weeks or months at a time. Among the most remarkable of the respiratory manifestations are the hysterical cries. These may mimic the sounds produced by animals, such as barking, mewing, or grunting, and in France epidemics of them have been repeatedly observed. Extraordinary cries may be produced, either inspiratory or expiratory. Attacks of gaping, yawning, and sneezing may also occur.

The hysterical cough is a frequent symptom, particularly in young girls. It may occur in paroxysms, but is often a dry, persistent, croaking cough, extremely monotonous and unpleasant to hear. Sir Andrew Clark has called attention to a loud, barking cough (*cynobex hebetica*) occurring about the time of puberty, chiefly in boys belonging to neurotic families. The attacks, which last about a minute, recur frequently.

A peculiar form of hysterical hæmoptysis may be very deceptive and lead to the diagnosis of pulmonary disorders. The sputum is a pale-red fluid, not so bright in color as in ordinary hæmoptysis, and on settling presents a reddish-brown sediment. It contains particles of food, pavement epithelium, red corpuscles, and micrococci, but no cylindrical or ciliated epithelium. It probably comes from the mouth or pharynx.

Digestive System.—Disturbed or depraved appetite, dyspepsia, and gastric pains are common in hysterical patients. The patient may have difficulty in swallowing the food, apparently from spasm of the gullet. There are instances in which the food seems to be expelled before it reaches the stomach. In other cases there is incessant gagging. In the hysterical vomiting the food is regurgitated without much effort and without nausea. This feature may persist for years without great disturbance of nutrition. The most striking and remarkable digestive disturbance in hysteria is the *anorexia nervosa* described by Sir William Gull. "To call it loss of appetite—anorexia—but feebly characterizes the symptom. It is rather an annihilation of appetite, so complete that it seems in some cases impossible ever to eat again. Out of it grows an antagonism to food which results at last and in its worst forms in spasm on the approach of food, and this in turn gives rise to some of those remarkable cases of survival for long periods without food" (Mitchell). There are three special features in anorexia nervosa: *First,* and most important, a psychical state, usually depressant, occasionally excited and restless. It is not always hysterical. *Secondly,* stomach symptoms, loss of appetite, regurgitation, vomiting, and the whole series of phenomena associated with nervous dyspepsia. *Thirdly,* emaciation, which reaches a grade seen only in cancer and dysentery. The patient finally takes to bed, and in extreme cases lies upon one side with the thighs and legs flexed, and contractures may occur. Food is either not taken at all or only upon urgent compulsion. The skin becomes wasted, dry, and covered with bran-like scales. No food may be taken for several weeks at a time, and attempts to feed may be followed by severe spasms. Although the condition looks so alarming, these cases, when removed from their home surroundings and treated by Weir Mitchell's method, sometimes recover in a remarkable way. It may take many months before any improvement is noted. Death, however, may follow with extreme emaciation. In a fatal case under my care the girl weighed only 49 pounds. No lesions were found post mortem.

Hysterical tympanites is a common feature, caused usually by tonic contraction of the diaphragm and retraction of the other abdominal muscles. It may be associated with the condition of peristaltic unrest (Kussmaul). Frequent discharges of fæces may be due to disturbance in either the small or large bowel. An obstinate form of diarrhœa is found in some hysterical patients, which proves very intractable and is associated especially with the taking of food. It seems an aggravated form of the looseness of bowels to which so many nervous people are subject on emotion or of the tendency which some have to diarrhœa immediately after eating. An entirely different form is that produced by what Mitchell calls the irritable rectum, in which scybala are passed frequently during the day, sometimes with great violence. Constipation is more frequent, however, and may be due to a loss of power in the muscles of the bowel, or in the abdominal muscles. In extreme cases the bowels may not be moved for two or three weeks, leading to great accumulation of fæces. Other disturbances are ano-spasm or intense pain in the rectum apart from any fissure. Hysterical ileus and fæcal vomiting are among the most remarkable of hysterical phenomena. Following a shock there are constipation, tympanites, vomiting, sometimes hæmatemesis. The constipation grows worse, everything taken by the mouth is rejected, the vomitus becomes fæcal in character, even scybala are brought up, and suppositories and enemata are vomited. The symptoms may continue for weeks and then gradually subside. Laparotomy—even thrice in one patient—has shown a perfectly normal-looking condition of the bowels (Parkes Weber).

Cardio-vascular.—Rapid action of the heart on the slightest emotion, with or without the subjective sensation of palpitation, is often a source of great distress. A slow pulse is less frequent. Pains about the heart may simulate angina. Flushes in various parts are among the most common symptoms. Sweating may occur, or the *seborrhœa nigricans*, causing a darkening of the skin of the eyelids.

Among the more remarkable vaso-motor phenomena are the so-called stigmata or hæmorrhages in the skin, such as were present in the celebrated case of Louise Lateau. In many cases these are undoubtedly fraudulent, but if, as appears credible, such bleeding may exist in the hypnotic trance, there seems no reason to doubt its occurrence in the trance of prolonged religious ecstasy.

(*d*) *Joint Affections.*—To Sir Benjamin Brodie and Sir James Paget we owe the recognition of these extraordinary manifestations of hysteria. Perhaps no single affection has brought more discredit upon the profession, for the cases are very refractory, and finally fall into the hands of a charlatan or faith-healer, under whose touch the disease may disappear at once. Usually it affects the knee or the hip, and may follow a trifling injury. The joint is usually fixed, sensitive, and swollen. The surface may be cool, but sometimes the local temperature is increased. To the touch it is very sensitive and movement causes great pain. In protracted cases the muscles about the joint are somewhat wasted, and in consequence it looks larger. The pains are often nocturnal, at which time the local temperature may be much increased. While, as a rule, neuromimetic joints yield to proper management, there are interesting instances in the literature in which organic change has succeeded the functional disturbance.

Intermittent hydrarthrosis may be a manifestation of hysteria, occurring in the knee or other joints, sometimes with transient paresis.

(*e*) *Mental Symptoms.*—Mental perversions of all kinds are common in hysterical patients and not much dependence can be placed on statements either about themselves or about others. A morbid craving for sympathy may lead to the commission of all sorts of bizarre and foolish acts.

Hallucinations and delirium may alternate with emotional outbursts of an aggravated character. There is an interesting condition which may be spoken of as the *status hystericus*. For weeks or months they may be confined to bed, entirely oblivious to their surroundings, with a dilirium which may simulate that of delirium tremens, particularly in being associated with loathsome and unpleasant animals. The nutrition may be maintained, but there is always a very heavy, foul breath. With seclusion and care recovery usually takes place within three or four months. At the onset of these attacks and during convalescence the patients must be incessantly watched, as a suicidal tendency is by no means uncommon.

Of hysterical manifestations in the higher centres that of trance is the most remarkable. This may develop spontaneously without any convulsive seizure, but more frequently it follows hysteroid attacks. Catalepsy may be present, a condition in which the limbs are plastic and remain in any position in which they are placed.

(*f*) *The Metabolism in Hysteria.*—In the ordinary forms of hysteria the urine does not show quantitative or qualitative changes, but in the severer types, characterized by convulsions, etc., there are important modifications; reduction in the urates and phosphates; the ratio of the earthy to the alkaline phosphates, normally 1:3, is 1:2, or even 1:1. The urine is also reduced in amount.

(*g*) *Self inflicted wounds,* more particularly burns, are sometimes met with in hysterical patients. I saw at the Hôtel Dieu, Paris, the remarkable condition described by Dieulafoy under the term Pathomimia, in which a young woman supposed to be the subject of a severe trophic disorder submitted to the amputation of the left arm before the confession was obtained that the lesions were self-inflicted! It is to be borne in mind that in Japan and other Eastern countries spontaneous tears occur in the soft parts, usually of the legs—the so-called Kamitachi disease, believed to be due to variations in atmospheric conditions, particularly during thunderstorms.

(*h*) *Hysterical Fever.*—In hysteria the temperature, as a rule, is normal. The cases with fever may be grouped as follows: (1) Instances in which the fever is the sole manifestation. These are rare, but I have seen cases in which the chronic course, the retention of the nutrition, and the entirely negative condition of the organs left no other diagnosis possible. In one case the patient had for four or five years an afternoon rise of temperature, reaching usually to 102° or 103°. She was well nourished and presented no pronounced hysterical symptoms, beyond a form of interrupted sighing respiration so often seen in hysteria. There was a marked neurotic history on one side of the family.

(2) Cases of hysterical fever with spurious local manifestations. These are very troublesome and deceptive cases. The patient may be suddenly taken ill with pain in various regions and elevation of temperature. The case may simulate meningitis. There may be pain in the head, vomiting, contracted pupils, and retraction of the neck—symptoms which may persist for weeks—and some anomalous manifestation during convalescence may alone indicate to the physician that he has had to deal with a case of hysteria, and has not, as he perhaps flattered himself, cured a case of meningitis. Mary Putnam Jacobi, in an article on hysterical fever, mentions a case in the service of Cornil which was admitted with dyspnœa, slight cyanosis, and a temperature of 39° C. The condition proved to be hysterical. There is also an hysterical pseudo-phthisis with pain in the chest, slight fever, and the expectoration of a blood-stained mucus. The cases of hysterical peritonitis may also show fever.

(3) *Hysterical Hyperpyrexia.*—It is a suggestive fact that the cases of paradoxical temperatures reported of late years, in which the thermometer has registered 112° to 120° or more, have been in women. Fraud has been practised in nearly all these cases.

Diagnosis.—Inquiry into the occurrence of previous manifestations and the mental conditions may give important information. These questions, as a rule, should not be asked the mother, who of all others is least likely to give satisfactory information about the patient's condition. The occurrence of the globus hystericus, of emotional attacks, of weeping and crying is always suggestive. The points of difference between the convulsive attacks and true epilepsy were referred to in their description, and, as a rule, little difficulty is experienced in distinguishing between the two conditions. The hysterical paralyses are very variable and apt to be associated with anæsthesia. The contractures may at times be very deceptive, but the occurrence of areas of anæsthesia, of retraction of the visual field, and the development of minor hysterical manifestations give valuable indications. The contractures disappear under full anæsthesia. Special care must be taken not to confound the spastic paraplegia of hysteria with lateral sclerosis.

The visceral manifestations are usually recognized without much difficulty. The practitioner has constantly to bear in mind the strong tendency in hysterical patients to practice deception.

Treatment.—The prophylaxis in hysteria may be gathered from the remarks on the relation of education to the disease. The successful treatment of hysteria demands qualities possessed by few physicians. The first element is a due appreciation of the nature of the disease on the part of the physician and friends. It is pitiable to think of the misery which has been inflicted on these unhappy victims by the harsh and unjust treatment which has resulted from false views of the nature of the trouble; on the other hand, worry and ill health, often the wrecking of mind, body, and estate, are entailed upon the near relatives in the nursing of a protracted case of hysteria. The minor manifestations, attacks of the vapors, the crying and weeping spells, are not of much moment and rarely require treatment. The physical condition should be carefully looked into and the mode of life regulated so as to insure system and order in everything. A congenial occupation offers the best remedy for many of these manifestations. Any functional disturbance should be attended to and a course of tonics prescribed. Special attention should be paid to the action of the bowels.

PSYCHOTHERAPY, in which the important features are hypnosis, suggestion, and reëducation.

Hypnosis.—The majority of hysterical patients can be hypnotized, but the general opinion now of those who know most on the subject is that by hypnosis alone hysteria is rarely cured. Sometimes a brilliant miracle is wrought in the case of hysterical paraplegia or hemiplegia, but as a routine treatment it has fallen into disfavor even in France.

Suggestion.—Babinski defines suggestion as "the action by which one endeavors to make another accept or realize an idea which is manifestly unreasonable." On the other hand, persuasion is applied when the ideas are reasonable, or at least are not in opposition to good sense. Most writers, however, use the word "suggestion" as meaning the introduction of mental associations and modifications of the patient's mental state leading to betterment. In proper hands it is a most powerful instrument, particularly when the patient has faith in the person who makes it. After a careful and sympathetic examination and testing the electrical reactions of the muscles of a paralyzed limb the suggestion to the hysteric, "Now I think you will be able to move it" may be all-sufficient. A strong, imperative command may sometimes have the same effect.

Reëducation.—In both hysteria and neurasthenia this should be the aim of all reasonable practice, but we must remember it is not always feasible: some of our patients would have to be rebuilt from the blastoderm. With patience and method much may be done, and the special merit of Weir Mitchell's work and of his system (which is not simply a rest cure, as many suppose) is that it is an elaborate plan of reëducation. The essentials are that the patient should be isolated from his friends and under the charge of an intelligent nurse. The physical condition is carefully studied and a rigid daily régime carried out: A milk diet of three to four quarts daily, rising to five or six, varying the food as the patient improves, and as the weight increases. This may be followed by a rapid gain in weight and the disappearance of all the unpleasant abdominal symptoms. Massage, hydrotherapy, and electricity are brought in as adjuncts, but very much depends upon the tact, patience, and, above all, the personality of the physician; the man counts more than the method. The mental condition has to be carefully studied and the patient's attitude toward life influenced by specially selected literature, careful conversation, and the suggestion of topics for thought.

THE ANALYTICAL OR CATHARTIC METHOD.—Introduced by Breuer and extended by Freud, it is in reality the old method of the confessional, in which the sinner poured out his soul in the sympathetic ear of the priest. It is a difficult procedure, not for all to attempt, exhausting alike to patient and doctor, and, when thoroughly carried out, time consuming. In the hands of those who have practised it, very good results have been obtained, particularly in young and carefully selected cases. The following statement of the method I take from Jelliffe ("System of Medicine," Vol. VII, page 866):

"His (Freud's) general procedure is to place the patient in a recumbent position, the physician sitting behind the patient's head at the end of the lounge. The physician thus remains practically out of sight of the patient, who is then asked to give a detailed account of his troubles, and to say everything that comes to the mind irrespective of its seeming logic or sense, and apart from disturbing, mortifying, or unnice suggestions. In all such histories gaps are inevitable. These the patient is urged to fill in by thinking closely of the attendant circumstances, speaking aloud all of the flitting thoughts that pass during this search ('free association'). All the thoughts are requested to be uttered, notwithstanding their disagreeable nature. The patient must exercise no critique and remain passive. It will be found that the disagreeable thoughts are pushed back with the greatest resistance. This is made all the more striking since the hysterical reaction, i. e., the symptom, is the symbolic expression of the realization of a repressed wish and gives the patient some gratification. A great effort is made to retain the symptom, especially as its origin is not really perceived, and since it represents, in symbol, the individual's former conscious strivings. In psycho-analysis one attempts to overcome all of these resistances, and by a series of judicious and tactful probings reconduct into the patient's consciousness the hidden thoughts which underlie these symptoms. Every symptom has some meaning; behind it there lies some associated mechanism, the origin of which the patient unconsciously or partly consciously represses. In the psycho-neurotic symbol may be read the cryptic expression of the original thought driven back and hidden.

"To slowly analyze and pick apart the mechanism is the object of the analytical method. One needs not only special tact for such excursions into the subtleties of the mental life of some individuals, but also a developed method of interpretation. Every act, every symbolic expression or action, lapse in speech, mannerism, needs to be carefully noted and its bearing coördinated. Freud lays particular emphasis on the analysis of dreams, since he believes that in the dream the subconscious, or the 'repressed conscious' is more apt to reveal itself. Hence a careful reading of Freud's 'Significance of Dreams' is of the greatest value in this study, also his 'Psychopathology of Every-day Life.' In his work on dreams he has developed to the full the chief directions along which his mind has traveled in the psychoanalytical method.

"It is of the utmost importance to trace back into the earliest years the striking emotional influences that have come into experience, as, for Freud, the hysterical reaction consists in a perverted type of reaction to these experiences. As is known, the blurring, or loss of an emotional influence—an affect, in short—is due to a number of factors. In normal life forgetting is the commonest type of a corrective adaptation, and forgetting is carried out with special ease if the emotional stress has not been excessive. Forgetting, however, is only a secondary phenomenon, and usually is more successful if the immediate reaction has been an adequate one. Such immediate reactions express themselves as tears, as anger, as impulsive acts, etc., and in such reactions the effect is discharged. In every-day life one calls it giving vent to one's feelings. If, however, the reaction is suppressed, the effect becomes united to the memory of the experience, and an emotional complex, or, to use a rather broad simile, a psychic boil, results, which must heal by absorption, by discharge, or by other means. Freud uses the term ab-react (abreagieren) to signify the adequate reaction, or discharge of such effects or their resulting complexes. Talking the whole thing over, giving vent to one's secrets and confessions are well-known abreactions.

"In hysteria certain of these complexes remain prominent; they are neither reacted too promptly, nor is their unpleasant feeling tone diminished by the blurring process of forgetting, although it is characteristic of the Freud point of view that the actual experience which gives rise to them becomes forgotten and the cause of the affect disturbance which becomes later converted, it may be into physical signs, remains apparently unknown to the patient. It must be dug out by psycho-analysis, and when once discovered catharsis takes place and the patient becomes cured."

Hydrotherapy is of great value, especially wet packs, salt baths, and various douches. General tonics, such as arsenic and iron, may be helpful, especially if the patients are nervous and anæmic. Sedatives are rarely indicated. Occasionally bromides may be necessary, but for the relief of sleeplessness all possible measures should be resorted to before the employment of drugs. The wet pack given hot or cold at night will usually suffice.

X. NEURASTHENIA

(*Psychasthenia*)

Definition.—A condition of weakness or exhaustion of the nervous system, giving rise to various forms of mental and bodily inefficiency.

The term, an old one, but first popularized by Beard, covers an ill-defined, motley group of symptoms, which may be either general and the expression of derangement of the entire system, or local, limited to certain organs; hence, the terms cerebral, spinal, cardiac, and gastric neurasthenia.

Etiology.—The causes may be grouped as hereditary and acquired.

(*a*) Hereditary.—We do not all start in life with the same amount of nerve capital. Parents who have led irrational lives, indulging in excesses of various kinds, or who have been the subjects of nervous complaints or of mental trouble, may transmit to their children an organization which is defective in what, for want of a better term, we must call "nerve force." Such individuals start handicapped with a neuropathic predisposition, and furnish a considerable proportion of our neurasthenic patients. As van Gieson sonorously puts it, "the potential energies of the higher constellations of their association centres have been squandered by their ancestors." So long as these individuals are content to transact a moderate business with their life capital, all may go well, but there is no reserve, and in the exigencies of modern life these small capitalists go under and come to us as bankrupts.

(*b*) Acquired.—The functions, though perverted most readily in persons who have inherited a feeble organization, may also be damaged in persons with no neuropathic predisposition by exercise which is excessive in proportion to the strength—i. e., by strain. The cares and anxieties attendant upon the gaining of a livelihood may be borne without distress, but in many persons the strain becomes excessive and is first manifested as *worry*. The individual loses the distinction between essentials and non-essentials, trifles cause annoyance, and the entire organism reacts with unnecessary readiness to slight stimuli, and is in a state which the older writers called irritable weakness. If such a condition be taken early and the patient given rest, the balance is quickly restored. In this group may be placed a large proportion of the neurasthenia which we see among business men, teachers, and journalists. Neurasthenia may follow the infectious diseases, particularly influenza, typhoid fever, and syphilis. The abuse of certain drugs, alcohol, tobacco, morphine may lead to a high grade of neurasthenia, though the drug habit is more often a result rather than a cause of the neurasthenia.

(*c*) Sexual Causes.—Undoubtedly the part played in the production of hysteria and allied neuroses by sexual factors is of the first importance. As already stated, Freud regards sexual trauma as the basis of hysteria, and he also regards neurasthenia as largely a product of disturbance in the sexual sphere. For him and his school the sexual impulses furnish the basis of the psychoneuroses. Repressed as they have to be in so many in our modern civilization, without normal outlet, the thought formations, retained in the unconscious state, express themselves by means of somatic phenomena—the objective features of hysteria and neurasthenia. *Cherchez la femme* is a safe rule in investigating a neurotic case. Freud may have ridden his hobby too hard, particularly in the insistence upon the importance of infantile sexuality, but in recognizing the rôle of the younger Aphrodite in the lives of men and women he has but followed the great master, Plato, who saw, while he deplored, the havoc wrought by her universal dominance.

The traumatic forms, especially those following upon railway accidents, will be separately considered.

Symptoms.—These are extremely varied, and may be general or localized; more often a combination of both. The appearance of the patient is suggestive, sometimes characteristic, but difficult to describe. Important information can be gained by the physician if he observes the patient closely as he enters the room—the way he is clothed, the manner in which he holds his body, his facial expression, and the humor which he is in. Loss of weight and slight anæmia may be present. The physical debility may reach a high grade and the patient may be confined to bed. Mentally the patients are usually low-spirited and despondent; women are frequently emotional.

The local symptoms may dominate the situation, and there have accordingly been described a whole series of types of the disease—cerebral, spinal, cardio-vascular, gastric, and sexual. In all forms there is a striking lack of accordance between the symptoms of which the patient complains and the objective changes discoverable by the physician. In nearly every clinical type of the disease the predominant symptoms are referable to pathological sensations and the psychic effects of these. Imperfect sleep is also complained of by a majority of patients, or, if not complained of, is found to exist on inquiry.

In the cerebral or psychic form the symptoms are chiefly connected with an inability to perform the ordinary mental work. Thus, a row of figures can not be correctly added, the dictation or the writing of a few letters is a source of the greatest worry, the transaction of petty details in business is a painful effort, and there is loss of power of fixed attention. With this condition there may be no headache, the appetite may be good, and the patient may sleep well. As a rule, however, there are sensations of fulness and weight or flushes, if not actual headache. Sleeplessness is a frequent concomitant of the cerebral form, and may be the first manifestation. Some of these patients are good-tempered and cheerful, but a majority are moody, irritable, and depressed.

Hyperæsthesia, especially to sensations of pain, is one of the main characteristics of almost all neurasthenic individuals. The sensations are nearly always referred to some special region of the body—the skin, eye muscles, the joints, the blood-vessels, or the viscera. It is frequently possible to localize a number of points painful to pressure (Valleix's points). In some patients there is marked vertigo, occasionally even resembling that of Ménière's disease.

If such pathological sensations continue for a long time the mood and character of the patient gradually alter. The so-called "irritable humor" develops. Many obnoxiously egoistic individuals met with in daily life are in reality examples of psychic neurasthenia. Everything is complained of. The patient demands the greatest consideration for his condition; he feels that he has been deeply insulted if his desires are not always immediately granted. He may at the same time have but little consideration for others. Indeed, in the severer forms of the disease he may show a malicious pleasure in attempting to make people who seem happier than himself uncomfortable. Such patients complain frequently that they are "misunderstood" by their fellows.

In many cases the so-called "anxiety conditions" gradually come on; one scarcely ever sees a case of advanced neurasthenia without the existence of some form of "anxiety." In the simpler forms of anxiety (nosophobic) there may be only a fear of impending insanity or of approaching death or of apoplexy. More frequently the anxious feeling is localized somewhere in the body —in the præcordial region, in the head, in the abdomen, in the thorax, or more rarely in the extremities.

In some cases the anxiety becomes intense and the patients are restless, and declare that they do not know what to do with themselves. They may throw themselves upon a bed, crying and complaining, and making convulsive movements with the hands and feet. Suicidal tendencies are not uncommon in such cases, and the patients may in desperation actually take their own lives.

Involuntary mental activity may be very troublesome; the patient complains that when he is overtired thoughts which he cannot stop or control run through his head with lightning-like rapidity. In other cases there is marked absence of ideas, the individual's mind being so filled up owing to the overexcitability of latent memory pictures that he is unable to form the proper associations for ideas called up by external stimuli. Sometimes a patient complains that a definite word, a name, a number, a melody, or a song keeps running in his head in spite of all he can do to abolish it.

In the severer cases the so-called "phobias" are common. The most frequent form perhaps is *agoraphobia,* in which patients the moment they come into an open space are oppressed by an exaggerated feeling of anxiety. They seem "frightened to death," and commence to tremble all over; they complain of compression of the thorax and palpitation of the heart. They may break into profuse perspiration and assert that they feel as though chained to the ground or that they can not move a step. It is remarkable that in some such cases the open space can be crossed if the individual be accompanied by some one, even by a child, or if he carry a stick or an umbrella! Other people are afraid to be left alone (monophobia), especially in a closed compartment (claustrophobia).

The fear of people and of society is known as anthropophobia. A whole series of other phobias have been described—batophobia, or the fear that high things will fall; pathophobia, or fear of disease; siderodromophobia, or fear of a railway journey; siderophobia or astrophobia, fear of thunder and lightning. Occasionally we meet with individuals who are afraid of everything and every one—victims of the so-called pantophobia.

The *special senses* may be disturbed, particularly vision. An aching or weariness of the eyeballs after reading a few minutes or flashes of light are common symptoms. The "irritable eye," the so-called nervous or neurasthenic asthenopia, is familiar to every family physician.

There may be acoustic disturbances—hyperalgesia and even true hyperacusia.

One of the most common of all the symptoms of neurasthenia is the *pressure in the head* complained of by these patients. This symptom, variously described, may be diffuse, but is more frequently referred to some one region—frontal, temporal, parietal, or occipital.

When the *spinal symptoms* predominate—spinal irritation or spinal neurasthenia—in addition to many of the features just mentioned, the patients complain of weariness on the least exertion, of weakness, pain in the back, intercostal neuralgiform pains, and of aching pains in the legs. There may be spots of local tenderness on the spine. The rachialgia may be spontaneous, or may be noticed only on pressure or movement. Occasionally there may be disturbances of sensation, particularly a feeling of numbness and tingling, and the reflexes may be increased. Visceral neuralgias, especially in connection with the genital organs, are frequently met with. The aching pain in the back or in the back of the neck is the most constant complaint in these cases. In women it is often impossible to say whether this condition is one of neurasthenia or hysteria. It is in these cases that the disturbances of muscular activity are most pronounced, and in the French writings *amyosthenia* particularly plays an important rôle. The symptoms may be irritative or paretic, or a combination of both. Disturbances of coördination are not uncommon in the severer forms. These are particularly prone to involve the associated movements of the eye muscles, leading to asthenopic lack of accommodation. Drooping of one eyelid is very common, probably owing to insufficient innervation on the part of the sympathetic rather than to paresis of the oculómotor nerve. Occasionally Romberg's symptom may be present, and the patient, or even his physician, may fear a beginning tabes. More rarely there is disturbance of such finely coördinated acts as writing and articulation, not unlike those seen at the onset of general paresis. Such symptoms are always alarming, and the greatest care must be taken in establishing a diagnosis. That they may be the symptoms of pure neurasthenia, however, can no longer be doubted.

The reflexes in neurasthenia are usually increased, the deep reflexes especially never being absent. The condition of the superficial reflexes is less constant, though these, too, are usually increased. The pupils are often dilated, and the reflexes are usually normal. There may be inequality of the pupils in neurasthenia. Errors in refraction are common, the correction of which may give great relief.

In another type of cases the muscular weakness is extreme, and may go on even to complete motor helplessness. Very thorough examination is necessary before deciding as to the nature of the affection, since in some instances serious mistakes have been made. Here belong the *atremia* of Neftel, the *akinesia algera* of Möbius, and the neurasthenic form of *astasia abasia* described by Binswanger.

In other cases the *cardio-vascular* symptoms are the most distressing, and may occur with only slight disturbance of the cerebro-spinal functions, though the conditions are nearly always combined. Palpitation of the heart, irregular and very rapid action (neurasthenic tachycardia), and pains and oppressive feelings in the cardiac region are the most common symptoms. The slightest excitement may be followed by increased action of the heart, sometimes associated with sensations of dizziness and anxiety, and the patients frequently have the idea that they suffer from serious disease of this organ. Attacks of pseudo-angina may occur.

Vaso-motor disturbances constitute a special feature of many cases. Flushes of heat, especially in the head, and transient hyperæmia of the skin may be very distressing symptoms. Profuse sweating may occur, either local or general, and sometimes nocturnal. The pulse may show interesting features, owing to the extreme relaxation of the peripheral arterioles. The arterial throbbing may be everywhere visible, almost as much as in aortic insufficiency. The pulse, too, may under these circumstances have a somewhat water-hammer quality. The capillary pulse may be seen in the nails, on the lips, or on the margins of a line drawn upon the forehead, and I have on several occasions seen pulsation in the veins of the back of the hand. A characteristic symptom in some cases is the *throbbing aorta.* This "preternatural pulsation in the epigastrium," as Allan Burns calls it, may be extremely forcible and suggest the existence of abdominal aneurism. The subjective sensations associated with it may be very unpleasant, particularly when the stomach is empty.

In women especially, and sometimes in men, the peripheral blood-vessels are contracted, the extremities are cold, the nose is red or blue, and the face has a pinched expression. These patients feel much more comfortable when the cutaneous vessels are distended, and resort to various means to favor this (wearing of heavy clothing, use of diffusible stimulants).

The general features of *gastro-intestinal neurasthenia* have been dealt with under the section of nervous dyspepsia. The connection of these cases with dilatation of the stomach, floating kidney, and the condition which Glénard calls *enteroptosis* has already been mentioned.

Sexual neurasthenia is a condition in which there is an irritable weakness of the sexual organs manifested by nocturnal emissions, unusual depression after intercourse, and often by a distressing dread of impotence. The mental condition of these patients is most pitiable, and they fall an easy prey to quacks and charlatans of all kinds. In males these symptoms are frequently due to diseased conditions in the deep urethra, especially of the verumontanum, and prostate.

Spermatorrhœa is the bugbear of the majority. They complain of continued losses, usually without accompanying pleasurable sensations. After defecation or micturition there may be seminal discharges. Microscopic examination sometimes reveals the presence of spermatozoa. Actual nervous impotence is not uncommon. The "painful testicle" is a well-known neurasthenic phenomenon. In the severer cases, especially those bearing the stigmata of degeneration, there may be evidence of sexual perversion.

In females it is common to find a tender ovary, and painful or irregular menstruation.

In all forms of neurasthenia the condition of the urine is important. Many cases are complicated with the symptoms of the condition known as lithæmia, and so marked may this be that some have indeed made a special form of lithæmic neurasthenia. Polyuria may be present, but is more common in hysteria. With disturbed digestion the urates and oxalates may be in excess.

Diagnosis.—*Psychasthenia.*—Under this term Janet would separate from neurasthenia the cases characterized by mental, emotional, and physical disturbances, imperative ideas, phobias of all sorts, doubts, enfeebled will, uncontrollable movements, and many of the borderland features of the insanity of young persons. It is really an inherited psychoneurosis, while neurasthenia is usually acquired. Obsessions of all sorts characterize the condition and there may be a feeling of unreality and even of loss of personality. How complicated the condition may be is shown from the following varieties distinguished by Janet: (1) The *doubter,* in whom obsessive ideas are not very precise, more of the nature of a general indication rather than a specific idea, such as a craze for research, for explanation, for computing. (2) The *scrupulous,* whose obsessions are of a moral nature. Their manias are of literalness of statement, of exact truth, of conjuration, of reparation, of symbols, etc. (3) The *criminal,* whose obsessive ideas are of homicide, theft, and other overt acts. The impulsive idea is stronger in this than in the other varieties. (4) The *inebriates,* dipsomaniac, morphinomaniac, etc., in whom the impulse seems to be least resistible. (5) The *genesically perverted.* (6) *Delirious psychasthenia,* a condition in which a delirious state of mind occurs, connected with the obsession.

The anxiety conditions and various phobias, as well as the different varieties of tic and the occupation neuroses when they accompany neurasthenia, are regarded as complications dependent in the majority of instances upon faulty heredity.

Neurasthenia is a disease above all others which has to be diagnosed from the subjective statements of the patient, and from an observation of his general behavior rather than from the physical examination. The physical examination is of the highest importance in excluding other diseases likely to be confounded with it. That somatic changes occur and that physical signs are often to be made out is very true, but there is nothing typical or pathognomonic in these objective changes.

The hypochondriac differs from the neurasthenic in the excessive psychic distortion of the pathological sensations to which he is subject. He is the victim of actual delusions regarding his condition.

The confusion of neurasthenia with hysteria is still more frequent; in women especially a diagnosis of hysteria is often made when in reality the condition is one of neurasthenia. In the absence of hysterical paroxysms, of crises, and of those marked emotional and intellectual characteristics of the hysterical individual the diagnosis of hysteria should not be made. Of course, in many of the cases of hysteria definite hysterical stigmata (hysterical paralyses, convulsions, contractures, anæsthesias, alterations in the visual field, etc.) are present, and the diagnosis is not difficult.

Epilepsy is not likely to be confounded with neurasthenia if there be definite epileptic attacks, but the cases of *petit mal* may be puzzling.

The onset of exophthalmic goitre may be mistaken for neurasthenia, especially if there be no exophthalmos at the beginning. The emotional disturbances and the irritability of the heart may mislead the physician. In pronounced cases of nervous prostration the differential diagnosis from the various psychoses may be extremely difficult.

The two forms of organic disease of the nervous system with which neurasthenia is most likely to be confounded are tabes and general paresis. The symptoms of the spinal form of neurasthenia may resemble those of the former disease, while the symptoms of the psychic or cerebral form of neurasthenia may be very similar to those of general paresis. The diagnosis, as a rule, presents no difficulty if the physician be careful to make a thorough routine examination. It is only the superficial study of a case that is likely to lead one astray. In tabes especially a consideration of the sensory disturbances, of the deep reflexes, and of the pupillary findings will always establish the presence or absence of the disease. In general paresis there is sometimes more difficulty. The onset of general paresis is often characterized by the appearance of symptoms quite like those of ordinary neurasthenia, and the family physician mav entirely overlook the grave nature of the malady. The mistake in the other direction is, however, perhaps just as common. A physician who once or twice has seen a case of general paresis arise out of what appeared to be one of pronounced neurasthenia is too prone afterward to suspect every neurasthenic to be developing the malign affection. The most marked symptoms, however, of psychic exhaustion do not justify a diagnosis of general paresis even when the history is suspicious, unless along with it there is a definite paresis of the pupils, of the facial muscles, or of the muscles of articulation. A history of syphilis or of chronic alcoholism or morphinism associated with severe psychic exhaustion should, of course, put one always on his guard, and the physician should be sharply on the lookout for the appearance of intellectual defects, paraphasia, facial paresis, and sluggishness of the pupils.

Treatment.—Prophylaxis.—Many patients come under our care a generation too late for satisfactory treatment, and it may be impossible to restore the exhausted capital. The greatest care should be taken in the rearing of children of neuropathic predisposition. From a very early age they should be submitted to a process of "psychic hardening," every effort being made to strengthen the bodily and mental condition. Even in infancy the child should not be pampered. Later on the greatest care should be exercised with regard to food, sleep, and school work. Complaints of children should not be too seriously considered.

Much depends upon the example set by the parents. A restless, emotional, constantly complaining mother will rack the nervous system of a delicate child. In some instances, for the welfare of a developing boy or girl, the physician may find it necessary to advise its removal from home.

Neurotic children are especially liable during development to fits of temper and of emotional disturbance. These should not be too lightly considered. Above all, violent chastisement in such cases is to be avoided, and loss of temper on the part of the parent or teacher is particularly pernicious for the nervous system of the child. Where possible, in such instances, the best treatment is to put the obstreperous child immediately to bed, and if the excitement and temper continue a warm bath followed by a cool douche may be effective. If he be put to bed after the bath sleep soon follows.

Special attention is necessary at puberty in both boys and girls. If there be at this period any marked tendency to emotional disturbance or to intellectual weakness the child should be removed from school and every care taken to avoid unfavorable influences.

Personal Hygiene.—Throughout life individuals of neuropathic predisposition should obey scrupulously certain hygienic and prophylactic rules. Intellectual work especially should be judiciously limited and should alternate frequently with periods of repose. Excitement of all kinds should of course be avoided, and such individuals will do well to be abstemious in the use of tobacco, tea, coffee, and alcohol, if, indeed, they be permitted to use these substances at all. The habit, happily becoming very common, of taking at least once a year a prolonged holiday away from the ordinary environment, in the woods, in the mountains, or at the seashore, should be urgently enjoined upon every neuropathic individual. In many instances it is found to be the greatest relief and rest if the patient can take his holiday away from his relatives.

During ordinary life nervous people should, during some portion of each day, pay rational attention to the body. Cold baths, swimming, exercises in the gymnasium, gardening, golf, lawn tennis, cricket, hunting, shooting, rowing, sailing, and bicycling are of value in maintaining the general nutrition. Such exercises are, of course, to be recommended only to individuals physically equal to them. If neurasthenia be once well established the greatest care must be observed in the ordering of exercise. Many nervous girls have been completely broken down by following injudicious advice with regard to long walks.

Treatment of the Condition.—The treatment of neurasthenia when once established presents a varied problem to the thoughtful physician. Every case must be handled upon its own merits, no two, as a rule, requiring exactly the same methods. In general it will be the aim of the medical adviser to remove the patient as far as possible from the influences which have led to his downfall, and to restore to normal the nervous mechanisms which have been weakened by injurious influences. The general character of the individual, his physical and social status, must of course be considered and the therapeutic measures carefully adjusted to these.

The diagnosis having been settled, the physician may assure the patient that with prolonged treatment, during which his coöperation with the physician is absolutely essential, he may expect to get well. He must be told that much depends upon himself and that he must make a vigorous effort to overcome certain of his tendencies, and that all his strength of will will be needed to further the progress of the cure. In the case of business or professional men, in whom the condition develops as a result of overwork or overstudy, it may be sufficient to enjoin absolute rest with change of scene and diet. A trip abroad, with a residence for a month or two in Switzerland, or, if there are symptoms of nervous dyspepsia, a residence at one of the Spas will usually prove sufficient. The excitement of the large cities abroad should be avoided. The longer the disease has lasted and the more intense the symptoms have been, the longer the time necessary for the restoration of health. In cases of any severity the patient must be told that at least six months' complete absence from business, under strict medical guidance, will be necessary. Shorter periods may of course be of benefit, which, however, as a rule, will be only temporary.

It will often be found advisable to make out a daily programme, which shall occupy almost the whole time of the patient. At first he need know nothing about this, the case being given over entirely to the nurse. As improvement advances, moderate physical and intellectual exercises, alternating frequently with rest and the administration of food, may be undertaken. Some one hour of the day may be left free for reading, correspondence, conversation, and games. In some instances the writing of letters is particularly harmful to the patient and must be prohibited or limited. Cultured individuals may find benefit from attention to drawing, painting, modelling, translating from a foreign language, the making of abstracts, etc., for short periods in the day.

In not a few cases, including a large proportion of neurasthenic women, a systematic Weir Mitchell treatment rigidly carried out should be tried. The patient must be isolated from his friends, and any regulations undertaken must be strictly adhered to, the consent of the patient and his family having first been gained. The treatment of the gastric and intestinal symptoms so important in this condition has already been considered. For the irregular pains, particularly in the back and neck, the thermo-cautery is invaluable.

Hydrotherapy is indicated in nearly every case if it can be properly applied. Much can be done at home or in an ordinary hospital, but for systematic hydrotherapeutic treatment residence in a suitable sanitarium is necessary. I have found the wet pack of especial value. Particularly at night, in cases of sleeplessness, it is perhaps the best remedy against insomnia we have. Salt baths are more helpful to some patients. The various forms of douches, partial packs, foot baths, etc., may be valuable in individual cases. Electro-therapy is of some value, though only in combination with psychic treatment and hydrotherapy.

Special care should be given to the recognition of local disease and proper measures instituted. Attention to the eyes is important. Infection of the naso-pharynx, sinus disease, visceroptosis, or anæmia should be corrected. In women the pelvic organs and in men the deep urethra and prostate may require treatment.

Treatment by drugs should be avoided as much as possible. They are of benefit chiefly in the combating of single symptoms. Alcohol, morphia, chloral, or cocaine should never be given. General tonics may be helpful, especially if the individual be anæmic. Arsenic and more often iron are then indicated. For the severer pains and nervous attacks some sedative may occasionally be necessary, especially at the beginning of the treatment. The bromides may here be given with advantage. An occasional dose of phenacetin or aspirin may be required, but the less of these substances we can get along with the better. For the relief of sleeplessness all possible measures should be resorted to before the employment of drugs. The wet pack will usually suffice. If absolutely necessary to give a drug, sulphonal, trional, or amylene hydrate may be employed.

In cases in which the anxiety conditions are disturbing the cautious use of opium in pill form may be necessary, since, as in the psychoses, opium here will sometimes yield permanent relief. A prolonged treatment with opium is, however, never necessary in neurasthenia.

Psychotherapy.—Hypnotism is rarely indicated. Carefully practiced suggestion is most helpful and the psycho-analytic method of Freud, as described under Hysteria, may be tried.

The use of religious ideas and practices may be most helpful, and this has come into vogue in various forms, as Christian Science, Emmanualism, Mental Healing, etc. It is an old story. In all ages, and in all lands, the prayer of faith, to use the words of St. James, has healed the sick; and we must remember that amid the Æsculapian cult, the most elaborate and beautiful system of faith healing the world has seen, scientific medicine took its rise. As a profession, consciously or unconsciously, more often the latter, *faith* has been one of our most valuable assets, and Galen expressed a great truth when he said, "He cures most successfully in whom the people have the greatest confidence." It is in these cases of neurasthenia and psychasthenia, the weak brothers and the weak sisters, that the personal character of the physician comes into play, and once let him gain the confidence of the patient, he can work just the same sort of miracles as Our Lady of Lourdes or Ste. Anne de Beaupré. Three elements are necessary: first, a strong personality in whom the individual has faith—Christ, Buddha, Æsculapius (in the days of Greece), one of the saints, or, what has served the turn of common humanity very well, a physician. Secondly, certain accessories—a shrine, a sanctuary, the services of a temple, or for us a hospital or its equivalent, with a skillful nurse. Thirdly, suggestion, either of the "only believe," "feel it," "will it" attitude of mind, which is the essence of every cult and creed, or of the active belief in the assurance of the physician that the precious boon of health is within reach.

XI. THE TRAUMATIC NEUROSES

(Railway Brain and Railway Spine; Traumatic Hysteria)

Definition.—A morbid condition following shock which presents the symptoms of neurasthenia or hysteria or of both. The condition is known as "railway brain" and "railway spine."

Erichsen regarded the condition as the result of inflammation of the meninges and cord, and gave it the name railway spine. Walton and J. J. Putnam, of Boston, were the first to recognize the hysterical nature of many of the cases, and to Westphal's pupils we owe the name traumatic neurosis.

Etiology.—The condition follows an accident, often in a railway train, in which injury has been sustained, or succeeds a shock or concussion, from which the patient may apparently not have suffered in his body. A man may appear perfectly well for several days, or even a week or more, and then develop the symptoms of the neurosis. Bodily shock or concussion is not necessary. The affection may follow a profound mental impression; thus, an engine-driver ran over a child, and received thereby a very severe shock, subsequent to which the most pronounced symptoms of neurasthenia developed. Severe mental strain combined with bodily exposure may cause it, as in a case of a naval officer who was wrecked in a violent storm and exposed for more than a day in the rigging before he was rescued. A slight blow, a fall from a carriage or on the stairs may suffice.

Symptoms.—The cases may be divided into three groups: simple neurasthenia, cases with marked hysterical manifestations, and cases with severe symptoms indicating or simulating organic disease.

(*a*) Simple Traumatic Neurasthenia.—The first symptoms usually develop a few weeks after the accident, which may or may not have been associated with an actual trauma. The patient complains of headache and tired feelings. He is sleepless and finds himself unable to concentrate his attention properly upon his work. A condition of nervous irritability develops, which may have a host of trivial manifestations, and the entire mental attitude of the person may for a time be changed. He dwells constantly upon his condition, gets very despondent and low-spirited, and in extreme cases melancholia may develop. He may complain of numbness and tingling in the extremities, and in some cases of much pain in the back. The bodily functions may be well performed, though such patients usually have, for a time at least, disturbed digestion and loss in weight. The physical examination may be entirely negative. The reflexes are slightly increased, as in ordinary neurasthenia. The pupils may be unequal; the cardio-vascular changes already described in neurasthenia may be present in a marked degree. According as the symptoms are more spinal or more cerebral, the condition is known as railway brain or railway spine.

(2) Cases with Marked Hysterical Features.—Following an injury of any sort, neurasthenic symptoms, like those described above, may develop, and in addition symptoms regarded as characteristic of hysteria. The emotional element is prominent, and there is but slight control over the feelings. The patients have headache, backache, and vertigo. A violent tremor may be present, and, indeed, constitutes the most striking feature of the case. In the case of an engineer who developed subsequent to an accident a series of nervous phenomenon the most marked feature was an excessive tremor of the entire body, which was specially manifest during emotional excitement. The most pronounced hysterical symptoms are the sensory disturbances. As first noted by Putnam and Walton, hemianæsthesia may occur as a consequence of traumatism. This is a common symptom in France, but rare in England and in the United States. Achromatopsia may exist on the anæsthetic side. A second, more common, manifestation is limitation of the field of vision, similar to that which occurs in hysteria.

(3) Cases in Which the Symptoms Suggest Organic Disease of the Brain and Cord.—As a result of spinal concussion, without fracture or external injury, there may subsequently develop symptoms suggestive of organic disease, which may come on rapidly or at a late date. In a case reported by Leyden the symptoms following the concussion were at first slight and the patient was regarded as a simulator, but finally the condition became aggravated and death resulted. The post mortem showed a chronic pachymeningitis, which had doubtless resulted from the accident. The cases in this group about which there is so much discussion are those which display marked sensory and motor changes. Following an accident in which the patient has not received external injury a condition of excitement may develop within a week or ten days; he complains of headache and backache, and on examination sensory disturbances are found, either hemianæsthesia or areas on the skin in which the sensation is much benumbed; or painful and tactile impressions may be distinctly felt in certain regions, and the temperature sense is absent. The distribution may be bilateral and symmetrical in limited regions or hemiplegic in type. Limitation of the field of vision is usually marked in these cases, and there may be disturbance of the senses of taste and smell. The superficial reflexes may be diminished; usually the deep reflexes are exaggerated. The pupils may be unequal; the motor disturbances are variable. The French writers describe cases of monoplegia with or without contracture, symptoms upon which Charcot lays great stress as a manifestation of profound hysteria. The combination of sensory disturbances—anæsthesia or hyperæsthesia—with paralysis, particularly if monoplegic, and the occurrence of contractures without atrophy and with normal electrical reactions, may be regarded as distinctive of hysteria.

In rare cases following trauma and succeeding to symptoms which may have been regarded as neurasthenic or hysterical there are organic changes which may prove fatal. That this sequence occurs is demonstrated clearly by recent post mortem examinations. The features upon which the greatest reliance can be placed as indicating organic change are optic atrophy, bladder symptoms, particularly in combination with tremor, paresis, and exaggerated reflexes.

The anatomical changes in this condition have not been very definite. When death follows spinal concussion within a few days there may be no apparent lesion, but in some instances the brain or cord has shown punctiform hæmorrhages. Edes has reported 4 cases in which a gradual degeneration in the pyramidal tracts followed concussion or injury of the spine; but in all these cases there was marked tremor and the spinal symptoms developed early, or followed immediately upon the accident.

Diagnosis.—A condition of fright and excitement following an accident may persist for days or even weeks, and then gradually pass away. The symptoms of neurasthenia or of hysteria which subsequently develop present nothing peculiar and are identical with those which occur under other circumstances. Care must be taken to recognize simulation, and, as in these cases the condition is largely subjective, this is sometimes extremely difficult. In a careful examination a simulator will often reveal himself by exaggeration of certain symptoms, particularly sensitiveness of the spine, and by increasing voluntarily the reflexes. Maunkopff suggests as a good test to take the pulse rate before, during, and after pressure upon an area said to be painful. If the rate is quickened, it is held to be proof that the pain is real. This is not, however, always the case. It may require a careful study of the case to determine whether the individual is honestly suffering from the symptoms of which he complains. A still more important question is, Has the patient organic disease? The symptoms given under the first two groups of cases may exist in a marked degree and may persist for several years without the slightest evidence of organic change. Hemianæsthesia, limitation of the field of vision, monoplegia with contracture, may all be present as hysterical manifestations, from which recovery may be complete. In our present knowledge the diagnosis of an organic lesion should be limited to those cases in which optic atrophy, bladder troubles, and signs of sclerosis of the cord are well marked—indications either of degeneration of the lateral columns or of multiple sclerosis. Examination by the X-rays is an important aid and has showed in some cases definite injury to the spine.

Prognosis.—A majority of patients with traumatic hysteria recover. In railway cases, so long as litigation is pending and the patient is in the hands of lawyers, the symptoms usually persist. Settlement is often the starting-point of a speedy and perfect recovery. On the other hand, there are a few cases in which the symptoms persist even after the litigation has been closed; the patient goes from bad to worse and psychoses develop, such as melancholia, dementia, or occasionally progressive paresis. And, lastly, in extremely rare cases organic lesions may occur as a sequence of the traumatic neurosis.

The function of the physician acting as medical expert in these cases consists in determining (*a*) the existence of actual disease, and (*b*) its character, whether simple neurasthenia, severe hysteria, or an organic lesion. The outlook for ultimate recovery is good except in cases which present the more serious symptoms above mentioned. Nevertheless it must be borne in mind that traumatic hysteria is one of the most intractable affections which we are called upon to treat. In the treatment of the traumatic neuroses the practitioner may be guided by the principles laid down in the preceding chapter, in which the treatment of neurasthenia in general has been described.

XII. OTHER FORMS OF FUNCTIONAL PARALYSIS

Periodical Paralysis.—The periodical paralysis of the ocular muscles, which may recur for years, has already been referred to. A periodical paralysis involving the general muscles, also a "family" affection, may return with great regularity. Goldflam described twelve cases in one family, the heredity being through the mother. In the United States E. W. Taylor described eleven cases in one family in five generations. Holtzapple, of York, Pa., reports 16 cases in one family. Six of the number died in an attack.

The clinical picture is similar in all recorded cases. The paralysis involves, as a rule, the arms and legs, but may be general below the neck. It comes on in healthy persons without apparent cause, and often during sleep. At first there may be weakness of the limbs, a feeling of weariness and sleepiness, but rarely sensory symptoms. The paralysis, beginning in the legs, to which it may be confined, is usually complete within the first twenty four hours. The neck muscles are sometimes involved, and occasionally those of the tongue and pharynx. The cerebral nerves and the special senses are, as a rule, unaffected. The temperature is normal or subnormal and the pulse slow. The deep reflexes are diminished, sometimes abolished, and the skin reflexes may be enfeebled. A most remarkable feature is the extraordinary reduction or complete abolition of the faradic excitability of both muscles and nerves.

Improvement begins within a few hours or a day or two, the paralysis disappearing completely and the patient becoming perfectly well. The attacks usually recur at intervals of one to two weeks, but they may return daily. They generally cease after the fiftieth year. There may be signs of acute dilatation of the heart during the attack. In the three cases reported by J. K. Mitchell, Flexner, and Edsall a diminished kreatinin excretion for several days before and at the beginning of a seizure was repeatedly found. There was a rise to normal after the attacks. Potassium citrate in full doses either shortened or aborted the paralyses.

Astasia; Abasia.—These terms, indicating respectively inability to stand and inability to walk, have been applied by Charcot and Blocq to diseased conditions characterized by loss of the power of standing or of walking, with retention of muscular power, coördination, and sensation. Blocq's definition is as follows: "A morbid state in which the impossibility of standing erect and walking normally is in contrast with the integrity of sensation, of muscular strength, and of the coördination of the other movements of the lower extremities." The condition forms a symptom group, not a morbid entity, and is probably a functional neurosis. Knapp analyzed 50 cases, of which half were in women. In 21 cases hysteria was present; in 3, chorea; in 2, epilepsy; and in 4, intention psychoses. As a rule, the patients, though able to move the feet and legs perfectly when in bed, are either unable to walk properly or can not stand at all. The disturbances have been very varied, and different forms have been recognized. The commonest, according to Knapp's analysis of the recorded cases, is the paralytic, in which the legs give out as the patient attempts to walk and "bend under him as if made of cotton." "There is no rigidity, no spasm, no incoördination. In bed, sitting, or even while suspended, the muscular strength is found to be good." Other cases are associated with spasm or ataxia; thus there may be movements which stiffen the legs and give to the gait a somewhat spastic character. In other instances there are sudden flexions of the legs, or even of the arms, or a saltatory, spring-like spasm. In a majority of the cases it is a manifestation of a neurosis allied to hysteria.

The cases, as a rule, recover, particularly in young persons. Relapses are not uncommon. The rest treatment and static electricity should be employed.

H. VASO-MOTOR AND TROPHIC DISORDERS

I. RAYNAUD'S DISEASE

Definition.—A vascular change, without organic disease of the vessels, chiefly seen in the extremities, but occurring also in the internal parts, in which a persistent ischæmia or a passive hyperæmia leads to disturbance of function or to loss of vitality with necrosis.

Etiology.—It is a comparatively rare disease. There were only 19 cases in about 20,000 medical patients admitted to the Johns Hopkins Hospital. Women are more frequently attacked than men—62.5 to 37.5 per cent. in Monro's series.

Sixty per cent. of the cases occurred in the second and third decades, but no age is exempt. A case has been reported in a six-months-old child and in a woman of 77 years.

Several members of a family may be affected. Neurotic and hysterical patients are more prone to the disease. Damp and cold weather, as in Great Britain, appears to favor its occurrence. Severe chilblain leading to superficial necrosis represents a type of the malady. In the infectious diseases areas of multiple necrosis occur, but, as a rule, the distribution is very different, and such cases should not be included under Raynaud's disease, nor should the local gangrene associated with arteritis.

Pathology.—According to the definition, cases are excluded in which organic disease of the vessels is present. In advanced cases sclerosis of the blood-vessels has been found; and neuritis has been described, but neither is an essential factor. Changes in the spinal cord have been reported, but in a majority of all cases the examination has been negative. The local syncope is an expression of a widespread constrictor influence causing spasm of the arteries and arterioles, so that not a drop of blood enters a part. This may be followed in an hour or two, or less, by active hyperæmia; the arteries and arterioles dilate widely and the dead-white finger becomes a bright pink. While hyperæmia may follow the ischæmia directly, more commonly there is an intervening period of asphyxia in which the finger becomes blue. In frost-bite, active hyperæmia, cyanosis, and local syncope is the order. In Raynaud's disease the order is usually syncope, asphyxia, and hyperæmia. In frost-bite it seems clear that the asphyxia is due to a backward flow from the veins, to which the local syncope yields as the part thaws, before the arteries passing to the part can be felt to pulsate. The asphyxia of Raynaud's disease may be due to the same cause; contraction of the veins has been seen by Barlow and by Weiss, but that was when the asphyxia already existed. The first thing must be the relaxation of the spasm of the venules and veins to permit of the blood entering the empty capillaries. In moderate grades of asphyxia some little blood trickles through the sluice gates, but in the deep purple skin of a typical example of Raynaud's disease the circulation has ceased and death of the part is imminent. The necrosis is a simple matter, as simple as if a string is tied tightly about the finger-tip.

The disease is the result of some as yet unknown instability of the vaso-motor centres.

Symptoms.—There are various grades of the disease, of which mild, moderate, and severe types may be recognized. In the mild forms the disease never gets beyond the stage of such vascular disturbance as is frequently seen in chilblains. The hands alone may be affected—more often the hands and feet. In the winter, on the slightest exposure, there is acro-cyanosis, which gives place in the warmth to active hyperæmia, sometimes with swelling, throbbing, and aching. The so-called "beefsteak" hand is often a great annoyance to women. It is a vaso-motor disturbance representing a potential case of Raynaud's disease. In these mild attacks I have seen one finger white and the adjacent ones red and blue.

The condition may persist for years and never pass on to necrosis. In a case of moderate severity a woman, aged say twenty or twenty five, after a period of worry or ill health, has pains in the fingers, or a numbness or tingling; then she notices that they are white and cold, and in an hour or so they become red and hot. Within a day or two a change occurs; they remain permanently blue perhaps as far as the second joint or to the knuckles. There is pain, sometimes severe enough to require morphia. The cyanosis persists and the tip of one finger or the terminal joint of another gets darker and a few blebs form. The other fingers show signs of restored circulation, but necrosis has occurred in the pad of one finger and perhaps the terminal inch of another. The necrotic parts gradually separate, and the patient may never have another attack, or in a year or two there is a recurrence.

The severer form is a terrible malady, and may affect fingers and toes at once and with them sometimes the tip of the nose and the ears. The pain is of great severity. Both feet may be swollen to the ankle with the toes black. It may look as if both feet would become gangrenous, but as a rule the process subsides, and in a case even of great severity only the tips of the toes are lost. A severe attack of this sort may last three or four months, when the patient recovers with the loss of two or three fingers or toes, a snip off the edge of both ears and a scar on the tip of the nose. Attacks of this severity may occur year by year, and there are terrible instances in which the patients have lost both hands and feet.

Of the parts affected Monro states that in 43 per cent. of the cases one or both of the upper extremities is involved. Parts other than the extremities may be attacked, as the chin, lips, nates, and eyelids.

Complications.—Temporary amblyopia due to spasm of the retinal vessels, transient aphasia, and transient hemiplegia have been met with. In a case which I have reported there were three attacks of aphasia with hemiplegia from which complete recovery took place. Associated with these were the features of Raynaud's disease. The patient died in a severe attack with pain in the right hand, gangrene to the elbow, and coma. Epilepsy has been reported in a great number of cases, and in one case in my clinic, reported by Thomas, the attacks only occurred in the winter when he had Raynaud's disease.

Albuminuria may occur during the attacks. Hæmoglobinuria has been present in a number of cases, and was well studied by the well-known surgeon, Druitt, in his own case. It is of the same nature as the paroxysmal hæmoglobinuria already described.

Scleroderma of the fingers may follow recurring attacks. Occasionally true generalized scleroderma begins with the features of Raynaud's disease. Arthritis has been present in certain cases.

Diagnosis.—There is rarely any difficulty in the diagnosis. One condition closely simulates it, namely, local gangrene of the toes associated with obliterative arteritis; but this occurs most frequently in older persons, in diabetic subjects, or in connection with well marked arterio-sclerosis. As a rule, the pulse in such cases is not to be felt in the dorsal artery. Allied to this form is a remarkable affection described by Buerger among the Russian Jews in New York—thrombotic phlebo-arteritis of the vessels of the leg with local gangrene. In the early stages the resemblance to Raynaud's disease is very close.

In the acute infections, particularly typhus fever, occasionally in epidemics of typhoid fever, and in malaria, areas of multiple gangrene occur. The distribution is usually different, and there is rarely any difficulty in distinguishing this form from Raynaud's disease.

Lastly, there are cases of multiple neurotic skin gangrene met with in hysterical and nervous patients, in the majority of which the lesions are self-inflicted. In military recruits local gangrene of the big toe has been caused by carbolic acid, and it seems probable that all of those so-called trophic and hysterical lesions are simulated.

Treatment.—In many cases the attacks recur for years uninfluenced by treatment. Mild attacks require no treatment. In the severer forms of local asphyxia, if in the feet, the patient should be kept in bed with the legs elevated. The toes should be wrapped in cotton wool. The pain is often very intense and may require morphia. Carefully applied, systematic massage of the extremities is sometimes of benefit. Galvanism may be tried. Barlow advises immersing the affected limb in salt water and placing one electrode over the spine and the other in the water. Nitroglycerin has been warmly recommended by Cates. Calcium lactate in 15 grain (1 gm.) doses, three or four times a day, is sometimes very effectual. It often relieves chilblains. Cushing has introduced a plan of treatment with the tourniquet which has proved very successful in several cases in my wards. The elastic bandage, or, better, one of his pneumatic tourniquets, is applied to an extremity tight enough to shut off the arterial circulation and left for some minutes. On releasing the constriction the member flushes brightly, owing to the vasomotor relaxation. The application in cases of severe spasm may have to be repeated at frequent intervals before the vascular constriction in the affected parts will be overcome, and the normal temperature and color return in them.

II. ERYTHROMELALGIA

(*Red Neuralgia*)

Definition.—"A chronic disease in which a part or parts—usually one or more extremities—suffer with pain, flushing, and local fever, made far worse if the parts hang down" (Weir Mitchell). The name signifies a painful, red extremity.

Symptoms.—In 1872 (Phila. Med. Times, November 23d), in a lecture on certain painful affections of the feet, Weir Mitchell described the case of a sailor, aged forty, who after an African fever began to have "dull, heavy pains, at first in the left and soon after in the right foot. There was no swelling at first. When at rest he was comfortable and the feet were not painful. After walking the feet were swollen. They scarcely pitted on pressure, but were purple with congestion; the veins were everywhere singularly enlarged, and the arteries were throbbing visibly. The whole foot was said to be aching and burning, but above the ankle there was neither swelling, pain, nor flushing." As the weather grew cool he got relief. Nothing seemed to benefit him. This brief summary of Mitchell's first case gives an accurate clinical picture of the disease. His second communication, On a Rare Vaso-Motor Neurosis of the Extremities, appeared in the Am. Jour. of the Medical Sciences for July, 1878, while in his Clinical Lessons on Nervous Diseases, 1897, will be found additional observations.

The disease is rare. The feet are much more often affected than the hands. The pain may be of the most atrocious character. It is usually, but not always, relieved by cool weather; in one of my cases the winter aggravates the trouble. In a few cases (Elsner, Dehio, Rolleston) the affection has been complicated with Raynaud's disease.

Mitchell speaks of it as a "painful nerve-end neuritis." Dehio suggests that there may be irritation in the cells of the ventral horns of the cord at certain levels. Excision of the nerves passing to the parts has been followed by relief. In one of Mitchell's cases gangrene of the foot followed excision of four inches of the musculo-cutaneous nerve and stretching of the posterior tibial. Sclerosis of the arteries was found. Of the 9 cases in which the local conditions were studied anatomically, the only constant change was a chronic endarteritis (Batty Shaw).

III. ANGIO-NEUROTIC ŒDEMA

(*Quincke's Disease*)

Definition.—An affection characterized by the occurrence of local œdematous swellings, more or less limited in extent, and of transient duration. Severe colic is sometimes associated with the outbreak. There is a marked hereditary disposition in the disease.

Symptoms.—The œdema appears suddenly and is usually circumscribed. It may appear in the face; the eyelid is a common situation; or it may involve the lips or cheek. The backs of the hands, the legs, or the throat may be attacked. Usually the condition is transient, associated perhaps with slight gastro-intestinal distress, and the affection is of little moment. There may be a remarkable periodicity in the outbreak of the œdema. In Matas' case this periodicity was very striking; the attack came on every day at eleven or twelve o'clock. The disease may be hereditary through many generations. In the family whose history I reported five generations had been affected, including twenty two members. The swellings appear in various parts; only rarely are they constant in one locality. The hands, face, and genitalia are the parts most frequently affected. Itching, heat, redness, or in some instances urticaria, may precede the outbreak. Sudden œdema of the larynx may prove fatal. Two members of the family just referred to died of this complication. In one member of this family, whom I saw repeatedly in attacks, the swellings came on in different parts; for example, the under lip would be swollen to such a degree that the mouth could not be opened. The hands enlarge suddenly, so that the fingers can not be bent. The attacks recur every three or four weeks. Accompanying them are usually gastro-intestinal attacks, severe colic, pain, nausea, and sometimes vomiting. It is quite possible that some of the cases of Leyden's intermittent vomiting may belong to this group. The colic is of great intensity and usually requires morphia. Arthritis apparently does not occur. Periodic attacks of cardialgia have also been met with during the outbreak of the œdema. Hæmoglobinuria has occurred in several cases.

The disease has affinities with urticaria, the giant form of which is probably the same disease. There is a form of severe purpura, often with urticarial manifestations, which is also associated with marked gastro-intestinal crises, and it is interesting to note that Schlesinger has reported a case in which a combination of erythromelalgia, Raynaud's disease, and acute œdema occurred. Quincke regards the condition as a vaso-motor neurosis, under the influence of which the permeability of the vessels is suddenly increased.

The **treatment** is very unsatisfactory. In the cases associated with anæmia and general nervousness, tonics, particularly large doses of strychnia, do good. I have seen great improvement follow the prolonged use of nitroglycerin; and calcium lactate may be tried, in doses of 15 grains (1 gm.) thrice daily.

IV. PERSISTENT HEREDITARY ŒDEMA OF THE LEGS

(*Milroy's Disease*)

This remarkable condition, first described by Milroy of Omaha, is characterized by persistent œdema of the legs, without any traceable cause, or any constitutional features. It is a fairly common complaint, affecting males and females equally. As many as 22 persons in Milroy's series were affected among 97 in six generations; in Hope and French's series 13 to 42 persons in five generations. The œdema is strictly limited to the lower limbs and varies very slightly. In some instances there are remarkable acute attacks, with chill, fever, and increase of swelling. Except mechanically the condition does not seriously interfere with health.

Here may be mentioned a remarkable familial affection described by Edgeworth of Bristol (*Lancet*, July 22, 1911), of a general subcutaneous œdema. Of six infants born of healthy parents, all but one died within the first few months, with general œdema, following upon diarrhœa. The cases differ essentially from those of œdema neonatorum.

V. FACIAL HEMIATROPHY

A rare affection characterized by progressive wasting of the bones and soft tissues of one side of the face. The atrophy starts in childhood, but in a few cases has not come on until adult life. Perhaps after a trifling injury or disease the process begins, either diffusely or more commonly at one spot on the skin. It gradually spreads, involving the fat, then the bones, more particularly the upper jaw, and last and least the muscles. The wasting is sharply limited at the middle line, and the appearance of the patient is very remarkable, the face looking as if made up of two halves from different persons. There is usually change in the color of the skin and the hair falls. Owing to the wasting of the alveolar processes the teeth become loose and ultimately drop out. The eye on the affected side is sunken, owing to loss of orbital fat. There is usually hemiatrophy of the tongue on the same side. Disturbance of sensation and muscle twitching may precede or accompany the atrophy. In a majority of the cases the atrophy has been confined to one side of the face, but there are instances on record in which the disease was bilateral, and a few cases in which there were areas of atrophy on the back and on the arm of the same side.

Of the autopsies, Mendel's alone is satisfactory. There was the terminal stage of an interstitial neuritis in all the branches of the trigeminus, from its origin to the periphery, most marked in the superior maxillary branch.

The disease is recognized at a glance. The facial asymmetry associated with congenital wryneck must not be confounded with progressive facial hemiatrophy. Other conditions to be distinguished are: Facial atrophy in anterior polio-myelitis, and more rarely in the hemiplegia of infants and adults; the atrophy following nuclear lesions and sympathetic nerve paralysis; acquired facial hemihypertrophy, such as in the case recorded by D. W. Montgomery, which may by contrast give to the other side an atrophic appearance; and, lastly, scleroderma (a closely related affection), if confined to one side of the face. The precise nature of the disease is still doubtful, but it is a suggestive fact that in many of the cases the atrophy has followed the acute infections. It is incurable.

VI. SCLERODERMA

Definition.—A condition of localized or diffuse induration of the skin.

Varieties.—Two forms are recognized: the circumscribed, which corresponds to the keloid of Addison, and to morphœa; and the diffuse, in which large areas are involved.

The disease affects females more frequently than males. The cases occur most commonly at the middle period of life. The *sclerema neonatorum* is a different affection, not to be confounded with it. The disease is more common in the United States than statistics indicate. I saw 20 cases in sixteen years.

In the *circumscribed form* there are patches, ranging from a few centimetres in diameter to the size of the hand or larger, in which the skin has a waxy or dead-white appearance, and to the touch is brawny, hard, and inelastic. Sometimes there is a preliminary hyperæmia of the skin, and subsequently there are changes in color, either areas of pigmentation or of complete atrophy of the pigment—leucoderma. The sensory changes are rarely marked. The secretion of sweat is diminished or entirely abolished. The disease is more common in women than in men, and is situated most frequently about the breasts and neck, sometimes in the course of the nerves. The patches may develop with great rapidity, and may persist for months or years; sometimes they disappear in a few weeks.

The *diffuse form*, though less common, is more serious. It develops first in the extremities or in the face, and the patient notices that the skin is unusually hard and firm, or that there is a sense of stiffness or tension in making accustomed movements. Gradually a diffuse, brawny induration develops and the skin becomes firm and hard, and so united to the subcutaneous tissues that it cannot be picked up or pinched. The skin may look natural, but more commonly is glossy, drier than normal, and unusually smooth. With reference to the localization, in Lewin and Heller's statistics in 66 observations the disease was universal; in 203, regions of the trunk were affected; in 193, parts of the head or face; in 287, portions of one or other of the upper extremities; and in 122, portions of the lower extremities. In 80 cases there were disturbances of sensation. The disease may gradually extend and involve the skin of an entire limb. When universal, the face is expressionless, the lips can not be moved, mastication is hindered, and it may become extremely difficult to feed the patient. The hands become fixed and the fingers immobile, on account of the extreme induration of the skin over the joints. Remarkable vaso-motor disturbances are common, as extreme cyanosis of the hands and legs. In one of my cases tachycardia was present. The disease is chronic, lasting for months or years. There are instances on record of its persistence for more than twenty years. Recovery may occur, or the disease may be arrested. One of my patients, with extensive involvement of the face, ears, and hands, improved very much. The patients are apt to succumb to pulmonary complaints or to nephritis. Arthritic troubles have been noticed in some instances; in others, endocarditis. Raynaud's disease may be associated with it. I have seen an instance of the diffuse form in which the primary symptoms were those of local asphyxia of the fingers, and in which, with extensive scleroderma of the arms and hands and face, there were cyanosis and swelling of the skin of the feet without any brawny induration. The pigmentation of the skin may be as deep as in Addison's disease, for which cases have been mistaken; scleroderma may occur as a complication of exophthalmic goitre.

The remarkable dystrophy known as *sclerodactylie* belongs to this disorder. There are symmetrical involvements of the fingers, which become deformed, shortened, and atrophied; the skin becomes thickened, of a waxy color, and is sometimes pigmented. Multiple calcareous nodules, not unlike tophi, but not uratic, may occur about the fingers. Bullæ and ulcerations have been met with in some instances, and a great deformity of the nails. The disease has usually followed exposure, and the patients are much worse during the winter, and are curiously sensitive to cold. There may be changes in the skin of the feet, but the deformity similar to that which occurs in the hand has not been noted. Some of the cases present in addition diffuse sclerodermatous changes of the skin of other parts. In Lewin and Heller's monograph there are 35 cases of isolated sclerodactylism, and 106 cases in which it was combined with scleroderma.

The **pathology** of the disease is unknown. It is usually regarded as a tropho-neurosis, probably dependent upon changes in the arteries of the skin leading to connective tissue overgrowth. The thyroid has been found atrophied.

Treatment.—The patients require to be warmly clad and to be guarded against exposure, as they are particularly sensitive to changes in the weather. Warm baths followed by frictions with oil should be systematically used. I have tried the thyroid feeding thoroughly in the diffuse form. In one case the disease appears to be arrested; the patient has taken the extract for seven years. In a second case, after a year the face became softer, and there has been permanent improvement. In a case of quite extensive localized scleroderma the patches became softer and the pigmentation much less intense. Salol in 15 grain (1 gm.) doses three times a day is stated to have been successful in several cases.

VII. AINHUM

Here a brief reference may be made to the remarkable trophic lesion described by Da Silva Lima, which is met with in negroes in Brazil, Africa, India, and occasionally in the Southern States. It is confined to the toes, usually the little toe, and begins as a furrow on the line of the digito-plantar fold. This gradually deepens, the end of the toe enlarges, and, usually without inflammation or pain, the toe falls off. The process may last some years. Cases have been reported in America by Hornaday, Pittman, F. J. Shepherd, and Morrison.

SECTION XII

DISEASES OF THE LOCOMOTOR SYSTEM

A. DISEASES OF THE MUSCLES

I. MYOSITIS

Definition.—Inflammation of the voluntary muscles.

A primary myositis occurs as an acute, subacute, or chronic affection. It is seen in two chief forms—the suppurative and non-suppurative.

I. Suppurative myositis, known also as infectious myositis, is especially frequent in Japan, where, according to Miyake, some 250 cases have been reported; but he claims that some of these examples belong to other affections. Miyake personally saw 33 cases in Japan during twenty one months' practice, and took cultures from all but one of them. In 2 cases the results were negative, but in 27 a pure culture of the staphylococcus pyogenes aureus was obtained, while in another the streptococcus and in 2 more the albus with the aureus was grown. The malady may involve one or many muscles, and is usually sudden in its onset. There are also high fever and marked prostration. Subsequently abscesses occur in the indurated muscles, and pyæmia may ensue if the implicated muscles are not thoroughly evacuated.

II. Dermato-myositis.—An acute or subacute inflammation of the muscles of unknown origin associated with œdema and dermatitis. Steiner collected 28 cases from the literature and reported two cases from my clinic. The muscle inflammation is here multiple, and is associated with œdema and a dermatitis. The case of E. Wagner may be taken as a typical example. A tuberculous but well-built woman entered the hospital, complaining of stiffness in the shoulders and a slight œdema of the back of the hands and forearms. There was paræsthesia, the arms became swollen, the skin tense, and the muscles felt doughy. Gradually the thighs became affected. The disease lasted about three months. The post mortem showed slight pulmonary tuberculosis; all the muscles except the glutei, the calf, and abdominal muscles were stiff and firm, but fragile, and there were serious infiltration, great proliferation of the interstitial tissue, and fatty degeneration. In the case reported by Jacoby the muscles were firm, hard, and tender, and there was slight œdema of the skin. The cases usually last from one to three months, though there are instances in which it has been longer. The swelling and tenderness of the muscles, the œdema, and the pain naturally suggest trichinosis, and, indeed, Hepp speaks of it as a pseudo-trichinosis. The nature of the disease is unknown. Of the 28 cases collected by Steiner 17 died. The anatomical changes are those just mentioned as found in E. Wagner's cases. One of

Senator's cases presented marked disorders of sensation and has been named neuro-myositis. Wagner suggests that some of these cases were examples of acute progressive muscular atrophy. The differentiation from trichinosis is possible only by removing a portion of the muscle. It has not yet been determined whether the eosinophilia described by Brown is peculiar to the trichinosis myositis.

III. Polymyositis Hæmorrhagica.—This form resembles the dermatomyositis in general features, but differs in the presence of hæmorrhages into and between the muscles. Of the ten cases analyzed by Thayer four recovered. Purpura and hæmorrhages from the mucous membranes may occur.

II. MYOSITIS OSSIFICANS PROGRESSIVA

This is a progressive inflammatory affection of the locomotor system of unknown origin, characterized by the gradual formation of bony masses in the fasciæ, muscles, aponeuroses, tendons, ligaments, and bones, with resulting ankylosis of most of the articulations (Steiner). About 100 cases have been reported. The process begins in the neck or back, usually with swelling of the affected muscles, redness of the skin, and slight fever, or with small nodules in the muscles which appear and disappear. After subsiding an induration remains, which becomes progressively harder as the transformation into bone takes place. The disease may ultimately involve a majority of the skeletal muscles. Nothing is known of the etiology. Malformation, microdactylism of the thumbs and big toes, is present in 75 per cent. of the cases.

III. MYALGIA

(*Fibrositis, Myositis*)

Definition.—A painful affection of the voluntary muscles and of the fasciæ and periosteum to which they are attached. It is probable that in many cases the fibrous tissue is especially affected—a fibrositis. It is by no means certain that the muscular tissues are the seat of the disease. Many writers claim that in some cases it is a neuralgia of the sensory nerves of the muscles. The affection has received various names, according to its seat, as torticollis, lumbago, pleurodynia, etc.

Etiology.—The attacks follow cold and exposure, and trauma is often a factor. It is most commonly met with in men, particularly those exposed to cold and whose occupations are laborious. It is apt to follow exposure to a draft of air, as from an open window in a railway carriage. A sudden chilling after heavy exertion may bring on an attack of lumbago. Persons of a gouty habit are certainly more prone to this affection, and one attack renders an individual more liable to another. It is usually acute, but may become subacute or even chronic, the last being more common in later life.

Pathology.—The changes are usually in the white fibrous tissue and are of an inflammatory nature. In acute cases there is a serous exudation in the affected parts and following this there may be proliferation of the fibrous tissue. This may extend between the muscle fibres and cause stiffness and pain. Disability with muscular atrophy may result from this. Nodules sometimes form which may be painful.

Symptoms.—In the acute forms the affection is entirely local. The constitutional disturbance is slight, and, even in severe cases, there may be no fever. Pain is a prominent feature and may be constant or occur only when the muscles are drawn into certain positions. It may be a dull ache, like the pain of a bruise, or sharp, severe, and cramp-like. It is often sufficiently intense to cause the patient to cry out. Pressure on the affected part usually gives relief. As a rule, myalgia is a transient affection, lasting from a few hours to a few days, although occasionally it is prolonged for several weeks. It is very apt to recur.

Much attention has been given of late to a form of myositis occurring chiefly in the muscles of the head and neck, causing at first swelling and puffiness, later indurations. They are found particularly in the muscles at the back of the neck, but they are occasionally present in the muscles of the abdomen and limbs. They may appear quite suddenly, sometimes in muscles that are over-worked, but in other instances they seem to be associated with changes in the weather. The affection of the muscles of the head and neck may be associated with headache, the so-called indurative headache. Some of the cases have a picture very similar to migraine. In the abdominal muscles these limited swellings may cause pain and suggest appendicitis.

The following are the principal varieties of myalgia:

(1) Lumbago, one of the most common and painful forms, affects the muscles of the loins and their tendinous attachments. Some patients are subject to attacks at short intervals. It occurs chiefly in workingmen and often after a strain in lifting. It comes on suddenly, and in very severe cases completely incapacitates the patient, who may be unable to turn in bed or to rise from the sitting posture. There may be difficulty in distinguishing this from arthritis of the spine or sacro-iliac joint disease. In these conditions the symptoms are more persistent. The restriction of motion in the spine is an aid in recognizing arthritis and the special features of sacro-iliac joint involvement should be looked for. The X-ray plates are a great aid.

(2) Stiff neck or torticollis affects the muscles of the antero-lateral or back region of the neck. It is very common, often unilateral, and occurs most frequently in the young. The patient holds the head in a peculiar manner turned to one side, and rotates the whole body in attempting to turn it.

(3) Pleurodynia involves the intercostal muscles on one side, and in some instances the pectorals and serratus magnus. This is, perhaps, the most painful form of the disease, as the chest can not be at rest. It is more common on the left than on the right side. A deep breath, or coughing, causes a very intense pain on pressure, sometimes over a very limited area. It may be difficult to distinguish from intercostal neuralgia, in which affection, however, the pain is usually more circumscribed and paroxysmal, and there are tender points along the course of the nerves. It is sometimes mistaken for pleurisy, but careful physical examination readily distinguishes between the two affections.

(4) Among other forms which may be mentioned are cephalodynia, affecting the muscles of the head; scapulodynia, omodynia, and dorsodynia, af-

fecting the muscles about the shoulder and upper part of the back. Myalgia may also occur in the abdominal muscles and in the muscles of the extremities. The chronic forms are distinguished by soreness or pain associated with varying degrees of disability. There may be marked stiffness of the muscles, which are sometimes painful on pressure and may show definite tender areas of induration.

Treatment.—Rest of the affected muscles is of the first importance, and it is well to protect them from cold by a covering of flannel. Strapping of the side will sometimes completely relieve pleurodynia. No belief is more widespread among the public than in the efficacy of porous plasters for muscular pains of all sorts, particularly those about the trunk. If the pain is severe and agonizing, a hypodermic of morphia gives immediate relief. For lumbago acupuncture is, in acute cases, the most efficient treatment. Needles of from three to four inches in length (ordinary bonnet-needles, sterilized, will do) are thrust into the lumbar muscles at the seat of pain, and withdrawn after five or ten minutes. In many instances the relief is immediate, and I can corroborate fully the statements of Ringer, who taught me this practice, as to its extraordinary and prompt efficacy in many instances. The constant current is sometimes very beneficial. In many forms of myalgia the thermo-cautery gives great relief and in obstinate cases blisters may be tried. Hot fomentations are soothing, and at the outset a Turkish bath may cut short the attack. The bowels should be freely opened and large amounts of water taken. The salicylates are usually effectual; sodium salicylate (gr. x to xv, 0.6 to 1 gm.), aspirin (gr. x, 0.6 gm.), or salol (gr. v, 0.3 gm.) may be given. Some patients respond well to colchicum (♏ xv, 1 c.c. of the wine). In chronic cases potassium iodide may be used, and both guaiacum and sulphur have been strongly recommended. Persons subject to this affection should be warmly clothed, and avoid, if possible, exposure to cold and damp. In gouty persons the diet should be restricted and the alkaline mineral waters taken freely. Large doses of nux vomica are sometimes beneficial. Massage sometimes gives relief; it should be given gently at first and more vigorously later.

IV. MYOTONIA

(*Thomsen's Disease*)

Definition.—An affection characterized by tonic cramp of the muscles on attempting voluntary movements. The disease received its name from the physician who first described it, in whose family it existed for five generations.

While the disease is in a majority of cases hereditary, hence the name myotonia congenita, there are other forms of spasm very similar which may be acquired, and others still which are quite transitory.

Etiology.—All the typical cases have occurred in family groups; a few isolated instances have been described in which similar symptoms have been present. Males are much more frequently affected than females. In 102 recorded cases, 91 were males and only 11 females (Hans Koch). The disease is rare in America and in England; it seems more common in Germany and in Scandinavia.

Symptoms.—The disease comes on in childhood. It is noticed that on account of the stiffness the children are not able to take part in ordinary games. The peculiarity is noticed only during voluntary movements. The contraction which the patient wills is slowly accomplished; the relaxation which the patient wills is also slow. The contraction often persists for a little time after he has dropped an object which he has picked up. In walking, the start is difficult; one leg is put forward slowly, it halts from stiffness for a second or two, and then after a few steps the legs become limber and he walks without any difficulty. The muscles of the arms and legs are those usually implicated; rarely the facial, ocular, or laryngeal muscles. Emotion and cold aggravate the condition. In some instances there is mental weakness. The sensation and the reflexes are normal. G. M. Hammond has reported three remarkable cases in one family, in which the disease began at the eighth year and was confined entirely to the arms. It was accompanied with some slight mental feebleness. The condition of the muscles is interesting. The patients appear and are muscular, and there is sometimes a definite hypertrophy of the muscles. The force is scarcely proportionate to the size. Erb has described a characteristic reaction of the nerve and muscle to the electrical currents—the so-called myotonic reaction, the chief feature of which is that normally the contractions caused by either current attain their maximum slowly and relax slowly, and vermicular, wave-like contractions pass from the cathode to the anode.

The disease is incurable, but it may be arrested temporarily. The nature of the affection is unknown. Dejerine and Sottas have found hypertrophy of the primitive fibres with multiplication of the nuclei of all the muscles, including the diaphragm, but not the heart. The spinal cord and the nerves were intact. From Jacoby's latest studies it is doubtful whether these changes in the muscles are in any way characteristic or peculiar to the disease. J. Koch, however, has found, in addition to the muscle hypertrophy, degenerative and regenerative changes present, which he considers sufficient to account for the myotonic disorder. Karpinsky and von Bechterew, from careful urinary examinations, regard the affection as due to an auto-intoxication of the muscle tissue, caused by some faulty metabolism. No treatment for the condition is known.

V. PARAMYOCLONUS MULTIPLEX

(*Myoclonia*)

Definition.—An affection, described by Friedreich, characterized by clonic contractions, chiefly of the muscles of the extremities, occurring either constantly or in paroxysms.

The cases have been chiefly in males, and the disease has followed emotional disturbance, fright, or straining. The contractions are usually bilateral and may vary from fifty to one hundred and fifty in the minute. Occasionally tonic spasms occur. They are not accompanied by any sensory disturbances. In the intervals between the attacks there may be tremors of the muscles. In the severe spasms the movements may be very violent; the body is tossed about, and it is sometimes difficult to keep the patient in bed. Gucci has described a family in which the affection has occurred in three generations. Weiss has also noted heredity in four generations. According to this author the essential symptoms are continuous or paroxysmal contractions, usually symmetrical and rhythmical, of muscles otherwise normal, which cease during sleep. There are neither psychical nor sensory disturbances. The condition is most common in young males, and is unaffected by treatment. Raymond groups this disease with fibrillary tremors, electric chorea (Dubini's disease), tic non douloureux of the face, and the convulsive tic, under the name of *myoclonics,* believing that it is only one link in a chain of pathological manifestations in the degenerate. Dana, in 1903, divided the myoclonias into five groups. In the first he placed paramyoclonus multiplex, and considered the names of four somewhat similar affections as synonyms of the same.

VI. MYASTHENIA GRAVIS

(*Asthenic Bulbar Paralysis; Erb-Goldflam's Symptom-Complex*)

Definition.—A disease with fatigue symptoms referable to the muscular system, due to failure of innervation without definite changes in muscles or nerves.

Of 180 cases collected by McCarthy, 83 were males and 96 females. The disease is most frequent in the third decade. The etiology is unknown.

The muscles innervated by the bulb are first affected—those of the eyes, the face, of mastication, and of the neck. After effort the muscles show fatigue, and if persisted in they fail to act and a condition of paresis or complete paralysis follows. All the voluntary muscles may become involved. After rest the power is recovered. In severe cases paralysis may persist. The myasthenic reaction of Jolly is the rapid exhaustion of the muscles, by faradism, not by galvanism. There are marked remissions and fluctuations in the severity of the symptoms.

Examination of the nervous system has revealed no abnormality. Weigert found a thymus tumor with metastatic growths in the muscles. Hun, Bloomer, and Streeter have described an infiltration of the muscles and of the thymus gland with lymphoid cells and a proliferation of the glandular elements of the thymus.

The diagnosis is easy—from the ptosis, the facial expression, the nasal speech, the rapid fatigue of the muscles, the myasthenic reaction, the absence of atrophy, tremors, etc., and the remarkable variations in the intensity of the symptoms. Of the 180 collected cases 72 proved fatal. The patient may live many years; recovery may take place. Rest, strychnia in full doses, massage, and alternate courses of iodide of potassium and mercury may be tried.

VII. AMYOTONIA CONGENITA

(*Oppenheim's Disease*)

A congenital affection characterized by general or local hypotonus of the voluntary muscles. Oppenheim called the disease *myatonia,* but this is phonetically so similar to *myotonia* (Thomsen's disease) that the name amyotonia of English writers is preferable.

Collier and Wilson, who have analyzed the recorded cases, give the following definition: "A condition of extreme flaccidity of the muscles, associated with an entire loss of the deep reflexes, most marked at the time of birth and always showing a tendency to slow and progressive amelioration. There is great weakness, but no absolute paralysis of any of the muscles. The limbs are most affected; the face is almost always exempt. The muscles are small and soft, but there is no local wasting. Contractures are prone to occur in the course of time. The faradic excitability in the muscles is lowered and strong faradic stimuli are borne without complaint. No other symptoms indicative of lesions of the nervous system occur."

In Spiller's case no lesions were found, but in an autopsy by Baudouin the cells of the anterior horns were found to be small, and there were extensive changes in the muscle fibres, similar to those in the myopathies.

B. DISEASES OF THE JOINTS

I. ARTHRITIS DEFORMANS

Definition.—A disease of the joints of doubtful etiology, but probably the result of infection, characterized by changes in the synovial membranes, cartilage, and peri-articular structures, and in some cases by atrophic and hypertrophic changes in the bones. A tendency to a chronic course is the rule.

Long believed to be intimately associated with gout and rheumatism (whence the names rheumatic gout and rheumatoid arthritis), this relationship seems disproved. By the studies of the Boston orthopedic surgeons (Bradford, Goldthwaite, and Lovett) and of Strangeways and his pupils at Cambridge (England) we are gradually getting a more accurate knowledge of the anatomical and clinical forms of this common disease. There is a difference of opinion as to whether there are two distinct diseases or varying forms of the same disease included under this heading. Those who hold the former view consider that in one disease the synovial membranes and the peri-articular tissues are particularly affected (rheumatoid arthritis) and in the other disease the cartilage and bone (osteo-arthritis). The disease occurs frequently and to it belong many of the cases termed "chronic rheumatism."

Etiology.—Age.—A majority of the cases are between the ages of twenty and fifty. In A. E. Garrod's analysis of 500 cases there were only 25 under twenty years of age. In 40 per cent. of the series of 500 cases studied by T. McCrae, the onset was before the age of thirty years. In the group with peri-articular changes predominating the age of onset is usually lower than in the group with special cartilaginous and bony changes.

Sex.—Among Garrod's cases there were 411 in women. Practically half of the series of McCrae were males. The incidence as to sex is influenced by the inclusion of the cases of spondylitis, of which a large majority is in males. In women a close association with the menopause has been noted.

Predisposition.—In 216 in Garrod's series there was a family history of joint trouble; in McCrae's series only in 114 among 500. Two or three children in a family may be affected. In America the incidence in the negro is relatively much less than in the white. Occupation and the station in life do not seem to have any special influence.

Exposure to cold, wet and damp, errors in diet, worry and care, and local injuries are all spoken of as possible exciting causes, but probably play but a small part.

As regards the views of the etiology of arthritis deformans, the one that it is of nervous origin is only of historical interest, and the modern opinion is that it is a result of some infectious process, certainly in the majority of cases.

Arthritis Deformans as a Chronic Infection.—This view is steadily gaining ground and the evidence suggests certain varieties of streptococci as the causal organism. This seems more probable than that the disease is due to a specific organism. The arthritis is secondary to a focus of infection somewhere. The possible sources are many but infection of the mouth and throat probably takes first place. Abscesses about the teeth should always be searched for (X-ray study) and the tonsils carefully examined. Other sources are: infection of the nose or sinuses, pyorrhœa alveolaris, otitis media, chronic bronchitis, infection of the urinary tract, pelvic disease in women, and infection of the prostate and seminal vesicles in men. The possibility of chronic infection from the intestinal tract must be considered although this is difficult to prove.

The acute onset, with fever in many cases, the polyarthritis, the presence of enlarged glands, the frequent enlargement of the spleen, the occurrence of pleurisy, endocarditis, and pericarditis in some cases are all suggestive of an infection. The likeness of the lesions to those due to arthritis from a specific cause, such as the gonococcus, is suggestive, and also the association of the arthritis with definite foci of infection in some cases. Lastly, a consideration of the form in children described by Still lends weight to this view, particularly in the widespread enlargement of the lymph glands and the swelling of the spleen.

Metabolic.—While the nutrition suffers in many cases there does not seem any evidence to support the view that the disease is primarily due to disturbance of metabolism. Metabolic changes are probably secondary just as are the trophic changes.

Morbid Anatomy.—The usual descriptions are of the late stages of the disease when extensive damage has occurred, for there have been few opportunities to study the early changes, although more frequent operations have extended our knowledge of them and radiographs have aided much. There are three main forms of change: (1) Lesions principally in the synovial membranes and peri-articular tissues (the so-called rheumatoid arthritis), (2) with atrophic changes in the cartilage and bones predominating, and (3) with hypertrophy and overgrowth of bone (so-called osteo-arthritis). The first and second are seen most frequently in the joints of the extremities, the third in the spine. Whether these are distinct diseases or different manifestations of the same disease it is difficult to say. In many cases all forms of change are found, which speaks against the view that there are two distinct diseases. The changes in general are: (1) Effusion, which is not constant and shows no special features. (2) Changes in the synovial membrane. These are inflammatory and often hæmorrhagic at the onset. There may be marked thickening and proliferation of the synovial fringes with the formation of villi—villous arthritis. (3) The capsule and surrounding tissues may be infiltrated and much swollen. The peri-articular tissues show infiltration and swelling, and the enlargement of the joint is more often due to swelling about it than to bony changes. (4) Cartilage. This may show erosion, ulceration, atrophy, or proliferation. The cartilage may disappear entirely, but the changes are often very irregular and uneven and the cartilage may be replaced by fibrous tissue or by bone, the latter being most common at the edge of the cartilage. The cartilages may be soft and gradually absorbed or thinned (this often begins opposite the point of greatest involvement of the synovial membrane). (5) Bone. This may show atrophy of varying grade. If the cartilage is completely absorbed the surface of the bone often becomes hard and eburnated. In the form spoken of as *hypertrophic* there is new bone formation which is most common at the edge of the articular surfaces. In the hip joint this may form an irregular ring of bone about the joint cavity. The commonest example of overgrowth of bone is seen on the so-called "Heberden's nodes," which are bony outgrowths at the terminal interphalangeal joints. There may be deposit of new bone in the ligaments, particularly in the spine. Proliferation of bone usually occurs at the margins of the joints in the form of irregular nodules—the osteophytes—which may lock the joints. The formation of bone may also occur in ligaments, especially of the spine, which may be converted into a rigid bony column. Bony ankylosis rarely occurs in the peripheral joints, but is common in the spine.

There may be extensive secondary changes. Muscular atrophy is common and may appear with great rapidity. Subluxation may occur, especially in the knee and finger joints. The hands often show great deformity, particularly ulnar deflection. Contractures may follow and the joints become fixed in a flexed position. Neuritis and trophic disturbances may be associated; the neuritis is sometimes due to direct extension of the inflammatory process. Subcutaneous fibroid nodules occasionally occur.

The radiographs show the changes very well. Erosion of the cartilage is easily seen. In the type with predominant peri-articular changes the cartilage and bone often show little alteration. The occurrence of various changes in different joints or even in the same joint is common and bony change may occur with marked involvement of the peri-articular tissues.

Symptoms.—The onset may be acute or gradual. In the acute form a number of joints may be involved, there may be high fever and the whole condition be suggestive of rheumatic fever. In other cases the onset is acute in one joint and others are involved a few days later. With the gradual onset one joint is attacked and others follow. Some cases are between and may be termed subacute. In cases with an acute onset the attack may not persist very long; with the chronic onset the duration is usually prolonged. The acute onset occurs more frequently in the form in which changes in the soft parts predominate.

Arthritis.—In the acute form the joints are swollen, tender, and hot to the touch, but do not often show marked redness. There may be effusion in the larger joints. Pain is a marked feature and is increased by movement, the patient usually taking the position in which he has the greatest ease.

When a joint is once attacked, the process does not subside quickly, and when the arthritis lessens some change remains in the joint which, however, may be very slight. The joints of the spine, especially in the cervical region, are often involved in the more acute forms, and in these there is rarely any permanent change. The temporo-maxillary joint is often involved, and arthritis here is always suggestive of this disease. The hands, when involved, show very characteristic changes. The knuckle joints are red, swollen, tender, and show limitation of motion. The fingers are often involved; swelling of the interphalangeal joints is common with a resulting thickening which gives a fusiform appearance to the finger. Partial dislocation, particularly at the terminal joint, is common. The knee joints are often involved with pain, effusion, limitation of motion, and later villous arthritis or subluxation. Thickening of the capsule usually occurs early.

In the hypertrophic (osteo-arthritis form) the process is rarely as acute as when the peri-articular parts are particularly involved (rheumatoid arthritis), but is usually polyarticular. The terminal finger joints, the hip joint, and the spine are especially affected. Pain is usually a marked feature, and the local features are not so marked. The process is more likely to be chronic.

Heberden's Nodes.—These are small bony outgrowths ("little hard knobs"—Heberden) at the terminal phalangeal joints, which develop gradually at the sides of the distal phalanges. They are much more common in women than in men. Heberden says "they have no connection with gout, being found in persons who have never had it," yet they are often regarded as indicating gout. In the early stage the joints may be swollen, tender, and slightly red, particularly when injured. The attacks of pain and swelling may come on in the joints at long intervals or follow injury. Sometimes they are the first manifestation of a general arthritis. Their distribution is not always regular and they are often largest on the fingers most used. They are often found in patients, the arthritis in whose other joints is of the other form. The condition is not curable; but there is this hopeful feature—the subjects whose arthritis begins in this way rarely have severe involvement of the larger joints. They have been regarded, too, as an indication of longevity.

The mon-articular form affects chiefly old persons, and is seen particularly in the hip and shoulder. It is identical with the general disease in its anatomical features. The muscles show wasting early and in the hip the condition ultimately becomes that described as *morbus coxæ senilis*. These cases seem not infrequently to follow an injury. They differ from the polyarticular form in occurring chiefly in men and at a later period of life.

The Vertebral Form (*Spondylitis*).—This may occur alone or with involvement of the peripheral joints. With the acute polyarthritis of the peripheral joints the spine may be involved, but there is usually no permanent change. With the hypertrophic form there is often bony proliferation and some spinal rigidity results which may involve the whole spine or only a part; in the latter case the lower dorsal and lumbar regions suffer most frequently. The condition may not involve more than a few vertebræ. The features are as variable as in the peripheral joints and there may be repeated acute attacks or a steady progressive process. In the general spine involvement the ribs may be fixed, the thorax immobile, and the breathing abdominal. There are two varieties of the general involvement which are sometimes regarded as special diseases. In one (von Bechterew) the spine alone is involved, and there are pronounced nerve-root symptoms—pain, anæsthesia, atrophy of the muscles, and ascending degeneration of the cord. Von Bechterew thinks it begins as a meningitis, leads to compression of the nerve roots, loss of function of the spinal muscles, atrophy of the intervertebral disks, and gradually ankylosis of the spine. In the other—Strümpell-Marie type—the hip and shoulder joints may be involved (spondylose rhizomélique), and the nervous symptoms are less prominent. Both appear to be forms of arthritis deformans, and should neither be regarded nor described as separate diseases. Spondylitis deformans is more frequent in males than in females, and trauma probably plays an important part in its etiology. Local involvement is particularly common in the lumbar region and may cause sciatica and a great variety of referred pains. Pressure on the nerve-roots cause great pain, paræsthesia, and atrophy of the muscles. Movement of the spine is usually restricted.

Arthritis Deformans in Children.—Some cases resemble closely the disease in adults, in others there are very striking differences. A very interesting variety has been differentiated by Still, in which the general enlargement of the joints is associated with swelling of the lymph glands and of the spleen. The onset is almost always before the second dentition, and girls are more frequently affected than boys. The symptoms complained of are usually slight stiffness in one or two joints; gradually others become involved. The onset may be acute with fever or even with chills. The enlargement of the joints is due rather to a general thickening of the soft tissues than to a bony enlargement. The limitation of movement may be extreme, owing to the fixation of the joints, and there may be much muscular wasting. The enlargement of the lymph glands is most striking, increases with fever, and may be general; even the epitrochlear glands may be as large as hazelnuts. The edge of the spleen can usually be felt below the costal margin. Sweating is often profuse and there may be anæmia, but heart complications are rare. The children look puny and generally show arrest of development.

General Features.—*Temperature.*—In the acute attacks this may rise to 102° or 103° F., but is frequently lower and often persists for weeks with a maximum about 100° F. The *pulse* is usually rapid in proportion to the fever, the most frequent range being from 90 to 110. Cardiac changes are found in a small proportion of cases. *Glandular enlargement* is common and may be general or especially marked in the glands related to the affected joints. The *spleen* is enlarged in some cases, the frequency being greater in the younger patients. *Subcutaneous nodules* occur in a few cases and are sometimes tender. The *blood* often shows a slight anæmia, which is not as marked as might be expected from the appearance of the patients. There is rarely much increase in the leucocytes and the differential count shows no peculiarity. The *urine* does not show any change of moment. The *skin* sometimes shows irregular areas of yellow pigmentation, especially on the face and arms. It may have a glossy appearance over the affected joints. Profuse sweating of the hands and feet is common. The *reflexes* are usually increased in acute cases and a return to normal is of good significance. They are sometimes absent. Muscular *atrophy* is common and sometimes advances very rapidly. It is most marked in the hands. Twitching of the muscles is not uncommon.

In some patients the bony atrophy is very marked. This is most common in females. In these disorganization of the joints occurs and the cartilage rapidly disappears. These cases usually progress rapidly downward. This atrophy is to be distinguished from that due to disuse.

Course.—*General Progressive Form.*—This occurs in two varieties, acute and chronic. The *acute* form may resemble, at its outset, ordinary rheumatic fever. There is involvement of many joints; swelling, particularly of the synovial sheaths and bursæ, but not often redness; there is moderate fever which is often persistent and may be from 99° to 100° F. for weeks. The pulse rate is usually high in proportion to the fever. In this form there may be repeated acute attacks, perhaps at intervals of years, or there may be repeated attacks in various joints. These usually leave definite changes, which may be slight at first, but tend to increase with subsequent attacks. Acute cases may occur at the menopause. Some cases progress very rapidly; they lose weight and strength; atrophy and arthritic deformity are marked; and they suggest a progressive septic process without suppuration.

The *chronic* form is the most common, although most of these have had at some time an acute attack, especially at the onset. The first symptoms are pain on movement and slight swelling, which may be in the joint itself or in the peri-articular sheaths. In some cases the effusion is marked, in others slight. The local conditions vary greatly, and periods of improvement alternate with attacks of swelling, redness, and pain. At first only one or two joints are affected; gradually other articulations are involved, and in extreme cases every joint in the body is affected. Pain is an extremely variable symptom. Some cases proceed to the most extreme deformity without severe pain; in others the suffering is very great, particularly at night and during exacerbations of the disease. There are cases in which pain of an agonizing character is an almost constant symptom, quite apart from the occurrence of acute disturbances. Pain has an important influence in the production of deformity, as it hinders movement and the joints are kept in the position of greatest ease.

Gradually the shape of the joints is greatly altered, partly by the thickening of the capsule and surrounding tissues, perhaps by the pressure of osteophytes, and often by the muscular contraction. In moving the affected joint crepitus may be felt. Ultimately the joints may be completely immobile, not by a true bony anchylosis, although it may be by the osteophytes which form around the articular surfaces like ringbone in the horse, but more often from adhesions, and peri-articular thickening. There is often an acute atrophy of the muscles about the joints and atrophy from disuse usually supervenes, so that contractures tend to flex the thigh upon the abdomen and the leg upon the thigh. There are cases with rapid muscular wasting, symmetrical involvement of the joints, increased reflexes, and trophic changes, which strongly suggest a central origin. Numbness, tingling, pigmentation or glossiness of the skin, and onychia may be present. In extreme cases the patient is completely helpless, and lies with the legs drawn up, the arms fixed, and all the articulations of the extremities fixed. Fortunately, it often happens in these severe general cases that the joints of the hand are not so much affected, and the patient may be able to knit or write, though unable to walk or use the arms. In many cases, after involving two or three joints, the disease becomes arrested, and no further development occurs. A majority of the patients finally reach a quiescent stage, in which they are free from pain and enjoy excellent health, suffering only from the inconvenience and crippling necessarily associated with the disease. Coincident affections are not uncommon. In the active stage the patients often suffer from dyspepsia, which may recur at intervals. A small percentage show cardiac lesions, and the pulse rate is usually higher than normal.

Diagnosis.—The cases with an acute onset may be difficult to distinguish from *rheumatic fever*. The affected joints are rarely as tender as in rheumatic fever, and the smaller joints are more often involved. The presence of thickening in a joint, rapid muscular atrophy, a relatively high pulse rate in relation to the fever (in the absence of endocarditis), and the absence of marked response to salicylate medication speak against rheumatic fever. The diagnosis from *gonorrhœal arthritis* may be difficult, but in this the small joints are usually not attacked so often, and after an onset with polyarthritis the majority of the affected joints usually clear, leaving one joint particularly involved. This rarely occurs in arthritis deformans. A careful search for gonococci is a great aid in diagnosis. In the chronic stage there may be considerable difficulty in distinguishing this disease from *gout*. This is particularly marked in either disease without marked joint changes. The study of the radiographs is particularly helpful and marked peri-articular changes speak for arthritis deformans. The finding of tophi or the estimation of the uric acid excretion may give the diagnosis of gout. It is important to distinguish *sub-deltoid bursitis* from the mon-articular form in the shoulder; the radiographs are a great aid. They are also important in the recognition of disease of the *sacro-iliac* joint and *tuberculosis* of the *hip-joint*. Special importance attaches to the diagnosis of the spinal forms. There is no difficulty in the case of general involvement, but with local changes in the lower spine it is not so easy. Pain on and restriction of movement are important; the patient is careful to limit any motion of the spine. Tuberculosis of the spine rarely offers any difficulty, especially with skiagrams.

Prognosis.—The age, general circumstances, character of the patient, the extent of damage to the joints, and the variety of change are all important. The outlook is not as dark as it is usually described. If the source of infection can be found and properly treated the prognosis is encouraging. In many patients the disease runs a certain course, and, if they can be brought through it with a minimum of damage, the ultimate outlook is good. In the form with peri-articular changes predominating, early diagnosis, treatment of the point of infection, the preservation of good nutrition, and a patient who is willing to fight are all encouraging factors. The outlook in the cases with the acute attacks is usually better than in those with a more chronic progressive course. Rapid muscular atrophy is of grave import. Cases in women beginning about the menopause should always have a grave prognosis. Rapid advancement in the joint changes is serious. In the form in children the outlook is not good, but some recover entirely. The group with marked hypertrophic changes (osteo-arthritis) usually do well. Heberden's nodes are permanent, but in the larger joints it is rare for the condition to advance to absolute crippling, although there may be considerable interference with function. Spondylitis rarely advances to complete immobility of the whole spine. The outlook is good in the local cases, but depends somewhat on the occupation and possibility of further trauma. The general condition of the patient is always of importance in estimating the outlook in any case. In those with marked nervous features the prognosis is not good.

Treatment.—Much depends on proper management and the pessimistic attitude is not justified. Certain things are important: early diagnosis so that treatment can be begun early, the avoidance of harmful measures, careful attention to the general condition, and every effort to limit the damage to the joints. Too much stress can not be placed on the need of early diagnosis; the disease is often regarded as "rheumatic" and the treatment directed to this (especially restriction of diet and the giving of salicylates for long periods) is usually harmful.

SOURCE OF INFECTION.—This should be carefully searched for and, if found, properly treated. If the tonsils are diseased they should be removed. Antistreptococcus serum has been used, and in some cases with benefit.

GENERAL MEASURES.—The patient should be kept out of doors as much as possible and every effort made to improve the general health. The *diet* should be the most nourishing possible. The mistake of cutting down the proteins is often made. Regard must be had to the digestion, and it is more often the carbohydrates which should be reduced. Water should be freely given, as elimination is important. The bowels should be kept open, and for this the salines are useful. It is important to see that the patients are warmly clad in cold weather and guarded against chilling. *Hydrotherapy* is useful locally in the form of compresses, but the hot bath treatment, so often given, more frequently does harm than good, particularly in acute cases. Baths, when taken, should be of very short duration. In more chronic cases bathing is sometimes of value. *Massage* is especially useful in the cases with synovial and peri-articular changes, and in them passive motion should be used early. *Climate* is of value in so far as patient is able to be out of doors and is saved from rapid changes of temperature.

MEDICINAL.—There is no drug which essentially influences the disease. The salicylates may be an aid in relieving pain, but should not be given for long periods. Iron, arsenic, and iodine are often useful. The iodide of iron in half drachm (2 c. c.) doses should be given persistently and alternated with Fowler's solution in five drop doses. Iodine may be given as the tincture in doses of two or three drops. Potassium iodide is sometimes of value when given for a long period. Thyroid and thymus gland extracts given persistently are sometimes beneficial. For the *pain* it is necessary to give drugs, although local measures should be used as much as possible. There are many which are available. Aspirin (gr. x, 0.6 gm.), guaiacol carbonate (gr. v, 0.3 gm.), antipyrin (gr. iii, 0.2 gm.), and sometimes codeia (gr. ½) are useful. Morphia should not be given on account of the danger of a habit.

LOCAL.—(*a*) Use of the joints must be governed by the condition. When the cartilage and bones are not involved, passive motion and massage are useful, followed later by active motion. The patient should be taught simple exercises. When the cartilages and bones are involved, *rest* is usually advisable for a time. Every effort should be made to avoid contracture and displacement, and in this the use of splints during the night is often valuable.

Caution should be exercised in advising complete fixation. This is sometimes useful for short periods in the osteo-arthritic form, but may result in fixation in the other form and is usually not advisable for it. (*b*) *Counter-irritation.* This is usually an aid, and the Paquelin cautery, blisters, mustard, and iodine may be used. It is usually better to use light counter-irritation frequently than severe at longer intervals. (*c*) *Hyperœmia.* This may be active, and baking is a favorite method, but it should not be given for more than thirty minutes at a time. The temperature should be as high as the patient can stand. Passive hyperæmia may be used for a short period at first, and later for many hours at a time. (*d*) *Hydrotherapy.* The persistent use of compresses is often of value. They may be put on in the evening and left on all night.

SURGICAL MEASURES.—These are useful for the correction of deformities. In the case of villous arthritis operation is usually indicated. In the group with marked hypertrophy of bone removal of the outgrowths may be helpful.

SPECIAL FORMS.—(*a*) *Heberden's nodes.* Avoidance of irritation and injury is important, and in the case of pain the use of compresses is helpful. (*b*) *Spondylitis.* During the acute stages rest is essential and should be secured by a plaster jacket or simple apparatus. In the milder forms firm strapping may give relief. Trauma should be especially avoided. (*c*) *Knee joint.* In many cases a simple elastic support is useful and may save the joint from injury.

VACCINES.—These have not proved of great value, but in a few cases the use of a polyvalent antistreptococcus serum has been of benefit.

Arthritis Secondary to Acute Infection.—While the majority of cases of arthritis are secondary to some form of infection, it is important to recognize that there are various forms. (1) Those with a definite bacterial cause, such as gonorrhœal or tuberculous arthritis. These usually have fairly well defined features. (2) Those secondary to infections of doubtful etiology, such as scarlet fever or measles. In some of these the arthritis is due to a secondary infection, but in others it appears to be due to the specific cause of the disease. (3) Arthritis secondary to definite infections in which there is no evidence of any organism in the joint. These are comparatively common and are difficult to designate. For example, arthritis, which may not be severe and subsides rapidly, occurs with an attack of tonsillitis or influenza. It has been suggested that these might be termed "toxic" or "toxæmic" arthritis. The term "infectious" arthritis, sometimes applied, is not a satisfactory one. The cases in this group usually clear without leaving permanent damage, but it is possible that if long continued they may result in the changes included under the heading of arthritis deformans.

"Chronic Rheumatism."—This term deserves mention because it is so commonly used, but it is a question whether its retention is justified. There is no uniformity in its usage and it is applied without discrimination to all kinds of arthritis and frequently to conditions which have nothing to do with the joints. Painful conditions of the joints, muscles, fasciæ, bones, and nerves are all termed "rheumatism." There is no disease entity to which the term can be applied, and it would be an advantage to give it up entirely.

II. INTERMITTENT HYDRARTHROSIS

The condition was described by Perrin in 1845, and there are about 70 cases on record (Garrod). The affection is characterized by a remarkable periodic swelling of one or several of the joints without fever. The swelling may take place with great rapidity, and there may even be a sensation of water rushing into the joint. There are usually pain and stiffness. The periods may be from ten to twelve days, or a month or even three months. Many of the cases have been in women and sometimes with marked hysterical symptoms. While some of the cases are secondary and only represent a phase in the evolution of various articular lesions, there appears to be a primary form characterized by a periodic swelling and nothing else. It is sometimes the joint equivalent to Quincke's œdema and may be associated with erythema, with angio-neurotic œdema, and in one of Garrod's patients there was at the same time circumscribed œdema of the lips and eyelids. A mother and daughter have been affected. The prognosis is not good; the attacks are apt to recur in spite of all forms of treatment.

C. DISEASES OF THE BONES

I. HYPERTROPHIC PULMONARY ARTHROPATHY

Definition.—A symmetrical enlargement of the bones of the hands and feet, and of the distal ends of the long bones, occurring in association with certain chronic diseases, particularly affections of the lungs.

Bamberger in 1889 reported a condition of abnormal thickening of the long bones in bronchiectasis, and the next year Marie described other cases and named the condition.

Etiology.—Clubbing of the fingers, or the Hippocratic fingers, represent a minor manifestation of this condition. Many varieties occur; indeed, there is a monograph with sketches of some thirty or forty forms. It is met with perhaps most constantly in congenital disease of the heart, in tuberculosis and in other affections of the lungs, particularly bronchiectasis, in congenital syphilis, in chronic jaundice, and in other chronic affections. In thoracic aneurism it may involve only the fingers of one hand. It usually comes on very slowly, but cases have been described of an acute appearance within a week or a fortnight. It may disappear. There is no bony alteration, but there is a fibrous thickening of the connective tissues with turgescence of the vessels. The condition is by no means easy to explain. The mechanical effect of congestion, the usual feature, explains the heart and lung cases, but not those of congenital syphilis and diseases of the liver, in which this is not present. Others have attributed it to a toxin.

Marie's syndrome is met with: (1) In diseases of the lungs and pleura. This was the case in 43 out of 55 cases collected by Thayer, and in 68 of Wynn's 100 cases. Bronchiectasis is the most common, then pulmonary tuberculosis and empyema.

(2) Other affections, such as chronic diarrhœa, chronic jaundice, nephritis, and congenital syphilis.

Marie regards the process as resulting from the absorption of toxins causing a periostitis; others have regarded it as a low form of tuberculous infection. The bones most frequently involved are the lower ends of the radius and ulna and the metacarpals, more rarely the lower end of the humerus, and the lower ends of the tibia and fibula.

Symptoms.—The affection comes on gradually, unnoticed by the patient. In other cases there is great sensitiveness of the ends of the long bones and of the fingers and toes. In one of my cases this was present in an extreme degree. The fully developed condition is easily recognized. The hands are large, the terminal phalanges swollen, the nails large and much curved. Similar changes occur in the toes, and the feet look large, especially the toes and the malleoli. The bones of the fore-arms are diffusely thickened, particularly near the wrist, and the tibiæ and fibulæ are greatly enlarged. Sometimes in advanced cases both ankles and knee-joints stand out prominently. The hypertrophy rarely affects the other long bones, though occasionally the extremities of the humerus and femur may be involved. The bones of the head are not attacked. Kyphosis may occur.

Diagnosis.—There is rarely any difficulty, as the picture presented by the hands and feet differs from that in acromegaly, and in practically all cases it is a secondary condition.

II. OSTEITIS DEFORMANS

(*Paget's Disease*)

Definition.—A chronic affection of the bones characterized by enlargement of the head, dorso-cervical kyphosis, enlargement of the clavicles, spreading of the base of the thorax and an outward and forward bowing of the legs.

The affection was described first by Sir James Paget, in 1877.

Etiology.—In the generalized form it is a rare disease, only two cases occurring among about 20,000 medical cases at the Johns Hopkins Hospital. I have seen three or four instances in private practice. The etiology of the disease is unknown. Mother and daughter have been affected. Some have regarded it as luetic, others as due to the arterio-sclerosis, which is a constant lesion. It may possibly be due to perversion of some internal secretion.

Pathology.—The skull, spine, and long bones are chiefly affected, those of the face, hands and feet are less involved. The skull may be as much as three quarters of an inch in thickness, and its circumference is increased. In one of Paget's cases it measured 71 cm. The shafts of the long bones are greatly thickened and they may weigh twice as much as a healthy bone of the same length. The femur is bent, the convexity forward; the tibiæ may be huge and very much bowed anteriorly. The bones of the upper extremities are less often involved, the spine shows a marked kyphosis, sometimes partial ankylosis; the pelvis is broadened.

The process is a rarefying osteitis which gradually involves the centre of the bones with the formation of Howship's lacunæ, Haversian spaces, and perforating canals. There is also new bone formation, both subperiosteal and myelogenous; the latter process gradually gains, and so the bones thicken.

Symptoms.—The disease begins, as a rule, in the sixth decade, sometimes with rheumatoid pains, but more frequently the patient notices first that the head begins to enlarge, so that he has to buy a larger hat. Then his friends notice that he is growing shorter, and that the legs are getting more and more bowed.

There is a painful variety of the disease with great soreness of the arms and legs, which may be much worse at night. Headache, bronchitis, pigmentation of the skin, have been noted. The reduction in stature is very remarkable; one of my patients lost 13 inches in height.

Diagnosis.—The disease is readily recognized. The face differs from acromegaly, in which it is ovoid or egg-shaped with the large end down, while in Paget's disease the face is triangular with the base upward. In a few cases the disease may be limited to a few bones. There is a variety, of which I have seen three examples, involving the tibiæ and fibulæ alone, and in one to a slight extent the femurs. These bones gradually enlarge, are bowed anteriorly and laterally, so that the only obvious features are a reduction in height with bowing of the legs.

There is also a variety which is sometimes known as tumor-forming osteitis deformans, in which the bones are much deformed with multiple hyperostosis and new growths. The relation of this to Paget's disease is doubtful.

III. LEONTIASIS OSSEA

In a remarkable condition known as *leontiasis ossea* there is hyperostosis of the bones of the cranium, and sometimes those of the face. The description is largely based upon the skulls in museums, but Allen Starr has recently reported an instance in a woman, who presented a slowly progressing increase in the size of the head, face, and neck, the hard and soft tissues both being affected. He has applied to the condition the term *megalo-cephaly*. Putnam states that the disease begins in early life, often as a result of injury. There may be osteophytic growths from the outer or inner tables, which in the latter situation may give the symptoms of tumor.

IV. OSTEOGENESIS IMPERFECTA

(*Fragilitas Ossium*)

This is a systemic disease of the fetus in which the normal osseous development does not occur. At birth there is marked fragility of all the bones. There may have been intra-uterine fractures which have united and show large calluses. The extremities are often bent and deformed. The main features are defective development of the cranium and fragility of all the bones. It was thought that death always occurred, but Nathan has shown that some of the patients survive and that the bones become firmer as the child grows older. Treatment consists in using every protection against injury. Fractures usually unite readily.

V. OSTEOPSATHYROSIS

(Fragilitas Ossium, Lobstein's Disease)

Definition.—A rare affection characterized by abnormal brittleness of the bones.

In the aged the bones get thin and fragile, and the same happens in many chronic wasting diseases and in the insane. In osteopsathyrosis the general health of the patient is excellent and the fractures follow very trifling injuries, as a slight blow, or pull, turning over in bed, or in the simple act of chewing the patient may fracture the jaw. It is more common in the early period of life, and many of the cases in children represent the condition just spoken of—osteogenesis imperfecta—but there are cases in which it has continued until old age. The number of fractures which a patient may have may amount to one hundred or more. The fractures may be painless and heal readily; there are rarely any complications, and in a case reported by B. Sachs the condition was associated with general muscular atrophy and polyuria.

VI. ACHONDROPLASIA

(Chondrodystrophia Fetalis)

Definition.—A dystrophy of the epiphyseal cartilages due to connective tissue invasion from the periosteum, in consequence of which the epiphyses and diphyses are prematurely united and there is failure of the normal growth of the long bones. In consequence the subjects become dwarfs with normal heads and trunks, but short, stumpy extremities.

Description.—Achondroplasic dwarfs are easily recognized. They are well nourished and strong, and of average intelligence. Their height varies from 3 to 4 feet; the head and trunk are of about normal size, but the extremities are very short, the fingers, when the arms are at the sides, reaching little below the crest of the ilium. The important point in diagnosis is that in the shortness of the limbs it is the proximal segments which are specially involved, the humerus and femur being even shorter than the ulna and tibia (rhizomelia). The limbs are considerably bent, but this is more an exaggeration of normal curves and abnormalities in the joints than pathological curves as in rickets. The features of rickets are absent. The hand is short, and has a trident shape, since the fingers, which are of almost equal length, often diverge somewhat. The root of the nose is depressed, the back flat, and the lumbar lordosis abnormally deep, owing to a tilting forward of the sacrum. The scapulæ are short, the fibulæ longer than the tibiæ, and the pelvis is contracted; hence, the number of these cases reported by obstetricians. Heredity plays little part.

Pathology.—Anatomically it is a dystrophy of the epiphyseal cartilages, the cells of which are irregularly scattered, and the ground substances invaded by connective tissues from the periosteum, which sends in bands of tissues across the end of the diaphysis. The development of the **bones** with a membranous matrix seems normal.

Virchow described the disease as fetal cretinism, others as fetal rickets. Of late naturally its origin has been associated with disturbance of the pituitary function, or of its hormonic relations. On the other hand, Murk Jansen of Leyden, in a recent monograph (1912), brings forward evidence to show that it results from a disturbance of the direct and indirect amniotic pressure, and he brings it into relationship with a number of other fetal malformations. He states, too, that the anatomical evidence is against changes in the sella turcica in the disease. But it is an argument in favor of some associated disturbance of the pituitary gland that achondroplasics often show precocious sexual development.

VII. OXYCEPHALY

Definition.—A cranial deformity associated with exophthalmos and impairment of vision.

Description.—The condition, known as *tower* or *steeplehead,* is characterized by great height of the forehead, sloping to a pointed vertex, with feebly marked supraorbital ridges, and the hairy scalp may be raised above the normal level, looking as if perched on the top of a comb. The intelligence is unimpaired. The condition is usually present at birth, though in some instances it develops from the second to the sixth year. As this curious growth of the head proceeds, headache may be present, exophthalmos develops, and the vision becomes impaired, due to progressive optic atrophy. Smell is often completely lost. The deformity appears to be due to premature synostosis of certain sutures, notably the sagittal and coronal. As a result of the premature union of these two sutures the growth of the vault of the skull is restricted in both its antero-posterior and tranverse diameters, and to accommodate the increasing bulk of the brain a compensatory increase in height takes place. Eventually the anterior fontanelle closes, but there is reason to think that this occurs at a later date than the normal, and its former site is marked by a slight protuberance with thinning of the bone. (Morley Fletcher, *Quarterly Jour. Med.,* IV, 1911.)

The optic neuritis and atrophy are the result of direct pressure exerted by the growing brain and may be compared to that of cerebral tumor. As yet we do not know the cause of this premature synostosis. The condition is one for which a decompression operation is indicated.

INDEX

A

C

E

F

G

H

I

J

K

L

M

N

O

P

Q

R

T

U

V

W

X

Y

Z

THE END